THE COMPLETE

PILL GUIDE

2nd Edition

Covering more than 1,500 brand-name and generic drugs, the revised 2nd edition of *The Complete Pill Guide* is the reference you'll turn to when your doctor prescribes a new medication. Up-to-date, easy-to-read entries tell you everything you need to know about the medications, including:

- **GENERIC and BRAND NAMES**
- **ABOUT THIS DRUG**
- **SIDE EFFECTS**
- **IMPORTANT PRECAUTIONS**
- **DRUG INTERACTIONS**
- **FOOD, VITAMIN, AND HERBAL INTERACTIONS**
- **RECOMMENDED DOSAGES**
- **SYMPTOMS OF OVERDOSE AND WHAT TO DO**
- **SPECIAL INFORMATION FOR PREGNANT OR NURSING WOMEN**
- **SPECIAL INFORMATION FOR SENIORS**
- **OPEN QUESTIONS OR CONTROVERSIES**
- **450 COLOR PHOTOGRAPHS**

With an informative introduction that explains how to minimize your risks when taking medications, how to communicate with your health-care provider, what to do in an emergency, and much more, *The Complete Pill Guide* is the perfect resource for all your questions about the medications your doctor prescribes.

THE COMPLETE PILL GUIDE

2nd Edition

The Latest Information About Generic and Brand-Name Prescription Drugs

---

Medical Editor:
Lewis A. Opler, M.D., Ph.D.

Editorial Director:
Lynn Sonberg

Project Manager:
Deborah Mitchell

Pharmaceutical Editors:
Lisa E. Davis, Pharm.D. and
Steven G. Ottariano, R.Ph.

Research:
Shelagh Masline and Deborah Mitchell

Production Editor:
Judith Gitenstein

BARNES & NOBLE BOOKS
NEW YORK

A BARNES & NOBLE BOOK

ISBN 0-7607-6553-7

1 2 3 4 5 6 7 8 9 10

Digital photography: Christopher Bain

Printed in the USA

ABOUT THE CONSULTANTS
Lewis A. Opler, M.D., Ph.D. is Clinical Professor of Psychiatry, New York University School of Medicine and Adjunct Professor of Psychiatry, Columbia University College of Physicians and Surgeons; **Lisa E. Davis, Pharm.D.** is Associate Professor of Clinical Pharmacy, University of the Sciences in Philadelphia; **Steven G. Ottariano, R.Ph.** is the Clinical Staff Pharmacist at the Veteran's Administration Medical Center in Manchester, New Hampshire.

DISCLAIMER
This book was written to provide selected information to consumers concerning frequently prescribed medications. Research about prescription drugs is an ongoing process; side effects and adverse reactions sometimes continue to be reported to the FDA after a drug has been approved for use in the general market. Efforts have been made to include up-to-date information in this book, however there can be no guarantee that what we know about particular drugs won't change with time and further research. **Readers should bear in mind that this book is not intended to be used for self-diagnosis or self-treatment; they should consult appropriate health professionals regarding all medical problems. Readers should never stop taking a prescription drug or alter the dosage or dosing schedule without first consulting their physicians or health-care practitioners.** Neither the publisher, the producer, the consultants, nor the writers take any responsibility for any possible consequences arising from any treatment, action, or application of medicine or preparation by any person reading or following the information in this book.

This book includes drugs approved by the FDA through June 2004.

The photographs appearing in this book, which show brand-name and generic medications, were included for information only. They were accurate at the time of publication, but from time to time manufacturers change the appearance of the medications they produce. All issues relating to the appearance and use of these drugs should be discussed with a qualified health professional.

Contents

How to Use This Book

You have in your hands a significant tool in your quest for better health care. Now, more than ever, it is necessary to share in the responsibility for your own safe and effective medical care. One reason for this is the unfortunate state of managed care in America. Health-care practitioners are pressured to see more and more patients and to spend less time with each patient. This pressure is passed along to you, the consumer. The result may be that you do not ask your health-care practitioner questions you would ask if you felt less rushed.

When your visit with your health-care practitioner is over and you have been handed your prescription, it is likely you do not know all you need to know about that prescription. It is up to you to make sure you will be using the drug safely, correctly, and efficiently.

This book can help you take some control of your health care by providing you with relevant information about more than 1,300 brand-name prescription drugs and more than 500 generic medications. These drugs were chosen based on the number of times they are prescribed and the frequency of the conditions they treat. New drugs approved by the Food and Drug Administration (FDA) as of June 1, 2002, that fit these criteria have been included as well.

The information in this book is not a substitute for professional advice from your health-care practitioner or pharmacist, but it *is* a source that will inform you about the drugs you have been prescribed. Once you have reliable information, you will be better equipped to ask questions of your health-care practitioner or pharmacist. With that in mind, we'd like to explain how you can easily navigate your way through this book to find information about the medications that concern you.

The entries are arranged alphabetically by generic name. The generic name of the drug you are looking for may be on your prescription container. If it isn't, the brand name in the index in the back of the book is cross-referenced to the proper generic name.

Each drug entry follows the same format and includes information in eleven (sometimes twelve, when applicable) key categories:

- **Generic Name.** A drug's generic name is its common, non-brand name. Some drugs are better known by their generic names; aspirin, morphine, and lithium are a few examples. In a few cases, the name of the drug class, such as cephalosporin antibiotics, is listed along with the generic names in that class. This has been done in cases where the drugs in that class are similar. All the information has been gathered in one place for all the drugs.
- **Brand Name(s).** The brand names listed are those most commonly associated with the generic drug. Not all name brands may be listed, since some drugs have dozens of brand names. Inclusion of a brand name does not suggest the drug is recommended; exclusion does not suggest a drug is less effective.
- After the brand name is an annotation as to whether or not the drug is available as a generic. Some drugs have patent restrictions that protect the manufacturer of the drug, and so that drug is available only by brand name.
- **About This Drug.** This section gives general background information, including the most common medical conditions for which the drug is prescribed, the class of drug it belongs to, and how the drug works in the body.
- **Side Effects.** A listing of common, less common, and rare side effects (where applicable) associated with the drug's use. The side effects listed are not all-inclusive. If you experience a side effect that has not been listed, contact your health-care practitioner immediately.
- **Important Precautions.** Information on various situations and conditions to be aware of when using the specific drug. This information may include, but not be limited to, medical conditions which may be counterindications for taking the drug, whether driving precautions should be followed, things you should tell your health-care practitioner before taking the drug, and any allergies that may not be compatible with the drug's use.
- **Drug Interactions.** Serious complications can occur when taking two or more drugs at the same time or within the same day. This section provides information on drug-drug interactions. However, it is always necessary to tell your health-care practitioner about any medications you are taking, prescription or nonprescription, before starting a new treatment drug because of the potential for a drug-drug reaction.
- **Food, Vitamin, and Herbal Interactions.** Though less frequent than drug-drug interactions, there are certain food-, vitamin-, and herb-drug interactions that have been reported or are suspected. This section identifies what we know about these interactions and what you should watch for.

- **Recommended Dosage.** The typical dosages for children (if applicable) and for adults for the most commonly prescribed forms of the drug. Information is also included on how to take the doses (e.g., with food or beverages or on an empty stomach) and how to handle a missed dose. This information is given as a guideline only. Only your health-care practitioner can determine the most appropriate dose for you.
- **Symptoms of Overdose and What to Do.** A list of the symptoms associated with an overdose of the drug, along with information on what to do if an overdose occurs.
- **Special Information for Pregnant or Nursing Women.** This section contains basic information on what experts know about the possible risks a specific drug poses to unborn or nursing children. The prevailing medical opinion is that pregnant or nursing women should take drugs only if the benefits clearly outweigh the possible risks to the child.
- **Special Information for Seniors.** Older adults often react differently to medications because of changes in some bodily functions as we age. Information on special precautions for seniors is given here.
- **Open Questions or Controversies.** This boxed section is included when there is a lack of consensus on the benefits versus the risks of a particular medication, when there is debate over a drug's safety, or if there is some other controversy surrounding the use of a specific drug about which the public should be aware.

Following "The Prescription Drug Profiles" you will find "A Primer of Drug Classifications." Drugs that have similar chemical makeups or similar therapeutic effects are grouped into classes. Generally, most drugs in any given class provide similar benefits—cause similar side effects, drug-drug interactions, and drug-herb interactions. This Primer is helpful if, for example, you are told under "Drug Interactions" that the medication you are taking interacts with drugs in certain drug classes. Each drug classification in the Primer lists the drugs that belong to that class.

NOTE: Because the names for drug classes are not standardized, classes listed in other references may vary. We have included alternative class names in parentheses in the Primer to help clear up any confusion.

Also included at the back of this book is a comprehensive index of both generic and brand names, cross-referenced for your convenience.

Everything You Need to Know About Prescription Drugs

Taking medication, whether it is prescription or over-the-counter, should never be done lightly. A drug is a potent substance, designed and administered for a reason: to offer relief from symptoms or to promote recovery. Because drugs are powerful substances, it is important to know the advantages they can provide us and the risks they may present. In the following pages, we talk about the things we need to respect about drugs, and ways in which to take medications safely.

SIDE EFFECTS AND ADVERSE REACTIONS

If we had to define the "perfect" drug, it might be one that (1) relieves all your symptoms and (2) causes no side effects. Unfortunately, no such drug exists. Even those that come close to accomplishing the first criterion don't meet the second. The truth is, even the safest and most effective medications can cause undesirable reactions.

Side effects are adverse reactions to drugs that can occur if you take the recommended dosage or too high a dosage, or if the drug is not eliminated from your body and accumulates over time. (Reactions that occur because two or more drugs are used together are "drug interactions" and are discussed separately in this chapter.)

How Serious Are Side Effects? According to a comprehensive study published in *The Journal of the American Medical Association* (JAMA), more than 106,000 deaths occur in American hospitals each year from side effects of medications. That means about 300 people a day die from an adverse reaction to a drug that had been administered to help them.

In addition, the study reported that 2,216,000 severe drug reactions occur in U.S. hospitals per year. These numbers include only people who suffered permanent disability, hospitalization, or death; they do not include anyone who was disabled for weeks or months, anyone who suffered falls or automobile accidents because their medications made them dizzy or sleepy, or people classified as outpatients. That means, says Jay S. Cohen, M.D., author of *Overdose: The Case Against the Drug Companies*, that the researchers "excluded side effects that occur far more often than the ones they included."

What Can You Do about Side Effects? Just because every drug has the potential to cause side effects doesn't mean you will necessarily experience them. However, because side effects can be dangerous, it is important to pay attention to ways in which your body responds to any drugs you take. If you experience anything unusual or if a current symptom has worsened soon after taking a drug, contact your health-care practitioner right away.

For example, nausea isn't an unusual symptom, but if it isn't the condition you are treating and if it started after you took the medication, you may be reacting to the drug. Or, if you were experiencing nausea before taking a drug and it gets worse after taking the medication, let your health-care practitioner know immediately.

It doesn't matter whether the symptoms you experience are listed under "Side Effects" or on any information you got from your health-care practitioner or pharmacist. Because each of us has a unique biochemical makeup, we can react differently to medications. Let your health-care practitioner know when side effects occur.

Many of the most common side effects and adverse reactions fall into the following categories. Keep these in mind the next time you take a prescription drug.

Appetite and Weight Changes. Several responses fall into this category, including loss of appetite, increase in appetite, fluid retention, and change in your sense of taste (a diminished or complete loss of taste; a metallic or bad taste). Any of these factors can affect weight.

Any drug that causes nausea or vomiting can cause a loss of appetite. There are many drugs, including antibiotics, that can have that effect. Sometimes taking a drug with food (if indicated) can help you avoid nausea.

Antipsychotics (e.g., haloperidol, risperidone) and steroids (e.g., cortisone, hydrocortisone) can increase appetite, while drugs from various drug categories can alter taste. Contact your health-care practitioner if you experience any changes in appetite, weight, or sense of taste.

Behavioral Changes. Some medications can cause significant changes in your behavior and mood. Such changes may not be as noticeable to you as they are to the people around you. Family, friends, or coworkers may ask why you seem more irritable, depressed, or anxious, or a partner may ask about your mood swings. If your behavior or mood seems to have changed since you've started taking a certain medication, contact your health-care practitioner. Some types of drugs known to cause behavioral and mood changes include amphetamines, analgesics, antibiotics, anticonvulsants, antihistamines, antiparkinsonians, asthma medications, antidepressants, cardiac drugs, some high blood pressure drugs, nasal decongestants, sedatives, thyroid hormones, and tranquilizers.

Drug Allergies. One way to avoid an allergic reaction to a drug is to tell your health-care practitioner and pharmacist about allergic reactions you may have had to any drug in the past, including over-the-counter drugs. This is no guarantee, however, that you will not experience an allergic reaction to a new medication. It is even possible to begin to experience a reaction to a drug you had been taking for some time with no problem.

Allergic drug reactions typically occur within minutes to hours of taking the drug. Symptoms can include a rash, hives, cough, wheezing, palpitations, difficulty breathing, nausea, watery eyes, and swelling in the throat. In more extreme cases, breathing difficulties can lead to cold sweats, low blood pressure, cardiac arrest, shock, and collapse. These are symptoms that occasionally occur with use of penicillin, cephalosporin antibiotics, insulin, or local anesthetics.

If someone has a severe allergic reaction (called *anaphylaxis*) to a drug, it can be life-threatening. What should you do?

IF THE INDIVIDUAL IS UNCONSCIOUS AND NOT BREATHING:

- Stay with the person and yell for help.
- If the victim is a child, try mouth-to-mouth breathing for one minute, then dial "911" or "0" (operator) for emergency medical assistance. If the individual is an adult, dial "911" or "0" first, then begin mouth-to-mouth.
- If there is no heartbeat, begin external cardiac massage.
- Continue mouth-to-mouth and massage (cardiopulmonary resuscitation, or CPR) until medical assistance arrives.
- Bring the prescription or medicine container with you to the hospital.

IF THE INDIVIDUAL IS UNCONSCIOUS AND BREATHING:

- Dial "911" or "0" (operator) for emergency medical help.
- If emergency help is not readily available or if it is faster for you to bring the person to an emergency room, do so.
- Bring the prescription or medicine container with you to the hospital.

Nutritional Deficiencies. Some drugs cause the body to lose essential nutrients or hinder its ability to absorb and use them. Diuretics are a good example. Some diuretics reduce the amount of potassium (a mineral that is critical for heart, kidney, and muscle function) through increased urination. Antibiotics can interfere with the body's ability to convert nutrients into forms the body can use. Additional drugs that may hinder normal absorption of nutrients include antacids, anticholinergics, anticonvulsants, cathartics, clofibrate, isoniazid, methotrexate, and neomycin sulfate. If you are using any of these drugs, talk to your health-care practitioner about any dietary or supplement changes you may need to make.

Sexual Changes. Changes that occur in this category usually include impotence or ejaculation problems in men, difficulty reaching orgasm in women, and a reduction in or loss of sex drive in both men and women. Drugs that can cause these difficulties include antianxiety drugs, antidepressants, antihypertensives, birth control pills, ulcer medications, and vasodilators. Talk to your health-care practitioner if you experience a change in your sexual desires, responses, or performance.

Skin Sensitivity. Many drugs can make your skin more sensitive to ultraviolet light from the sun, which can result in sunburn. This reaction, called photosensitivity, is often associated with antidepressants, antipsychotics, barbiturates, cough and cold remedies, diuretics, gastrointestinal drugs, some oral contraceptives, sulfa drugs, and tetracycline drugs. Verteporfin, a drug used in the laser treatment of macular degeneration, is one of the latest drugs on the market that can significantly increase photosensitivity.

If you are taking a drug that can cause photosensitivity, protect yourself by wearing sunscreen with an SPF—sun protective factor—of at least 15. It is important also to wear protective clothing, such as long sleeves, long pants, and a hat. There are several mail-order houses that sell specially made clothing with fabrics that offer SPF protection.

Vision Changes. Some commonly prescribed drugs, such as antidepressants, steroids, and thiazide diuretics, are known to cause blurred vision. Many drugs are reported to cause double vision, among them antidepressants, antidiabetic drugs, sedatives, and tranquilizers, while others may cause nearsightedness (e.g., oral contraceptives, thiazide diuretics), changes in color vision (e.g., acetaminophen, cortisone-like drugs, erythromycin, sulfonamides), cataracts (e.g., chlorpromazine, pilocarpine), and sensitivity to light (e.g., antidiabetic drugs, atropinelike drugs, tetracyclines). Immediately report any vision changes to your health-care practitioner.

DRUG INTERACTIONS

Drug interactions are responses that can occur when you take two or more drugs either at the same time or at different times during the same day. Such interactions can occur between two or more prescription or over-the-counter drugs, including alcohol and tobacco, and are a serious concern, because so many people take more than one medication.

Drug interactions can be positive—one drug may enhance the therapeutic benefits of another one—or they may be negative. We are concerned here primarily with the negative interactions, because they can be serious and even life-threatening.

Several problems can arise with drug interactions. Your chances of experiencing a drug interaction increase with the number of drugs you are taking. One drug may enhance the toxic effects of another drug, or one drug may cancel the benefits of a second or third one. If new or worsened symptoms result from a drug interaction and your health-care practitioner does not recognize them as such, he or she may prescribe yet another drug to treat those symptoms, thinking they represent a new illness. This new drug can then cause even more interactions to occur.

To help prevent drug interactions, make sure all your health-care practitioners and your pharmacist know about all medications you are taking—prescription and over-the-counter—as well as your alcohol, tobacco, and recreational drug use. Alcohol, for example, can be deadly when combined with tranquilizers or many other drugs. Ask your health-care practitioner whether you can consume alcohol when being treated with a specific drug.

This is not the time to hide alcohol or recreational drug use from health professionals; the consequences could be serious, even deadly. Pharmacists now have computer programs that can immediately identify which drugs and other substances may cause dangerous reactions, but the information *they* provide is only as accurate as the information *you* provide.

Food, Vitamin, and Herbal Interactions. Like drug-drug interactions, food-, vitamin-, or herb-drug interactions can sometimes be positive. This is more likely to be true with vitamin-drug interactions, because some drugs can deplete your body of essential nutrients, and taking vitamin supplements can help correct any deficiencies. When applicable, these benefits are mentioned in this book.

The realm of drug-herb interactions is not as well researched as other drug interactions, but new information is being added all the time. Each drug listing in this book includes this new dimension in drug interactions and tells you the latest in what is known about herb-drug relationships. With about 50 percent of Americans using some type of herbal supplement at one time or another, and about $15.7 billion in sales estimated in the year 2000, this information can be invaluable to your good health.

Although many drugs can be taken with food, there are some cases in which certain foods should not be eaten. Monoamine oxidase (MAO) inhibitors, for example, when combined with aged cheeses, liver, pickled foods, sauerkraut, yeast extract, or yogurt may cause severe headache, brain hemorrhage, or death. If you are taking certain anticoagulants, excessive consumption of foods high in vitamin K, such as green leafy vegetables and liver, can interfere with the drugs' effectiveness. You may need to stay clear of soybeans, brussel sprouts, and other foods that contain goitrogens if you are taking thyroid drugs, because goitrogens can interfere with production of the thyroid hormone and produce goiter.

If you are taking an antihypertensive drug, you may need to avoid herbs known to raise blood pressure, such as licorice. Herbs such as comfrey and chaparral, when taken with acetaminophen, may increase the risk of liver damage. St. John's wort can lower blood levels and may reduce the effectiveness of many important medications, including indinavir and other drugs used to treat HIV infection, drugs used to treat heart disease (such as digoxin, diltiazem, or nifedipine), antidepressants (such as amitriptyline, imipramine, or amoxapine), antiseizure drugs (such as carbamazepine, phenytoin, or phenobarbital), certain anticancer drugs (such as irinotecan, cyclophosphamide, tamoxifen, paclitaxel, or etoposide) or drugs to prevent transplant rejection (such as cyclosporine, rapamycin, or tacrolimus) or pregnancy (ethinyl estradiol).

The bottom line: inform your health-care practitioner and pharmacist about any herbs or other supplements you are taking.

DRUG DEPENDENCE

Drug dependence can creep up on you. It can begin innocently enough: you're prescribed a narcotic painkiller for back pain or arthritis or pain from an automobile accident. You may be having trouble sleeping and your health-care practitioner gives you a prescription for sleeping pills. You use the drugs regularly over a period of weeks and months. You notice that you need increasing amounts of the drug to experience its benefits. Then, if you try to stop using the drug, you experience withdrawal symptoms, such as sweating, nervousness, tremors, nausea, vomiting, and possibly seizures and hallucination. These are all signs of a physical dependence. In contrast, addiction, a disorder that is characterized by compulsive drug use and craving, represents more of a psychological dependence. Whereas experts agree that most individuals who take these drugs regularly for several weeks or more will develop a physical dependence, few actually develop an addictive behavior.

Drugs that Can Cause Physical Dependence. Some drugs, like antianxiety drugs, sleeping pills, and tranquilizers, which belong to a larger drug group called benzodiazepines, can cause physical dependence after only one to two months of regular use. Drugs commonly prescribed for pain relief and inflammation, including narcotic analgesics such as meperidine, morphine, and oxycodone, as well as drug combinations that contain these narcotics, also cause dependence. Other drugs to be aware of include amphetamines, which are used in diet pills; barbiturates, used to treat epilepsy, insomnia, and sometimes nervousness; and codeine, which is often combined with aspirin or acetaminophen.

Narcotics Used in Terminal Illness. A subject of much debate and controversy has been the use of narcotics with people who have terminal illnesses, such as late-stage cancer. Because narcotics can be physically and psychologically addictive, some health-care practitioners are reluctant to prescribe them to patients who have chronic pain, even though they can clearly benefit the patient. Fortunately, more and more health-care practitioners are realizing that prescribing narcotics to patients who suffer with significant, chronic pain will not turn their patients into "addicts." According to Russell Portenoy, M.D., a pain specialist at Memorial Sloan-Kettering Cancer Center in New York, "There is growing literature showing that opioids [narcotics] can be used for a long time with few side effects and that abuse and addiction are not a problem." Studies also show that patients who are prescribed these medications return to normal functioning within a week, after a period of adjustment to the drug.

Sandra Johnson, former president of the American Society of Law, Medicine and Ethics, and an expert on pain management and elder-care, says, "The risk of addiction for someone who is receiving end-of-life care is irrelevant and side effects aren't severe and eventually clear up." Those side effects can include blurred vision, constipation, and lethargy.

There has also been some question about the use of narcotics shortening the life of terminally ill patients. A new study published in the July 29, 2000, issue of *Lancet* states that "increasing use of pain-killing opioids such as morphine in terminally ill patients does not shorten life."

PREGNANT WOMEN AND DRUGS

Pregnancy is a unique situation: whatever substances ingested by the mother are passed along, in varying amounts, to the developing fetus, a life that does not have all the tools it needs to adequately fight off infections and other assaults to the system, such as drugs. Two of the best-known tragedies involving prescription drug use in pregnant women—thalidomide in the 1960s and diethylstilbestrol (DES) in the 1970s—have shown us the harm drugs can do when taken during pregnancy. More than 8,000 children were born with birth defects caused by use of thalidomide, and countless numbers of women developed vaginal cancer from DES use. These lessons taught us that a woman of childbearing age should take drugs only if they are critical to the preservation of her health, unless she has documented evidence that she is not pregnant.

How Drugs Affect the Fetus. Because it would be unethical to conduct studies of the effects of drugs on pregnant women, we rely on studies done on pregnant animals. This is why, in most of the entries in this book, you will read that studies have not been done on humans, or that adequate research is not available. Sometimes there have been case studies in which pregnant women have taken a specific drug and certain birth defects or other abnormalities were noted and reported after delivery. Such cases provide a warning to other women who may be planning to become pregnant or who are pregnant and who may need certain medications.

Research shows that, if a mother takes a drug, it will be detected in the fetus at nearly the same levels found in the mother's bloodstream. Some drugs, such as alcohol, aspirin, diazepam (Valium), penicillin G, and tetracycline, pass through the placenta and into the fetus' bloodstream within minutes. Diazepam is also an example of a drug that reaches higher levels in the fetus than it does in the mother.

Think of the placenta as a pipeline that carries whatever a pregnant woman ingests directly to her developing fetus. This includes caffeine, nicotine, vitamins, herbs, and medications. If you think you're pregnant, or if you plan to become pregnant soon, talk to your health-care practitioner before you take any prescription or over-the-counter drugs, as well as vitamins, herbs, and other supplements.

Impact of Drugs on Breastfeeding. If the placenta is one pipeline, the breast is another. Drugs are transmitted to nursing infants in varying amounts and can have different effects. Oral contraceptives, for example, can reduce milk production and change the protein, fat, and vitamin content of the milk. It is also possible that the hormones in contraceptives will cause feminization of male infants. Diazepam, an antipsychotic drug, is eliminated more slowly in infants than it is in adults, which means it can accumulate in the child and cause adverse reactions.

If you are breastfeeding, talk to your health-care practitioner before you take any drug. Together you can discuss the potential benefits weighed against the potential risks to your child. In many cases, women are advised to switch to bottle feeding while they are undergoing treatment, to help ensure the safety of the child.

CHILDREN AND DRUGS

When your children get sick, you naturally want the best care and medication you can get. When the health-care practitioner hands you a prescription and you read the warnings, you will probably notice that it says "safety and dosage have not been established for pediatric use." Does that mean the drug is not safe for your child?

The dose your health-care practitioner has recommended is likely one that other health-care practitioners have found to be effective and safe. However, more likely than not, the drug has not undergone any research to document that it is safe for children. According to the American Academy of Pediatrics, only about 25 percent of the prescription drugs marketed in the U.S. have been approved for children.

Testing Drugs for Children. In 1997, the Pediatric Exclusivity Provision of the Food and Drug Administration Modernization Act (FDAMA) was put into play. Before this provision, very few clinical trials were conducted to determine whether or not a drug was safe for children. Since the regulations were implemented in 1998, more than 58 studies of pediatric use have been carried out. The trials continue. In time, all drugs with relevance to children should have documented information to back up their use, or recommended nonuse, in children.

Antibiotics Overprescribed. Despite the fact that antibiotics don't do anything to help viral infections such as the common cold or flu, health-care practitioners still overprescribe antibiotics, especially for children. One survey, for example, conducted by the Centers for Disease Control and Prevention (CDC) showed that 86 percent of pediatricians surveyed in Georgia regularly prescribe antibiotics for bronchitis, even though it was rarely appropriate, and that 42 percent prescribe them for the common cold.

Parents are a key factor in the overprescribing of antibiotics. In a study published in 1999 in *Pediatrics*, 40 percent of pediatricians said that at least 10 times during the preceding month, a parent had requested an antibiotic even though it was not indicated. Forty-eight percent of the health-care practitioners said that parents always, most of the time, or often pressure them to prescribe an antibiotic when such drugs are not appropriate. Approximately 33 percent of these health-care practitioners occasionally or more frequently gave into those requests.

An inappropriately prescribed antibiotic can do your child more harm than good. Antibiotic resistance is a major problem, and it typically starts in childhood when antibiotics are given when not needed. If your child does not have a bacterial infection, antibiotics will not help. Furthermore, taking an antibiotic when it is not needed makes your child susceptible to potential side effects. Talk to your health-care practitioner about alternative medications or approaches when your child is ill with a viral condition.

Safety First. Children are not little adults. Their body systems and organs are not completely mature, they have lower body mass and fluid levels, and they metabolize substances at a different rate; thus they are at greater risk for experiencing side effects. For this reason, health-care practitioners typically give children doses based on their body weight.

If your child has been given a prescription, ask your health-care practitioner if the prescription is necessary (remember the warning about antibiotics). If it is, ask what side effects to expect and what you should do if they occur. Tell the health-care practitioner about any over-the-counter medications or supplements the child may be taking.

DRUGS AND THE ELDERLY

It's a fact that older adults take more and more kinds of medications than younger people. People between the ages of 55 and 64, for example, are given an average of eight different prescriptions in a given year. Those older than 70 take an average of 6.5 drugs daily. And that's just prescription drugs: according to the Food and Drug Administration (FDA), the average older person is also taking two over-the-counter medications as well. Thus the potential for side effects and drug interactions in older people is high, and increases as the number of drugs used increases. Taking many drugs can tax the body at any age, and among older adults, it can be a particular problem for several reasons. One is that the organs of older people do not function as efficiently as they did during their younger years. Kidney function, for example, can decrease by as much as 50 percent by the time people reach age 70. This means drugs are eliminated from the body at a slower rate, resulting in an accumulation that can cause or worsen side effects or other problems. Liver function also declines, and this is important because the liver cleanses and detoxifies the blood. If this system is not working optimally, too-high levels of the drug may accumulate and cause toxicity.

The digestive system also changes as we age. Drugs are absorbed mainly in the stomach and small intestine. With age, these organs do not always metabolize food and medications as well as they once did, which means greater amounts of a drug can remain in the bloodstream for longer periods of time. This is the main reason why older people often need lower dosages of medications.

Drug Misuse Among the Elderly. Misprescribing drugs for older adults—whether they are given too high a dose, drugs for problems they could treat with lifestyle changes, or medications to treat side effects of another drug that are masquerading as a disease—is a major problem. Although people older than 60 make up about 19 percent of the U.S. population, they account for 51 percent of all deaths and 39 percent of all hospitalizations related to medication reactions. Nine percent of the side effects, reports *The Journal of the American Board of Family Practice*, occurred even though individuals were given what is considered to be standard doses.

Some researchers believe that the 9 percent figure is low. According to a report in *The New England Journal of Medicine*, "The overall incidence of adverse drugs reactions in the elderly is two to three times that found in young adults," and that "the incidence is probably underestimated, because adverse drug reactions are less readily recognized by the elderly themselves and because the reactions may mimic the characteristics of disease states."

You may have heard the expression "Start low and go slow" when referring to the way in which medications should be prescribed and administered to older individuals. Yet according to many medical professionals, including Jay S. Cohen, M.D., author of *Overdose*, there are at least 86 top-selling prescription drugs for which drug manufacturers do not provide lower starting doses for older people. The list includes drugs that are prescribed often for older adults, including antidepressants (e.g., trazodone, venlafaxine), anti-inflammatories (e.g., celecoxib, sulindac), antihistamines (e.g., fexofenadine, loratadine), antihypertensives (e.g., quinapril, metoprolol), and cholesterol-lowering agents (e.g., fluvastatin, atorvastatin), among others. This means it is up to your health-care practitioner to prescribe a lower initial dose, and it is up to you to ask questions of your health-care practitioner and pharmacist when you are given a prescription.

Another problem is that many elderly people see more than one health-care practitioner and then receive multiple prescriptions for the same medical condition. One health-care practitioner may prescribe a loop diuretic, for example, while another gives a thiazide diuretic. An added complication is that many elderly people decide to self-medicate, using over-the-counter drugs, and fail to let their health-care practitioners know. Two categories of drugs that older patients frequently overuse are laxatives and analgesics, such as acetaminophen. Because they are over-the-counter (OTC) medications, people mistakenly believe they are safer than prescription drugs, and can often get into trouble if they are also taking prescription or other OTC medications.

Drug-Induced Conditions in the Elderly. Along with misprescribed medications comes the risk of experiencing drug-induced conditions. This problem then becomes part of another cycle common among older patients: being treated with more drugs for a "disease" that is actually a drug-induced condition.

For example, among older adults, urinary incontinence is a common reaction to some antidepressants, antiparkinsonian drugs, diuretics, and sedatives. Depression is often the result of taking antianxiety drugs, beta-blockers, clonidine, levodopa, or digoxin. Constipation is especially bothersome among those taking tricyclic antidepressants, quinidine, benztropine, or meclizine, while delirium can be a side effect of diuretics, digoxin, cimetidine, and nonsteroidal anti-inflammatory drugs. Rather than being prescribed yet another drug to treat these "new illnesses," it may be better to talk to your health-care practitioner about changing your current prescription and trying lifestyle modifications.

Special Needs. Medical conditions common among the elderly, such as arthritis, memory lapses, and vision problems, can make it difficult for some to take their medications correctly. In fact, up to 75 percent of older adults take the wrong amount of a drug or take it at the wrong time. If you need help in taking your medications, see "Guidelines for Safe Drug Use" in this chapter for some tips.

QUESTIONS AND CONTROVERSIES

In recent years, it's become commonplace to open a magazine or newspaper and see advertisements for prescription drugs. Every other television commercial seems to be telling us to ask our health-care practitioner about such-and-such a medication. When we turn on the news, we often hear about how a certain medication is being investigated, how a drug is being misused or overprescribed, or how some individuals or special interest groups are filing a lawsuit, claiming that a particular drug is unsafe.

News and information about drugs are all around us, and it can become difficult, even impossible, to separate the noise from the facts. Often there's just too much information for us to process. When we go to our health-care practitioners and pharmacists, we depend on them to prescribe and dispense the drugs we need, but as we've mentioned, many of us don't ask questions or don't ask the right ones.

In this book, you will see a box called "Open Questions and Controversies" in some of the drug entries. These boxes highlight individual drugs that have been the subject of debate or questions in recent years. What follows here is a broader look at some of the drug categories that have sparked controversy.

Antidepressants. Depression is the most common psychiatric disorder among adults. It can range from mild and temporary to chronic and severe, with suicidal thoughts and attempts.

Antidepressants, when prescribed and used properly, can be effective in treating many forms of depression. However, some health-care practitioners and other health professionals have expressed concern that antidepressants are being overprescribed, and that health-care practitioners and patients also have a tendency to overestimate the benefits of the drugs while minimizing the risks and side effects. The manufacturers of the most widely prescribed antidepressants, the selective serotonin reuptake inhibitors (SSRIs), admit that their products can trigger mania. More common side effects of these drugs include restlessness, difficulty sleeping, headache, nausea, decreased appetite, and decreased sexual drive. Side effects with tricyclic antidepressants can include dry mouth, drowsiness, changes in heart rate, and sudden drops in blood pressure. If combined with alcohol, antidepressants can cause lack of coordination, poor judgment, and diminished alertness.

Also of concern is the evidence from several studies indicating that for a significant percentage of patients a placebo is just as effective as an antidepressant. This indicates the possibility that antidepressants may be overprescribed, and that they may be inappropriately prescribed.

One more caution: if you are diagnosed with depression, it's important that your health-care practitioner knows about any drugs you are taking. Many commonly prescribed drugs, including antibiotics, antihypertensives, beta-blockers, and ulcer drugs, can cause depression. Rather than take a drug to treat a *side effect* of another drug, your health-care practitioner may be able to change the offending medication and avoid prescribing an antidepressant at all.

Antipsychotic Drugs. Drugs in this category are also known as major tranquilizers or neuroleptic drugs. Included in this category are clozapine (Clozaril), haloperidol (Haldol), loxapine (Loxitane), risperidone (Risperdal), and thiothixene (navane). Although they are meant to be used to treat psychotic disorders, such as schizophrenia, they are frequently misused when given to residents of nursing homes or mental institutions for other conditions or simply to help control their behavior.

Antipsychotic drugs can cause a serious side effect called tardive dyskinesia, an often irreversible condition in which people experience involuntary movements of the lips, tongue, fingers, toes, and trunk. Although it is difficult to accurately determine the number of cases of tardive dyskinesia associated with antipsychotic drugs, it is estimated that up to 60 percent of patients who take these medications over a long period of time will experience some degree of this disorder. This situation suggests that extreme caution should be exercised by any health-care practitioner who prescribes these drugs and that patients need to be monitored closely.

Benzodiazepines. Drugs in this category are used to treat anxiety, depression, insomnia, and various other disorders, including coronary heart disease. They are controversial for several reasons: they can be addictive, even when taken for only a short time. They can be fatal if taken with alcohol use. This is a particular problem because some people being treated for emotional disorders also drink alcohol regularly. Withdrawal symptoms can be especially serious, even more so than stopping heroin "cold turkey." Drugs in the benzodiazepine category include alprazolam (Xanax), chlordiazepoxide (Librium), diazepam (Valium), lorazepam (Ativan), oxazepam (Serax), and triazolam (Halcion), among others.

COX-2 Inhibitors. COX-2 inhibitors are a type of nonsteroidal anti-inflammatory drug (NSAID) designed to block inflammation and pain as effectively as traditional NSAIDs, such as ibuprofen and aspirin, but while causing fewer gastrointestinal problems and stomach ulcers. Unlike traditional NSAIDs, the COX-2 inhibitors inhibit the actions of a natural enzyme called cyclooxygenase-2 (COX-2), which has been linked to inflammation, but do not affect the activity of cyclooxygenase-1 (COX-1), which protects the lining of the stomach. Thus COX-2 inhibitors are less likely to cause stomach ulcers, stomach bleeding, and other gastrointestinal problems associated with traditional NSAIDs.

As of September 2004, there were three drugs in the COX-2 category: Bextra (valdecoxib), Celebrex (celecoxib) and Vioxx (rofecoxib). On September 30, 2004, Merck & Company, Inc., makers of Vioxx, voluntarily withdrew the drug from the worldwide market because of safety concerns. The withdrawal of Vioxx was based on data from a trial that was evaluating the efficacy of the drug in the prevention of recurring colorectal polyps in patients who had a history of colorectal adenomas. The study showed an increased risk for cardiovascular events, such as heart attack and stroke, in patients who had been taking Vioxx for 18 months or longer when compared with those who were taking a placebo. Raymond V. Gilmartin, chairman, president, and chief executive officer of Merck, said, "Although we believe it would have been possible to continue to market Vioxx with labeling that would incorporate these new data, given the availability of alternative therapies, and the questions raised by the data, we concluded that a voluntary withdrawal is the responsible course to take." Individuals who have a history of heart attack or stroke, or who are at risk for these conditions, are encouraged to discuss their use of COX-2 inhibitors with their health-care practitioner.

Oral Contraceptives. Oral contraceptives—"the Pill"—usually contain two hormones, estrogen and progesterone (and its synthetic version, progestin). Despite widespread use, much debate continues about the safety and benefits versus risks of taking the Pill. On the positive side, some studies show that oral contraceptives that contain both estrogen and progestin protect against endometrial and ovarian cancer, and that even after you stop taking the Pill the benefits seem to continue for about 15 years. Another benefit of the Pill is that it seems to reduce the frequency of benign breast lumps and cysts, and offers protection against endometriosis, pelvic inflammatory disease, and iron-deficiency anemia. Some of the newer oral contraceptives also improve mild acne conditions.

On the negative side, you are at risk for complications from the pill (including heart problems and stroke) if you smoke, have a history of blood clots, or have asthma, diabetes, high blood pressure, liver disease, unexplained vaginal bleeding, or cancer of the breast, uterus, or ovaries. Women who take the Pill for many years may develop gallstones or have difficulty becoming pregnant. Among women who take progestin-only (synthetic progesterone) contraceptives, there has been reported to be a 30 percent increase in the risk of breast cancer. However, included in these reports were findings involving contraceptives that are not used anymore. While the risk of developing breast cancer with oral contraceptives remains controversial, certain factors, such as the type and amount of hormones used, the woman's age when the contraceptive was started, duration of use, and personal risk of breast cancer, including family history of breast cancer, may influence this risk.

Hormone Replacement Therapy. Two types of hormone replacement therapy—estrogen replacement therapy (ERT) and hormone replacement therapy (HRT; using both estrogen and progesterone/progestin)—are typically prescribed for menopausal symptoms or to help prevent postmenopausal osteoporosis. Both therapies are controversial, and both have benefits and risks. For example, when it comes to women who use ERT, in 1995 the Harvard Nurses' Health Study reported a 30 to 70 percent increased risk of breast cancer. A later study (1997) in the *New England Journal of Medicine* that looked at data from 60,000 postmenopausal women found a 43 percent increased risk of death from breast cancer.

Use of HRT also raises concerns. In January 2000, *The Journal of the American Medical Association* reported on the results of the Breast Cancer Detection Demonstration Project, which followed more than 46,000 postmenopausal women. The study found that HRT may increase the risk of breast cancer even more than that of estrogen treatment alone. A National Cancer Institute study published shortly after the Breast Cancer Detection Demonstration Project revealed that five years of HRT increases the risk of breast cancer by 24 percent, which is four times the risk from ERT alone. Recently, a large study of HRT from the Women's Health Initiative was stopped early due to findings that indicate an increased risk of invasive breast cancer, strokes, heart attacks, and cardiovascular disease. Although women using HRT had a reduction in hip fractures, total fractures, and colorectal cancer, the increased risks do not appear to justify its use for these purposes.

Clearly, a woman's decision to use either ERT or HRT, or neither one, should be made after careful consideration and with the advice of a medical professional.

How to Minimize Your Risks When Taking Drugs

COMMUNICATING WITH YOUR HEALTH-CARE PRACTITIONER

Are you afraid to ask your health-care practitioner questions about your prescriptions because you feel like you're bothering him or that your questions are stupid? Does your health-care practitioner hand you a prescription without giving you complete instructions about how to use it and warning you of its possible side effects? Does your health-care practitioner understand your lifestyle and individual needs so that he or she can prescribe the best medication for you?

Maintaining clear communication with your health-care practitioner about your medication use and needs is critical to your health. Your health-care practitioner may prescribe the very best drug for your specific condition, yet if you don't understand how to take it, it may do you no good at all or make your condition worse. This is an example of poor communication between patients and health-care practitioners, and it can be harmful to your health.

What to Tell Your Health-Care Practitioner. A study conducted by Wayne State University found that "most people are interrupted by their health-care practitioners within the first 18 seconds of beginning to explain what is wrong with them." If this has happened to you, did you feel uncomfortable or intimidated? Did you forget what you wanted to say? Did you believe you didn't have the right to continue with your explanation?

You can help prevent such situations by being prepared. That preparation can come in handy when filling out medical forms as well as talking with the health-care practitioner. One of the first things we do when we visit a new health-care practitioner is provide written information about our health, medical history, and lifestyle habits. Because it can be difficult to remember everything, it's a good idea to prepare for the visit by making notes beforehand at home, jotting down dates of past accidents or hospitalizations, names and dosages of medications, vitamins, or herbs you may be taking, and any other relevant health information.

You may need to ask family members about illnesses that run in your family or the cause of death of close relatives. If necessary, keep a diary of symptoms, reactions to foods or other substances, or anything else you think may relate to your health or current medical problem. If you have difficulty remembering when certain things happened, try to link them with holidays or other significant events in your life, like a wedding, birthday, or vacation.

It's also important to keep your regular health-care practitioners up to date on any changes in any of these areas.

Questions to Ask Your Health-Care Practitioner. Your health-care practitioner just handed you a prescription or a few samples along with your prescription. You know you should ask questions, but they've all slipped your mind. Here's a list to get you started. Take this list with you on your visit. You may want to add some of your own questions after reading through these and the drug profiles in the second part of this book.

- How long should I take this medication?
- What's the best way to take this medication: with food, between meals, with liquids?
- If I have trouble swallowing this medication, can I crush it or take it in another form?
- Is there a generic brand of this drug? Is the generic version as effective as the name brand? (See "Brand-Name vs. Generic Drugs" on page 34.)
- What benefits can I expect from this drug?
- What side effects might I expect? Ask your health-care practitioner to be specific. You'll want to know if it will affect your vision (especially if you will be driving or operating machinery), balance, appetite, concentration, mood, sex life, and so on.
- Does this drug interact with _____? Here you will make sure your health-care practitioner knows which medications you are already taking, if any, including over-the-counter drugs such as aspirin or ibuprofen.
- Does this medication interact with caffeine, alcohol, vitamins, herbs, or other supplements? Should I avoid any of these substances while taking this medication?

- Are there any non-drug alternatives to taking this drug, such as dietary changes, exercise, stress management techniques, nutritional supplements, or therapy?
- Is this the lowest possible dosage I can take? Can I reduce the dosage?
- Does this medication have the potential to make me physically or psychologically dependent on it?

Don't Leave the Office Yet. It's not enough to ask the questions; make sure you jot down the answers. Don't expect to remember everything your health-care practitioner tells you; there can be a lot of information to digest.

Look at the prescription before you leave the office. Make sure the name and dosage are clearly written. According to a report in *The Journal of the American Medical Association* in 1979, about 50 percent of health-care practitioners' handwritten prescriptions are difficult to interpret, and things haven't changed much since then. A clearly written prescription also saves time, because the pharmacist doesn't have to call your health-care practitioner for clarification.

E-Mail, Anyone? Some health-care practitioners use E-mail to stay in touch with their patients. If you have E-mail, ask your health-care practitioner if he or she uses it to answer nonemergency questions, and how often the messages are checked and answered. Obviously E-mail isn't the best method of communication for all circumstances, but you may call in a question and then have your health-care practitioners answer via E-mail, when they have time after office hours.

The American Medical Association has drawn up guidelines for health-care practitioners to follow concerning E-mail. Health-care practitioners should not share patients' E-mail addresses with marketers or family members and should never send group E-mails where other recipients are listed. The guidelines require that health-care practitioners ask their patients what method of communication they prefer and to mark the preference on patients' charts.

PHARMACISTS: YOUR BEST RESOURCE

Next to your health-care practitioner, your pharmacist is your best resource for information about prescription and nonprescription drugs. In fact, some people feel more comfortable talking with and asking questions of their pharmacist, although we hope you can establish a good relationship with your health-care practitioners as well.

What a Good Pharmacist Can Do for You. One of the best things you can do is have all your prescriptions filled at the same pharmacy by a pharmacist you know and trust. Pharmacies are computerized today, which means they have information about you and your medication history at their fingertips. This make it easy for your pharmacist to identify quickly any drug interactions or allergies you have and whether any new prescriptions may cause a problem.

Your pharmacist also has the authority to contact your health-care practitioner about any medication he or she believes may be dangerous for you. Pharmacists have about six years of scientific training behind them, and they are fully qualified to answer questions about side effects and drug interactions that concern you.

Questions to Ask Your Pharmacist. About 50 percent of the nearly 2 billion prescriptions dispensed every year are used incorrectly. Why? Again, people don't ask questions. When you're at the pharmacy, take advantage of the situation. You may not have asked your health-care practitioner all the questions you had in mind. Maybe you didn't ask any at all. Or you may just need some clarification. In any event, your pharmacist is there for you. Here are some questions to get you started:

- Is this drug available in generic form? What is the difference in cost? Is the generic bioequivalent to the brand name?
- How should I store this drug?
- If I have trouble swallowing the tablet or capsule, may I crush the tablet or open the capsule?
- Is this drug available in a form that is easier to take?
- What side effects may I expect?
- What should I do if I experience side effects? Which ones should concern me, and which ones usually go away, and how soon?
- When should I take this medication—between or with meals, at bedtime?
- What should I do if I miss a dose?
- Are there any foods, beverages, or other medications I should not take while I take this drug?
- For people who have difficulty opening prescription bottles or who have vision problems: can this medication be placed in an easy-to-open container? Do you have large-print instructions?
- For people with English-language difficulties: can instructions be provided in another language?

ONLINE PHARMACIES: ARE THEY SAFE?

It seems that you can buy just about anything over the Internet. That may be a good thing when it comes to purchasing CDs and watches, but it may not be so good when it comes to prescription medications.

Convenience and lower cost are the two main reasons people say they like to get their prescriptions from online pharmacies. If you don't want to drive to a drugstore to get your prescription and you can wait a few days or a week to get your prescription in the mail, then you may find online pharmacy services convenient. However, if your child develops an earache and you want antibiotics immediately, an online pharmacy won't be able to help you.

If you are homebound or live far from a pharmacy, online drug availability can be very convenient. Online pharmacies also allow you to comparison shop for price and availability. When it comes to cost, you must consider the cost of shipping. Once you tack on postage and handling fees, the cost of your prescription may meet or exceed your neighborhood pharmacy.

The Food and Drug Administration (FDA) warns consumers that they should beware of shady websites, undocumented claims, and illegal deals when it comes to online prescription drugs. Here are some of the factors you should consider before you make an online purchase.

Suspect any online pharmacy that does not require you to mail in your prescription, or one that does not verify your prescription with your prescriber. These practices suggest that these pharmacies have little or no regard for their customers' health or welfare, because they do not bother to make sure individuals are getting the proper prescription and that the drugs are indeed going to the person for whom they were intended.

Suspect any online pharmacy that dispenses drugs based solely on a questionnaire you are asked to complete online. There is no way the recipients of your questionnaire will know whether you are telling the truth, and basically anyone can fill out a questionnaire and say they need a particular drug. Some state medical boards are taking action against health-care practitioners who prescribe medications over the Internet. Why? Because these health-care practitioners do not know you or the condition of your health. They can only rely on what you tell them.

- Make sure the website offers a street address for the pharmacy service and a toll-free number you can call. If these are not available, do not use the site.

- The pharmacy should have a pharmacist available to answer your questions, either via phone or E-mail correspondence. Preferably this service should be free. If no pharmacist is available, do not purchase from that site.
- Be wary of websites that offer only a few drugs, especially "lifestyle" drugs—those that help you lose weight, improve your sexual performance, or grow hair. Such sites may not be legitimate.
- Review the pharmacy's guidelines regarding confidentiality of patient health-care information.
- Do not patronize any website that makes unrealistic claims about "magic cures" or quick-fix medications for serious medical conditions.
- Question any site that claims to be backed by well-known medical institutions or government agencies without first checking to see if their claims are true. This means you'll need to contact the institutions or agencies named (which can be done easily online via their public information offices), but it's better to be safe than sorry.
- Buy from nationally recognized chains (e.g., CVS, Walgreen's, Drug Emporium) or established prescription businesses (e.g., American Association of Retired Persons Pharmacy Service).
- Beware of foreign websites. They may be dispensing subpotent, outdated, contaminated, or counterfeit products. Even though the Food and Drug Administration contacts foreign pharmacy sites and questions their activities, many continue to operate.
- Look for a site that offers a money-back guarantee and promises reasonable delivery times.
- Look for the Verified Internet Pharmacy Practices Site seal on the websites you visit. This seal is an endorsement from the National Association of Boards of Pharmacy (NABP), an organization that can tell you whether a particular online pharmacy is in good standing. You can contact the NABP by accessing their website at *www.nabp.net* or calling them at (847) 698-6227.
- You can also contact each state board of pharmacy (the state in which the online pharmacy is physically located) to verify the pharmacy's legitimacy.
- If you think a website may be operating illegally, contact the Food and Drug Administration (FDA) by sending an E-mail to *webcomplaints@ora.fda.gov*.

BRAND-NAME VS. GENERIC DRUGS

Generic drugs are medications that are identified by their chemical composition rather than their brand, or trade, name. Most people, for example, recognize the brand name Valium, yet the generic name of this antianxiety drug is diazepam. You can ask for the brand name or the generic if your health-care practitioner prescribes this drug for you, although if you have a prescription drug plan, your insurance company may only pay for the cost of the generic drug.

Why Brand-Name Drugs Cost More Than Generics. In the majority of cases, generic drugs are equally as effective as brand-name medications. They also are typically less expensive than brand names, often as much as 50 percent or more. Why is this so?

Pharmaceutical companies spend a great deal of time (usually a decade or more) and money—typically more than $300 million—researching, developing, producing, and marketing a new drug. The result of all that time and effort is, if all goes well, a brand-name drug that is patented and sold exclusively under a single trade name for 17 years, which allows the company to make back the money it invested. Once a patent expires, or if there is no patent, other companies can manufacture and sell that drug under the drug's generic name or under different brand names. These other companies don't have to invest all that time and money to bring the original drug to market. Therefore, they can sell the drug at a lower cost.

Are Generic Drugs Really Any Good? If you've been reluctant to ask your health-care practitioner or pharmacist for the generic equivalents of drugs you are taking, or if someone has told you that brand-name medications are superior to generics, consider this: did you know that major drug companies produce an estimated 70 to 80 percent of the generic drugs on the market? And did you know that the Food and Drug Administration (FDA) approves generic drugs only if they act in the body the same way as the original brand-name drug? So what are you waiting for?

True, there isn't a generic form available for every brand name. Your health-care practitioner or pharmacist can tell you if generics are available, or you can check in the drug entries in the second part of this book. There are also a few rare exceptions in which the same active ingredient, produced by different manufacturers, is absorbed by the body at a different rate. This difference can mean one drug may be slightly more or less effective than another one.

For example, generic conjugated estrogens are slightly different from Premarin, a brand-name estrogen hormone, and the difference may make the generic less effective at preventing osteoporosis. If you have any questions about the bioequivalence of any generic, ask your health-care practitioner or pharmacist about it.

WHEN PRESCRIPTION DRUGS ARE SOLD OVER-THE-COUNTER

More than 600 ingredients or dosages that once were available by prescription only are now available over-the-counter (OTC). During the past twenty-five years, the FDA has authorized the over-the-counter sale of more than fifty drugs that previously were sold by prescription. Most of those drugs fall into the categories of decongestants, antihistamines, analgesics (painkillers), antiulcer, and anti-itch medications.

Drug companies like to market a prescription drug as OTC because it means more profits for them. But there is also an advantage for consumers: convenience. You don't need to go to your health-care practitioner and get a prescription for your medications. That's where you *may* also save money, depending on the type of insurance coverage you have. Some OTC versions of prescription drugs are less expensive, but in many cases they are not. And while some insurance plans pay most or all of a prescription's cost, you must foot the bill for OTC drugs.

Making the Transition to OTC. Not just any drug can make the transition from prescription to OTC. The FDA has criteria a prescription drug must meet before it can make the transition.

- The prescription drug must have at least a three-year history of safe use
- The OTC drug cannot cause serious side effects if it is misused
- The medical condition the OTC drug will treat must be self-diagnosable. That's why you can buy OTC drugs for the common cold or a headache but not for high cholesterol or Alzheimer's disease
- The OTC drug should relieve symptoms

In 2000, Merck & Co., maker of lovastatin (Mevacor), and Bristol-Myers Squibb, maker of pravastatin (Pravachol), petitioned the FDA to sell these two cholesterol-lowering prescription drugs over-the-counter. However, in 1997, the FDA had clearly stated in its "Guidance for Industry" statement that cholesterol-lowering drugs should be available by prescription only. One reason is that these drugs are used to treat a condition that is not self-recognizable. You must be tested for your cholesterol level, and your levels need to be monitored by a health-care practitioner. Thus cholesterol-lowering drugs do not meet one of the criteria set forth by the FDA, and Merck and Bristol-Myers Squibb were turned down.

The Safety Factor. Just because a drug is OTC does not mean it can't cause serious side effects if it isn't taken properly. For example: aspirin, the "wonder drug," can cause bleeding of the stomach if taken in too high doses and, among a small percentage of people, even when taken at recommended doses. Thus any drug, prescription or OTC, should be taken according to directions or your healthcare practitioner's instructions, and regarded with caution.

COMPOUNDING PHARMACIES

When it comes to getting your prescription filled, you have more than one option: you can go to a standard pharmacy or drugstore, or you can go to a compounding pharmacy. A compounding pharmacy prepares a specialized drug product to fulfill an individual's specific needs that cannot be met by a standard prescription.

For example: if you have difficulty swallowing a tablet or capsule, you can get your prescription prepared into a solution. Many drugs contain dyes and fillers such as lactose (e.g., decongestants, antibiotics) that can cause allergic reactions in a small percentage of people. If you are one of those people, you can get a compounding pharmacist to prepare your prescription without the offending ingredient. And if your child refuses to take a bad-tasting medication, flavoring it with cherry or grape can make the medicine go down.

The Food and Drug Administration (FDA) defined the limits of legitimate compounding under the FDA Modernization Act of 1997. However, although compounding pharmacists begin with an FDA-approved drug, changes they make to any given drug may convert an approved drug into an unapproved one. That means there is the potential for reactions to occur between ingredients because of the change that was made.

Compounding pharmacies are an option. Pharmacist and former FDA pharmacy compounding steering committee member Robert Tonelli said, "Whenever possible, FDA would recommend that patients use an approved drug. We have more data and reporting requirements on those to assure us of their safety and effectiveness." (Rules for compounding can be seen at the FDA website: *http://www.fda.gov/fdac/features/2000/400_compound.html*)

GUIDELINES FOR SAFE DRUG USE

Until the day the perfect drug exists—one that relieves all your symptoms and causes no side effects—we must recognize that every drug has potential benefits as well as potential risks. To maximize the first and minimize the latter, you need to follow some guidelines concerning everything from storing drugs properly to understanding the dosage instructions.

Storing Your Medications. This seems obvious: in the bathroom medicine cabinet, right? Wrong. The heat and humidity generated in the bathroom can change the chemical composition of some drugs. The same goes for the kitchen. Because not all drugs are alike, here are some storage guidelines.

- Ask your pharmacist how to store your prescription. The instructions should be on the prescription, but ask anyway.
- Some medications need to be refrigerated. Make sure, however, that you only refrigerate those that should be.
- If a drug should be refrigerated, don't keep it at the back of the refrigerator, as some units tend to be much colder in the back and may freeze your prescription.
- Keep medications away from excess heat and light. For example, don't leave your prescriptions on a bureau that gets direct sunlight.
- Keep your medications in their original containers to help prevent deterioration or losing their labels.
- Many medications, such as narcotics and sedatives, are subject to theft. Make sure you keep all medications in a safe and perhaps unlikely place (e.g., a linen closet, pantry, or utensil drawer), especially if you have repair people or other "stranger traffic" in your home. Drugs left in bathroom medicine cabinets, for example, can easily be lifted by individuals who ask to use your bathroom.

Safeguards Against Tampering. Pharmacists know how different drugs and their packaging should look. If you suspect there is something wrong with either the appearance, smell, or consistency of a drug or the packaging, bring it to the attention of your pharmacist. Here's what you should look for:

- Tablets should be all the same size, color, thickness, texture, and shape. Check that all the imprints are the same.
- Capsules should be fully intact and uniform in appearance, color, and odor, and have the same imprint.
- Tubes, jars, and eye drop containers should be properly sealed.
- Ointments, lotions, and creams should be smooth and consistent, without separation of the ingredients.

Drug Labels. Prescription labels should contain the following information: your first and last name, the name of the prescriber, the drug name (brand and generic if applicable), the pharmacy's address and telephone number, the prescription number, use directions, and the date it was dispensed. Also make sure there's an expiration date for the drug on the label. Medications can lose their effectiveness and breakdown into harmful substances over time. If you cannot find the expiration date, ask your pharmacist to get the information for you.

With so much information on a label, it can be difficult to see. If you have difficulty reading the label, ask the pharmacist if you can get the information in larger print. Also, make sure you understand any abbreviations on the label (see "Latin Lesson").

Take Your Medications Correctly. Ninety-six percent of patients do not ask questions about their prescriptions. Twenty percent of patients cannot read well enough to follow a medical treatment program effectively at home. Many people don't realize the consequences of taking their prescriptions incorrectly. These are major reasons why individuals fail to comply with drug treatment instructions.

Whether you don't take the drug at all, you miss doses, you double up on doses, or you take the wrong amount or at the wrong times, these behaviors can have a serious negative impact on your health. If you don't understand the dosage instructions or you miss a dose, call your health-care practitioner or pharmacist immediately for guidance.

LATIN LESSON: READING ABBREVIATIONS ON YOUR PRESCRIPTION LABEL

Abbreviation	Latin for	Meaning
ac	*ante cibum*	before meals
bid	*bis in die*	twice a day
hs	*hora somni*	at bedtime
od	*oculus dexter*	right eye
os	*oculus sinister*	left eye
po	*per os*	by mouth (orally)
pc	*post cibum*	after meals
prn	*pro re nata*	as needed
q3h	*quaque 3 hora*	every 3 hours
qd	*quaque die*	every day (daily)
qid	*quater in die*	4 times a day
tid	*ter in die*	3 times a day

Sometimes it's difficult or impossible to take a medication if you can't swallow the pill or capsule, or the taste is especially offensive. In such situations, ask your health-care practitioner if you can have a different form of the drug (see "Compounding Pharmacies").

Timing Is Everything. Taking your medications at the right time can have a significant impact on their effectiveness and safety. Make sure you understand the dosing instructions: does four times a day mean every six hours, or with breakfast, lunch, and dinner and at bedtime? Should you take the medication with food? If you drive to work and your medication makes you drowsy, should you take your morning dose after you arrive at the office?

Timing is especially important if you are taking two or more drugs. Some drugs interact if they are taken together; others are safe. Discuss your drug dosing schedule with your health-care practitioner or pharmacist. Then choose a way to make sure you remember it accurately. You may want to use a scheduling chart or calendar, on which you can mark off each dose as soon as you take it.

Side Effects. When you get your prescription, you should be given information about possible side effects. This does not mean, however, that you will experience any of them; it also does not mean that you won't develop some that aren't on the list. Everyone reacts to drugs differently. If you experience any unusual reactions to a drug, contact your health-care practitioner.

Discontinuing a Drug. You should never stop taking a drug without first consulting with your health-care practitioner. Some drugs, such as tranquilizers, antidepressants, and sleeping pills, can cause adverse reactions such as nausea and vomiting if you stop taking them suddenly. Certain high blood pressure medications can cause abnormal blood pressures or heart rate if they are stopped suddenly. Others that can cause dependence, such as antianxiety drugs and narcotics, can cause severe withdrawal symptoms, including tremors, vomiting, and hallucinations, if stopped abruptly.

Old Prescriptions. Old prescriptions that you never used up should not be saved unless you consult your health-care practitioner and he determines that you may be able to use them again in the near future. Remember, however, that drugs lose their potency over time, so check the expiration dates. Unneeded, unused drugs should be flushed down the toilet, especially if there are small children in the home who may find them.

Prevent Poisonings and Overdoses. Hopefully you will never need to institute any of the emergency procedures discussed in the section "What to Do in an Emergency" on page 43. One way to ensure that is to prevent poisonings or overdoses.

- If there are children in the home, lock all medications out of sight and reach.
- Make sure there are childproof tops on all medication containers.
- Never leave medications around where children can reach them. As soon as you take your own dose or give your child a dose, put the medication out of reach.
- Never refer to medications as candy or "tastes good."
- Dispose of unwanted or unneeded drugs by emptying pill and capsule bottles, crushing the contents, and flushing them down the toilet. Pour liquid medications down the sink.
- Stress upon your children that they should never take any kind of medicine without your help. Draw a big "X" on prescription bottles so they can identify which containers they should always avoid.
- If a medication looks or smells like it has deteriorated (changes in color or consistency), do not take it. Contact your health-care practitioner or pharmacist immediately.
- If you need to take medications during the night, turn on the light and use your glasses if you need them for reading.
- Never take someone else's medication.
- If you take two or more medications a day, it can be difficult to remember how and when to take each one. You may actually take too many of any one or more drugs and cause serious reactions. Devise a plan that helps you, such as a chart, calendar, or weekly pill boxes.

YOUR STAY IN THE HOSPITAL

If you are hospitalized for any reason, bring your medications with you, as well as any OTC drugs and supplements you may take regularly. Studies show that hospital patients consume an average of nine drugs during their hospital stay, while some take as many as twenty. The result is that about one-third of hospitalized patients experience adverse drug reactions.

To help safeguard yourself against medication errors and reactions, consider the following guidelines:

- Keep a list of all the drugs you are taking, and each time a new one is added, add it to the list.
- Tell the health-care practitioners about any drug allergies you have and make sure they are noted on your chart.

- When a new drug is given to you, make sure you know what it is, what it's for, and how it may interact with other drugs you are taking.
- You have the right to refuse any medication. If you do not understand why a drug is being given to you or what the benefits are, you can say no. You may also ask if there are any alternatives to that specific drug.
- Before you are discharged from the hospital, make sure you understand all about the drugs you will be taking at home, and ask for the information in writing.

What to Do in an Emergency

Accidental poisoning usually occurs in young children who are curious and swallow drugs that have not been properly locked away. Adults typically overdose on a drug either because they've been careless or they don't have the proper instructions.

If an overdose or poisoning has occurred:

- Contact a poison control center, emergency department, or paramedics immediately, even if symptoms have not yet appeared. The telephone numbers for these emergency options should be next to all your telephones at all times, especially if you have small children at home.
- Have the prescription container handy so you can read the label information to the medical professionals you contact.
- Never induce vomiting or force liquids unless you've been instructed to do so by medical professionals or the label, especially if the individual is unconscious or not breathing. You should keep a bottle of syrup of ipecac handy (for inducing vomiting) in your home for such emergencies. If you don't have syrup of ipecac available, you may be instructed to get the individual to drink as much water as possible, which will help dilute the drug in the stomach.
- If you have been instructed by a medical professional to induce vomiting, save the vomit for analysis at the hospital.

The Prescription Drug Profiles

GENERIC NAME
Acarbose

BRAND NAME
Precose
No generic available

ABOUT THIS DRUG
Acarbose is an antidiabetic drug that is prescribed for people who have type II (non-insulin-dependent) diabetes who cannot control their high glucose (sugar) levels by diet alone. It can be safely combined with sulfonylurea drugs if diet and sulfonylurea drugs together don't adequately control glucose levels (see Sulfonylurea Antidiabetes Drugs).

Acarbose differs from most other antidiabetic drugs in that it interferes with enzymes in the intestinal tract (intestinal alpha glucosidase and pancreatic alpha amylase) that metabolize (break down) complex carbohydrates into simple sugars, including glucose. The result is a delay in the absorption of glucose into the bloodstream after eating and a more controlled, lower blood sugar level.

SIDE EFFECTS
About 75 percent of people who take acarbose experience stomach gas when they first start taking the drug. This side effect usually diminishes or goes away after a few weeks. However, if you develop this or any other side effect when taking acarbose, contact your health-care practitioner immediately. He or she will determine whether or not you should continue to take the drug.

- *Common:* abdominal pain, diarrhea
- *Rare:* liver irritation, minor abnormalities in blood tests, especially those associated with liver enzymes

IMPORTANT PRECAUTIONS
Use this drug only under a health-care practitioner's supervision. Do not take acarbose if you are allergic or sensitive to it, or if you have diabetic ketoacidosis, cirrhosis, severe kidney disease, inflammatory bowel disease, ulcers in your colon, intestinal obstruction, absorption diseases, or severe digestive diseases, or if you tend to experience severe gas.

When taken without other antidiabetic drugs, acarbose does not cause abnormally low blood sugar (hypoglycemia). It can, however, cause hypoglycemia if you take it in combination with insulin or other antidiabetic medications. If you are combining acarbose with other antidiabetic drugs, talk with your health-care practitioner first.

DRUG INTERACTIONS

Tell your health-care practitioner and pharmacist about any prescription or over-the-counter medications you are taking, as well as any vitamins, herbs, and other supplements. Possible drug interactions with acarbose may include the following:

- The effects of warfarin and sulfonylureas (e.g., glipizide, glyburide) may be increased and result in hypoglycemia.
- Amylase may reduce the benefits of acarbose.
- Digestive enzyme preparations that contain lipase or amylase may cause loss of blood sugar control.
- Digoxin may lower blood levels of digoxin and loss of benefits.
- Insulin increases the risk of hypoglycemia.
- Sulfonamide antibiotics may increase the risk for hypoglycemia.
- These drugs may decrease the effects of acarbose: adrenocorticosteroids (e.g., cortisone, prednisone), beta-blockers (e.g., acebutolol, propranolol), calcium channel blockers (e.g., diltiazem, verapamil), furosemide, bumetanide, isoniazid, monoamine oxidase inhibitors (e.g., phenelzine), nicotinic acid, phenytoin, rifampin, theophylline, thiazide diuretics (e.g., chlorothiazide), and thyroid hormones.
- Clofibrate, disopyramide, high doses of aspirin or other salicylates, and some nonsteroidal anti-inflammatory drugs (talk to your health-care practitioner about specific ones) may cause hypoglycemia when taken concurrently with acarbose.

FOOD, VITAMIN, AND HERBAL INTERACTIONS

Acarbose does not interact negatively with food; however, it must be taken with the first bite of food if it is to be effective. Because chromium supplements can change the way your body uses glucose, you should talk to your health-care practitioner before taking chromium and acarbose. Herbs that may alter your blood glucose levels include garlic, ginger, ginseng, hawthorn, and nettle. Discuss use of these herbs and acarbose with your health-care practitioner before you take any of them.

RECOMMENDED DOSAGE

Acarbose is available in tablets: 25-, 50-, and 100-mg strength. Your health-care practitioner will determine the dosage that is right for you. The typical dosage is:

- *Children:* The safety and effectiveness of acarbose has not been established for individuals younger than 18 years.
- *Adults 18 to 65 Years of Age:* One 25-mg tablet three times daily, taken with your first bite of food. Your health-care practitioner will monitor your progress and make adjustments at 4- to 8-week intervals as needed to achieve blood sugar control. If you weigh less than 132 pounds, the maximum dosage you can take is 50 mg three times daily; if you weigh more, then the maximum dosage is 100 mg three times a day.
- *Over 65 Years of Age:* No special instructions unless you have limited kidney function. Then your health-care practitioner will determine if this drug is appropriate for you.

If you miss a dose, skip it and take your next scheduled dose at your next meal. Taking acarbose between meals provides no benefit because there must be food digesting in the intestines for it to work. Never stop taking acarbose without first consulting your health-care practitioner.

SYMPTOMS OF OVERDOSE AND WHAT TO DO

In case of overdose, symptoms will be similar to typical side effects: gas, abdominal discomfort, and diarrhea. They will disappear quickly. An overdose of acarbose alone will not cause hypoglycemia.

SPECIAL INFORMATION FOR PREGNANT OR NURSING WOMEN

The effects of acarbose on pregnant women have not been studied adequately. Therefore, if you are pregnant or plan to become pregnant, tell your health-care practitioner before taking this medication. Because it is important to maintain normal blood sugar levels during pregnancy, your health-care practitioner may prescribe injected insulin for that purpose. It's not known whether acarbose passes into breast milk; therefore your health-care practitioner may advise you either not to use this drug if you are breastfeeding or not to nurse.

SPECIAL INFORMATION FOR SENIORS

Older individuals who have severe kidney disease should not use this drug.

GENERIC NAME

Acebutolol

BRAND NAME

Sectral

Generic available

ABOUT THIS DRUG

Acebutolol is an antihypertensive drug (type, beta-blocker) used primarily to treat mild-to-moderate high blood pressure (hypertension) and abnormal heart rhythms.

Acebutolol, like other beta-blockers, reduces the rate and force of the heart's contractions, which results in lower blood pressure. It helps ease some heart rhythm problems by slowing down the nerve impulses that move through the heart.

SIDE EFFECTS

Side effects associated with this drug are generally mild and usually occur soon after you first start taking it. However, you should tell your health-care practitioner immediately if you experience them.

- *Less Common:* abnormal vision, chest pain, constipation, cough, depression, diarrhea, frequent urination, gas, headache, indigestion, joint pain, nasal inflammation, nausea, difficulty breathing, fluid retention and swelling, sleep problems, weakness, strange dreams
- *Rare:* abdominal pain, anxiety, back pain, burning or painful eyes, cold extremities, conjunctivitis, fever, heart failure, itching or rash, loss of appetite, low blood pressure, muscle pain, nervousness, painful or difficult urination, excessive urination at night, dark urine, slow heartbeat, inflamed throat, vomiting, wheezing

IMPORTANT PRECAUTIONS

Tell your health-care practitioner if you are sensitive or allergic to this drug or any other drugs, especially other beta-blockers.

Before taking acebutolol, inform your health-care practitioner if you have asthma, severe heart failure, poor circulation or circulatory disease, chronic bronchitis, emphysema, hyperthyroidism (overactive thyroid), diabetes, depression, kidney disease, liver disease, any type of seizure disorder, myasthenia gravis, heart block, or a very slow heart rate (bradycardia).

If you have angina, you risk aggravating your angina if you suddenly stop taking this drug. Your health-care practitioner will gradually decrease your dosage over 1 to 2 weeks.

Because this drug can cause lightheadedness, make sure you know how you react to the drug before you drive or operate any type of dangerous equipment.

DRUG INTERACTIONS

Tell your health-care practitioner and pharmacist about any prescription or over-the-counter medications you are taking, as well as any vitamins, herbs, and other supplements. When acebutolol is taken along with other drugs, the effects of any of the medications may be reduced, increased, or changed in some other way. Possible drug interactions include the following:

- Albuterol and acebutolol together results in a loss of effect from both drugs.
- Alcohol may increase the drug's sedative effect and exaggerate the reduction in blood pressure.
- Amiodarone, phenytoin, or digitalis drugs may result in severe slowing of the heart.
- Blood pressure medications such as clonidine, guanabenz, and reserpine may excessively lower blood pressure.
- Calcium-channel blockers (e.g., verapamil) may lead to an increased risk of abnormal heart rhythm.
- Some over-the-counter cold and nasal remedies, such as Afrin and Sudafed, can interfere with acebutolol.
- Indomethacin and other NSAIDs (e.g., diclofenac) can decrease the effects of acebutolol.
- Ergots (e.g., pergolide) and acebutolol together increases the risk of getting gangrene and also increases the chance of experiencing cold hands and feet.
- Methyldopa may result in a sudden increase in blood pressure.
- Acebutolol can interfere with the effects of antiasthma drugs such as theophylline, aminophylline, ephedrine, and isoproterenol.
- Acebutolol may cover up signs of inadequate thyroid hormone replacement.
- Cimetidine increases the amount of acebutolol the body absorbs.

FOOD, VITAMIN, AND HERBAL INTERACTIONS

Acebutolol does not interact negatively with any food. However, it is best to avoid excessive salt intake if you have high blood pressure. If you plan to take or are taking any herbs or supplements, talk with your health-care practitioner before starting acebutolol. Ginseng, goldenseal, licorice, ephedra (ma huang), and saw palmetto may raise your blood pressure; garlic and calcium may help lower it.

RECOMMENDED DOSAGE

Acebutolol is available in 200- and 400-mg capsules. Your health-care practitioner will determine the most appropriate dosage and schedule for your needs. Typical dosage ranges are as follows.

- *Children:* Not indicated for children younger than 18 years.
- *Adults to 65 Years:* For mild-to-moderate hypertension, 200 to 800 mg daily in divided doses. For severe hypertension, up to 1,200 mg may be taken in two divided doses. Acebutolol can be taken alone or with another antihypertensive drug approved by your health-care practitioner. For irregular heartbeat, 400 mg daily taken in two divided doses 12 hours apart. Your health-care practitioner may gradually increase your dosage to 800 or 1,200 mg daily.
- *Over 65 Years:* Lower doses are generally effective, and total daily intake should not exceed 800 mg.

Never stop taking acebutolol suddenly or without first talking with your health-care practitioner. If you miss a dose, take the forgotten dose as soon as you remember. If it's within 4 hours of your next scheduled dose, do not take the missed dose. Return to your dosing schedule. Never take two doses at the same time. You can take acebutolol with or without food, and you can open the capsule if you prefer. Take it at the same time every day.

SYMPTOMS OF OVERDOSE AND WHAT TO DO

Although there is no specific information available about symptoms of overdose for acebutolol, the effects associated with an overdose of other beta-blockers include cold, sweaty skin, congestive heart failure, weakness, extremely slow heart rate, low blood pressure, fainting, difficulty breathing, and seizures. Seek emergency medical help immediately and bring the prescription bottle with you.

SPECIAL INFORMATION FOR PREGNANT OR NURSING WOMEN

Information about the effects of acebutolol on pregnant women is inadequate, but infants born to women who took beta-blockers while pregnant have been born with low birth weights, low blood pressure, and reduced heart rates. If you are pregnant or plan to become pregnant, talk with your health-care practitioner before starting this drug. It should be avoided during pregnancy.

Acebutolol does pass into breast milk and could affect your nursing infant. If acebutolol is necessary for your health, your health-care practitioner may advise you to stop breastfeeding until your treatment is complete.

SPECIAL INFORMATION FOR SENIORS

Older individuals are more likely than younger ones to experience cold extremities, chest pain, breathing difficulties, increased sweating, heartbeat changes, and lower body temperature. Frequent blood pressure checks are recommended.

GENERIC NAME

Acetaminophen

BRAND NAMES

Acephen, Aceta, Acetaminophen Uniserts, Apacet, Aspirin Free Anacin Maximum Strength, Childrens' Pain Reliever, Dapacin, Dynafed, Feverall, Genapap, Genebs, Halenol, Infants' Pain Reliever, Liquiprin, Mapap, Maranox, Meda Cap/Tab, Neopap, Oraphen-PD, Panadol, Redutemp, Ridenol, Silapap, Tapanol, Tempra, Tylenol, Uni-Ace

Generic available; also available over-the-counter

ABOUT THIS DRUG

Acetaminophen is an analgesic and antipyretic (anti-fever) medication available by prescription and over-the-counter. It is used by individuals who either do not want to use or who are sensitive or allergic to aspirin or other nonsteroidal anti-inflammatory drugs (NSAIDs).

Acetaminophen is most commonly used to relieve fever and pain associated with the common cold, flu, other viral infections, and other conditions characterized by pain and fever. Many people also take it to relieve headache, menstrual cramps, arthritis pain, and toothache, even though it is not effective against inflammation. Children are given acetaminophen to relieve fever and for pain and discomfort associated with the common cold, flu, immunizations, teething, and tonsillectomy.

SIDE EFFECTS

Acetaminophen rarely causes side effects when taken as directed. If you do develop side effects, stop taking the drug and contact your health-care practitioner immediately.

- *If Taken Long-Term or in Large Doses:* liver damage, itching, fever, rash, low blood sugar, yellowing of the whites of the eyes or the skin, changes in the composition of your blood
- *Rare:* allergic reactions (difficulty breathing, hives, rash, swelling)

IMPORTANT PRECAUTIONS

Always follow the prescribing directions from your health-care practitioner or those on the package. Do not take acetaminophen if you are sensitive or allergic to it. Do not take this drug for more than 10 days in a row for pain (five for children) or three days for fever unless your health-care practitioner prescribes it. If you have liver or kidney disease or a viral infection of the liver, do not take acetaminophen until you talk to your health-care practitioner.

Long-term use of large amounts of acetaminophen (e.g., 3,000 to 4,000 mg daily for a year) can cause liver damage. See your health-care practitioner immediately if you have been taking high amounts of the drug for a long time.

DRUG INTERACTIONS

Let your health-care practitioner and pharmacist know of any prescription or over-the-counter drugs you are taking, as well as any vitamins, herbs, or other supplements. Possible drug interactions with acetaminophen may include the following:

- Large doses or long-term use of barbiturates, carbamazepine, phenytoin and similar drugs, rifampin, and sulfinpyrazone may reduce the effects of acetaminophen. They may also increase your risk of liver toxicity.
- Check with your health-care practitioner before combining acetaminophen with any of the following drugs: cholestyramine, isoniazid, any nonsteroidal anti-inflammatory drug (e.g., ibuprofen, naproxen), oral contraceptives, warfarin, and zidovudine.
- Alcohol and acetaminophen are not a good mix: alcohol increases the risk of liver toxicity and liver failure. If you use acetaminophen regularly, avoid alcohol use. If you usually have three or more alcoholic drinks daily, talk to your health-care practitioner before starting acetaminophen.

FOOD, VITAMIN, AND HERBAL INTERACTIONS

There are no food interactions reported for acetaminophen. If you use or plan to use the herbs chaparral, comfrey, or coltsfoot while taking acetaminophen, talk with your health-care practitioner before taking any of these remedies together. These herbs can cause liver damage, and when combined with acetaminophen may increase the risk of liver problems. There is also some evidence that high doses of vitamin C (3,000 mg daily) may raise the levels of acetaminophen in the body, thus increasing the risk of drug toxicity.

RECOMMENDED DOSAGE

Acetaminophen is available in tablets, caplets, elixir (a special cup is provided for measuring), and drops (for infants). Follow your health-care practitioner's directions or those on the package. The typical dose ranges are as follows:

- *Children Younger than 4 Months:* 40 mg 4-5 times daily
- *Children 4 to 11 Months:* 80 mg 4-5 times daily
- *Children 1 to 2 Years:* 120 mg 4-5 times daily
- *Children 3 Years:* 160 mg 4-5 times daily
- *Children 4 to 5 Years:* 240 mg 4-5 times daily
- *Children 6 to 8 Years:* 320 mg 4-5 times daily
- *Children 9 to 10 Years:* 400 mg 4-5 times daily
- *Children 11 Years:* 480 mg 4-5 times daily
- *Children 12 Years and Older and Adults:* 300-600 mg 4-6 times daily; or 1,000 mg 3-4 times daily. Do not exceed a maximum dosage of 4,000 mg daily.

If you miss a dose, take it as soon as you remember. However, if it is within an hour of your next dose, do not take the skipped dose; continue with your regular dosing schedule. Do not take a double dose.

SYMPTOMS OF OVERDOSE AND WHAT TO DO

Acute acetaminophen overdose may cause abdominal tenderness, abnormal heart rhythms, appetite loss, confusion, drowsiness, kidney or liver failure, low blood pressure, nausea, sweating, vomiting, and yellowing of the eyes. If overdose occurs, contact your local poison control office or emergency department. You will be instructed to take syrup of ipecac (available at drug stores and pharmacies) to induce vomiting. You will then be told to go to the emergency room. Bring the acetaminophen bottle with you.

SPECIAL INFORMATION FOR PREGNANT OR NURSING WOMEN

When taken in recommended doses and according to package directions, acetaminophen is considered safe during pregnancy and breastfeeding. However, you should check with your health-care practitioner before taking any medication when pregnant or nursing. Regular use of high doses of acetaminophen may cause birth defects or hinder fetal development.

SPECIAL INFORMATION FOR SENIORS

Lower doses may be advisable. Adverse reactions may be more likely and more severe among older individuals.

GENERIC NAME

Acetaminophen plus narcotic: codeine phosphate, hydrocodone, or oxycodone

BRAND NAMES

Acetaminophen + codeine phosphate: Aceta with Codeine, Capital with Codeine, Phenaphen with Codeine No. 3, Phenaphen with Codeine No. 4, Tylenol with Codeine No. 2, Tylenol with Codeine No. 3, Tylenol with Codeine No. 4

Generic available

Acetaminophen + hydrocodone bitartrate: Anexsia (5/500, 7.5/650, and 10/660), Bancap HC, Cta-Plus, Co-Gesic, Dolacet, Duocet, Hydrocet, Hydrogesic, Hy-Phen, Lorcet (HD, Plus, 10/650), Lortab (also 2.5/500, 5/500, 7.5/500, 10/500), Margesic H, Norco, Panacet 5/500, Stagesic, T-Gesic, Vicodin (also ES, HP), Zydone

Acetaminophen + oxycodone: Endocet, Percocet, Roxicet, Roxicet 5/500, Roxilox, Tylox

ABOUT THIS DRUG

Acetaminophen plus codeine, hydrocodone, or oxycodone is a narcotic analgesic (painkiller) used to treat mild-to-moderately-severe pain. The acetaminophen portion of each medication reduces pain and fever. The narcotic component is used to reduce moderate to severe pain, induce a calming effect, and, in the case of codeine and hydrocodone, control cough as well.

These drugs work by suppressing certain brain functions, which in turn suppress pain perception and emotional response to pain. Both codeine and hydrocodone also help suppress the cough reflex.

SIDE EFFECTS

If you experience any side effects when taking any of these drugs, contact your health-care practitioner immediately. Only a health-care practitioner can determine whether it is safe for you to continue taking them.

- *Common:* drowsiness, dry mouth, urinary retention, constipation, dizziness, lightheadedness, nausea, sedation, shortness of breath, vomiting
- *Less Common:* abdominal pain, allergic reactions (hives, swelling, difficulty breathing), depression, exaggerated sense of well-being, itching. At high doses, decreased breathing may occur.

IMPORTANT PRECAUTIONS

These drugs should be taken exactly as prescribed by your health-care practitioner. Before taking these drugs, tell your health-care practitioner about any problems you have had with alcohol or drug addiction. If you have ever had adrenal, kidney, liver, or thyroid disease, difficulty urinating, or an enlarged prostate, talk to your health-care practitioner before taking these drugs. Narcotics can cover up symptoms of stomach problems; therefore, if you have a stomach condition, talk to your health-care practitioner before taking any of these drugs. Because of an increased risk of liver damage when alcohol and acetaminophen are combined, check with your health-care practitioner before taking any of these drugs if you usually drink three or more alcoholic beverages daily.

Narcotics may make you drowsy and impair your ability to drive a vehicle or operate potentially dangerous machinery. Monitor the effects of the drug on you for several days before you participate in such activities.

If you have had a head injury, talk to your health-care practitioner before taking any of these drugs. Narcotics can increase the pressure of the fluid in the skull and interfere with recovery from the injury.

DRUG INTERACTIONS

Tell your health-care practitioner and pharmacist about any prescription or over-the-counter drugs you are taking, as well as any vitamins, herbs, or other supplements. Possible drug interactions with acetaminophen may include the following:

- Acetaminophen + narcotic may increase the effects of antianxiety drugs (e.g., diazepam), antidepressants (e.g., amitriptyline, phenelzine), tranquilizers (e.g., haloperidol, chlorpromazine), antihistamines (e.g., clemastine), other narcotic analgesics (e.g., meperidine), antispasmodics (e.g., benztropine, dicyclomine), and other drugs that depress the central nervous system (e.g., temazepam, phenobarbital).

- Acetaminophen + narcotic increases the effects of atropinelike drugs and increases the risk of urinary retention and constipation.
- Tramadol may increase the risk of breathing difficulties.
- Ritonavir and perhaps other protease inhibitors may reduce effects of codeine and oxycodone and lead to toxicity with hydrocodone.
- Cimetidine may increase the risk of breathing difficulties and suppression of the central nervous system.

FOOD, VITAMIN, AND HERBAL INTERACTIONS

The herbs valerian root and kava may cause drowsiness if taken along with any of these drugs. If St. John's wort is taken along with medications that contain hydrocodone, extreme photosensitivity may result.

RECOMMENDED DOSAGE

Your health-care practitioner will determine your actual dosage and schedule, based on the severity of your pain and how the drugs affect you. There are many different brands of acetaminophen + narcotic, and each has its own specific dosing regimen. The dosages given below are typical ONLY FOR THE BRAND NAME INDICATED. If your health-care practitioner prescribes a different brand, the dosing may differ.

For Acetaminophen + Codeine (Brand: Tylenol with Codeine)

- *Children 3 to 6 Years:* 1 teaspoon elixir 3 or 4 times daily
- *Children 7 to 12 Years:* 2 teaspoons elixir 3 or 4 times daily
- *Adults:* 15 to 60 mg of codeine and 300 to 1,000 mg acetaminophen per dose (tablets). The maximum dose per 24-hour period is 360 mg codeine and 4,000 mg acetaminophen. Your dose will be determined by your health-care practitioner. If you take the elixir, the typical adult dose is 1 tablespoon every 4 hours as needed.

For Acetaminophen + Hydrocodone (Brand: Vicodin)

- *Children:* This drug is not indicated for children.
- *Adults:* 1 or 2 tablets every 4 to 6 hours as needed. The maximum daily dose is 8 tablets.

For Acetaminophen + Oxycodone (Brand: Percocet)

- *Children:* This drug is not indicated for children.
- *Adults:* 1 tablet every 6 hours as needed.

Acetaminophen + narcotic may be taken with food or with milk. If you miss a dose of any of these medications, take it as soon as you remember, unless it is nearly time for your next dose. In that case, do not take the missed dose, and stay with your regular dosing schedule. Never take two doses at once.

SYMPTOMS OF OVERDOSE AND WHAT TO DO

If an overdose occurs, seek emergency medical attention. Symptoms of an overdose may include blood disorders, bluish skin, cold and clammy skin, general bodily discomfort, heart problems, excessive sweating, kidney problems, limp muscles, liver failure, low blood pressure, nausea, slow heartbeat, difficulty breathing, vomiting, and extreme sleepiness that can progress to coma.

SPECIAL INFORMATION FOR PREGNANT OR NURSING WOMEN

Use of any narcotic during pregnancy may result in physical addiction of the infant. If you are pregnant or plan to become pregnant, or if you are breastfeeding or plan to breastfeed, talk to your healthcare practitioner before starting any of the acetaminophen + narcotic drugs. He or she can determine whether the potential benefits outweigh the potential dangers. Use of any narcotic painkillers shortly before delivery may compromise the breathing of the mother and infant.

SPECIAL INFORMATION FOR SENIORS

Older individuals should exercise great caution when taking these drugs. This population is more susceptible to drowsiness, dizziness, falling, urinary retention, constipation (possibly leading to fecal impaction), and unsteadiness.

GENERIC NAME

Acetazolamide

BRAND NAMES

Dazamide, Diamox, Diamox Sequels
Generic available

ABOUT THIS DRUG

Acetazolamide is used primarily to treat glaucoma (excessive pressure in the eye), epileptic seizures, and fluid buildup caused by congestive heart failure or medication. It is considered to be a diuretic and a sulfonamide.

This drug blocks an enzyme called carbonic anhydrase, which results in a slowing of fluid accumulation in the eye and an increase in urination. It also helps controls epileptic seizures, although exactly how acetazolamide does this is not known.

SIDE EFFECTS

Contact your health-care practitioner if you develop side effects while taking this drug. Only he or she can determine if you should continue to take acetazolamide.

- *Common:* diarrhea, increased urination, loss of appetite, nausea, ringing in the ears, vomiting, metallic taste, tingling or pins and needles in the extremities, mouth, or anus
- *Less Common or Rare:* anemia, bloody or black stools, blood in urine, confusion, convulsions, drowsiness, fever, hives, liver problems, nearsightedness, paralysis, rash, photosensitivity, severe allergic reaction, peeling skin

This medication has the chemical characteristics of sulfonamide drugs. In rare cases, severe side effects, including bruises, sore throat, fever, and rash, have been reported. If these reactions occur, see your health-care practitioner immediately.

IMPORTANT PRECAUTIONS

Tell your health-care practitioner if you are sensitive or allergic to acetazolamide or any other drugs.

You should not take this drug if you have low potassium or sodium levels, or if you have serious kidney, liver, or Addison's disease. If you have emphysema or another type of breathing disorder, use this drug with caution.

Although this drug is for treatment of glaucoma, it should not be used for prolonged treatment of the type known as chronic noncongestive angle-closure glaucoma.

Like all sulfonamides, acetazolamide can cause blood reactions. Before starting this drug, your health-care practitioner should administer baseline complete blood and platelet counts and monitor your blood throughout your treatment for significant changes.

DRUG INTERACTIONS

Tell your health-care practitioner and pharmacist if you are taking any prescription or over-the-counter drugs, as well as any vitamins, herbs, or other supplements. Possible drug interactions with acetazolamide may include the following:

- High doses of aspirin can result in various reactions, from loss of appetite to rapid breathing or even death.
- Acetazolamide may prevent or delay absorption of primidone.
- Diflunisal may cause excessive lowering of eye pressure.
- Acetazolamide may increase the blood levels of cyclosporine.
- Acetazolamide may decrease the amount of lithium in your blood.
- Acetazolamide may enhance the therapeutic reactions or the side effects of amphetamines (e.g., methylphenidate, phenmetrazine), anticholinergics (e.g., atropine, scopolamine), mecamylamine, and quinidine.
- Acetazolamide may reduce the response to insulin or oral antidiabetic drugs.
- Adrenocorticoids (e.g., amcinonide, cortisone) may increase the risk of hypernatremia or edema.

FOOD, VITAMIN, AND HERBAL INTERACTIONS

Acetazolamide is a diuretic and thus can cause potassium loss. Therefore, take it with potassium-rich foods such as bananas, citrus, melons, and tomatoes.

RECOMMENDED DOSAGE

Acetazolamide is available in tablets and extended release capsules. Although the doses given below are typical, only your health-care practitioner can determine which dose and schedule is most appropriate for you.

For Glaucoma

- *Children:* This drug is not indicated for children with this condition.
- *Adults:* For open-angle glaucoma, the dose can range from 250 mg to 1 g daily.

For Epilepsy

- *Children:* Although the safety and effectiveness of acetazolamide has not been determined for children, some health-care practitioners prescribe it for various types of epilepsy: 8 to 30 mg per 2.2 pounds of body weight is the typical dose.

- *Adults:* 8 to 30 mg per 2.2 pounds of body weight in 2 or more doses. The typical range is 375 to 1,000 mg daily.

For Congestive Heart Failure

- *Children:* This drug is not indicated for children with this condition.
- *Adults:* Typical starting dose is 250 to 375 mg per day or 5 mg per 2.2 pounds of body weight, taken in the morning. Your health-care practitioner may tell you to take this dose every other day or for 2 days and then 1 day off.

Acetazolamide can be taken with food to help reduce the risk of stomach upset. If you are unable to swallow the tablets, you can crush them and mix in 2 teaspoons of water and 2 teaspoons of honey and take it immediately. If you miss a dose, take it as soon as you remember. However, if it is nearly time for your next scheduled dose, do not take the missed dose. Follow your regular dosing schedule. Never take a double dose.

SYMPTOMS OF OVERDOSE AND WHAT TO DO

No specific information on overdosing with acetazolamide is available. However, symptoms that may occur include dizziness, drowsiness, decreased appetite, nausea, vomiting, numbness or tingling in the extremities, tremors, and ringing in the ears. If overdose does occur, seek medical attention immediately, and bring the prescription bottle with you to the hospital.

SPECIAL INFORMATION FOR PREGNANT OR NURSING WOMEN

No studies have adequately investigated the effects of acetazolamide during pregnancy or breastfeeding. If you are pregnant or plan to become pregnant, or if you are breastfeeding or plan to do so, talk with your health-care practitioner before starting this drug. Only a health-care practitioner can determine whether the potential benefits will outweigh the potential dangers.

SPECIAL INFORMATION FOR SENIORS

No special instructions are provided for seniors. However, adverse reactions may be more likely and severe.

GENERIC NAME

Acetohexamide

see Sulfonylurea Antidiabetes Drugs, page 971

GENERIC NAME

Acitretin

BRAND NAME

Soriatane
No generic available

ABOUT THIS DRUG

Acitretin is an antipsoriatic drug that is related to vitamin A. It is used to treat severe psoriasis, a skin condition characterized by thick, reddened skin. It should only be used for cases that have not responded to other treatments because its use is associated with many risks.

It is uncertain how acitretin works, and it typically does not produce significant results until after about 2 to 3 months of treatment.

SIDE EFFECTS

If you experience side effects when taking acitretin, contact your health-care practitioner immediately. He or she will determine whether you should continue to use it.

- *Most Common:* peeling skin, hair loss, inflamed lips
- *Common:* dry eyes, chills, stiffness, dry skin, itching, rash, tingling in the hands or feet, sticky skin, loss of patches of skin, runny nose, fingernail problems
- *Less Common:* constipation, diarrhea, fatigue

IMPORTANT PRECAUTIONS

If you are a woman, you must not take this drug while you are pregnant and you must not get pregnant for three years after you finish treatment because of the high risk of birth defects. It is not known whether men who take acitretin before conception occurs place the fetus at risk.

This drug should be used with caution if you have liver or kidney problems. If you have bone or spine problems, use of this drug can make those conditions worse. Use of acitretin can make it difficult to control glucose levels if you have diabetes.

Tell your health-care practitioner if you have ever had an allergic reaction to acitretin, etretinate, isotretinoin, tretinoin, or any vitamin A preparations, including supplements, as well as to any foods, preservatives, or dyes.

Up to 50 percent of people who take acitretin experience a rise in their blood fat levels. This can be a significant problem if you have diabetes, are obese, have a history of either condition, or drink excessive amounts of alcohol. Before you start taking acitretin, your health-care practitioner should take your blood fat levels and monitor them periodically throughout your treatment.

Do not donate blood while you are taking acitretin or for up to three years after completing treatment. Your blood could be given to a pregnant woman and affect her fetus.

Avoid excessive exposure to wind, cold, and sunlight, especially during the first few weeks of treatment, because your skin will be especially sensitive to drying, irritation, and sunburn. Protective measures (e.g., sunscreen, long sleeves, hats) should be taken.

Use of acitretin can cause a sudden reduction in night vision as well as increased sensitivity to sunlight. These reactions may make it dangerous to operate a vehicle or machinery.

DRUG INTERACTIONS

Tell your health-care practitioner and pharmacist if you are taking any prescription or over-the-counter drugs, as well as any vitamins, herbs, or other supplements. Possible drug interactions with acitretin may include the following:

- Glyburide may result in abnormally low blood glucose levels. Your health-care practitioner may need to adjust your diabetic treatment while you are taking acitretin.
- Etretinate, isotretinoin, tretinoin, or any other vitamin A–type formulations may result in toxicity, characterized by severe headache, cracked lips, sparse, coarse hair, and other symptoms.
- Methotrexate can increase the risk of liver damage.
- Acitretin may reduce the effectiveness of low-progestin oral contraceptives. You will need to switch to another birth control method and use it for at least three years after you complete treatment.
- Tetracyclines (e.g., doxycycline, minocycline) may increase the risk of severe pressure buildup in the brain.
- Alcohol along with acitretin produces etretinate, a compound that is related to acitretin and which remains in the body longer. Because etretinate can also affect a fetus, alcohol should be avoided when taking acitretin and for at least 2 months after treatment.

FOOD, VITAMIN, AND HERBAL INTERACTIONS

Because acitretin is related to vitamin A, and too much vitamin A can cause toxicity, you must not take more than 1,000 mg of a vitamin A supplement while being treated with acitretin.

RECOMMENDED DOSAGE

Acitretin is available in capsules. The dosages given here are typical. Your health-care practitioner will determine the best dosage for your needs.

- ➤ *Children:* This drug is not indicated for children.
- ➤ *Adults:* 25 to 50 mg daily with your main meal.

If you miss a dose, take it as soon as you remember. However, if it is nearly time for your next scheduled dose, do not take the missed dose. Follow your regular dosing schedule. Never take a double dose.

SYMPTOMS OF OVERDOSE AND WHAT TO DO

If overdose occurs, seek medical attention immediately. Symptoms of overdose may include drowsiness, severe, continuing headache, irritability, itchy skin, and severe, persistent nausea or vomiting.

SPECIAL INFORMATION FOR PREGNANT OR NURSING WOMEN

This drug causes birth defects. Women who take acitretin must not be pregnant before they begin taking this drug, and they must take a pregnancy test within one week of starting treatment. To ensure pregnancy does not occur, women must use two forms of birth control throughout treatment and for three years after stopping the drug. Women also should not breastfeed while taking this drug.

SPECIAL INFORMATION FOR SENIORS

There are no special precautions for seniors. Older individuals may experience more pronounced side effects than younger users.

GENERIC NAME

Acrivastine *see Antihistamine-Decongestant Combinations, page 132*

GENERIC NAME
Acyclovir

BRAND NAME
Zovirax
Generic available

ABOUT THIS DRUG
Acyclovir is an antiviral drug used to treat various types of herpes viral infections, including genital herpes, shingles, nongenital herpes infections, and chicken pox. It does not cure any of these conditions, but it does reduce symptoms and speed up healing time.

Acyclovir interferes with the reproduction of DNA in the herpes viruses and slows down the growth rate of existing viruses.

SIDE EFFECTS
If any side effects occur while you are taking this drug, contact your health-care practitioner. She or he will decide whether it is safe for you to continue to take acyclovir.

- *More Common* (oral doses): diarrhea, general bodily discomfort, nausea, vomiting
- *Less Common or Rare* (oral doses): headache, loss of appetite, constipation, leg pain, sore throat, sleeplessness, fever
- *Common* (ointment): burning, itching, rash, stinging, mild pain, vaginal inflammation

IMPORTANT PRECAUTIONS
Do not take this drug if you have ever had an allergic reaction to it or similar drugs. The ointment contains polyethylene glycol; do not use this form of the drug if you are sensitive to this compound. Do not use the ointment inside the vagina or in the eyes.

If you have a kidney, nerve, or liver disorder, talk to your health-care practitioner before starting this drug. It is important to drink 2 to 3 quarts of liquids daily (unless your health-care practitioner says otherwise) when taking this drug.

To prevent the spread of genital herpes to your partner, you should avoid sexual intercourse when lesions are present.

DRUG INTERACTIONS
If you are taking any prescription or over-the-counter drugs, or any vitamins, herbs, or other supplements, talk to your health-care prac-

titioner and pharmacist before you start to take acyclovir. Possible drug interactions with acyclovir may include the following:

- Any other ointment or topical medication could cause a reaction and thus should not be used along with acyclovir.
- Cyclosporine may increase the risk of kidney toxicity.
- Probenecid (oral form) may elevate blood levels of acyclovir and thus increase the risk of side effects.
- Meperidine may cause neurological problems.
- Phenytoin and valproic acid may cause a loss of control over epileptic seizures.
- Zidovudine may cause lethargy and severe drowsiness.

FOOD, VITAMIN, AND HERBAL INTERACTIONS

The herbs ephedra (ma huang), ginseng, saw palmetto, and licorice may elevate blood pressure and reduce the effects of acyclovir. Garlic and calcium may lower blood pressure. If you use or plan to use any of these supplements, talk to your health-care practitioner.

RECOMMENDED DOSAGE

Acyclovir is available in tablets, capsules, suspension, and ointment. The dosages given here are typical. However, your health-care practitioner will determine the dosage and schedule that is best for your needs.

For Genital Herpes

- *Adults (oral):* one 200-mg capsule or 1 teaspoon liquid (1 teaspoon = 200 mg) every 4 hours, 5 times daily for 10 days. For recurrent herpes, 400 mg twice daily or 200 mg 2 to 5 times daily. To suppress chronic herpes, 400 to 800 mg daily every day.
- *Adults (ointment):* Apply every 3 hours, 6 times daily for 7 days.

For Shingles (Herpes Zoster)

- *Adults:* 800 mg every 4 hours, 5 times daily for 7 to 10 days.

For Chicken Pox

- *Children Younger than 2 Years:* Although the safety and efficacy of this drug have not been established for this age group, your health-care practitioner may prescribe the oral form if he or she determines that the benefits outweigh the potential risks.

- *Children 2 Years and Older:* 20 mg per 2.2 pounds of body weight taken 4 times daily for 5 days. Children who weigh more than 88 pounds should take the adult dose.
- *Adults:* 800 mg, 4 times daily for 5 days.

You may take acyclovir with food if it upsets your stomach. If you miss a dose, take it as soon as you remember. However, if it is nearly time for your next dose, don't take the skipped dose; stay on your regular dosing schedule. Do not take a double dose. If you miss a dose of ointment, take it as soon as you remember, and then continue with your regular schedule.

When applying the ointment, use gloves or a finger cot to prevent spreading the infection. The optimal amount of ointment to use is about 1/2-inch strip of the drug, which should cover about 4 square inches of lesions.

If you have kidney disease, your health-care practitioner should make the appropriate dosage adjustments.

SYMPTOMS OF OVERDOSE AND WHAT TO DO

If overdose occurs, seek medical attention immediately. An overdose of oral acyclovir may cause kidney damage. If the ointment form is ingested, contact your poison control center immediately.

SPECIAL INFORMATION FOR PREGNANT OR NURSING WOMEN

The effects of acyclovir on a fetus have not been studied adequately, but it has been shown to pass into breast milk. If you are pregnant or plan to become pregnant, or if you are breastfeeding or plan to do so, talk to your health-care practitioner before starting this drug. Together you can weigh the potential benefits versus the potential risks.

SPECIAL INFORMATION FOR SENIORS

Your health-care practitioner will likely start your treatment at the lower end of the dosage range, especially if you have kidney problems. Shingles, which most often affects people older than 50, should be treated with acyclovir within 48 to 72 hours of the appearance of the rash.

Adverse reactions may be more common in older individuals. To help minimize them, drink at least 2 to 3 quarts of liquid (not alcohol) daily.

GENERIC NAME
Adalimumab

BRAND NAME
Humira
No generic available

ABOUT THIS DRUG
Adalimumab is a disease-modifying antirheumatic drug (DMARD) used to treat symptoms of moderate to severe rheumatoid arthritis.

This drug is a tumor necrosis factor (TNF) antagonist, a substance that blocks the action of TNF, which is a naturally occurring protein that helps cause inflammation. Adalimumab blocks the effects of TNF, thus slowing down the inflammation process and inhibiting joint deterioration. It can be given along with methotrexate.

SIDE EFFECTS
Be sure to tell your health-care practitioner if you experience any side effects while taking adalimumab. Only your health-care practitioner can determine whether it is safe for you to continue taking this drug.

- *Most Common:* at the injection site: bruising, itching, rash, redness, swelling; also sinus infection, headache, nausea
- *Rare:* dizziness, numbness or tingling, vision problems, weakness in legs

IMPORTANT PRECAUTIONS
Tell your health-care practitioner if you are sensitive or allergic to adalimumab or any of its ingredients (citrate, citric acid, mannitol, polysorbate 80, sodium phosphate), or to any other drugs. The needle cover of the syringe contains latex. People who are allergic to this substance should not handle the needle cover.

In rare cases, certain kinds of cancer have developed in people who take adalimumab or other TNF blockers. Individuals who have had more serious rheumatoid arthritis for a prolonged time may have a greater than average risk of getting cancer that affects the lymph system (lymphoma).

If you develop a swollen face, have breathing difficulties, or experience a severe rash while taking adalimumab, contact your health-care practitioner immediately.

Tuberculosis and other opportunistic fungal infections have been noted in people who take TNF-blocking drugs. You should not take adalimumab if you have an active infection, either chronic or localized. Your health-care practitioner should monitor you closely if you develop a new infection while taking adalimumab. Use of adalimumab should be discontinued if you develop a serious infection.

Do not take adalimumab if you are scheduled for major surgery or within 2 weeks prior to or 3 months following getting any type of vaccination.

DRUG INTERACTIONS

Tell your health-care practitioner and pharmacist if you are taking any prescription or nonprescription drugs, as well as any vitamins, herbs, or other supplements. No specific drug interactions have been noted.

FOOD, VITAMIN, AND HERBAL INTERACTIONS

No food, vitamin, or herbal interactions have been noted.

RECOMMENDED DOSAGE

Adalimumab is available in a single-dose, pre-filled glass syringe with a fixed needle, designed to be self-administered subcutaneously (under the skin). The dosages given here are typical. However, your health-care practitioner will determine the most appropriate dose and schedule for your needs.

- *Children:* not recommended for children
- *Adults:* One self-injection every two weeks. Each dose is premeasured at 40 mg.

If you miss a dose, take it as soon as you remember, then take your next dose when it is scheduled. Never take a double dose.

You should rotate the injection site. Never give yourself an injection in an area that is tender or bruised.

SYMPTOMS OF OVERDOSE AND WHAT TO DO

Symptoms of overdose include dizziness, headache, nausea, numbness or tingling, vision problems, and weakness in legs. If overdose occurs, seek immediate medical attention and bring the prescription container with you to the hospital.

SPECIAL INFORMATION FOR PREGNANT OR NURSING WOMEN

No adequate studies of the effects of adalimumab on pregnant or nursing women have been done. If you are pregnant or plan to become pregnant and this drug is crucial for your health, you and your health-care practitioner must weigh the potential benefits against the potential risks to the fetus.

Adalimumab may pass into breast milk. If you are breastfeeding, your health-care practitioner may advise you to stop until your treatment is complete.

SPECIAL INFORMATION FOR SENIORS

Because there is a higher incidence of infection and malignancy in older adults, they should use caution when taking this drug.

GENERIC NAME

Adapalene

BRAND NAME

Differin

No generic available

ABOUT THIS DRUG

Adapalene is an anti-acne medication that is similar to retinoids, which are related to vitamin A. It is a gel that works primarily on the visible acne lesions. Very little of the drug is absorbed through the skin.

Adapalene slows down production of the substance that accumulates in acne lesions and reduces inflammation.

SIDE EFFECTS

If side effects occur, they usually develop during the first 2 to 4 weeks of treatment and then subside. If you experience any adverse reactions, contact your health-care practitioner as soon as possible. Depending on their severity, your health-care practitioner may change how you use the drug or advise you to stop.

➤ *Common:* burning, dryness, irritation, itching, redness, scaling, stinging, sunburn, flare-up of acne

➤ *Rare:* stinging sunburn, worsening acne

IMPORTANT PRECAUTIONS

Do not use this drug if you are sensitive or allergic to it, or if you have sunburn. Never apply it to abrasions, cuts, eczema, mucous membranes, or your lips.

Adapalene increases sensitivity to sunlight, as well as cold weather and wind. While using adapalene, protect yourself from overexposure to these factors: use sunscreen or protective clothing over treated areas.

Avoid using adapalene along with products that can irritate the skin, including cosmetics that can dry the skin, medicated soaps, and products that contain alcohol, spices, astringents, or lime.

DRUG INTERACTIONS

Tell your health-care practitioner and pharmacist if you are using any skin products that contain resorcinol, salicylic acid, or sulfur. These products may react if used along with adapalene. If you are using such items or used them recently, do not start treatment with adapalene until you are no longer experiencing the effects of those products.

FOOD, VITAMIN, AND HERBAL INTERACTIONS

No interactions are reported.

RECOMMENDED DOSAGE

- *Children Younger than 12 Years:* Not indicated for this age group.
- *Adults:* Wash the affected area, then apply a thin layer of adapalene at bedtime.

If you miss a dose, apply it as soon as you remember. If it is nearly time for your next dose, do not apply the dose you skipped, and continue with your regular schedule. It may take 2 to 3 months to see significant results from use of this drug.

SYMPTOMS OF OVERDOSE AND WHAT TO DO

Overuse of adapalene can cause discomfort and peeling, red skin. If overuse occurs, contact your health-care practitioner immediately.

SPECIAL INFORMATION FOR PREGNANT OR NURSING WOMEN

The effects of adapalene during pregnancy and breastfeeding have not been studied adequately. If you are pregnant or plan to become pregnant, or if you are breastfeeding or plan to do so, talk to your health-care practitioner before using this drug. He or she can advise you about using adapalene.

SPECIAL INFORMATION FOR SENIORS

There are no special precautions for seniors.

GENERIC NAME

Albendazole

BRAND NAME

Albenza
No generic available

ABOUT THIS DRUG

Albendazole is an anthelmintic, which means it kills parasitic intestinal worms. It is used to treat infections of the nervous system that are caused by tapeworms from pigs and cysts caused by tapeworms from dogs.

This drug disrupts the normal functioning of tapeworms, causing them to die and pass out of the body in feces.

SIDE EFFECTS

If you experience adverse reactions while taking albendazole, contact your health-care practitioner immediately. She or he can decide whether you should continue with treatment.

- *Common:* inflamed liver, headache, abdominal pain, nausea, vomiting
- *Less Common:* dizziness, fainting, hair loss (reverses when the drug is stopped), increased pressure in the head
- *Rare:* fever, drop in blood cell count, itching, rash, kidney failure, drug allergy

IMPORTANT PRECAUTIONS

Liver inflammation is a common reaction of this drug, but it usually reverses once the drug is stopped. If you have liver obstruction, abnormally high levels of albendazole may be detected in your blood. Your health-care practitioner should monitor your blood levels and liver function while you take this drug.

Although albendazole is rarely used in children younger than 6 years, no unusual problems have been noted.

DRUG INTERACTIONS

Talk to your health-care practitioner and pharmacist about any prescription or over-the-counter drugs you are taking, as well as any vitamins, herbs, or other supplements.

Use of albendazole along with dexamethasone, praziquantel, cimetidine, or corticosteroids increases the amount of albendazole in the blood and may increase effects and/or adverse reactions.

FOOD, VITAMIN, AND HERBAL INTERACTIONS

Albendazole should be taken with a high-fat meal (about 40 g) to promote absorption.

RECOMMENDED DOSAGE

Albendazole is available in tablets. The dosages given here are typical, but your health-care practitioner will determine the best dosage for your condition.

- *Children and Adults (under 130 pounds):* about 7 mg per pounds of body weight daily, divided into two doses, with meals. The total daily dose should not exceed 800 mg.
- *Children and Adults (130 pounds and greater):* 400 mg twice daily with meals.

If you are treating pork tapeworm, take the dose prescribed by your health-care practitioner for 8 to 30 days. For dog tapeworm, take the prescribed dose for 28 days and stop for 2 weeks. This schedule can be repeated three times.

If you miss a dose, take it as soon as you remember unless it is nearly time for your next dose. In that case, do not take the skipped dose. Continue with your regular schedule. Never take a double dose.

SYMPTOMS OF OVERDOSE AND WHAT TO DO

There is little information about the effects of albendazole overdose. If overdose occurs, seek immediate medical attention, and bring the prescription bottle with you.

SPECIAL INFORMATION FOR PREGNANT OR NURSING WOMEN

Albendazole may cause birth defects. If you are a woman of childbearing age, you must take a pregnancy test, and have a negative result, before you can start treatment with albendazole. While taking this drug, and for one month after stopping, you must avoid becoming pregnant. If you become pregnant while being treated, you must stop the drug at once.

If you are breastfeeding or plan to breastfeed, talk to your health-care practitioner before starting albendazole. Only a health-care practitioner can weigh the potential benefits versus the potential risks.

SPECIAL INFORMATION FOR SENIORS

No special precautions are needed for seniors. However, adverse reactions may be more severe.

GENERIC NAME

Albuterol (also levalbuterol)

BRAND NAMES

Proventil HFA, Proventil Inhaler, Proventil Repetabs, Proventil Tablets, Ventolin Inhaler, Ventolin Nebules, Ventolin Rotacaps, Ventolin Syrup, Ventolin Tablets, Volmax Controlled Release Tablets, Volmax Extended Release Tablets (also Xopenex)
Generic available

ABOUT THIS DRUG

Albuterol is a bronchodilator used to relieve acute bronchial asthma and reduce the frequency and severity of chronic, recurrent asthma attacks. It is also used to help prevent exercise-induced bronchospasm. Levalbuterol is a type of albuterol that is used for the same purposes; however, it has a lower risk of side effects.

Albuterol and levalbuterol relax constricted air passages, which in turn makes it easier to breathe and relieves wheezing. The inhaled forms of albuterol usually produce results within 15 minutes; the oral forms can take about 30 minutes.

SIDE EFFECTS

If you experience any side effects while using this drug, contact your health-care practitioner immediately. A health-care practitioner can determine whether you should continue to use the drug or change your treatment program.

- *Common:* aggression, agitation, appetite changes, cough, diarrhea, dizziness, excitement, general discomfort, headache, heartburn, increased difficulty breathing, irritated throat, muscle cramps, nausea, nervousness, nightmares, nosebleed, palpitations, rash, ringing in the ears, sleeplessness, stuffy nose, tremors, vomiting, wheezing
- *Common for Proventil HFA:* allergic reaction, back pain, fever, inflamed nasal passages, respiratory infection, urinary problems
- *Less Common:* chest pain or discomfort, difficulty urinating, drowsiness, dry mouth, dry throat, flushing, high blood pressure, muscle spasm, restlessness, sweating, vertigo, weakness

- *Less Common for Proventil HFA:* anxiety, belching, chills and fever, coordination difficulties, depression, difficulty speaking, diabetes, dizziness, fluid retention, gas, palpitations, leg cramps, ringing in the ears, sleepiness
- *Rare (with use of inhaled products):* hoarseness, increased wheezing, rapid heartbeat, rash or hives, unusual swelling of the throat or mouth

IMPORTANT PRECAUTIONS

When using albuterol inhalation aerosol, you should not use any other inhaled medications without your health-care practitioner's permission. Talk to your health-care practitioner before using any form of albuterol if you have any type of heart condition, high blood pressure, diabetes, an overactive thyroid gland, or a seizure disorder. If you are sensitive or allergic to albuterol or other bronchodilators, do not use this drug. Do not take albuterol if you are taking any monoamine oxidase (MAO) inhibitors, or if you took one in the past two weeks.

Albuterol can cause an immediate, life-threatening allergic reaction when the first dose is taken. Seek emergency medical treatment if this occurs.

DRUG INTERACTIONS

Let your health-care practitioner and pharmacist know about any prescription or over-the-counter drugs you are taking, as well as any vitamins, herbs, or other supplements. Possible drug interactions with albuterol may include the following:

- Albuterol may reduce the amount of digoxin in the blood.
- Amphetamines, dopamine, ephedrine, isoproterenol, and phenylephrine may worsen adverse effects on the heart.
- Beta-blockers (e.g., propranolol) can antagonize the effects of albuterol and result in a loss of effects of both drugs.
- Monoamine oxidase (MAO) inhibitors can cause very high blood pressure and heart stimulation.
- Theophylline may result in rapid loss of the drug from the body and a loss of its benefits.
- Thiazide and loop diuretics (e.g., bendroflumethiazide, furosemide) may cause additive lowering of blood potassium levels.
- Tricyclic antidepressants may cause a dramatic rise in blood pressure.

FOOD, VITAMIN, AND HERBAL INTERACTIONS

Avoid excessive intake of caffeine from beverages and foods, including coffee, tea, colas, and chocolate. Use of the herbs St. John's wort, ephedra (ma huang), or kola may result in abnormal stimulation of the central nervous system.

RECOMMENDED DOSAGE

Albuterol comes in tablets (regular and sustained release), inhalation capsules, inhalation solution, inhalation aerosol, and syrup. The doses given here are typical. However, use of albuterol is highly individualized. Your health-care practitioner will determine the best dosage and schedule for your particular condition.

Inhalation Solution

- *Albuterol—Children 2 to 12 Years:* Based on body weight, but should not exceed 2.5 mg taken 3 to 4 times daily.
- *Albuterol—Adults and Children 12 Years and Older:* 2.5 mg 3 to 4 times daily by nebulizer.
- *Levalbuterol—Adults and Children 12 Years and Older:* 0.63 mg 3 times daily by nebulizer, every 6 to 8 hours.

Inhalation Aerosol

- *Adults and Children 4 Years and Older:* Ventolin, 2 inhalations every 4 to 6 hours for sudden or severe bronchial spasm or prevention of asthmatic symptoms.
- *Adults and Children 12 Years and Older:* Proventil and Proventil HFA, 2 inhalations every 4 to 6 hours for sudden or severe bronchial spasm or prevention of asthmatic symptoms.

Tablets

- *Children 6 to 12 Years:* 2 mg, 3 or 4 times daily as a starting dose. Your health-care practitioner may increase the dose. Maximum daily dose should not exceed 32 mg.
- *Adults and Children 12 Years and Older:* 2 or 4 mg, 3 to 4 times daily as a starting dose. Your health-care practitioner may increase the dose. Maximum daily dose should not exceed 32 mg.
- *Adults Older Than 60 Years:* 2 mg, 3 or 4 times daily starting dose. May be increased up to 8 mg, 3 or 4 times daily.

Proventil Repetabs and Volmax Extended-Release Tablets

- *Children 6 to 12 Years:* For Proventil Repetabs, starting dose is 4 mg every 4 hours. Your health-care practitioner may increase the dosage, but it should not exceed 24 mg daily.
- *Adults and Children 12 Years and Older:* 8 mg every 12 hours.

Syrup

- *Children 2 to 6 Years:* 0.1 mg per 2.2 pounds of body weight, to a maximum of 4 mg, 3 times daily.
- *Children 6 to 14 Years:* 1 teaspoon, 3 to 4 times daily starting dose.
- *Adults and Children 14 Years and Older:* 1 or 2 teaspoons, 3 to 4 times daily starting dose.
- *Adults Older than 60 Years:* 2 mg, 3 or 4 times daily. May be increased up to 8 mg, 3 or 4 times daily.

When using the inhalational form of this drug, inhale it during the second half of your intake breath. If you are directed to take more than 1 puff per dose, wait 5 minutes between puffs. If the amount of drug that worked previously fails to provide relief, contact your health-care practitioner immediately. Do not take more than the prescribed number of inhalations without your health-care practitioner's permission.

Never inhale albuterol if you have anything else in your mouth.

If you miss a dose, take it as soon as you remember. However, if it is nearly time for your next dose, do not take the missed dose. Continue with your regular schedule. Do not take a double dose.

SYMPTOMS OF OVERDOSE AND WHAT TO DO

An overdose of inhaled albuterol can cause chest pain, high blood pressure, and, in rare cases, death. If this type of overdose occurs, seek emergency medical attention. Overdose of oral albuterol may cause palpitations, unusual heart rhythm or heartbeat, chest pain, high blood pressure, fever, chills, cold sweats, nausea, vomiting, dilation of the pupils, convulsions, tremors, or collapse. If the overdose occurred within the past 30 minutes, syrup of ipecac can be used to induce vomiting, but only if the individual is not unconscious or convulsing. Seek emergency medical treatment. If symptoms have already appeared, seek emergency medical treatment, and bring the prescription container with you.

SPECIAL INFORMATION FOR PREGNANT OR NURSING WOMEN

If you are pregnant or plan to become pregnant, talk to your health-care practitioner before starting this drug. Albuterol can delay or slow natural labor, cause high blood pressure or rapid heartbeat in the mother, and cause low blood sugar and rapid heartbeat in the infant. Your health-care practitioner will weigh the potential benefits versus the potential risks of your using this drug during pregnancy.

It's not known whether albuterol passes into breast milk. If your health-care practitioner determines that this drug is necessary for your health, together you will need to weigh the potential benefits against the potential risks.

SPECIAL INFORMATION FOR SENIORS

Older individuals can be susceptible to the effects of albuterol. Common reactions may include nervousness, muscle tremors, irregular heart rhythms, and palpitations. Avoid excessive or continual use.

GENERIC NAME

Alclometasone dipropionate

see Corticosteroids, Topical, page 337

GENERIC NAME

Alefacept

BRAND NAME

Amevive
No generic available

ABOUT THIS DRUG

Alefacept is an antipsoriatic medication used to treat adults who have moderate to severe chronic plaque psoriasis and who are candidates for systemic treatment or phototherapy.

Psoriasis is believed to be caused by an increase in the production of T-lymphocytes in response to stimulation. Stimulated T-lymphocytes cause skin cells to grow rapidly, and rapid growth of skin cells produces skin plaques of psoriasis. Alefacept reduces stimulation and production of T-lymphocytes.

SIDE EFFECTS

Be sure to tell your health-care practitioner if you experience any side effects while taking alefacept. Only your health-care practitioner can determine whether it is safe for you to continue taking this drug.

- *Most Common:* chills, cough, fever, hoarseness, low back pain, painful or difficult urination; at injection site (IM): pain, inflammation
- *Less Common:* body aches, congestion, runny nose, serious infections, sore throat, swallowing difficulties, swollen glands in neck, voice changes
- *Rare:* arm, back, and/or jaw pain, chest pain, chest tightness, irregular heartbeat, nausea, shortness of breath, sweating, vomiting

IMPORTANT PRECAUTIONS

Tell your health-care practitioner if you are sensitive or allergic to alefacept or to any other drugs.

While taking this drug, your health-care practitioner will likely conduct weekly blood tests to check your T-lymphocyte levels. You should not take alefacept if your blood lymphocyte count is less than 250/microliter.

Talk to your health-care practitioner before getting a vaccination during treatment with alefacept. Alefacept may reduce the action of vaccines that use live strains of virus (e.g., measles, mumps, rubella).

Use of alefacept may increase your risk of malignancies and infection. You should not use this drug if you have a history of systemic malignancy or if you have a clinically important infection. If signs of a new infection appears while taking alefacept, you should report them to your health-care practitioner immediately.

DRUG INTERACTIONS

Tell your health-care practitioner and pharmacist if you are taking any prescription or nonprescription drugs, as well as any vitamins, herbs, or other supplements. Studies of drug-drug interactions have not been done, but because alefacept suppresses the immune system, it should not be used with other drugs or therapies (e.g., phototherapy) that have the same effect.

FOOD, VITAMIN, AND HERBAL INTERACTIONS

No food, vitamin, or herbal interactions have been noted.

RECOMMENDED DOSAGE

Alefacept is available as an intramuscular injection and intravenous infusion and is administered by a health-care practitioner. The dosages given here are typical. However, your health-care practitioner will determine the most appropriate dose and schedule for your needs.

- *Children:* not recommended for children
- *Adults:* One 15-mg dose intramuscularly taken once per week for 12 weeks; or one 7.5-mg dose intravenously taken once per week for 12 weeks

If you miss an appointment to get your weekly dose, make an appointment to get it as soon as possible. Talk to your health-care practitioner about maintaining your regular dosing schedule.

SYMPTOMS OF OVERDOSE AND WHAT TO DO

Overdose is unlikely, as alefacept is administered by a health-care practitioner in a medical setting. Symptoms of overdose include chills, headache, joint ache, low white blood cell count, and sinusitis. If you believe an overdose has occurred, seek immediate medical attention.

SPECIAL INFORMATION FOR PREGNANT OR NURSING WOMEN

Adequate studies of the effects of alefacept on pregnant or nursing women have not been done. If you are pregnant or plan to become pregnant, talk to your health-care practitioner.

It is not known whether alefacept passes into breast milk. If you are breastfeeding, your health-care practitioner may advise you to stop until your treatment is complete.

SPECIAL INFORMATION FOR SENIORS

The incidence of infections and certain malignancies is higher in seniors, so caution should be exercised when prescribing this drug.

GENERIC NAME

Alendronate *see Bisphosphonates, page 200*

GENERIC NAME

Alfuzosin

BRAND NAME

Uroxatral

No generic available

ABOUT THIS DRUG

Alfuzosin blocks alpha-adrenergic receptors in the urinary tract and is used to ease urinary tract symptoms due to benign prostatic hyperplasia (BPH), an enlarged prostate.

This drug works by relaxing the muscles in the prostate gland and the opening of the bladder, thus improving the flow of urine and decreasing symptoms of BPH.

SIDE EFFECTS

Be sure to tell your health-care practitioner if you experience any side effects while taking alfuzosin. Only your health-care practitioner can determine whether it is safe for you to continue using/taking this drug.

- ➤ *Most Common:* dizziness, fatigue, headache
- ➤ *Less Common:* chest pain, lightheadedness or faintness (especially when getting up quickly from a seated or lying position)

IMPORTANT PRECAUTIONS

Tell your health-care practitioner if you are sensitive or allergic to alfuzosin, especially other alpha-blockers such as doxazosin, quanadrel, prazosin, or terazosin, or to any other drugs.

Because alfuzosin can cause dizziness, make sure you know how you respond to it before you drive or operate dangerous equipment.

Do not take alfuzosin if you have liver or kidney problems. Before taking this drug, talk to your health-care practitioner if you have severe heart disease (including a personal or family history of a rare heart condition called congenital prolongation of the QT interval), kidney disease, low blood pressure, or chest pain.

DRUG INTERACTIONS

Tell your health-care practitioner and pharmacist if you are taking any prescription or nonprescription drugs, as well as any vitamins, herbs, or other supplements. Possible drug interactions include the following:

- ➤ Do not take ketoconazole, itraconazole, or protease inhibitors (e.g., ritonavir) when using alfuzosin.
- ➤ Talk to your health-care practitioner before taking other alpha-blockers (e.g., doxazosin, quanadrel, prazosin, terazosin) or diltiazem when taking alfuzosin.

FOOD, VITAMIN, AND HERBAL INTERACTIONS
No food, vitamin, or herbal interactions have been reported.

RECOMMENDED DOSAGE
Alfuzosin is available in 10-mg tablets. The dosages given here are typical. However, your health-care practitioner will determine the most appropriate dose and schedule for your needs.

- *Children:* This drug is not recommended for children.
- *Adults:* 10 mg as a single dose once daily.

Alfuzosin should be taken with food and immediately after the same meal each day. Never take this drug on an empty stomach. Do not crush or chew the tablet.

If you miss a dose, take it as soon as your remember. If it is nearly time for your next dose, skip the missed dose. Return to your regular dosing schedule. Never take a double dose.

SYMPTOMS OF OVERDOSE AND WHAT TO DO
Symptoms of overdose include dizziness, extremely low blood pressure, fatigue, headache, palpitations, and weakness. If overdose occurs, seek immediate medical attention and bring the prescription container with you to the hospital.

SPECIAL INFORMATION FOR PREGNANT OR NURSING WOMEN
Alfuzosin is approved for use by men only.

SPECIAL INFORMATION FOR SENIORS
Side effects are more likely to occur and may be more severe in older adults.

GENERIC NAME
Allopurinol

BRAND NAMES
Aloprim, Lopurin, Zyloprim
Generic available

ABOUT THIS DRUG
Allopurinol belongs to the class of anti-gout drugs. It is used primarily as long-term treatment to prevent acute gout (a form of arthritis characterized by elevated blood levels of uric acid that form crys-

tals), and to control high blood levels of uric acid in people who have uric acid or calcium oxalate kidney stones. It will not stop an active gout attack, but it will, if taken regularly for a few months, reduce symptoms.

This drug reduces production of uric acid by blocking the enzyme xanthine oxidase, which in turn prevents crystals from forming.

SIDE EFFECTS

The most common side effect associated with allopurinol is a skin reaction, which, in the majority of cases, is not serious. However, in rare cases it can become severe or even life-threatening. If you notice the beginnings of a rash, stop taking the drug and contact your health-care practitioner immediately. The rash may begin as itching and scaling, or your skin can peel off in sheets. The rash may be accompanied by fever, aching joints, jaundice, or chills.

If you experience any other side effects when using allopurinol, call your health-care practitioner. A decision can then be made about whether you should continue to take the drug.

- *Common:* acute attacks of gout, diarrhea, rash, nausea
- *Less Common or Rare:* abdominal pain, bruising, chills, fever, hair loss, headache, hepatitis, hives, indigestion, itching, jaundice, joint pain, kidney failure, loose nails, muscle disease, nosebleed, severe blistering and bleeding on the lips, eyes, or nose, skin peeling, dark skin spots, taste change, tingling or pins and needles, vomiting

IMPORTANT PRECAUTIONS

Do not take allopurinol if you have had an allergic reaction to it in the past, including a rash, or if you are having an acute gout attack. Before starting this drug, tell your health-care practitioner if you have a family history of hemochromatosis (an iron metabolism disorder), or liver or kidney disease, if you have a blood or bone marrow disorder or epilepsy, or if you are on a low-protein diet.

Drink 10 to 12 eight-ounce glasses of liquid (preferably water; no alcohol) a day while taking allopurinol, unless your health-care practitioner instructs you otherwise. This helps prevent the formation of crystals in the urine or kidneys.

Allopurinol is not for use in children unless they have high uric acid levels associated with rare metabolic conditions or neoplastic disease.

During treatment with allopurinol, your health-care practitioner should periodically check your kidney and liver function, as a few cases of liver toxicity have been reported. If your kidney function is severely compromised, you should take lower doses of this drug.

DRUG INTERACTIONS

Let your health-care practitioner and pharmacist know if you are taking any prescription or over-the-counter drugs, as well as vitamins, herbs, or other supplements. Possible drug interactions with allopurinol may include the following:

- ➤ Alcohol, diazoxide, mecamylamine, and pyrazinamide can raise uric acid levels, necessitating higher doses of allopurinol.
- ➤ Allopurinol increases the effects of azathioprine and mercaptopurine.
- ➤ Ampicillin, amoxicillin, bacampicillin, or hetacillin are more likely to cause a rash in susceptible individuals.
- ➤ Antacids that contain aluminum may decrease the therapeutic effect of allopurinol.
- ➤ Anticoagulants (e.g., warfarin) may break down slower in the body, necessitating a lower dose.
- ➤ Cyclophosphamide may result in cyclophosphamide toxicity.
- ➤ Dacarbazine, probenecid, and sulfinpyrazone may cause an excessive reduction in uric acid levels.
- ➤ Tamoxifen may increase allopurinol levels and an increased risk of liver toxicity.
- ➤ Thiazide diuretics (e.g., bendroflumethiazide, chlorothiazide) and angiotensin-converting enzyme (ACE) inhibitors increase the risk of allergic reactions.
- ➤ Vidarabine may increase the risk of neurotoxic effects and anemia, nausea, pain, and itching.
- ➤ Theophylline, along with more than 600 mg of allopurinol daily, may result in increased side effects and toxic reactions to theophylline.

FOOD, VITAMIN, AND HERBAL INTERACTIONS

A low-protein diet may increase your risk of toxicity unless your dosage of allopurinol is reduced. A diet low in purine is recommended to reduce the risk of gout attacks. Foods high in purines, which should be avoided, include anchovies, poultry, legumes, sardines, liver, and other organ meats.

Do not take more than 2,000 mg of vitamin C per day while on allopurinol, as the combination may increase your risk of kidney stone formation.

RECOMMENDED DOSAGE

Allopurinol is available in 100-, 200-, and 300-mg tablets. The dosages given here are typical. However, your health-care practitioner will determine the dosage and schedule that meets your needs and reevaluate it periodically to make sure it is adequately controlling your uric acid levels.

- *Children under 6 Years:* 150 mg daily.
- *Children 6 to 10 Years:* 300 to 600 mg daily.
- *Adults and Children 11 Years and Older:* 100 to 800 mg daily, based on the disease and response to medication. The usual starting dose is 100 mg daily, with increases made at one-week intervals until the desired results are reached.

To help prevent stomach irritation, allopurinol can be taken with food or a full glass of water, or immediately after meals. If you miss a dose, take it as soon as you remember. However, if it is nearly time for your next dose, do not take the missed dose, and remain on your regular schedule. Never take a double dose.

SYMPTOMS OF OVERDOSE AND WHAT TO DO

No specific information is available about taking an overdose of allopurinol. However, the expected symptoms would be exaggerated side effects. If an overdose occurs, seek medical attention immediately, and take the prescription container with you.

SPECIAL INFORMATION FOR PREGNANT OR NURSING WOMEN

Adequate information about the effects of this drug on pregnant or nursing women is not available. Generally, avoid use of allopurinol during the first three months of pregnancy. During the latter six months, this drug should be used only if your health-care practitioner believes it is necessary for your health.

Allopurinol passes into breast milk. If allopurinol is important for your health, your health-care practitioner may advise you to avoid breastfeeding.

SPECIAL INFORMATION FOR SENIORS

Lower starting and ongoing doses should be prescribed because of reduced kidney function among older individuals.

GENERIC NAME
Almotriptan malate *see Triptan-Type Antimigraine Drugs, page 1083*

GENERIC NAME
Alprazolam

BRAND NAMES
Alprazolam Intensol, Xanax
Generic available

ABOUT THIS DRUG
Alprazolam is a benzodiazepine, or antianxiety drug, used mainly for short-term relief of mild-to-moderate anxiety and nervous tension, and for the treatment of panic disorder.

Like other benzodiazepines, alprazolam enhances the activity of the nerve transmitter gamma-aminobutyric acid (GABA), which then blocks the action of higher brain areas and results in a calming effect.

SIDE EFFECTS
Contact your health-care practitioner if you experience any side effects while taking alprazolam. Side effects, especially drowsiness, most often occur at the start of treatment and disappear as treatment continues. However, they may return or are more likely if your dosage is increased.

- *More Common:* abdominal discomfort, abnormal involuntary movement, agitation, allergies, anxiety, blurred vision, chest pain, confusion, constipation, change in sex drive, change in appetite, abnormal dreams, drowsiness, dry mouth, fainting, fatigue, fluid retention, headache, hyperventilation, inability to fall asleep, impaired memory, irritability, lack of coordination, lightheadedness, low blood pressure, menstrual problems, muscle twitching, nausea and vomiting, nervousness, palpitations, rash, restlessness, ringing in the ears, salivation changes, skin inflammation, speech difficulties, stiffness, stuffy nose, sweating, tremors, upper respiratory infections, weakness, weight gain or loss
- *Less Common or Rare:* abnormal muscle tone, concentration difficulties, decreased coordination, dizziness, double vision, fear, hallucinations, decreased control over urination or bowel movements, infection, itching, jaundice, loss of appetite, muscle cramps or spasticity, rage, sedation, seizures, sleep problems, slurred speech, stimulation, talkativeness, taste changes, memory loss, tingling or pins

and needles, uninhibited behavior, urine retention, muscle and bone weakness

IMPORTANT PRECAUTIONS

Do not take this drug if you have ever had an allergic reaction to it or another benzodiazepine, or if you have acute narrow-angle glaucoma or myasthenia gravis. Talk to your health-care practitioner before you take alprazolam if you have a history of palpitations, tachycardia (abnormally slow heartbeat), depression or serious mental illness, alcoholism, or drug abuse. Also, if you have impaired liver or kidney function, a seizure disorder, severe chronic lung disease, or open-angle glaucoma, you should tell your health-care practitioner before starting alprazolam.

This drug can cause physical and/or psychological dependence if it is used for a prolonged period. Alprazolam is typically meant to be taken for no more than 8 weeks unless otherwise advised by your health-care practitioner.

Because use of this drug can impair mental alertness, judgment, reaction time, and physical coordination, you should avoid all hazardous activities, including driving, when taking this drug.

DRUG INTERACTIONS

Inform your health-care practitioner and pharmacist about any prescription and over-the-counter medications you are taking, as well as any vitamins, herbs, or other supplements. Alprazolam should never be taken with itraconazole or ketoconazole, because the combination can cause an abnormally high accumulation of alprazolam in the body. Possible drug interactions with alprazolam may include the following:

- Alcohol may decrease coordination and mental functioning.
- Alprazolam may decrease the effects of levodopa.
- Antihistamines (e.g., clemastine, doxylamine), antipsychotics (e.g., haloperidol, risperidone), antidepressants (e.g., amitriptyline, imipramine), buspirone, and narcotics (e.g., morphine) can result in increased depression of the central nervous system.
- Benzodiazepines (e.g., diazepam, temazepam) can cause increased central nervous system depression.
- Carbamazepine, rifampin, and theophylline may decrease the effects of alprazolam.
- Cimetidine, disulfiram, fluoxetine, fluvoxamine, isoniazid, macrolide antibiotics (e.g., erythromycin, clarithromycin), omeprazole, oral

contraceptives, paroxetine propoxyphene, ritonavir, sertraline, and valproic acid may increase the effects of alprazolam.

- ➤ Digoxin may result in digoxin toxicity.
- ➤ Phenytoin may result in phenytoin toxicity.

FOOD, VITAMIN, AND HERBAL INTERACTIONS

Avoid use of beverages and foods that contain caffeine, such as coffee, tea, colas, and chocolate, because they can counteract the effects of alprazolam.

Herbs that have a sedative effect may cause excessive physical depression, sedation, and impairment if taken along with alprazolam. These herbs include ashwagandha, calendula, catnip, hops, kava, lady's slipper, lemon balm, passionflower, sassafras, skullcap, valerian, and herba mansa.

RECOMMENDED DOSAGE

Alprazolam is available in tablets (0.25-, 0.5-, 1-, and 2-mg strength) and oral solution (0.25-, 0.5-, and 1 mg/5 ml; and 0.25 mg/2.5 ml). The dosages given here are typical. However, your actual dose and schedule must be determined by your health-care practitioner to meet your particular needs.

For Anxiety

- ➤ *Children:* Only your health-care practitioner can determine if it is appropriate for your child.
- ➤ *Adults:* Start at 0.25 to 0.5 mg three times daily. Your health-care practitioner may increase your dose if needed. Maximum daily dose is usually 4 mg.
- ➤ *Adults Older than 60 Years:* Start at 0.25 mg two or three times daily. Your health-care practitioner may increase your dose if needed.

For Panic

- ➤ *Children:* Only your health-care practitioner can determine if it is appropriate for your child.
- ➤ *Adults:* Start at 0.5 mg three times daily. Your health-care practitioner may increase your dose if needed. Maximum daily dose is usually 10 mg.
- ➤ *Adults Older than 60 Years:* Start at 0.25 mg two or three times daily. Your health-care practitioner may increase your dose if needed.

When taking the concentrated oral solution, mix it in water, juice, soda, or soft food such as pudding or applesauce. The tablets can be taken with or without food, and they can be crushed. If you miss a dose, take it if you are less than one hour late. However, if it is more than one hour late, do not take the missed dose and return to your regular schedule. Never take a double dose.

Do not suddenly stop taking this drug, as it may cause withdrawal symptoms. Only your health-care practitioner can advise you on how and when to stop or change your dose.

SYMPTOMS OF OVERDOSE AND WHAT TO DO

If an overdose occurs, seek emergency medical treatment, and bring the prescription container with you. Symptoms of overdose include confusion, sleepiness, poor coordination, lack of response to pain, loss of reflexes, shallow breathing, low blood pressure, and coma.

SPECIAL INFORMATION FOR PREGNANT OR NURSING WOMEN

Although there are no adequate studies of alprazolam in pregnant women, a closely related benzodiazepine shows evidence of human fetal risk. Therefore, do not take this drug if you are pregnant or plan to become pregnant. Infants are at increased risk of respiratory problems, muscular weakness, and withdrawal symptoms if the drug is used during pregnancy. Alprazolam may pass into breast milk. Your health-care practitioner may advise you to stop breastfeeding while you take this drug.

SPECIAL INFORMATION FOR SENIORS

Dizziness and falling are more likely to occur among older individuals who take benzodiazepines. Your health-care practitioner will likely start you on a lower dose, especially if you have liver or kidney disease.

GENERIC NAME

Alprostadil

BRAND NAMES

Caverject, Edex, Muse
Generic available

ABOUT THIS DRUG

Alprostadil is a smooth muscle relaxant and prostaglandin E1 (PGE1) used primarily to treat erectile dysfunction (impotence). It is classified as an anti-impotence drug.

Alprostadil dilates the blood vessels that supply blood to the penis and relaxes the muscles in the penis to help keep the blood there. To accomplish this, alprostadil must be injected into the penis (Caverject, Edex) or inserted into the urethra in the form of a tiny suppository (pellet; Muse).

SIDE EFFECTS

The most common side effect for both forms of the drug is penile pain, which is reported by about one-third of users. If you experience any side effects when using this drug, contact your health-care practitioner. Your health-care practitioner can determine whether it is safe for you to continue to use the drug.

- *More Common (suppository form):* extremely low blood pressure, flu symptoms, headache, infection, burning sensation in the penis, penis bleeding, testicular pain
- *Less Common (suppository form):* back pain, dizziness, leg pain, pelvic pain, rapid pulse, runny nose, swelling of leg veins, pain behind the testicles
- *More Common (injection):* prolonged erection (lasting for more than six hours, known as priapism), deformity of the penis (causing hardened tissue in the penis or erections at an unusual angle), blood blister at the injection site, upper respiratory infection, pain in the penis, discoloration of the head of the penis
- *Less Common (injection):* abnormal vision, back pain, bruising at the injection site, dizziness, cough, flu symptoms, headache, heart attack, high blood pressure, inflammation of the prostate gland, leg pain, nasal congestion, redness, sinus inflammation, skin disorders
- *Rare (injection):* abnormal ejaculation, bleeding at the urethra, blood in the urine, dizziness, fainting, urgent, frequent, or impaired urination, itching, lack of sensation in the penis, leg cramps, low blood pressure, nausea, numbness, painful erection, pelvic pain, extreme sweating, rash on the penis, redness, sensitivity, swollen scrotum, testicular pain, tight foreskin, weakness, yeast infection

IMPORTANT PRECAUTIONS

This drug is for use in adult males only. Do not use this drug if your health-care practitioner has advised you not to have sex. If you have sickle cell anemia, high levels of red blood cells and platelets, a tumor of the bone marrow, a penile implant, or an unusually formed penis, you should not use the injectable form of alprostadil. You should not use either form of the drug if it causes an allergic reaction or if you have ever had a reaction to any prostaglandin drug.

Alprostadil does not offer any protection against sexually transmitted diseases; therefore a condom should be used. Even a small amount of bleeding at the injection or suppository site can increase your risk of transmitting a blood-borne disease such as human immunodeficiency virus (HIV).

If you take the suppository, avoid driving or operating hazardous equipment after taking it, because this form may cause fainting or a sudden drop in blood pressure.

DRUG INTERACTIONS

Let your health-care practitioner and pharmacist know about any prescription and over-the-counter medications you are taking, as well as any vitamins, herbs, or other supplements. No drug interactions have been reported; however, the following interactions are possible:

- Alprostadil may increase the effect of anticoagulants (blood-thinning drugs) such as heparin.
- Drugs that affect the blood vessels, such as high blood pressure medication, may cause reactions. Talk to your health-care practitioner before using any of these medications.
- Cyclosporine levels may decrease when used along with alprostadil.

FOOD, VITAMIN, AND HERBAL INTERACTIONS

No food, vitamin, or herbal interactions have been reported.

RECOMMENDED DOSAGE

Alprostadil is available in an injectable form, which is administered directly into the penis; and as a suppository, which is inserted into the urethra. The doses given here are typical. However, your health-care practitioner will determine the exact dose of the injection or suppository that is best for you. To make that determination, your health-care practitioner will give you your first dose in the office and instruct you on the proper technique. You will also be given written instructions.

- *Caverject:* Start at 1.25 or 2.5 mcg. Your health-care practitioner will increase the dose as needed to produce an erection that lasts about one hour.
- *Edex:* Start at 1 to 40 mcg given over 5 to 10 seconds. After injecting Edex, place finger pressure on the injection site for 5 minutes or until bleeding stops.
- *Muse:* Start at 125 or 250 mcg. Your health-care practitioner will increase the dose as needed to produce an erection that lasts about one hour.

If you choose the injectable form of alprostadil, never use it more than three times a week, and always wait at least 24 hours between uses. Alternate the side of the penis and the site of the injection each time you use the drug, and avoid visible veins when choosing the injection site. Each needle/syringe and vial should be used only once and then discarded.

The suppository should never be used more than two times in each 24-hour period. Throw away each applicator after a single use.

An injection results in an erection in 5 to 20 minutes and in about 90 percent of cases; the suppository causes an erection in about 5 minutes, but the success rate is lower, about 65 percent.

SYMPTOMS OF OVERDOSE AND WHAT TO DO

No overdoses of alprostadil (injectable form) have been reported. However, the main symptom of an overdose would be priapism (prolonged erection lasting 6 hours or more). If this occurs, seek medical assistance immediately.

SPECIAL INFORMATION FOR PREGNANT OR NURSING WOMEN

Alprostadil is for use by men only. If you are using alprostadil and have sexual intercourse with a pregnant woman, you must wear a condom, because the drug passes into the semen and can adversely affect the heart of a developing fetus.

SPECIAL INFORMATION FOR SENIORS

No special instructions are needed for older users.

GENERIC NAME

Amantadine

BRAND NAME

Symmetrel
Generic available

ABOUT THIS DRUG

Amantadine is classified as an antiviral and antiparkinsonian drug. It is used primarily to treat respiratory tract infections caused by flu viruses (type A), and for Parkinson's disease. It is up to 90 percent effective in preventing type A flu and in reducing its symptoms if it is taken within 2 days after symptoms appear, but it is not useful against other types of flu or other viral infections, or the common cold.

It is not clear how amantadine works against flu viruses, but it appears to prevent the virus from entering the body's cells. Amantadine also improves muscle control and reduces stiffness in people with Parkinson's disease by increasing the level of the nerve transmitter dopamine.

SIDE EFFECTS

If side effects occur, contact your health-care practitioner immediately. She or he can determine whether it is safe for you to continue to take this drug.

- *More Common:* lightheadedness, dizziness, weakness, feeling faint, dry mouth, constipation, patchy skin discoloration on legs or feet (temporary)
- *Less Common:* depression, anxiety, irritability, hallucinations, confusion, loss of appetite, weakness, swelling in extremities, headache, heart failure, urinary difficulties, vomiting, slurred speech, visual disturbances
- *Rare:* convulsions, eczema-type rash, eye spasms and uncontrollable eye movements, increased white blood cell count

IMPORTANT PRECAUTIONS

Do not take amantadine if you are sensitive or allergic to it. Before taking amantadine, you should talk to your health-care practitioner if you have any type of seizure disorder, kidney or liver disease, eczema or similar rashes, or a history of heart disease, heart failure, peptic ulcer disease, serious mental or emotional disorder, low white blood cell count, or orthostatic hypotension (lowering of blood pressure when standing). You should also inform your health-care practitioner if you are currently taking medication for emotional or mental disorders.

Avoid excessive exposure to cold when taking amantadine, because it may cause livedo reticularis, reddish-blue patchy skin discoloration that appears on the legs or feet. Congestive heart failure is also possible in people who are predisposed to this condition.

Amantadine has a potential for abuse because it can cause hallucinations and feelings of detachment in some people.

Because amantadine can cause dizziness, lightheadedness, blurred vision, and confusion, avoid driving and other potentially hazardous activities if these side effects occur.

DRUG INTERACTIONS

Talk to your health-care practitioner and pharmacist about any prescription and over-the-counter drugs you are taking, as well as any vitamins, herbs, or other supplements. Possible drug interactions with amantadine may include the following:

- Alcohol may worsen amantadine's side effects and hinder your ability to concentrate, drive, or operate machinery.
- Amantadine may increase the effects of levodopa and may cause acute mental disturbances.
- Amphetamine and amphetamine-like drugs may cause adverse behaviors.
- Anticholinergic drugs like benztropine can increase amantadine's side effects.
- Co-trimoxazole, sulfamethoxazole, or trimethoprim may increase the risk of central nervous system stimulation or heart arrhythmia.
- Hydrochlorothiazide-triamterene (a diuretic combination drug) may interfere with elimination of amantadine from the body and result in amantadine toxicity.

FOOD, VITAMIN, AND HERBAL INTERACTIONS

No interactions have been reported.

RECOMMENDED DOSAGE

Amantadine is available in tablets, capsules, and syrup. The dosages given here are typical. However, your health-care practitioner will determine the dosage that is most appropriate for you.

- *Children 1 to 9 Years:* 2 to 4 mg per pound of body weight daily, up to 150 mg
- *Adults and Children 10 Years and Older:* 100 to 300 mg daily
- *Adults 65 Years and Older:* 100 mg daily

Take amantadine with or after meals. If you miss a dose, take it as soon as you remember. However, if it is nearly time for your next dose, do not take the forgotten dose, and resume your regular dosing schedule. Do not take a double dose.

If you are taking the syrup, be sure to use the measuring spoon that comes with your prescription to get the proper dose.

If you are using amantadine to treat parkinsonism, suddenly stopping the drug may cause an acute parkinsonian crisis. Talk to your health-care practitioner if you want to stop taking this drug. If you are using this drug to treat influenza A infections, continue taking it for 48 hours after your symptoms disappear to ensure effectiveness.

SYMPTOMS OF OVERDOSE AND WHAT TO DO
If overdose occurs, seek emergency medical treatment and take the prescription container with you. Symptoms of overdose include nausea, vomiting, loss of appetite, excitability, tremors, weakness, blurred vision, slurred speech, tiredness, and convulsions. Potentially fatal abnormal heart rhythms are also possible.

SPECIAL INFORMATION FOR PREGNANT OR NURSING WOMEN
If you are pregnant or plan to become pregnant, talk to your health-care practitioner before starting amantadine. Pregnant women should take this drug only if their health-care practitioner determines it is absolutely critical for their health and all possible risks to the fetus have been explained. Amantadine passes into breast milk; thus women should not breastfeed when taking this drug.

SPECIAL INFORMATION FOR SENIORS
Because seniors typically have reduced kidney function, lower doses of amantadine are given. Seniors are also especially sensitive to this drug's effects. Common side effects include confusion, difficult urination, blurred vision, constipation, and dry mouth, nose, and throat.

GENERIC NAME
Amcinonide

see Corticosteroids, Topical, page 337

GENERIC NAME
Amiloride

BRAND NAME
Midamor
Generic available

ABOUT THIS DRUG
Amiloride is a potassium-sparing diuretic, which means it helps eliminate excessive fluid associated with congestive heart failure without

causing the body to lose a lot of potassium. Potassium is a nutrient that is essential for heart function and other critical bodily activities.

This drug promotes loss of salt (sodium) and water from the body while retaining potassium by altering enzymes in the kidneys.

SIDE EFFECTS

If you experience side effects while taking amiloride, contact your health-care practitioner to see if you should continue taking it or if your dose needs to be changed. Do not make any dosage changes without your health-care practitioner's supervision.

- *More Common:* abnormally high blood potassium levels, abnormally low blood sodium level, dehydration, constipation, dizziness on standing
- *Less Common:* rash, itching, headache, decreased ability to taste salt, dry mouth, nausea, vomiting, stomach pains, diarrhea, depression, visual disturbances, ringing in the ears, tremors
- *Rare:* loss of scalp hair, liver or kidney toxicity, increased internal eye pressure, palpitations and arrhythmias, decreased libido, impotence

IMPORTANT PRECAUTIONS

You should not take this drug if you are sensitive or allergic to it, if your blood potassium level is above normal, if you have diabetic nerve damage, or if you have acute kidney failure or you are unable to produce urine.

Talk to your health-care practitioner before taking amiloride if you are allergic to similar drugs, if you have glaucoma, diabetes, kidney disease, impaired kidney function, or liver disease, or if you are taking diuretics, blood pressure medication, digitalis, or lithium.

Avoid exposure to heat while taking this drug, as excessive sweating may cause you to lose too much water, sodium, and potassium.

Because this drug may cause dizziness or visual disturbances, avoid hazardous activities, including driving, if these symptoms occur.

DRUG INTERACTIONS

Tell your health-care practitioner and pharmacist about any prescription and over-the-counter drugs you are taking, as well as any vitamins, herbs, or other supplements. Possible drug interactions with amiloride may include the following:

- Amiloride may increase the effects of blood pressure lowering drugs, requiring dose adjustments.

- Digoxin may be less effective in treating heart failure if used along with amiloride.
- Angiotensin-converting enzyme (ACE) inhibitors (e.g., benazepril) or angiotensin II antagonists (e.g., valsartan) may cause abnormally high blood potassium levels.
- Lithium may result in lithium toxicity.
- Metformin may raise this drug's levels and increase lactic acidosis.
- Nonsteroidal anti-inflammatory drugs (NSAIDs) (e.g., diclofenac, ibuprofen) may reduce therapeutic effect.
- Spironolactone or triamterene may result in dangerously high potassium levels. Do not combine these drugs with amiloride.

FOOD, VITAMIN, AND HERBAL INTERACTIONS

Avoid excessive salt intake and high potassium foods (e.g., bananas) while taking amiloride.

Because this drug helps the body hold onto potassium, do not take potassium supplements while using amiloride. It may also cause the body to retain magnesium, so magnesium supplements also should be avoided unless directed by your health-care practitioner.

The herb white willow, which has properties similar to aspirin, should be avoided when taking amiloride. Ginseng may raise blood pressure and blunt the benefits of amiloride. Goldenseal, ephedra (ma huang), licorice, and saw palmetto also may raise blood pressure. Taking supplements of calcium or garlic may help lower blood pressure; talk to your health-care practitioner.

RECOMMENDED DOSAGE

Amiloride is available in 5-mg tablets. The dosage given here is typical; however, your health-care practitioner will determine the dosage best suited for your needs.

- *Children:* Your health-care practitioner will determine whether this drug is appropriate for your child.
- *Adults:* One 5-mg tablet daily, preferably in the morning. Your health-care practitioner may increase your dosage up to 15 mg as needed.
- *Adults Older than 60 Years:* The dose must be reduced and determined by your health-care practitioner.

Taking amiloride with food may help prevent nausea or stomach upset. You may crush the tablet and mix with soft food if desired.

Do not suddenly stop taking this drug unless your health-care practitioner tells you to do so.

SYMPTOMS OF OVERDOSE AND WHAT TO DO

If an overdose occurs, seek immediate medical attention and bring the prescription container with you. Symptoms of overdose may include thirst, drowsiness, fatigue, weakness, nausea, vomiting, confusion, numbness and tingling in the extremities and face, shortness of breath, and irregular heart rhythm.

SPECIAL INFORMATION FOR PREGNANT OR NURSING WOMEN

No adequate studies have been done of the effects of this drug on pregnant or nursing women. If you are pregnant, plan to become pregnant, or are breastfeeding or plan to do so, consult with your health-care practitioner before using amiloride. Your health-care practitioner will determine whether the potential benefits outweigh the potential risks.

SPECIAL INFORMATION FOR SENIORS

A decrease in kidney function usually seen in older individuals makes it likely that potassium levels may rise. Use of this drug in seniors should not exceed 2 to 3 weeks, and the dose should be lower than the normal adult amounts. Use of amiloride may cause excessive loss of water and an increased risk of clots and thus stroke, thrombosis, and heart attack.

GENERIC NAME

Aminolevulinic acid

BRAND NAME

Levulan Kerastick
No generic available

ABOUT THIS DRUG

Aminolevulinic acid is a photodynamic therapy sensitizer, which means it is used as part of a light treatment for a skin disorder called actinic keratoses. These skin lesions usually appear in older adults who have fair skin. The drug is applied by a health-care practitioner in the office, and 14 to 18 hours later the treated skin is exposed to a special blue light, which does not heat the skin, for about 17 minutes.

Aminolevulinic acid causes skin cells to become much more sensitive to certain types of light. When the blue light is directed on the treated areas, the acid causes the diseased skin cells to slough off.

SIDE EFFECTS

No side effects usually occur from application of the drug before it is treated with the blue light. If for any reason you do not return for the blue light treatment during the 14- to 18-hour period, call your health-care practitioner. You then must avoid exposing the treated areas to sunlight or prolonged or intense lighting, including indoor lights, for at least 40 hours.

Once your skin is treated with the light therapy, side effects may occur.

- *More Common:* tingling, stinging, prickling, or burning. These feelings usually improve by the end of the light treatment.
- *Less Common:* pain, tenderness, swelling, skin ulcers, small blisters, oozing, loss of sensation in the treated area, scabs

IMPORTANT PRECAUTIONS

Do not use this drug if you have a bleeding or blood disorder, if you are allergic to it or porphyrins, or if you have porphyria (a skin disorder). Aminolevulinic acid should not be applied around the eyes or inside the mouth or nose.

Use of this drug greatly increases your sensitivity to the sun and bright indoor lights. Wearing sunscreen does not prevent this sensitivity; therefore, you need to wear protective clothing, a hat, and sunglasses for adequate protection.

DRUG INTERACTIONS

Tell your health-care practitioner and pharmacist about any prescription or over-the-counter drugs you are taking, as well as herbs, vitamins, and other supplements. Taking aminolevulinic acid along with other drugs that have the potential to increase your sensitivity to light may then increase the effects of aminolevulinic acid. They include griseofulvin, phenothiazines, sulfonamides, sulfonylureas, tetracycline, and thiazide diuretics.

FOOD, VITAMIN, AND HERBAL INTERACTIONS

No interactions with foods, vitamins, or herbs are documented.

RECOMMENDED DOSAGE

Your health-care practitioner will apply the drug to your lesions in the office, as needed.

SYMPTOMS OF OVERDOSE AND WHAT TO DO

Overuse of this topical drug is not documented. Because only qualified medical professionals should administer this drug, ingestion should not occur. If the drug is accidentally ingested, emergency medical attention is needed.

SPECIAL INFORMATION FOR PREGNANT OR NURSING WOMEN

If you are pregnant or breastfeeding, talk to your health-care practitioner before undergoing this treatment approach. The safety of this drug in pregnant or breastfeeding women is not known; therefore your health-care practitioner must weigh the potential benefits versus the potential risks.

SPECIAL INFORMATION FOR SENIORS

There are no special precautions for seniors. Because aging skin tends to be more sensitive, side effects may be more severe.

GENERIC NAME

Aminophylline *see Xanthine Bronchodilators, page 1116*

GENERIC NAME

Amiodarone

BRAND NAMES

Cordarone, Pacerone
No generic available

ABOUT THIS DRUG

Amiodarone is an antiarrhythmic drug used to prevent and treat heartbeat irregularities, such as atrial fibrillation and ventricular tachycardia. It should be given only to individuals who have a life-threatening condition and who do not respond to other drug treatments.

This drug slows and regulates the nerve impulses in the heart, which makes the heart less responsive to abnormal stimulation.

SIDE EFFECTS

Amiodarone causes side effects in about 75 percent of people who take 400 mg or more daily. About 18 percent of them stop taking the drug because of these effects. Up to 9 percent of people who take this drug experience abnormalities in liver function. If you experience any side effects while taking amiodarone, contact your health-care practitioner immediately. She or he can decide whether it is safe for you to continue to take it.

- *More Common:* Nausea, vomiting, constipation, loss of appetite, low-grade fever, photosensitivity, trembling or shaking, unsteadiness when walking, headache, tingling or numbness in the fingers or toes
- *Less Common:* odd taste in the mouth, vision disturbances, dry eyes, chills, dizziness, nervousness or restlessness, lowered sex drive in males, scrotal pain and swelling, slowed heartbeat, excessive sweating, insomnia, fatigue, unexpected change in weight, blue-gray discoloration of the skin
- *Rare:* lung inflammation, changes in thyroid function, bloating, changes in blood clotting, fibrous deposits in the lungs, heart failure, reduced heart rate

IMPORTANT PRECAUTIONS

Do not take amiodarone if you are allergic or sensitive to this drug or if you have heart block. Tell your health-care practitioner if you have an allergy to iodine, as this drug contains 75 mg of iodine.

Because amiodarone has the potential to cause heart block, worsen abnormal heart rhythms (2 to 5% of users), and cause fatal lung and respiratory problems (in 10% or more of people when taken at high doses), thyroid abnormalities (up to 10% of users), and fatal liver failure (rare), it should only be used when other treatment attempts have failed.

Partial or total loss of vision can occur. Most people who take amiodarone for six months or longer develop deposits in their cornea, which can cause blurred vision in up to 10 percent of users. Because of the high incidence (10%) of photosensitivity, sunscreen should be used regularly.

This drug can cause dizziness or unsteadiness; therefore don't drive or perform hazardous tasks if you experience these symptoms.

Before any type of medical or dental procedure that requires general anesthesia, tell your health-care practitioner or dentist that you are taking amiodarone.

DRUG INTERACTIONS

Before starting amiodarone, tell your health-care practitioner and pharmacist about any prescription and over-the-counter drugs you are taking, as well as any vitamins, herbs, or other supplements. Amiodarone may interact with many drugs, including the following:

- Amiodarone increases the effects of beta-blockers (e.g., metoprolol), digoxin, flecainide, procainamide, quinidine, theophylline, and warfarin and other anticoagulants.
- Cholestyramine hinders the absorption of amiodarone.
- Cimetidine and ritonavir interfere with the metabolism of amiodarone, which can lead to high blood levels and enhanced side effects.
- Phenytoin can antagonize amiodarone, and amiodarone can increase the effect of phenytoin.
- Note that drug interactions with amiodarone can still occur up to several months after you stop taking the drug because it stays in the body for a long time.

FOOD, VITAMIN, AND HERBAL INTERACTIONS

No food interactions are documented. A test tube study suggests that taking 100 to 400 IU of vitamin E daily may help prevent amiodarone's toxic effects on the lungs. This study has not been done in humans, however.

Use of the herbs chaparral, comfrey, or coltsfoot, which have the potential to cause liver damage, should be avoided. Use of St. John's wort may increase photosensitivity.

RECOMMENDED DOSAGE

Amiodarone is available in 200-mg tablets. The dosages given here are typical; however, your health-care practitioner will identify the best dose and dosage schedule for your particular needs.

- *Children:* Dosage varies case to case and is determined by your health-care practitioner.
- *Adults:* 800 to 2,400 mg daily in 3 or 4 equally divided doses. This regimen is usually then reduced to 60 to 800 mg daily for 30 days; then 200 to 400 mg daily.

Amiodarone works best if taken on an empty stomach, because food delays its absorption into the bloodstream. If you experience stomach upset, it can be taken with food.

If you take amiodarone once a day and miss a dose, you can take it as soon as you remember if it is within 12 hours of your last dose. If it is longer, do not take the missed dose, and remain on your regular schedule. If you take the drug twice daily and skip a dose, take it if it is within 6 hours of your regular dose. If you forget to take 2 or more doses in a row, call your health-care practitioner. Never take a double dose of this drug.

SYMPTOMS OF OVERDOSE AND WHAT TO DO

If overdose occurs, seek emergency medical treatment and bring the prescription container with you. Symptoms include seizures, irregular or very slow heartbeat, and loss of consciousness.

SPECIAL INFORMATION FOR PREGNANT OR NURSING WOMEN

Studies suggest that amiodarone may cause heart and thyroid problems in the fetus. If you are pregnant, your health-care practitioner will weigh the potential benefits versus the potential risks of your taking this drug.

Amiodarone passes into breast milk. If you are nursing, your health-care practitioner may advise you to stop breastfeeding while taking this drug.

SPECIAL INFORMATION FOR SENIORS

A lower dose is indicated for older individuals who have poor liver function. Seniors are also more likely to experience side effects, and they may be more severe. Common reactions include thyroid problems, difficulty walking, and numbness, tingling, trembling, or weakness in the feet and hands.

GENERIC NAME

Amitriptyline *see Tricyclic Antidepressants, page 1076*

GENERIC NAME

Amlexanox

BRAND NAME

Aphthasol

No generic available

ABOUT THIS DRUG

Amlexanox is a topical skin-ulcer medication used to treat mouth ulcers (canker sores) in people who have a normal immune system.

Amlexanox speeds up the healing of mouth ulcers and slows the production or release of substances that cause inflammation, but the exact way it accomplishes these benefits is not known.

SIDE EFFECTS

Side effects occur infrequently, but if you do experience adverse reactions, contact your health-care practitioner.

- *Less Common:* stinging, pain, or burning after application
- *Rare:* irritated mouth, diarrhea, nausea

IMPORTANT PRECAUTIONS

Do not use amlexanox if you are sensitive or allergic to it or any of the ingredients in the medication.

The safety and effectiveness of this drug has not been determined for people with a compromised immune system. If you have acquired immunodeficiency syndrome (AIDS), are taking immunosuppressant drugs, or are receiving chemotherapy, talk to your health-care practitioner before using this drug.

Wash your hands immediately after you apply amlexanox. If paste gets into your eyes, wash them out immediately with cool water.

DRUG INTERACTIONS

No drug interactions have been documented.

FOOD, VITAMIN, AND HERBAL INTERACTIONS

No interactions with foods, vitamins, or herbs have been documented.

RECOMMENDED DOSAGE

Amlexanox is available as an adhesive oral paste that is applied to each mouth ulcer, using your finger or a cotton swab. The dosage given here is typical; however, your health-care practitioner may suggest a different schedule for you.

- *Children:* Talk to your health-care practitioner about using this drug in children.
- *Adults:* The typical dose is 1/4 inch applied to each ulcer after breakfast, lunch, and dinner, and at bedtime.

Begin to apply amlexanox as soon as you notice a mouth ulcer is forming and use it until the ulcers heal. Contact your health-care practitioner if your mouth ulcers do not clear up or your pain does not disappear after 10 days of treatment.

If you miss a dose, apply the medication as soon as you remember. If it is nearly time for your next dose, do not apply the skipped dose, and continue with your regular application schedule. Do not apply more than the recommended amount at any time.

SYMPTOMS OF OVERDOSE AND WHAT TO DO

If amlexanox were ingested by mistake, it would likely cause nausea, diarrhea, and vomiting. If this occurs, call your poison control center or seek emergency medical assistance, and bring the container with you.

SPECIAL INFORMATION FOR PREGNANT OR NURSING WOMEN

The effect of amlexanox on pregnant or nursing women is not known. If you are pregnant or breastfeeding, discuss use of this drug with your health-care practitioner, who can weigh the potential benefits versus the potential risks.

SPECIAL INFORMATION FOR SENIORS

There are no special precautions for older adults.

GENERIC NAME

Amlodipine

BRAND NAME

Norvasc
No generic available

ABOUT THIS DRUG

Amlodipine is prescribed for angina, a condition in which individuals experience crushing chest pain, and for high blood pressure. It is classified as a calcium channel blocker, an anti-angina drug, and an antihypertensive drug.

Like other calcium channel blockers, amlodipine interferes with the movement of calcium into heart muscle, which in turn relaxes the blood vessels and reduces heart rate. It also results in a lowering of blood pressure and reduced chest pain.

SIDE EFFECTS

If you experience side effects while taking amlodipine, contact your health-care practitioner. Only your health-care practitioner can determine whether you should continue to take this drug.

- *More Common:* dizziness, fatigue, flushing, fluid retention, headache, palpitations
- *Less Common:* abdominal pain, nausea, sleepiness
- *Rare:* abnormal dreams, agitation, anxiety, apathy, back pain, change in sense of taste or smell, change in appetite, chest pain, cold and clammy skin, conjunctivitis, constipation, cough, depression, diarrhea, difficulty breathing, difficult or painful urination, difficulty swallowing, dizziness, double vision, dry mouth, dry skin, eye pain, fainting, gas, hair loss, heart failure, hives, hot flashes, increased sweating, indigestion, inflamed skin, irregular heartbeat or pulse, itching, joint pain, lack of coordination, loose stools, memory loss, low blood pressure, migraine, muscle cramps or weakness, nervousness, nosebleed, purple or red spots on the skin, rash, ringing in the ears, sexual problems, slow heartbeat, thirst, tingling or pins and needles, tremors, twitching, vertigo, vision problems, vomiting, weight gain

IMPORTANT PRECAUTIONS

Avoid this medication if you are sensitive or allergic to it.

Amlodipine must be used with caution if you have certain heart conditions, liver or kidney disease, or high blood pressure, so be sure to give your health-care practitioner an accurate medical history. In rare cases, people with severe heart disease may experience more frequent angina attacks or even a heart attack when starting this drug.

Tell your health-care practitioner if you have ever had a negative reaction to any calcium blocker, or if you are currently taking digitalis, a beta-blocker, or drugs that lower blood pressure.

Because this drug may cause dizziness, do not drive or operate hazardous machinery until you know how the drug affects you.

The safety and effectiveness of this drug has not been determined for children.

DRUG INTERACTIONS

Let your health-care practitioner and pharmacist know about any prescription and nonprescription drugs you are taking, as well as any vitamins, herbs, or other supplements. Possible drug interactions include the following:

- Adenosine, beta-blockers (e.g., acebutolol, metoprolol), or digitalis may cause heart rate and rhythm problems.
- Some antifungals (e.g., fluconazole, itraconazole) may result in toxic levels of amlodipine.
- Delavirdine may cause increased amlodipine levels and toxicity.

- Cimetidine may increase the effects of amlodipine.
- Cyclosporine may result in increased levels of cyclosporine and a greater risk of toxicity.
- Nonsteroidal anti-inflammatory drugs (NSAIDs; e.g., etodolac, naproxen) or oral anticoagulants (e.g., warfarin) may increase the risk of gastrointestinal bleeding.
- Rifampin may reduce the therapeutic effect of amlodipine.
- Ritonavir and probably other protease inhibitors (e.g., nelfinavir) may cause amlodipine toxicity.

FOOD, VITAMIN, AND HERBAL INTERACTIONS

Avoid taking this medication with grapefruit or grapefruit juice, and do not ingest either of these foods for at least one hour after taking your dose.

Avoid herbs that can increase blood pressure, including ginseng, goldenseal, ephedra (ma huang), licorice, and saw palmetto. Calcium and garlic can be beneficial as they help lower blood pressure. Be sure to talk to your health-care practitioner before taking these supplements.

RECOMMENDED DOSAGE

Amlodipine is available in 2.5-, 5-, and 10-mg tablets. The dosages given here are typical; however, your health-care practitioner will determine the dosage and schedule that is best for your needs.

- *Children up to 12 Years:* This drug is not indicated for children younger than 12 years.
- *Children 12 Years and Older and Adults to Age 60:* For chronic angina: 5 to 10 mg daily. For congestive heart failure: 5 mg once daily for 2 weeks, with an increase to 10 mg as needed and tolerated. For high blood pressure: 2.5 to 10 mg daily in a single dose.
- *Adults Older than 60 Years:* Lower doses (2.5 for high blood pressure and 5 mg for angina) are suggested.

This medication was designed to be taken once daily. It can be taken with or following food to help reduce stomach irritation. The tablet may be crushed if needed.

Take this medication exactly as prescribed, even if your symptoms disappear. Consult with your health-care practitioner before stopping this drug.

If you miss a dose, take it as soon as you remember. If it is nearly time for your next dose, do not take the skipped dose, and continue with your regular dosing schedule. Never take a double dose.

SYMPTOMS OF OVERDOSE AND WHAT TO DO

If an overdose occurs, seek immediate medical attention, and bring the prescription container with you. Symptoms will likely include a dramatic drop in blood pressure and a rapid heartbeat.

SPECIAL INFORMATION FOR PREGNANT OR NURSING WOMEN

Adequate studies of the effects of this drug on pregnant or nursing women are not available. If you are pregnant or planning to become pregnant, talk to your health-care practitioner before taking amlodipine. Your health-care practitioner can determine whether the potential benefits outweigh the potential risks.

Amlodipine may pass into breast milk. Your health-care practitioner may tell you to stop breastfeeding until you have completed treatment.

SPECIAL INFORMATION FOR SENIORS

Seniors may be started on a lower dose. They are also more likely to experience adverse reactions and ones of more severity.

OPEN QUESTIONS OR CONTROVERSIES

Amlodipine, along with other calcium channel blockers, have been found in some studies to increase the risk of cancer, including breast cancer in postmenopausal women (Fitzpatrick, AL et al. *Cancer* 1997; 80:1438-47) and increased risk of gastrointestinal bleeding (Pahor, *Lancet* 1996; 347).

There is also a question about its use in treating hypertension. This is being investigated in a study whose results should be available by the end of 2002 or early 2003. The Antihypertensive and Lipid-Lowering Treatment to Prevent Heart Attack Trial (ALLHAT) is a multicenter clinical trial of more than 42,000 high-risk patients aged 55 years and older who have high blood pressure. Researchers are determining whether the occurrence of fatal coronary heart disease and/or nonfatal myocardial infarction is different between individuals who take a diuretic (chlorthalidone), a calcium channel blocker (amlodipine), an angiotensin-converting enzyme inhibitor (lisinopril), or an alpha-adrenergic blocker (doxazosin; this medication was eventually dropped from the study). The outcome of this trial may help clarify the safety of amlodipine in older hypertensive patients.

GENERIC NAME

Amlodipine/atorvastatin

BRAND NAME

Caduet
No generic available

ABOUT THIS DRUG

The drug combination of amlodipine/atorvastatin brings together two commonly prescribed heart medications. It is the first drug to treat high blood pressure and high cholesterol and is used primarily in the treatment of hypertension and chronic stable angina.

Atorvastatin is a statin drug that blocks the effects of an enzyme known as HMG-CoA reductase, which in turn blocks the production of cholesterol and triglycerides. Amlodipine (a calcium channel blocker) interferes with the movement of calcium into heart muscles, which in turn relaxes the blood vessels, reduces heart rate, and results in a lowering of blood pressure and reduced chest pain.

SIDE EFFECTS

Be sure to tell your health-care practitioner if you experience any side effects while taking amlodipine/atorvastatin. Only your health-care practitioner can determine whether it is safe for you to continue taking this drug.

- *Most Common:* chest pain, dizziness, edema, fatigue, flushing, headache, insomnia, nausea, palpitations
- *Rare:* allergic reaction (closing of the throat, difficulty breathing, hives, swelling of the lips, tongue, or face), chest pain, severe dizziness or fainting, swelling of the ankles or legs (moderate to severe), unusually slow or fast heartbeat

IMPORTANT PRECAUTIONS

Tell your health-care practitioner if you are sensitive or allergic to amlodipine/atorvastatin or to any other drugs, especially other calcium channel blockers or statins.

Amlodipine must be used with caution if you have certain heart conditions, liver or kidney disease, or high blood pressure, so be sure to give your health-care practitioner an accurate medical history. In rare cases, people with severe heart disease may experience more frequent angina attacks or even a heart attack when starting amlodipine.

Tell your health-care practitioner if you are taking any other HMG-CoA reductase inhibitors, such as fluvastatin, lovastatin, pravastatin, rosuvastatin, or simvastatin; if you drink alcohol; if you have another heart or blood vessel disease such as aortic stenosis, heart failure, low blood pressure, sick sinus syndrome, or coronary artery disease; or if you have any other chronic medical condition.

Because use of this drug may cause dizziness, make sure you know how it affects you before you drive or operate hazardous equipment. Also, rise slowly from a sitting or lying position, as dizziness and a possible fall may occur.

Contact your health-care practitioner immediately if you experience unexplained muscle pain, weakness, or tenderness, especially if you also have a fever, abdominal pain, unexplained fatigue, dark urine, pale-colored stools, or yellowing of the skin or eyes, as these may be early symptoms of muscle or liver problems.

DRUG INTERACTIONS

Tell your health-care practitioner and pharmacist if you are taking any prescription or nonprescription drugs, as well as any vitamins, herbs, or other supplements. No studies of interactions have been conducted with this combination drug and other drugs. However, studies have been done on the individual components. Known drug-drug interactions with amlodipine include the following:

- Adenosine, beta-blockers (e.g., acebutolol, metoprolol), or digitalis may cause heart rate and rhythm problems.
- Some antifungals (e.g., fluconazole, itraconazole) may result in toxic levels of amlodipine.
- Delavirdine may cause increased amlodipine levels and toxicity.
- Cimetidine may increase the effects of amlodipine.
- Cyclosporine may result in increased levels of cyclosporine and a greater risk of toxicity.
- Nonsteroidal anti-inflammatory drugs (NSAIDs; e.g., etodolac, naproxen) or oral anticoagulants (e.g., warfarin) may increase the risk of gastrointestinal bleeding.
- Rifampin may reduce the therapeutic effect of amlodipine.
- Ritonavir and probably other protease inhibitors (e.g., nelfinavir) may cause amlodipine toxicity.

Known drug-drug interactions with atorvastatin (statins in general) include the following:

- Statins should be taken with caution, if at all, with cyclosporine, erythromycin, gemfibrozil, or niacin. These combinations increase the risk of muscle problems.
- Statins increase the absorption of digoxin.
- Itraconazole and cholesyramine may increase the effects of statins.
- Propranolol may reduce the effects of statins.
- Statins may increase the effects of warfarin.
- Separate doses of antacids and atorvastatin by at least one hour.
- Atorvastatin increases blood levels of oral contraceptives.
- Using alcohol with statins increases the risk of liver damage.

FOOD, VITAMIN, AND HERBAL INTERACTIONS

It is very important to follow your health-care practitioner's dietary recommendations. A low-fat, low-cholesterol diet will help control cholesterol and triglyceride levels.

Avoid taking this medication with grapefruit or grapefruit juice, and do not ingest either of these foods for at least one hour after taking your dose, as their interaction could lead to potentially dangerous effects.

Avoid herbs that can increase blood pressure, including ginseng, goldenseal, ephedra (ma huang), licorice, and saw palmetto. Calcium and garlic can be beneficial as they help lower blood pressures. Be sure to talk to your health-care practitioner before taking these supplements. Do not take St. John's wort, as its interaction with atorvastatin can cause heightened sensitivity to the sun.

RECOMMENDED DOSAGE

The combination of amlodipine/atorvastatin is available in tablets in the following formulations of amlodipine-to-atorvastatin: 5 mg/10 mg, 5 mg/20 mg, 5 mg/40 mg, 5 mg/80 mg, 10 mg/10 mg, 10 mg/20 mg, 10 mg/40 mg, and 10 mg/80 mg. The dosages given here are typical. However, your health-care practitioner will determine the most appropriate dose and schedule for your needs.

- *Children:* not recommended for children
- *Adults:* The maximum dose of the amlodipine component is 10 mg once daily; maximum of the atorvastatin component is 80 mg once daily. Your health-care practitioner will determine the most appropriate starting dose for you, based on whether or not you are already taking one of the components and the condition to be treated.

This drug combination should be taken with 8 ounces of water and either with or without food. It is best to take your dose at the same time each day.

If you miss a dose, take it as soon as you remember. If it is nearly time for your next dose, do not take the missed dose. Continue with your regular dosing schedule. Never take a double dose.

SYMPTOMS OF OVERDOSE AND WHAT TO DO

Symptoms of overdose have not been noted. However, they will likely include a dramatic drop in blood pressure and a rapid heartbeat. If overdose occurs, seek immediate medical attention and bring the prescription container with you to the hospital.

SPECIAL INFORMATION FOR PREGNANT OR NURSING WOMEN

This drug combination should not be used if you are pregnant or plan to become pregnant, as it is known to cause birth defects if taken during pregnancy.

Although it is not known whether amlodipine/atorvastatin passes into breast milk, your health-care practitioner may recommend that you discontinue this medication while nursing, or recommend you switch to bottle feeding if you are taking this medication.

SPECIAL INFORMATION FOR SENIORS

Seniors are more sensitive to the effects of these drugs, so lower doses should be prescribed.

GENERIC NAME

Amoxapine *see Tricyclic Antidepressants, page 1076*

GENERIC NAME

Amoxicillin *see Penicillin Antibiotics, page 812*

GENERIC NAME

Amphetamine *see Dextroamphetamine, page 355*

GENERIC NAME

Ampicillin *see Penicillin Antibiotics, page 812*

GENERIC NAME
Amprenavir

BRAND NAME
Agenerase
No generic available

ABOUT THIS DRUG
Amprenavir is a protease inhibitor which, when combined with other drugs, reduces the levels of HIV (human immunodeficiency virus) in the blood of people infected with the organism. Amprenavir is always taken as part of a drug "cocktail" consisting of two or three drugs against the virus.

Amprenavir, like other protease inhibitors, prevents the mature HIV virus from forming by interfering with the activity of a viral protease, an enzyme needed by HIV to reproduce. This drug is not a cure for HIV infection or AIDS (acquired immunodeficiency syndrome).

SIDE EFFECTS
Because amprenavir is always taken along with other drugs, the side effects are associated with multidrug treatment. The drugs most often taken with amprenavir include AZT, ddI, ddC, or 3TC. Report any side effects you experience while taking any of these drug combinations.

➤ *Most Common:* nausea, vomiting, diarrhea, mild rash, itching, high blood sugar, high blood triglycerides

➤ *More Common:* changes in sense of taste, tingling in the hands or feet or around the mouth

➤ *Less Common:* depression, high blood cholesterol levels

➤ *Rare:* life-threatening rash, diabetes, buffalo hump

IMPORTANT PRECAUTIONS
Do not take this drug if you are sensitive or allergic to it. If you are allergic to sulfa drugs, you may also be allergic to amprenavir.

People with liver disease may need a lower dosage. Individuals who have hemophilia may have an increased risk of bleeding.

In rare instances, protease inhibitors can cause a redistribution of body fat and result in a moon-shaped face, buffalo hump, enlarged breasts, or abnormal thinness. Severe, life-threatening skin reactions are also a rare occurrence.

Amprenavir can worsen active cases of diabetes or bring out latent cases. Use of an oral diabetes drug or insulin may be needed.

DRUG INTERACTIONS

Let your health-care practitioner and pharmacist know about any prescription and nonprescription drugs you are taking, as well as any vitamins, herbs, or other supplements. Amprenavir can interact with other drugs.

- Amprenavir can significantly reduce the effectiveness of birth control pills. You will need to use another form of birth control while taking amprenavir.
- Antacids should be taken at least one hour before or one hour after taking amprenavir.
- Astemizole, bepridil, cisapride, dihydroergotamine, ergotamine, lidocaine injections, midazolam, triazolam, tricyclic antidepressants, and quinidine can cause severe, life-threatening reactions if taken with amprenavir. Do not combine these drugs.
- Amiodarone, lidocaine injections, warfarin, and tricyclic antidepressants may need dosage adjustments before you begin to take amprenavir.
- Carbamazepine, phenytoin, and phenobarbital reduce the effectiveness of amprenavir.
- Statin cholesterol-lowering drugs (e.g., simvastatin, fluvastatin) combined with amprenavir can increase the risk of drug toxicity.
- Sildenafil's side effects are dramatically enhanced when combined with amprenavir.
- Other drugs that should be used with caution include alprazolam, calcium channel blockers, carbamazepine, clozapine, corticosteroids, clorazepate, dapsone, delavirdine, diazepam, efavirenz, erythromycin, estrogens, flurazepam, itraconazole, loratadine, nevirapine, pimozide, and progesterone.

FOOD, VITAMIN, AND HERBAL INTERACTIONS

High-fat foods may reduce the effectiveness of amprenavir.

Amprenavir capsules contain high amounts of vitamin E. Do not take a vitamin E supplement while using this form of the drug.

The herb St. John's wort can decrease the blood levels of this drug by up to 57 percent, which can significantly reduce its effectiveness. Do not use St. John's wort along with amprenavir.

RECOMMENDED DOSAGE

Amprenavir is available in 125-mg capsules and in solution. The dosages given here are typical; however, your health-care practitioner must determine the best dosage and schedule for your needs.

Capsules

- *Children Younger than 4 Years:* Not recommended.
- *Children 4 to 12 Years:* 9 mg per pound of body weight, twice daily or 6.8 mg per pound of body weight three times a day along with other anti-HIV drugs. Maximum 2,400 mg daily. This dosage also applies to older children who weigh less than 110 pounds.
- *Children 13 to 16 Years and Adults:* 1,200 mg twice a day along with other anti-HIV drugs. Adults who have moderate to severe liver disease should take 300 to 450 mg twice daily.

Oral Solution

- *Children Younger than 4 Years:* Not recommended.
- *Children 4 to 12 Years:* 10.2 mg per pound of body weight twice daily or 7.7 mg per pound of body weight three times daily along with other anti-HIV drugs. Maximum 2,800 mg daily. This dosage also applies to older children who weigh less than 110 pounds.

Do not switch from the capsules to the oral solution or vice versa, because the oral solution is not absorbed as well as the capsules and so is less efficient at the same milligram levels. If you miss a dose, take it as soon as you remember if no more than four hours have passed since you were scheduled to take it. If it is longer, do not take the forgotten dose, and stay on your regular dosing schedule. Never take a double dose.

SYMPTOMS OF OVERDOSE AND WHAT TO DO

No cases of overdose have been documented. If, however, an overdose occurs, seek emergency medical assistance. Take the prescription container with you.

SPECIAL INFORMATION FOR PREGNANT OR NURSING WOMEN

Amprenavir causes birth defects in animals, but studies in pregnant women have not been conducted. If you are pregnant or plan to become pregnant, talk to your health-care practitioner for guidance. He or she can determine whether the potential benefits outweigh the potential risks. There is no evidence that amprenavir reduces the risk of transmitting the virus from the mother to the fetus.

It is not known whether amprenavir is transmitted in breast milk. However, women with HIV should not breastfeed because they can pass the virus to an uninfected child.

SPECIAL INFORMATION FOR SENIORS

It is not known whether older adults will experience more or different side effects than younger users.

GENERIC NAME

Anagrelide

BRAND NAME

Agrylin
No generic available

ABOUT THIS DRUG

Anagrelide is a platelet count–reducing agent, used to reduce the risk of blood clots in people who have too many platelets in their blood. This condition, known as thrombocytosis, occurs mainly in adults.

SIDE EFFECTS

Report any side effects to your health-care practitioner so he or she can determine whether it is safe for you to continue to take the drug.

- ➤ *Most Common:* headache (affects more than 40%), diarrhea, abdominal pain, edema, palpitations, nausea, dizziness, pain, flatulence, weakness
- ➤ *More Common:* cough, chest pain, loss of appetite, fever, severe itching, malaise, heartburn, rash, slow heartbeat, vomiting
- ➤ *Less Common or Rare:* back pain, canker sores, confusion, constipation, fever or chills, joint or muscle pain, mental depression, sudden, severe headache or weakness, symptoms of a heart attack (anxiety, cold sweating, increased heart rate, nausea or vomiting, shortness of breath, severe pain or pressure in the chest and/or arms, back, jaw, or neck), bloody urine, blurred or double vision, painful or difficult urination, swelling of lower legs or feet, unusual bleeding or bruising, unusual tiredness, stuffy or runny nose, ringing in the ears, nervousness, photosensitivity, temporary loss of hair

IMPORTANT PRECAUTIONS

Do not take anagrelide if you are sensitive or allergic to it.

Inform your health-care practitioner if you have known or suspected heart disease, kidney disease, or liver disease. Anagrelide may have a negative effect on the heart, liver, and kidneys.

You will need to have your blood monitored before starting treatment, every two days during the first week of treatment, and then at least once weekly thereafter until you reach the desired maintenance dosage.

Inform your health-care practitioner or dentist before undergoing any surgical procedures.

Safety and efficacy in people age 16 years and younger have not been determined.

DRUG INTERACTIONS

No interactions between anagrelide and other drugs have been documented. However, you should still tell your health-care practitioner and pharmacist about any prescription and nonprescription drugs you are taking, as well as any vitamins, herbs, or other supplements. The drugs used most often along with anagrelide are acetaminophen, allopurinol, aspirin, furosemide, hydroxyurea, iron, and ranitidine. So far, there is no clinical evidence that anagrelide interacts with any of these medications. One case report suggests that sucralfate may hinder absorption of anagrelide.

FOOD, VITAMIN, AND HERBAL INTERACTIONS

No food, vitamin, or herbal interactions have been documented.

RECOMMENDED DOSAGE

Anagrelide is available in 0.5- and 1.0-mg capsules. The dosages given here are typical; however, your health-care practitioner will determine the most appropriate dosage for your needs.

➤ *Children 16 Years and Younger:* Your health-care practitioner will determine if it is appropriate.

➤ *Adults:* 0.5 mg four times daily, or 1 mg twice daily, for at least seven days. Thereafter, your health-care practitioner will adjust your dosage.

Take each dose with a full glass of water. If you miss a dose, take it as soon as you remember. However, if it is nearly time for your next dose, do not take the missed dose. Remain on your regular dosing schedule, and never take a double dose.

SYMPTOMS OF OVERDOSE AND WHAT TO DO

Symptoms of an anagrelide overdose are not known, but would likely include bleeding and blood in the stool or in vomit. If an overdose occurs, seek immediate medical attention, and bring the prescription container with you.

SPECIAL INFORMATION FOR PREGNANT OR NURSING WOMEN

No adequate studies have been done on the effect of anagrelide on pregnant or nursing women. If you are pregnant, plan to become pregnant, or are nursing, talk to your health-care practitioner. He or she will determine whether the potential benefits outweigh the potential risk of taking this drug.

SPECIAL INFORMATION FOR SENIORS

There are no special precautions for seniors. Older adults may experience more severe or frequent side effects.

GENERIC NAME

Anakinra

BRAND NAME

Kineret
No generic available

ABOUT THIS DRUG

Anakinra is an antirheumatic medication used to reduce the signs and symptoms of moderate to severe rheumatoid arthritis in people 18 years or older. It should only be used by those who have not responded to one or more other disease-modifying antirheumatic drugs (DMARDs).

Interleukin-1 is a substance that is produced in response to inflammatory stimuli and plays a role in various activities, such as degradation of cartilage and promotion of bone resorption. Anakinra blocks the activity of interleukin-1.

SIDE EFFECTS

If you experience any side effects while taking anakinra, contact your health-care practitioner. She or he can determine whether it is safe for you to continue taking the drug.

- *Most Common:* mild, transient reaction (e.g., pain, inflammation, skin discoloration) at the injection site that lasts 14 to 28 days. Nearly 75 percent of patients experience this side effect.
- *Less Common:* serious infection (2% of users), decrease in absolute neutrophil blood count, platelets, and total white blood cell count

IMPORTANT PRECAUTIONS

Do not take anakinra if you are sensitive or allergic to it. Anakinra also should not be used if you have an active infection. If you have asthma, you may be at higher risk of developing an infection.

The safety and efficacy of this drug in patients with a compromised immune system has not been determined.

If you have liver or kidney dysfunction, consult with your health-care practitioner before using this drug.

DRUG INTERACTIONS

Anakinra entered the market in 2001, and at that time no drug-drug interaction studies had been done. However, always tell your health-care practitioner and pharmacist about any prescription and nonprescription drugs you are taking, as well as any vitamins, herbs, or other supplements.

The safety of anakinra used in combination with tumor necrosis factor (TNF) blocking agents, which are also used to treat rheumatoid arthritis, has not been determined. Preliminary research suggests that there is a higher rate of serious infection (7%) when anakinra is used along with the TNF blocking agent etanercept. Therefore, this drug combination should only be used if no other alternatives exist.

FOOD, VITAMIN, AND HERBAL INTERACTIONS

No interactions with food, vitamins, or herbal products have been documented.

RECOMMENDED DOSAGE

Anakinra is available in prefilled syringes. The dosages given here are typical; however, your health-care practitioner will determine the dosage most appropriate for you.

- *Children:* This drug is not indicated for children under age 18 years.
- *Adults:* 100 mg injected subcutaneously at the same time each day.

Your health-care practitioner will instruct you or your caregiver on how to make the injections at home. Always visually inspect the solution for discoloration, cloudiness, or particulates before using it. If you observe any of these conditions, do not use the prefilled syringe. If you miss a dose, take it as soon as you remember. However, if it is nearly time for your next dose, do not take the missed dose. Continue on your regular dosing schedule. Never take a double dose.

SYMPTOMS OF OVERDOSE AND WHAT TO DO

No overdoses have been documented. If an overdose occurs, seek immediate medical attention, and bring the prescription container with you.

SPECIAL INFORMATION FOR PREGNANT OR NURSING WOMEN

No adequate studies have been conducted on pregnant or nursing women. If you are pregnant or plan to become pregnant, or you are breastfeeding, consult with your health-care practitioner. This drug should be used only if the potential benefits outweigh the potential risks.

SPECIAL INFORMATION FOR SENIORS

Older adults may be more susceptible to side effects. Because this drug is substantially eliminated by the kidney, special care should be taken if anakinra is taken by seniors, who often have impaired renal function.

GENERIC NAME

Anastrozole

BRAND NAME

Arimidex

No generic available

Note: This entry contains information that applies to letrozole (brand name: Femara).

ABOUT THIS DRUG

Anastrozole is an antiestrogen, antineoplastic (anticancer) drug. It is normally given to postmenopausal women with advanced breast cancer who have used other antiestrogen drugs such as tamoxifen.

A type of estrogen called estradiol stimulates breast tumors. Anastrozole reduces the blood levels of estradiol and thus inhibits the growth of the tumors.

SIDE EFFECTS

If you experience side effects while using this drug, report them to your health-care practitioner. Because this drug may prolong survival and improve quality of life, health-care practitioners often suggest ways to relieve any bothersome adverse reactions. Only your health-care practitioner can determine whether it is safe for you to continue taking anastrozole.

- *Most Common:* abdominal pain, back pain, bone pain, chest pain, constipation, cough, depression, diarrhea, dizziness, dry mouth, headache, hot flashes, nausea, pelvic pain, pins and needles, rash, shortness of breath, sore throat, weakness
- *Less Common:* anxiety, blood clots, breast pain, bronchitis, confusion drowsiness, fever, flu-like symptoms, fractures, thinning hair, high blood pressure, infection, insomnia, itching, joint pain, muscle pain, neck pain, sweating, urinary tract infection, vaginal bleeding, weight loss

IMPORTANT PRECAUTIONS

Do not take anastrozole if you are sensitive or allergic to it.

Because anastrozole can cause dizziness, make sure you are not affected by this side effect before you drive or operate hazardous machinery.

Anastrozole can raise your blood cholesterol levels; therefore you health-care practitioner may regularly check your cholesterol levels.

DRUG INTERACTIONS

No drug-to-drug interactions have been documented. However, you should still tell your health-care practitioner and pharmacist about any prescription and nonprescription drugs you are taking, as well as any vitamins, herbs, or other supplements.

FOOD, VITAMIN, AND HERBAL INTERACTIONS

No food, vitamin, or herbal interactions have been documented.

RECOMMENDED DOSAGE

Anastrozole is available in 1-mg tablets. Letrozole is available in 2.5 mg tablets. The dosages given here are typical; however, your health-care practitioner will determine the dose most appropriate for your needs.

- *Children:* Not indicated for children.
- *Adults:* For anastrozole, one 1-mg tablet taken once daily; for letrozole, one 2.5-mg tablet taken once daily.

If you miss a dose, take it if you remember within 12 hours of your last dose. If it is beyond 12 hours, do not take the missed dose and continue with your regular dosing schedule. Never take a double dose.

SYMPTOMS OF OVERDOSE AND WHAT TO DO

There are no reports of overdose with anastrozole. However, if overdose does occur, seek immediate medical attention, and bring the prescription container with you.

SPECIAL INFORMATION FOR PREGNANT OR NURSING WOMEN

If you are pregnant or plan to become pregnant, do not take anastrozole. This drug causes birth defects in animals and could be toxic to your unborn child. Your chances of having a miscarriage or a stillborn infant also increase if you take this drug.

Anastrozole may pass through your breast milk; therefore your health-care practitioner will probably advise you not to breastfeed while taking this drug.

SPECIAL INFORMATION FOR SENIORS

No special precautions are noted for older adults. However, seniors may experience more severe side effects.

GENERIC NAME

Class: Angiotensin II Blockers

Generics: (1) candesartan; (2) eprosartan; (3) irbesartan; (4) losartan; (5) olmesartan; (6) telmisartan; (7) valsartan

BRAND NAMES

(1) Atacand; (2) Teveten; (3) Avapro; (4) Cozaar; (5) Benicar; (6) Micardis; (7) Diovan
No generic available

ABOUT THIS DRUG

The drugs in the angiotensin II blocker family, also referred to as angiotensin II receptor antagonists, are prescribed for individuals who have high blood pressure and, in the case of losartan, also for left ventricular hypertrophy (an abnormally sized left ventricle).

These drugs block the effects of angiotensin II, a substance that causes the blood vessels to constrict and thus raise blood pressure. Thus angiotensin II blockers help the blood vessels remain open and thus keep blood pressure down. None of these drugs are a cure for hypertension; they merely help control it.

SIDE EFFECTS

Report any side effects you may experience to your health-care practitioner. Only a health-care practitioner can decide whether it is safe for you to continue to take the drug. It is possible to experience an excessive lowering of blood pressure with the first dose. Symptoms include lightheadedness or faintness.

The side effect profiles for each drug in this class differ.

Candesartan

➤ *Less Common or Rare:* chills, cough or hoarseness, fever, lower back or side pain, difficult or painful urination, dizziness, joint pain, nosebleed or bleeding gums, swelling of feet or lower legs

Eprosartan

➤ *Less Common or Rare:* abdominal pain, burning or painful urination, changes in urinary frequency, cough, dizziness, fever, joint pain, sore throat, swollen face, lips, limbs, or tongue, unusual tiredness

Irbesartan

➤ *Less Common or Rare:* anxiety and/or nervousness, belching, cold-like symptoms, confusion, dark urine, diarrhea, dizziness, headache, heartburn, hive-like swelling on face, eyelids, lips, tongue, throat, hands, legs, feet, or sex organs, irregular heartbeat, itching, jaundice, loss of appetite, muscle or bone pain, numbness or tingling in hands, feet, or lips, shortness of breath, unusual tiredness, weakness or heaviness in the legs

Losartan

➤ *Common:* headache

➤ *Less Common:* back pain, fatigue, diarrhea, nasal congestion

➤ *Rare:* difficulty breathing or swallowing, hoarseness, swelling of the face, mouth, hands, or throat, dizziness, cough, fever, sore throat

Olmesartan

➤ *Common:* dizziness. This is the only side effect reported from the clinical trials by the manufacturer at the time of this writing. See "Open Questions or Controversies."

Telmisartan

➤ *Less Common or Rare:* abdominal pain, back pain, changes in urinary frequency, changes in vision, changes in appetite, coughing, diarrhea, dry mouth, dizziness, ear congestion or pain, fever, head congestion, headache, heartburn, increased sweating, muscle pain or spasm, nasal congestion, nausea, nervousness, painful urination, rapid heartbeat, rash, runny nose, sneezing, sore throat, swelling in hands, lower legs, and feet

Valsartan

➤ *Less Common:* abdominal pain, anxiety, constipation, cough, dizziness, dry mouth, edema, fatigue, gas, impotence, heart palpitations, insomnia, joint pain, nausea, rash, sinusitis, viral infection, upper respiratory infection

IMPORTANT PRECAUTIONS

Do not take angiotensin II blocker drugs if you are sensitive or allergic to them.

If you have kidney or liver disease, a history of coronary artery disease, or a history of circulation problems in the brain, inform your health-care practitioner of these conditions before you take these drugs. If you plan to take losartan, tell your health-care practitioner if you have a history of allergy to aspirin or penicillin.

Because these drugs may cause confusion, do not drive or operate hazardous machinery until you know how you will react to the medication.

These drugs may cause excessive dizziness, lightheadedness, or fainting with the first dose. This side effect may be made worse by alcohol, dehydration, fever, prolonged sitting or standing, exercise, or hot weather.

DRUG INTERACTIONS

Before you take any of the angiotensin II blockers, tell your health-care practitioner and pharmacist about any prescription and nonprescription drugs you are taking, as well as any vitamins, herbs, and other supplements.

➤ Potassium-sparing diuretics (e.g., amiloride, spironolactone) used along with any of the angiotensin II blockers may abnormally raise blood potassium levels.

➤ Irbesartan may interact with tolbutamide.

➤ Telmisartan along with digoxin may cause high levels of digoxin.

➤ Telmisartan along with warfarin may cause a slight increase in the level of warfarin.

FOOD, VITAMIN, AND HERBAL INTERACTIONS

Excessive caffeine intake should be avoided. If you are taking losartan, consult your health-care practitioner if you are taking potassium supplements or using salt substitutes or low-salt milk.

Ginseng, goldenseal, licorice, ephedra (ma huang), and saw palmetto may raise blood pressure and blunt the effects of these medications. Avoid these herbs while taking angiotensin II blockers. Calcium and garlic can be beneficial as they help lower blood pressure. Be sure to talk to your health-care practitioner before taking these supplements.

RECOMMENDED DOSAGE

The dosage recommendations given here are typical. However, your health-care practitioner will determine the most appropriate dosage and schedule to fit your needs.

Candesartan

Available in 16-mg tablets

- *Children:* Not recommended for children under age 18.
- *Adults:* Starting dose is 16 mg once daily if you are not already taking hydrochlorothiazide. The usual maintenance dose is 8 to 32 mg daily, taken once or divided into 2 doses.

Eprosartan

Available in 400- and 600-mg tablets

- *Children:* Not recommended for children under age 18.
- *Adults:* 400 to 800 mg daily in one dose or two divided doses.

Irbesartan

Available in 75-, 100-, and 300-mg tablets

- *Children Younger than 6 Years:* Use to be determined by your health-care practitioner.
- *Children 6 to 12 Years:* 75 mg once daily. Your health-care practitioner may increase the dose if needed.
- *Children 13 Years and Older and Adults:* Starting dose of 150 mg daily if you are not already taking hydrochlorothiazide. Your health-care practitioner may increase it up to 300 mg as tolerated. Starting dose of 75 mg daily if you are also taking hydrochlorothiazide.

Losartan

Available in 25- and 50-mg tablets

➤ *Children:* Not recommended for children under age 18.

➤ *Adults:* Starting dose is 25 to 50 mg daily. Maintenance dose is 25 to 100 mg taken once daily or divided into 2 doses.

Olmesartan

➤ *Children:* Not recommended for children under age 18.

➤ *Adults:* 20 or 40 mg once daily.

Telmisartan

Available in 40- and 80-mg tablets

➤ *Children:* Use to be determined by your health-care practitioner.

➤ *Adults:* 40 mg once daily. Your health-care practitioner may increase the dose if needed.

Valsartan

Available in 80- and 160-mg capsules

➤ *Children:* Not recommended for children under age 18.

➤ *Adults:* Starting dose is 80 mg daily; maximum is 320 mg once daily.

SYMPTOMS OF OVERDOSE AND WHAT TO DO

Symptoms of an overdose may include dizziness, fainting, rapid heartbeat, slowed heartbeat, nausea, vomiting, and chest pain. If an overdose occurs, seek emergency medical attention, and bring the prescription container with you.

SPECIAL INFORMATION FOR PREGNANT OR NURSING WOMEN

Angiotensin II blockers should not be taken during pregnancy or breastfeeding. Discuss safer alternatives to lower your blood pressure with your health-care practitioner if you are pregnant, plan to become pregnant, or are breastfeeding. If you become pregnant while taking any of these drugs, inform your health-care practitioner immediately.

SPECIAL INFORMATION FOR SENIORS

No special precautions are needed for older adults. However, side effects may be more likely and more severe.

OPEN QUESTIONS OR CONTROVERSIES

Telmisartan, eprosartan, and olmesartan are the newest additions to the angiotensin II blocker family (November 2000, November 2001, and April 2002, respectively). Studies suggest that blacks may have a smaller response to the blood pressure lowering effects of telmisartan, while losartan is less effective in most blacks.

For treatment of high blood pressure, the drug treatment of choice, according to Sidney M. Wolf, M.D., author of *Worst Pills, Best Pills,* is hydrochlorothiazide, a diuretic (water pill), along with proper diet, losing weight, exercise, and decreasing your intake of alcohol and salt. Hydrochlorothiazide is considerably less expensive than other blood pressure medications.

Both losartan and irbesartan are available combined with hydrochlorothiazide. Dr. Wolf suggests that if you also need to take hydrochlorothiazide along with either losartan or irbesartan, buy the angiotensin drug and your hydrochlorothiazide separately until your health-care practitioner has stabilized both of your doses. If your optimal dose is the same as the one available in the combination losartan HCT or irbesartan HCT product, then you may want to buy the combination product. He recommends comparing the prices of buying them separately and together for the best savings.

GENERIC NAME

Class: Antiemetics (5HT$_3$ type)

Generics: (1) dolasetron; (2) granisetron; (3) ondansetron; (4) palonosetron

BRAND NAMES

(1) Anzemet; (2) Kytril; (3) Zofran; (4) Aloxi
No generic available

ABOUT THIS DRUG

This class of antiemetics (antinausea) drugs is used to prevent nausea and vomiting caused by radiation treatment and chemotherapy for cancer, as well as to prevent these symptoms following surgery.

These drugs interfere with the nerve transmissions and the chemical receptor sites that stimulate nausea and induce vomiting.

SIDE EFFECTS

Let your health-care practitioner know about any side effects you experience while taking these drugs. Only a health-care practitioner can determine whether it is safe for you to continue treatment.

Dolasetron

- *Most Common:* headache, fatigue, diarrhea, slow heartbeat, dizziness, rapid heartbeat, chills, indigestion, fever, hypertension
- *Less Common or Rare:* hypotension, rash, taste changes, abnormal vision flushing, vertigo

Granisetron

- *Common:* headache, constipation, weakness, diarrhea, abdominal pain, nausea, vomiting
- *Less Common:* dizziness, insomnia, anxiety, fever, loss of appetite, hair loss

Ondansetron

- *More Common:* headache, fever, constipation, diarrhea
- *Less Common:* abdominal pain or cramps, dizziness, drowsiness, dry mouth, feeling cold, itching, unusual weakness
- *Rare:* chest pain, shortness of breath, rash, hives, tight chest, wheezing

Palonosetron

- *More Common:* constipation, diarrhea, dizziness, fatigue, headache
- *Less Common or Rare:* allergic reaction (closing of the throat, difficulty breathing, hives, swelling of the face, throat, and lips), irregular heartbeat

IMPORTANT PRECAUTIONS

Do not take these drugs if you are sensitive or allergic to them.

Tell your health-care practitioner if you have liver disease or heart disease, or if you have had abdominal surgery recently.

Because these drugs can cause dizziness and drowsiness, do not drive or engage in potentially dangerous activities until you know how you react to them.

DRUG INTERACTIONS

Inform your health-care practitioner and pharmacist about any prescription and nonprescription medications you are taking, as well as any vitamins, herbs, or other supplements. No drug-drug interactions have been noted for granisetron; however, the following may occur:

- Cimetidine may cause blood levels of dolasetron to rise.
- Rifampin may cause blood levels of dolasetron to drop.
- Cimetidine and phenobarbital may interact with ondansetron.

FOOD, VITAMIN, AND HERBAL INTERACTIONS

No food, vitamin, or herbal interactions have been noted.

RECOMMENDED DOSAGE

The doses given here are typical. (Doses for the injectable forms are not provided here; talk to your health-care practitioner for more information. Palonosetron is administered by IV only.) However, your health-care practitioner will determine the most appropriate dose and schedule for your particular needs.

Dolasetron

Available in solution, in 50- and 100-mg tablets, and by injection

- *Children Younger than 2 Years:* Safety has not been determined for this age group.
- *Children 2 to 16 Years:* 1.8 mg/kg within one hour before chemotherapy of solution or tablets. When given after surgery, 1.2 mg/kg is the typical dose.
- *Adults:* 100 mg within one hour before chemotherapy. When given to prevent postsurgical nausea, 100 mg within 2 hours before surgery is the typical dose.

Granisetron

Available in 1-mg tablets

- *Children:* No information available on the use of oral granisetron in children.
- *Adults:* 1 mg twice daily: one tablet taken up to 1 hour before chemotherapy and the second 12 hours after the first tablet, only on days chemotherapy is given.

Ondansetron

Available in oral solution, 4- and 8-mg tablets, and oral disintegrating tablets

- *Children 4 to 12 Years:* 4 mg or 1 teaspoon, 30 minutes before chemotherapy. Repeat this dose 4 and 8 hours later, than again every 8 hours for 1 to 2 days.
- *Children 12 Years and Older and Adults:* 8 mg or 2 teaspoons of solution, 30 minutes before chemotherapy. Repeat this dose 8 hours

after the first dose, then again every 12 hours for 1 to 2 days. To prevent nausea and vomiting after surgery, the typical dose is 16 mg or 4 teaspoons, 1 hour before anesthesia.

If you miss a dose of dolasetron or granisetron, take it as soon as you remember. However, if it is nearly time for your next dose, do not take the skipped dose, and remain on your regular dosing schedule. Never take a double dose.

If you miss a dose of ondansetron and you do not feel nauseated, do not take the missed dose, and remain on your regular dosing schedule. If, however, you miss a dose and you feel nauseated or you vomit, take the missed dose as soon as possible. If vomiting continues, call your health-care practitioner. Do not take a double dose.

These medications should be taken with food to help prevent stomach upset. When taking the oral disintegrating dose of ondansetron, allow the tablet to dissolve on your tongue. No liquids are needed unless desired.

SYMPTOMS OF OVERDOSE AND WHAT TO DO

No specific symptoms of overdose to these drugs have been reported. Likely symptoms may include hypotension and dizziness. If an overdose occurs, seek immediate medical attention, and bring the prescription container with you.

SPECIAL INFORMATION FOR PREGNANT OR NURSING WOMEN

No adequate studies have been done on pregnant or nursing women. If you are pregnant or plan to become pregnant, talk to your health-care practitioner. Only your health-care practitioner can determine whether the potential benefits outweigh the potential risks.

These drugs may pass into breast milk. If you are breastfeeding, your health-care practitioner will advise you to stop until your treatment is completed.

SPECIAL INFORMATION FOR SENIORS

No special precautions are needed for older adults.

OPEN QUESTIONS OR CONTROVERSIES

A novel use for ondansetron may be for treatment of early onset alcoholism. Several studies have suggested that ondansetron, or ondansetron along with the opioid antagonist naltrexone,

(continued from page 131)
reduces cravings among people with early onset alcoholism better than placebo. One of the studies, published in *The Journal of the American Medical Association* (2000; vol. 284), used ondansetron alone and found that while it was effective in early onset alcoholism, it was not useful in people who had later onset disease. Another study, published in *Psychopharmacology* (2001; vol. 154), reported that the combination of ondansetron and naltrexone was effective. Whether ondansetron proves to be helpful in the treatment of people who have early onset alcoholism remains an open question and one that researchers continue to investigate.

GENERIC NAME

Class: Antihistamine-decongestant combination

Generics: (1) acrivastine and pseudoephedrine; (2) azatadine and pseudoephedrine; (3) brompheniramine and pseudoephedrine; (4) dexbrompheniramine and pseudoephedrine; (5) carbinoxamine and pseudoephedrine; (6) chlorpheniramine and pseudoephedrine; (7) chlorpheniramine and phenylephrine; (8) chlorpheniramine and phenyltoloxamine and phenylephrine; (9) chlorpheniramine and pyrilamine and phenylephrine; (10) fexofenadine and pseudoephedrine; (11) loratadine and pseudoephedrine; (12) promethazine and phenylephrine

BRAND NAMES

(1) Semprex-D; (2) Trinalin Repetabs; (3) Allent, Bromfed, Dallergy-JR, Endafed, Lodrane LD, Respahist, Rondec, Touro A & H, ULTRAbrom; (4) Disobrom, Dexaphen-SA; (5) Carbiset, Carbiset TR, Carbodec, Carbodec TR, Cardec-S, Rondec, Rondec-TR; (6) Anamine, Anamine TD, Anaplex, Arohist Pediatric, Brexin LA, Chlordrine SR, Chlorphedrine SR, Codimal LA, Colfed-A, Cophene No 2, Deconamine, Deconomed SR, Duralex, Dur-Tap/PD, Fedahist Gyrocaps, Fedahist Timecaps, Histalet, Klerist-D, Kronofed-A, Kronofed-A Jr, ND Clear, Novafed A, Rescon, Rescon ED, Rescon JR, Rinade BID, Tanafed, Time-Hist; (7) Dallergy-D, Ed A-Hist, Histor-D, Prehist, Rolatuss Plain, Ru-Tuss; (8) Comhist; (9) Atrohist Pediatric, Rhinatate, R-Tannate,

R-Tannamine, Rynatan, Tanoral, Triotann, Tritan, Tri-Tannate; (10) Allegra-D; (11) Claritin-D 12-Hour, Claritin-D 24-Hour; (12) Phenergan VC, Promethazine VC, Promethazine VC Plain, Prometh VC Plain
Some available as generic; ask your pharmacist

ABOUT THIS DRUG

The combination of antihistamine and decongestant is used to treat symptoms of upper respiratory conditions, seasonal allergies such as hayfever, and the common cold.

The antihistamine portion of these drugs relieves allergy symptoms (sneezing, itching, watery eyes, hives, swelling, and other symptoms of allergic reactions). The decongestant portion constricts the blood vessels, which reduces the blood flow to swollen nasal passages. This in turn improves the flow of air in the passages, relieves swelling, and reduces nasal secretions.

SIDE EFFECTS

Despite the large number of drug combinations in this category, the side effects tend to be similar. Ask your health-care practitioner or pharmacist for information about side effects for the specific prescription you receive.

If you experience side effects while taking any of these drugs, contact your health-care practitioner. He or she will determine whether you should continue to take the medication.

➤ *More Common:* dizziness, drowsiness, dry mouth, excitation, nervousness, poor coordination, restlessness, sedation, sleeplessness, upset stomach

➤ *Less Common or Rare:* abnormal heartbeat, abnormal movements, agitation, anxiety, back pain, bloated stomach, change in taste, change in tear production, chest pain, conjunctivitis, constipation, convulsions, depression, diarrhea, difficulty breathing, earache, eye pain, facial swelling, fatigue, flu-like symptoms, flushing, gas, high blood pressure, increased sweating, indigestion, itching, leg cramps, migraine, mood disorders, muscle pain or stiffness, nasal congestion, nosebleed, painful menstrual periods, pneumonia, ringing in the ears, thirst, toothache, tremor, upper respiratory infection, urinary difficulties, vaginal swelling, viral infections, vision problems, vomiting, weakness, weight loss, wheezing

IMPORTANT PRECAUTIONS

Do not take any of these medications if you are sensitive or allergic to any of the antihistamines or decongestants in them. Also avoid these products if you have narrow-angle glaucoma, prostate disease, severe heart disease, bladder obstruction, overactive thyroid, or some types of stomach ulcers, if you are experiencing asthma attacks, or if you are taking monoamine oxidase inhibitor (MAOI) drugs for high blood pressure or depression. If you have severe liver disease, do not use loratadine and pseudoephedrine.

The antihistamine portion of these medications can cause drowsiness and dizziness. Therefore, do not drive or operate hazardous equipment until you know how you will react to the drug.

If you have a history of liver or kidney problems, if you have asthma, or if you are at risk for fainting or drowsiness, talk to your health-care practitioner before using any of these medications.

If you have diabetes, the decongestant may put you at greater risk of having blood vessel or heart disease. The decongestant can also raise blood pressure and increase heart rate if you have hypertension.

DRUG INTERACTIONS

Tell your health-care practitioner and pharmacist about any prescription and over-the-counter medications you are taking, as well as any vitamins, herbs, or other supplements. Antihistamine-decongestant combination drugs may interact with other medications. Generally, do not use any prescription antihistamine-decongestant drugs along with any over-the-counter antihistamines, decongestants, or combination drugs.

- Alcohol, along with an antihistamine-decongestant, can significantly increase drowsiness. Do not drink alcohol when taking any of these drugs.
- Aspirin, in large amounts, can cause ringing of the ears. This symptom may be masked by regular antihistamine use.
- Cimetidine may significantly raise blood levels of loratadine and may lead to toxicity.
- Disopyramide and other drugs that prolong the QT interval should be avoided because of potential heart problems.
- Fluvoxamine, indinavir, itraconazole (and perhaps other antifungals), and macrolide antibiotics (e.g., clarithromycin, erythromycin) may raise the blood levels of loratadine.
- Maprotiline and tricyclic antidepressants (e.g., amitriptyline, clomipramine) may make the side effects of the antihistamines more severe.
- Monoamine oxidase inhibitors (MAOI) (e.g., furazolidone, phenelzine) may cause the side effects of antihistamines to become more se-

vere. MAOIs should not be taken within 2 weeks of taking any antihistamine-decongestant medication.

- Quinidine may change the effects of quinidine and result in negative effects on the heart.
- Sotalol may cause heart problems and should be avoided.

FOOD, VITAMIN, AND HERBAL INTERACTIONS

Do not take loratadine with grapefruit or grapefruit juice. Avoid beverages and foods that contain caffeine (e.g., coffee, tea, chocolate, colas) because they may cause jitters, nervousness, rapid heartbeat, and anxiety.

The herbs kava and valerian root may significantly increase drowsiness. Use of St. John's wort may increase photosensitivity.

RECOMMENDED DOSAGE

Dosages of combination antihistamine-decongestant drugs vary. Follow the dosing instructions given to you by your health-care practitioner or pharmacist.

If you miss a dose, take it as soon as you remember. However, if it is nearly time for your next dose, do not take the missed dose. Continue to follow your regular dosing schedule. Do not take a double dose.

SYMPTOMS OF OVERDOSE AND WHAT TO DO

Symptoms of overdose can include chest pain, chills, drowsiness, dry mouth, fever, irregular or rapid heartbeat, nausea, nervousness, and urinary problems. In case of overdose, seek immediate medical attention, and bring the prescription container with you to the hospital.

SPECIAL INFORMATION FOR PREGNANT OR NURSING WOMEN

The effects of antihistamine-decongestant drugs on pregnant and breastfeeding women have not been adequately studied. Before starting any of these drugs, tell your health-care practitioner if you are pregnant or plan to become pregnant.

Some of these drugs are known to pass into breast milk, while others have not been adequately studied. If you are breastfeeding or plan to do so, talk to your health-care practitioner. She or he can determine whether the drug is essential to your health and weigh the risks and benefits of its use. Your health-care practitioner may advise you to stop breastfeeding until your treatment is completed.

SPECIAL INFORMATION FOR SENIORS

Older individuals are more prone to experience side effects, and they can be more severe.

GENERIC NAME

Antipyrine/benzocaine/glycerin

BRAND NAMES

Allergen Ear Drops, Auralgan Otic, Auroto Otic, Otocalm Ear
Generic available

ABOUT THIS DRUG

This three-drug combination is used to treat severe earache in children and adults, most commonly a condition known as "swimmer's ear," in which water accumulates in the ear canal. The drug is classified as an analgesic. Although it can relieve symptoms, it cannot cure the infection.

The antipyrine provides pain relief, while the benzocaine deadens the nerves inside the ear, and the glycerin absorbs any water that is in the ear.

SIDE EFFECTS

Report any side effects you may experience when using this drug. The only side effect reported has been local irritation.

IMPORTANT PRECAUTIONS

Do not use this medication if you are sensitive or allergic to any of its ingredients.

Do not use this drug if you have a punctured ear drum unless directed to do so by your health-care practitioner.

DRUG INTERACTIONS

This drug combination is not known to interact with other medications. Do not use other ear medications with an antipyrine/ benzocaine/glycerin combination.

FOOD, VITAMIN, AND HERBAL INTERACTIONS

No food, vitamin, or herbal interactions have been documented.

RECOMMENDED DOSAGE

All antipyrine/benzocaine/glycerin combination drugs are available in a liquid and are applied using a dropper. The method of application given here is typical for both children and adults. However, your health-care practitioner will determine the best dosage and schedule for your needs.

- ➤ Warm the bottle by holding it in your hands for several minutes until the medication is at body temperature.
- ➤ Shake the bottle.
- ➤ Lie on your side or tilt your head so the affected ear is facing up.
- ➤ Pull the ear lobe up and administer the needed number of drops.
- ➤ Do not touch the ear with the dropper.
- ➤ Moisten a piece of gauze with the medication and insert it into the ear opening.
- ➤ Keep your head tilted for 5 to 7 minutes.
- ➤ Repeat this process every 1 to 2 hours until the pain and congestion are gone.

If you miss a dose, use it as soon as you remember. However, if it is nearly time for your next dose, do not use the missed dose, and remain on your regular schedule.

SYMPTOMS OF OVERDOSE AND WHAT TO DO

No reports of overdose with this drug have been reported. If it is accidentally ingested, seek immediate medical attention, and bring the prescription container with you.

SPECIAL INFORMATION FOR PREGNANT OR NURSING WOMEN

No adequate studies of the use of this drug in pregnant or nursing women have been done. If you are pregnant or plan to become pregnant, or if you are breastfeeding or plan to do so, talk with your health-care practitioner before starting this drug. Only a health-care practitioner can determine whether the potential benefits will outweigh the potential dangers.

SPECIAL INFORMATION FOR SENIORS

No special restrictions are required for older individuals.

GENERIC NAME
Apraclonidine

BRAND NAME
Iopidine
No generic available

ABOUT THIS DRUG
Apraclonidine is used to reduce inner eye pressure in people with glaucoma, and both before and after eye surgery. It is classified as a sympathomimetic.

Although experts are not sure exactly how apraclonidine works, it appears to reduce eye pressure by decreasing production of eye fluid. It takes effect about 1 hour after application and provides maximum effect at 3 to 5 hours.

SIDE EFFECTS
If you experience any side effects when using this medication, contact your health-care practitioner. Only he or she can determine whether it is safe for you to continue using the drug.

➤ *Most Common:* red, itchy, tearing eye, eye discomfort, lid swelling, dry mouth, headache, weakness

➤ *Less Common:* blanching of the eye, upper lid elevation, dilated pupils, blurred vision, allergic reactions, crusty eyelid, dizziness, abnormal vision, eye pain, abdominal pain, diarrhea, vomiting, nasal burning, runny nose, sore throat, worsening asthma, constipation and nausea, slow heartbeat, abnormal heart rhythms, chest pain, fainting, swelling, difficulty sleeping, irritability, pain, numbness, or tingling in the hands or feet, taste changes, rash

IMPORTANT PRECAUTIONS
Do not use apraclonidine if you are sensitive or allergic to it or to clonidine.

Because apraclonidine can cause dizziness or impair your vision, make sure you know how you react to this medication before you drive or operate hazardous machinery.

Before using apraclonidine, inform your health-care practitioner if you have any of the following conditions: depression, heart or blood vessel disease, kidney or liver disease, or high blood pressure. Also inform your health-care practitioner if you have ever had an unusual reaction to a medication that reduces the pressure within the eye.

Apraclonidine may cause your eyes to be more sensitive to light. Wear sunglasses and avoid exposure to bright light while using this drug.

If you wear soft contacts, remove them before administering this drug. Apraclonidine contains a preservative that can discolor soft contacts.

DRUG INTERACTIONS

Tell your health-care practitioner and pharmacist about any prescription or over-the-counter drugs you are taking, as well as any vitamins, herbs, or other supplements. Possible drug interactions with apraclonidine may include the following:

- Drugs used to treat high blood pressure or cardiovascular problems, which can include diuretics, beta-blockers, and antihypertensives, may reduce your heart rate or blood pressure.
- Monoamine oxidase inhibitors (MAOIs) (e.g., phenelzine, isocarboxazid) can reduce the breakdown of apraclonidine and increase the risk of side effects.

FOOD, VITAMIN, AND HERBAL INTERACTIONS

No interactions with food, vitamins, or herbs have been reported.

RECOMMENDED DOSAGE

Apraclonidine is a liquid that is dispensed in an eyedropper and is available in two strengths: 0.5% and 1.0%. The 0.5% potency is typically used for people who have glaucoma; the 1.0% potency is usually given to people before and after eye surgery. The dosage information provided here is typical. However, your health-care practitioner will determine the most appropriate dose and schedule for you.

For Glaucoma

- *Children:* Your health-care practitioner will determine if it is appropriate.
- *Adults:* 1 drop in each eye 2 or 3 times daily.

Before and After Eye Surgery

- *Children:* Your health-care practitioner will determine if it is appropriate.
- *Adults:* 1 drop in the affected eye one hour before surgery, then 1 drop immediately after surgery.

Always wash your hands before administering this drug. Tilt back the head, press your finger gently on the skin just beneath the lower eyelid, and pull the lower eyelid away from the eye gently. Drop the medicine into the eye and close your eye. Do not touch the dropper to the eye. Do not blink. Apply light pressure to the inner corner of the eye with your finger for 1 to 2 minutes.

If you use this drug regularly and you miss a dose, take it as soon as you remember. However, if it is nearly time for your next application, do not take the missed dose, and remain on your regular schedule. Do not take double doses.

SYMPTOMS OF OVERDOSE AND WHAT TO DO

Symptoms of overdose may include exaggerated side effects, especially those that affect the nervous system. If overdose occurs, flush the eye with cool water and seek immediate medical attention. Bring the prescription container with you.

SPECIAL INFORMATION FOR PREGNANT OR NURSING WOMEN

Apraclonidine has not been studied in pregnant or breastfeeding women. If you are pregnant or plan to become pregnant, or if you are breastfeeding or plan to do so, talk with your health-care practitioner before starting this drug. Only a health-care practitioner can determine whether the potential benefits will outweigh the potential dangers.

SPECIAL INFORMATION FOR SENIORS

Older individuals do not need to follow any special precautions.

GENERIC NAME

Aprepitant

BRAND NAME

Emend

No generic available

ABOUT THIS DRUG

Aprepitant is an antiemetic (antinausea) drug used to prevent nausea and vomiting associated with cancer chemotherapy. Aprepitant is always used along with other antiemetics.

Aprepitant works by blocking P/neurokinin 1 (NK1), a key receptor in the brain stem that is involved with nausea and vomiting. This drug is unlike $5HT_3$ type antiemetics (see page 128) in how it prevents these symptoms.

SIDE EFFECTS

Let your health-care practitioner know about any side effects you experience while taking aprepitant. Only a health-care practitioner can determine whether it is safe for you to continue treatment.

- *Most Common:* dehydration, diarrhea, dizziness, hiccups, weakness

IMPORTANT PRECAUTIONS

Do not take aprepitant if you are sensitive or allergic to it or if you are taking astemizole, cisapride, pimozide, or terfenadine.

Talk to your health-care practitioner before taking aprepitant if you have liver problems.

Use of aprepitant may reduce the effectiveness of birth control pills. If you are using birth control pills, you should talk to your health-care practitioner about using a back-up birth control method during treatment.

Because aprepitant can cause dizziness, you should be certain of your response to it before you drive or operate hazardous machinery.

DRUG INTERACTIONS

Inform your health-care practitioner and pharmacist about any prescription and nonprescription medications you are taking, as well as any vitamins, herbs, or other supplements. Possible drug interactions with aprepitant include the following:

- Astemizole, cisapride, pimozide, and terfenadine may increase the risk of serious side effects and should not be used when taking aprepitant.
- Benzodiazepines (e.g., alprazolam, midazolam, triazolam) may increase the risk of side effects.
- Doses of dexamethasone and methylprednisolone may need to be reduced if taken along with aprepitant.
- Caution and monitoring is recommended if aprepitant is taken along with docetaxel, etoposide, ifosfamide, imatinib, irinotecan, paclitaxel, vinblastine, vincristine, or vinorelbine.
- The effectiveness of oral contraceptives may be reduced when taken along with aprepitant.
- Aprepitant may decrease the anticoagulant effectiveness of warfarin.

FOOD, VITAMIN, AND HERBAL INTERACTIONS

No food, vitamin, or herbal interactions have been noted.

RECOMMENDED DOSAGE

Aprepitant is available in 80- and 125-mg tablets. The dosages given here are typical. However, dosing of this drug is different for different people. Therefore, your health-care practitioner will determine the most appropriate dose and schedule for your needs.

- *Children:* to be determined by your health-care practitioner
- *Adults:* 125 mg one hour before chemotherapy on day 1 and 80 mg once per day on days 2 and 3

Aprepitant should be taken with 8 ounces of water and either with or without food. The first dose should be taken 1 hour before chemotherapy, with subsequent doses taken once per day. If you miss a dose, take it as soon as you remember. If it is nearly time for your next dose, do not take the missed dose. Continue with your regular dosing schedule. Do not take a double dose.

SYMPTOMS OF OVERDOSE AND WHAT TO DO

Symptoms of overdose are not known; however, they might include headache and drowsiness. If overdose occurs, seek immediate medical attention and bring the prescription container with you to the hospital.

SPECIAL INFORMATION FOR PREGNANT AND NURSING WOMEN

No adequate studies of the effects of aprepitant on pregnant or nursing women have been done. If you are pregnant or plan to become pregnant, you and your health-care practitioner must weigh the potential benefits against the potential risks to the fetus.

Aprepitant may pass into breast milk. If you are breastfeeding, your health-care practitioner may advise you to stop until your treatment is done.

SPECIAL INFORMATION FOR SENIORS

Older adults are more likely to experience side effects, and those reactions may be more severe.

GENERIC NAME

Aripiprazole

BRAND NAME

Abilify
No generic available

ABOUT THIS DRUG

Aripiprazole is an antipsychotic drug used as short-term treatment of schizophrenia. Although aripiprazole cannot cure schizophrenia, it can help people live a more normal life.

This drug works by changing the actions of dopamine and, to a lesser degree, serotonin in the brain.

SIDE EFFECTS

Be sure to tell your health-care practitioner if you experience any side effects while taking aripiprazole. Only your health-care practitioner can determine whether it is safe for you to continue taking this drug.

- *Most Common:* anxiety, constipation, headache, lightheadedness, nausea, problems sleeping, rash, restlessness, sleepiness, vomiting, weakness, mild weight gain
- *Less Common:* blurred vision, cough, fever, rhinitis, tremor, signs of increased blood sugar or diabetes mellitus (increased urination, thirst, weakness)
- *Rare:* neuroleptic malignant syndrome (symptoms include high fever, muscle rigidity, confusion, change in pulse, blood pressure, or heartbeat, and sweating), tardive dyskinesia (symptoms include involuntary and abnormal muscle movements; the risk increases with increasing duration of use)

IMPORTANT PRECAUTIONS

Tell your health-care practitioner if you are sensitive or allergic to aripiprazole or to any other drugs. Before taking aripiprazole, you should inform your health-care practitioner if you have heart problems, have had a heart attack or stroke, or have or have had seizures. Aripiprazole can make you more likely to experience a seizure, especially if you have a history of seizures or a medical condition that increases the risk of having a seizure.

Use of aripiprazole can impair judgment, thinking, and motor skills. Therefore, until you know how aripiprazole affects you, do not drive a car, operate machinery, or perform other tasks that require concentration.

This drug may cause swallowing difficulties and can cause choking. These problems have led to aspiration pneumonia in some patients.

Contact your health-care practitioner immediately if you experience uncontrollable movements of the jaw, tongue, arms, mouth, or legs while taking this drug; also if you have fever, sweating, irregular pulse or heartbeat, or muscle rigidity.

Avoid getting overheated or dehydrated when taking aripiprazole, as this drug can lower body temperature.

Hyperglycemia, in some cases extreme and associated with ketoacidosis or death, has been reported in patients who have been treated with atypical antipsychotic medications such as aripiprazole. If you have diabetes and start this medication, you should be monitored regularly for worsening glucose control.

DRUG INTERACTIONS

Tell your health-care practitioner and pharmacist if you are taking any prescription or nonprescription drugs, as well as any vitamins, herbs, or other supplements. Possible drug interactions include the following:

- Carbamazepine can reduce blood levels of aripiprazole.
- Ketoconazole, quinidine, fluoxetine, and paroxetin can increase blood levels of aripiprazole.
- Aripiprazole may increase the effect of antihypertensive medications, such as acebutolol, bexaxolol, clonidine, guanabenz, and others.

FOOD, VITAMIN, AND HERBAL INTERACTIONS

Grapefruit and grapefruit juice may increase aripiprazole levels, so you should avoid these foods while taking aripiprazole.

Do not combine aripiprazole with herbs that produce sedative effects, such as catnip, elecampane, goldenseal, gotu kola, hops, kava, lemon balm, skullcap, St. John's wort, and valerian.

Avoid alcohol use while taking aripiprazole.

RECOMMENDED DOSAGE

Aripiprazole is available in 2-, 5-, 10-, 15-, 20-, and 30-mg tablets. The dosages given here are typical. However, your health-care practitioner will determine the most appropriate dose and schedule for your needs.

- *Children:* Not recommended for children younger than 18

- *Adults:* Typical dose is 10 to 15 mg taken once daily. Your health-care practitioner will determine whether a higher dose is necessary. Dose increases should not be made before 2 weeks of treatment have been completed.

Aripiprazole can be taken with or without food. If you forget a dose, take it as soon as you remember. If it is almost time for the next dose, skip the missed dose and resume your normal schedule. Never take a double dose. It takes at least one week, and often two, for the beneficial effects of this drug to be evident.

SYMPTOMS OF OVERDOSE AND WHAT TO DO

Symptoms of overdose include drowsiness and vomiting. If overdose occurs, seek immediate medical attention and bring the prescription container with you to the hospital.

SPECIAL INFORMATION FOR PREGNANT OR NURSING WOMEN

No studies have adequately investigated the effects of aripiprazole during pregnancy or breastfeeding. If you are pregnant or plan to become pregnant, talk with your health-care practitioner before starting this drug. Only a health-care practitioner can determine whether the potential benefits outweigh the potential dangers.

Do not breastfeed while taking aripiprazole. Your health-care practitioner will likely advise you to switch to bottle feeding until your treatment is complete.

SPECIAL INFORMATION FOR SENIORS

Aripiprazole should be used cautiously in patients who are at risk for aspiration pneumonia, such as those with Alzheimer's disease.

GENERIC NAME

Aspirin, Buffered Aspirin

BRAND NAMES

Aspergum, Bayer, Bufferin, Easprin, Ecotrin, Empirin, Genprin, Genuine Bayer, Halfprin, Magnaprin, ZORprin
Generic available

ABOUT THIS DRUG

Aspirin is a nonsteroidal anti-inflammatory drug (NSAID) used to relieve mild-to-moderate pain and inflammation, to reduce fever, and to prevent the formation of blood clots.

Aspirin inhibits the release of substances called prostaglandins, which play a role in inflammation and pain. It also affects the temperature-regulation center in the brain to reduce fever, and prevents the production of thromboxane in blood platelets, which inhibits the formation of blood clots.

SIDE EFFECTS

Tell your health-care practitioner about any side effects you may experience when using aspirin. Your health-care practitioner will let you know if it is safe for you to continue taking this drug.

- *Most Common:* rash, nasal discharge, stomach irritation, heartburn, nausea, vomiting, ringing in the ears, drowsiness
- *Less Common or Rare:* insomnia, bruising, fever, weakness, sore throat, abnormal bleeding. Symptoms of Reye's syndrome, a rare but serious disorder that affects children 16 years and younger, include vomiting, agitation, extreme fatigue, confusion, difficulty breathing, swelling of the face, itching, and redness of the face. Seek immediate medical attention.

IMPORTANT PRECAUTIONS

Do not take aspirin if you are sensitive or allergic to it. Also avoid aspirin if you have a bleeding disorder (e.g., hemophilia), active peptic ulcer disease, or a history of urticaria.

Before taking aspirin, consult your health-care practitioner if you are taking an anticoagulant or an oral antidiabetic drug, if you have a history of peptic ulcer disease, kidney or liver disease, or gout, if you have asthma, carditis, nasal polyps, or lupus erythematosus, or if you plan to have any type of surgery.

Children age 16 years and younger should not take aspirin if they have flu, chicken pox, or similar infections, as an often fatal condition called Reye's syndrome may develop. Consult your health-care practitioner before giving aspirin to children.

DRUG INTERACTIONS

Tell your health-care practitioner and pharmacist if you are taking any prescription or over-the-counter medications, as well as any vitamins, herbs, or other supplements. Possible drug interactions with aspirin may include the following:

- Acetazolamide, cimetidine, and para-aminobenzoic acid may increase the effects of aspirin.
- Adrenocortical steroids (e.g., amcinonide, budesonide) may result in additive stomach irritation and bleeding.

- Alcohol may increase the risk of stomach damage and increase bleeding time.
- Alendronate may result in increased risk of stomach irritation and diarrhea and decreased absorption of alendronate.
- Antacids (continued use) and cholestyramine may decrease the effects of aspirin.
- Aspirin may increase the risk of bleeding when used with heparin and oral anticoagulants (e.g., warfarin).
- Aspirin may increase the effects of methotrexate, tiludronate, and valproic acid.
- Insulin may require dosage adjustments.
- Lithium levels may increase.
- Zafirlukast levels may increase and increase adverse effects.
- The effects of ACE inhibitors (e.g., captopril, enalapril), beta-blockers (e.g., atenolol, labetalol), furosemide, other NSAIDs (e.g., ketorolac, naproxen), phenytoin, probenecid, spironolactone, sulfinpyrazone, and tiludronate may be decreased by aspirin.

FOOD, VITAMIN, AND HERBAL INTERACTIONS

Taking aspirin with food helps prevent stomach irritation, but it also reduces the amount of aspirin absorbed.

The herbs dong quai, feverfew, garlic, ginkgo, ginger, horse chestnut, and red clover may cause an increased risk of bleeding or stomach irritation if taken with aspirin.

The supplement arginine (an amino acid) may increase stomach irritation, while vitamin E, even in small amounts (50 mg daily), may lead to a significantly increased risk of bleeding. Fish oil supplements and OPCs (oligomeric proanthocyanidins) may also increase the risk of bleeding.

Cayenne (*Capsicum annuum* and *C. frutescens*), which is derived from hot peppers, and licorice root (*Glycyrrhiza glabra*) can protect the stomach against the irritation caused by aspirin. Talk to your health-care practitioner before taking these supplements.

RECOMMENDED DOSAGE

Aspirin is available in capsules (enteric-coated), tablets (regular, gum, enteric-coated, chewable), and suppositories, and in different strengths. The dosage information given here is typical. However, your health-care practitioner will determine the dosage and schedule that is best for you.

- *Children Ages 2 to 4 Years:* 160 mg every four hours, up to 5 doses daily
- *Children Ages 4 to 6 Years:* 240 mg every four hours, up to 5 doses daily
- *Children Ages 6 to 9 Years:* 320 mg every four hours, up to 5 doses daily
- *Children Ages 9 to 11 Years:* 400 mg every four hours, up to 5 doses daily
- *Children Ages 11 to 12 Years:* 480 mg every four hours, up to 5 doses daily
- *Adults:* For pain and fever, 325 to 650 mg every four hours, as needed. For prevention of blood clots, 80 to 100 mg daily or every other day (but see "Open Questions or Controversies"), and for arthritis, 3,600 to 5,400 mg daily (only under a health-care practitioner's supervision).

For children, do not exceed 5 days of continual use without first consulting with your health-care practitioner. Both children and adults should take all doses with food or a full glass of water to help prevent stomach irritation.

If you miss a dose, take it as soon as you remember. However, if it is nearly time for your next dose, do not take the missed dose. Continue with your regular dosing schedule. Do not take a double dose.

SYMPTOMS OF OVERDOSE AND WHAT TO DO

Symptoms of an overdose include nausea, vomiting, disorientation, fever, seizures, rapid breathing, dizziness, ringing in the ears, delirium, convulsions, and impaired hearing. If overdose occurs, seek immediate medical attention and bring the drug container with you.

SPECIAL INFORMATION FOR PREGNANT OR NURSING WOMEN

Studies show that regular use of aspirin during pregnancy can be detrimental to the mother and her fetus and has been associated with an increase in stillbirths and newborn deaths. Aspirin should be avoided completely during the last three months of pregnancy. If you are pregnant or plan to become pregnant, talk to your health-care practitioner about using aspirin. Only a health-care practitioner can determine whether the potential benefits will outweigh the potential dangers.

Aspirin does pass into breast milk. If you are breastfeeding or plan to do so, your health-care practitioner will likely advise you to stop if you take aspirin.

SPECIAL INFORMATION FOR SENIORS

Older individuals are more likely to experience stomach irritation, ringing in the ears, confusion, and nausea when taking aspirin. Sudden hemorrhaging can occur; people 60 years and older should look out for black- or gray-colored stools, which indicates stomach bleeding. Seniors who have liver disease should not take aspirin.

OPEN QUESTIONS OR CONTROVERSIES

Studies indicate that a dose of aspirin daily can decrease the risk of heart attack by 28% in people who are at risk of heart disease. Those at risk include people who have high cholesterol, men older than 40, postmenopausal women, people who smoke, and individuals who have high blood pressure. A study in the *British Medical Journal* (12 January 2002) by the Antithrombotic Trialists' Collaboration reported that 75 to 150 mg daily is effective for long-term use, but that an initial dose of at least 150 mg may be needed for acute cases.

But Dr. Alfred Berg from the University of Washington says that the risks of aspirin can overshadow the benefits for people whose risk of heart disease is low. In the *Annals of Internal Medicine* (15 January 2002), researchers reported that for 1,000 patients with a 5% risk for coronary heart disease over 5 years, aspirin would prevent 6 to 20 heart attacks but would cause up to 2 strokes and up to 4 major gastrointestinal bleeding episodes. For people with a 1% risk over 5 years, aspirin would prevent up to 4 heart attacks but would cause up to 2 strokes and up to 4 major gastrointestinal bleeding episodes.

So while the net benefit of taking aspirin daily increases as the risk of cardiovascular risk increases, you and your health-care practitioner should discuss the feasibility of your taking aspirin in light of your relative risk and possible adverse effects. Daily aspirin therapy is clearly not for everyone.

GENERIC NAME

Aspirin combinations *see Codeine, Morphine, Oxycodone, page 313*

GENERIC NAME
Atazanavir

BRAND NAME
Reyataz
No generic available

ABOUT THIS DRUG
Atazanavir is an antiviral drug used to treat human immunodeficiency virus (HIV) infection. It is taken with other drugs as part of a "drug cocktail."

This drug blocks the activity of a protease, an enzyme that forms new proteins and enzymes that contribute to the growth and spread of HIV.

SIDE EFFECTS
Be sure to tell your health-care practitioner if you experience any side effects while taking atazanavir. Only your health-care practitioner can determine whether it is safe for you to continue taking this drug.

- *Most Common:* abdominal pain, diarrhea, headache, nausea, rash, vomiting
- *Less Common:* dizziness, extreme weakness or tiredness, fever, increase in blood glucose levels, increase or redistribution of body fat, jaundice, numbness or tingling in arms or legs, rash
- *Rare:* decreased heart rate, lactic acidosis (accumulation of acid in the blood; symptoms include difficulty breathing, persistent nausea, vomiting, and weakness)

IMPORTANT PRECAUTIONS
Tell your health-care practitioner if you are sensitive or allergic to atazanavir or to any other drugs.

Before you take atazanavir, tell your health-care practitioner if you have diabetes mellitus, hyperglycemia, heart conduction problems, hemophilia, hepatitis, elevated transaminase, or liver disease.

Before undergoing surgery, including dental surgery, tell your health-care practitioner or dentist that you are taking atazanavir.

Because atazanavir can cause dizziness, make sure you know how you react to the drug before you drive or operate hazardous equipment.

Atazanavir does not prevent the risk of transmitting HIV to others. Appropriate preventive measures need to be taken.

DRUG INTERACTIONS

Tell your health-care practitioner and pharmacist if you are taking any prescription or nonprescription drugs, as well as any vitamins, herbs, or other supplements. Possible drug interactions include the following:

- The following drugs should not be taken with atazanavir: bepridil, cisapride, dihydroergotamine, ergonovine, ergotamine, indinavir, irinotecan, lovastatin, methylergonovine, midazolam, pimozide, esomeprazole, lansoprazole, omeprazole, pantoprazole, rabeprazole, rifampin, simvastatin, triazolam.
- If you take antacids or didanosine, you should take atazanavir two hours before or one hour after these medications.
- If you take any of the following drugs with atazanavir, your health-care practitioner may need to change the doses of your medications or monitor you for side effects: amiodarone, antidepressants (e.g., amitriptyline, amoxapine, clomipramine, desipramine, doxepin, imipramine, nortriptyline, protriptyline, trimipramine), beta-blockers (e.g., atenolol, labetalol, metaprolol, nadolol, propranolol), calcium channel blockers (e.g., diltiazem, felodipine, nicardipine, nifedipine, verapamil), statin drugs (e.g., atorvastatin), cimetidine, clarithromycin, cyclosporine, digoxin, efavirenz, famotidine, sirolimus, tacrolimus, nizantadine, oral contraceptives, quinidine, ranitidine, rifabutin, ritonavir, saquinavir, sirolimus, tacrolimus, tenofovir, and warfarin.
- Atazanavir may increase blood concentrations of phosphodiesterase inhibitors (PDE5) used for erectile dysfunction (e.g., vardenafil, tadalafil), leading to an increased risk for side effects.

FOOD, VITAMIN, AND HERBAL INTERACTIONS

Talk to your health-care practitioner before consuming grapefruit or grapefruit juice when taking this drug. Do not use St. John's wort or products containing St. John's wort because they can decrease blood concentrations and effectiveness of atazanavir.

RECOMMENDED DOSAGE

Atazanavir is available in 100-, 150-, and 200-mg capsules. The dosages given here are typical. However, your health-care practitioner will determine the most appropriate dose and schedule for your needs.

- *Children:* use and dose to be determined by your health-care practitioner
- *Adults:* starting dose is 400 mg once daily. If atazanavir is administered with ritonavir, your health-care practitioner may reduce your dose of atazanavir to 300 mg daily. If you are taking both atazanavir

and efavirenz, your health-care practitioner may add 100 mg of ritonavir to keep your atazanavir levels acceptable.

Atazanavir should be taken with food. If you miss a dose, take it as soon as you remember. If it is within 6 hours of your next dose, do not take the missed dose. Continue with your regular dosing schedule. Never take a double dose.

SYMPTOMS OF OVERDOSE AND WHAT TO DO
Symptoms of overdose include abdominal or stomach pain, chills, dark urine, dizziness or lightheadedness, fever, headache, itching, loss of appetite, nausea, rash, unpleasant breath odor, unusual tiredness or weakness, vomiting of blood, and yellow eyes or skin. If overdose occurs, seek immediate medical attention and bring the prescription container with you to the hospital.

SPECIAL INFORMATION FOR PREGNANT OR NURSING WOMEN
Adequate studies of the effects of atazanavir on pregnant or nursing women have not been done. If you are pregnant or plan to become pregnant, talk to your health-care practitioner.

It is not known whether atazanavir passes into breast milk. However, women who have HIV should not breastfeed because they may pass the infection on to their infant.

SPECIAL INFORMATION FOR SENIORS
No special information for seniors has been noted.

GENERIC NAME
Atenolol

BRAND NAME
Tenormin
Generic available

ABOUT THIS DRUG
Atenolol is a beta-blocker used to treat mild-to-moderate high blood pressure as well as angina and cardiac arrhythmias (irregular heartbeat). Treatment with this drug can be lifelong. Atenolol does not cure high blood pressure, but merely keeps it under control.

Atenolol blocks certain nerve impulses, which slows the rate and contraction force of the heart and lowers blood pressure.

SIDE EFFECTS

If you experience any side effects when taking atenolol, contact your health-care practitioner. Only a health-care practitioner can determine whether it is safe for you to continue taking this drug.

- *Most Common:* decreased ability to engage in physical activities, dizziness, drowsiness, fatigue, weakness, insomnia, decreased libido
- *Less Common or Rare:* anxiety, chest pain, constipation, depression, diarrhea, dry eyes, itching, irritability, nausea or vomiting, nightmares, numbness, tingling, or other unusual sensations in the toes and fingers, shortness of breath, slow heartbeat, wheezing, nasal congestion

IMPORTANT PRECAUTIONS

Do not take atenolol if you are sensitive or allergic to it.

If you have any of the following medical conditions, talk to your health-care practitioner before taking atenolol: a history of severe congestive heart failure or overactive thyroid function (hyperthyroidism), asthma, seasonal allergies, other bronchial conditions, coronary artery disease, myasthenia gravis, or kidney or liver disease.

If you have diabetes, this medication may mask symptoms of low blood sugar or change your blood sugar levels.

If you have a medical emergency or are planning surgery or dental surgery, inform your health-care practitioner or dentist that you are taking atenolol.

Inform your health-care practitioner if you are taking clonidine, digitalis, quinidine, reserpine, or any calcium blocker (e.g., diltiazem, nifedipine).

Atenolol can cause drowsiness and dizziness; therefore be sure you are fully aware of how you react to the drug before you drive or operate hazardous machinery.

If you have high blood pressure, it is important for you to take atenolol regularly for it to be effective, even if you feel better.

DRUG INTERACTIONS

Tell your health-care practitioner and pharmacist about any prescription and nonprescription drugs you are taking, as well as any vitamins, herbs, or other supplements. Possible drug interactions with atenolol may include the following:

- Amiodarone may cause cardiac arrest.
- Ampicillin or bacampicillin may cause lower blood levels of atenolol.

- Aspirin-containing drugs, fluvoxamine, indomethacin, sulfinpyrazone, and estrogen drugs may interfere with the ability of atenolol to lower blood pressure.
- Cimetidine increases the amount of atenolol absorbed by the body.
- Digoxin may cause very slow heart rates.
- Insulin and oral antidiabetic drugs (e.g., acarbose, glipizide) may cause undetectable or prolonged low blood sugar.
- Phenothiazines (e.g., chlorpromazine, promazine) may increase the effects of both atenolol and the phenothiazines.
- Quinidine may cause additive lowering of blood pressure.
- Verapamil can cause excessively low blood pressure and significant slowing of the heart rate.

FOOD, VITAMIN, AND HERBAL INTERACTIONS

Avoid excessive salt intake while using atenolol.

Calcium may cause a significant reduction in the amount of atenolol the body absorbs. This effect appears to disappear after a few days. Taking calcium supplements at a different time of the day than atenolol can reduce this situation.

Herbs that can increase blood pressure, including ginseng, goldenseal, licorice, ephedra (ma huang), and saw palmetto, should be avoided.

RECOMMENDED DOSAGE

Atenolol is available in 25-, 50-, and 100-mg tablets. The dosages given here are typical. However, your health-care practitioner will determine the best dosage and schedule for your particular needs.

- *Children:* The safety and effectiveness of atenolol has not been determined in children.
- *Adults:* For hypertension and angina, the usual starting dose is 50 mg daily, which your health-care practitioner may gradually increase up to 100 mg over 7 to 10 days. The maximum daily dose is 100 mg. In some cases, health-care practitioners prescribe a single 200-mg dose for people who have angina.
- *Adults 60 Years and Older:* Your health-care practitioner will determine your dosage.

Atenolol can be taken with or without food. However, taking it with food can reduce the amount absorbed by the body by up to 20%.

Do not suddenly stop taking atenolol. It can cause heart attack and increased chest pain.

If you miss a dose, take it as soon as you remember. However, if it's within 8 hours of your next scheduled dose, do not take the missed dose. Stay on your regular dosing schedule, and never take a double dose.

SYMPTOMS OF OVERDOSE AND WHAT TO DO

Symptoms of overdose include congestive heart failure, constricted airways, convulsions, low blood sugar, low blood pressure, slow heartbeat, sluggishness, weakness, and wheezing. If an overdose occurs, seek immediate medical attention, and bring the prescription container with you.

SPECIAL INFORMATION FOR PREGNANT OR NURSING WOMEN

If you are pregnant or plan to become pregnant, talk to your health-care practitioner before using this drug. Atenolol, and other beta-blockers, can cause infants to be born with lower birth weights, reduced heart rates, and low blood pressure. Use of this drug should be avoided during pregnancy.

Atenolol passes into breast milk. If atenolol is essential to your health, your health-care practitioner may advise you to stop breast-feeding while you are under treatment.

SPECIAL INFORMATION FOR SENIORS

Your health-care practitioner will determine the best dosage for your needs. Older individuals who take atenolol are more likely to experience chest pain, sudden breathing difficulties, cold hands and feet, reduced body temperature, and increased sweating.

GENERIC NAME

Atomoxetine

BRAND NAME

Strattera

No generic available

ABOUT THIS DRUG

Atomoxetine is a selective norepinephrine reuptake inhibitor that is used to treat attention deficit hyperactivity disorder (ADHD) in children and adults. It is used as part of a total treatment program that may include psychological, educational, and social strategies.

Atomoxetine is believed to work by boosting levels of norepinephrine, a brain chemical that regulates activity.

SIDE EFFECTS

Be sure to tell your health-care practitioner if you experience any side effects while taking atomoxetine. Only your health-care practitioner can determine whether it is safe for you to continue taking this drug.

- *More Common in Children:* appetite loss, constipation, cough, crying, diarrhea, dizziness, drowsiness, dry mouth, ear infection, fatigue, headache, indigestion, influenza, irritability, mood swings, nausea, runny nose, skin inflammation, stomach pain, vomiting, weight loss
- *More Common in Adults:* abnormal dreams, abnormal orgasms, appetite loss, chills, constipation, diminished sex drive, dizziness, dry mouth, fatigue or sluggishness, fever, flatulence, headache, hot flushes, impotence, indigestion, insomnia, menstrual problems, muscle pain, nausea, palpitations, prostate inflammation, sinusitis, skin inflammation, sweating, tingling, urinary problems, weight loss
- *Less Common:* allergic reactions (edema, hives, rash)

IMPORTANT PRECAUTIONS

Tell your health-care practitioner if you are sensitive or allergic to atomoxetine or to any other drugs.

Because this drug can cause dizziness, make sure you know how you react to it before you drive or operate hazardous equipment.

No studies of the effectiveness or safety of this drug or its effects on height and weight have been done beyond 10 weeks. Thus if you require longer-term treatment, your health-care practitioner should monitor you or your child closely.

Before taking atomoxetine, talk to your health-care practitioner if you have a liver disorder. Also use this drug with caution if you have high blood pressure, tachycardia (abnormally rapid heartbeat), urinary retention or hesitancy, cardiovascular disease, or cerebrovascular disease. If you have narrow-angle glaucoma, you should not take atomoxetine.

During trials, atomoxetine slowed children's average rate of growth. It is not known whether final adult height and weight are affected. Your health-care practitioner may interrupt use of atomoxetine for your child if he or she is not growing or gaining weight at the expected rate.

DRUG INTERACTIONS

Tell your health-care practitioner and pharmacist if you are taking any prescription or nonprescription drugs, as well as any vitamins, herbs, or other supplements. Possible drug interactions include the following:

- Atomoxetine should not be used while you are taking a monoamine oxidase inhibitor (MAOI) antidepressant, nor should you take it within two weeks of discontinuing use of an MAOI.
- Your health-care practitioner may prescribe a lower dose of atomoxetine if you are also taking fluoxetine, paroxetine, or quinidine.
- Use of albuterol and similar asthma medications, as well as any drug that causes an increase in blood pressure, such as phenylephrine, which is found in some over-the-counter cold formulas, may increase the effects of atomoxetine.

FOOD, VITAMIN, AND HERBAL INTERACTIONS

No food, vitamin, or herbal interactions have been noted.

RECOMMENDED DOSAGE

Atomoxetine is available in 10-, 18-, 25-, 40-, and 60-mg capsules. The dosages given here are typical. However, your health-care practitioner will determine the most appropriate dose and schedule for your needs.

- *Children Younger Than 6 Years:* Atomoxetine has not been tested in this age group.
- *Children and Adolescents Weighing Up to 154 Pounds:* Usual starting dosage is 0.5 mg/2.2 lb of body weight per day. After at least 3 days, your health-care practitioner may increase the daily total to a recommended level of 1.2 mg/2.2 lb. Daily doses should not exceed 1.4 mg/2.2 lb or a total of 100 mg, whichever is less.
- *Children, Adolescents, and Adults Weighing More Than 154 Pounds:* Usual starting dosage is 40 mg/day. After at least 3 days, your health-care practitioner may increase the daily total to a recommended level of 80 mg. After 2 to 4 weeks, dosage may be increased to a maximum of 100 mg/day.

Atomoxetine may be taken with or without food. If you miss a dose, take it as soon as you remember. If it is nearly time for your next dose, skip the missed dose and return to your regular dosing schedule. Never take a double dose.

SYMPTOMS OF OVERDOSE AND WHAT TO DO

Symptoms of overdose are not known. If you believe an overdose has occurred, seek immediate medical attention and bring the prescription container with you to the hospital.

SPECIAL INFORMATION FOR PREGNANT OR NURSING WOMEN

Adequate studies of the effects of atomoxetine on pregnant or nursing women have not been done. If you are pregnant or plan to become pregnant, talk to your health-care practitioner. Only a health-care practitioner can determine whether the potential benefits outweigh the risks.

It is not known whether atomoxetine passes into breast milk. If you are breastfeeding, your health-care practitioner will likely advise you to switch to bottle feeding until your treatment is complete.

SPECIAL INFORMATION FOR SENIORS

Side effects are more likely to occur and to be more severe in older adults.

GENERIC NAME

Atorvastatin

see Statin Cholesterol-Lowering Drugs, page 959

GENERIC NAME

Atovaquone

BRAND NAME

Mepron
No generic available

ABOUT THIS DRUG

Atovaquone is an anti-infective agent used to treat mild-to-moderately-severe pneumocystis carinii pneumonia (PCP). This condition is common among people who have AIDS (acquired immunodeficiency syndrome). Atovaquone is for individuals who cannot take the standard therapy for PCP, which is the antibiotic combination trimethoprim and sulfamethoxazole.

Atovaquone prevents the infectious organisms from manufacturing DNA and other substances they need to reproduce and grow.

SIDE EFFECTS

Always talk to your health-care practitioner about any side effects that develop while you are taking atovaquone. Only a health-care practitioner can decide if it is safe for you to continue taking the drug.

- *More Common:* abdominal pain, anxiety, constipation, cough, diarrhea, dizziness, fatigue, fever, headache, insomnia, loss of appetite, nausea, rash, sleeplessness, vomiting, weakness
- *Less Common:* changes in sense of taste, low blood sugar, low blood pressure

IMPORTANT PRECAUTIONS

Do not take atovaquone if you are sensitive or allergic to it or any of its components.

If you have any type of gastrointestinal condition, such as colitis, talk to your health-care practitioner before using this drug, as absorption may be compromised.

To be absorbed properly, atovaquone requires that it be taken with high-fat foods. If you are unable to eat enough or the right foods twice a day to take this medication, you may need to take it intravenously.

DRUG INTERACTIONS

Tell your health-care practitioner and pharmacist about any prescription and nonprescription drugs you are taking, as well as any vitamins, herbs, or other supplements. Possible drug interactions with atovaquone include the following:

- Atovaquone may increase the blood levels of digoxin, warfarin, oral antidiabetic drugs (e.g., acarbose, glipizide), and other drugs that bind to blood proteins. Talk to your health-care practitioner.
- Rifabutin and rifampin may reduce the blood levels of atovaquone and could lessen its effectiveness.
- Zidovudine along with atovaquone can result in a dramatic reduction in the rate at which zidovudine is eliminated from the body. This may cause problems in some individuals.

FOOD, VITAMIN, AND HERBAL INTERACTIONS

Atovaquone should be taken with a high-fat meal, which can increase the amount of drug absorbed by 300%. No vitamin or herbal interactions have been documented.

RECOMMENDED DOSAGE

Atovaquone is available in an oral suspension. The dosages given here are typical. However, your health-care practitioner will determine the best dosage and schedule for your needs.

- *Children Younger than 12 Years:* Your health-care practitioner will determine if this drug is appropriate.

- *Children 12 Years and Older and Adults:* 750 mg of oral suspension twice daily for 21 days.

Atovaquone should be taken with a high-fat meal to help the body better absorb it.

Do not stop taking this drug, even if you feel better, without first consulting your health-care practitioner. Stopping too soon may cause the infection to return or slow your recovery. The usual length of treatment is 21 days.

If you miss a dose, take it as soon as you remember. However, if it is nearly time for your next dose, do not take the missed dose. Resume your regular dosage schedule and do not take a double dose.

SYMPTOMS OF OVERDOSE AND WHAT TO DO

No cases of atovaquone overdose have been documented. If overdose occurs, seek immediate medical attention, and bring the prescription container with you.

SPECIAL INFORMATION FOR PREGNANT OR NURSING WOMEN

Atovaquone has caused fetal abnormalities in animal studies. If you are pregnant or plan to become pregnant, talk to your health-care practitioner. Only you and your health-care practitioner can weigh the potential benefits against the potential risks.

If you are breastfeeding, your health-care practitioner will likely advise you to stop while you are being treated. Atovaquone has an affinity for fat, and so is likely to pass into breast milk.

SPECIAL INFORMATION FOR SENIORS

Older individuals may be more sensitive to the side effects of atovaquone.

GENERIC NAME

Augmented betamethasone dipropionate

see Corticosteroids, Topical, page 337

GENERIC NAME

Azatadine

see Antihistamine-Decongestant Combinations, page 132

GENERIC NAME
Azelaic acid

BRAND NAME
Finacea
No generic available

ABOUT THIS DRUG
Azelaic acid is a topical medication for treatment of the inflammatory bumps and lesions associated with mild to moderate rosacea.

Although it is not clearly understood how this medication works, it reduces the number of inflamed lesions.

SIDE EFFECTS
Be sure to tell your health-care practitioner if you experience any side effects while using azelaic acid. Only your health-care practitioner can determine whether it is safe for you to continue using this drug.

- *Most Common:* burning, itchiness, scaling or dry skin, stinging, tingling
- *Less Common:* acne, inflammation, irritation, rash, swelling, sensitivity to light
- *Rare:* bleaching of skin, excessive hair growth, worsening asthma, worsening cold sores

IMPORTANT PRECAUTIONS
Tell your health-care practitioner if you are sensitive or allergic to azelaic acid, propylene glycol (additive that is found in many facial products), or to any other drugs.

Keep using azelaic acid as prescribed by your health-care practitioner even if you don't see immediate improvement. It can take up to four weeks to see results.

Avoid contact of azelaic acid with your eyes, mouth, or nose. If azelaic acid does get into your eyes, wash them out with a large amount of water and see your health-care practitioner if irritation persists.

DRUG INTERACTIONS
No drug-drug interactions have been reported. However, still tell your health-care practitioner and pharmacist if you are taking any prescription or nonprescription drugs, as well as any vitamins, herbs, or other supplements.

FOOD, VITAMIN, AND HERBAL INTERACTIONS

No food, vitamin, or herbal interactions have been reported. You are advised to avoid spicy foods, hot food or beverages, and alcoholic beverages.

RECOMMENDED DOSAGE

Azelaic acid is available as a gel. The dosages given here are typical. However, your health-care practitioner will determine the most appropriate dose and schedule for you.

- *Children:* to be determined by your health-care practitioner
- *Adults:* apply the gel two times per day, once in the morning and once in the evening

Before applying azelaic acid, wash the area to be treated with a soapless cleaning lotion, pat skin dry, and apply the gel, rubbing it in until it is evenly spread and transparent. Avoid using alcohol cleansers or astringents, abrasives, and peeling agents with azelaic acid.

If you miss an application, apply it as soon as you remember. If it is nearly time for your next application, do not apply the missed dose. Continue with your regular application schedule.

SYMPTOMS OF OVERDOSE AND WHAT TO DO

Overdose is unlikely. However, if your skin becomes severely irritated after using azelaic acid, stop using it and contact your health-care practitioner as soon as possible.

SPECIAL INFORMATION FOR PREGNANT OR NURSING WOMEN

No adequate studies of the effects of azelaic acid have been done with pregnant or nursing women. If you are pregnant or plan to become pregnant, talk to your health-care practitioner.

It is not known whether azelaic acid passes into breast milk. If you are breastfeeding, your health-care practitioner will likely advise you to stop until your treatment is complete.

SPECIAL INFORMATION FOR SENIORS

No special instructions are needed for older adults.

GENERIC NAME
Azelastine

BRAND NAMES
Astelin (nasal), Optivar (ophthalmic)
No generic available

ABOUT THIS DRUG
Azelastine is a histamine blocker (antihistamine) that is used to relieve or treat symptoms of hay fever (seasonal allergic rhinitis) and vasomotor rhinitis (nasal form) or itchy eyes caused by allergic conjunctivitis (ophthalmic form).

Azelastine blocks the effects of histamine, a substance that occurs naturally in the body and causes itching, sneezing, swelling, watery eyes, hives, and other allergic reactions.

SIDE EFFECTS
Inform your health-care practitioner if you experience any side effects while using azelastine. He or she can let you know if it is safe for you to continue using this drug. The following side effects are attributed to both forms of the medication; those associated with the ophthalmic form only are noted as such.

- *Most Common:* bitter taste in the mouth, drowsiness, headache, weight gain; temporary eye burning or stinging—ophthalmic form only
- *Less Common:* abdominal pain, anxiety, back pain, blood in the urine, blurred vision (ophthalmic form only), breast pain, constipation, coughing, depression, dizziness, dry mouth, fatigue, flu-like symptoms, flushing, high blood pressure, increased appetite, laryngitis, loss of sensitivity to touch, mouth and tongue sores, muscle pain, nausea, nasal burning, nervousness, nosebleeds, pinkeye, rapid heartbeat, sleep disturbances, sore throat, sneezing, swelling of eye, eyelid, or inner lining of eyelid (ophthalmic form only), taste loss, vertigo, vomiting, watery eyes, wheezing

IMPORTANT PRECAUTIONS
Do not use azelastine if you are sensitive or allergic to this drug.

Azelastine can cause drowsiness and dizziness; therefore make sure you know how you will react to this drug before you drive or operate hazardous equipment.

Tell your health-care practitioner if you have kidney disease, as levels of azelastine may be elevated in the blood.

Close your eyes when administering this drug to avoid getting it into your eyes. Azelastine can cause blurred vision if sprayed into the eyes.

DRUG INTERACTIONS

Tell your health-care practitioner and pharmacist about any prescription and nonprescription drugs you are taking, as well as any vitamins, herbs, and other supplements. Possible drug interactions with azelastine may include the following:

- Alcohol, sedatives (e.g., temazepam, zolpidem), and tricyclic antidepressants (e.g., amitriptyline, imipramine) may increase the risk of drowsiness.
- Cimetidine may cause elevated blood levels of azelastine, which may result in increased side effects.

FOOD, VITAMIN, AND HERBAL INTERACTIONS

Use of any of the following herbs may increase the sedative effects of azelastine: calendula, capsicum, catnip, goldenseal, gotu kola, hops, kava, lady's slipper, lemon balm, passionflower, sage, sassafras, Siberian ginseng, skullcap, St. John's wort, stinging nettle, and valerian, among others.

RECOMMENDED DOSAGE

Azelastine is a nasal spray that comes in a pump container. The dosage given here is typical. However, your health-care practitioner will determine the best dosage and schedule for your needs.

For Hay Fever

- *Children Younger Than 5 Years:* The safety and effectiveness of azelastine in children has not been established
- *Children 5 to 11 Years:* 1 spray per nostril no more than twice daily
- *Children 12 Years and Older and Adults:* 2 sprays per nostril no more than twice daily

For Vasomotor Rhinitis

- *Children Younger than 12 Years:* To be determined by your health-care practitioner
- *Children 12 Years and Older and Adults:* 2 sprays per nostril no more than twice daily

For Allergic Conjunctivitis

- *Children Younger than 3 Years:* Use and dose will be determined by your health-care practitioner
- *Children 3 Years and Older and Adults:* 1 drop in the affected eye twice daily

The first time you use the nasal form, or if you have not used the pump for several days, prime it by depressing it several times until a fine mist appears. When using azelastine, blow your nose gently before spraying. When inhaling the spray, keep your head upright and sniff sharply while spraying.

If you are using the ophthalmic form and you wear contacts, remove your contacts before you use this medication. Wait at least 10 minutes after you use the medicine before you put your contacts back in.

For both forms, if you miss a dose, take it as soon as you remember. However, if it is nearly time for your next dose, do not take the missed dose. Remain on your regular schedule, and never take a double dose.

SYMPTOMS OF OVERDOSE AND WHAT TO DO

An overdose is very unlikely, and the only symptom would probably be extreme drowsiness. If an overdose occurs, seek medical assistance immediately.

SPECIAL INFORMATION FOR PREGNANT OR NURSING WOMEN

The effects of azelastine on pregnancy or breastfeeding have not been studied adequately. If you are pregnant or plan to become pregnant, tell your health-care practitioner immediately. He or she may advise you to stop treatment while you are pregnant.

It is not known whether azelastine passes into breast milk. Your health-care practitioner may advise you to stop breastfeeding while you use this drug.

SPECIAL INFORMATION FOR SENIORS

No special precautions have been noted. Older individuals may experience more drowsiness.

GENERIC NAME

Azithromycin

BRAND NAME

Zithromax

No generic available

ABOUT THIS DRUG

Azithromycin is an antibiotic that is used to treat upper and lower respiratory tract infections, skin infections, middle ear infections, tonsillitis, sexually transmitted diseases, and pharyngitis.

Azithromycin belongs to a subgroup of antibiotics (a macrolide antibiotic) that either kills bacteria or inhibits their growth.

SIDE EFFECTS

Tell your health-care practitioner about any side effects you may experience while taking azithromycin. Only a health-care practitioner can determine whether it is safe for you to continue taking the drug.

- *Most Common:* diarrhea, nausea, stomach cramps, stomach gas, vomiting
- *Less Common:* blood in the stools, chest pain, dizziness, fainting, hairy tongue, headache, heart palpitations, jaundice, kidney inflammation, rash, swelling, tiredness, vaginal irritation, yeast infections
- *Other Common Side Effects Sometimes Seen in Children:* agitation, constipation, fever, insomnia, loss of appetite, nervousness, overactivity, pinkeye, stomach inflammation

IMPORTANT PRECAUTIONS

Do not use this drug if you are sensitive or allergic to it or to any macrolide antibiotic. If you develop a serious allergic reaction (e.g., swelling of the face, lips, and neck, difficulty breathing), stop taking the drug and seek immediate medical help.

If you have liver disease or liver damage, kidney problems, or chronic bronchitis, consult your health-care practitioner before taking this drug.

Bowel inflammation (colitis) is associated with azithromycin as well as other antibiotics.

This drug should be taken exactly as prescribed. Do not stop taking it before your health-care practitioner tells you to, even if you feel better. The drug's effectiveness may be severely compromised if you stop taking it too soon.

Like some other antibiotics, in rare cases azithromycin may cause a potentially fatal form of diarrhea called pseudomembranous colitis. This condition may go away spontaneously if treatment is stopped; however, see your health-care practitioner immediately if diarrhea develops.

Azithromycin should not be taken by individuals who have pneumonia or any of the following: cystic fibrosis, nosocomially acquired illness, known or suspected bacteremia; or by people who have pneumonia and who are elderly, debilitated, or who have underlying medical conditions that may compromise their ability to heal (e.g., immunodeficiency).

DRUG INTERACTIONS

Tell your health-care practitioner and pharmacist about any prescription and nonprescription drugs you are taking, as well as any vitamins, herbs, or other supplements. Possible drug interactions with azithromycin may include the following:

- Antacids that contain aluminum or magnesium (e.g., Maalox, Mylanta) may hinder the absorption of azithromycin. Antacids and azithromycin should be taken at least one hour apart.
- Cyclosporin blood levels may increase and cause kidney damage.
- Pimozide taken along with azithromycin may cause death in rare cases.
- Statin cholesterol-lowering drugs (e.g., atorvastatin, lovastatin) may increase the risk of developing a potentially fatal condition that involves destruction of muscle and muscle pain.

FOOD, VITAMIN, AND HERBAL INTERACTIONS

Two well-recognized side effects of antibiotics are yeast infections and diarrhea, which result because the antibiotic kills not only bad but also beneficial bacteria. Supplements of probiotics, such as *Lactobacillus acidophilus* or *Bifidobacterium longum,* while taking antibiotics and for a week or two after stopping can help prevent these reactions.

RECOMMENDED DOSAGE

Azithromycin is available in tablets, capsules, and powder packets (to be mixed in water and drunk). The dosages given here are typical. However, your health-care practitioner will determine the dosage and schedule that is best for you.

- *Children 6 Months and Older:* For treatment of middle ear infections and pneumonia, 10 mg of oral suspension per 2.2 pounds of body weight in a single dose on day 1, followed by 5 mg per 2.2 pounds of body weight for the next 4 days

- *Children 2 Years and Older:* For strep throat and tonsillitis, 12 mg per 2.2 pounds of body weight once daily for 5 days
- *Adults:* For respiratory disease, tonsillitis, strep throat, and skin infections, 500 mg in a single dose on day 1, then 250 mg once daily for the next 4 days. For genital ulcer disease, 1,000 mg one time only; and for sexually transmitted diseases, 2,000 mg one time only.

Azithromycin capsules and the powder should be taken at least one hour before or two hours after a meal. If you use the powder, mix the contents of the packet with 2 ounces of water in a glass and drink it immediately. Add 2 more ounces of water to the glass, stir, and drink to make sure you've taken all the medication. The tablets can be taken with food.

If you miss a dose, take it as soon as you remember. However, if it is nearly time for your next dose, do not take the missed dose. Continue on your regular dosing schedule, and never take a double dose.

SYMPTOMS OF OVERDOSE AND WHAT TO DO

No cases of overdose have been reported. If overdose occurs, seek immediate medical attention, and bring the prescription container with you. Symptoms may include nausea, vomiting, stomach cramps, and diarrhea.

SPECIAL INFORMATION FOR PREGNANT OR NURSING WOMEN

No adequate studies of the effects of azithromycin on pregnant or nursing women have been done. If you are pregnant or plan to become pregnant, talk to your health-care practitioner before using this medication. Your health-care practitioner can weigh the potential benefits against the potential risks.

Although it is not known whether azithromycin passes into breast milk, other macrolide antibiotics do. If you are breastfeeding, your health-care practitioner will likely advise you to stop while you are being treated.

SPECIAL INFORMATION FOR SENIORS

Azithromycin should be used with caution in seniors who have liver problems. Older individuals who have pneumonia or other serious illnesses should probably be treated with other antibiotics.

GENERIC NAME

Bacampicillin

see Penicillin Antibiotics, page 812

GENERIC NAME

Baclofen

BRAND NAME

Lioresal
Generic available

ABOUT THIS DRUG

Baclofen is a muscle relaxant prescribed to relax muscles and to relieve the pain caused by muscle cramps and spasms. It is typically taken by individuals who have multiple sclerosis, spinal cord injuries or disease, or other nervous system conditions.

Baclofen appears to interfere with nerve impulses that travel from the spinal cord to the muscles, thus relieving pain and spasms.

SIDE EFFECTS

Be sure to tell your health-care practitioner if you experience any side effects while taking baclofen. Only your health-care practitioner can determine whether it is safe for you to continue taking this drug.

- *Most Common:* dizziness, drowsiness, headache, low blood pressure, lightheadedness, nausea and vomiting, sleeplessness, weakness
- *Less Common:* ankle swelling, clumsiness, constipation, difficult or painful urination, diarrhea, euphoria, loss of appetite, muscle or joint pain, numbness or tingling in hands or feet, trembling, stomach pain, weight gain
- *Rare:* bloody urine or blood in stool, blurred vision, chest pain, fainting, hallucinations, rash or itching, ringing or buzzing in the ears, slurred speech, seizures

IMPORTANT PRECAUTIONS

Tell your health-care practitioner if you are sensitive or allergic to baclofen or to other drugs.

Because baclofen can cause drowsiness and dizziness, do not drive or operate hazardous equipment until you are sure how you react to the drug.

Baclofen should not be taken for muscle spasms that are associated with stroke, cerebral palsy, Parkinson's disease, or rheumatic disease because its benefits have not been proven in these disorders. People who have epilepsy or psychotic disorders should not take baclofen because it can worsen their condition.

Inform your health-care practitioner if you have a history of diabetes, stroke, emotional or mental problems, or kidney disease before you take baclofen.

Baclofen may increase your blood sugar levels. If you have diabetes, your health-care practitioner may need to adjust your antidiabetic medication to take this into account.

Do not suddenly stop taking baclofen unless your health-care practitioner instructs you to do so. Abruptly stopping baclofen can lead to seizures and hallucinations.

DRUG INTERACTIONS

Inform your health-care practitioner and pharmacist if you are taking any prescription or nonprescription drugs, as well as any vitamins, herb, or other supplements. Possible drug interactions with baclofen may include the following:

- Alcohol and other nervous system depressants (e.g., antihistamines, sedatives, barbiturates, muscle relaxants) can increase the severity of drowsiness, dizziness, and other central nervous system effects.
- Drugs that lower blood pressure, such as antihypertensive drugs (e.g., clonidine, enalapril), beta-blockers (e.g., atenolol, carteolol), and diuretics (e.g., amiloride, furosemide) may increase the risk of fainting or dizziness.
- Monoamine oxidase inhibitor (MAOI) drugs (e.g., phenelzine, tranylcypromine) may cause drowsiness, nervous system depression, and low blood pressure.
- Tricyclic antidepressants (e.g., amitriptyline, imipramine) may cause severe muscle weakness and increase the severity of other side effects.

FOOD, VITAMIN, AND HERBAL INTERACTIONS

Herbs that may produce sedative effects (e.g., calendula, catnip, goldenseal, gotu kola, hops, kava, lady's slipper, passionflower, skullcap, St. John's wort, and valerian, among others) along with baclofen may increase the severity of the sedative reactions.

RECOMMENDED DOSAGE

Baclofen is available in tablets. The dosages given here are typical. However, your health-care practitioner will determine the best dose and schedule for your needs.

- *Children Younger than 12 Years:* Your health-care practitioner will determine whether this drug is appropriate for your child.
- *Children 12 years and Older and Adults:* 15 mg daily for three days, gradually increased by your health-care practitioner to 40 to 80 mg daily.

Baclofen can be taken with or without food.

If you miss a dose and it's within 1 hour of your scheduled dose, take it immediately. If you don't remember to take the missed dose until more than 1 hour later, do not take the skipped dose. Continue with your regular dosing schedule. Never take a double dose.

SYMPTOMS OF OVERDOSE AND WHAT TO DO

Symptoms of overdose include loss of muscle tone, twitching, convulsions, blurred or double vision, breathing difficulties, seizures, vomiting, and coma. If an overdose occurs, seek immediate medical attention, and bring the prescription container with you.

SPECIAL INFORMATION FOR PREGNANT OR NURSING WOMEN

Baclofen can cause birth defects in animals. If you are pregnant or plan to become pregnant, talk to your health-care practitioner. You and your health-care practitioner can weigh the potential benefits against the potential risks.

Baclofen taken orally passes into breast milk. If you are breastfeeding, your health-care practitioner will likely advise you to stop until your treatment is done.

SPECIAL INFORMATION FOR SENIORS

Mood changes, severe drowsiness, hallucinations, depression, and confusion may be more likely to occur in older adults.

GENERIC NAME

Balsalazide

BRAND NAME

Colazal

No generic available

ABOUT THIS DRUG

Balsalazide is a gastrointestinal agent and anti-inflammatory drug used to treat mild-to-moderate ulcerative colitis.

This drug reduces inflammation in the colon by blocking production of chemicals that cause the bowel to become overactive and inflamed.

SIDE EFFECTS

Contact your health-care practitioner if you develop side effects while taking this drug. Only he or she can determine whether it is safe for you to continue taking it.

- *More Common:* diarrhea, headache, stomach pain
- *Less Common:* blood in urine, constipation, coughing, cramps, dry mouth, fever, gas, heartburn, joint pain, loss of appetite, lower back pain, muscle pain, pain while urinating, stuffy nose, sleep difficulties, unusual tiredness or weakness, yellowish skin

IMPORTANT PRECAUTIONS

Tell your health-care practitioner if you are sensitive or allergic to balsalazide or to other drugs.

If you have liver or kidney problems, tell your health-care practitioner before you take this medication. If you have pyloric stenosis, it may take longer for the drug to reach your colon.

DRUG INTERACTIONS

Tell your health-care practitioner and pharmacist if you are taking any prescription or over-the-counter drugs, as well as any vitamins, herbs, or other supplements. To date, no drug-drug interaction studies have been conducted. However, it is possible that antibiotics could interfere with the release of balsalazide in the colon. It is also recommended that you avoid this drug if you are allergic to aspirin or aspirin-like drugs.

FOOD, VITAMIN, AND HERBAL INTERACTIONS

No food, vitamin, or herbal interactions have been noted.

RECOMMENDED DOSAGE

Balsalazide is available in 750-mg capsules. Although the doses given below are typical, only your health-care practitioner can determine which dose and schedule is most appropriate for you.

- *Children:* Your health-care practitioner will determine whether balsalazide is appropriate for your child.
- *Adults:* Three 750-mg capsules three times daily (for a maximum of 6.75 g daily) for 8 weeks. This dosage can be taken for up to 12 weeks as ordered by your health-care practitioner.

If you miss a dose, take it as soon as you remember. However, if it is nearly time for your next dose, do not take the missed dose. Continue with your regular dosing schedule. Never take a double dose.

SYMPTOMS OF OVERDOSE AND WHAT TO DO

No specific information about overdosing with balsalazide is available. Likely symptoms would include severe side effects, such as nausea, vomiting, diarrhea, and cramps. If overdose occurs, seek immediate medical attention and bring the prescription bottle with you.

SPECIAL INFORMATION FOR PREGNANT OR NURSING WOMEN

No adequate studies of the effects of balsalazide on pregnant or nursing women have been conducted. If you are pregnant or plan to become pregnant, or if you are breastfeeding, talk to your health-care practitioner. You and your health-care practitioner can weigh the potential benefits against the potential risks.

SPECIAL INFORMATION FOR SENIORS

No special information is available for seniors.

GENERIC NAME

Becaplermin

BRAND NAME

Regranex
No generic available

ABOUT THIS DRUG

Becaplermin is a topical gel that is used to treat diabetic ulcers that develop on the lower legs. It belongs to a drug class called recombinant human growth factor.

Becaplermin is a genetically engineered form of human platelet-derived growth factor that occurs naturally in the body. It attracts and promotes the growth of cells involved in new tissue production and wound repair.

SIDE EFFECTS

Contact your health-care practitioner if you experience side effects while taking becaplermin. Only he or she can determine whether it is safe for you to continue taking it.

- *Common:* irritation at the site of application

IMPORTANT PRECAUTIONS

Tell your health-care practitioner if you are sensitive or allergic to becaplermin or to any other drugs.

Becaplermin is not recommended for use in children younger than 16 years.

If you have cancerous or other unusual growths in the area being treated, consult your health-care practitioner before applying becaplermin.

DRUG INTERACTIONS

Tell your health-care practitioner and pharmacist if you are taking any prescription or nonprescription drugs, as well as any vitamins, herbs, or other supplements. No drug-drug interactions have been documented.

FOOD, VITAMIN, AND HERBAL INTERACTIONS

No food, vitamin, or herbal interactions have been noted.

RECOMMENDED DOSAGE

Becaplermin is available as a topical gel. Although the doses given here are typical, your health-care practitioner will determine the dose and schedule that are best for you.

- *Children:* Not recommended for children younger than 16 years.
- *Adults:* Apply a thin, continuous layer to the affected area, as directed by your health-care practitioner. Cover the treated area with a saline-moistened dressing for 12 hours. After 12 hours, remove the dressing, rinse the area with water or saline, and cover the area again with another saline-moistened dressing. Do not apply gel.

If you miss a dose, apply it as soon as you remember. If it is nearly time for your next dose, do not apply the missed dose. Continue with your regular dosing schedule on the next day. Applying extra gel does not make your wound heal any faster.

When applying the gel, do not allow the tip of the tube to touch your skin or any other surface.

SYMPTOMS OF OVERDOSE AND WHAT TO DO

No overdose cases have been reported. If too much gel is applied or if it is accidentally ingested, seek immediate medical attention. Bring the prescription container with you.

SPECIAL INFORMATION FOR PREGNANT OR NURSING WOMEN

No adequate studies of the effects of becaplermin on pregnant or nursing women have been conducted. If you are pregnant or plan to become pregnant, or if you are breastfeeding, talk to your health-care practitioner. You and your health-care practitioner can weigh the potential benefits against the potential risks to the fetus.

SPECIAL INFORMATION FOR SENIORS

No special instructions are needed for older adults.

GENERIC NAME

Beclomethasone dipropionate

see Corticosteroids, Nasal Inhalation, *page 327;* Corticosteroids, Oral Inhalers, *page 334*

GENERIC NAME

Benazepril

BRAND NAME

Lotensin
No generic available

ABOUT THIS DRUG

Benazepril is used primarily to control high blood pressure. It belongs to a class of drugs called angiotensin-converting enzyme (ACE) inhibitors.

Benazepril, like other ACE inhibitors, prevents the conversion of a hormone (angiotensin I) to another hormone, angiotensin II. Because the conversion does not occur, blood vessels relax and blood pressure is reduced.

SIDE EFFECTS

Contact your health-care practitioner if you experience side effects while taking benazepril. Only a health-care practitioner can determine whether you should continue to take this drug.

- *Common:* persistent dry cough
- *Less Common:* dizziness, drowsiness, headache, loss of taste, muscle weakness, nausea, numbness or tingling in the hands, feet, or lips, rash, unusual fatigue
- *Rare:* abdominal pain, ankle swelling, chest pain or palpitations, confusion, decreased urination, fever and chills, intense itching, sudden difficulty breathing or swallowing, swelling of the face, mouth, or extremities, yellow eyes or skin. Contact your health-care practitioner immediately if these symptoms occur.

IMPORTANT PRECAUTIONS

Tell your health-care practitioner if you are sensitive or allergic to benazepril or to other drugs, especially other ACE inhibitors.

Benazepril can cause a sudden drop in blood pressure. For this reason, and because it can also cause dizziness, do not drive or operate hazardous equipment until you know how you will react to this drug.

Kidney function can be affected by benazepril. Your health-care practitioner should monitor your urine for protein content while you are being treated with this drug.

Periodic monitoring of your blood count is recommended, as benazepril can affect white blood cell counts and may increase your susceptibility to infection.

If you have any of the following medical conditions, tell your health-care practitioner before you take benazepril: scleroderma, systemic lupus, any form of heart or liver disease, diabetes, elevated potassium levels, renal artery stenosis, or a blood cell disorder.

Contact your health-care practitioner if you experience excessive sweating, dehydration, severe diarrhea, fever, or vomiting. These conditions may cause you to lose a great deal of water and cause your blood pressure to become abnormally low.

DRUG INTERACTIONS

Tell your health-care practitioner and pharmacist if you are taking any prescription or over-the-counter drugs, as well as any vitamins, herbs, or other supplements. Possible drug interactions include the following:

- Antacids should be taken at least 2 hours apart from benazepril.
- Beta-blockers (e.g., acebutolol, nadolol) and diuretics (e.g., amiloride, indapamide) may increase the blood pressure lowering effects of benazepril.
- Capsaicin may trigger or stimulate cough.
- Lithium's effects can be increased.
- Indomethacin may reduce the ability of benazepril to lower blood pressure.
- Allopurinol increases the chance of side effects for both drugs.
- Benazepril increases the blood levels of digoxin, which may result in increased digoxin-related side effects.

FOOD, VITAMIN, AND HERBAL INTERACTIONS

Discuss your salt intake with your health-care practitioner when taking this medication. Also avoid using salt substitutes or drinking low-salt milk, as these substances can cause abnormally high potassium levels, which can lead to heart problems.

If you plan to or are taking any herbs or supplements, talk with your health-care practitioner before starting benazepril. Ginseng, goldenseal, licorice, ephedra (ma huang), and saw palmetto may raise your blood pressure; garlic and calcium may help lower it.

Do not take potassium supplements while taking benazepril unless directed to do so by your health-care practitioner.

RECOMMENDED DOSAGE

Benazepril is available in 5-, 10-, 20-, and 40-mg tablets. The dosages given here are typical; however, your health-care practitioner will determine which dose and schedule is most appropriate for you.

- *Children Younger than 12 Years:* Dosage has not been established for children.
- *Adults:* 10 mg once daily if not taking a diuretic; 5 mg daily if taking a diuretic. Typical maintenance dose is 20 to 40 mg daily either as a single dose or divided into 2 equal doses. Your health-care practitioner will monitor you to determine if you need to take a diuretic to control your blood pressure or whether benazepril alone is sufficient.
- *Adults 60 Years and Older:* dosing can be the same as in the 12- to 60-year age group unless kidney function is compromised. In that case, your health-care practitioner may reduce your dose by 50 percent (see "Special Information for Seniors").

Benazepril can be taken with or without food and should be taken at the same time every day.

If you miss a dose, take it as soon as you remember. If it is nearly time for your next dose, do not take the missed dose. Continue on your regular dosing schedule. Never take a double dose.

SYMPTOMS OF OVERDOSE AND WHAT TO DO

Symptoms of overdose include lightheadedness, dizziness, and fainting. If overdose occurs, seek immediate medical attention and bring the prescription bottle with you to the hospital.

SPECIAL INFORMATION FOR PREGNANT OR NURSING WOMEN

Benazepril can cause birth defects or death to a developing fetus, especially during the second and third trimesters of pregnancy. If you are pregnant or plan to become pregnant, talk to your health-care practitioner about the potential risks to your unborn child.

Small amounts of benazepril pass into breast milk. If you are breastfeeding, your health-care practitioner may advise you to stop while you are under treatment.

SPECIAL INFORMATION FOR SENIORS

If kidney function is significantly impaired, dosing is usually reduced by 50 percent. Total daily dose should not exceed 40 mg.

GENERIC NAME

Bendroflumethiazide

see Thiazide Diuretics, page 1020

GENERIC NAME

Benzonatate

BRAND NAME

Tessalon
No generic available

ABOUT THIS DRUG

Benzonatate is an oral, antitussive (anticough) agent used to treat cough due to cold or flu. It is not for chronic cough related to asthma, smoking, or emphysema or cough that produces large amounts of mucus or phlegm.

Benzonatate acts directly on the lungs and breathing passages, and may also affect the cough center in the brain.

SIDE EFFECTS

Contact your health-care practitioner if you develop side effects while taking benzonatate. Only he or she can determine if you should continue to take this drug.

- *Less Common:* burning sensation in the eyes, constipation, dizziness, drowsiness, headache, itching, nausea or vomiting, rash, stuffy nose
- *Rare:* confusion, difficulty breathing, difficulty speaking, hallucinations

IMPORTANT PRECAUTIONS

Tell your health-care practitioner if you are sensitive or allergic to benzonatate or any other drugs, especially local anesthetics.

Benzonatate should be swallowed whole; never chew this medication, as it can cause numbness of the mouth and throat and may result in choking or a severe allergic reaction. If this occurs, seek immediate medical attention.

Tell your health-care practitioner if you have any medical condition that produces mucus or phlegm. Because benzonatate decreases cough, it may be difficult for you to eliminate mucus, which can then collect in your lungs.

DRUG INTERACTIONS

Tell your health-care practitioner and pharmacist about any prescription and nonprescription drugs you are taking, as well as any vitamins, herbs, or other supplements. No drug-drug interactions have been documented.

FOOD, VITAMIN, AND HERBAL INTERACTIONS

No food, vitamin, or herbal interactions have been documented.

RECOMMENDED DOSAGE

Benzonatate is available as 500-mg softgel capsules. Typical doses are given here. However, your health-care practitioner will determine the most appropriate dose and schedule for you.

- *Children Up to 10 Years:* Your health-care practitioner will determine whether this drug is appropriate for your child.

- *Children Older than 10 Years and Adults:* 100 mg three times daily, as needed. The maximum dose is 600 mg daily.

It is essential to take benzonatate exactly as prescribed. If you forget a dose, take it as soon as you remember. If it's nearly time for your next dose, do not take the missed dose. Continue with your regular dosing schedule, and do not take a double dose.

SYMPTOMS OF OVERDOSE AND WHAT TO DO

Symptoms of overdose include restlessness, convulsions, and tremors. If overdose occurs, seek immediate medical attention and bring the prescription container with you to the hospital.

SPECIAL INFORMATION FOR PREGNANT OR NURSING WOMEN

No adequate studies of the effects of benzonatate on pregnant or nursing women have been done. If you are pregnant or plan to become pregnant, talk to your health-care practitioner. Together you can weigh the potential benefits against the potential risks to the fetus.

If you are breastfeeding, your health-care practitioner may advise you to stop while you are under treatment.

SPECIAL INFORMATION FOR SENIORS

No special precautions are needed for older adults.

GENERIC NAME

Benzthiazide *see Thiazide Diuretics, page 1020*

GENERIC NAME

Benztropine

BRAND NAME

Cogentin

Generic available

ABOUT THIS DRUG

Benztropine is an anticholinergic (controls spasms) used to treat the symptoms of Parkinson's disease. It is not a cure for the disease.

Benztropine counteracts the activity of acetylcholine, a naturally occurring transmitter of nerve impulses that provokes muscle spasms. This drug can reduce muscle spasms by about 20 percent.

SIDE EFFECTS

Be sure to tell your health-care practitioner if you experience any side effects while taking benztropine. Only your health-care practitioner can determine whether it is safe for you to continue taking this drug.

➤ *Most Common:* constipation, blurred vision, increased sensitivity to bright light, urinary difficulties

➤ *Less Common:* rash, disorientation, memory loss, hallucinations, agitation, nervousness, delirium, listlessness, depression, drowsiness, euphoria, dizziness, headache, weakness, tingling or heaviness in the hands or feet, rapid heartbeat, low blood pressure, dry mouth, swollen glands, nausea, vomiting, upset stomach, double vision, muscle weakness or cramping, flushing, decreased sweating, impotence

IMPORTANT PRECAUTIONS

Tell your health-care practitioner if you are sensitive or allergic to benztropine or other drugs.

Benztropine can reduce your ability to sweat. This makes it easy for you to overheat if you exercise, are exposed to excessive sun, or are in a hot environment. Overheating, which can lead to heat exhaustion, heatstroke, or even death, is especially a problem among the elderly, people with nervous system disease, chronically ill individuals, and alcoholics.

Do not take benztropine if you have angle-closure glaucoma, heart disease, high blood pressure, tardive dyskinesia, gastrointestinal tract obstructions, prostatitis, myasthenia gravis, or stomach ulcers.

Because benztropine can cause drowsiness and impair mental functioning, make sure you know how you react to the drug before you drive or operate hazardous equipment.

This drug should not be taken by children younger than 3 years.

DRUG INTERACTIONS

Tell your health-care practitioner and pharmacist about any prescription and nonprescription drugs you are taking, as well as any vitamins, herbs, or other supplements. Possible drug interactions include the following:

➤ Antihistamines (e.g., cetirizine, loratadine), phenothiazines (e.g., chlorpromazine, thioridazine), antidepressants (e.g., fluoxetine, amitriptyline), monoamine oxidase inhibitor (MAOI) drugs, and other anticholinergic drugs (e.g., atropine, scopolamine) may increase the side effects of benztropine.

- Antacids (e.g., Maalox, Mylanta) may decrease the effects of benztropine. Take antacids at least one hour before or after you take benztropine.
- Benztropine may decrease the effects of cisapride and haloperidol.
- Clozapine may cause elevated temperatures, bowel obstruction, and neurological side effects.
- Amantadine may cause increased confusion and hallucinations.
- Procainamide may increase the risk of heart conduction difficulties.

FOOD, VITAMIN, AND HERBAL INTERACTIONS

Herbs that produce a sedative effect may cause potentially dangerous depressant interactions when used with benztropine. Some of those herbs include calendula, capsicum, catnip, goldenseal, gotu kola, hops, kava, lady's slipper, passionflower, sage, Siberian ginseng, skullcap, St. John's wort, and valerian.

RECOMMENDED DOSAGE

Benztropine is available in 0.5- and 1-mg tablets and capsules. The dosages given here are typical; however, your health-care practitioner will determine the most appropriate dose and schedule for you.

- *Children 3 Years and Younger:* Benztropine should not be used in this age group.
- *Children Up to 18 Years:* Your health-care practitioner will determine if the drug is appropriate.
- *Adults:* 0.5 to 2 mg daily in a single dose at bedtime. The dose can range up to 6 mg under a health-care practitioner's supervision.
- *Adults Older than 60 Years:* Low starting doses are recommended.

Benztropine can be taken with food or after eating to help reduce stomach irritation. The tablet may be crushed.

If you miss a dose, take it as soon as you remember. If it's nearly time for your next dose, do not take the missed dose. Continue with your regular dosing schedule. Never take a double dose.

SYMPTOMS OF OVERDOSE AND WHAT TO DO

Symptoms of overdose include weakness, drowsiness, stupor, impaired vision, confusion, hallucinations, rash, dilated pupils, rapid pulse and dry, hot skin. If overdose occurs, seek immediate medical attention, and bring the prescription container with you to the hospital.

SPECIAL INFORMATION FOR PREGNANT OR NURSING WOMEN

No adequate studies have been done on the effects of taking benztropine during pregnancy or nursing. If you are pregnant or plan to become pregnant, or if you are breastfeeding, talk to your health-care practitioner about the potential risks and benefits of taking this drug.

SPECIAL INFORMATION FOR SENIORS

Seniors are at increased risk of experiencing confusion, hallucinations, nightmares, glaucoma, and impaired urination associated with enlargement of the prostate gland (prostatitis).

GENERIC NAME

Bepridil

BRAND NAME

Vascor
No generic available

ABOUT THIS DRUG

Bepridil is a calcium-channel blocker that is used to treat angina. Because it can cause serious heart rhythm problems, it should be reserved for individuals who have not responded well to other anti-angina medications.

Bepridil blocks certain channels in blood vessels, which results in relaxed vessels, a reduction in blood pressure, and an increased flow of blood to the heart, thus reducing chest pain.

SIDE EFFECTS

Be sure to tell your health-care practitioner if you experience any side effects while taking bepridil. Only your health-care practitioner can determine whether it is safe for you to continue taking this drug.

- *Most Common:* nausea, indigestion, diarrhea, loss of strength, dizziness
- *Less Common:* dry mouth, tremor, abnormal heart rhythms, breathing difficulties, very slow or very rapid heartbeat, coughing or wheezing, constipation, headache, unusual tiredness or weakness

- *Rare:* low blood pressure, fainting, swelling of the ankles, feet, or legs

IMPORTANT PRECAUTIONS

Tell your health-care practitioner if you are sensitive or allergic to bepridil or to any other drugs.

Use this drug with extreme caution if you have a history of problems with heart rhythm or if you have heart failure.

Research shows that people who take calcium channel blockers more than once a day are at greater risk of having a heart attack than people who take other types of drugs for the same medical conditions. Talk to your health-care practitioner about whether a calcium channel blocker is the best drug for your situation.

Do not suddenly stop taking this drug; your health-care practitioner will gradually reduce your dosage.

DRUG INTERACTIONS

Tell your health-care practitioner and pharmacist about any prescription and nonprescription drugs you are taking, as well as any vitamins, herbs, or supplements. Possible drug interactions with bepridil may include the following:

- Beta-blockers (e.g., acebutolol, nadolol) may cause very low blood pressure, heart failure, or an increased incidence of angina.
- Bepridil may increase the effects of anticoagulant drugs (e.g., warfarin).
- Acetazolamide, amphotericin B by injection, corticosteroids (e.g., amcinonide, budesonide), dichlorphenamide, diuretics, or methazolamide can cause very low potassium levels, which can worsen the effects of bepridil.

FOOD, VITAMIN, AND HERBAL INTERACTIONS

Magnesium may increase the chance of side effects, such as dizziness, leg swelling, and nausea. Talk to your health-care practitioner if you are taking magnesium supplements.

RECOMMENDED DOSAGE

Bepridil is available in 200- and 300-mg tablets. The dosages given here are typical; however, your health-care practitioner will determine the most appropriate dosage and schedule for you.

- *Children:* Your health-care practitioner will determine if this drug is appropriate for your child.
- *Adults:* 200-300 mg once daily

Bepridil can be taken with or without food. If bepridil causes stomach upset, taking it with food can eliminate that symptom.

If you miss a dose, take it as soon as you remember. If it is nearly time for your next dose, do not take the missed dose. Continue with your regular dosing schedule. Never take a double dose.

SYMPTOMS OF OVERDOSE AND WHAT TO DO

Symptoms of overdose include nausea, dizziness, weakness, confusion, slurred speech, very low blood pressure, drowsiness, and unusual heart rhythms. If overdose occurs, seek immediate medical attention, and bring the prescription container with you to the hospital.

SPECIAL INFORMATION FOR PREGNANT OR NURSING WOMEN

High doses of bepridil affect the development of animal fetuses. If you are pregnant or plan to become pregnant, talk to your health-care practitioner before using this drug. Bepridil should not be used unless the benefits clearly outweigh the potential risks to the fetus.

Bepridil passes into breast milk. If you are breastfeeding, your health-care practitioner will likely advise you to stop until your treatment is complete.

SPECIAL INFORMATION FOR SENIORS

Older adults may require dosage adjustments and more frequent monitoring by their health-care practitioners.

GENERIC NAME

Betaine

BRAND NAME

Cystadane

No generic available

ABOUT THIS DRUG

Betaine is a homocysteine antagonist used to treat homocysteinuria—a condition in which the amino acid homocysteine is dangerously high and levels of it can be detected in the urine. Homocysteinuria can lead to the formation of blood clots, osteoporosis and other bone diseases, and an increased risk of heart disease and heart attack.

The prescription drug betaine contains the ingredient betaine, a naturally occurring substance in the body that aids in the proper processing of homocysteine. Betaine is usually prescribed along with vitamin B_6, vitamin B_{12}, and folate, which all work together to process homocysteine and thus bring the levels down.

SIDE EFFECTS

Be sure to tell your health-care practitioner if you experience any side effects while taking betaine. Only your health-care practitioner can determine whether it is safe for you to continue taking this drug.

- *Less Common:* nausea, diarrhea, stomach and intestinal problems, bad odor, possible mental changes

IMPORTANT PRECAUTIONS

Tell your health-care practitioner if you are sensitive or allergic to betaine or any other drugs.

Do not use the powder if it will not completely dissolve in water or if the solution has color.

DRUG INTERACTIONS

Tell your health-care practitioner and pharmacist about any prescription or nonprescription drugs you are taking, as well as any vitamins, herbs, or supplements. No drug-drug interactions have been noted.

FOOD, VITAMIN, AND HERBAL INTERACTIONS

No interactions with food, vitamins, or herbs have been noted.

RECOMMENDED DOSAGE

Betaine comes in a powder that must be mixed with water. The dosages given here are typical. Your health-care practitioner will determine the most appropriate dosage and schedule for you.

- *Children Younger than 3 Years:* 100 mg per 2.2 pounds of body weight daily. Your health-care practitioner will increase the dosage as needed until homocysteine levels are normal.
- *Children Older than Age 3 and Adults:* 3 grams (3 scoops) mixed with 4 to 6 ounces of water twice daily. Mix completely and drink immediately. Your health-care practitioner will increase the dosage as needed until homocysteine levels are normal.

Use the scoop provided with the prescription when using this drug. Make sure the powder is completely dissolved in water before you drink it.

If you miss a dose, take it as soon as you remember. If it is nearly time for your next dose, do not take the missed dose. Continue with your regular dosing schedule. Never take a double dose.

SYMPTOMS OF OVERDOSE AND WHAT TO DO

No cases of betaine overdose have been reported. Some people are safely treated with up to 20 grams daily. If an overdose occurs, call your poison control center or go to the emergency room. Bring the prescription container with you to the hospital.

SPECIAL INFORMATION FOR PREGNANT OR NURSING WOMEN

No adequate studies have been done on the effects of betaine on pregnant or nursing women. If you are pregnant or plan to become pregnant, talk to your health-care practitioner. This drug should not be used during pregnancy unless the benefits of therapy clearly outweigh the potential risks to the fetus.

If you are breastfeeding, your health-care practitioner may advise you to stop until you have completed treatment.

SPECIAL INFORMATION FOR SENIORS

No special precautions are needed.

GENERIC NAME

Betamethasone

see Corticosteroids, Oral, page 330; Corticosteroids, Topical, page 337

GENERIC NAME

Betaxolol

BRAND NAMES

Betoptic, Betoptic S, Kerlone

No generic available

ABOUT THIS DRUG

Betaxolol is a beta-blocker and antihypertensive drug used to treat open-angle glaucoma (high pressure in the eye) and high blood pressure.

The ophthalmic form of betaxolol reduces the production of fluids in the eye and slightly increases the rate at which the fluids leave the eye. The oral form reduces blood pressure by reducing the rate and force of the heart's contractions, which results in lower blood pressure.

SIDE EFFECTS

Be sure to tell your health-care practitioner if you experience any side effects while taking betaxolol. Only your health-care practitioner can determine whether it is safe for you to continue taking this drug. Even though the ophthalmic form of betaxolol is administered into the eye, the drug does get into the bloodstream, so it can affect other parts of the body.

Ophthalmic Form

- ➤ *More Common:* temporary eye discomfort
- ➤ *Less Common:* blurred vision, poor night vision, increased sensitivity to light, headache, insomnia, sinus irritation, taste changes

Oral Form

- ➤ *More Common:* impotence, dizziness or lightheadedness, especially when rising suddenly from a lying or sitting position, palpitations, frequent headaches
- ➤ *Less Common:* unusual tiredness or weakness, slow heartbeat, congestive heart failure, depression, constipation, diarrhea, nausea, vomiting, upset stomach, urinary problems, blurred vision, rash, hair loss, stuffy nose, chest pain, joint or back pain, liver toxicity, drug allergy (fever, sore throat), nervousness

IMPORTANT PRECAUTIONS

Tell your health-care practitioner if you are sensitive or allergic to betaxolol or any other drugs.

Betaxolol should be used with caution if you have asthma or other respiratory problems, diabetes, decreased heart function, or other heart problems.

If you will be undergoing surgery, your health-care practitioner may advise you to stop taking betaxolol several days before the procedure, as surgical anesthesia can increase the risk of heart problems during surgery.

This medication can lose some of its effectiveness for glaucoma if you have been taking it for a long time.

Call your health-care practitioner immediately if you experience depression, back or joint pain, breathing difficulties, rash, cold hands or feet, fainting, dizziness, or irregular heartbeat.

Because betaxolol can cause drowsiness, dizziness, or eye problems, make sure you know how you react to the drug before you take it and drive or operate hazardous equipment.

DRUG INTERACTIONS

Be sure to tell your health-care practitioner and pharmacist about any prescription and nonprescription drugs you are taking, as well as any vitamins, herbs, and other supplements. Betaxolol may interact with the following drugs.

(Note: These interactions are more likely when using the oral rather than the ophthalmic form.)

- Betaxolol can interfere with the actions of oral antidiabetic drugs (e.g., glipizide, glyburide).
- Betaxolol may increase the blood-pressure-lowering effects of other antihypertensive drugs, including clonidine, guanabenz, and reserpine, and calcium channel blockers, such as nifedipine.
- Betaxolol may increase the effects of verapamil and increase the risk of congestive heart failure and slow heart rate.
- Aspirin-containing drugs, estrogen drugs, indomethacin, and sulfinpyrazone may hinder the ability of betaxolol to lower blood pressure.
- Fluoroquinolone antibiotics (e.g., ciprofloxacin, levofloxacin) may elevate betaxolol blood levels and lead to toxicity.
- Fluvoxamine and venlafaxine may drastically reduce heart rate and blood pressure.
- Amiodarone may cause an extremely slow heart rate and heart attack.
- Betaxolol may counteract the effects of thyroid hormone replacement therapy.
- Cimetidine increases the amount of betaxolol that is absorbed into the bloodstream.
- The effects of some antiasthma drugs (e.g., ephedrine, isoproterenol, theophylline, aminophylline) may be reduced by betaxolol.
- Digitalis and phenytoin along with betaxolol can cause excessive slowing of the heart.

FOOD, VITAMIN, AND HERBAL INTERACTIONS

Betaxolol does not interact negatively with food. However, it is best to avoid excessive salt intake if you have high blood pressure. If you plan to or are taking any herbs or supplements, talk with your health-care practitioner before starting betaxolol. Ginseng, goldenseal, licorice, ephedra (ma huang), and saw palmetto may raise your blood pressure; garlic and calcium may help lower it.

RECOMMENDED DOSAGE

Betaxolol is available as eyedrops (2.8 and 5.6 mg/ml) and as 10- and 20-mg tablets. The dosages given here are typical. Your health-care practitioner will determine the most appropriate dosage and schedule for you.

For Glaucoma

- *Children Younger than 12 Years:* The safety and effectiveness for children has not been determined.
- *Adults:* 1 drop in the affected eye twice daily.

For Hypertension

- *Children Younger than 12 Years:* The safety and effectiveness for children has not been determined.
- *Adults:* 10 mg once daily (5 mg for those who have kidney failure). Your health-care practitioner may increase your dose as needed up to 20 mg every 24 hours.

If you miss a dose of the ophthalmic form, take it as soon as you remember. If it is nearly time for your next dose, do not take the missed dose. Continue with your regular dosing schedule. Never take a double dose.

If you miss a dose of the oral form, take it as soon as you remember. If it is within 8 hours of your next dose and you take the drug once daily, do not take the missed dose. Continue with your regular dosing schedule. If it is within 4 hours of your next dose and you take the drug twice a day, do not take the missed dose. Continue with your regular dosing schedule. Never take a double dose.

If taking the oral form, do not suddenly stop taking it unless directed to do so by your health-care practitioner. Abrupt withdrawal from the drug may cause breathing difficulties, increased sweating, unusually irregular heartbeat, and chest pain.

SYMPTOMS OF OVERDOSE AND WHAT TO DO

Symptoms of overdose include irregular heartbeat, severe dizziness or fainting, seizures, bluish fingernails or palms, and breathing difficulties. If overdose occurs, seek immediate medical attention, and bring the prescription container with you to the hospital.

SPECIAL INFORMATION FOR PREGNANT OR NURSING WOMEN

Although the effects of betaxolol on pregnant or breastfeeding women have not been adequately studied, infants born to women who took other beta-blockers while pregnant had low blood pressure, lower birth weights, and reduced heart rates. If you are pregnant or plan to become pregnant, talk to your health-care practitioner. Betaxolol should be avoided during pregnancy.

Beta-blockers pass into breast milk. If you are breastfeeding, your health-care practitioner will likely advise you to stop until your treatment is complete.

SPECIAL INFORMATION FOR SENIORS

Older adults may need less of the drug to achieve the desired results. Side effects such as cold hands and feet, chest pain, breathing difficulties, increased sweating, changes in heartbeat, and reduced body temperature are more likely to affect seniors.

GENERIC NAME

Bevacizumab

BRAND NAME

Avastin
No generic available

ABOUT THIS DRUG

Bevacizumab is an anticancer drug used in the treatment of colorectal cancer that has metastasized (spread) to other parts of the body. It is used in combination with 5-fluorouracil.

This drug prevents the growth of tumor cells by reducing new blood vessel growth (angiogenesis). This is the first angiogenesis inhibitor approved for marketing in the United States.

SIDE EFFECTS

Side effects are common. Consult your health-care practitioner if they are persistent or severe. Only he or she can determine whether it is safe for you to continue receiving bevacizumab.

- *Most Common:* abdominal pain, constipation, diarrhea, fainting, hypertension, leukopenia (low white blood cell levels), low neutrophil levels, weakness

- *Less Common/Rare:* gastrointestinal perforation that requires surgery, impaired wound healing, blood clots resulting in stroke or heart attack, bleeding, congestive heart failure, and protein in urine.

IMPORTANT PRECAUTIONS

Tell your health-care practitioner if you are sensitive or allergic to bevacizumab or to any other drugs, or to mouse protein.

You should not have surgery during the month of or in the month following treatment with bevacizumab, as wound healing may be poor and result in bleeding or infection.

Before being treated with bevacizumab, talk to your doctor if you have liver or kidney disease, heart disease, high blood pressure, a history of stroke or transient ischemic attack (TIA), or bleeding in the brain, or if you have an open wound.

Stop using bevacizumab at least three weeks before elective surgery, and do not resume treatment until your surgical incision has healed completely.

DRUG INTERACTIONS

No drug-drug interactions have been documented. However, you should still tell your health-care practitioner and pharmacist if you are taking any prescription or nonprescription drugs, as well as any vitamins, herbs, or other supplements.

FOOD, VITAMIN, AND HERBAL INTERACTIONS

No food, vitamin, or herbal interactions have been reported.

RECOMMENDED DOSAGE

Bevacizumab is administered by intravenous infusion under the supervision of a qualified health-care practitioner experienced in the use of cancer chemotherapy. It is typically given in combination with 5-fluorouracil at a dose of 5 mg/kg once every 14 days until progress is detected. Your health-care practitioner will determine the most appropriate dose and schedule for your needs.

SYMPTOMS OF OVERDOSE AND WHAT TO DO

Symptoms of overdose are not known, but may include headache. If overdose occurs, seek immediate medical attention.

SPECIAL INFORMATION FOR PREGNANT OR NURSING WOMEN

Adequate studies of the effects of bevacizumab on pregnant or nursing women have not been done. Discuss the appropriate use of birth control methods with your health-care practitioner if you plan to be treated with bevacizumab.

It is not known whether bevacizumab passes into breast milk. However, your health-care practitioner will likely recommend you switch to bottle feeding while you take this drug.

SPECIAL INFORMATION FOR SENIORS

Side effects are more likely to occur and are more severe in older adults.

GENERIC NAME

Bicalutamide

BRAND NAME

Casodex
No generic available

ABOUT THIS DRUG

Bicalutamide is an antiandrogen (an androgen is a male hormone) that is given to men who have prostate cancer. It is typically prescribed along with another hormone product.

Bicalutamide competes with the hormone testosterone, which promotes cancer growth. When bicalutamide binds to receptors where testosterone normally attaches itself, it prevents the hormone from reaching the cancer cells so they grow more slowly or not at all.

SIDE EFFECTS

Be sure to tell your health-care practitioner if you experience any side effects while taking bicalutamide. Only your health-care practitioner can determine whether it is safe for you to continue taking this drug.

- *Most Common:* hot flashes, diarrhea, constipation, nausea, pain, back pain, weakness, and pelvic pain. About 40% of patients who take bicalutamide experience breast tenderness, pain, or swelling.
- *Less Common:* abdominal pain, anemia, chest pain, flu symptoms, high blood pressure, high blood sugar, blood in the urine, impotence, difficulty breathing, bone pain, headache, vomiting, rash
- *Rare:* Rare side effects can occur anywhere in the body and include liver damage (pain or tenderness in upper right side of abdomen, yellow eyes or skin). Contact your health-care practitioner if you experience any side effects not listed here.

IMPORTANT PRECAUTIONS

Tell your health-care practitioner if you are sensitive or allergic to bicalutamide or any other drugs.

Bicalutamide may reduce sperm count.

DRUG INTERACTIONS

Tell your health-care practitioner and pharmacist about any prescription and nonprescription drugs you are taking, as well as any vitamins, herbs, or other supplements. If you take oral anticoagulant drugs (e.g., warfarin), bicalutamide may increase the effects of these drugs. Your health-care practitioner may need to adjust your dosage.

FOOD, VITAMIN, AND HERBAL INTERACTIONS

No food, vitamin, or herbal interactions have been noted.

RECOMMENDED DOSAGE

Bicalutamide is available in 50-mg tablets. The dosage given here is typical. However, your health-care practitioner will determine the most appropriate dosage and schedule for you.

- *Children:* This drug is not indicated for children
- *Adults:* 50 mg once daily, in the morning or evening

Treatment with bicalutamide should always be started along with a luteinizing hormone-releasing hormone drug (e.g., goserelin, leuprolide). Both drugs should be taken exactly as prescribed by your health-care practitioner, and they should be taken at the same time each day.

If you miss a dose, take it as soon as you remember. If it is nearly time for your next dose, do not take the missed dose. Continue with your regular dosing schedule. Never take a double dose.

SYMPTOMS OF OVERDOSE AND WHAT TO DO

Symptoms of overdose include teariness, loss of appetite, vomiting, tiredness, slow breathing, and poor muscle coordination. If overdose occurs, seek immediate medical attention. Bring the prescription container with you to the hospital.

SPECIAL INFORMATION FOR PREGNANT OR NURSING WOMEN

This drug is not used by women.

SPECIAL INFORMATION FOR SENIORS

No special information is needed for older adults.

GENERIC NAME

Bimatoprost

BRAND NAME

Lumigan
No generic available

ABOUT THIS DRUG

Bimatoprost is a prostamide (a synthetic analog of prostaglandin) that is used to treat open-angle glaucoma and ocular hypertension. It is primarily for individuals who are intolerant of or have not responded to other treatments.

This drug lowers pressure in the eye by imitating the effects of prostamides, which are naturally occurring substances in the body. Bimatoprost increases the flow of fluids from the eye, thus lowering intraocular pressure.

SIDE EFFECTS

Be sure to tell your health-care practitioner if you experience any side effects while taking bimatoprost. Only your health-care practitioner can determine whether it is safe for you to continue taking this drug.

- *Most Common:* conjunctival hyperemia (blood congestion), ocular pruritis (severe itching), growth of eyelashes (occurs in up to 45% of patients)
- *Less Common:* eye dryness, visual disturbance, eye burning, eye pain, sensation as if something is in the eye, darkening eyelashes, cataracts, inflamed eye (iritis), headache

IMPORTANT PRECAUTIONS

Tell your health-care practitioner if you are sensitive to bimatoprost or any other drugs.

Bimatoprost can cause eye color to change by increasing the number of brown pigments in the iris. The long-term effect of this change is not known. Eye color change can occur over months or even years and may be permanent. Other changes that may occur include eyelid skin darkening and change to eyelashes (increase in number, thickness, length, and pigmentation).

Do not administer bimatoprost while wearing contacts. Remove your contacts before putting in the drops and keep them out for 15 minutes after administering the drops.

Contact your health-care practitioner immediately if you experience any ocular (eye) side effects while using this drug.

Do not allow the dropper to touch the eye or any other surface. Contamination of the medication may result in an infection and serious eye problems.

DRUG INTERACTIONS

Tell your health-care practitioner and pharmacist about any prescription and nonprescription drugs you are taking, as well as any vitamins, herbs, or other supplements. Bimatoprost is not known to interact with other drugs. If you are using another eye medication along with bimatoprost, allow at least 5 minutes between the administration of the different drugs.

FOOD, VITAMIN, AND HERBAL INTERACTIONS

No food, vitamin, or herbal interactions have been noted.

RECOMMENDED DOSAGE

Bimatoprost is available as an ocular solution in an eyedropper bottle. The dosage give here is typical. Your health-care practitioner will determine the most appropriate dosage for your needs.

- *Children:* This drug is not indicated for children.
- *Adults:* 1 drop in each affected eye once daily

If you miss a dose, take it as soon as you remember. If it is nearly time for your next dose, do not take the missed dose. Continue with your regular dosing schedule. Never take a double dose.

Administer the medication without allowing the dropper to touch the eye or any other surface. Do not rinse the dropper with water or any other substance.

SYMPTOMS OF OVERDOSE AND WHAT TO DO

No cases of overdose have been reported. If overdose occurs, or if the drug is ingested, call your health-care practitioner or poison center for instructions. Tests in animals have shown no toxic effects at amounts equal to 70 times higher than an accidental dose of one container taken by a 22-pound child.

SPECIAL INFORMATION FOR PREGNANT OR NURSING WOMEN

No adequate studies of bimatoprost have been done in pregnant or nursing women. If you are pregnant or plan to become pregnant, talk to your health-care practitioner. Do not use this drug unless the benefits of therapy clearly outweigh the potential risks to the fetus.

If you are breastfeeding, your health-care practitioner will likely advise you to stop until you have completed treatment with bimatoprost.

SPECIAL INFORMATION FOR SENIORS

No special instructions are needed for older adults.

OPEN QUESTIONS OR CONTROVERSIES

Bimatoprost has been in the news several times since it was approved by the Food and Drug Administration (FDA) in 2001. In the 2001 Annual Report of the FDA's Office of Drug Safety, bimatoprost was approved as a second- rather than a first-line treatment for glaucoma because of concerns about deaths and cardiovascular events associated with a related ophthalmic product, latanoprost. This does not mean, however, that bimatoprost will cause the same effects.

Also in 2001, the FDA took issue with the manufacturer of Lumigan (Allergan) for overstating the efficacy of their product. In particular, the FDA asked Allergan to discontinue use of its materials that suggested Lumigan was superior to latanoprost (Xalatan) and travoprost (Travatan) at reducing intraocular pressure in both black and nonblack patients.

In November 2001, the results of a trial comparing bimatoprost and latanoprost were released at the annual meeting of the American Academy of Ophthalmology. The study involved 232 patients who received either latanoprost (119) or bimatoprost (113) once daily for three months. Bimatoprost was as effective, if not more effective, than latanoprost at relieving intraocular pressure. Both drugs were deemed to be equally safe, but individuals who took latanoprost complained of headache much more than people who took bimatoprost.

GENERIC NAME

Bisoprolol

BRAND NAME

Zebeta

No generic available

ABOUT THIS DRUG

Bisoprolol is a beta-blocker that is used primarily to treat high blood pressure.

This drug slows the heart rate and the force of heart contractions by blocking certain nerve impulses. This results in a reduction in blood pressure.

SIDE EFFECTS

Be sure to tell your health-care practitioner if you experience any side effects while taking bisoprolol. Only your health-care practitioner can determine whether it is safe for you to continue taking this drug.

- ➤ *Most Common:* impotence, dizziness, especially when rising suddenly to a standing position, rapid heartbeat, fatigue, weakness, drowsiness, insomnia
- ➤ *Less Common or Rare:* anxiety, irritability, nervousness, constipation, diarrhea, dry eyes, itching, nausea, vomiting, nightmares, numbness or tingling in the fingers, toes, or scalp, shortness of breath, wheezing, chest pain, swelling of the ankles and lower legs, depression

IMPORTANT PRECAUTIONS

Tell your health-care practitioner if you are sensitive or allergic to bisoprolol or any other drugs, especially other beta-blockers.

If you have angina, you risk aggravating your angina if you suddenly stop taking this drug. Your health-care practitioner will gradually decrease your dosage over 1 to 2 weeks.

Bisoprolol should be used with caution if you have liver or kidney disease, thyroid disease, blood vessel disease, asthma, or a history of heart disease.

If you have diabetes, consult your health-care practitioner before using this drug. Bisoprolol may mask symptoms of low blood sugar (hypoglycemia).

If you plan to undergo major surgery, your health-care practitioner may ask you to stop taking bisoprolol at least 2 days before your surgery.

DRUG INTERACTIONS

Tell your health-care practitioner and pharmacist about any prescription and nonprescription drugs you are taking, as well as any vitamins, herbs, and other supplements. Possible drug interactions include the following:

- Bisoprolol may increase the blood-pressure-lowering effects of other blood-pressure-reducing drugs such as clonidine, guanabenz, reserpine, and calcium-channel blockers (e.g., nifedipine).
- Aspirin and aspirin-containing drugs, estrogen drugs, indomethacin, and sulfinpyrazone may hinder the blood-pressure-reducing effect of bisoprolol.
- Bisoprolol and ergot alkaloids (e.g., pergolide) may result in a worsening of cold hands and feet. Gangrene is also possible.
- Bisoprolol may cover up signs of inadequate thyroid hormone replacement.
- Bisoprolol may reduce the effectiveness of some antiasthma drugs, including aminophylline, ephedrine, isoproterenol, and theophylline.
- Digitalis or phenytoin along with bisoprolol may cause excessive slowing of the heart and possibly cause heart block.
- Calcium-channel blockers, flecainide, haloperidol, hydralazine, oral contraceptives, phenothiazine tranquilizers (e.g., molindone), propafenone, quinidine, and quinolone antibacterial drugs may elevate the amount of bisoprolol in the bloodstream and increase its effects.
- Cimetidine increase the amount of bisoprolol that is absorbed.

FOOD, VITAMIN, AND HERBAL INTERACTIONS

Bisoprolol does not interact negatively with any food. However, it is best to avoid excessive salt intake if you have high blood pressure. If you plan to or are taking any herbs or supplements, talk with your health-care practitioner before starting bisoprolol. Ginseng, goldenseal, licorice, ephedra (ma huang), and saw palmetto may raise your blood pressure; garlic and calcium may help lower it.

RECOMMENDED DOSAGE

Bisoprolol is available in 2.5-, 5-, and 10-mg tablets. The dosages given here are typical; however, only your health-care practitioner can determine the most appropriate dosage and schedule for you.

- *Children Up to 18 Years:* Not indicated for children.
- *Adults Up to Age 65:* Starting dose is 5 mg once daily, which may be gradually increased up to 20 mg daily. Individuals who have kidney or liver disease may need only 2.5 mg daily to start.
- *Adults 65 and Older:* Lower doses may be appropriate; your health-care practitioner will determine the dosage.

If you miss a dose, take it as soon as you remember. If it is nearly time for your next dose, do not take the missed dose. Continue with your regular dosing schedule. It is best to take bisoprolol at the same time every day. Never take a double dose.

Do not suddenly stop taking bisoprolol unless advised to do so by your health-care practitioner. Bisoprolol can be taken with or without food.

SYMPTOMS OF OVERDOSE AND WHAT TO DO

Symptoms of overdose include severe dizziness or fainting, breathing difficulties, seizures, bluish-colored fingernails or palms, and unusually slow, unusually fast, or irregular heartbeat. If overdose occurs, seek immediate medical attention and bring the prescription container with you to the hospital.

SPECIAL INFORMATION FOR PREGNANT OR NURSING WOMEN

Infants born to women who took beta-blockers while pregnant have been born with low birth weights, low blood pressure, and reduced heart rates. If you are pregnant or plan to become pregnant, talk with your health-care practitioner before starting bisoprolol. It should be avoided during pregnancy.

It's not known whether bisoprolol passes into breast milk. If bisoprolol is necessary for your health, your health-care practitioner may advise you to stop breastfeeding until your treatment is complete.

SPECIAL INFORMATION FOR SENIORS

Seniors are more likely to experience cold hands and feet, reduced body temperature, sudden breathing difficulties, chest pain, changes in heartbeat, and increased sweating.

GENERIC NAME

Class: Bisphosphonates

Generics: (1) alendronate, (2) etidronate, (3) ibandronate, (4) risedronate, (5) tiludronate

BRAND NAMES

(1) Fosamax, (2) Didronel, (3) Boniva, (4) Actonel, (5) Skelid
No generic available

ABOUT THIS DRUG

The bisphosphonates are bone resorption inhibitors that are used primarily to treat osteoporosis in postmenopausal women and Paget's disease (rapid breakdown and reformation of bone).

Bisphosphonates help prevent the loss of bone mass and can help make bones stronger, although experts are not sure how they accomplish these goals.

SIDE EFFECTS

Be sure to tell your health-care practitioner if you experience any side effects while taking bisphosphonates. Only your health-care practitioner can determine whether it is safe for you to continue taking these drugs.

Alendronate

- *Most Common:* pain, indigestion, nausea
- *Common:* abdominal pain, gas, back pain, stomach ulcers
- *Less Common or Rare:* constipation, diarrhea, difficulty swallowing, headache, flu-like symptoms, upset stomach, swelling in legs and arms, vomiting, change in taste

Etidronate

- *Most Common:* fever
- *Common:* nausea, flu-like symptoms
- *Less Common or Rare:* allergic reactions (itching, rash, sudden swelling that goes away by itself), convulsions, constipation, inflamed lining of the mouth, low blood levels of phosphate or magnesium, breathing difficulties, changes in taste

Ibandronate

- *Most Common:* back pain, heartburn, upper respiratory infection
- *Common:* diarrhea, headache, high cholesterol, muscle pain, pain in extremities, urinary tract infection

Risedronate

- *Most Common:* abdominal pain, headache, diarrhea, severe joint pain
- *Common:* chest pain, constipation, dizziness, nausea, bone pain, sinus irritation, swelling in the arms or legs
- *Less Common or Rare:* bronchitis, buzzing or ringing in the ears, infection, rash, tooth problems, leg cramps, weakness, poor vision in one eye, dry eyes, fatigue, vitamin D deficiency

Tiludronate

- *Most Common:* diarrhea, nausea
- *Common:* headache, fluid in the lungs, respiratory infection, runny nose, sinus irritation, upset stomach
- *Less Common or Rare:* cough, dizziness, aches and pains, cataracts, eye redness, glaucoma, rash, tooth problems, tingling in the hands or feet, vitamin D deficiency, muscle aches, fatigue, high blood pressure, fainting, appetite loss, constipation, abdominal pain, sleeplessness, vomiting

IMPORTANT PRECAUTIONS

Tell your health-care practitioner if you are sensitive or allergic to any of the bisphosphonates or any other drugs.

To reduce the risk of throat or stomach irritation, do not lie down for at least 30 minutes after you take alendronate or risedronate.

Bisphosphonates are generally not given to children. Men with osteoporosis may benefit from these drugs.

If you have severe kidney disease or active stomach or intestinal disease, do not take bisphosphonates because they can worsen your condition.

Alendronate is not recommended for women who are taking hormone replacement therapy. If you have low blood calcium levels and/or vitamin D deficiency, they must be treated before you begin taking alendronate.

DRUG INTERACTIONS

Tell your health-care practitioner and pharmacist about any prescription and nonprescription drugs you are taking, as well as any vitamins, herbs, or other supplements. Possible drug interactions with bisphosphonates may include the following:

- Antacids can interfere with the absorption of bisphosphonates. Take these two types of drugs at least 30 minutes apart.
- Aluminum-containing antacids should be taken at least 1 hour before or after tiludronate.
- Aspirin or other nonsteroidal anti-inflammatory drugs (NSAIDs; e.g., ibuprofen, naproxen) taken along with alendronate increase the risk of developing intestinal or stomach side effects.
- Aspirin can interfere with the absorption of tiludronate.
- Indomethacin can increase the blood levels of tiludronate by 2 to 4 times.

- Warfarin may interact with etidronate; talk to your health-care practitioner.

FOOD, VITAMIN, AND HERBAL INTERACTIONS

Any kind of food or drink, even mineral water, can interfere with the absorption of these drugs. See "Recommended Dosage" for directions on how to take these drugs. Consumption of supplements that contain calcium, vitamin D, iron, magnesium, or aluminum, as well as foods high in calcium (e.g., milk, cheese, yogurt), should be consumed at least 2 hours before or after taking bisphosphonates.

RECOMMENDED DOSAGE

Bisphosphonates are available in tablet form. The dosages given here are typical; however, your health-care practitioner will determine the most appropriate dosage and schedule for you.

Alendronate

- *Children:* Not recommended for children
- *Adults:* 10 to 40 mg daily; or 70 mg once weekly

Etidronate

- *Children:* Not recommended for children
- *Adults:* Starting dose, up to 4.5 mg per pound of body weight, gradually increasing to no more than 9 mg per pound of body weight, daily

Ibandronate

- *Children:* Not recommended for children
- *Adults:* 2.5 mg tablet once daily

Risedronate

- *Children:* Not recommended for children
- *Adults:* 30 mg daily

Tiludronate

- *Children:* Not recommended for children
- *Adults:* 480 mg daily

Bisphosphonates should be taken with 6 to 8 ounces of plain water only. Alendronate and risedronate should be taken every morning at least 30 minutes before eating, drinking, or taking any type of medications or supplements, or once weekly if taking the 70-mg dosage, following the same guidelines. Etidronate should be taken at least 2 hours before a meal on an empty stomach. Tiludronate should be taken immediately after getting up in the morning, and you must wait at least 4 hours before eating. Ibandronate should be taken at least 60 minutes before the first food or drink of the day and before you take any oral medications or supplements.

If you miss a dose, take it as soon as you remember. If it is nearly time for your next dose, do not take the missed dose. Continue with your regular schedule. Never take a double dose. If you forget to take a morning dose and you take it later that day, you must follow the dosing instructions concerning intake of food or other substances.

SYMPTOMS OF OVERDOSE AND WHAT TO DO

There is little information about overdosing with bisphosphonates. Symptoms include very low blood-calcium levels, upset stomach, heartburn, irritation of the esophagus, and ulcers. If overdose occurs, seek immediate medical attention. Bring the prescription container with you to the hospital.

SPECIAL INFORMATION FOR PREGNANT OR NURSING WOMEN

Bisphosphonates cause abnormal bone structure in animal fetuses and are toxic to pregnant animals. If you are pregnant or plan to become pregnant, talk to your health-care practitioner. If any of these drugs are considered to be crucial for your health, you and your health-care practitioner will need to weigh the potential benefits against the potential risks to the fetus.

It is not known whether bisphosphonates pass into breast milk. If you are breastfeeding, your health-care practitioner may advise you to stop until your treatment is completed.

SPECIAL INFORMATION FOR SENIORS

No special instructions are needed for seniors.

OPEN QUESTIONS OR CONTROVERSIES

Several recent studies have indicated that once-weekly administration of alendronate and risedronate are as effective as daily treatments. At the 83rd Annual Meeting of the Endocrine Soci-

(continued from page 204)
ety in June 2001, Dr. Sunil J. Wimalawansa of the Robert Wood Johnson Medical School in New Brunswick, New Jersey, reported that postmenopausal women who took alendronate once a week for four years (two years at 60 mg once weekly and then either 60 or 40 mg once weekly for two more years) showed the same increase in bone density as women who took 10 mg daily for four years. The women in the once-weekly group also experienced fewer upper gastrointestinal side effects than the once-daily group.

In another study, reported in November 2001, 35 mg of risedronate given once weekly to postmenopausal women with osteoporosis was as effective as 5 mg taken daily. The one-year study also showed a similar incidence of side effects in both groups.

Compliance is better when individuals take a medication weekly rather than daily. Women who are prescribed either alendronate or risedronate should discuss the once-weekly option with their health-care practitioners.

GENERIC NAME

Bitolterol

BRAND NAME

Tornalate

No generic available

ABOUT THIS DRUG

Bitolterol is a bronchodilator used to treat asthma, bronchospasm, and chronic obstructive pulmonary disease (COPD). It can be used as needed to treat asthma attacks or regularly to help prevent them.

Bitolterol relaxes the smooth muscles that surround the bronchial airways, which opens up constricted air passages and makes breathing easier.

SIDE EFFECTS

Be sure to tell your health-care practitioner if you experience any side effects while taking bitolterol. Only your health-care practitioner can determine whether it is safe for you to continue taking this drug.

- *Most Common:* cough, dry or sore throat, tremors
- *Common:* restlessness, weakness, anxiety, nausea, vomiting, nervousness, dizziness, sweating, muscle cramps
- *Less Common or Rare:* angina, abnormal heart rhythm, heart palpitations, breathing problems, bronchospasm, flushing, lightheadedness, abnormal liver tests and urine protein tests

IMPORTANT PRECAUTIONS

Tell your health-care practitioner if you are sensitive or allergic to bitolterol or to other drugs.

If you use this drug too often, you may develop severe, persistent breathing difficulties, such as wheezing, coughing, and shortness of breath, plus an inability to speak, confusion, and bluish color to the lips or fingernails. Heart attacks have occurred in extreme cases. Seek immediate medical assistance.

Because this drug can cause dizziness and nervousness, make sure you know how you react to the drug before you drive or operate hazardous equipment.

If you have a history of angina, diabetes, heart disease, high blood pressure, glaucoma, stroke, seizures, or prostate disease, use this drug with caution.

DRUG INTERACTIONS

Let your health-care practitioner and pharmacist know about any prescription and nonprescription drugs you are taking, as well as any vitamins, herbs, or other supplements. Possible drug interactions include the following:

- Monoamine oxidase inhibitors (MAOIs; e.g., phenelzine), thyroid drugs, other bronchodilators, and some antihistamines may increase the effects of bitolterol.
- Theophylline along with bitolterol may increase the risk of heart damage.
- Bitolterol may antagonize the effects of guanethidine, reserpine, methyldopa, and other blood-pressure-lowering drugs.
- Beta-blockers (e.g., propranolol, acebutolol) may antagonize bitolterol.
- If you are also taking a steroid inhaler, take bitolterol first. Wait about 15 minutes before you use the steroid inhaler.

FOOD, VITAMIN, AND HERBAL INTERACTIONS

No food, vitamin, or herbal interactions have been noted.

RECOMMENDED DOSAGE

Bitolterol is available as an inhalant. The dosages given here are typical. However, your health-care practitioner will determine the most appropriate dosage and schedule for your needs.

- *Children Younger than Age 12:* Not recommended for children under age 12.
- *Children Age 12 and Older and Adults:* To treat an attack, take 2 inhalations at least 1 to 3 minutes apart, followed by a third inhalation if needed. To prevent an attack, take 2 inhalations every 8 hours. The maximum is 3 inhalations in 6 hours or 2 every 4 hours.

Inhale the drug during the second half of your inward breath to allow the medication to reach deeper into your lungs.

If you miss a dose, take it as soon as you remember. If it is nearly time for your next dose, do not take the missed dose. Continue with your regular dosing schedule. Never take a double dose.

SYMPTOMS OF OVERDOSE AND WHAT TO DO

Symptoms of overdose include exaggerated side effects as well as chest pain and high blood pressure. If overdose occurs, seek immediate medical attention, and bring the prescription container with you to the hospital.

SPECIAL INFORMATION FOR PREGNANT OR NURSING WOMEN

No adequate studies of the effects of bitolterol on pregnant or nursing women have been done. If you are pregnant or plan to become pregnant, talk to your health-care practitioner. You and your health-care practitioner need to weigh the potential benefits against the potential risks.

Bitolterol passes into breast milk. If you are breastfeeding, your health-care practitioner will advise you to stop until your treatment is complete.

SPECIAL INFORMATION FOR SENIORS

Older adults are more likely to experience side effects, and they may be more severe.

GENERIC NAME
Brimonidine

BRAND NAME
Alphagan
No generic available

ABOUT THIS DRUG
Brimonidine is an alpha agonist used to treat glaucoma, an eye disorder characterized by increased pressure within the eyeball. Severe or complete loss of vision can result.

This drug reduces the production of fluids in the eye and promotes the flow of fluids out of the eye, which reduces intraocular pressure.

SIDE EFFECTS
Be sure to tell your health-care practitioner if you experience any side effects while taking brimonidine. Only your health-care practitioner can determine whether it is safe for you to continue taking this drug.

- *Most Common:* burning, redness, and stinging of the eyes, dry mouth, headache, blurred vision, drowsiness, eye allergy and itching
- *Common:* unusual sensitivity to bright light, eyelid swelling and redness, eye pain, dry eye, respiratory symptoms, dizziness, upset stomach, weakness, abnormal vision, muscle pain
- *Less Common:* crusty eyelids, abnormal taste, eye bleeding, sleeplessness, high blood pressure, heart palpitations, dry nose, fainting, anxiety

IMPORTANT PRECAUTIONS
Tell your health-care practitioner if you are sensitive or allergic to brimonidine or to any other drugs.

If you have cardiovascular disease, kidney or liver disease, depression, cerebral or coronary insufficiency, or Raynaud's disease, or if you experience dizziness or fainting when you rise from a lying or sitting position, you should exercise caution when using this drug.

Because brimonidine's effectiveness can diminish over time, you need to have periodic checkups to make sure the drug is still working.

If you wear soft contacts, take them out before you administer the drops. Wait at least 15 minutes after you put in the drops before you put your lenses back in.

DRUG INTERACTIONS

Tell your health-care practitioner and pharmacist about any prescription or over-the-counter drugs you are taking, as well as any vitamins, herbs, or other supplements. Possible drug interactions include the following:

- Tricyclic antidepressants (e.g., amitriptyline, imipramine) may increase the breakdown of brimonidine.
- Brimonidine may increase the effects of alcohol, barbiturates, sedatives, anesthetics, beta-blockers, blood-pressure-lowering medications, and cardiac glycosides.

FOOD, VITAMIN, AND HERBAL INTERACTIONS

No food, vitamin, or herbal interactions have been noted.

RECOMMENDED DOSAGE

Brimonidine is available in eye drops. The dosage given here is typical. However, your health-care practitioner will determine the most appropriate dosage and schedule for you.

- *Children:* Not recommended for children younger than 12 years
- *Children Older than 12 Years and Adults:* 1 drop in the affected eye every 8 hours, three times daily

If you miss a dose, take it as soon as you remember. If it is nearly time for your next dose, do not take the missed dose. Continue with your regular dosing schedule. Never take a double dose.

To avoid contamination and spread of infection, do not allow the dropper to touch the eye or any surface. Do not rinse the dropper with water or any other substance.

SYMPTOMS OF OVERDOSE AND WHAT TO DO

No cases of overdose have been reported. If you accidentally put too much of the medication in your eye, flush the eye with cool water. If the liquid is ingested, seek immediate medical assistance. Bring the prescription container with you to the hospital.

SPECIAL INFORMATION FOR PREGNANT OR NURSING WOMEN

No adequate studies of the effects of brimonidine on pregnant or nursing women have been conducted. If you are pregnant or plan to become pregnant, talk to your health-care practitioner before you use this drug. You and your health-care practitioner must weigh the potential risks against the potential benefits.

If you are breastfeeding, your health-care practitioner may advise you to stop until your treatment is complete.

SPECIAL INFORMATION FOR SENIORS
Older adults are more likely to experience side effects, and they may be more severe.

GENERIC NAME
Brompheniramine *see Antihistamine-Decongestant Combination, page 000*

GENERIC NAME
Budesonide *see also* ***Corticosteroids, Nasal Inhalation****, page 327;* ***Corticosteroids, Oral Inhalers****, page 334*

BRAND NAMES
Rhinocort, Pulmicort Turbuhaler, Rhinocort Nasal Inhaler, Pulmicort Respules, Entocort EC
No generic available

ABOUT THIS DRUG
Budesonide is a corticosteroid that is used to reduce inflammation in two different types of medical conditions. One is respiratory-related disorders, including bronchial asthma that does not respond to bronchodilators; and both seasonal and perennial rhinitis (allergies). The other is mild-to-moderate, active Crohn's disease, an inflammatory condition of the intestinal tract.

In respiratory cases, budesonide reduces or prevents inflammation of the lining of the airways and reduces allergic response to inhaled allergens. In Crohn's disease, it reduces inflammation of the small and large intestines.

SIDE EFFECTS
Be sure to tell your health-care practitioner if you experience any side effects while taking budesonide. Only your health-care practitioner can determine whether it is safe for you to continue taking this drug.

- *Most Common:* fungus infections of the mouth and throat (thrush), stinging sensation in the nose (when using nasal form), suppressed adrenal gland function

- *Less Common or Rare:* dry mouth, sore throat, cough, headache, nausea, hoarseness, rash, nosebleed, weight gain, osteoporosis, slowed growth (in children), increased susceptibility to chicken pox, increased risk of cataracts, allergic pneumonitis (lung inflammation), bronchospasm, asthmatic wheezing, nose perforation

IMPORTANT PRECAUTIONS

Tell your health-care practitioner if you are sensitive or allergic to budesonide or to any other drugs.

Do not take budesonide if you have severe acute asthma or status asthmaticus for which you need more intense treatment; if you can control your asthma with other antiasthmatic drugs that are not related to cortisone; or if you need cortisone-like drugs infrequently to control your asthma.

If you have a history of tuberculosis of the lungs, have recently been exposed to chicken pox or other viral illnesses, or have nose ulcers, chronic bronchitis, bronchiectasis, any type of respiratory infection, herpes of the eye, or liver damage, talk to your health-care practitioner before taking budesonide.

Tell your health-care practitioner if you are taking or recently took any cortisone-related drugs for any condition.

DRUG INTERACTIONS

Tell your health-care practitioner and pharmacist about any prescription and nonprescription drugs you are taking, as well as any vitamins, herbs, or other supplements. Possible drug interactions include the following:

- Oral bronchodilators (e.g., aminophylline, ephedrine), inhalant bronchodilators (e.g., epinephrine, isoetharine), methylphenidate, and some antiepileptic drugs (e.g., phenytoin) may increase the effects of budesonide.
- Methylphenidate and budesonide together can cause increased growth suppression in children.
- Some antiepileptic drugs can increase the risk of osteoporosis.

FOOD, VITAMIN, AND HERBAL INTERACTIONS

The oral and nasal forms of budesonide are not known to react with foods or vitamins. If you take the capsule form (Entocort EC), do not take it with grapefruit juice, and do not consume grapefruit juice anytime while you are on budesonide, because toxic reactions may occur.

Because both St. John's wort and budesonide are metabolized by the liver, there is a possibility that budesonide may be less effective if you take it with St. John's wort.

RECOMMENDED DOSAGE

Budesonide comes in the following forms and strengths: nasal inhaler, oral inhaler, spacer form, Turbuhaler, nebulized form (jet nebulizer), and capsules. The dosages listed below are typical; however, your health-care practitioner will determine the actual dose and schedule that best fits your needs.

- *Infants and Children 1 to 8 Years:* For maintenance treatment of asthma and preventive therapy, budesonide inhalation suspension is a nebulized formulation. The recommended dose ranges from 0.5 to 1 mg daily in one or two doses, based on your health-care practitioner's assessment.
- *Children 6 Years and Older:* For seasonal rhinitis, use the nasal inhaler: 2 inhalations in each nostril twice daily (morning and evening) or 4 inhalations in each nostril in the morning (256 mcg maximum daily).
- For perennial allergic rhinitis, use the same dosage, but check with your health-care practitioner as the inhaler actually releases 50 mcg rather than the 32 mcg recommended dose.
- For asthma: oral inhaler (dosage to be determined based on prior treatment): (1) bronchodilators alone, 200 mcg twice daily; (2) oral corticosteroids, 400 mcg twice daily; (3) inhaled corticosteroids, 200 mcg twice daily. Children younger than 12 years receive one puff or 0.2 mg twice daily (maximum, 2 puffs daily, or 0.8 mg).
- *Adults:* For seasonal rhinitis, use the nasal inhaler, 2 inhalations in each nostril twice daily (morning and evening) or 4 inhalations once in the morning (maximum, 256 mcg daily). Your health-care practitioner should check the effectiveness of the treatment after 3 to 7 days. If you are not getting a significant response after 3 weeks of treatment, you should stop the drug.
- For perennial rhinitis, take the same dose as for seasonal rhinitis. Consult with your health-care practitioner, because the inhaler actually releases 50 mcg rather than the 32 mcg recommended. The dose can be adjusted, with the guidance of your health-care practitioner, as your symptoms improve or if they return.
- For asthma (actual dosage based on prior treatment): if you are receiving (1) bronchodilators alone, take 200 to 400 mcg twice daily; (2) oral corticosteroids, 400 to 800 mcg twice daily; or (3) inhaled corticosteroids, 200 to 400 mcg twice daily. If you can control your asthma using oral corticosteroids, the budesonide inhaler must be used at the same time as the oral corticosteroids for about 7 days, after which you can gradually reduce the oral corticosteroids.
- *Adults 65 Years and Older:* Use dosing similar to that used for children.

- For treatment of Crohn's disease in adults, the recommended dosage is three 3-mg capsules taken in the morning for 8 weeks. See "Open Questions and Controversies."

Budesonide can be taken with or without food. After each use, always rinse your mouth and gargle with water.

If you miss a dose, take it as soon as you remember. If it is nearly time for your next dose, do not take the missed dose. Continue with your regular dosing schedule. Never take a double dose.

SYMPTOMS OF OVERDOSE AND WHAT TO DO

Symptoms of overdose include fluid retention, stomach irritation, nervousness, and flushing of the face. If overdose occurs, seek immediate medical attention and bring the prescription container with you to the hospital.

SPECIAL INFORMATION FOR PREGNANT OR NURSING WOMEN

No adequate studies of the effects of budesonide on pregnant or nursing women have been done. If you are pregnant or plan to become pregnant, talk to your health-care practitioner. You and your health-care practitioner need to weigh the potential risks against the potential benefits of this drug.

If you are breastfeeding, your health-care practitioner may advise you to stop while you are under treatment.

SPECIAL INFORMATION FOR SENIORS

If you are older than 60 years and you have bronchiectasis, you should be monitored closely by your health-care practitioner if you take budesonide. If you have osteoporosis or cataracts or are at risk for these conditions, use of this drug increases the risk of both problems. Tell your health-care practitioner if you have a bone disease, a gastrointestinal disorder, diabetes, glaucoma, fungal or herpes infection, high blood pressure, high cholesterol, hypothyroid, or heart, kidney, or liver disease.

OPEN QUESTIONS OR CONTROVERSIES

Entocort EC was approved by the FDA in October 2001 for the treatment of mild-to-moderate Crohn's disease, based on the results of five clinical trials involving a total of approximately 1,000 patients whose Crohn's disease involved the ileum and/or

(continued from page 213)
ascending colon. Between 48 and 69 percent of the patients treated with Entocort EC (9 mg once daily) improved clinically after eight weeks. No longer-term studies have been done. Therefore, as of February 2002, there was no research to validate the safety or efficacy of Entocort EC past 8 weeks of treatment.

GENERIC NAME

Bumetanide

see Loop Diuretics, page 622

GENERIC NAME

Bupropion

BRAND NAMES

Wellbutrin, Wellbutrin-SR, Zyban
No generic available

ABOUT THIS DRUG

Bupropion serves two primary purposes. One is as an antidepressant in the treatment of major depression. The other is as a nicotine-free agent to help people stop smoking.

In the treatment of depression, bupropion appears to help balance the levels of brain chemicals (neurotransmitters) that are likely associated with emotions, mental state, and mood. As a smoking deterrent, it seems to help reduce the desire for nicotine.

SIDE EFFECTS

Be sure to tell your health-care practitioner if you experience any side effects while taking bupropion. Only your health-care practitioner can determine whether it is safe for you to continue taking this drug. The side effects differ depending on whether the drug is used for depression or smoking cessation.

- *Most Common:* For depression: nausea, vomiting, constipation, unusual weight loss, dry mouth, loss of appetite, dizziness, increased sweating, trembling. For smoking cessation: dry mouth, insomnia, abdominal pain, anxiety, constipation, diarrhea, dizziness, joint pain, itching, nasal inflammation
- *Less Common or Rare:* For depression: acne, blisters in the mouth and eyes, chills, fever, difficulty concentrating, drowsiness, fatigue,

blurred vision, impotence, indigestion, ringing in the ears, sexual dysfunction, unusual euphoria, hostility, hallucinations, irregular heartbeat, confusion, rash, insomnia, severe headache, seizures. For smoking cessation: rash, tremor, chest pain, thirst, swelling of the face, increased blood pressure, mouth ulcers, bronchitis, changes in taste, dry skin, throbbing heartbeat

IMPORTANT PRECAUTIONS

Tell your health-care practitioner if you are sensitive or allergic to bupropion or to any other drugs.

Bupropion should not be taken if you have a history of seizures, anorexia nervosa, bulimia, or addiction to narcotics, cocaine, or alcohol.

Talk to your health-care practitioner before using this drug if you have a brain or spinal cord tumor, heart disease, liver or kidney disease, or head injury.

Because bupropion can cause dizziness or shaking, make sure you know how you react to this drug before you drive or operate hazardous equipment.

About 28 percent of people who take bupropion for depression lose 5 pounds or more. If weight loss can be injurious to your health, bupropion may not be the proper antidepressant drug for you.

DRUG INTERACTIONS

Tell your health-care practitioner and pharmacist about any prescription and nonprescription drugs you are taking, as well as any vitamins, herbs, or other supplements. Possible drug interactions include the following:

- Bupropion should not be taken with any other medications that contain bupropion (e.g., Zyban to stop smoking and Wellbutrin for depression).
- Carbamazepine may reduce the blood levels of bupropion.
- Levodopa can increase the side effects of both levodopa and bupropion.
- Phenelzine (a monoamine oxidase inhibitor; MAOI) increases the risk of bupropion's side effects. Allow at least 2 weeks between stopping phenelzine or any other MAOI and starting bupropion.
- Haloperidol, lithium, loxapine, molindone, phenothiazine tranquilizers (e.g., chlorpromazine, promazine), thioxanthene tranquilizers (e.g., thiothixene), and tricyclic antidepressants (e.g., imipramine, amitriptyline) increase the risk of seizures.

- Nicotine patches can raise your blood pressure. Tell your health-care practitioner if you plan to use both a nicotine patch and bupropion to stop smoking.

FOOD, VITAMIN, AND HERBAL INTERACTIONS

No food, vitamin, or herb interactions have been reported.

RECOMMENDED DOSAGE

Bupropion is available in tablets and extended release tablets. The dosages given here are typical. However, your health-care practitioner will determine the most appropriate dose and schedule for you.

For Depression

- *Children:* The safety and effectiveness have not been determined.
- *Adults:* Starting dose is 100 mg twice daily, increased by your health-care practitioner to 100 mg three times daily. The maximum is 150 mg three times daily. If you use the extended release tablets, starting dose is 150 mg daily, increased to 150 mg twice daily. The maximum recommended dose is 200 mg twice daily.

For Smoking Cessation

- *Children:* The safety and effectiveness have not been determined.
- *Adults:* Starting dose is 150 mg in the morning, increased to 150 mg twice daily (morning and early evening). The maximum recommended dose is 300 mg. This program can continue for 7 to 12 weeks.

If you miss a dose, take it as soon as you remember. If it is nearly time for your next dose, do not take the missed dose. Continue with your regular dosing schedule. Never take a double dose.

SYMPTOMS OF OVERDOSE AND WHAT TO DO

Symptoms of overdose when treating for depression include hallucinations, seizures, chest pain, breathing difficulties, rapid heartbeat, and loss of consciousness. When treating for smoking cessation, reported symptoms of overdose include blurred vision, confusion, nausea, jitteriness, hallucinations, seizures, drowsiness, and vomiting. If overdose occurs, seek immediate medical attention, and bring the prescription container with you to the hospital.

SPECIAL INFORMATION FOR PREGNANT OR NURSING WOMEN

No adequate studies have been done on the effects of bupropion on pregnant or nursing women. If you are pregnant or plan to become pregnant, talk to your health-care practitioner. You and your health-care practitioner can weigh the potential risks against the potential benefits of this drug.

Bupropion passes into breast milk. If you are breastfeeding, your health-care practitioner may advise you to stop until you complete treatment.

SPECIAL INFORMATION FOR SENIORS

Older adults who have liver or kidney conditions may need a lower dose.

OPEN QUESTIONS OR CONTROVERSIES

In June 2004, the Food and Drug Administration asked manufacturers of bupropion to include in their labeling a warning statement that recommends close observation of adult and pediatric patients for clinical worsening of depression or the emergence of suicidality when being treated with this drug, especially when beginning the drug, or at the time of dose changes, either increases or decreases.

GENERIC NAME

Buspirone

BRAND NAME

BuSpar
Generic available

ABOUT THIS DRUG

Buspirone is a mild tranquilizer and an antianxiety drug used to treat anxiety.

This drug affects the activity of brain chemicals (especially serotonin and dopamine) that are associated with emotions, mental state, and mood. Unlike many other drugs used to treat anxiety, buspirone does not appear to cause physical dependence.

SIDE EFFECTS

Be sure to tell your health-care practitioner if you experience any side effects while taking buspirone. Only your health-care practitioner can determine whether it is safe for you to continue taking this drug.

- *Most Common:* dizziness, nausea, headache, fatigue, nervousness, excitement
- *Common:* rash, clamminess, sweating, heart palpitations, muscle aches and pains
- *Less Common:* chest pain, low blood pressure, fainting, stroke, heart attack, heart failure, euphoria, sleeplessness, anger, depression, depersonalization, fear, stupor, slurred speech, intolerance to cold

IMPORTANT PRECAUTIONS

Tell your health-care practitioner if you are sensitive or allergic to buspirone or any other medications.

If you have liver or kidney disease, talk to your health-care practitioner before using buspirone.

Because buspirone may cause dizziness or fainting, make sure you know how you react to this drug before you drive or operate hazardous equipment.

DRUG INTERACTIONS

Tell your health-care practitioner and pharmacist about any prescription and nonprescription drugs you are taking, as well as any vitamins, herbs, or other supplements. Possible drug interactions include the following:

- Monoamine oxidase inhibitors (e.g., phenelzine) may cause severe hypertension and other dangerous side effects.
- The effects of central nervous system drugs (e.g., sedatives, antianxiety drugs, tranquilizers) on buspirone are unknown. These drugs should not be combined unless prescribed by your health-care practitioner.
- Alcohol may enhance drowsiness and dizziness.
- Buspirone may increase the side effects of haloperidol.
- Trazodone may cause liver inflammation.

FOOD, VITAMIN, AND HERBAL INTERACTIONS

Herbs that have a sedative effect may cause excessive physical depression, sedation, and impairment if taken along with buspirone. These herbs include ashwagandha, calendula, catnip, hops, kava, lady's slipper, lemon balm, passionflower, sassafras, skullcap, valerian, and herba mansa.

RECOMMENDED DOSAGE

Buspirone is available as a tablet. The dosages given here are typical. However, your health-care practitioner will determine the most appropriate dose and schedule for your needs.

- *Children Younger than 18 Years:* The safety and effectiveness have not been determined for children younger than 18.
- *Adults:* 5 mg three times daily. The maximum dosage is 60 mg daily.

If you miss a dose, take it as soon as you remember. If it is nearly time for your next dose, do not take the missed dose. Continue with your regular dosing schedule. Never take a double dose.

SYMPTOMS OF OVERDOSE AND WHAT TO DO

Symptoms of overdose include severe drowsiness, dizziness, nausea, vomiting, and pinpoint pupils. If overdose occurs, seek immediate medical attention and bring the prescription container with you to the hospital.

SPECIAL INFORMATION FOR PREGNANT OR NURSING WOMEN

No adequate studies of the effects of buspirone on pregnant or nursing women have been done. If you are pregnant or plan to become pregnant, talk to your health-care practitioner. You and your health-care practitioner can weigh the potential risks against the potential benefits of this drug.

Buspirone passes into breast milk. If you are breastfeeding, your health-care practitioner may advise you to stop until you have completed treatment.

SPECIAL INFORMATION FOR SENIORS

Side effects may be more common and more severe in older adults.

GENERIC NAME

Butalbital/acetaminophen/caffeine

BRAND NAMES

Esgic, Esgic-Plus, Femcet, Fioricet, Fiorpap, Isocet, Repan
Generic available

ABOUT THIS DRUG

Butalbital/acetaminophen/caffeine is a combination nonnarcotic analgesic used to treat headache and migraine that do not respond to nonprescription pain relievers.

Butalbital is a barbiturate that causes sedation and relieves pain; acetaminophen interferes with prostaglandins, naturally occurring substances that cause inflammation; and caffeine enhances the effectiveness of pain relievers.

SIDE EFFECTS

Be sure to tell your health-care practitioner if you experience any side effects while taking butalbital/acetaminophen/caffeine. Only your health-care practitioner can determine whether it is safe for you to continue taking this drug combination.

- *Most Common:* abdominal pain, lightheadedness, drowsiness, dizziness, nausea, vomiting, sweating, appetite loss
- *Less Common or Rare:* weakness, headache, upset stomach, agitation, tremor, hallucinations, disorientation, euphoria, dry mouth, constipation, sleeplessness, palpitations, urinary difficulties, rash, itching, confusion, rapid breathing, diarrhea

IMPORTANT PRECAUTIONS

Tell your health-care practitioner if you are sensitive or allergic to any of the components of this drug or to any other drugs.

Butalbital can cause physical dependence. Talk to your health-care practitioner about this possibility.

Long-term use of acetaminophen can cause liver damage.

DRUG INTERACTIONS

Tell your health-care practitioner and pharmacist about any prescription and nonprescription drugs you are taking, as well as any vitamins, herbs, or other supplements. The butalbital/ acetaminophen/ caffeine combination can interact with other drugs.

- Alcohol may cause symptoms of overdose.
- Alcohol, barbiturates, sleeping pills, tranquilizers, and other central nervous system depressants may cause drowsiness, tiredness, and concentration difficulties. Talk to your health-care practitioner before you take any other drugs with butalbital/acetaminophen/caffeine.

FOOD, VITAMIN, AND HERBAL INTERACTIONS

Herbs that have a sedative effect may cause excessive physical depression, sedation, and impairment if taken along with butalbital/ acetaminophen/caffeine combination. These herbs include ashwagandha, calendula, catnip, hops, kava, lady's slipper, lemon balm, passionflower, sassafras, skullcap, and valerian, among others.

RECOMMENDED DOSAGE

Butalbital/acetaminophen/caffeine combinations are available in tablets and capsules. The dosages given here are typical. However, your health-care practitioner will determine the most appropriate dose and schedule for you.

- *Children Younger than 12 Years:* The safety and effectiveness of this drug combination has not been established in children younger than 12 years.
- *Adults:* 1 to 2 tablets or capsules every 4 hours or as needed, according to your health-care practitioner's instructions.

The butalbital/acetaminophen/caffeine combination is most effective if taken on an empty stomach. However, it can be taken with food if it upsets your stomach.

If you miss a dose, take it as soon as you remember. If it is nearly time for your next dose, do not take the missed dose. Continue with your regular dosing schedule. Never take a double dose.

SYMPTOMS OF OVERDOSE AND WHAT TO DO

Symptoms of overdose include nervousness that progresses to stupor or coma, breathing difficulties, pinpoint pupils, cold and clammy skin, low blood pressure, nausea, vomiting, dizziness, ringing in the ears, facial flushing, sweating, and thirst. If overdose occurs, seek immediate medical attention and bring the prescription container with you to the hospital.

SPECIAL INFORMATION FOR PREGNANT OR NURSING WOMEN

The butalbital/acetaminophen/caffeine combination is associated with birth defects, delayed delivery, prolonged labor, and breathing problems for the newborn. If you are pregnant or plan to become pregnant, talk to your health-care practitioner immediately. Regular use of this drug combination during the last 3 months of pregnancy can result in drug dependency in the newborn.

This drug combination passes into breast milk. If you are breastfeeding, your health-care practitioner will likely advise you to stop until you have completed treatment. Infants who breastfeed with women who are taking butalbital/acetaminophen/caffeine may experience shortness of breath, slow heartbeat, or tiredness.

SPECIAL INFORMATION FOR SENIORS

Side effects may be more common and more severe in older adults. Especially troublesome may be lightheadedness, dizziness, or fainting when rising suddenly from a lying or sitting position.

GENERIC NAME

Butalbital/aspirin/caffeine

BRAND NAMES

Amaphen, Anoquan, Endolor, Esgic, Femcet, Fiorinal, Lanorinal, Margesic, Medigesic, Triad
Generic available

ABOUT THIS DRUG

Butalbital/aspirin/caffeine is a combination of a barbiturate (butalbital) and an analgesic (aspirin) used to relieve migraine and headache.

Butalbital is a barbiturate that causes sedation and relieves pain; aspirin interferes with prostaglandins, naturally occurring substances that cause inflammation; and caffeine enhances the effectiveness of pain relievers.

SIDE EFFECTS

Be sure to tell your health-care practitioner if you experience any side effects while taking butalbital/aspirin/caffeine. Only your health-care practitioner can determine whether it is safe for you to continue taking this drug combination.

- *Most Common:* lightheadedness, dizziness, sedation, nausea, vomiting, sweating, appetite loss, upset stomach
- *Less Common or Rare:* headache, sleeplessness, agitation, tremor, weakness, hallucinations, disorientation, euphoria, dry mouth, constipation, facial flushing, palpitations, urinary problems, rash, itching, confusion, rapid breathing, diarrhea

IMPORTANT PRECAUTIONS

Tell your health-care practitioner if you are sensitive or allergic to any of the components of this drug combination or to any other drugs.

Because it contains aspirin, this drug combination should not be taken by anyone younger than age 16 or if you develop dizziness, hearing loss, or ringing in the ears.

Butalbital/aspirin/caffeine should not be used if you have liver damage. Use it with extreme caution if you have asthma or other respiratory problems.

Long-term use of this drug combination can lead to drug dependence and addiction.

This drug combination may cause drowsiness and dizziness. Therefore, make sure you know how you react to the drug before you drive or operate hazardous equipment.

This drug contains aspirin, which may interfere with blood clotting. If you are planning to undergo surgery, tell your health-care practitioner or dentist you are taking this drug combination.

DRUG INTERACTIONS

Tell your health-care practitioner and pharmacist if you are taking any prescription or nonprescription drugs, as well as any vitamins, herbs, or other supplements. Possible drug interactions include the following:

- Corticosteroids (e.g., cortisone, prednisone), phenylbutazone, or alcohol may irritate your stomach and increase your risk of getting an ulcer.
- Butalbital/aspirin/caffeine may counteract the blood-pressure-lowering effects of angiotensin-converting enzymes inhibitors (e.g., captopril, enalapril) and beta-blockers (e.g., acebutolol, nadolol).
- Nonsteroidal anti-inflammatory drugs (NSAIDs; e.g., ibuprofen, naproxen) may increase the risk of side effects, especially stomach irritation.
- Butalbital/aspirin/caffeine may increase the side effects of methotrexate and valproic acid.
- Alcohol, barbiturates, sleeping pills, tranquilizers, and other central nervous system depressants may cause drowsiness, tiredness, and concentration difficulties.
- Nitroglycerine may lead to a sudden drop in blood pressure.

FOOD, VITAMIN, AND HERBAL INTERACTIONS

Herbs that have a sedative effect may cause excessive physical depression, sedation, and impairment if taken along with a butalbital/aspirin/caffeine combination. These herbs include ashwagandha, calendula, catnip, hops, kava, lady's slipper, lemon balm, passionflower, sassafras, skullcap, and valerian, among others.

RECOMMENDED DOSAGE

The butalbital/aspirin/caffeine combination drugs are available in tablets and capsules. The dosages given here are typical. However, your health-care practitioner will determine the most appropriate dose and schedule for you.

- *Children Younger than 16 Years:* This drug combination is not recommended for children younger than 16.
- *Adults:* 1 to 2 tablets or capsules every 4 hours or as needed and directed by your health-care practitioner.

Butalbital/aspirin/caffeine is most effective if taken on an empty stomach. However, take it with food if it causes stomach upset.

If you miss a dose, take it as soon as you remember. If it is nearly time for your next dose, do not take the missed dose. Continue with your regular dosing schedule. Never take a double dose.

SYMPTOMS OF OVERDOSE AND WHAT TO DO

Symptoms of overdose include nervousness that progresses to stupor or coma, pinpoint pupils, cold and clammy skin, breathing difficulties, low blood pressure, nausea, vomiting, dizziness, ringing in the ears, flushing, sweating, convulsions, liver or kidney failure, and thirst. If overdose occurs, seek immediate medical attention and bring the prescription container with you to the hospital.

SPECIAL INFORMATION FOR PREGNANT OR NURSING WOMEN

The butalbital/aspirin/caffeine combination is associated with birth defects, delayed delivery, prolonged labor, and breathing problems for the newborn. If you are pregnant or plan to become pregnant, talk to your health-care practitioner immediately. Regular use of this drug combination during the last 3 months of pregnancy can result in drug dependency in the newborn.

This drug combination passes into breast milk. If you are breastfeeding, your health-care practitioner will likely advise you to stop until you have completed treatment. Infants who breastfeed with women who are taking butalbital/aspirin/caffeine may experience shortness of breath, slow heartbeat, or tiredness.

SPECIAL INFORMATION FOR SENIORS

Side effects may be more common and more severe in older adults. Especially troublesome may be lightheadedness, dizziness, or fainting when rising suddenly from a lying or sitting position.

GENERIC NAME
Butalbital/aspirin/caffeine/codeine

BRAND NAMES
Ascomp with Codeine No. 3, Butalbital Compound with Codeine, Fiorinal with Codeine, Idenal with Codeine, Isollyl with Codeine
Generic available

ABOUT THIS DRUG
Butalbital/aspirin/caffeine/codeine is a combination of a barbiturate (butalbital), an analgesic (aspirin), and a narcotic analgesic (codeine) to treat migraine and headache.

The butalbital is a barbiturate that causes sedation and relieves pain; aspirin interferes with prostaglandins, naturally occurring substances that cause inflammation; caffeine enhances the effectiveness of pain relievers; and codeine blocks pain signals to the brain.

SIDE EFFECTS
Be sure to tell your health-care practitioner if you experience any side effects while taking butalbital/aspirin/caffeine/codeine. Only your health-care practitioner can determine whether it is safe for you to continue taking this drug combination.

- *Most Common:* drowsiness, flushed face, lightheadedness, depression, increased urination
- *Less Common or Rare:* insomnia, headache, constipation, increased sweating, unusual fatigue, nightmares, wheezing, tight chest, pinpoint pupils, vomiting blood, sore throat, fever, mouth sores, hearing loss, blood in urine

IMPORTANT PRECAUTIONS
Tell your health-care practitioner if you are sensitive or allergic to any of the components of this drug combination or to any other drugs.

Because it contains aspirin, this drug combination should not be taken by anyone younger than age 16 or if you develop dizziness, hearing loss, or ringing in the ears.

Butalbital/aspirin/caffeine/codeine should not be used if you have liver damage. Use it with extreme caution if you have asthma or other respiratory problems.

Long-term use of this drug combination can lead to drug dependence and addiction.

This drug combination may cause drowsiness and dizziness.

Therefore, make sure you know how you react to the drug before you drive or operate hazardous equipment.

This drug contains aspirin, which may interfere with blood clotting. If you are planning to undergo surgery, tell your health-care practitioner or dentist you are taking this drug combination.

DRUG INTERACTIONS

Tell your health-care practitioner and pharmacist about any prescription and nonprescription drugs you are taking, as well as any vitamins, herbs, and other supplements. Possible drug interactions include the following:

- Corticosteroids (e.g., cortisone, prednisone), phenylbutazone, or alcohol may irritate your stomach and increase your risk of getting an ulcer.
- Butalbital/aspirin/caffeine may counteract the blood-pressure-lowering effects of angiotensin-converting enzyme inhibitors (e.g., captopril, enalapril) and beta-blockers (e.g., acebutolol, nadolol).
- Nonsteroidal anti-inflammatory drugs (NSAIDs; e.g., ibuprofen, naproxen) may increase the risk of side effects, especially stomach irritation.
- Butalbital/aspirin/caffeine may increase the side effects of methotrexate and valproic acid.
- Alcohol, barbiturates, sleeping pills, tranquilizers, and other central nervous system depressants may cause drowsiness, tiredness, and concentration difficulties.
- Nitroglycerine may lead to a sudden drop in blood pressure.

FOOD, VITAMIN, AND HERBAL INTERACTIONS

Herbs that have a sedative effect may cause excessive physical depression, sedation, and impairment if taken along with a butalbital/aspirin/caffeine/codeine combination. These herbs include ashwagandha, calendula, catnip, hops, kava, lady's slipper, lemon balm, passionflower, sassafras, skullcap, and valerian, among others.

RECOMMENDED DOSAGE

Butalbital/aspirin/caffeine/codeine combinations are available in tablets and capsules. The dosages given here are typical. However, your health-care practitioner will determine the most appropriate dose and schedule to suit your needs.

- *Children Younger than 16 Years:* This drug combination is not recommended for children younger than 16.
- *Adults:* 1 or 2 tablets or capsules every 4 hours or as prescribed by your health-care practitioner.

Butalbital/aspirin/caffeine/codeine is most effective when taken on an empty stomach. However, you can take it with food if it causes stomach upset.

If you miss a dose, take it as soon as you remember. If it is nearly time for your next dose, do not take the missed dose. Continue with your regular dosing schedule. Never take a double dose.

SYMPTOMS OF OVERDOSE AND WHAT TO DO

Symptoms of overdose include nervousness that progresses to stupor or coma, pinpoint pupils, nausea, vomiting, dizziness, low blood pressure, cold clammy skin, ringing in the ears, flushing, sweating, thirst, breathing problems, convulsions, kidney or liver failure, and confusion. If overdose occurs, seek immediate medical attention and bring the prescription container with you to the hospital.

SPECIAL INFORMATION FOR PREGNANT OR NURSING WOMEN

The butalbital/aspirin/caffeine/codeine combination is associated with birth defects and may cause bleeding and breathing problems in the newborn. Pregnant women may experience prolonged labor, delayed delivery, and bleeding difficulties. If you are pregnant or plan to become pregnant, talk to your health-care practitioner immediately. Regular use of this drug combination during the last 3 months of pregnancy can result in drug dependency in the newborn.

This drug combination passes into breast milk. If you are breastfeeding, your health-care practitioner will likely advise you to stop until you have completed treatment. Infants who breastfeed with women who are taking butalbital/aspirin/ caffeine/codeine may experience shortness of breath, slow heartbeat, or tiredness.

SPECIAL INFORMATION FOR SENIORS

Side effects are more common and more severe in older adults. Especially be aware of lightheadedness, dizziness, or fainting when rising from a lying or seated position.

GENERIC NAME

Butenafine

BRAND NAME

Mentax

No generic available

ABOUT THIS DRUG

Butenafine is an antifungal medication used to treat tinea pedis (athlete's foot).

This medication prevents fungal organisms from producing the substances they need to reproduce and grow. Butenafine is effective only against fungi; it cannot kill bacteria or viruses.

SIDE EFFECTS

Be sure to tell your health-care practitioner if you experience any side effects while using butenafine. Only your health-care practitioner can determine whether it is safe for you to continue taking this drug.

- *Most Common:* burning, itching, redness, swelling, irritation at the application site

IMPORTANT PRECAUTIONS

Tell your health-care practitioner if you are sensitive or allergic to butenafine or to any other drugs, or if you have any medical conditions.

When applying butenafine, avoid all contact with your eyes, nose, and mouth. Wash your hands after applying the medication. If you don't notice some improvement within a few days, tell your health-care practitioner. The fungus causing your condition may be resistant to this drug.

Follow the full course of treatment prescribed by your health-care practitioner, even if your symptoms improve before treatment is done. Stopping too soon may cause the infection to return.

DRUG INTERACTIONS

Tell your health-care practitioner and pharmacist about any prescription and nonprescription drugs you are taking, as well as any vitamins, herbs, and other supplements. When you apply butenafine, do not combine it with any other medications.

FOOD, VITAMIN, AND HERBAL INTERACTIONS

No food, vitamin, or herbal interactions have been noted.

RECOMMENDED DOSAGE

Butenafine is available in a cream. The dosages given here are typical. However, your health-care practitioner will determine the most appropriate dose and schedule for you.

- *Children Younger than 12 Years:* Not recommended.

- ➤ *Children Older than 12 and Adults:* Apply enough cream to cover the affected area and the surrounding skin once daily for 4 weeks.

If you miss a dose, apply it as soon as you remember. If it is nearly time for your next dose, do not apply the missed dose. Continue with your regular dosing schedule. Do not apply a double dose.

SYMPTOMS OF OVERDOSE AND WHAT TO DO

No cases of overdose have been reported. If butenafine is accidentally ingested, seek immediate medical assistance and bring the prescription container with you to the hospital.

SPECIAL INFORMATION FOR PREGNANT OR NURSING WOMEN

No adequate studies of the effects of butenafine on pregnant or nursing women have been done. If you are pregnant or plan to become pregnant, talk to your health-care practitioner. You and your health-care practitioner can weigh the potential benefits against the potential risks.

It is not known whether butenafine passes into breast milk. If you are breastfeeding, your health-care practitioner may advise you to stop until your treatment is complete.

SPECIAL INFORMATION FOR SENIORS

No special instructions are needed for seniors.

GENERIC NAME

Butoconazole *see Miconazole, page 694*

GENERIC NAME

Calcitonin

BRAND NAMES

Calcimar, Miacalcin, Osteocalcin, Salmonine
No generic available

ABOUT THIS DRUG

The calcitonin in these drugs is a synthetic form of the naturally occurring hormone by the same name that is produced by the thyroid gland. Calcitonin is used primarily to prevent bone loss in postmenopausal women who have osteoporosis, and to treat Paget's disease, a disorder in which bone is broken down and restored too rapidly, causing fragile bone and malformation.

Calcitonin reduces the rate of calcium that is lost from bone and slows down the rate at which bone is broken down before it is replaced.

SIDE EFFECTS

Be sure to tell your health-care practitioner if you experience any side effects while taking calcitonin. Only your health-care practitioner can determine whether it is safe for you to continue taking this drug.

- *Most Common:* diarrhea, nausea, vomiting, loss of appetite, stomach pain, flushing or redness of the hands, feet, face, or ears
- *Less Common:* headache, dizziness, pressure in the chest, breathing problems, stuffy nose, tingling of the hands or feet, weakness, back pain, joint pain, chills, increased output of urine, rash, hives

IMPORTANT PRECAUTIONS

Tell your health-care practitioner if you are sensitive or allergic to calcitonin or to any other drugs.

This drug is administered using a nasal inhaler and can affect the lining of your nose. Periodic examination of your nasal passages by your health-care practitioner is recommended.

Contact your health-care practitioner if you develop severe nose irritation or nose ulcers.

Do not take calcitonin if you have a recently healed bone fracture.

DRUG INTERACTIONS

Tell your health-care practitioner and pharmacist if you are taking any prescription or nonprescription drugs, as well as any vitamins, herbs, or other supplements. No drug-drug interactions have been reported for calcitonin.

FOOD, VITAMIN, AND HERBAL INTERACTIONS

No food, vitamin, or herb interactions have been reported.

RECOMMENDED DOSAGE

Calcitonin is available in a nasal spray and as an injection. Only the nasal spray dosage is given here. This dosage is typical; however, your health-care practitioner will determine the most appropriate dose and schedule for you.

- *Children:* No information is available on the use of calcitonin in children.
- *Adults:* 1 spray (200 IU) in one nostril each day. Alternate nostrils daily.

If you miss a dose, take it as soon as you remember. If it is nearly time for your next dose, do not take the missed dose. Continue with your regular dosing schedule. Never take a double dose. Call your health-care practitioner if you miss two or more doses.

SYMPTOMS OF OVERDOSE AND WHAT TO DO

Symptoms of overdose may include spasms. If overdose occurs, seek immediate medical attention and bring the prescription container with you to the hospital.

SPECIAL INFORMATION FOR PREGNANT OR NURSING WOMEN

Calcitonin does not cross the placenta, but the injectable form can cause low birth weight in animals. If you are pregnant or plan to become pregnant, talk to your health-care practitioner. Do not use this drug unless the potential benefits outweigh the potential risks.

It is not known whether calcitonin passes into breast milk. If you are breastfeeding, your health-care practitioner may advise you to stop until your treatment is complete.

SPECIAL INFORMATION FOR SENIORS

There are no special precautions for older adults.

GENERIC NAME

Candesartan *see Angiotensin II Blockers, page 123*

GENERIC NAME

Capecitabine

BRAND NAME

Xeloda

No generic available

ABOUT THIS DRUG

Capecitabine is an antimetabolite that is used to treat breast cancer and colorectal cancer that has spread to other parts of the body, despite other cancer treatments.

Once capecitabine enters the body, it is converted into an anticancer agent called 5-FU (5-flurouracil), a substance that binds to enzymes in cancer cells and prevents their growth.

SIDE EFFECTS

Be sure to tell your health-care practitioner if you experience any side effects while taking capecitabine. Only your health-care practitioner can determine whether it is safe for you to continue taking this drug.

- *Most Common:* constipation, diarrhea, abdominal pain, mouth sores, hand-and-foot syndrome, skin inflammation, tingling or pain in the feet or hands, fatigue, loss of appetite, eye irritation, fever, nausea, vomiting, low blood-cell counts
- *Common:* headache, nail problems, upset stomach, dizziness, sleeplessness, dehydration, swelling, muscle aches, arm and leg pain
- *Less Common or Rare:* Various side effects can affect nearly any part of the body.

IMPORTANT PRECAUTIONS

Tell your health-care practitioner if you are sensitive or allergic to capecitabine or to any other drugs.

Contact your health-care practitioner if you have 4 to 6 more bowel movements daily than normal, if you are very nauseous, or if you vomit 2 or more times in one day. He or she will likely adjust your dosage.

If you experience swelling, pain, or sores in your mouth or on your tongue, stop taking capecitabine immediately and call your health-care practitioner.

If you experience symptoms of hand-and-foot syndrome (i.e., numbness, tingling, pain, redness, swelling, skin loss, and blistered hands or feet), stop taking the drug and call your health-care practitioner immediately.

Call your health-care practitioner (but continue taking capecitabine) if you develop a fever of 100.5 degrees or higher or you develop other signs of infection.

DRUG INTERACTIONS

Tell your health-care practitioner and pharmacist if you are taking any prescription or nonprescription drugs, as well as any vitamins,

herbs, or other supplements. Possible drug interactions include the following:

- Capecitabine may increase the effects of amphotericin B (by injection), antithyroid agents (e.g., methimazole), chloramphenicol, colchicine, flucytosine, ganciclovir, interferon, plicamycin, and zidovudine.
- Anticoagulants (e.g., warfarin) may increase the risk of bleeding.
- Antacids (e.g., Maalox, Mylanta) can increase by 20% the amount of capecitabine your body absorbs. Take antacids and capecitabine at least 2 hours apart.
- Leucovorin increases the side effects of 5-FU. Never combine leucovorin and capecitabine.

FOOD, VITAMIN, AND HERBAL INTERACTIONS

Inform your health-care practitioner if you are taking folic acid supplements while taking capecitabine, because this vitamin can increase the side effects of the drug.

RECOMMENDED DOSAGE

Capecitabine is available in 150- and 500-mg tablets. The dosages given here are typical. However, your health-care practitioner will determine the most appropriate dose and schedule for you.

- *Children:* The safety and effectiveness in children younger than 18 have not been established.
- *Adults:* Starting dose is usually 2,500 mg per square meter of body surface daily, divided into 2 doses, taken about 12 hours apart and within 30 minutes after finishing a meal. Your health-care practitioner will adjust the dosage depending on the side effects you experience.

If you miss a dose, do not take that skipped dose at all. Continue with your regular dosing schedule. Never take a double dose.

SYMPTOMS OF OVERDOSE AND WHAT TO DO

Symptoms of overdose include nausea, vomiting, diarrhea, stomach irritation, bleeding, and reduced blood-cell counts. If overdose occurs, seek immediate medical attention, and bring the prescription container with you to the hospital.

SPECIAL INFORMATION FOR PREGNANT OR NURSING WOMEN

Capecitabine crosses the placenta, and it can harm the fetus. If the drug is essential for your health, you and your health-care practitioner must weigh the potential risks against the potential benefits of this drug. You should not get pregnant while taking capecitabine.

It is not known whether capecitabine crosses into breast milk. If you are breastfeeding, your health-care practitioner may advise you to stop until your treatment is complete.

SPECIAL INFORMATION FOR SENIORS

Women 80 and older are more likely to experience severe diarrhea, nausea, and vomiting. Patients 60 and older who are also taking an anticoagulant (blood thinner) are more likely to experience blood clotting difficulties.

GENERIC NAME

Captopril

BRAND NAME

Capoten
Generic available

ABOUT THIS DRUG

Captopril is an angiotensin-converting enzyme (ACE) inhibitor drug used to treat high blood pressure and congestive heart failure.

Like other ACE inhibitors, captopril prevents the conversion of the hormone angiotensin I to another hormone, angiotensin II. Prevention of this transformation allows the blood vessels to relax, which reduces blood pressure and relieves symptoms of heart failure.

SIDE EFFECTS

Tell your health-care practitioner if you experience any side effects while taking captopril. Only your health-care practitioner can determine whether it is safe for you to continue taking this drug.

- *Most Common:* cough, rash, itching
- *Less Common:* chest pain, headache, dizziness, fatigue, sleep problems, tingling in hands or feet, palpitations, abdominal pain, nausea, vomiting, diarrhea, appetite loss, dry mouth, hair loss, breathing difficulties
- *Rare:* Rare side effects can occur throughout the body.

IMPORTANT PRECAUTIONS

Tell your health-care practitioner if you are sensitive or allergic to captopril or to any other drugs.

Rarely, captopril causes very low blood pressure. It may also cause dizziness or fainting. Until you know how you respond to the drug, do not drive or operate hazardous equipment.

Captopril may cause a reduction in kidney function, especially if you have heart failure. Your health-care practitioner may need to adjust your dosage if you have kidney problems.

Captopril may increase your risk of getting an infection. Your health-care practitioner should periodically check your blood count.

If you are taking captopril for your heart, do not increase physical activity too quickly. Discuss your exercise program with your health-care practitioner.

If you develop swelling of your tongue, throat, face, arms, or legs while taking captopril, stop taking the drug and contact your health-care practitioner immediately.

DRUG INTERACTIONS

Tell your health-care practitioner and pharmacist if you are taking any prescription or nonprescription drugs, as well as any vitamins, herbs, or other supplements. Possible drug interactions include the following:

- Diuretics (e.g., amiloride, furosemide) and beta-blockers (e.g., acebutolol, metoprolol) increase the blood-pressure-lowering effect of captopril.
- Captopril may increase blood potassium levels when it is taken with potassium-sparing diuretics (e.g., amiloride, triamterene).
- Probenecid, phenothiazine tranquilizers (e.g., chlorpromazine, promazine), and antivomiting agents (e.g., ondansetron, dolasetron) may increase the effects of captopril.
- Antacids (e.g., Maalox, Mylanta) should be taken at least 2 hours before or after taking captopril.
- Captopril may raise blood levels of digoxin and increase the risk of digoxin-related side effects.
- Indomethacin may lower the blood-pressure-lowering effect of captopril.
- Allopurinol increases the risk of adverse drug reactions.

FOOD, VITAMIN, AND HERBAL INTERACTIONS

Discuss your salt intake with your health-care practitioner when taking captopril. Avoid using salt substitutes or drinking low-salt milk, as these substances can cause abnormally high potassium levels, which can lead to heart problems. Also avoid foods high in potassium, such as bananas and citrus, unless you are also taking medications that reduce potassium levels. Do not take potassium supplements while taking captopril unless directed to do so by your health-care practitioner.

If you plan to take or are taking any herbs or supplements, talk with your health-care practitioner before starting captopril. Ginseng, goldenseal, licorice, ephedra (ma huang), and saw palmetto may raise your blood pressure; garlic and calcium may help lower it.

Capsaicin (derived from chili peppers) may trigger or aggravate the cough associated with captopril. Iron supplements can hinder the absorption of captopril. If you are taking iron supplements, do so 2 to 3 hours before or after taking your captopril dose.

RECOMMENDED DOSAGE

Captopril is available in tablets. The dosages given here are typical. However, your health-care practitioner will determine the most appropriate dose and schedule for you.

- ➤ *Children:* Consult your health-care practitioner.
- ➤ *Adults:* For high blood pressure, starting dose is 25 mg 2 to 3 times daily. Your health-care practitioner may increase your dose up to 150 mg 2 or 3 times daily. For congestive heart failure, 25 mg three times daily. In both cases, 450 mg is the maximum daily dose.

Captopril should be taken on an empty stomach 1 hour before meals.

If you miss a dose, take it as soon as you remember. If it is nearly time for your next dose, do not take the missed dose. Continue with your regular dosing schedule. Never take a double dose.

SYMPTOMS OF OVERDOSE AND WHAT TO DO

Symptoms of overdose include dizziness, fainting, nausea, vomiting, chest pain, and weak, rapid pulse. If overdose occurs, seek immediate medical attention and bring the prescription container with you to the hospital.

SPECIAL INFORMATION FOR PREGNANT OR NURSING WOMEN

Captopril can cause birth defects or death to a developing fetus, especially during the second and third trimesters of pregnancy. If you are pregnant or plan to become pregnant, talk to your health-care practitioner about the potential risks to your unborn child.

Small amounts of captopril pass into breast milk. If you are breastfeeding, your health-care practitioner may advise you to stop while you are under treatment.

SPECIAL INFORMATION FOR SENIORS

Side effects are more likely to occur and to be more severe among older adults.

GENERIC NAME

Carbamazepine

BRAND NAMES

Atretol, Carbatrol, Epitol, Tegretol, Tegretol-XR
Generic available

ABOUT THIS DRUG

Carbamazepine is an anticonvulsant substance used to control certain types of epileptic seizures. It is especially used in people whose seizures cannot be controlled with phenytoin, phenobarbital, or primidone.

This medication inhibits the neurons from uncontrollable firing, which results in seizures.

SIDE EFFECTS

Be sure to tell your health-care practitioner if you experience any side effects while taking carbamazepine. Your health-care practitioner will let you know whether it is safe for you to continue taking this drug.

- *Most Common:* dizziness, drowsiness, nausea, vomiting
- *Less Common or Rare:* mood and behavioral changes, especially in children; breathing difficulties, hives, itching, rash, and other allergic reactions. Side effects can also affect other parts of the body.

IMPORTANT PRECAUTIONS

Tell your health-care practitioner if you are sensitive or allergic to carbamazepine or to any other drugs, especially to tricyclic antidepressants (e.g., amitriptyline, imipramine).

Potentially deadly side effects are associated with this drug. If you experience fever, rash, mouth ulcers, easy bruising, reddish or purplish spots on your skin, or sore throat, contact your health-care practitioner immediately. These symptoms suggest a blood disorder.

If you have a history of heart, liver, or kidney damage or have glaucoma, talk to your health-care practitioner before using this drug.

Do not use carbamazepine if you have a history of bone marrow depression or if you are taking monoamine oxidase inhibitors.

If you are taking carbamazepine to control seizures, do not stop taking it suddenly. Only your health-care practitioner can determine how to gradually cease taking this drug.

Because carbamazepine may cause drowsiness and dizziness, do not drive or operate dangerous equipment until you know how you will react to the drug.

Carbamazepine may cause potentially life-threatening blood reactions. It can also aggravate glaucoma in people who have this condition, and it may activate underlying confusion, agitation, or psychosis.

DRUG INTERACTIONS

Tell your health-care practitioner and pharmacist if you are taking any prescription or nonprescription drugs, as well as any vitamins, herbs, or other supplements. Possible drug interactions with carbamazepine may include the following:

- Cimetidine, clarithromycin, danazol, diltiazem, isoniazid, propoxyphene, erythromycin-type antibiotics, fluoxetine, fluvoxamine, mexiletine, nicotinamide, terfenadine, troleandomycin, valproate, and verapamil may increase blood levels of carbamazepine and could lead to carbamazepine toxicity.
- Cisplatin, doxorubicin, felbamate, rifampin, and theophylline may reduce the effectiveness of carbamazepine.
- Carbamazepine may reduce the effectiveness of birth control pills and may cause spotting.
- Barbiturates (e.g., phenobarbital), phenytoin, primidone, and charcoal tablets or powder may decrease the absorption of carbamazepine.
- Carbamazepine counteracts the effects of acetaminophen, warfarin, theophylline, cyclosporine, dacarbazine, digitalis drugs, disopyramide, doxycycline, haloperidol, levothyroxine, and quinidine.
- Use of other antiseizure drugs (e.g., felbamate, hydantoins) may cause unpredictable side effects.
- Lithium may increase nervous system side effects.

FOOD, VITAMIN, AND HERBAL INTERACTIONS

No food, vitamin, or herbal interactions have been noted.

RECOMMENDED DOSAGE

Carbamazepine is available in tablets, capsules, and oral suspension. The dosages given here are typical. However, your health-care practitioner will determine the most appropriate dose and schedule for you.

- *Children Younger than 6 Years:* 10 to 20 mg per 2.2 pounds of body weight. Total daily dose should not exceed 35 mg per 2.2 pounds of body weight.
- *Children Ages 6 to 12 Years:* 200 mg twice daily or one-half teaspoon 4 times daily. Your health-care practitioner may increase the dose gradually. Maximum daily dosage is 1,000 mg.
- *Children 13 and Older and Adults:* 400 to 1,200 mg daily in 3 to 4 divided doses.

Carbamazepine should always be taken with food; do not take it on an empty stomach. If you miss a dose, take it as soon as you remember. If it is nearly time for your next dose, do not take the missed dose. Continue with your regular dosing schedule. Never take a double dose.

SYMPTOMS OF OVERDOSE AND WHAT TO DO

Symptoms of overdose appear 1 to 3 hours after ingestion. They include coma, convulsions, dizziness, drowsiness, inability to urinate, irregular breathing, lack of coordination, twitching muscles, nausea, dilated pupils, restlessness, severe muscle spasm, shock, tremors, vomiting, and voluntary rapid eye movements. If overdose occurs, seek immediate medical assistance and bring the prescription container with you to the hospital.

SPECIAL INFORMATION FOR PREGNANT OR NURSING WOMEN

No adequate studies of the effects of carbamazepine on pregnant or nursing women have been done. Birth defects in infants have been reported, however. If you are pregnant or plan to become pregnant, talk to your health-care practitioner. You and your health-care practitioner should weigh the potential benefits against the potential risks.

Carbamazepine passes into breast milk. If you are breastfeeding, your health-care practitioner may advise you to switch to bottle feeding.

SPECIAL INFORMATION FOR SENIORS

Your health-care practitioner should periodically monitor the level of carbamazepine in your blood.

GENERIC NAME

Carbenicillin indanyl sodium

see Penicillin Antibiotics, page 812

GENERIC NAME

Carbidopa

see also Levodopa, page 610

BRAND NAME

Lodosyn
Generic available

ABOUT THIS DRUG

Carbidopa is an enzyme inhibitor designed to be used along with levodopa/carbidopa or levodopa to help control the symptoms of Parkinson's disease when either of the other medications does not provide sufficient control. It does not have any antiparkinsonian effects when taken alone.

Carbidopa reduces the amount of levodopa patients need to control symptoms and also helps patients tolerate levodopa. It minimizes the breakdown of levodopa in the body, which then makes it more accessible to the brain.

SIDE EFFECTS

Be sure to tell your health-care practitioner if you experience any side effects while taking carbidopa. Only your health-care practitioner can determine whether it is safe for you to continue taking this drug. Carbidopa itself causes very few side effects. Most of those listed here are associated with the use of both levodopa and carbidopa.

- *Most Common* (carbidopa alone): involuntary movements, nausea; (combined treatment) nausea, vomiting, drowsiness, dizziness, muscle twitches, dry mouth, blurred vision, insomnia, confusion, nightmares, fatigue
- *Less Common:* none for carbidopa alone. Combined treatment: seizures, persistent nausea, vomiting, or diarrhea, suicidal thoughts, allergic reactions (e.g., swelling of the lips, face, or tongue, difficulty breathing, hives), uncontrollable movements, mood and behavior changes

IMPORTANT PRECAUTIONS

Tell your health-care practitioner if you are sensitive or allergic to carbidopa or to any other drugs.

Do not take carbidopa if you have narrow-angle glaucoma or malignant melanoma (a type of skin cancer).

Before using carbidopa, tell your health-care practitioner if you have any type of heart disease, kidney disease, respiratory disease, hormonal disorder, stomach or intestinal ulcers, depression or any type of psychiatric condition, or wide-angle glaucoma.

DRUG INTERACTIONS

Tell your health-care practitioner and pharmacist if you are taking any prescription or nonprescription drugs, as well as any vitamins, herbs, or other supplements. Possible drug interactions include the following:

- Antacids may increase the effects of carbidopa and levodopa.
- Antiseizure drugs (e.g., phenytoin, ethotoin), papaverine, antidepressants (e.g., amitriptyline, doxepin), and medications used to treat psychiatric conditions (e.g., chlorpromazine, fluphenazine) may decrease the effects of carbidopa and levodopa.
- Do not take levodopa/carbidopa if you are taking or you did take monoamine oxidase inhibitors (MAOIs) within the past 14 days.

FOOD, VITAMIN, AND HERBAL INTERACTIONS

Vitamin B6 may decrease the effects of carbidopa and levodopa. A high-protein diet can reduce the effectiveness of levodopa, and thus carbidopa. Protein intake should be limited; talk to your health-care practitioner.

RECOMMENDED DOSAGE

Carbidopa is available in tablets. The dosages given here are typical. However, your health-care practitioner will determine the most appropriate dose and schedule for your needs.

- *Children:* Your health-care practitioner will determine the appropriate dosage.
- *Adults:* Carbidopa is added in steps of up to 25 mg daily until the desired effect is attained.

If you miss a dose, take it as soon as you remember. If it is nearly time for your next dose, do not take the missed dose. Continue with your regular dosing schedule. Never take a double dose.

SYMPTOMS OF OVERDOSE AND WHAT TO DO

Because carbidopa is always taken along with levodopa, the symptoms of overdose are associated with the use of both drugs. Symptoms of overdose include sudden or severe confusion, hallucinations, and delirium. If overdose occurs, seek immediate medical attention and bring all the prescription containers with you.

SPECIAL INFORMATION FOR PREGNANT OR NURSING WOMEN

No adequate studies of the effects of carbidopa and levodopa have been done on pregnant or nursing women, but both substances are known to cause birth defects in animals. If you are pregnant or plan to become pregnant, talk to your health-care practitioner. If these drugs are crucial for your health, the potential benefits must be weighed against the potential risks.

Carbidopa and levodopa may pass into breast milk. If you are breastfeeding, your health-care practitioner may advise you to stop breastfeeding.

SPECIAL INFORMATION FOR SENIORS

Older adults may need lower doses. Seniors are also more likely to develop abnormal heart rhythms or other heart problems, especially those who have heart disease.

GENERIC NAME

Carbinoxamine

see Antihistamine-Decongestant Combination, page 132

GENERIC NAME

Carisoprodol

BRAND NAME

Soma

Generic available

ABOUT THIS DRUG

Carisoprodol is a muscle relaxant that is used to relieve the pain and discomfort associated with sprains, strains, and back pain.

This drug is believed to relieve pain by interfering with the nerve signals that cause the muscles to go into spasm.

SIDE EFFECTS

Be sure to tell your health-care practitioner if you experience any side effects while taking carisoprodol. Only your health-care practitioner can determine whether it is safe for you to continue taking this drug.

- *Most Common:* drowsiness
- *Less Common:* dizziness or lightheadedness, fainting, depression, hives, breathing difficulties, rapid heartbeat, tight chest, wheezing, allergic fever, stinging or burning eyes, headache, unusual stimulation, upset stomach, hiccups, nausea, vomiting
- *Rare:* Rare side effects can affect various parts of the body.

IMPORTANT PRECAUTIONS

Tell your health-care practitioner if you are sensitive or allergic to carisoprodol or to any other drugs, especially meprobamate. Do not take carisoprodol if you have acute intermittent porphyria (rare condition characterized by abdominal pain and neurological disturbances).

On rare occasions, unusual side effects such as extreme muscle weakness, dizziness, temporary loss of use of the legs and arms, double vision, temporary loss of vision, joint pain, euphoria, confusion, disorientation, agitation, and dilated pupils occur in individuals within a few minutes to hours of taking their first dose.

This drug should be used with extreme caution if you have liver or kidney disease.

Because carisoprodol causes drowsiness and dizziness, make sure you know how you react to the drug before you drive or operate dangerous equipment.

DRUG INTERACTIONS

Tell your health-care practitioner and pharmacist if you are taking any prescription or nonprescription drugs, as well as any vitamins, herbs, or other supplements. Possible interactions include the following:

- Carisoprodol increases the effects of alcohol.
- Sleeping pills, tranquilizers, and other central nervous system depressants should be avoided when taking carisoprodol because they intensify the sedative effect.

FOOD, VITAMIN, AND HERBAL INTERACTIONS

No food, vitamin, or herbal interactions have been noted.

RECOMMENDED DOSAGE

Carisoprodol is available in tablets. The dosages given here are typical. However, your health-care practitioner will determine the most appropriate dose and schedule for your needs.

- *Children Younger than 12*: not recommended
- *Children Older than 12 and Adults:* 350 mg 3 to 4 times daily and at bedtime

Carisoprodol can be taken with food to help prevent stomach irritation.

If you miss a dose, take it as soon as you remember if it's only about an hour since your scheduled dose. If it is later, do not take the missed dose. Continue with your regular dosing schedule. Never take a double dose.

SYMPTOMS OF OVERDOSE AND WHAT TO DO

Symptoms of overdose include slurred speech, stupor, coma, shock, and breathing problems. An overdose of carisoprodol can be fatal. If overdose occurs, seek immediate medical assistance, and bring the prescription container with you to the hospital.

SPECIAL INFORMATION FOR PREGNANT OR NURSING WOMEN

No adequate studies of the effects of carisoprodol on pregnant or nursing women have been done. If you are pregnant or plan to become pregnant, tell your health-care practitioner. You and your health-care practitioner should weigh the potential benefits against the potential risks for the fetus.

Large amounts of carisoprodol pass into breast milk. If you are breastfeeding, your health-care practitioner will likely advise you to stop until your treatment is complete.

SPECIAL INFORMATION FOR SENIORS

Older adults with liver or kidney disease may experience sleepiness or impaired concentration when using this drug.

GENERIC NAME

Carteolol

BRAND NAMES

Cartrol, Ocupress

No generic available

ABOUT THIS DRUG

Carteolol is a beta-blocker that is used to treat high blood pressure and angina (oral form) and glaucoma (increased pressure inside the eye; ophthalmic form).

The ophthalmic form of carteolol reduces the production of fluids in the eye and slightly increases the rate at which the fluids leave the eye. The oral form reduces blood pressure by reducing the rate and force of the heart's contractions, which results in lower blood pressure.

SIDE EFFECTS

Be sure to tell your health-care practitioner if you experience any side effects while taking carteolol. Only your health-care practitioner can determine whether it is safe for you to continue taking this drug.

- *Most Common* (oral form): impotence, dizziness, rapid heartbeat, unusual fatigue, weakness, drowsiness, muscle cramps, insomnia; (ophthalmic form) temporary eye irritation, tearing, inflamed eye, burning, swelling
- *Less Common or Rare* (oral form): anxiety, irritability, nervousness, constipation, diarrhea, dry eyes, itching, nausea, vomiting, nightmares, tingling in the fingers, toes, or scalp, shortness of breath, wheezing, irregular heartbeat, chest pain, swelling of the ankles, feet, and lower legs, depression; (ophthalmic form) blurred vision, poor night vision, increased sensitivity to light, headache, insomnia, sinus irritation, odd taste in the mouth, palpitations, breathing problems, dizziness caused by low blood pressure

IMPORTANT PRECAUTIONS

Tell your health-care practitioner if you are sensitive or allergic to carteolol or to any other drugs.

Inform your health-care practitioner if you have asthma, severe heart failure, very slow heart rate, or heart block before taking this drug, because it can aggravate these conditions.

If you have angina and take carteolol for high blood pressure, do not suddenly stop taking this drug because you may aggravate the angina.

Carteolol should be used with extreme caution if you have liver or kidney disease, poor circulation, circulatory disease, chronic bronchitis, diabetes, low blood sugar, myasthenia gravis, overactive thyroid, or chronic obstructive pulmonary disease.

If you plan to undergo major surgery, your health-care practitioner may ask you to stop taking carteolol two days before surgery, because this drug can interact with surgical anesthetics and increase heart problems.

DRUG INTERACTIONS

Tell your health-care practitioner and pharmacist if you are taking any prescription or nonprescription drugs, as well as any vitamins, herbs, or other supplements. Carteolol may interact with other drugs.

- Carteolol can interfere with the actions of oral antidiabetic drugs (e.g., glipizide, glyburide).
- Carteolol may increase the blood-pressure-lowering effects of other antihypertensive drugs, including clonidine, guanabenz, and reserpine, and calcium channel blockers, such as nifedipine.
- Carteolol may worsen the symptoms of cold hands and feet associated with ergot alkaloids and lead to gangrene.
- Calcium channel blockers (e.g., amlodipine, verapamil), flecainide, haloperidol, hydralazine, oral contraceptives, phenothiazine tranquilizers (e.g., molindone), quinolone antibacterials (e.g., fleroxacin, ofloxacin), and quinidine may increase the amount of carteolol in the blood and increase the effects of carteolol.
- Aspirin-containing drugs, estrogen drugs, indomethacin, and sulfinpyrazone may hinder the ability of carteolol to lower blood pressure.
- Carteolol may counteract the effects of thyroid hormone replacement therapy.
- Cimetidine increases the amount of oral carteolol that is absorbed into the bloodstream.
- The effects of some antiasthma drugs (e.g., ephedrine, theophylline, aminophylline) may be reduced by carteolol.
- Digitalis and phenytoin along with carteolol can cause excessive slowing of the heart.

FOOD, VITAMIN, AND HERBAL INTERACTIONS

If you plan to or are taking any herbs or supplements, talk with your health-care practitioner before starting carteolol. Ginseng, goldenseal, licorice, ephedra (ma huang), and saw palmetto may raise your blood pressure; garlic and calcium may help lower it.

RECOMMENDED DOSAGE

Carteolol is available in tablets and as an ophthalmic solution. The dosages given here are typical. However, your health-care practitioner will determine the most appropriate dose and schedule for you.

Ophthalmic Dose

- *Children:* one drop twice daily
- *Adults:* one drop twice daily

Oral Dose

- *Children Younger than 12 Years:* Your health-care practitioner will determine the appropriate dose.
- *Children Older than 12 and Adults:* 2.5 mg once daily, increased to 5 to 10 mg daily as needed. If you have impaired kidney function, your dose may be 2.5 mg once every 1 to 3 days as needed.

If you miss a dose, take it as soon as you remember. If it is nearly time for your next dose, do not take the missed dose. Continue with your regular dosing schedule. Never take a double dose.

SYMPTOMS OF OVERDOSE AND WHAT TO DO

Symptoms of overdose include slow heartbeat, severe dizziness, fainting, irregular or fast heartbeat, difficulty breathing, seizures, and bluish-colored fingernails or palms. If overdose occurs, seek immediate medical attention and bring the prescription container with you to the hospital.

SPECIAL INFORMATION FOR PREGNANT OR NURSING WOMEN

No adequate studies of the effects of carteolol on pregnant or nursing women have been done. Animal studies have not revealed any birth defects. If you are pregnant or plan to become pregnant, talk to your health-care practitioner. You and your health-care practitioner should weigh the potential benefits against the potential risks to the fetus.

Carteolol may pass into breast milk. If you are breastfeeding, your health-care practitioner may advise you to stop until your treatment is complete.

SPECIAL INFORMATION FOR SENIORS

Side effects may be more likely and more severe in older adults. When taking the oral form, your health-care practitioner may need to reduce the dose.

GENERIC NAME

Carvedilol

BRAND NAME

Coreg
No generic available

ABOUT THIS DRUG

Carvedilol is a beta-blocker used to treat mild-to-moderate congestive heart failure and high blood pressure. It is typically used in conjunction with digitalis, diuretics, or angiotensin-converting enzyme inhibitors.

Carvedilol blocks certain areas of the central nervous system, which reduces the amount of blood pumped and reduces the risk of very rapid heartbeat.

SIDE EFFECTS

Be sure to tell your health-care practitioner if you experience any side effects while taking carvedilol. Only your health-care practitioner can determine whether it is safe for you to continue taking this drug.

➤ *Most Common:* dizziness or lightheadedness especially when getting up suddenly from a sitting or lying position, impotence, unusual fatigue, weakness, drowsiness, insomnia, diarrhea, nausea, vomiting

➤ *Less Common or Rare:* anxiety, irritability, nervousness, constipation, dry eyes, itching, nightmares, numbness, tingling or other sensations in your fingers, toes, or scalp, wheezing, shortness of breath, irregular or slow heartbeat, chest pain, swelling of the feet, ankles, and lower legs, depression

IMPORTANT PRECAUTIONS

Tell your health-care practitioner if you are sensitive or allergic to carvedilol or to any other drugs.

Because carvedilol causes severe liver damage in about 1 percent of people who take it, you should not take this drug if you have severe liver disease. Call your health-care practitioner immediately if you develop symptoms of liver damage, including severe itching, dark-colored urine, appetite loss, and yellowish skin and eyes.

Carvedilol can disguise signs of low blood sugar and may increase the effects of oral antidiabetic drugs or insulin. Consult with your health-care practitioner if you have diabetes and plan to take carvedilol.

Carvedilol can also mask symptoms of an overactive thyroid gland. However, if you suddenly stop taking carvedilol, you may trigger an attack of hyperthyroidism.

If you have plans to receive general anesthesia, tell your health-care practitioner you are taking carvedilol. Heart function may be compromised if you receive anesthetics while taking carvedilol.

Do not suddenly stop taking this drug, as it may cause angina and possibly a heart attack in people who have advanced heart disease.

DRUG INTERACTIONS

Tell your health-care practitioner and pharmacist if you are taking any prescription or nonprescription drugs, as well as any vitamins, herbs, or other supplements. Possible interactions may include the following:

- Carvedilol increases the effects of oral antidiabetic drugs and insulin. You will need to monitor your blood sugar levels regularly.
- Carvedilol increases the effects of calcium channel drugs (e.g., verapamil, diltiazem) and the blood-pressure-lowering effect of clonidine.
- Carvedilol increases the amount of digoxin in the blood; thus you may need to adjust your dosage of digoxin.
- Cimetidine increases by 30 percent the amount of carvedilol your body absorbs. However, this interaction does not appear to have any negative effects.
- Rifampin reduces by about 70 percent the amount of carvedilol absorbed into the bloodstream. Your rifampin dose will need to be adjusted.

FOOD, VITAMIN, AND HERBAL INTERACTIONS

Carvedilol should be taken with food to avoid dizziness or a sudden drop in blood pressure. It is also best to avoid excessive salt intake if you have high blood pressure.

If you plan to or are taking any herbs or supplements, talk with your health-care practitioner before starting carvedilol. Ginseng, goldenseal, licorice, ephedra (ma huang), and saw palmetto may raise your blood pressure; garlic and calcium may help lower it.

RECOMMENDED DOSAGE

Carvedilol is available in tablets. The dosages given here are typical. However, your health-care practitioner will determine the most appropriate dose and schedule for your situation.

For High Blood Pressure

- *Children:* not recommended for children
- *Adults:* Starting dose is 6.25 mg twice daily, increased to 25 mg twice daily if needed.

For Heart Failure

➤ *Children:* not recommended for children

➤ *Adults:* 3.125 mg twice daily for 2 weeks. The dose may be doubled every 2 weeks to a maximum daily dosage of 25 mg twice daily if you weigh less than 187 pounds and 50 mg twice daily if you weigh more.

Carvedilol should be taken at the same time each day. If you miss a dose, take it as soon as you remember. If it is within 4 hours of your next scheduled dose, do not take the missed dose. Continue with your regular dosing schedule. Never take a double dose.

SYMPTOMS OF OVERDOSE AND WHAT TO DO

Symptoms of overdose include unusually slow heartbeat, vomiting, breathing problems, seizures, and severe dizziness or fainting. If overdose occurs, seek immediate medical assistance and bring the prescription container with you to the hospital.

SPECIAL INFORMATION FOR PREGNANT OR NURSING WOMEN

Animal studies indicate that carvedilol crosses the placenta and may interfere with the fetus. If you are pregnant or plan to become pregnant, talk to your health-care practitioner. If carvedilol is essential for your health, you and your health-care practitioner will need to weigh the potential benefits against the potential risks to the fetus. Infants born to women who took other beta-blockers while pregnant have had low blood pressure, lower birth weights, and reduced heart rates.

Small amounts of carvedilol pass into human breast milk. If you are breastfeeding, your health-care practitioner will likely advise you to stop until your treatment is complete.

SPECIAL INFORMATION FOR SENIORS

Older adults usually need lower doses. They also are more likely to experience side effects, especially dizziness. Frequent blood pressure monitoring is recommended.

GENERIC NAME

Caspofungin

BRAND NAME

Cancidas

No generic available

ABOUT THIS DRUG

Caspofungin is an antifungal medication used to help the body overcome invasive aspergillosis that has not responded to other antifungal treatment.

Caspofungin blocks the synthesis of a primary component in the cell wall of fungi.

SIDE EFFECTS

Be sure to tell your health-care practitioner if you experience any side effects while taking caspofungin. Only your health-care practitioner can determine whether it is safe for you to continue taking this drug.

- *Less Common:* pain or redness at the injection site, redness, vomiting, fever, nausea

IMPORTANT PRECAUTIONS

Tell your health-care practitioner if you are sensitive or allergic to caspofungin or to any other drugs.

Let your health-care practitioner know if you have any medical problems, especially liver disease.

DRUG INTERACTIONS

Tell your health-care practitioner and pharmacist if you are taking any prescription or nonprescription drugs, as well as any vitamins, herbs, or other supplements. Possible interactions may include the following:

- Cyclosporin may increase the chance of liver problems.
- Caspofungin may decrease the effects of tacrolimus.
- Carbamazepine, dexamethasone, efavirenz, nevirapine, rifampicin, and phenytoin may reduce blood levels of caspofungin.

FOOD, VITAMIN, AND HERBAL INTERACTIONS

No food, vitamin, or herbal interactions have been noted.

RECOMMENDED DOSAGE

Caspofungin is only available through medical professionals and is given intravenously. The dosages given here are typical. However, your health-care practitioner will determine the most appropriate dose and schedule for your needs.

- *Children:* use and dosage to be determined by your health-care practitioner

➤ *Adults:* starting dose is 70 mg intravenously, thereafter usually 50 mg daily intravenously

SYMPTOMS OF OVERDOSE AND WHAT TO DO

No reports of overdose with caspofungin have been documented. If an overdose were to occur, you would likely be at a medical facility, because this drug must be administered by medical personnel.

SPECIAL INFORMATION FOR PREGNANT OR NURSING WOMEN

No adequate studies have been done on the effects of caspofungin in pregnant or nursing women. If you are pregnant or plan to become pregnant, talk to your health-care practitioner. You and your health-care practitioner should weigh the potential benefits against the potential risks to the fetus.

It's not known whether caspofungin passes into breast milk. If you are breastfeeding, your health-care practitioner may advise you to stop until your treatment is complete.

SPECIAL INFORMATION FOR SENIORS

No special information is needed for older adults.

GENERIC NAMES

Cefaclor *see Cephalosporin antibiotics, page 256*

Cefadroxil *see Cephalosporin antibiotics, page 256*

Cefdinir *see Cephalosporin antibiotics, page 256*

Cefditoren pivoxil *see Cephalosporin antibiotics, page 256*

Cefixime *see Cephalosporin antibiotics, page 256*

Cefpodoxime proxetil *see Cephalosporin antibiotics, page 256*

Cefprozil *see Cephalosporin antibiotics, page 256*

Ceftibuten *see Cephalosporin antibiotics, page 256*

Cefuroxime axetil *see Cephalosporin antibiotics, page 256*

GENERIC NAME
Celecoxib

BRAND NAME
Celebrex
No generic available

ABOUT THIS DRUG
Celecoxib is a type of nonsteroidal anti-inflammatory drug (NSAID) called a COX-2 inhibitor. It is used to relieve the pain and inflammation associated with osteoarthritis and rheumatoid arthritis.

Celecoxib inhibits the actions of a natural enzyme called COX-2, but unlike other NSAIDs, it does not influence the activity of COX-1, which protects the lining of the stomach. Therefore celecoxib is less likely to cause stomach bleeding and ulcers than older NSAIDs.

SIDE EFFECTS
Be sure to tell your health-care practitioner if you experience any side effects while taking celecoxib. Only your health-care practitioner can determine whether it is safe for you to continue taking this drug.

➤ *Most Common:* abdominal pain, diarrhea, headache, indigestion, inflamed sinuses, nausea, respiratory infection

➤ *Less Common or Rare:* back pain, dizziness, gas, insomnia, rash, runny nose, sore throat, swelling, allergic reactions (difficulty breathing, swelling of the face or throat, rash, hives), blurred vision, bronchitis, chest pain, constipation, difficult urination, drowsiness, dry mouth, dry skin, earache, eye infection or pain, fatigue, fever, hives, hot flashes, increased blood pressure, increased heart rate, joint pain, kidney stones, leg cramps, liver problems, mouth ulcers, muscle ache, urinary tract infections, vaginal problems, weakness, weight gain

IMPORTANT PRECAUTIONS
Tell your health-care practitioner if you are sensitive or allergic to celecoxib or to any other drugs, especially other NSAIDs, aspirin, sulfonamide drugs (e.g., sulfadiazine, sulfisoxazole), and salicylates.

Do not take celecoxib if you have ever had an asthma attack or experienced facial and throat swelling or skin eruptions after taking aspirin or other NSAIDs.

Before using this drug, tell your health-care practitioner if you have a history of stomach ulcers, stomach bleeding, alcohol abuse, or tobacco use.

If you have asthma, liver or kidney disease, or are prone to anemia, celecoxib should be used with caution.

If you develop symptoms of liver poisoning while taking celecoxib, stop taking the drug immediately and contact your health-care practitioner. Symptoms include nausea, fatigue, itching, flu-like symptoms, yellowish skin, and pain in the right side of the stomach.

If you have heart failure, high blood pressure, or swelling, celecoxib should be used with caution, as it can cause water retention, which can aggravate these conditions.

DRUG INTERACTIONS

Tell your health-care practitioner and pharmacist if you are taking any prescription or nonprescription drugs, as well as any vitamins, herbs, or other supplements. Celecoxib may interact with other drugs.

- Lithium can cause higher levels of celecoxib and an increased risk of side effects.
- Aspirin, ibuprofen, and other prescription or over-the-counter NSAIDs may increase the risk of bleeding.
- Amiodarone, fluoxetine, fluconazole, ritonavir, and sertraline may increase the effects of celecoxib.
- Warfarin may increase the risk of bleeding.
- Rifampin, carbamazepine, and phenytoin may decrease the effects of celecoxib.
- Alcohol can increase the risk of stomach complications.

FOOD, VITAMIN, AND HERBAL INTERACTIONS

Do not combine celecoxib with herbs such as clove oil, feverfew, garlic, ginkgo, or ginseng, as these substances may affect clotting.

RECOMMENDED DOSAGE

Celecoxib is available in 100- and 200-mg capsules. The dosages given here are typical. However, your health-care practitioner will determine the most appropriate dose and schedule for your needs.

- *Children Younger than 18 Years:* The safety and effectiveness of celecoxib have not been determined for children younger than 18.

- *Adults:* For osteoarthritis, 100 mg taken twice daily, or 200 mg once daily. For rheumatoid arthritis, 100 to 200 mg twice daily.

If you miss a dose, take it as soon as you remember. If it is nearly time for your next dose, do not take the missed dose. Continue with your regular dosing schedule. Never take a double dose.

SYMPTOMS OF OVERDOSE AND WHAT TO DO

Symptoms of overdose include breathing problems, coma, drowsiness, fainting, gastrointestinal bleeding, hives, itching, nausea, stomach pain, and vomiting. If overdose occurs, seek immediate medical attention and bring the prescription container with you to the hospital.

SPECIAL INFORMATION FOR PREGNANT OR NURSING WOMEN

Celecoxib can harm the fetus if the drug is taken during the third trimester, although experts are unsure about its effects earlier in pregnancy. If you are pregnant or plan to become pregnant, talk to your health-care practitioner. You and your health-care practitioner should weigh the potential benefits against the potential risks to the fetus.

It is uncertain whether celecoxib passes into breast milk. If you are breastfeeding, your health-care practitioner may advise you to switch to bottle feeding.

SPECIAL INFORMATION FOR SENIORS

Older adults may be more sensitive to the side effects.

OPEN QUESTIONS OR CONTROVERSIES

On September 30, 2004, the COX-2 inhibitor Vioxx (rofecoxib) was voluntarily withdrawn from the marketplace by the manufacturer, Merck & Company, Inc., because studies showed that use of the drug for 18 months or longer placed patients at significant risk of cardiovascular events, such as heart attack and stroke. As of October 2004, it had not been determined whether use of Celebrex (Celecoxib), also a COX-2 inhibitor, is associated with the same risks as Vioxx. However, the findings of the Vioxx studies launched investigations into the safety of celecoxib. Before taking celecoxib, you should consult with your health-care practitioner.

GENERIC NAME

Cephalexin

see Cephalosporin antibiotics, page 256

GENERIC NAME

Cephalexin hydrochloride

see Cephalosporin antibiotics, page 256

GENERIC NAME

Class: Cephalosporin antibiotics

Generics: (1) cefaclor, (2) cefadroxil, (3) cefdinir, (4) cefixime, (5) cefpodoxime, (6) cefprozil, (7) ceftibuten, (8) cefuroxime axetil, (9) cephalexin, (10) cephalexin hydrochloride, (11) cephradine, (12) loracarbef

BRAND NAMES

(1) Ceclor, Ceclor CD, Ceclor Pulvules; (2) Duricef; (3) Omnicef; (4) Suprax; (5) Vantin; (6) Cefzil; (7) Cedax; (8) Ceftin; (9) Keflex; (10) Keftab; (11) Velosef; (12) Lorabid

ABOUT THIS DRUG

The cephalosporin antibiotics are related to cephalosporin C, an antibiotic that is similar to penicillin. These antibiotics are used to treat various common bacterial infections, and each one has certain infections for which it is best suited. (All the information in this profile refers to the oral forms of these drugs. They are all also available in injectable form.)

All of the cephalosporin antibiotics prevent the bacteria from building cell walls, which they need for survival.

SIDE EFFECTS

Be sure to tell your health-care practitioner if you experience any side effects while taking any of these medications. Only your health-care practitioner can determine whether it is safe for you to continue taking these drugs.

- *Most Common:* abdominal pain, gas, nausea, vomiting, diarrhea, rash, itching
- *Less Common:* dizziness, tingling in the hands or feet, seizures, confusion, headache, tiredness, muscle aches and swelling, loss of ap-

petite, changes in taste, colitis. Serum sickness (rash, joint pain, fever) is associated with cefaclor.

- *Rare:* kidney problems, inflamed liver, jaundice

IMPORTANT PRECAUTIONS

Tell your health-care practitioner if you are sensitive or allergic to any of the cephalosporins or to any other drugs. About 15 percent of people who are allergic to penicillin are also allergic to cephalosporins. Symptoms of an allergic reaction include hives, rash, fever, and joint aches and pains. Allergic reactions typically begin several days after treatment has started and go away several days after treatment is stopped.

Prolonged or frequent use of cephalosporins can cause a secondary infection that will not respond to the antibiotic being taken.

Report any signs of anemia (paleness, weakness, tiredness, breathing difficulties, and abnormal heart rhythms) to your health-care practitioner.

DRUG INTERACTIONS

Tell your health-care practitioner and pharmacist if you are taking any prescription or nonprescription drugs, as well as any vitamins, herbs, or other supplements. Possible drug interactions with cephalosporin antibiotics include the following:

- Antacids can reduce the amount of cefaclor, cefdinir, and cefpodoxime in the bloodstream. To avoid this situation, take antacids at least 2 hours before or after taking the antibiotics.
- Cimetidine, famotidine, nizatidine, and ranitidine can reduce the effectiveness of cefpodoxime and cefuroxime. These drugs should not be combined.
- Probenecid may raise increase the blood levels of some cephalosporins.
- Cephalosporins may cause false-positive test results for sugar in urine (diabetes test) in some products.
- Potent loop diuretics (e.g., furosemide, bendroflumethiazide) may lead to kidney damage.

FOOD, VITAMIN, AND HERBAL INTERACTIONS

Iron supplements and iron-fortified foods may interfere with the absorption of cefdinir. Consume these items at least 2 hours before or after you take your cephalosporin dose.

RECOMMENDED DOSAGE

Cephalosporins are available in tablets and capsules. The dosages given here are typical. However, your health-care practitioner will determine the most appropriate dose and schedule for your needs.

Cefaclor

- *Children Up to 12 Years:* 9 mg per pound of body weight daily in 2 to 3 equal doses
- *Adults:* 250 mg every 8 hours, or 375 to 500 mg every 12 hours

Cefadroxil

- *Children Up to 12 Years:* 13 mg per pound of body weight daily, in 1 to 2 doses
- *Adults:* 1 to 2 g daily, in 1 to 2 doses

Cefdinir

- *Children Up to 13 Years:* 3 to 6.5 mg per pound of body weight daily for 5 to 10 days
- *Adults:* 300 to 600 mg daily

Cefixime

- *Children Up to 12 Years:* 3.5 mg per pound of body weight daily, in 1 to 2 doses
- *Adults:* 400 mg daily, in 1 to 2 doses

Cefpodoxime Proxetil

- *Children 5 Months to 12 Years:* 2.5 to 5 mg per pound of body weight daily. Maximum for middle ear infections, 400 mg daily; for sore throat or tonsillitis, 200 mg daily.
- *Adults:* 200 to 400 mg daily, in 1 to 2 doses

Cefprozil

- *Children 6 Months to 12 Years:* 13 mg per pound of body weight every 12 hours
- *Adults:* 250 to 1,000 mg daily

Ceftibuten

- *Children Up to 12 Years:* 4 mg per pound of body weight, once daily for 10 days
- *Adults:* 400 mg once daily for 10 days

Cefuroxime

- *Children Up to 12 Years:* 125 to 250 mg every 12 hours
- *Adults:* 125 to 500 mg every 12 hours

Cephalexin

- *Children Up to 12 Years:* 11 to 23 mg per pound of body weight daily. For middle ear infections, the dose can be increased to 46 mg per pound of body weight.
- *Adults:* 250 to 1,000 mg every 6 hours. For urinary infections, up to 500 mg every 12 hours.

Cephradine

- *Children 9 Months and Older:* 11 to 45 mg per pound of body weight daily, in 2 to 4 doses
- *Adults:* 250 to 500 mg every 6 to 12 hours

Loracarbef

- *Children 6 Months to 12 Years:* 6.5 to 13 mg per pound of body weight daily
- *Adults:* 200 to 400 mg every 12 hours

Cephalosporin antibiotics can be taken with food or milk to reduce the chance of stomach upset. Food increases the absorption of cefpodoxime and cefuroxime.

If you miss a dose that you take once daily, take it as soon as you remember. If it is nearly time for your next dose, take the missed dose immediately and take your next dose 10 to 12 hours later. Then return to your regular dosing schedule. If you take the medication twice daily, take the dose you forgot immediately and the next dose 5 to 6 hours later. Then return to your regular schedule. If you take the medication three or more times daily, take the missed dose immediately and your next dose 2 to 4 hours later. Then return to your regular schedule. Never take a double dose.

SYMPTOMS OF OVERDOSE AND WHAT TO DO

Symptoms of overdose include seizures, severe abdominal pain, bloody diarrhea, and vomiting. Overdoses with cephalosporin are usually not serious and can be treated with antacids or milk. However, contact your local poison control center or hospital emergency room for information.

SPECIAL INFORMATION FOR PREGNANT OR NURSING WOMEN

Adequate studies of the effects of cephalosporin antibiotics on pregnant and nursing women have not been done. If you are pregnant or plan to become pregnant, talk to your health-care practitioner before using these drugs.

Cephalosporin antibiotics pass into breast milk and may affect nursing infants. If you are breastfeeding, your health-care practitioner may advise you to stop until you have completed treatment.

SPECIAL INFORMATION FOR SENIORS

Older adults may require lower doses because of reduced kidney function.

GENERIC NAME

Cephradine

see Cephalosporin antibiotics, page 256

GENERIC NAME

Cerivastatin

see Statin Cholesterol-lowering Drugs, page 959

GENERIC NAME

Cetirizine

BRAND NAME

Zyrtec

No generic available

ABOUT THIS DRUG

Cetirizine is an antihistamine prescribed for treatment of seasonal and year-round allergies.

Like other antihistamines, cetirizine blocks the release of histamines (chemicals released by the body during allergic reactions). Unlike older antihistamines, it appears to cause less sedation while being as effective.

SIDE EFFECTS

Be sure to tell your health-care practitioner if you experience any side effects while taking cetirizine. Only your health-care practitioner can determine whether it is safe for you to continue taking this drug.

- *Most Common* (in Adults): drowsiness, dry mouth, fatigue
- *Most Common* (in Children Ages 6 to 11): abdominal pain, cough, diarrhea, headache, nosebleed, sleepiness, sore throat, wheezing
- *Less Common* (in Adults): dizziness, sore throat
- *Less Common* (in Children Ages 6 to 11): nausea, vomiting

IMPORTANT PRECAUTIONS

Tell your health-care practitioner if you are sensitive or allergic to cetirizine or to any other drugs, especially hydroxyzine.

Because cetirizine can cause drowsiness, be sure you know how you react to the drug before you drive or operate hazardous equipment.

Before taking cetirizine, tell your health-care practitioner if you have liver or kidney disease. He or she may reduce your dose.

DRUG INTERACTIONS

Tell your health-care practitioner and pharmacist if you are taking any prescription or nonprescription drugs, as well as any vitamins, herbs, or other supplements. Significant drug-drug interactions involving cetirizine have not been reported. However, cetirizine may increase the depressive effects of alcohol, sedatives, tranquilizers, painkillers, muscle relaxants, barbiturates, and other antihistamines.

FOOD, VITAMIN, AND HERBAL INTERACTIONS

The herbs kava and valerian root may intensify drowsiness.

RECOMMENDED DOSAGE

Cetirizine is available in tablets and syrup. The dosages given here are typical. However, your health-care practitioner will determine the most appropriate dose and schedule for your needs.

- *Children 2 to 5 Years:* Starting dose is 1/2 teaspoon syrup (2.5 mg) once daily. The dosage may be increased to a maximum of 1 teaspoon (5 mg) once daily or 1/2 teaspoon (5 to 10 mg) every 12 hours. Children with liver or kidney disease should not take cetirizine.
- *Children 6 to 11 Years:* Starting dose is 1 to 2 teaspoons syrup (5 to 10 mg) once daily. Children with kidney or liver conditions usually get a lower dose.

- *Children 12 Years and Older and Adults:* 5 to 10 mg once daily. Individuals with kidney or liver disease usually take 5 mg daily.

If you miss a dose, take it as soon as you remember. If it is nearly time for your next dose, do not take the missed dose. Continue with your regular dosing schedule. Never take a double dose.

SYMPTOMS OF OVERDOSE AND WHAT TO DO

Symptoms of overdose in adults is extreme sleepiness, while in children extreme drowsiness is preceded by irritability and restlessness. If overdose occurs, seek immediate medical assistance and bring the prescription container with you to the hospital.

SPECIAL INFORMATION FOR PREGNANT OR NURSING WOMEN

The effects of cetirizine on pregnant or nursing women have not been adequately studied. If you are pregnant or plan to become pregnant, tell your health-care practitioner. You and your health-care practitioner should weigh the potential benefits against the potential risks to the fetus.

Cetirizine passes into breast milk. If you are breastfeeding, your health-care practitioner may advise you to stop until your treatment is complete.

SPECIAL INFORMATION FOR SENIORS

No special instructions are needed for older adults.

OPEN QUESTIONS OR CONTROVERSIES

In early 2002, U.S. drug regulators recommended that cetirizine (Zyrtec, made by American Home Products and Johnson & Johnson) along with fexofenadine (Allegra, made by Aventis) be made available in an over-the-counter form. These drugs may have reached OTC status by the time this book is released.

GENERIC NAME

Cetuximab

BRAND NAME

Erbitux

No generic available

ABOUT THIS DRUG

Cetuximab is the first monoclonal antibody drug approved to treat advanced colorectal cancer that has metastasized (spread to other parts of the body). It is used as a combination treatment intravenously (IV) along with irinotecan, another anticancer drug for colorectal cancer, or alone if patients cannot tolerate irinotecan.

This drug is believed to work by targeting a protein called epidermal growth factor receptor on the surface of cancer cells and inhibiting their growth. Cetuximab has been shown to shrink tumors and delay tumor growth in some patients whose cancer expresses the epidermal growth factor receptor protein.

SIDE EFFECTS

Be sure to tell your health-care practitioner if you experience any side effects while receiving cetuximab. Only your health-care practitioner can determine whether it is safe for you to continue receiving this drug.

- *Most Common:* abdominal pain, acne-like rash, constipation, diarrhea, dry skin, fever, tiredness or weakness
- *Less Common or Rare:* allergic reaction (difficulty breathing, low blood pressure, itching, or rash, usually during the first infusion), interstitial lung disease (symptoms include sudden onset or worsening of cough, fever, shortness of breath)

IMPORTANT PRECAUTIONS

Tell your health-care practitioner if you are sensitive or allergic to cetuximab, murine (mouse) proteins, to any components of cetuximab, or to any other drugs.

Always wear sunscreen and a hat and limit your exposure to the sun while receiving cetuximab, as sunlight can exacerbate any skin reactions that may occur.

DRUG INTERACTIONS

Tell your health-care practitioner and pharmacist if you are taking any prescription or nonprescription drugs, as well as any vitamins, herbs, or other supplements. No drug-drug interactions have been reported.

FOOD, VITAMIN, AND HERBAL INTERACTIONS

No food, vitamin, or herbal interactions have been noted.

RECOMMENDED DOSAGE

Cetuximab is administered intravenously by a trained health-care professional. The dosages given here are typical. However, your health-care practitioner will determine the most appropriate dose and schedule for your needs.

- *Children:* Not recommended for children
- *Adults:* Usual first infusion is 400 mg/m^2, and then 250 mg/m^2 weekly

Cetuximab is usually administered along with irinotecan, or given alone to patients who cannot tolerate irinotecan. Pretreatment with an intravenous antihistamine (diphenhydramine) is recommended to decrease the chance of allergic reaction during the infusion.

SYMPTOMS OF OVERDOSE AND WHAT TO DO

Symptoms of overdose are not known. If you believe an overdose has occurred, seek immediate medical attention.

SPECIAL INFORMATION FOR PREGNANT OR NURSING WOMEN

Adequate studies of the effects of cetuximab on pregnant or nursing women have not been done. However, animal studies suggest it has the potential to be transmitted to the fetus. If you are pregnant or plan to become pregnant, talk to your health-care practitioner. Only a health-care practitioner can determine whether the potential benefits outweigh the risks.

If you are breastfeeding, your health-care practitioner will likely advise you to switch to bottle feeding during treatment and for 60 days following your last dose of cetuximab.

SPECIAL INFORMATION FOR SENIORS

There are no special instructions for seniors.

GENERIC NAME

Chlordiazepoxide

BRAND NAMES

Libritabs, Librium

Generic available

ABOUT THIS DRUG

Chlordiazepoxide is a benzodiazepine tranquilizer and antianxiety agent used primarily to treat anxiety and agitation.

This drug produces mild sedation by enhancing the effect of a chemical (gamma-ainobutyric acid, or GABA), which in turn dampens the transmission of nerve signals and reduces nerve excitation.

SIDE EFFECTS

Be sure to tell your health-care practitioner if you experience any side effects while taking chlordiazepoxide. Only your health-care practitioner can determine whether it is safe for you to continue taking this drug.

- *Most Common:* mild drowsiness during the initial days of treatment, weakness, confusion
- *Less Common:* depression, lethargy, disorientation, headache, slurred speech, stupor, dizziness, tremor, constipation, dry mouth, nausea, impotence, altered heart rhythm, low blood pressure, fluid retention, blurred or double vision, itching, rash, hiccups, inability to control urination

IMPORTANT PRECAUTIONS

Tell your health-care practitioner if you are sensitive or allergic to chlordiazepoxide or to any other drugs in the benzodiazepine group of drugs.

Chlordiazepoxide may aggravate narrow-angle glaucoma, but is safe to take if you have open-angle glaucoma.

Do not take chlordiazepoxide if you have severe depression, psychosis, severe lung disease, sleep apnea, kidney or liver disease, or alcohol addiction.

This drug should not be taken for longer than 3 to 4 months continuously, at which time your health-care practitioner should reevaluate you. Chlordiazepoxide can also lose its effectiveness with prolonged use.

Chlordiazepoxide may be addictive, and withdrawal symptoms can occur after only 4 weeks of use.

Because chlordiazepoxide can cause drowsiness, make sure you know how the drug affects you before you drive or operate hazardous equipment.

DRUG INTERACTIONS

Tell your health-care practitioner and pharmacist if you are taking any prescription or nonprescription drugs, as well as any vitamins, herbs, or other supplements. Possible drug interactions include the following:

- Alcohol, other tranquilizers, narcotics, barbiturates, monoamine oxidase inhibitors, sleeping pills, antihistamines, and antidepressants may result in excessive depression, sleepiness, breathing difficulties, tiredness, and related symptoms.

- Cimetidine, oral contraceptives, disulfiram, fluoxetine, isoniazid, ketoconazole, metoprolol, probenecid, propoxyphene, propranolol, rifampin, and valproic acid may prolong the effects of chlordiazepoxide.
- Theophylline may reduce the sedative effects of chlordiazepoxide.

FOOD, VITAMIN, AND HERBAL INTERACTIONS

Herbs that produce a sedative effect may cause potentially dangerous depressant interactions when used with chlordiazepoxide. Some of those herbs include calendula, capsicum, catnip, goldenseal, gotu kola, hops, kava, lady's slipper, passionflower, sage, Siberian ginseng, skullcap, St. John's wort, and valerian, among others.

RECOMMENDED DOSAGE

Chlordiazepoxide is available in 5-, 10-, and 25-mg tablets and capsules. The doses given here are typical. However, your health-care practitioner will determine the most appropriate dose and schedule for your needs.

- *Children Up to Age 6 Years:* not recommended
- *Children 6 to 16 Years:* Your health-care practitioner will decide if it is appropriate. Typical starting dose is 5 mg 2 to 4 times daily, with a maintenance dose of up to 30 to 40 mg daily.
- *Adults:* 5 to 100 mg daily, depending on age, weight, severity of the disease, and other factors

If you miss a dose, take it as soon as you remember. If it is nearly time for your next dose, do not take the missed dose. Continue with your regular dosing schedule. Never take a double dose.

SYMPTOMS OF OVERDOSE AND WHAT TO DO

Symptoms of overdose include convulsions, weakness, breathing difficulties, tremor, muscle contractions, blurred vision, depression, bluish skin, dizziness, and coma. If overdose occurs, seek immediate medical attention. If you call a poison control center, they may instruct you to induce vomiting, unless the individual is having convulsions or is unconscious, using ipecac syrup or charcoal. Follow their instructions. If you go to an emergency room, bring the prescription container with you.

SPECIAL INFORMATION FOR PREGNANT OR NURSING WOMEN

Chlordiazepoxide can cause birth defects if taken during the first trimester. If you are pregnant or plan to become pregnant, talk to your health-care practitioner. This drug should not be taken during pregnancy.

This drug may pass into breast milk. If you are breastfeeding, your health-care practitioner may advise you to stop until your treatment is complete.

SPECIAL INFORMATION FOR SENIORS

Older adults usually need lower doses, especially those who have liver or kidney disease. Seniors are also more sensitive to the effects of chlordiazepoxide.

GENERIC NAME

Chlorothiazide *see Thiazide Diuretics, page 1020*

GENERIC NAME

Chlorotrianisene *see Estrogens, page 436*

GENERIC NAME

Chlorpheniramine *see Antihistamine-Decongestant Combination, page 132*

GENERIC NAME

Chlorpromazine

BRAND NAME

Thorazine

Generic available

Note: This entry contains information that applies to another phenothiazine antipsychotic medication, mesoridazine (brand names: Serentil; Serentil Concentrate).

ABOUT THIS DRUG

Chlorpromazine is a phenothiazine antipsychotic drug used to treat psychotic disorders, such as schizophrenia, and moderate to severe depression with anxiety.

This drug and other phenothiazines affect the hypothalamus, a portion of the brain that controls body temperature, alertness, muscle tone, hormone balance, vomiting, and metabolism.

SIDE EFFECTS

Be sure to tell your health-care practitioner if you experience any side effects while taking chlorpromazine. Only your health-care practitioner can determine whether it is safe for you to continue taking this drug.

- *Most Common:* drowsiness, especially during the first few weeks of treatment; dry mouth, lightheadedness, decreased sweating
- *Less Common:* blood changes (e.g., anemia), abnormal heart rate, heart attack, blood pressure changes, sexual dysfunction, breast pain, swelling, blurred vision
- *Rare:* Jaundice (yellowing of the skin and eyes) may occur during the first 2 to 4 weeks of treatment. Also extreme and persistent restlessness, uncontrolled movements, loss of coordination, shuffling gait, trembling, weakness in the extremities, uncontrolled chewing, lip-smacking, or tongue movements, rash, absence of facial expression, difficulty urinating, increased skin sensitivity to the sun

People taking antipsychotic drugs may experience a rare but life-threatening set of side effects known as neuroleptic malignant syndrome (NMS). Symptoms include fever, difficulty breathing, rapid heartbeat, rigid muscles, mental changes, increased sweating, irregular blood pressure, and convulsions. Immediate medical attention is required.

Side effects such as lip-smacking, wormlike movements of the tongue, and slow, rhythmical, involuntary movements are characteristic of a disorder known as tardive dyskinesia. Older adults (especially women) are more susceptible to this condition, which may become permanent. If you experience tardive dyskinesia, your health-care practitioner will probably advise you to stop taking this drug.

IMPORTANT PRECAUTIONS

Tell your health-care practitioner if you are sensitive or allergic to chlorpromazine or to any other drugs, including other phenothiazines.

Do not take chlorpromazine if you have very low blood pressure, Parkinson's disease, or heart, liver, kidney, or blood disease.

Chlorpromazine should be used under strict medical supervision if you have glaucoma, epilepsy, urinary problems, breast cancer, benign prostatic hyperplasia, or ulcers.

This drug can depress the cough reflex, causing you to accidentally choke to death. Because chlorpromazine helps prevent vomiting, it can mask symptoms of conditions caused by an overdose of another drug.

Avoid exposure to extreme heat, because chlorpromazine affects the temperature control center of your brain.

DRUG INTERACTIONS

Tell your health-care practitioner and pharmacist if you are taking any prescription or nonprescription drugs, as well as any vitamins, herbs, or other supplements. Possible drug interactions include the following:

- Alcohol and other drugs that depress the central nervous system (e.g., barbiturates, sleeping pills, narcotics, tranquilizers) may produce additional sedative effects.
- Antacids that contain aluminum may reduce the effectiveness of phenothiazine drugs.
- Bromocriptine and appetite suppressants may be less effective.
- Guanethidine's ability to lower blood pressure may be reduced.
- Lithium may cause disorientation, loss of consciousness, or uncontrolled muscle movements.
- Propranolol may result in very low blood pressure.
- Tricyclic antidepressants (e.g., amitriptyline, imipramine) may cause antidepressant side effects.

FOOD, VITAMIN, AND HERBAL INTERACTIONS

Herbs that produce a sedative effect may cause potentially serious depressant interactions when used with chlorpromazine. Some of those herbs include calendula, capsicum, catnip, goldenseal, gotu kola, hops, kava, lady's slipper, passionflower, sage, Siberian ginseng, skullcap, St. John's wort, and valerian, among others.

RECOMMENDED DOSAGE

Chlorpromazine is available in capsules, tablets, liquid concentrate, syrup, and suppositories. The dosages given here are typical. However, your health-care practitioner will determine the most appropriate dose and schedule for your needs.

- *Children Up to 6 Months:* not recommended
- *Children Older than 6 Months:* Dosages are based on the child's weight. Oral doses are given at 0.25 mg per pound of body weight, taken every 4 to 6 hours, as needed; suppositories are given at 0.5 mg per pound of body weight every 6 to 8 hours.
- *Adults:* Starting dose for psychotic disorders can range from 30 to 75 mg daily, taken in 3 to 4 divided doses. Your health-care practitioner may increase the dosage semiweekly.

Chlorpromazine can be taken with food if it upsets your stomach. The liquid form should be taken with fruit juice or another nonalcoholic liquid.

If you miss a dose, take it as soon as you remember. If it is nearly time for your next dose, do not take the missed dose. Continue with your regular dosing schedule. Never take a double dose.

SYMPTOMS OF OVERDOSE AND WHAT TO DO

Symptoms of overdose include agitation, coma, convulsions, breathing difficulties, dry mouth, extreme sleepiness, fever, intestinal blockage, irregular heart rate, low blood pressure, restlessness, and swallowing difficulties. If an overdose occurs, seek immediate medical attention and bring the prescription container with you to the hospital.

SPECIAL INFORMATION FOR PREGNANT OR NURSING WOMEN

Adequate studies of the effects of chlorpromazine on pregnant or nursing women have not been done. If you are pregnant or plan to become pregnant, talk to your health-care practitioner. This drug should not be used during pregnancy unless your health-care practitioner determines it is essential for your health.

Chlorpromazine may pass into breast milk. Your health-care practitioner may advise you to stop breastfeeding until you have finished treatment.

SPECIAL INFORMATION FOR SENIORS

Older adults generally need lower doses of chlorpromazine. Because seniors are at greater risk of low blood pressure, health-care practitioners need to monitor it regularly. Older women are especially at higher risk for tardive dyskinesia, a condition characterized by involuntary muscle spasms and twitches.

GENERIC NAME

Chlorpropamide *see Sulfonylurea Antidiabetes Drugs, page 971*

GENERIC NAME

Chlorthalidone *see Thiazide Diuretics, page 1020*

GENERIC NAME

Chlorzoxazone

BRAND NAMES

EZE-DS, Paraflex, Parafon Forte DSC, Relax-Ds, Relaxazone, Remular-S

Generic available

ABOUT THIS DRUG

Chlorzoxazone is a muscle relaxant used to relieve severe, painful muscle spasms, strains, sprains, and other muscle problems.

Chlorzoxazone suppresses the activity in the central nervous system, which then interferes with the transmission of nerve signals from the spinal cord to the muscles. It is not a substitute for other treatment approaches, such as physical therapy, rest, and surgery.

SIDE EFFECTS

Be sure to tell your health-care practitioner if you experience any side effects while taking chlorzoxazone. Only your health-care practitioner can determine whether it is safe for you to continue taking this drug.

- *Most Common:* dizziness, drowsiness, lightheadedness
- *Less Common:* headache, diarrhea, constipation, heartburn, nausea, vomiting, stomach cramps or pain
- *Rare:* liver problems, internal bleeding, severe allergic reactions, breathing difficulties

IMPORTANT PRECAUTIONS

Tell your health-care practitioner if you are sensitive or allergic to chlorzoxazone or to any other drugs.

Do not take chlorzoxazone if you have porphyria, a rare metabolic condition.

If you have kidney or liver disease, chlorzoxazone should be taken with caution.

Because chlorzoxazone can lead to physical dependence, anyone with a history of substance abuse should use this medication with extreme caution.

Treatment should generally be limited to 10 days. Periodic liver tests are recommended during treatment.

Drowsiness and dizziness are common side effects. Make sure you know how you react to this drug before you drive or operate dangerous equipment.

Chlorzoxazone may cause your urine to turn orange or purple-red. This is not dangerous.

DRUG INTERACTIONS

Tell your health-care practitioner and pharmacist if you are taking any prescription or nonprescription drugs, as well as any vitamins, herbs, or other supplements. Chlorzoxazone may interact with various drugs:

- Central nervous system depressants (e.g., alcohol, sleeping pills, tranquilizers, barbiturates) may enhance the depressive effects of chlorzoxazone. Do not combine these drugs.

FOOD, VITAMIN, AND HERBAL INTERACTIONS

Herbs that produce a sedative effect may cause potentially dangerous depressant interactions when used with chlorzoxazone. Some of those herbs include calendula, capsicum, catnip, goldenseal, gotu kola, hops, kava, lady's slipper, passionflower, sage, Siberian ginseng, skullcap, St. John's wort, and valerian, among others.

RECOMMENDED DOSAGE

Chlorzoxazone is available in tablets and caplets. The dosages given here are typical. However, your health-care practitioner will determine the most appropriate dose and schedule for your needs.

- *Children Up to 12 Years:* not recommended
- *Adults:* 250 to 750 mg, 3 to 4 times daily

Chlorzoxazone can be taken with food to reduce stomach irritation. You can crush the tablets and mix the medication with food if desired.

If you miss a dose, take it as soon as you remember. If it is nearly time for your next dose, do not take the missed dose. Continue with your regular dosing schedule. Never take a double dose.

SYMPTOMS OF OVERDOSE AND WHAT TO DO

Symptoms of overdose include nausea, vomiting, loss of appetite, headache, severe weakness, increased sweating, fainting, breathing problems, irritability, convulsions, and loss of consciousness. If overdose occurs, seek immediate medical attention and bring the prescription container with you to the hospital.

SPECIAL INFORMATION FOR PREGNANT OR NURSING WOMEN

No adequate studies of the effects of chlorzoxazone on pregnant or nursing women have been done. If you are pregnant or plan to become pregnant, talk to your health-care practitioner. You and your health-care practitioner should weigh the potential benefits against the potential risks to the fetus.

Chlorzoxazone may pass into breast milk. If you are breastfeeding, your health-care practitioner may advise you to bottle feed while you are undergoing treatment.

SPECIAL INFORMATION FOR SENIORS

Older adults may be more sensitive to the effects of chlorzoxazone, and they may experience more severe side effects.

GENERIC NAME

Cholestyramine

BRAND NAMES

LoCHOLEST Prevalite, LoCHOLEST Light, Questran, Questran Light
Generic available

ABOUT THIS DRUG

Cholestyramine is an anti-hyperlipidemic (blood-fat reducer) used primarily to treat primary hypercholesterolemia (abnormally high low-density lipoprotein cholesterol). It should be used along with exercise and a sensible diet recommended by your health-care practitioner.

This drug reduces blood cholesterol levels by absorbing bile acids in the intestinal tract. The body needs cholesterol to produce bile acids, which digest fat; thus fat digestion requires more bile acid from cholesterol.

SIDE EFFECTS

Be sure to tell your health-care practitioner if you experience any side effects while taking cholestyramine. Only your health-care practitioner can determine whether it is safe for you to continue taking this drug.

- *Most Common:* constipation
- *Less Common or Rare:* abdominal pain, bloating, bleeding disorders, nausea, vomiting, diarrhea, heartburn, appetite loss, fatty stool, anxiety, asthma, backache, dizziness, drowsiness, fainting, fatigue, hiccups, hives, inflamed eye, irritation in the anal area, muscle pain, ringing in the ears, shortness of breath, sour taste, swollen glands, tingling sensation, wheezing

IMPORTANT PRECAUTIONS

Tell your health-care practitioner if you are sensitive or allergic to cholestyramine or to any other drugs.

Do not take cholestyramine without your health-care practitioner's permission if you are being treated for gallbladder obstruction or if you are receiving treatment for any condition that contributes to increased blood cholesterol (e.g., hyperthyroidism, diabetes, obstructive liver disease, or alcoholism).

Cholestyramine can alter acidity in the blood, especially in younger and smaller individuals. Therefore regular monitoring by your health-care practitioner is recommended.

Brush and floss often while taking this medication, as it can stain or erode the teeth.

DRUG INTERACTIONS

Tell your health-care practitioner and pharmacist if you are taking any prescription or nonprescription drugs, as well as any vitamins, herbs, or other supplements. Possible drug interactions include the following:

- Cholestyramine interferes with absorption of most drugs taken orally, including but not limited to acetaminophen, amiodarone, aspirin, cephalexin, clindamycin, clofibrate, corticosteroids, diclofenac, digitalis, furosemide, gemfibrozil, glipizide, hydrocortisone, imipramine, methyldopa, nicotinic acid, penicillin, phenobarbital, phenytoin, propranolol, tetracycline, thiazide diuretics, thyroid medications, tolbutamide, trimethoprim, warfarin, and other anticoagulants. To avoid this problem, take other drugs at least 1 hour before or 4 to 6 hours after you take cholestyramine.

FOOD, VITAMIN, AND HERBAL INTERACTIONS

Cholestyramine hinders the digestion and absorption of fats and fat-soluble vitamins, including vitamins A, D, E, and K, as well as folate (folic acid), iron, and calcium. Take these supplements at least 1 hour before or 4 to 6 hours after you take cholestyramine.

RECOMMENDED DOSAGE

Cholestyramine is available in a powder that can be mixed with water, juice, soda, or soft foods such as applesauce or pudding. The dosages given here are typical. However, your health-care practitioner will determine the most appropriate dose and schedule for your needs.

- *Children:* use and dose to be determined by your health-care practitioner
- *Adults:* 4 g (1 packet of powder) taken 1 to 6 times daily

Do not take the powder in its dry form; follow mixing direction carefully, and take cholestyramine before meals.

If you miss a dose, take it as soon as you remember. If it is nearly time for your next dose, do not take the missed dose. Continue with your regular dosing schedule. Never take a double dose.

SYMPTOMS OF OVERDOSE AND WHAT TO DO

The primary symptom of overdose includes bowel impaction. If an overdose occurs, seek immediate medical attention and bring the prescription container with you to the hospital.

SPECIAL INFORMATION FOR PREGNANT OR NURSING WOMEN

Cholestyramine may indirectly affect the fetus because it reduces the absorption of vitamins A, D, E, and K, as well as folate (folic acid), iron, and calcium, all of which are necessary for normal fetal development. If cholestyramine is essential for your health, you and your health-care practitioner must weigh the potential benefits against the potential risks to the fetus.

Cholestyramine does not pass into breast milk. However, because of its effect on vitamin absorption, breast milk may be less nutritious. If you are breastfeeding, your health-care practitioner may advise you to switch to bottle feeding.

SPECIAL INFORMATION FOR SENIORS

Older adults are more likely to experience side effects, especially constipation.

GENERIC NAME
Ciclopirox

BRAND NAMES
Loprox, Peniac Nail Lacquer
Generic available

ABOUT THIS DRUG
Ciclopirox is an antifungal used to treat fungal and yeast infections that affect the nails and skin, such as candida, jock itch, and athlete's foot.

Ciclopirox penetrates skin, sweat glands, hair, and hair follicles and either interferes with the growth of fungus and yeast or kills them.

SIDE EFFECTS
Be sure to tell your health-care practitioner if you experience any side effects while using ciclopirox. Only your health-care practitioner can determine whether it is safe for you to continue using this drug.

➤ *Most Common:* burning, itching, and stinging at the site of application

IMPORTANT PRECAUTIONS
Tell your health-care practitioner if you are sensitive or allergic to ciclopirox or to any other drugs.

Ciclopirox is for external use only. Do not apply an airtight dressing over the affected area unless told to do so by your health-care practitioner.

DRUG INTERACTIONS
Tell your health-care practitioner and pharmacist if you are taking any prescription or nonprescription drugs, as well as any vitamins, herbs, or other supplements. Ciclopirox is not known to cause any drug interactions.

FOOD, VITAMIN, AND HERBAL INTERACTIONS
No food, vitamin, or herbal interactions have been noted.

RECOMMENDED DOSAGE
Ciclopirox is available in cream, gel, and lotion. The dosage given here is typical. However, your health-care practitioner will determine the most appropriate dose and schedule for your needs.

- *Children Up to Age 10 or 16:* The safety and effectiveness of cream and lotion ciclopirox have not been determined for children up to age 10; for gel, up to age 16.
- *Adults:* Apply enough of the topical medication to cover the affected areas. Massage it into the skin twice daily. If using the nail lacquer, apply to infected nails once daily.

Follow your health-care practitioner's instructions for use for the entire 2- to 4-week treatment course, even if your symptoms have cleared up earlier. When using the nail lacquer, apply it only to nails, as it can irritate the skin.

If you miss a dose, apply it as soon as you remember. If it is nearly time for your next dose, do not apply the missed dose. Continue with your regular dosing schedule. Never apply a double dose.

SYMPTOMS OF OVERDOSE AND WHAT TO DO

Application of too much cream or lotion is not likely to cause a significant reaction. If ciclopirox is accidentally ingested, nausea and stomach upset may occur. Seek immediate medical assistance and bring the prescription container with you to the hospital.

SPECIAL INFORMATION FOR PREGNANT OR NURSING WOMEN

Ciclopirox may cross the placenta; however, high doses given to animals have not shown any harm to the fetus. If you are pregnant or plan to become pregnant, talk to your health-care practitioner. You and your health-care practitioner should weigh the potential benefits against the potential risks to the fetus.

It is not known whether ciclopirox passes into breast milk. If you are breastfeeding, your health-care practitioner may advise you to stop until you have finished treatment.

SPECIAL INFORMATION FOR SENIORS

Older adults have no special restrictions when using this drug.

GENERIC NAME

Cilostazol

BRAND NAME

Pletal

No generic available

ABOUT THIS DRUG

Cilostazol is an antiplatelet drug used to reduce the symptoms of leg pain and spasms that are induced by walking and caused by reduced blood flow.

Cilostazol helps maintain blood flow by preventing blood clots and relaxing the blood vessels.

SIDE EFFECTS

Be sure to tell your health-care practitioner if you experience any side effects while taking cilostazol. Only your health-care practitioner can determine whether it is safe for you to continue taking this drug.

- *Most Common:* diarrhea, headache, muscle aches, increased risk of infection
- *Common:* rapid heartbeat, dizziness, fainting, upset stomach, nausea, back pain, swelling in the arms and legs, sore throat, runny nose
- *Less Common or Rare:* gas, cough, abdominal pain. Other side effects not listed may occur.

IMPORTANT PRECAUTIONS

Tell your health-care practitioner if you are sensitive or allergic to cilostazol or to any other drugs.

The safety and effectiveness of cilostazol have not been determined when used beyond 6 months, nor have they been established for children younger than 18 years.

Because of the risk of dizziness and fainting, make sure you know how you react to cilostazol before you drive or operate hazardous equipment.

DRUG INTERACTIONS

Tell your health-care practitioner and pharmacist if you are taking any prescription or nonprescription drugs, as well as any vitamins, herbs, or other supplements. The following drugs can interact with cilostazol:

- Fluconazole, fluvoxamine, fluoxetine, itraconazoe, ketoconazole, miconazole, nefazodone, and sertraline may reduce the breakdown of cilostazole and result in prolonged effects. Your health-care practitioner may prescribe half the typical dose of cilostazole if you are also taking any of these other drugs.
- Aspirin can increase the blood-thinning effect of cilostazol. Your health-care practitioner may prescribe half the typical dose of cilostazole if you are also taking aspirin or any other antiplatelet or anticoagulant drugs.

- Diltiazem as well as erythromycin and similar antibiotics increase the blood levels of cilostazole. Your health-care practitioner may prescribe half the typical dose of cilostazole if you are also taking any of these drugs.
- Smoking causes the liver to break down cilostazol faster, thus reducing the drug's effectiveness.

FOOD, VITAMIN, AND HERBAL INTERACTIONS

Do not drink grapefruit juice anytime during your treatment with cilostazole because it can interfere with breakdown of the drug. Because cilostazole affects blood clotting, herbs that should be avoided include feverfew, garlic, ginkgo, and ginseng.

RECOMMENDED DOSAGE

Cilostazole is available in tablets. The dosages given here are typical. However, your health-care practitioner will determine the most appropriate dose and schedule for your needs.

- *Children Up to 18 Years:* not recommended
- *Adults:* 100 mg twice daily, or 50 mg twice daily if you are taking any of the drugs named under "Drug Interactions" or if so instructed by your health-care practitioner

Cilostazole should be taken on an empty stomach at least 1 hour before or 2 hours after meals.

If you miss a dose, take it as soon as you remember. If it is nearly time for your next dose, do not take the missed dose. Continue with your regular dosing schedule. Never take a double dose.

SYMPTOMS OF OVERDOSE AND WHAT TO DO

Symptoms of overdose can include severe headache, diarrhea, dizziness, fainting, and irregular heartbeat. If overdose occurs, seek immediate medical attention, and bring the prescription container with you to the hospital.

SPECIAL INFORMATION FOR PREGNANT OR NURSING WOMEN

Animal studies show that cilostazol harms the fetus, but no adequate studies have been done in pregnant women. If your health-care practitioner determines that this drug is critical for your health, you and he or she must weigh the potential benefits against the potential risks to the fetus.

Cilostazol may pass into breast milk. If you are breastfeeding, your health-care practitioner will likely advise you to stop until your treatment is complete.

SPECIAL INFORMATION FOR SENIORS

No special instructions are needed for older adults.

GENERIC NAME

Cimetidine

BRAND NAMES

Tagamet, Tagamet HB
Generic available

ABOUT THIS DRUG

Cimetidine is a histamine H_2 antagonist (blocker) used to treat stomach and duodenum ulcers, upset stomach, gastroesophageal reflux disease, and other symptoms of stomach distress.

This drug blocks the activity of histamine, which in turn reduces the production of stomach acid and other stomach secretions. Once stomach acid production has decreased, the body can better heal itself.

SIDE EFFECTS

Be sure to tell your health-care practitioner if you experience any side effects while taking cimetidine. Only your health-care practitioner can determine whether it is safe for you to continue taking this drug.

➤ *Most Common:* drowsiness, abdominal pain, diarrhea, headache, fatigue, nausea, vomiting

➤ *Less Common:* blurred vision, breast swelling, depression, hallucinations, insomnia, rash, hives, decreased sexual desire or function, temporary hair loss, leaking nipples

➤ *Rare:* unusual bleeding or bruising, unusual tiredness, weakness, abnormal heart rhythms, heart attack, reversible muscle or joint pain

IMPORTANT PRECAUTIONS

Tell your health-care practitioner if you are sensitive or allergic to cimetidine or to any other drugs, especially other histamine H_2 antagonists (e.g., ranitidine, nizatidine).

Use cimetidine with caution if you have liver or kidney disease.

Rarely, cimetidine causes confusion, agitation, hallucinations, depression, anxiety, or disorientation within 2 or 3 days of starting therapy. Contact your health-care practitioner immediately if these occur. These symptoms, which usually appear in people who are very ill, are elderly, or have kidney disease, usually disappear several days after stopping treatment.

Symptoms associated with gastrointestinal problems that cimetidine typically is prescribed to treat may also indicate stomach cancer. Your health-care practitioner should screen for possible malignancy.

Cimetidine is not for use in children younger than 16 years.

DRUG INTERACTIONS

Tell your health-care practitioner and pharmacist if you are taking any prescription or nonprescription drugs, as well as any vitamins, herbs, or other supplements. Possible drug interactions include the following:

- Cimetidine may increase the side effects of alcohol, aminophylline, benzodiazepine tranquilizers, sleeping pills (except lorazepam, oxazepam, and temazepam), oral antidiabetes drugs, caffeine, calcium channel blockers, carbamazepine, carmustine, chloroquine, flecainide, fluorouracil, labetolol, lidocaine, metoprolol, metronidazole, mexiletine, narcotics, ondansetron, phenytoin, procainamide, propafenone, propranolol, quinine, quinidine, tacrine, theophylline drugs (except dyphylline), triamterene, tricyclic antidepressants (e.g., amitriptyline, imipramine), valproic acid, and warfarin.
- Cimetidine may decrease absorption of fluconazole, indomethacin, ketoconazole, and tetracycline antibiotics.
- Antacids reduce the effectiveness of cimetidine. To prevent this reaction, take antacids at least 3 hours before or after your cimetidine dose.
- Cimetidine may reduce the effects of digoxin and tocainide.
- Enteric-coated tablets should not be taken along with cimetidine because the latter causes a change in stomach acidity and thus makes the tablets dissolve prematurely.
- Metoclopramide and anticholinergic drugs (e.g., oxybutynin, benztropine) may reduce the effectiveness of cimetidine.
- Smoking cigarettes reverses the healing benefits of cimetidine on ulcers.

FOOD, VITAMIN, AND HERBAL INTERACTIONS

Cimetidine may decrease the absorption of iron, folate (folic acid), vitamin B_{12}, vitamin D, and zinc. Talk to your health-care practitioner about possibly taking a multivitamin-mineral supplement.

RECOMMENDED DOSAGE

Cimetidine is available in tablets, oral solution, and oral suspension. The dosages given here are typical. However, your health-care practitioner will determine the most appropriate dose and schedule for your needs.

➤ *Children Up to 16 Years:* not recommended

➤ *Adults:* For treatment of ulcers, 400 to 800 mg at bedtime, or 300 mg 4 times daily with meals and at bedtime, or 400 mg twice daily. For prevention of ulcers: 300 mg twice daily or 400 mg once at bedtime. For heartburn and acid indigestion: 200 mg when symptoms start, then 200 mg within the next 24 hours for a maximum of 400 mg in a 24-hour period. For gastroesophageal reflux disease: 800 to 1,600 mg daily in 2 to 4 divided doses for about 12 weeks.

Cimetidine should be taken with meals (as directed) or with water at bedtime.

If you miss a dose, take it as soon as you remember. If it is nearly time for your next dose, do not take the missed dose. Continue with your regular dosing schedule. Never take a double dose.

SYMPTOMS OF OVERDOSE AND WHAT TO DO

Little is known about cimetidine overdose, but you can expect side effects to be exaggerated. If overdose occurs, contact your poison control center, which will likely advise you to induce vomiting with ipecac syrup. You can also go to your local emergency department and bring the prescription container with you.

SPECIAL INFORMATION FOR PREGNANT OR NURSING WOMEN

Cimetidine crosses the placenta, although animal studies have not revealed any damage to the fetus. If you are pregnant or plan to become pregnant, talk to your health-care practitioner about the potential benefits and risks to the fetus.

Large amounts of cimetidine pass into breast milk. If you are breastfeeding, you should switch to bottle feeding until your treatment is complete.

SPECIAL INFORMATION FOR SENIORS

Older adults may need lower doses because they typically have reduced kidney function. They may also be more susceptible to side effects, especially confusion and other nervous system symptoms.

GENERIC NAME

Ciprofloxacin *see Fluoroquinolone Antibiotics, page 468*

GENERIC NAME

Citalopram

BRAND NAME

Celexa
No generic available

ABOUT THIS DRUG

Citalopram is a selective serotonin reuptake inhibitor (SSRI), a type of antidepressant used to treat depression. This class of antidepressants is not related to older tricyclic and tetracyclic antidepressants.

Citalopram and other SSRIs prevent the movement of serotonin (a neurohormone) into the nerve endings, which forces this substance to remain outside the nerve endings. This is where it is effective in improving mood, mental alertness, and physical activity.

SIDE EFFECTS

Be sure to tell your health-care practitioner if you experience any side effects while taking citalopram. Only your health-care practitioner can determine whether it is safe for you to continue taking this drug.

- *Most Common:* dry mouth, dizziness, diarrhea or loose stools, fatigue, sexual dysfunction, headache, tremors, nausea, sleeplessness
- *Common:* excessive sweating, upset stomach, agitation, constipation
- *Less Common or Rare:* chest pain, nervousness, anxiety, tingling or numbness in the hands or feet, twitching, palpitations, muscle spasms, confusion, rash, gas, changes in appetite, vision changes, frequent urination, fever, back pain, chills, confusion, reduced skin sensation, nightmares, weight gain, vomiting, taste changes, ringing in the ears, urinary difficulties, menstrual difficulties, depersonalization

IMPORTANT PRECAUTIONS

Tell your health-care practitioner if you are sensitive or allergic to citalopram or to any other drugs, especially other SSRIs.

Potentially deadly reactions may occur if you take citalopram and a monoamine oxidase inhibitor (e.g., phenelzine, furazolidone).

If you have liver or kidney disease or a seizure disorder, you should exercise caution when using this drug.

If you have mania or hypomania, citalopram may activate your condition.

Severely depressed individuals should have access to limited amounts of citalopram at one time to reduce the risk of overdose and suicide.

DRUG INTERACTIONS

Tell your health-care practitioner and pharmacist if you are taking any prescription or nonprescription drugs, as well as any vitamins, herbs, or other supplements.

- Citalopram may increase the effect of metoprolol, warfarin, and tricyclic antidepressants (e.g., doxepin, imipramine).
- Carbamazepine may reduce the effect of citalopram.
- Cimetidine may increase the effect of citalopram.
- Monoamine oxidase inhibitors (MAOIs) should never be used with citalopram, as the combination may cause a life-threatening reaction.

FOOD, VITAMIN, AND HERBAL INTERACTIONS

Natural substances that have a known or an apparent effect on serotonin levels, including 5-HTP (5-hydroxytryptophan), SAM-e (S-adenosylmethionine), and St. John's wort, when combined with citalopram or other SSRIs, may cause a toxic condition known as serotonin syndrome. This syndrome is characterized by restlessness, confusion, weakness, tremor, muscle twitching, high fever, profuse sweating, rapid heartbeat, and anxiety. These drug-supplement combinations should be avoided.

RECOMMENDED DOSAGE

Citalopram is available in tablets and oral solution. The dosages given here are typical. However, your health-care practitioner will determine the most appropriate dose and schedule for your needs.

- *Children Up to 18 Years:* The safety and effectiveness of citalopram has not been determined for this age group.

- *Adults:* 40 mg once daily, morning or night.
- *Adults 60 and Older:* 20 mg daily, morning or night. This dose is also recommended for adults who have liver disease.

Citalopram should be taken on an empty stomach at least 1 hour before or 2 hours after meals to help maintain consistent blood levels.

If you miss a dose, take it as soon as you remember. If it is nearly time for your next dose, do not take the missed dose. Continue with your regular dosing schedule. Never take a double dose.

SYMPTOMS OF OVERDOSE AND WHAT TO DO

Symptoms of overdose include nausea, vomiting, rapid heartbeat, anxiety, dilated pupils, tiredness, and changes in electrocardiogram results. If overdose occurs, seek immediate medical attention and bring the prescription container with you to the hospital.

SPECIAL INFORMATION FOR PREGNANT OR NURSING WOMEN

No adequate studies of the effects of citalopram on pregnant or nursing women have been done. If you are pregnant or plan to become pregnant, talk to your health-care practitioner. Do not use this drug unless the benefits of therapy clearly outweigh the potential risks to the fetus.

Citalopram passes into breast milk. If you are breastfeeding, your health-care practitioner may advise you to stop until you have completed therapy.

SPECIAL INFORMATION FOR SENIORS

Older adults typically start with half the normal adult beginning dose. Side effects are also more likely to occur and to be more severe in seniors.

OPEN QUESTIONS OR CONTROVERSIES

In June 2004, the Food and Drug Administration asked manufacturers of citalopram to include in their labeling a warning statement that recommends close observation of adult and pediatric patients for clinical worsening of depression or the emergence of suicidality when being treated with this drug, especially when beginning the drug, or at the time of dose changes, either increases or decreases.

GENERIC NAME

Clarithromycin

BRAND NAME

Biaxin
No generic available

ABOUT THIS DRUG

Clarithromycin is a macrolide antibiotic used to treat mild-to-moderate infections of the lower and upper respiratory tract, and for duodenal ulcers caused by the bacterium *Helicobacter pylori.*

Clarithromycin fights bacterial infections by either killing the bacteria or inhibiting their growth, depending on the organism involved and the amount of antibiotic present.

SIDE EFFECTS

Be sure to tell your health-care practitioner if you experience any side effects while taking clarithromycin. Only your health-care practitioner can determine whether it is safe for you to continue taking this drug. Most side effects are mild and go away when you stop taking the drug.

- *Most Common:* nausea, vomiting, upset stomach, taste changes, gas, headache
- *Rare:* colitis (severe abdominal cramps and severe, possibly bloody diarrhea), allergic reactions (swelling of the lips, tongue, face, and throat, breathing problems, rash, hives), blood clotting disorders, heartbeat irregularities in people with heart conditions

IMPORTANT PRECAUTIONS

Tell your health-care practitioner if you are sensitive or allergic to clarithromycin or to any other drugs, especially other macrolide antibiotics.

This drug should be taken with caution if you have severe kidney disease or liver disease. Dosage adjustments may be required.

DRUG INTERACTIONS

Tell your health-care practitioner and pharmacist if you are taking any prescription or nonprescription drugs, as well as any vitamins, herbs, or other supplements. Possible drug interactions include the following:

- Clarithromycin may increase the blood-thinning effects of warfarin in individuals who take it regularly.

- Taking clarithromycin with omeprazole, carbamazepine, or ranitidine bismuth-sulfate can raise the blood levels of both drugs.
- Rifabutin and rifampin can hinder the effects of clarithromycin and increase the risk of intestinal side effects.
- Pimozide has caused at least two deaths when taken with clarithromycin. Avoid this combination.
- Clarithromycin may prolong the effects of alprazolam, diazepam, midazolam, and triazolam and lead to serious nervous system depression.
- Theophylline levels may be increased by clarithromycin and lead to a theophylline overdose.
- Fluconazole increases the blood levels of clarithromycin.
- Clarithromycin increases the effects of buspirone and causes adverse reactions.
- Clarithromycin may affect the amount of zidovudine in the blood.
- Cyclosporine, digoxin, ergot drugs (e.g., ergotamine, methysergide), tacrolimus, and triazolam may cause drug side effects.
- Statin-lowering drugs (e.g., simvastatin, fluvastatin) along with clarithromycin may lead to a potentially deadly condition characterized by severe muscle pain and destruction.

FOOD, VITAMIN, AND HERBAL INTERACTIONS

No food, vitamin, or herbal interactions have been noted.

RECOMMENDED DOSAGE

Clarithromycin is available as tablets and in oral suspension. The dosages given here are typical. However, your health-care practitioner will determine the most appropriate dose and schedule for your needs.

- *Children Up to 6 Months:* not recommended
- *Children 6 Months to 12 Years:* 3.4 mg per pound of body weight, up to 500 mg every 12 hours for 10 days
- *Adults:* For infections, 250 to 500 mg every 12 hours for 1 to 2 weeks. For ulcers, 500 mg three times daily along with the ulcer medication prescribed by your health-care practitioner (e.g., ranitidine, omeprazole)

Clarithromycin can be taken with or without food. If you take the suspension form, shake it well before using. Clarithromycin should be taken at the same time each day.

If you miss a dose, take it as soon as you remember. If it is within

4 hours of your next dose, do not take the missed dose, and return to your regular schedule. Never take a double dose.

SYMPTOMS OF OVERDOSE AND WHAT TO DO

Symptoms of overdose include severe nausea, vomiting, stomach cramps, and diarrhea. If overdose occurs, seek immediate medical attention and bring the prescription container with you to the hospital.

SPECIAL INFORMATION FOR PREGNANT OR NURSING WOMEN

Clarithromycin has caused birth defects in animals. If you are pregnant or plan to become pregnant, talk to your health-care practitioner. Do not use this drug unless the benefits of therapy clearly outweigh the potential risks to the fetus.

It is not known whether clarithromycin passes into breast milk, but other macrolide antibiotics do. If you are breastfeeding, your health-care practitioner will likely advise you to stop until your treatment is complete.

SPECIAL INFORMATION FOR SENIORS

Older adults, especially those who have severe kidney disease, will need a dose adjustment.

GENERIC NAME

Clemastine

BRAND NAMES

Contac 12 Hour Allergy, Tavist, Tavist-1, Tavist-D
Generic available

ABOUT THIS DRUG

Clemastine is an antihistamine used to relieve stuffy and runny nose, itchy eyes, and scratchy throat associated with seasonal allergies (hayfever).

This drug blocks the release of histamine (a chemical released by the body during an allergic reaction). Histamine is responsible for the symptoms associated with seasonal allergies, as well as itching, rash, and hives.

SIDE EFFECTS

Be sure to tell your health-care practitioner if you experience any side effects while taking clemastine. Only your health-care practitioner can determine whether it is safe for you to continue taking this drug.

- *Most Common:* dry mouth, nose, and throat, nosebleed, headache, weakness, nervousness, stomach upset, nausea, vomiting, cough, stuffy nose, bowel habit changes
- *Less Common:* drowsiness, hair loss, depression, sleeplessness, menstrual irregularities, aching muscles, sweating, visual disturbances, frequent urination, tingling in the feet or hands, allergic reactions (rash, itching, hives, breathing difficulties)

IMPORTANT PRECAUTIONS

Tell your health-care practitioner if you are sensitive or allergic to clemastine or to any other drugs, especially other antihistamines.

Because clemastine can make you drowsy, make sure you know how you react to this drug before you drive or operate dangerous equipment.

Do not take clemastine if you have asthma or other deep-breathing problems, glaucoma, enlarged prostate, obstructed bladder, intestinal blockage, stomach ulcers, or other stomach conditions because the drug can aggravate these problems.

If you have heart disease, circulatory problems, high blood pressure, or an overactive thyroid, use clemastine with caution.

DRUG INTERACTIONS

Tell your health-care practitioner and pharmacist if you are taking any prescription or nonprescription—drugs, as well as any vitamins, herbs, or other supplements. Possible drug interactions include the following:

- Alcohol, tranquilizers, sleeping pills, or other central nervous system depressants may increase the sedative effects of clemastine.
- Clemastine may increase the effects of anticoagulants (blood-thinning drugs such as warfarin).
- Monoamine oxidase inhibitor (MAOI) antidepressants and anticholinergics (e.g., atropine, scopolamine) may increase the side effects of clemastine and also cause urinary difficulties.

FOOD, VITAMIN, AND HERBAL INTERACTIONS

Herbs that produce a sedative effect may cause significant depressant interactions when used with clemastine. Some of those herbs include calendula, capsicum, catnip, goldenseal, gotu kola, hops, kava, lady's slipper, passionflower, sage, Siberian ginseng, skullcap, St. John's wort, and valerian, among others.

RECOMMENDED DOSAGE

Clemastine is available as tablets, syrup, and extended-release tablets and caplets. The dosages given here are typical. However, your health-care practitioner will determine the most appropriate dose and schedule for your needs.

- *Children 6 to 11 Years:* For hayfever, 0.67 mg twice daily, or as instructed by your health-care practitioner. For hives and swelling, 1.34 mg twice daily up to 4.02 mg daily, or as instructed by your health-care practitioner. Children in this age group should take syrup only.
- *Children 12 Years and Older and Adults:* For hayfever, 1.34 mg twice daily up to a maximum of 8.04 mg daily (60 ml syrup or 6 tablets) or 2.68 mg up to 3 times daily. For hives and swelling, 2.68 mg 1 to 3 times daily up to 8.04 mg daily.

Clemastine should be taken on an empty stomach at least 1 hour before or 2 hours after eating. If, however, clemastine causes stomach irritation, it can be taken with food.

If you miss a dose, take it as soon as you remember. If it is nearly time for your next dose, do not take the missed dose. Continue with your regular dosing schedule. Never take a double dose.

SYMPTOMS OF OVERDOSE AND WHAT TO DO

Symptoms of overdose in adults include seizures, drowsiness, lethargy, hallucinations, and coma. Among children, overdose symptoms may include bluish color to the skin, convulsions, dry mouth, excitement, fever, fixed and dilated pupils, flushing, hallucinations, severe heart problems, tremors, twitching, coma, and uncoordinated movements. If overdose occurs, seek immediate medical attention and bring the prescription container with you to the hospital.

SPECIAL INFORMATION FOR PREGNANT OR NURSING WOMEN

Adequate studies of the effects of clemastine on pregnant or nursing women have not been done. If you are pregnant or plan to become pregnant, talk to your health-care practitioner. Antihistamines used during the last three months of pregnancy can cause severe reactions in newborns.

Clemastine passes into breast milk. If you are breastfeeding, your health-care practitioner will likely advise you to stop until your treatment is done.

SPECIAL INFORMATION FOR SENIORS

Side effects are more likely to occur and are more severe in older adults.

GENERIC NAME

Clindamycin

BRAND NAMES

Cleocin, Cleocin-T, Cleocin Pediatric, Cleocin T Gel, Cleocin T Topical Solution, Cleocin Vaginal Ovules, Clinda-Derm
Generic available

ABOUT THIS DRUG

Clindamycin is used to treat serious bacterial infections, including acne and vaginal infections. It is one of the few oral antibiotic drugs that works against anaerobic bacteria, which prosper in the absence of oxygen, such as in wounds, lung abscesses, infections of the female genital tract, and abdominal infections.

This drug inhibits the production of protein that bacteria need to grow and reproduce.

SIDE EFFECTS

Be sure to tell your health-care practitioner if you experience any side effects while taking clindamycin. Only your health-care practitioner can determine whether it is safe for you to continue taking this drug.

Oral Doses

- *Most Common:* diarrhea (in up to 30% of patients), stomach pain, nausea, vomiting, painful swallowing
- *Less Common:* itching, rash, drug sensitivity (e.g., breathing difficulties, yellowing of the skin or eyes), joint pain, colitis

Topical Lotion

- *Most Common:* dry skin, red, burning, or peeling skin, oily skin, itching
- *Less Common:* diarrhea, abdominal pain, colitis, gastrointestinal upset

Vaginal Cream

- *Most Common:* irritation, vaginitis, cervicitis (inflamed cervix)
- *Less Common:* nausea, vomiting, diarrhea, constipation, abdominal pain, dizziness, headache, fainting, vaginal discharge

IMPORTANT PRECAUTIONS

Tell your health-care practitioner if you are sensitive or allergic to clindamycin or to any other drugs, especially lincomycin and other antibiotics.

Clindamycin can cause colitis, a severe, potentially fatal intestinal condition that is characterized by diarrhea, bloody stool, and abdominal cramps. Therefore, clindamycin should be reserved for serious infections or those that do not respond to or cannot be treated by other drugs.

If you experience diarrhea while taking clindamycin, do not take diarrhea medication until you talk with your health-care practitioner. He or she will recommend the most appropriate medication.

If you have kidney or liver disease, clindamycin should be used with caution.

Do not take clindamycin if you have a history of intestinal inflammation, ulcerative colitis, or antibiotic-associated colitis unless you have permission from your health-care practitioner.

When using the vaginal cream, avoid sexual intercourse.

DRUG INTERACTIONS

Tell your health-care practitioner and pharmacist if you are taking any prescription or nonprescription drugs, as well as any vitamins, herbs, or other supplements. Possible drug interactions include the following:

- Erythromycin should not be taken with clindamycin.
- Kaolin-Pectin Suspension, prescribed for diarrhea, can delay the absorption of clindamycin capsules into the bloodstream. If these two drugs are necessary, they should be taken at least 1 hour apart.

FOOD, VITAMIN, AND HERBAL INTERACTIONS

No food, vitamin, or herb interactions have been noted. Your health-care practitioner may recommend that you take probiotics, "friendly" bacteria supplements that can help reduce the diarrhea associated with use of antibiotics. Suggested supplements include *Lactobacillus acidophilus, Bifidobacterium longum, L. bulgaricus, L. thermophilus, L. reuteri,* and *B. bifidus*, taken during and for several weeks after treatment.

RECOMMENDED DOSAGE

Clindamycin is available in capsules, as an oral solution, as a topical cream and gel, and as a vaginal cream. The dosages given here are typical. However, your health-care practitioner will determine the most appropriate dose and schedule for your needs.

Oral Forms

- *Children 1 Month and Older:* 0.9 to 2.3 mg per per pound of body weight daily every 6 hours, or as directed by your health-care practitioner
- *Adults:* 150 to 300 mg every 6 hours

Topical Forms

- *Children Up to 12 Years:* dose to be determined by your health-care practitioner
- *Adults:* apply twice daily, using just enough to cover the affected areas

Vaginal Cream

- *Children Up to 12 Years:* dose to be determined by your health-care practitioner
- *Adults (nonpregnant):* 100 mg inserted into the vagina once daily at bedtime for 3 or 7 days, as prescribed by your health-care practitioner

The oral forms should be taken with a full glass of water or with food to prevent stomach and intestinal irritation.

If you miss a dose, take it as soon as you remember. If it is nearly time for your next dose, do not take the missed dose. Continue with your regular dosing schedule. Never take a double dose.

SYMPTOMS OF OVERDOSE AND WHAT TO DO

Symptoms of overdose include severe diarrhea or other drug side effects. If overdose occurs, seek immediate medical attention and bring the prescription container with you to the hospital.

SPECIAL INFORMATION FOR PREGNANT OR NURSING WOMEN

Clindamycin crosses the placenta. If you are pregnant or plan to become pregnant, talk to your health-care practitioner. If this drug is considered to be crucial for your health, you and your health-care practitioner must weigh the potential benefits against the potential risks to the fetus.

Clindamycin passes into breast milk. If you are breastfeeding, your health-care practitioner will likely advise you to stop until your treatment is done.

SPECIAL INFORMATION FOR SENIORS

Older adults who have other illnesses may not be able to tolerate the side effects of clindamycin, especially diarrhea. Other treatments should be considered.

GENERIC NAME

Clobetasol propionate

see Corticosteroids, Topical, page 337

GENERIC NAME

Clocortolone pivalate

see Corticosteroids, Topical, page 337

GENERIC NAME

Clofibrate

BRAND NAMES

Abitrate, Atromid-S

Generic available

ABOUT THIS DRUG

Clofibrate is an anti-hyperlipidemic (blood-fat reducing) agent used to treat high blood levels of triglycerides and cholesterol. It is usually prescribed for people who have not responded to changes in diet, weight control, and exercise.

This medication interferes with the body's production of cholesterol and triglycerides and increases the rate at which these fats are metabolized.

SIDE EFFECTS

Be sure to tell your health-care practitioner if you experience any side effects while taking clofibrate. Only your health-care practitioner can determine whether it is safe for you to continue taking this drug.

- *Most Common:* nausea
- *Less Common:* vomiting, loose stools, upset stomach, gas, weakness, rash, headache, mouth sores, dizziness, tiredness, muscle cramps, itching, brittle hair or hair loss, abnormal heart rhythms, gallstones, especially with long-term use, impotence, enlarged liver, reduced urinary output, bloody urine. There are also claims that clofibrate can cause blurred vision, breast enlargement, stomach ulcers, stomach bleeding, arthritis-like symptoms, and uncontrollable muscle spasm.

IMPORTANT PRECAUTIONS

Tell your health-care practitioner if you are sensitive or allergic to clofibrate or to any other drugs.

If you have kidney disease, your clofibrate dose will need to be adjusted.

Clofibrate should be used with caution if you have heart disease, gallstones, cirrhosis, liver disease, stomach ulcer, or an underactive thyroid.

If you undergo blood tests for any reason, tell the health-care practitioner you are taking clofibrate, as this drug can interfere with some blood test results.

DRUG INTERACTIONS

Tell your health-care practitioner and pharmacist if you are taking any prescription or nonprescription drugs, as well as any vitamins, herbs, or other supplements. Possible drug interactions include the following:

- Anticoagulant (e.g., warfarin) dosages may need to be reduced by 50 percent. Be sure your health-care practitioner knows if you are taking both an anticoagulant and clofibrate.
- Rifampin may reduce the effectiveness of clofibrate.
- Statin-lowering drugs (e.g., simvastatin, fluvastatin) may cause skeletal muscle destruction.
- Clofibrate may reduce the effect of chenodiol.
- Clofibrate may increase the effects of oral antidiabetic drugs (e.g., glipizide, glyburide) and other drugs used to treat diabetes insipidus (e.g., carbamazepine, desmopressin, diuretics, and hormone replacement agents).
- Contraceptive drugs may affect the effectiveness of clofibrate.
- Probenecid may increase both the effectiveness and the side effects of clofibrate.

FOOD, VITAMIN, AND HERBAL INTERACTIONS

Clofibrate hinders the digestion and absorption of fats and fat-soluble vitamins, including vitamins A, D, E, and K, as well as folate (folic acid), iron, and calcium. Take these supplements at least 1 hour before or 4 to 6 hours after you take clofibrate.

RECOMMENDED DOSAGE

Clofibrate is available as capsules. The dosage given here is typical. However, your health-care practitioner will determine the most appropriate dose and schedule for your needs.

- *Children:* to be determined by your health-care practitioner
- *Adults:* 1,500 to 2,000 mg daily, taken in 2 to 4 divided doses

Clofibrate can be taken with food or milk to help prevent stomach irritation.

If you miss a dose, take it as soon as you remember. If it is nearly time for your next dose, do not take the missed dose. Continue with your regular dosing schedule. Never take a double dose.

SYMPTOMS OF OVERDOSE AND WHAT TO DO

Symptoms of overdose will likely be severe side effects. If overdose occurs, seek immediate medical attention and bring the prescription container with you to the hospital.

SPECIAL INFORMATION FOR PREGNANT OR NURSING WOMEN

Large amounts of clofibrate cross the placenta and can affect the fetus. If you are pregnant or plan to become pregnant, talk to your health-care practitioner. Clofibrate should be stopped several months before trying to conceive.

Clofibrate passes into breast milk. If you are breastfeeding, your health-care practitioner will likely advise you to stop until treatment is complete. Also, because of the effect of clofibrate on vitamin absorption, breast milk may be less nutritious.

SPECIAL INFORMATION FOR SENIORS

Older adults who have compromised kidney function may need dosage adjustments.

GENERIC NAME

Clomipramine

see Tricyclic Antidepressants, page 1076

GENERIC NAME

Clonazepam

BRAND NAME

Klonopin

Generic available

ABOUT THIS DRUG

Clonazepam is an anticonvulsant and benzodiazepine tranquilizer used to treat seizure disorders, anxiety, and panic attacks. It should be reserved for people who have not responded to other drug treatments for these conditions.

This drug produces mild sedation by enhancing the effect of a chemical (gamma-ainobutyric acid, or GABA), which in turn dampens the transmission of nerve signals and reduces nerve excitation.

SIDE EFFECTS

Be sure to tell your health-care practitioner if you experience any side effects while taking clonazepam. Only your health-care practitioner can determine whether it is safe for you to continue taking this drug.

- *Most Common:* drowsiness, poor muscle control, behavioral changes, slurred speech
- *Less Common:* constipation, nausea, vomiting, urinary problems, unusual fatigue, change in sexual desire or ability
- *Rare:* difficulty concentrating, depression, hallucinations, low blood pressure, rash, sore throat, fever and chills, sores in throat or mouth, unusual bruising or bleeding, yellowish tinge to eyes or skin

IMPORTANT PRECAUTIONS

Tell your health-care practitioner if you are sensitive or allergic to clonazepam or to any other drugs, especially other benzodiazepines (e.g., alprazolam, diazepam).

When stopping treatment with clonazepam, do so gradually. Suddenly stopping can cause withdrawal symptoms, including seizures, tremors, vomiting, increased sweating, and abdominal or muscle cramps.

Do not use clonazepam if you have severe depression, severe lung disease, sleep apnea, alcoholism, kidney disease, or liver disease. This drug can aggravate your condition and increase the depressive effects of benzodiazepines.

Do not use clonazepam if you have narrow-angle glaucoma, but the drug is safe if you have open-angle glaucoma.

Clonazepam should be used with caution if you have chronic respiratory illness, because the drug can increase salivation and other secretions that can make breathing difficult.

Because clonazepam can cause drowsiness, make sure you know how you react to the medication before you drive or operate dangerous equipment.

DRUG INTERACTIONS

Tell your health-care practitioner and pharmacist if you are taking any prescription or nonprescription drugs, as well as any vitamins, herbs, or other supplements. Possible drug interactions include the following:

- Alcohol, antihistamines (e.g., clemastine, cetirizine), other anticonvulsants, narcotic pain relievers, tranquilizers and sleeping pills (e.g., alprazolam, lorazepam), monoamine oxidase inhibitors (e.g., phenelzine), and tricyclic antidepressants (e.g., amitriptyline, doxepin) can increase the depressant effects of clonazepam.
- Valproic acid may cause severe petit mal seizures.
- Phenobarbital, phenytoin, and smoking may reduce the effectiveness of clonazepam.
- Cimetidine, oral contraceptives, disulfiram, fluoxetine, isoniazid, ketoconazole, metoprolol, probenecid, propoxyphene, propranolol, rifampin, and valproic acid may prolong the effects of clonazepam.
- Clonazepam may reduce the effect of levodopa.
- Theophyline may reduce the sedative effects of clonazepam.
- Antacids may interfere with the absorption of clonazepam. To prevent this reaction, take antacids at least 1 hour before or after taking clonazepam.
- Clonazepam may increase the blood levels of digoxin and increase the risk of digoxin toxicity.

FOOD, VITAMIN, AND HERBAL INTERACTIONS

Herbs that produce a sedative effect may cause significant depressant interactions when used with clonazepam. Some of those herbs include calendula, capsicum, catnip, goldenseal, gotu kola, hops, kava, lady's slipper, passionflower, sage, Siberian ginseng, skullcap, St. John's wort, and valerian, among others.

RECOMMENDED DOSAGE

Clonazepam is available in tablets and wafers. The dosages given here are typical. However, your health-care practitioner will determine the most appropriate dose and schedule for your needs.

- *Children Up to Age 10 (or Less than 66 Pounds):* Starting dose is 0.004 to 0.013 mg per pound of body weight daily. The dosage may be increased gradually to a maximum of 0.045 to 0.09 mg per pound of body weight.
- *Children Age 10 and Older and Adults:* Starting dose is 0.5 mg three times daily. The dose is increased by 0.5 to 1 mg every 3 days until control of seizures is achieved or side effects develop. Maximum daily dose is 20 mg.

Clonazepam is most effective when taken on an empty stomach. However, if it causes stomach irritation, you can take it with food.

If you miss a dose by less than one hour, take it as soon as you remember. If it is more than one hour past your scheduled dose, do not take the missed dose. Continue with your regular dosing schedule. Never take a double dose.

SYMPTOMS OF OVERDOSE AND WHAT TO DO

Symptoms of overdose include confusion, coma, sleepiness, low blood pressure, difficulty breathing, poor reflexes, and other depressive effects. If overdose occurs, seek immediate medical attention and bring the prescription container with you to the hospital.

SPECIAL INFORMATION FOR PREGNANT OR NURSING WOMEN

Clonazepam crosses the placenta and can affect the fetus. This drug should not be used during pregnancy unless it is considered to be crucial by your health-care practitioner. Then you and your health-care practitioner must weigh the potential benefits against the potential risks.

It is uncertain whether clonazepam passes into breast milk. If you are breastfeeding, your health-care practitioner may advise you to switch to bottle feeding.

SPECIAL INFORMATION FOR SENIORS

Older adults, especially those who have kidney or liver disease, are more likely to experience side effects, and perhaps more severe ones. Seniors may require lower doses.

GENERIC NAME

Clonidine

BRAND NAMES

Catapres, Catapres-TTS-1, Catapres-TTS-2, Catapres-TTS-3
Generic available

ABOUT THIS DRUG

Clonidine is an antihypertensive drug used to treat high blood pressure.

This drug reduces blood pressure by stimulating the alpha-adrenergic receptors in the brain and dilating blood vessels.

SIDE EFFECTS

Be sure to tell your health-care practitioner if you experience any side effects while taking clonidine. Only your health-care practitioner can determine whether it is safe for you to continue taking this drug.

Tablets

- *Most Common:* dry mouth, sedation, constipation, drowsiness
- *Common:* headache, fatigue, dizziness. These take about 4 to 6 weeks to disappear.
- *Less Common:* loss of appetite, nausea, vomiting, weight gain, breast pain or enlargement, swollen, painful glands in the throat, heart failure, palpitations, rapid heartbeat, dizziness when rising quickly from a lying or seated position, problems sleeping, hallucinations, anxiety, depression, nervousness, restlessness, rash, difficult or painful urination, dry nose, dry and burning eyes, fever, joint and muscle pain, leg cramps, thinning or loss of scalp hair, nightmares, reduced or loss of sex drive

Transdermal Patch

- *Most Common:* dry mouth, drowsiness
- *Less Common:* nausea, constipation, taste changes, dry throat, fatigue, headache, lethargy, nervousness, dizziness, impotence, mild skin reactions (itching, swelling, burning, peeling, white patches)

IMPORTANT PRECAUTIONS

Tell your health-care practitioner if you are sensitive or allergic to clonidine or to any other drugs.

Do not take clonidine if you have a recent history of heart attack or have chronic kidney failure, blood vessel disease in the brain, or cardiac insufficiency.

Do not stop taking clonidine without your health-care practitioner's supervision. Suddenly stopping clonidine can lead to a sudden rise in blood pressure, agitation, nervousness, headache, and possibly death.

If you have a history of mental depression or Raynaud's syndrome, clonidine can make them worse.

Use of the transdermal patch is not recommended if you have lupus, scleroderma, or polyarteritis nodosa as absorption of the drug into the body is blocked.

Tolerance to clonidine occurs in some people. If this happens, your blood pressure will rise and your health-care practitioner will need to adjust your dosage.

DRUG INTERACTIONS

Tell your health-care practitioner and pharmacist if you are taking any prescription or nonprescription drugs, as well as any vitamins, herbs, or other supplements. Possible drug interactions with clonidine include the following:

➤ Alcohol, barbiturates (e.g., phenobarbital), and sedatives and tranquilizers (e.g., diazepam, oxazepam) should be avoided because they heighten the depressive effects of clonidine.

➤ Antidepressants (e.g., amitriptyline, fluoxetine), appetite suppressants, estrogens, indomethacin and other nonsteroidal anti-inflammatory drugs (e.g., ibuprofen, naproxen), and prazosin may counteract the effects of clonidine.

➤ Beta-blockers (e.g., acebutolol, metoprolol) may increase the drug-withdrawal reaction and cause the blood pressure to rise.

➤ Verapamil may cause atrioventricular block (abnormal heartbeat patterns) and blood pressure to drop.

FOOD, VITAMIN, AND HERBAL INTERACTIONS

Herbs that produce a sedative effect may cause significantly depressant interactions when used with clonidine. Some of those herbs include calendula, capsicum, catnip, goldenseal, gotu kola, hops, kava, lady's slipper, passionflower, sage, Siberian ginseng, skullcap, St. John's wort, and valerian, among others.

RECOMMENDED DOSAGE

Clonidine is available in tablets and as a transdermal patch. The dosages given here are typical. However, your health-care practitioner will determine the most appropriate dose and schedule for your needs.

- *Children Up to Age 12*: safety and effectiveness have not been determined
- *Children 12 and Older and Adults:* Starting dose is 0.1 mg twice daily, in the morning and at bedtime. Your health-care practitioner will gradually increase the dosage until the desired response is achieved. The maintenance dose is usually 0.2 to 0.6 mg daily in divided doses. If using the transdermal patch, apply one patch per week, the same day each week.

Take clonidine tablets on an empty stomach unless you experience stomach irritation, in which case you can take them with food. Tablets should be taken at the same time each day; the patch should be applied at the same time and on the same day each week.

If you miss a dose, take it as soon as you remember. If it is nearly time for your next dose, do not take the missed dose. Continue with your regular dosing schedule. Never take a double dose. If you miss two or more doses of the tablets or forget to change the patch three days past when it was due, contact your health-care practitioner.

SYMPTOMS OF OVERDOSE AND WHAT TO DO

Symptoms of overdose include constriction of pupils, drowsiness, high blood pressure followed by a drop in pressure, seizures, agitation, nausea, vomiting, slowed breathing, slowed heartbeat, weakness, and low body temperature. If overdose occurs, seek immediate medical attention and bring the prescription container with you to the hospital.

SPECIAL INFORMATION FOR PREGNANT OR NURSING WOMEN

Clonidine crosses the placenta, and animal studies show that it can cause harmful effects to the fetus. If you are pregnant or plan to become pregnant and this drug is essential for your health, you and your health-care practitioner must weigh the potential benefits against the potential risks to the fetus.

Clonidine passes into breast milk. If you are breastfeeding, your health-care practitioner may advise you to stop until your treatment is done.

SPECIAL INFORMATION FOR SENIORS

Seniors should begin with a lower starting dose. They also are more susceptible to the side effects.

GENERIC NAME

Clopidogrel

BRAND NAME

Plavix
No generic available

ABOUT THIS DRUG

Clopidogrel is an antiplatelet drug used to help prevent heart attack and stroke in individuals who either have already had a heart attack or stroke or are at risk for them.

This drug helps prevent blood clot formation by making the platelets (cells that gather and form clots) less sticky. Some studies suggest that it is superior to aspirin in this regard.

SIDE EFFECTS

Be sure to tell your health-care practitioner if you experience any side effects while taking clopidogrel. Only your health-care practitioner can determine whether it is safe for you to continue taking this drug.

- *Most Common:* rash and other skin conditions
- *Common:* chest pain, flu-like symptoms, pain, dizziness, fever, abdominal pain, joint pain, back pain, respiratory infection, headache, black-and-blue marks
- *Less Common:* high blood pressure, diarrhea, nausea, bleeding, nosebleeds, breathing problems, tiredness, swollen arms or legs, cough, bronchitis, high blood cholesterol, urinary infection, depression
- *Rare:* stomach ulcer, bleeding in the brain

IMPORTANT PRECAUTIONS

Tell your health-care practitioner if you are sensitive or allergic to clopidogrel, ticlopidine (a similar antiplatelet), or to any other drugs.

If you have bleeding ulcers, liver problems, brain hemorrhage, or other bleeding conditions, clopidogrel should be used with caution.

DRUG INTERACTIONS

Tell your health-care practitioner and pharmacist if you are taking any prescription or nonprescription drugs, as well as any vitamins, herbs, or other supplements. Possible interactions with clopidogrel include the following:

- Clopidogrel may interfere with the body's ability to break down anti-inflammatory drugs (e.g., ibuprofen, etodolac), phenytoin, tamoxifen, tolbutamide, torsamide, warfarin, and fluvastatin.
- Use of nonsteroidal anti-inflammatory drugs can increase bleeding in the intestines and stomach.
- Other antiplatelet drugs and warfarin should not be used with clopidogrel unless you are under a health-care practitioner's supervision, as it may lead to dangerous bleeding problems.

FOOD, VITAMIN, AND HERBAL INTERACTIONS

Because clopidogrel affects blood clotting, herbs that should be avoided include feverfew, garlic, ginkgo, ginger, and ginseng.

RECOMMENDED DOSAGE

Clopidogrel is available in 75-mg tablets. The dosage given here is typical. However, your health-care practitioner will determine the most appropriate dose and schedule for your needs.

- *Children:* to be determined by your health-care practitioner
- *Adults:* 75 mg once daily

Clopidogrel can be taken with or without food.

If you miss a dose, take it as soon as you remember. If it is nearly time for your next dose, do not take the missed dose. Continue with your regular dosing schedule. Never take a double dose.

SYMPTOMS OF OVERDOSE AND WHAT TO DO

Little information is available about overdosing with clopidogrel. Reduced ability to clot blood is likely. If overdose occurs, seek immediate medical attention, and bring the prescription container with you to the hospital.

SPECIAL INFORMATION FOR PREGNANT OR NURSING WOMEN

No adequate studies of the effects of clopidogrel on pregnant or nursing women have been done. Other antiplatelet drugs, such as aspirin, are not recommended during pregnancy. You and your health-care practitioner need to weigh the potential benefits against the potential risks to the fetus.

Clopidogrel may pass into breast milk. If you are breastfeeding, your health-care practitioner will likely advise you to stop during treatment.

SPECIAL INFORMATION FOR SENIORS

No special precautions have been noted for older adults.

GENERIC NAME

Clorazepate

BRAND NAMES

Gen-Xene, Tranxene, Tranxene-SD
Generic available

ABOUT THIS DRUG

Clorazepate is a benzodiazepine tranquilizer used to treat anxiety disorders and panic attacks.

This drug produces mild sedation by enhancing the effect of a chemical (gamma-ainobutyric acid, or GABA), which in turn dampens the transmission of nerve signals and reduces nerve excitation.

SIDE EFFECTS

Be sure to tell your health-care practitioner if you experience any side effects while taking clorazepate. Only your health-care practitioner can determine whether it is safe for you to continue taking this drug.

- *Most Common:* mild drowsiness during the first few days of treatment
- *Less Common or Rare:* depression, confusion, lethargy, disorientation, headache, slurred speech, dizziness, tremors, constipation, dry mouth, nausea, urinary problems, sexual difficulties, low blood pressure, fluid retention, blurred or double vision, rash, nervousness, sleep difficulties, stomach and intestinal disorders

IMPORTANT PRECAUTIONS

Tell your health-care practitioner if you are sensitive or allergic to clorazepate or to any other drugs, especially other benzodiazepines.

Clorazepate is habit-forming if taken for a prolonged time. It can also cause withdrawal symptoms if you abruptly stop taking it, even after only 4 weeks of treatment.

Do not take clorazepate if you have a psychotic disorder or if you have severe lung disease, sleep apnea, liver disease, alcoholism, kidney disease, or narrow-angle glaucoma. (It is safe to take if you have open-angle glaucoma.)

Clorazepate should not be taken for longer than 3 to 4 months, at which time you should be reevaluated by your health-care practitioner.

Because clorazepate causes drowsiness, you should know how you react to the drug before you drive or operate dangerous equipment.

DRUG INTERACTIONS

Tell your health-care practitioner and pharmacist if you are taking any prescription or nonprescription drugs, as well as any vitamins, herbs, or other supplements. Possible drug interactions include the following:

- Alcohol, other tranquilizers, narcotics, barbiturates, monoamine oxidase inhibitors, antihistamines, and antidepressants should not be taken with clorazepate, because the result may be excessive tiredness, breathing difficulties, depression, and related symptoms.
- Cimetidine, disulfiram, fluoxetine, isoniazid, ketoconazole, metoprolol, oral contraceptives, probenecid, propoxyphene, propranolol, rifampin, and valproic acid can prolong the effects of clorazepate.
- Antacids should be taken at least 1 hour before or after you take clorazepate, as they can interfere with the absorption of clorazepate.
- Clorazepate may increase the blood levels of digoxin and phenytoin and the chance of toxicity of both drugs.
- Levodopa may be less effective.

FOOD, VITAMIN, AND HERBAL INTERACTIONS

Herbs that produce a sedative effect may cause potentially significant depressant interactions when used with clorazepate. Some of those herbs include calendula, capsicum, catnip, goldenseal, gotu kola, hops, kava, lady's slipper, passionflower, sage, Siberian ginseng, skullcap, St. John's wort, and valerian, among others.

RECOMMENDED DOSAGE

Clorazepate is available as tablets. The dosages given here are typical. However, your health-care practitioner will determine the most appropriate dose and schedule for your needs.

- *Children Up to 9 Years:* not recommended
- *Children 9 Years and Older and Adults:* 15 to 60 mg daily, with the average being 30 mg in divided doses. Your health-care practitioner will adjust your dose as needed.
- *Adults 60 and Older:* starting dose is 7.5 to 15 mg daily

Clorazepate works best if taken on an empty stomach, but if stomach irritation occurs, take it with food.

If you miss a dose, take it as soon as you remember. If it is nearly time for your next dose, do not take the missed dose. Continue with your regular dosing schedule. Never take a double dose.

SYMPTOMS OF OVERDOSE AND WHAT TO DO

Symptoms of overdose include low blood pressure, confusion, poor coordination, loss of reflexes, shallow breathing, sedation, and coma. If overdose occurs, seek immediate medical attention and bring the prescription container with you to the hospital.

SPECIAL INFORMATION FOR PREGNANT OR NURSING WOMEN

Clorazepate may cause birth defects if it is taken during the first trimester. If you are pregnant or plan to become pregnant, you should not take this drug.

This drug may pass into breast milk. If you are breastfeeding, your health-care practitioner may advise you to stop until your treatment is complete.

SPECIAL INFORMATION FOR SENIORS

Older adults, especially those who have kidney or liver disease, are more likely to experience side effects. Smaller doses are generally recommended.

GENERIC NAME

Clotrimazole

BRAND NAMES

Gyne-Lotrimin, Lotrimin, Mycelex Troches, Mycelex, Mycelex-7
Generic available

ABOUT THIS DRUG

Clotrimazole is an antifungal medication used to treat fungal infections of the skin (e.g., athlete's foot, jock itch, ringworm), mouth, and vaginal tract.

This drug prevents fungi from producing vital substances they need to grow and reproduce.

SIDE EFFECTS

Be sure to tell your health-care practitioner if you experience any side effects while taking clotrimazole. Only your health-care practitioner can determine whether it is safe for you to continue taking this drug.

- *Most Common:* none for the topical; diarrhea, stomach cramps, nausea, vomiting for the lozenge if swallowed; vaginal burning, itching, discharge, or other irritation for the vaginal cream
- *Less Common or Rare:* hives, itching, burning, peeling, stinging, redness or other skin irritation for the topical or lozenge; headache, stomach cramps, irritation for vaginal cream

IMPORTANT PRECAUTIONS

Tell your health-care practitioner if you are sensitive or allergic to clotrimazole or to any other drugs.

If you experience itching or irritation when using clotrimazole, stop using it.

If you are treating a vaginal infection, contact your health-care practitioner if your condition does not improve after 7 days of treatment.

If you use the vaginal cream or tablets, the drug may cause irritation to your sexual partner. Either avoid sex while being treated or have male partners use a condom.

Take clotrimazole for the full treatment course even if your symptoms disappear before then. If you stop too early, the infection may return.

DRUG INTERACTIONS

Tell your health-care practitioner and pharmacist if you are taking any prescription or nonprescription drugs, as well as any vitamins, herbs, or other supplements. No drug-drug interactions have been reported for clotrimazole. However, talk to your health-care practitioner before using any other antifungal medications.

FOOD, VITAMIN, AND HERBAL INTERACTIONS

No food, vitamin, or herbal interactions have been noted.

RECOMMENDED DOSAGE

Clotrimazole is available as a topical cream, lotion, and solution, oral lozenge, vaginal cream, and vaginal tablets. The dosages given here are typical. However, your health-care practitioner will determine the most appropriate dose and schedule for your needs.

Skin Infections

- *Children and Adults:* Apply topical cream, lotion, or solution twice daily, in the morning and evening.

Thrush (Mouth Infection)

- *Children 5 Years and Older and Adults:* Dissolve one 10-mg lozenge in the mouth 5 times daily for 14 days.

Vaginal Infection

- *Children 12 Years and Older and Adults:* Insert vaginal cream with an applicator, 50 mg of 1% cream for 6 to 14 nights, or 100 mg of 2% cream for 3 nights, or 500 mg of 10% cream for 1 night.
- *Nonpregnant Teenagers and Adults:* For vaginal tablets, insert one 100-mg tablet for 6 to 14 nights, or one 200-mg tablet for 3 nights, or one 500-mg tablet for 1 night.

The oral lozenge form is best taken on an empty stomach, at least 1 hour before or 2 hours after eating. If you experience stomach irritation, you can take it with food if you allow the lozenge to dissolve completely in your mouth.

If you miss a dose, take it as soon as you remember. If it is nearly time for your next dose, do not take the missed dose. Continue with your regular dosing schedule. Never take a double dose.

SYMPTOMS OF OVERDOSE AND WHAT TO DO

An overdose with clotrimazole is unlikely. If an overdose occurs, or if the vaginal tablets are accidentally ingested, call your poison control center or emergency department for instructions. If you go to the hospital, take the prescription container with you.

SPECIAL INFORMATION FOR PREGNANT OR NURSING WOMEN

No adequate studies of the effects of clotrimazole on pregnant or nursing women have been done, but no problems have been reported. If you are pregnant or plan to become pregnant, talk to your health-care practitioner.

Clotrimazole may pass into breast milk. If you are breastfeeding, your health-care practitioner will likely advise you to stop until your treatment is complete.

SPECIAL INFORMATION FOR SENIORS

No special precautions have been noted for older adults.

GENERIC NAME

Cloxacillin sodium

see Penicillin Antibiotics, page 812

GENERIC NAME

Clozapine

BRAND NAME

Clozaril

ABOUT THIS DRUG

Clozapine is an antipsychotic used to treat severe schizophrenia in people who have not responded to other treatments. Although clozapine is not a cure for schizophrenia, it can help people live a more normal life.

This drug inhibits the activity of dopamine, a chemical in the brain. Overstimulation of certain centers in the brain by dopamine is believed to be involved in some psychiatric conditions.

SIDE EFFECTS

Be sure to tell your health-care practitioner if you experience any side effects while taking clozapine. Only your health-care practitioner can determine whether it is safe for you to continue taking this drug.

- *Most Common:* abdominal discomfort, agitation, confusion, constipation, dizziness, drowsiness, dry mouth, fainting, fever, headache, heartburn, high blood pressure, abnormal muscle movement, low blood pressure, nausea, sleep problems, rapid heartbeat and other heart-related conditions, sweating, salivation, sedation, vertigo, vision problems, vomiting, weight gain. About 5 percent of individuals experience seizures.
- *Less Common:* anemia, angina, anxiety, increased appetite, blood clots, bluish tinge in the skin, breast pain, bronchitis, constant involuntary eye movements, cough, depression, diarrhea, breathing diffi-

culties, chills, fever, dilated pupils, disorientation, dry throat, fatigue, heart problems, hives, impotence, hallucinations, irritability, itching, jerky movements, joint pain, lethargy, loss of appetite, muscle spasm, painful menstruation, paranoia, poor coordination, skin inflammation, slurred speech, stuttering, swollen salivary glands, urinary difficulties, vaginal itch, weakness, wheezing, yellow skin and eyes. This is only a partial list; also contact your health-care practitioner if you experience side effects not listed here.

People taking antipsychotic drugs may experience a rare but life-threatening set of side effects known as neuroleptic malignant syndrome (NMS). Symptoms include fever, difficulty breathing, rapid heartbeat, rigid muscles, mental changes, increased sweating, irregular blood pressure, and convulsions. Immediate medical attention is required.

Side effects such as lip smacking, wormlike movements of the tongue, and slow, rhythmical, involuntary movements are characteristic of a disorder known as tardive dyskinesia. Older adults (especially women) are more susceptible to this condition, which may become permanent. If you experience tardive dyskinesia, your health-care practitioner will probably advise you to stop taking this drug.

IMPORTANT PRECAUTIONS

Tell your health-care practitioner if you are sensitive or allergic to clozapine or to any other drugs.

About 1 percent of people who take clozapine develop a potentially deadly condition called agranulocytosis, a rapid decline in their white blood cell count. Treatment must be stopped immediately if this condition occurs. Therefore, if you take clozapine you should undergo blood tests every week during treatment and for 4 weeks after stopping treatment to see if this condition develops.

You should not take clozapine if you have a bone marrow disease or uncontrolled epilepsy, or if you are taking a drug that could decrease your white blood cell count or affect your bone marrow (e.g., carbamazepine).

Use of clozapine is associated with a risk of fatal myocarditis (inflammation of the myocardium), especially during the first month of treatment, and other heart problems. If you have any type of heart disease, you should be monitored regularly while taking this drug.

This drug should be used with caution if you have glaucoma, prostate conditions, or liver, heart, or kidney disease.

Because clozapine can cause drowsiness, sedation, and some motor skills problems (e.g., poor coordination, jerky movements, muscle spasm), make sure you know how you react to this drug before you drive or operate dangerous equipment. These symptoms are typically most prominent during the first few weeks of therapy.

DRUG INTERACTIONS

Tell your health-care practitioner and pharmacist if you are taking any prescription or nonprescription drugs, as well as any vitamins, herbs, or other supplements. Possible drug interactions include the following:

- Anticholinergic drugs such as tricyclic antidepressants (e.g., amitriptyline, imipramine) can enhance anticholinergic effects, including blurred vision, confusion, and dry mouth.
- Alcohol and other central nervous system depressants (e.g., benzodiazepines, antipsychotics) may increase the sedative effects of clozapine. Do not use these drugs while taking clopazine.
- Drugs that help lower blood pressure (e.g., antihypertensives, diuretics, beta-blockers) may increase the blood-pressure-lowering effects of clozapine.
- Lithium and clozapine together may cause a condition called neuroleptic malignant syndrome, characterized by high fever, confusion, seizures, irregular pulse, muscle rigidity, increased sweating, and irregular blood pressure. It is potentially fatal.
- Clozapine may increase blood levels of digoxin, heparin, phenytoin, and warfarin.
- Cigarette smoking may alter your dosage needs. Consult with your health-care practitioner.

FOOD, VITAMIN, AND HERBAL INTERACTIONS

Herbs that produce a sedative effect may cause significant depressant interactions when used with clozapine. Some of those herbs include calendula, capsicum, catnip, goldenseal, gotu kola, hops, kava, lady's slipper, passionflower, sage, Siberian ginseng, skullcap, St. John's wort, and valerian, among others.

RECOMMENDED DOSAGE

Clozapine is available in tablets. The dosages given here are typical. However, your health-care practitioner will determine the most appropriate dose and schedule for your needs.

- *Children Up to Age 16*: safety and effectiveness have not been determined
- *Adults:* starting dose is 12.5 mg once or twice daily. Your health-care practitioner may gradually increase your dosage until you reach a daily dose of 300 to 450 mg daily

If you miss a dose, take it as soon as you remember. If it is nearly time for your next dose, do not take the missed dose. Continue with your regular dosing schedule. Never take a double dose.

SYMPTOMS OF OVERDOSE AND WHAT TO DO

Symptoms of overdose include delirium, drowsiness, excessive salivation, low blood pressure, fainting, pneumonia, rapid heartbeat, seizures, breathing difficulties, and coma. If overdose occurs, seek immediate medical assistance and bring the prescription container with you to the hospital.

SPECIAL INFORMATION FOR PREGNANT OR NURSING WOMEN

No adequate studies of the effects of clozapine on pregnant or nursing women have been done. If you are pregnant or plan to become pregnant, you and your health-care practitioner must weigh the potential benefits against the potential risks to the fetus. Clozapine should be used during pregnancy only if it is essential to your health.

Clozapine may pass into breast milk. If you are breastfeeding, your health-care practitioner will likely advise you to stop and to bottle feed.

SPECIAL INFORMATION FOR SENIORS

Older adults may be more seriously affected by the side effects of this drug, especially dizziness when rising from a lying or seated position. Excitability and confusion are also more likely to occur. Older men are at higher risk of developing prostate problems.

GENERIC NAME

Codeine, morphine, oxycodone

BRAND NAMES

Codeine is available as generic only. Morphine: Avinza, MS Contin, MS/L, MS/L Concentrate, MS/S, Oramorph SR. Oxycodone: Oxycontin, Oxy-R, OxyFAST Concentrate, Percolone, Roxicodone Solution

ABOUT THIS DRUG

Codeine, morphine, and oxycodone are opioid (narcotic) painkillers. Codeine is used to treat mild to moderate pain or to control severe cough; morphine is used to treat severe pain; and oxycodone is used to treat moderate to severe pain.

All of these drugs act on specific areas of the spinal cord and brain where pain signals are processed.

SIDE EFFECTS

Be sure to tell your health-care practitioner if you experience any side effects while taking codeine, morphine, or oxycodone. Only your health-care practitioner can determine whether it is safe for you to continue taking these drugs.

- *Most Common:* constipation, drowsiness, dizziness or lightheadedness, nausea, vomiting, loss of appetite, sweating
- *Less Common:* euphoria, headache, agitation, uncoordinated muscle movements, disorientation, visual disturbances, dry mouth, facial flushing, urinary difficulties, reduced sex drive, itching, rash, anemia, low blood sugar, yellowish skin or eyes

IMPORTANT PRECAUTIONS

Tell your health-care practitioner if you are sensitive or allergic to codeine, morphine, oxycodone, or any other drugs, especially other opioids.

Codeine, morphine, and oxycodone should be used with extreme caution if you have asthma or other respiratory problems.

Before taking opioids, consult with your health-care practitioner if you have any of the following: seizures, brain disorder, head injury, lung disease, prostate problems, urinary difficulties, gallstones, colitis, a history of alcohol or drug abuse, or heart, liver, kidney, or thyroid disease.

Long-term use of these drugs may cause addiction.

Use of opioids can make it difficult for your health-care practitioner to monitor your progress if you have suffered a head injury.

DRUG INTERACTIONS

Tell your health-care practitioner and pharmacist if you are taking any prescription or nonprescription drugs, as well as any vitamins, herbs, or other supplements. Possible interactions with codeine, morphine, or oxycodone may include the following:

- Alcohol, sleeping pills, tranquilizers, and other central nervous system depressant drugs should not be taken along with opioids, as serious depressant effects may occur.
- Drugs that lower blood pressure (e.g., antihypertensives, beta-blockers) may lead to abnormally low blood pressure. Avoid this combination.

- Cimetidine may lead to breathing problems, confusion, disorientation, and seizures.
- Morphine may increase the blood levels of zidovudine.

FOOD, VITAMIN, AND HERBAL INTERACTIONS

Herbs that produce a sedative effect may cause potentially serious depressant interactions when used with opioids. Some of those herbs include calendula, capsicum, catnip, goldenseal, gotu kola, hops, kava, lady's slipper, passionflower, sage, Siberian ginseng, skullcap, St. John's wort, and valerian, among others.

RECOMMENDED DOSAGE

Both codeine and oxycodone are available as tablets and an oral solution; morphine is also available in capsules. The dosages given here are typical. However, your health-care practitioner will determine the most appropriate dose and schedule for your needs.

Codeine

- *Children Up to Age 12*: for pain, 0.5 mg of oral solution per 2.2 pounds of body weight every 4 to 6 hours as needed
- *Children:* for cough (age 2), 3 mg every 4 to 6 hours; (age 3) 3.5 mg every 4 to 6 hours; (age 4) 4 mg every 4 to 6 hours; (age 5) 4.5 mg every 4 to 6 hours; (age 6 to 12) 5 to 10 mg every 4 to 6 hours
- *Adults:* for pain, 15 to 60 mg every 3 to 6 hours as needed. For cough: 10 to 20 mg every 3 to 6 hours as needed

Morphine

- *Children:* to be determined by your health-care practitioner
- *Adults:* to start, 10 to 30 mg every 4 to 6 hours. Your health-care practitioner will then adjust the dose based on your needs. Avinza is taken once daily, 30 to 120 mg, as prescribed by your health-care practitioner.

Oxycodone

- *Children:* to be determined by your health-care practitioner
- *Adults:* 5 to 15 mg every 4 to 6 hours

If you miss a dose, take it as soon as you remember. If it is nearly time for your next dose, do not take the missed dose. Continue with your regular dosing schedule. Never take a double dose.

SYMPTOMS OF OVERDOSE AND WHAT TO DO

Symptoms of overdose include difficulty breathing, extreme tiredness progressing to stupor and then coma, pinpoint pupils, cold, clammy skin, slowed heartbeat, low blood pressure, convulsions, and cardiac arrest. If overdose occurs, seek immediate medical attention and bring the prescription container with you to the hospital.

SPECIAL INFORMATION FOR PREGNANT OR NURSING WOMEN

These opioids cross the placenta, and excessive use during pregnancy may cause newborns to be drug dependent. Like all narcotics, codeine, morphine, and oxycodone may also cause breathing problems in infants during delivery. If you are pregnant or plan to become pregnant, and any of these drugs are crucial for your health, you and your health-care practitioner must weigh the potential benefits against the potential risks to the fetus.

All three of these opioids pass into breast milk. If you are breastfeeding, your health-care practitioner will likely advise you to bottle feed while you are under treatment.

SPECIAL INFORMATION FOR SENIORS

Older adults are more likely to be sensitive to the side effects of these drugs. Your health-care practitioner should choose the lowest effective dosage.

GENERIC NAME

Codeine phosphate

see Promethazine, page 879

GENERIC NAME

Colchicine

BRAND NAME

None; available as generic only

ABOUT THIS DRUG

Colchicine is an antigout medication used to treat gouty arthritis and to prevent attacks.

Colchicine appears to interfere with the body's ability to make uric acid, the substance associated with the pain and inflammation of gout, and reduces the inflammatory response to uric acid crystals that develop inside the joints.

SIDE EFFECTS

Be sure to tell your health-care practitioner if you experience any side effects while taking colchicine. Only your health-care practitioner can determine whether it is safe for you to continue taking this drug.

- *Most Common:* if you take the maximum doses for an acute gout attack, you may experience vomiting, abdominal pain, diarrhea, reduced urination, kidney damage, blood vessel damage, and bloody urine
- *Less Common or Rare:* rash, appetite loss, muscle and nerve weakness, hair loss, reduced platelet and white blood cell counts, blood clotting problems, rash, nerve inflammation

IMPORTANT PRECAUTIONS

Tell your health-care practitioner if you are sensitive or allergic to colchicine or to any other drugs.

If you experience vomiting, abdominal pain, diarrhea, nausea, kidney damage, or bloody urine, stop taking the drug immediately and contact your health-care practitioner.

Individuals who have poor kidney function are especially susceptible to feelings of weakness while taking colchicine. This goes away 3 to 4 weeks after stopping the drug.

If you take colchicine for prolonged periods, your health-care practitioner should conduct periodic blood counts to check for low levels of white blood cells and platelets.

Colchicine can interfere with sperm formation.

DRUG INTERACTIONS

Tell your health-care practitioner and pharmacist if you are taking any prescription or nonprescription drugs, as well as any vitamins, herbs, or other supplements. Possible drug interactions include the following:

- Sensitivity to central nervous system depressants (e.g., alcohol, tranquilizers) may increase
- Phenylbutazone increases the risk of side effects
- Anticancer drugs, bumetanide, diazoxide, ethacrynic acid, furosemide, mecamylamine, pyrazinamide, triamterene, and thiazide diuretics may reduce the effectiveness of colchicine

FOOD, VITAMIN, AND HERBAL INTERACTIONS

Long-term use of colchicine can interfere with the absorption of vitamin B_{12}. Talk to your health-care practitioner about taking a vitamin B_{12} supplement.

RECOMMENDED DOSAGE

Colchicine is available in tablets. The dosages given here are typical. However, your health-care practitioner will determine the most appropriate dose and schedule for your needs.

- *Children:* not recommended
- *Adults:* for acute gout attack, 0.5 to 1.2 mg immediately, followed by 0.5 to 1.2 mg every 1 to 2 hours until you get relief from pain, or you experience nausea, vomiting, or diarrhea. To prevent gout attacks, 0.5 to 1.8 mg daily, or as needed. Some people only require this dose every 3 to 4 days.

Colchicine can be taken with or without food.

If you miss a dose, take it as soon as you remember. If it is nearly time for your next dose, do not take the missed dose. Continue with your regular dosing schedule. Never take a double dose.

SYMPTOMS OF OVERDOSE AND WHAT TO DO

Symptoms of overdose can take 1 to 3 days to begin. They typically start with nausea, vomiting, stomach pain, and diarrhea (can be bloody), as well as burning in the throat or stomach or on the skin. If overdose occurs, seek immediate medical attention and bring the prescription container with you to the hospital.

SPECIAL INFORMATION FOR PREGNANT OR NURSING WOMEN

Colchicine crosses the placenta and can harm the fetus. If you are pregnant or plan to become pregnant, do not use this drug unless the benefits of therapy clearly outweigh the potential risks to the fetus.

It is not known whether colchicine passes into breast milk. If you are breastfeeding, your health-care practitioner may advise you to bottle feed while you are being treated.

SPECIAL INFORMATION FOR SENIORS

Older adults are more likely to experience side effects and should exercise caution when using this drug.

GENERIC NAME

Colesevelam

BRAND NAME
Welchol
No generic available

ABOUT THIS DRUG
Colesevelam is an antihyperlipidemic (blood-fat reducer) used to treat high cholesterol levels in the blood in people for whom exercise and diet have not produced good results.

This drug attaches to bile acids in the intestines and interferes with their absorption, which in turn sets off actions that result in a lowering of low-density lipoprotein cholesterol in the blood.

SIDE EFFECTS
Be sure to tell your health-care practitioner if you experience any side effects while taking colesevelam. Only your health-care practitioner can determine whether it is safe for you to continue taking this drug. Because is not absorbed by the body, it is associated with fewer side effects than other antihyperlipidemic drugs.

- *Most Common:* flatulence, constipation
- *Less Common:* diarrhea, abdominal pain, headache, belching, indigestion, acid stomach, dry or sore throat, congestion, muscle aches

IMPORTANT PRECAUTIONS
Tell your health-care practitioner if you are sensitive or allergic to colesevelam or to any other drugs.

Colesevelam is less effective if you are greatly overweight.

If you have a recent history of gastrointestinal surgery or if you have bowel obstruction, difficulty swallowing, or severe gastrointestinal motility problems, colesevelam can make these situations worse.

DRUG INTERACTIONS
Tell your health-care practitioner and pharmacist if you are taking any prescription or nonprescription drugs, as well as any vitamins, herbs, or other supplements. Possible drug interactions with colesevelam may include the following:

- Colesevelam can reduce the absorption of cephalexin, clindamycin, chenodiol, corticosteroids, penicillin G, phenylbutazone, tetracyclines, thyroid, thiazides, trimethoprim, and warfarin.

FOOD, VITAMIN, AND HERBAL INTERACTIONS

Colesevelam interferes with the digestion and absorption of fats and fat-soluble vitamins, including vitamins A, D, E, and K, as well as folate (folic acid), iron, and calcium. Take these supplements at least 1 hour before or 4 to 6 hours after you take colesevelam.

RECOMMENDED DOSAGE

Colesevelam is available in tablets. The dosage given here is typical. However, your health-care practitioner will determine the most appropriate dose and schedule for your needs.

- *Children:* not recommended
- *Adults:* 6 tablets daily, either in 1 or 2 divided doses

Colesevelam should be taken with food and liquid.

If you miss a dose, take it as soon as you remember. If it is nearly time for your next dose, do not take the missed dose. Continue with your regular dosing schedule. Never take a double dose.

SYMPTOMS OF OVERDOSE AND WHAT TO DO

Because colesevelam is not absorbed by the body, the changes of an overdose causing dangerous symptoms is low. However, if an overdose occurs, seek medical attention. Bring the prescription container with you.

SPECIAL INFORMATION FOR PREGNANT OR NURSING WOMEN

No adequate studies of the effects of colesevelam have been done with pregnant or nursing women, but animal studies have not shown it to cause birth defects or other abnormalities. Colesevelam may indirectly affect the fetus, because it reduces the absorption of vitamins A, D, E, and K, as well as folate, iron, and calcium, all of which are necessary for normal fetal development. If you are pregnant or plan to become pregnant, you and your health-care practitioner should weigh the potential benefits against the potential risks to the fetus.

Colesevelam may pass into breast milk. If you are breastfeeding, your health-care practitioner may advise you to stop until treatment is complete.

SPECIAL INFORMATION FOR SENIORS

Older adults are more likely to experience side effects, especially those involving the gastrointestinal tract (e.g., diarrhea, constipation).

GENERIC NAME

Colestipol

BRAND NAME

Colestid

No generic available

ABOUT THIS DRUG

Colestipol is an antihypolipidemic (blood-fat reducing) drug used to reduce cholesterol levels in individuals who have high blood levels of low-density lipoprotein (LDL).

Colestipol binds with bile acids in the intestinal tract, which then form an insoluble substance that is excreted in the stool, thus lowering bile acid levels. In response to the lower acid levels, the liver transforms more cholesterol into bile acids, which lowers the level of cholesterol in the blood.

SIDE EFFECTS

Be sure to tell your health-care practitioner if you experience any side effects while taking colestipol. Only your health-care practitioner can determine whether it is safe for you to continue taking this drug.

- *Most Common:* constipation, heartburn, bloating, belching, abdominal discomfort, irritated anal area
- *Less Common:* hives, gas, diarrhea, nausea, vomiting, gallstones, tarry stools

IMPORTANT PRECAUTIONS

Tell your health-care practitioner if you are sensitive or allergic to colestipol or to any other drugs.

If you experience severe abdominal pain while taking colestipol, immediately stop taking the drug and contact your health-care practitioner. You may have an intestinal obstruction, a very rare reaction to colestipol.

If you have gallstones, peptic ulcer, intestinal bleeding conditions, underactive thyroid, heart disease, hemorrhoids, constipation, or a malabsorption disorder, colestipol may make your condition worse.

Colestipol is less effective if you are greatly overweight.

DRUG INTERACTIONS

Tell your health-care practitioner and pharmacist if you are taking any prescription or nonprescription drugs, as well as any vitamins,

herbs, or other supplements. Possible drug interactions include the following:

- Colestipol may reduce the benefits of anticoagulants (e.g., warfarin).
- Digitalis, diuretics (e.g., amiloride, furosemide), penicillin G (oral), propranolol (oral), tetracyclines (e.g., doxycycline, minocycline), thyroid hormones, and vancomycin (oral) may be less effective if taken with colestipol. Take these drugs 4 to 5 hours before or after your colestipol dose.

FOOD, VITAMIN, AND HERBAL INTERACTIONS

Colestipol hinders the digestion and absorption of fats and fat-soluble vitamins, including vitamins A, D, E, and K, as well as folate (folic acid), iron, and calcium. Take these supplements at least 1 hour before or 4 to 6 hours after you take colestipol.

RECOMMENDED DOSAGE

Colestipol is available in tablets and as a powder. The dosages given here are typical. However, your health-care practitioner will determine the most appropriate dose and schedule for your needs.

- *Children:* to be determined by your health-care practitioner
- *Adults:* starting dose is 2 g once or twice daily before meals. Your health-care practitioner will gradually increase your dose. Typical maintenance dosage is up to 30 g daily, taken in divided doses before meals

If you use the powder, mix it thoroughly and let it stand for 15 minutes before drinking it.

If you miss a dose, take it as soon as you remember. If it is nearly time for your next dose, do not take the missed dose. Continue with your regular dosing schedule. Never take a double dose.

SYMPTOMS OF OVERDOSE AND WHAT TO DO

The primary symptom of an overdose is bowel impaction. If overdose occurs, seek immediate medical attention and bring the prescription container with you to the hospital.

SPECIAL INFORMATION FOR PREGNANT OR NURSING WOMEN

Colestipol may indirectly affect the fetus because it reduces the absorption of vitamins A, D, E, and K, as well as folate (folic acid), iron, and calcium, all of which are necessary for normal fetal development. If colestipol is essential for your health, you and your health-care practitioner must weigh the potential benefits against the potential risks to the fetus.

Colestipol does not pass into breast milk. However, because of the drug's effect on vitamin absorption, breast milk may be less nutritious. If you are breastfeeding, your health-care practitioner may advise you to switch to bottle feeding.

SPECIAL INFORMATION FOR SENIORS

Older adults are more likely to experience side effects, especially constipation.

GENERIC NAME

Conjugated Estrogens *see Estrogens, page 436*

GENERIC NAME

Class: Contraceptives, oral

Generics: (1) Desogestrel + ethinyl estradiol; (2) Ethynodiol diacetate + ethinyl estradiol; (3) Levonorgestrel + ethinyl estradiol; (4) Norethindrone + ethinyl estradiol; (5) Norethindrone + mestranol; (6) Norethindrone acetate + ethinyl estradiol; (7) Norgestimate + ethinyl estradiol; (8) Norgestrel + ethinyl estradiol

BRAND NAMES

(1) Desogen 28, Desogen Ortho-Cept, Marvelon, Ortho-Cept; (2) Demulen 1/35, Demulen 1/50, Demulen 30, Demulen 50, Nelulen 1/35E, Nelulen 1/50E, Zovia 1/35E, Zovia 1/50E; (3) Alesse, Levlen, Levlite, Levora, Min-Ovral, Nordette, Tri-Levlen, Triphasil, Triquilar, Trivora; (4) Brevicon, Brevicon 0.5/35, Brevicon 1/35, Estrostep, Estrostep Fe, GenCept 0.5/35, GenCept 1/35, GenCept 10/11, Genora 0.5/35, Genora 1/35, Genora 1/50, Jenest-28, Necon 0.5/35-21, Necon 0.5/35-28, Necon 1/35-21, Necon 1/35-28, Necon 1/50-21, Necon 1/50-28, NEE 1/35, NEE 1/50, Nelova 0.5/35E, Nelova 1/35E, Nelova 10/11, Norethin 1/35E, Norinyl 1+35, Ortho 0.5/35, Ortho 1/35, Ortho 7/7/7, Ortho 10/11, Ortho-Novum 0.5, Ortho-Novum 1/35, Ortho-Novum 2, Ortho-Novum 7/7/7, Ovcon-35, Ovcon-50, Symphasic, Tri-Norinyl; (5) Genora 1/50, Norethin 1/50M, Norinyl 1+50, Norinyl 1/50, Ortho-Novum 1/50, Ortho-Novum 1/80, Ortho-Novum 10/11, Ortho-Tri-Cyclen

21, Ortho-Tri-Cyclen 28; (6) Loestrin 1/20, Loestrin 1.5/30, Minestrin 1/20, Norcept-E 1/35, Noriestrin 1/50, Norlestrin 2.5/50; (7) Cyclen, Ortho-Cyclen, Tri-Cyclen; (8) Lo-Ovral, Ovral
No generic available

ABOUT THIS DRUG

Oral contraceptives are synthetic female sex hormones, used to prevent pregnancy and to regulate menstrual periods.

These drugs suppress the pituitary hormones, which stimulate ovulation; alter the uterine lining so that it resists implantation by a fertilized egg; and change the mucus at the cervix opening to prevent sperm from entering.

SIDE EFFECTS

Be sure to tell your health-care practitioner if you experience any side effects while taking oral contraceptives. Only your health-care practitioner can determine whether it is safe for you to continue taking these drugs. It often takes trying several different prescriptions before finding the best oral contraceptive for any given individual. The side effects tend to increase as the amount of hormone they contain increases.

- *Most Common:* vaginal discharge, brown patches on the skin, fluid retention, acne, breakthrough bleeding
- *Less Common:* headache, leg swelling (blood clots are possible), depression, muscle and joint pain, severe abdominal pain, bulging eyes, breast lumps, frequent urination, nausea, vomiting, changed sex drive, bloating, appetite changes
- *Rare:* rash, itch, fever, excess hair growth, change in voice, amenorrhea (absence of a period), insomnia, hair loss, jaundice

IMPORTANT PRECAUTIONS

Tell your health-care practitioner if you are sensitive or allergic to any of the ingredients in these combination drugs or to any other drugs.

You should not get pregnant for at least 6 months after stopping oral contraceptives.

Do not take oral contraceptives if you are pregnant or if you have heart disease, blood clots, stroke, liver disease, cancer of the breast, uterus, or ovaries, or unexplained vaginal bleeding.

Do not take oral contraceptives if you smoke, as it increases your risk of stroke, heart attack, and blood clots.

You are at an increased risk of heart attack if you take oral contraceptives for more than 10 years, or if you are between 40 and 49 and also have high blood pressure, diabetes, high blood cholesterol, or heart problems, or if you also smoke or are obese.

Consult with your health-care practitioner before starting oral contraceptives if you have any of the following: fibrocystic breast, migraine, uterine fibroid tumors, epilepsy, tuberculosis, varicose veins, depression, kidney problems, a strong family history of breast cancer, liver problems, asthma, high blood pressure, endometriosis, diabetes, or sickle-cell anemia, or you are older than 35. Talk to your health-care practitioner if within the next 2 months you are planning to have surgery (including dental surgery) that will require general or spinal anesthesia.

Oral contraceptives may increase your sensitivity to sunlight. Wear protective clothing and sunscreen.

If you wear contact lenses, you may experience some eye discomfort because oral contraceptives can cause minor changes in the shape of your eyeball.

If you are taking any drugs that reduce the effectiveness of oral contraceptives (see "Drug Interactions"), you should use another form of contraception as a backup to help prevent pregnancy.

DRUG INTERACTIONS

Tell your health-care practitioner and pharmacist if you are taking any prescription or nonprescription drugs, as well as any vitamins, herbs, or other supplements. Possible drug interactions include the following:

- Antibiotics (e.g., amoxicillin, ampicillin, and others; check with your health-care practitioner), anticonvulsants (e.g., acetazolamide, clonazepam), nonsteroidal anti-inflammatory drugs (e.g., etodolac, naproxen), antihistamines (e.g., cetirizine, loratadine), barbiturates (e.g., phenobarbital), carbamazepine, chloramphenicol, meprobamate, mineral oil, phenytoin, rifampin, tetracyclines (e.g., doxycycline, minocycline), sulfadoxine, pyrimethamine, and thiazolidinediones can reduce the contraceptive effects of oral contraceptives.
- Oral contraceptives can increase the effect of benzodiazepines (e.g., alprazolam, diazepam), cyclosporine, metoprolol, phenothiazines (e.g., chlorpromazine, promazine), theophylline, prednisolone, prednisone, and meperidine.
- Oral contraceptives may decrease the effects of terazosin, clofibrate, dextrothyroxine, guanethidine, oral antidiabetes drugs (e.g., glyburide, glipizide), and insulin.
- Oral contraceptives may increase the toxicity of tricyclic antidepressants (e.g., amitriptyline, imipramine).
- Aminocaproic acid and tranexamic acid may increase the possibility of blood clots.

FOOD, VITAMIN, AND HERBAL INTERACTIONS

Oral contraceptives may reduce the body's levels of vitamin C, vitamin B_2, zinc, and magnesium. Talk to your health-care practitioner about supplementation. Excessive vitamin C may increase the effectiveness of oral contraceptives.

Because oral contraceptives may increase levels of copper in the body, do not take supplements that contain copper while taking these drugs.

The herbs milk thistle, black cohosh, and St. John's wort may decrease the effectiveness of oral contraceptives, while licorice may worsen certain side effects associated with the drugs.

RECOMMENDED DOSAGE

Oral contraceptives are available in tablets. Because there are so many different kinds of oral contraceptives, you need to take your prescription as instructed by your health-care practitioner.

- Oral contraceptives are available in three main forms: single-phase, 2-phase, and 3-phase. The single-phase products provide constant amounts of estrogen and progestin throughout the entire month of treatment. The 2-phase products provide a steady level of estrogen with rising and then decreasing levels of progestin. The 3-phase pills, which are the newest on the market, provide even levels of estrogen and three different levels of progestin, which is meant to simulate the body's natural hormone cycle.
- If you miss a dose of a single- or 2-phase product, take 2 pills the following day. If you miss 2 consecutive days, take 2 pills for the next 2 days, then return to your regular schedule of 1 pill daily. If you miss 3 consecutive pills, stop taking the pills for the next 7 days and use another form of contraception. On the 8th day, begin a new cycle of treatment.
- For the 3-phase pills, if you miss 1 dose, take 2 pills the following day. If you miss 2 consecutive days, take 2 pills for the next 2 days, then return to your regular schedule. If you miss 3 consecutive days of pills, stop taking the pills and wait until your period begins. Use another form of contraception during this time.

SYMPTOMS OF OVERDOSE AND WHAT TO DO

Symptoms of overdose include nausea and breakthrough bleeding. If overdose occurs, seek immediate medical assistance and bring the prescription container with you to the hospital.

SPECIAL INFORMATION FOR PREGNANT OR NURSING WOMEN

Oral contraceptives may effect fetal development and can cause birth defects. They should not be used during pregnancy. If you become pregnant while taking oral contraceptives, stop taking them immediately and contact your health-care practitioner.

Oral contraceptives pass into breast milk and can reduce the amount of milk you produce. If you are breastfeeding, you should switch to bottle feeding.

SPECIAL INFORMATION FOR SENIORS

These drugs are not intended for women who have gone through menopause.

GENERIC NAME

Class: Corticosteroids, nasal inhalation

Generics: (1) beclomethasone; (2) budesonide (see Budesonide entry); (3) dexamethasone; (4) flunisolide; (5) fluticasone; (6) mometasone; (7) triamcinolone

BRAND NAMES

(1) Beconase, Beconase AQ, Vancenase, Vancenase AQ; (2) Rhinocort Aqua, Rhinocort Nasal Inhaler, Rhinocort Turbuhaler; (3) Dexacort Turbinaire; (4) Nasalide, Nasarel, Rhinalar; (5) Flonase; (6) Nasonex; (7) Nasacort, Nasacort AQ, Tri-Nasal

Generics available

ABOUT THIS DRUG

Nasally inhaled corticosteroids are used to treat severe symptoms of seasonal and chronic allergic rhinitis (hay fever) that have not responded to other medications.

These drugs reduce inflammation of the mucous membranes in the nasal passages.

SIDE EFFECTS

Be sure to tell your health-care practitioner if you experience any side effects while taking nasal corticosteroids. Only your health-care practitioner can determine whether it is safe for you to continue taking this drug.

- *Most Common:* irritation of the nasal passages and throat, burning, stinging, dryness, headache
- *Less Common:* nausea, nosebleed, nasal congestion, bronchial asthma, sneezing attacks, lightheadedness, loss of the sense of taste
- *Rare:* ulcers in the nasal passages, watery eyes, sore throat, wheezing, increased eye pressure, vomiting, hypersensitivity reaction (e.g., itching, rash, breathing difficulties, swelling)

IMPORTANT PRECAUTIONS

Tell your health-care practitioner if you are sensitive or allergic to any of the inhaled corticosteroids or to the propellants in the spray, which include benzalkonium chloride, disodium acetate, phenylethanol, fluorocarbones, and proplylene glycol; or to any other drugs.

In rare cases, *Candida* yeast infections can develop in the nose and throat.

DRUG INTERACTIONS

Tell your health-care practitioner and pharmacist if you are taking any prescription or nonprescription drugs, as well as any vitamins, herbs, or other supplements. No possible interactions with other drugs have been noted.

FOOD, VITAMIN, AND HERBAL INTERACTIONS

No food, vitamin, or herbal interactions have been noted.

RECOMMENDED DOSAGE

Nasally inhaled corticosteroids are available in nasal inhalers. The dosages given here are typical. However, your health-care practitioner will determine the dose and schedule that are most appropriate for you.

Beclomethasone

- *Children 6 to 12 Years:* 1 spray in each nostril 3 times daily
- *Children Age 13 and Older and Adults:* 1 spray in each nostril 2 to 4 times daily

Budesonide: see "Budesonide" entry

Flunisolide

- *Children 6 to 14 Years:* 1 spray in each nostril 3 times daily; or 2 sprays in each nostril 2 times daily

- *Children 15 Years and Older and Adults:* starting dose, 2 sprays in each nostril 2 times a day, which may be increased up to 8 sprays a day in each nostril

Fluticasone

- *Children 4 Years and Older:* 1 spray in each nostril once daily, which may be increased to 2 sprays per day in each nostril
- *Adults:* starting dose, 2 sprays in each nostril once daily or divided into 2 doses. Dosage may be reduced by half within a few days if appropriate.

Mometasone

- *Children 12 Years and Older and Adults:* 2 sprays in each nostril once daily. The dosage may be increased to 4 sprays daily in each nostril.

Triamcinolone

- *Children 6 to 12 Years:* 1 (Nasacort AQ) or 2 (Nasacort) sprays in each nostril once daily. The dosage may be increased to 2 sprays daily in each nostril if needed.
- *Children 13 Years and Older and Adults:* 2 sprays in each nostril once daily. The dosage may be increased to 4 sprays daily in each nostril.

If you miss a dose, take it as soon as you remember. If it is nearly time for your next dose, do not take the missed dose. Continue with your regular dosing schedule. Never take a double dose.

SYMPTOMS OF OVERDOSE AND WHAT TO DO

No specific symptoms of an overdose of inhaled corticosteroids are expected. If you suspect an overdose has occurred, or if someone has accidentally ingested any of these drugs, call your health-care practitioner, poison control center, or emergency room for instructions. Serious adverse effects related to overuse or ingesting these drugs are unlikely.

SPECIAL INFORMATION FOR PREGNANT OR NURSING WOMEN

Using large amounts of corticosteroids during pregnancy may suppress fetal growth. Although only small amounts of nasal corticosteroids enter the bloodstream, you and your health-care practitioner should weigh the potential risks against the potential benefits of using these drugs during pregnancy.

Dexamethasone passes into breast milk, and the other nasal corticosteroids may as well. If you are breastfeeding, your health-care practitioner will likely advise you to bottle feed until your treatment is done.

SPECIAL INFORMATION FOR SENIORS

No special precautions are noted for older adults.

GENERIC NAME

Class: Corticosteroids, oral

Generics: (1) betamethasone; (2) cortisone; (3) dexamethasone; (4) hydrocortisone; (5) methylprednisolone; (6) prednisolone; (7) prednisone; (8) triamcinolone

BRAND NAMES

(1) Celestone; (2) Cortone Acetate; (3) Decadron, Dexameth, Dexone, Hexadrol; (4) Cortef, Cortenema, Cortifoam, Hydrocortone; (5) Medrol; (6) DeltapCortef, Pediapred, Prelone; (7) Deltasone, Liquid Pred, Meticorten, Orasone, Panasol-S, Prednicen-M, Prednisone Intensol, Sterapred, Sterapred DS; (8) Aristocort, Atolone, Kenacort
Generics available

ABOUT THIS DRUG

Oral corticosteroids are used to treat a variety of conditions, including arthritis, adrenal disease, skin disorders, asthma and other severe respiratory diseases, gastrointestinal diseases, and inflammation of the heart, nerves, and other organs.

Synthetic corticosteroids are designed to work like the natural ones produced by the adrenal glands, which affect nearly every system in the body. Health-care practitioners prescribe individual corticosteroids based on the potency needed for a specific condition and the drug's past performance with that condition.

SIDE EFFECTS

Be sure to tell your health-care practitioner if you experience any side effects while taking oral corticosteroids. Only your health-care practitioner can determine whether it is safe for you to continue taking this drug.

- *Common:* indigestion, acne, nausea, vomiting, gas, headache, insomnia, dizziness, increased appetite, swollen legs or feet, poor wound healing

- *Less Common:* tarry or bloody stool, infections, blurred vision, fever, mood changes, restlessness, frequent urination, irregular menstrual periods, euphoria, muscle cramps, stomach or hip pain, thirst, fatigue
- *Rare:* irregular heartbeat, convulsions, leg or thigh pain, rash, joint pain, unusual hair growth on the body or face, hallucinations, confusion, skin color changes

IMPORTANT PRECAUTIONS

Tell your health-care practitioner if you are sensitive or allergic to any of the corticosteroids or to any other drugs. Generally, if you are sensitive or allergic to one corticosteroid, you will have a negative reaction to all of them. Also, oral corticosteroids often contain tartrazine dyes and sulfite preservatives, which cause allergic reactions in some people.

Corticosteroids compromise the immune system, making you more susceptible to infections. New infections that develop while you are taking corticosteroids for another condition can become serious.

If you want to stop taking corticosteroids, do so gradually and under your health-care practitioner's guidance. Stopping quickly may cause adrenal gland failure.

Long-term use of corticosteroids can increase your risk of glaucoma, eye infections, and cataracts.

Corticosteroids should be used with caution if you have severe kidney disease, ulcerative colitis, heart failure, high blood pressure, thrombophlebitis (vein inflammation associated with a blood clot, usually in the legs), Cushing's disease, myasthenia gravis, metastatic cancer, diabetes, underactive thyroid disease, stomach ulcers, cirrhosis, seizure disorder, osteoporosis, or an antibiotic-resistant infection.

If you take more than 40 mg daily of prednisone or high doses of other corticosteroids, you are at risk of corticosteroid psychosis, characterized by euphoria, sleeplessness, delirium, mood swings, personality changes, and severe depression. These symptoms typically develop 15 to 30 days after starting treatment and are more common among women.

DRUG INTERACTIONS

Tell your health-care practitioner and pharmacist if you are taking any prescription or nonprescription drugs, as well as any vitamins, herbs, or other supplements. Possible drug interactions include the following:

- Oral corticosteroids may reduce the effects of anticoagulants (e.g., warfarin), antidiabetics (e.g., glipizide, glyburide), salicylates (e.g., aspirin, salsalate), isoniazid, and mifepristone.
- Antacids may result in reduced effect of prednisone and dexamethasone.
- Anticholinergics (e.g., atropine, scopolamine) may cause glaucoma.
- Carbamazepine, cholestyramine, colestipol, cyclosporine, ephedrine, glutethimide, rifampin, primidone, phenytoin, phenobarbital, mitotane, and antihistamines (e.g., clemastine, cetirizine) may decrease the effects of oral corticosteroids.
- Tricyclic antidepressants (e.g., clomipramine, imipramine) may increase the risk of mental side effects.
- Nonsteroidal anti-inflammatory drugs (NSAIDs) may increase the risk of ulcers and also increase the effects of oral corticosteroids.
- Carbonic anhydrase inhibitors (e.g., acetazolamide, methazolamide) may result in an increased loss of calcium.
- Oral contraceptives may increase the effects of oral corticosteroids.
- Digoxin and digitoxin may result in severe potassium depletion and possibly digitalis toxicity.
- Diuretics (e.g., amiloride, indapamide) and foscarnet may cause potassium depletion.
- Sympathomimetics (e.g., barbiturates, ephedrine) may cause glaucoma.

FOOD, VITAMIN, AND HERBAL INTERACTIONS

If you are taking potassium supplements, oral corticosteroids may reduce their effect.

RECOMMENDED DOSAGE

Oral corticosteroids are available in tablets, syrup elixir, and oral solution. The dosages given here are typical. However, your healthcare practitioner will determine the most appropriate dose and schedule for you.

Betamethasone

- *Children Up to Age 12:* dose depends on body weight
- *Children 12 Years and Older and Adults:* 0.25 to 7.2 mg daily, 1 or 2 divided doses

Cortisone

- *Children Up to Age 12:* dose depends on body weight

- *Children 12 Years and Older and Adults:* 25 to 300 mg daily, 1 or 2 divided doses

Dexamethasone

- *Children Up to Age 12:* dose depends on body weight
- *Children 12 Years and Older and Adults:* 0.5 to 10 mg as determined by your health-care practitioner

Hydrocortisone

- *Children Up to Age 12:* dose depends on body weight
- *Children 12 Years and Older and Adults:* 20 to 800 mg every 1 or 2 days as a single or divided dose

Methylprednisolone

- *Children Up to Age 12:* dose depends on body weight
- *Children 12 Years and Older and Adults:* 4 to 160 mg every 1 or 2 days as a single or divided dose

Prednisolone

- *Children Up to Age 12:* dose depends on body weight
- *Children 12 Years and Older and Adults:* 5 to 200 mg as needed and determined by your health-care practitioner

Prednisone

- *Children Up to Age 12:* dose depends on body weight
- *Children 12 Years and Older and Adults:* 5 to 200 mg every 1 to 2 days as a single or divided dose

Triamcinolone

- *Children Up to Age 12:* dose depends on body weight
- *Children 12 Years and Older and Adults:* 2 to 60 mg as 1 or 2 divided doses

Oral corticosteroids should be taken with food or with an antacid to help prevent stomach irritation. If these measures don't help, contact your health-care practitioner.

If you miss a dose, take it as soon as you remember. If it is nearly time for your next dose, do not take the missed dose. Continue with your regular dosing schedule. Never take a double dose.

SYMPTOMS OF OVERDOSE AND WHAT TO DO

Symptoms of overdose include fluid retention, severe headache, convulsions, and heart failure. If overdose occurs, seek immediate medical attention and bring the prescription container with you to the hospital.

SPECIAL INFORMATION FOR PREGNANT OR NURSING WOMEN

Long-term use of high doses of corticosteroids, as well as chronic use during the first trimester, may cause birth defects. If you are pregnant or plan to become pregnant, and any of these drugs are considered crucial by your health-care practitioner, you and your health-care practitioner must weigh the potential risks against the potential benefits.

Oral corticosteroids may pass into breast milk. Although low doses of some oral corticosteroids may be taken for short periods of time while breastfeeding, you should consult with your health-care practitioner before using any of them. Your health-care practitioner may advise you to switch to bottle feeding until your treatment is done.

SPECIAL INFORMATION FOR SENIORS

Older adults may be more susceptible to side effects and experience more severe ones. Oral corticosteroids are more likely to aggravate edema, diabetes, or ulcers, and are more likely to cause osteoporosis (especially in women) and cataracts with prolonged use.

GENERIC NAME

Class: Corticosteroids, oral inhalers

Generics: (1) betaclomethasone; (2) budesonide, see Budesonide entry; (3) dexamethasone; (4) flunisolide; (5) fluticasone; (6) triamcinolone

BRAND NAMES

(1) Beclodisk, Becloforte, Beclovent, Beclovent Rotacaps, Qvar, Vanceril; (2) Pulmicort Nebuamp, Pulmicort Turbuhaler; (3) Decadron Respihaler; (4) Aerobid, Aerobid-M, Bronalide; (5) Flovent, Rotadisk; (6) Azmacort

Generics available

ABOUT THIS DRUG

Orally inhaled corticosteroids are used for the prevention of symptoms of chronic bronchial asthma. They are not effective in the treatment of acute asthma attacks.

These drugs help prevent inflammation in the lungs and breathing passages.

SIDE EFFECTS

Be sure to tell your health-care practitioner if you experience any side effects while taking oral corticosteroids. Only your health-care practitioner can determine whether it is safe for you to continue taking these drugs.

- *Most Common:* dry mouth, cough, throat irritation, hoarseness
- *Less Common:* dry throat, headache, nausea, bruising, pain when swallowing, thrush (yeast infection in the mouth or throat)
- *Rare:* difficulty breathing, pain or tight chest

IMPORTANT PRECAUTIONS

Tell your health-care practitioner if you are sensitive or allergic to orally inhaled corticosteroids, any other corticosteroids, or any other drugs.

Before you start using these corticosteroids, tell your health-care practitioner if you have osteoporosis or tuberculosis, or a history of tuberculosis.

Orally inhaled corticosteroids are not recommended for children younger than six years.

DRUG INTERACTIONS

Tell your health-care practitioner and pharmacist if you are taking any prescription or nonprescription drugs, as well as any vitamins, herbs, or other supplements. No possible interactions with other drugs have been noted.

FOOD, VITAMIN, AND HERBAL INTERACTIONS

No food, vitamin, or herbal interactions have been noted.

RECOMMENDED DOSAGE

Orally inhaled corticosteroids are available in oral inhalers. The dosages given here are typical. However, your health-care practitioner will determine the most appropriate dose and schedule for you.

Beclomethasone

- *Children Age 6 to 12 Years:* 1 to 2 inhalations 3 to 4 times daily
- *Children 13 Years and Older and Adults:* 2 inhalations 3 to 4 times daily; or 4 inhalations twice daily. If you have severe asthma, up to 16 inhalations daily can be taken.

Budesonide: see "Budesonide" entry

Flunisolide

- *Children 6 to 12 Years:* 2 inhalations morning and evening. Do not exceed 4 inhalations daily
- *Children 16 Years and Older and Adults:* 2 inhalations morning and evening. Do not exceed 8 inhalations daily

Fluticasone

- *Children 12 Years and Older and Adults:* 88 to 880 mcg twice daily
- *Children 12 Years and Older and Adults:* Rotadisk, 100 to 1,000 mcg twice daily

Triamcinolone

- *Children 6 to 12 Years:* 1 to 2 inhalations 3 to 4 times daily. Maximum 12 inhalations daily
- *Children 12 Years and Older and Adults:* 2 inhalations 3 to 4 times daily. Maximum 16 inhalations daily

Before using the inhaler, drink water to moisten your throat. Wait at least one minute between inhalations. Rinse your mouth after completing your dose to help prevent dry mouth and throat irritation.

If you miss a dose, take it as soon as you remember. If it is nearly time for your next dose, do not take the missed dose. Continue with your regular dosing schedule. Never take a double dose.

SYMPTOMS OF OVERDOSE AND WHAT TO DO

No specific symptoms of an overdose of orally inhaled corticosteroids are expected. If you suspect an overdose has occurred, or if someone has accidentally ingested any of these drugs, call your health-care practitioner, poison control center, or emergency room for instructions. Serious adverse effects related to overuse or ingesting these drugs are unlikely.

SPECIAL INFORMATION FOR PREGNANT OR NURSING WOMEN

Using large amounts of corticosteroids during pregnancy may suppress fetal growth. If you are pregnant or plan to become pregnant, you and your health-care practitioner should weigh the potential risks against the potential benefits of using these drugs during pregnancy.

Although oral corticosteroids pass into breast milk, it is not known whether orally inhaled corticosteroids do. If you are breastfeeding, your health-care practitioner may advise you to switch to bottle feeding until your treatment is done.

SPECIAL INFORMATION FOR SENIORS

No special precautions are noted for older adults.

GENERIC NAME

Class: Corticosteroids, topical

Generics: (1) alclometasone, (2) amcinonide, (3) betamethasone (augmented and regular), (4) clobetasol, (5) clocortolone, (6) desonide, (7) desoximetasone, (8) dexamethasone, (9) diflorasone, (10) fluocinolone, (11) fluocinonide, (12) flurandrenolide, (13) fluticasone, (14) halcinonide, (15) halobetasol, (16) hydrocortisone, (17) mometasone, (18) prednicarbate, (19) triamcinolone

BRAND NAMES

(1) Aclovate, (2) Cyclocort, (3) Alphatrex, Betatrex, Beta-Val, Diprosone, Dipropionate, Diprolene, Diprolene AF, Luxiq, Maxivate, Psorion Cream, Teladar, Valisone, (4) Cormax, Embeline, Embeline E, Temorate, Temorate E, (5) Cloderm, (6) DesOwen, (7) Topicort, (8) Aeroseb-Dex, Decadron, Decaspray, (9) Florone, Florone E, Maxiflor, Psorcon, (10) Fluonid, Flurosyn, FS Shampoo, Synalar, Synalar-HP, (11) Fluonex, Lidex, Lidex-E, (12) Cordran, Cordran SP, (13) Cutivate, (14) Halog, Halog-E, (15) Ultravate, (16) 1% HC, Acticort 100, Bactine hydrocortisone, Cetacort, Cortaid Intensive Therapy, Delcort, Gynecort, Hycort, Hydrocort, Lanacort-5, Nutracort, Penecort, Tegrin-HC, among others, (17) Elocon, (18) Dermatop, (19) Aristocort, Aristocort A, Delta-Tritex, Flutex, Kenalog, Kenonel, Triacet, Triderm

Generics available

ABOUT THIS DRUG

Topical corticosteroids are prescribed to treat inflammation, itching, and other skin problems. They are available in many strengths, and each one has conditions for which it is better suited than others. Your health-care practitioner will make that determination.

These drugs appear to interfere with the production of various natural substances in the body that cause inflammation, swelling, pain, and redness.

SIDE EFFECTS

Be sure to tell your health-care practitioner if you experience any side effects while taking topical corticosteroids. Only your health-care practitioner can determine whether it is safe for you to continue taking these drugs.

- *Most Common:* burning, itching, irritation, redness, dryness, acne, stinging and cracking, numbness or tingling in the extremities
- *Less Common:* with prolonged use, unusual bleeding or bruising, increased susceptibility to infection, and blistering and pus near hair follicles may occur

IMPORTANT PRECAUTIONS

Tell your health-care practitioner if you are sensitive or allergic to topical corticosteroids, to other forms of corticosteroids, or to any other drugs.

Do not apply topical corticosteroids to areas that have had other topical agents applied to them, especially those that contain alcohol (e.g., colognes, aftershave lotions, moisturizers). Irritation, dryness, or an increased risk of an allergic reaction may occur.

Before using these medications, consult with your health-care practitioner if you have diabetes, glaucoma, cataracts, skin infections or sores, tuberculosis, or infections elsewhere in your body.

Application of topical corticosteroids around the eyes for long periods may cause glaucoma or cataracts.

Topical corticosteroids should not be used for more than 2 weeks on children and teenagers unless your health-care practitioner has instructed you to do so. Specific drugs that should not be used at all on children's skin include augmented betamethasone, clobetasol, desoximetasone, fluticasone, and halobetasol.

After applying topical corticosteroids, do not cover the treated areas with bandages or other coverings unless specifically instructed to do so by your health-care practitioner. This includes diapers and plastic pants used on infants. All coverings may worsen the condition being treated.

Be careful not to get the drug into your eyes. Wash your hands immediately after applying the dose. If some of the drug gets into your eyes, flush them with water.

DRUG INTERACTIONS

Tell your health-care practitioner and pharmacist if you are taking any prescription or nonprescription drugs, as well as any vitamins, herbs, or other supplements. No significant drug interactions have been reported.

FOOD, VITAMIN, AND HERBAL INTERACTIONS

No food, vitamin, or herbal interactions have been noted.

RECOMMENDED DOSAGE

Topical corticosteroids are available in gel, cream, lotion, tape, aerosol, and ointment. The dosages are different for each different medication. Follow your health-care practitioner's directions or those on the label. Ask your pharmacist if you need help.

If you miss a dose, apply it as soon as you remember. If it is nearly time for your next dose, do not apply the missed dose. Continue with your regular dosing schedule. Never apply a double dose.

SYMPTOMS OF OVERDOSE AND WHAT TO DO

No symptoms of an overdose with topical corticosteroids have been reported. If someone accidentally ingests the drug or an overdose occurs, call your health-care practitioner, local poison control center, or emergency department for instructions.

SPECIAL INFORMATION FOR PREGNANT OR NURSING WOMEN

Topical corticosteroids applied for long periods of time or in large amounts during pregnancy may cause birth defects. If you are pregnant or plan to become pregnant and these drugs are considered to be crucial for your health, you and your health-care practitioner must weigh the potential benefits against the potential risks.

Topical corticosteroids may pass into breast milk. If you are breastfeeding, your health-care practitioner may advise you to bottle feed until your treatment is done. Nursing women should never use clobetasol.

SPECIAL INFORMATION FOR SENIORS

Older adults are more likely to have high blood pressure and osteoporosis. The risk of these effects is more likely with other forms of corticosteroids; however, high doses and prolonged use does increase their risk. Seniors also have thinner skin and are more susceptible to skin tearing or blood-containing blisters.

GENERIC NAME

Cortisone

see Corticosteroids, Oral, page 330

GENERIC NAME

Cromolyn

BRAND NAMES

Crolom, Cromoptic, Gastrocrom, Intal, Nasalcrom, Opticrom
Generic available for all forms except ophthalmic

ABOUT THIS DRUG

Cromolyn is an antiasthmatic and antiallergy agent used to help control symptoms of seasonal allergies, chronic bronchial asthma, and conjunctivitis (inflammation of the mucous membranes of the eyelids and whites of the eyes), which is associated with allergies.

This drug inhibits the release of histamine (chemicals released by the body during allergic reactions) from mast cells. Histamine, a natural substance produced by the body, causes sneezing, hives, itchy and watery eyes, swelling, and other allergic symptoms.

SIDE EFFECTS

Be sure to tell your health-care practitioner if you experience any side effects while taking cromolyn. Only your health-care practitioner can determine whether it is safe for you to continue taking this drug.

- *Most Common:* ophthalmic form: burning or stinging of the eyes; nasal and inhalant forms: dry throat, throat irritation, sneezing, burning, stinging, or irritation in nose
- *Less Common:* ophthalmic form: increased itching or watering of the eyes, dry or puffy around the eyes; nasal and inhalant forms: cough, headache, postnasal drip, unpleasant taste

IMPORTANT PRECAUTIONS

Tell your health-care practitioner if you are sensitive or allergic to cromolyn or to any other drugs.

Cromolyn is not effective against acute allergy attacks; it is only to be used to prevent or reduce the number of allergy attacks and their severity.

If you have kidney or liver disease, your health-care practitioner will likely prescribe a lower dose.

Exercise caution when using aerosol cromolyn if you have abnormal heart rhythm or diseased coronary blood vessels.

DRUG INTERACTIONS

Tell your health-care practitioner and pharmacist if you are taking any prescription or nonprescription drugs, as well as any vitamins, herbs, or other supplements. No significant drug interactions have been reported.

FOOD, VITAMIN, AND HERBAL INTERACTIONS

Oral or inhaled cromolyn products should not be mixed with food, juice, or milk. The ophthalmic and nasal forms can be taken without regard for these substances.

RECOMMENDED DOSAGE

Cromolyn is available as an aerosol, inhalation solution, nasal solution, and ophthalmic solution. The dosages given here are typical. However, your health-care practitioner will determine the most appropriate dose and schedule for you.

Inhalation Aerosol

- *Children 5 Years and Older and Adults:* to prevent asthma symptoms, 2 inhalations 4 times daily
- *Children 5 Years and Older and Adults:* to prevent bronchospasm, 2 inhalations at least 10 to 15 minutes before exercise or exposure to allergens

Inhalation Solution

- *Children 2 Years and Older and Adults:* 20 mg 4 times daily, 4 to 6 hours apart

Nasal Solution

- *Children 6 Years and Older and Adults:* 1 spray in each nostril 3 to 6 times daily

Ophthalmic Solution

- *Children Up to Age 4*: use and dosage to be determined by your health-care practitioner

➤ *Children 4 Years and Older and Adults:* 1 drop 4 to 6 times daily in evenly spaced intervals

If you miss a dose, take it as soon as you remember if it is within 2 hours of being late. If it is more than 2 hours past your scheduled dose, do not take the missed dose. Continue with your regular dosing schedule. Never take a double dose.

SYMPTOMS OF OVERDOSE AND WHAT TO DO

Symptoms of an overdose are increased side effects. If overdose occurs, contact your health-care practitioner, local poison control center, or emergency room for instructions.

SPECIAL INFORMATION FOR PREGNANT OR NURSING WOMEN

No adequate studies of the effects of cromolyn on pregnant or nursing women have been done. In animal studies, very large amounts of the drug affected the fetus but did not cause birth defects. If you are pregnant or plan to become pregnant, and your health-care practitioner deems this drug crucial to your health, the two of you will need to weigh the potential benefits against the potential risks.

Cromolyn may pass into breast milk. If you are breastfeeding, your health-care practitioner may advise you to stop until your treatment is done.

SPECIAL INFORMATION FOR SENIORS

Older adults who have reduced liver or kidney function may need lower dosages.

GENERIC NAME

Cyclobenzaprine

BRAND NAME

Flexeril

Generic available

ABOUT THIS DRUG

Cyclobenzaprine is a muscle relaxant that is used to treat pain and limited motion caused by muscle spasms.

This drug blocks the pain signals to the brain and may also provide sedation.

SIDE EFFECTS

Be sure to tell your health-care practitioner if you experience any side effects while taking cyclobenzaprine. Only your health-care practitioner can determine whether it is safe for you to continue taking this drug.

- *Most Common:* dizziness, dry mouth, drowsiness
- *Less Common:* blurred vision, fast heartbeat, insomnia, numbness in the extremities, bad taste, fatigue, nausea, sweating
- *Rare:* confusion, depression, unsteadiness, hallucinations, rash, itch, swelling, breathing problems

IMPORTANT PRECAUTIONS

Tell your health-care practitioner if you are sensitive or allergic to cyclobenzaprine or to any other drugs.

Do not take cyclobenzaprine if you had a heart attack within the past 6 weeks, or if you have congestive heart failure or an overactive thyroid.

Consult your health-care practitioner before starting cyclobenzaprine if you have glaucoma, a heart condition, prostate problems, urinary difficulties, or an overactive thyroid.

Because drowsiness and dizziness are common side effects, make sure you know how you react to the drug before you drive or operate dangerous equipment.

Persistent dry mouth may lead to dental or gum problems. Make sure you maintain adequate fluid intake and keep your mouth moist by sucking on ice chips or chewing sugarless gum.

DRUG INTERACTIONS

Tell your health-care practitioner and pharmacist if you are taking any prescription or nonprescription drugs, as well as any vitamins, herbs, or other supplements. Possible drug interactions include the following:

- Tricyclic antidepressants (e.g., imipramine, amitriptyline) and central nervous system depressants (e.g., barbiturates, narcotics, sedatives, tranquilizers, benzodiazepines) may increase sedation.
- Monoamine oxidase inhibitors (MAOIs) taken while you are taking cyclobenzaprine or within 2 weeks of taking it may increase the chance of serious side effects.
- Cyclobenzaprine may reduce the effects of clonidine, guanethidine, methyldopa, and rauwolfia alkaloids.
- Cyclobenzaprine may increase the effects of anticholinergics (e.g., atropine, scopolamine) and antihistamines (e.g., clemastine, cetirizine).

- Procainamide and quinidine may result in increased conduction disturbance.

FOOD, VITAMIN, AND HERBAL INTERACTIONS

No food, vitamin, or herbal interactions have been noted.

RECOMMENDED DOSAGE

Cyclobenzaprine is available in 10-mg tablets. The dosages given here are typical. However, your health-care practitioner will determine the most appropriate dose and schedule for you.

- *Children Up to 15 Years:* dose and use to be determined by your health-care practitioner
- *Children 15 Years and Older and Adults:* 10 mg three times daily. Your health-care practitioner may increase the total dose to a maximum of 60 mg daily.

If you miss a dose, take it as soon as you remember. If it is nearly time for your next dose, do not take the missed dose. Continue with your regular dosing schedule. Never take a double dose.

SYMPTOMS OF OVERDOSE AND WHAT TO DO

Symptoms of overdose include severe mental confusion, agitation, trouble with concentration, difficulty walking or standing, dilated pupils, severe drowsiness, and coma. If overdose occurs, seek immediate medical attention and bring the prescription container with you to the hospital.

SPECIAL INFORMATION FOR PREGNANT OR NURSING WOMEN

No adequate studies of the effects of cyclobenzaprine on pregnant or nursing women have been done. Animal studies have not revealed any birth defects or other effects on the fetus. If you are pregnant or plan to become pregnant, you and your health-care practitioner should weigh the potential benefits against the potential risks.

Cyclobenzaprine may pass into breast milk. If you are breastfeeding, your health-care practitioner may advise you to stop until your treatment is done.

SPECIAL INFORMATION FOR SENIORS

Older adults are more likely to experience side effects, and they may be more severe.

GENERIC NAME
Cyclosporine

BRAND NAMES

Ciclosporin, Neoral, Sandimmune
No generic available

ABOUT THIS DRUG

Cyclosporine is an immunosuppressant given to organ transplant recipients to treat donor organ transplant rejection as well as help prevent it.

This drug suppresses the body's natural tendency to reject donor organs, although exactly how it does this is not known.

SIDE EFFECTS

Be sure to tell your health-care practitioner if you experience any side effects while taking cyclosporine. Only your health-care practitioner can determine whether it is safe for you to continue taking this drug.

➤ *Most Common:* inflamed gums, tremors, increased hair growth, kidney damage, high blood pressure

➤ *Common:* abdominal discomfort, acne, breathing problems, convulsions, cough, diarrhea, flushing, headache, liver damage, muscle, bone, or joint pain, nausea, numbness or tingling, inflamed sinuses, vomiting, wheezing

➤ *Less Common:* abdominal distention, fever, fluid retention, bleeding gums, blood disorders, hearing loss, frequent urination, conjunctivitis, dizziness, hiccups, high blood sugar, indigestion, infection, insomnia, peptic ulcer, rash, vertigo

➤ *Rare:* anxiety, breast development in males, blood in the urine, chest pain, constipation, depression, heart attack, itching, mouth sores, sluggishness, gastrointestinal bleeding, tingling, visual disturbances, weakness

IMPORTANT PRECAUTIONS

Tell your health-care practitioner if you are sensitive or allergic to cyclosporine or to any other drugs.

Do not take cyclosporine if you have chicken pox or shingles.

Consult your health-care practitioner before taking cyclosporine if you have liver problems, kidney disease, or an infection.

Prolonged use may cause reduced kidney function.

Cyclosporine can cause hypertension. Your health-care practitioner should regularly monitor your blood pressure.

Never stop taking this drug without first consulting your health-care practitioner. Cyclosporine is typically taken for the rest of a person's life.

Because absorption of cyclosporine is not consistent, your health-care practitioner will need to regularly monitor your blood levels of the drug to make sure you are getting the correct amount.

Cyclosporine suppresses your immune system, making you more susceptible to infection and certain malignancies, including lymph system cancer and skin cancer.

DRUG INTERACTIONS

Tell your health-care practitioner and pharmacist if you are taking any prescription or nonprescription drugs, as well as any vitamins, herbs, or other supplements. Possible drug interactions include the following:

- Androgens (male hormones), cimetidine, danazol, diltiazem, potassium-sparing diuretics (e.g., amiloride, triamterene), erythromycin, estrogens, fluconazole, itraconazole, and zafirlukast may increase the effects of cyclosporine.
- Vancomycin may increase the chance of hearing loss or kidney damage.
- Tiopronin may increase the risk of toxicity to the kidneys.
- Anticonvulsants (e.g., carbamazepine, diazepam), modafinil, terbinafine, and rifampin may decrease the effect of cyclosporine.
- Itraconazole and nimodipine may increase cyclosporine toxicity.
- Virus vaccines may increase the adverse reactions to the vaccines.
- Immunosuppressants (e.g., azathioprine, cyclophosphamide) may increase the risk of infection.
- Alcohol may increase the possibility of toxicity. Do not use along with cyclosporine.

FOOD, VITAMIN, AND HERBAL INTERACTIONS

Avoid eating foods that are high in potassium, such as bananas, oranges, waffles, oatmeal, tomatoes, baked beans, and milk. Also avoid grapefruit and grapefruit juice while taking cyclosporine. Cyclosporine may deplete your body's supplies of magnesium. Talk to your health-care practitioner about taking a magnesium supplement.

Avoid use of the herbs mistletoe, oak bark, marshmallow root, licorice, and St. John's wort when taking cyclosporine.

RECOMMENDED DOSAGE

Cyclosporine is available in capsules, in oral solution, and by injection. Your health-care practitioner will determine the most appropriate dose based on various factors unique to you.

If you miss a dose and fewer than 12 hours have passed, take that dose as soon as you remember. If it is nearly time for your next dose, do not take the missed dose. Continue with your regular dosing schedule. Never take a double dose.

SYMPTOMS OF OVERDOSE AND WHAT TO DO

No specific information concerning overdosing with cyclosporine is available; however, kidney and liver problems can be expected. If an overdose occurs, seek immediate medical attention and bring the prescription container with you to the hospital.

SPECIAL INFORMATION FOR PREGNANT OR NURSING WOMEN

No adequate studies of the effects of cyclosporine on pregnant or nursing women have been done. Animal studies have revealed serious birth defects. If you are pregnant or plan to become pregnant, tell your health-care practitioner immediately. Cyclosporine should be used during pregnancy only if the benefits outweigh the potential risks to the fetus.

Cyclosporine passes into breast milk. If you are breastfeeding, your health-care practitioner will advise you to stop and switch to bottle feeding.

SPECIAL INFORMATION FOR SENIORS

No special precautions are noted for older adults.

GENERIC NAME

Delavirdine

BRAND NAME

Rescriptor

No generic available

ABOUT THIS DRUG

Delavirdine is an antiviral used to treat HIV (human immunodeficiency virus) in combination with other drugs.

This drug inhibits the activity of a specific enzyme that is necessary for the reproduction of HIV. However, delavirdine is not effective against HIV unless it is used in combination with other anti-HIV drugs.

SIDE EFFECTS

Be sure to tell your health-care practitioner if you experience any side effects while taking delavirdine. Only your health-care practitioner can determine whether it is safe for you to continue taking this drug.

- *Most Common:* nausea, rash (occurs in about 20% of patients)
- *Common:* headache, tiredness
- *Less Common:* diarrhea, vomiting, irritated liver, itching, abdominal cramps, back pain, chills, fatigue, stiff neck, rapid breathing, migraine, loss of appetite, bloody stools, gas, thirst, loss of coordination, amnesia, anxiety, disorientation, dizziness, hallucinations, insomnia, nightmares, tremor, cough, hair loss, dry eyes, ear pain

A side effect of combination therapy with delavirdine is fat redistribution/accumulation. This reaction can appear as loss of fat from the face, arms, and/or legs, accumulation of fat in the neck and upper back ("buffalo hump"), and breast enlargement.

IMPORTANT PRECAUTIONS

Tell your health-care practitioner if you are sensitive or allergic to delavirdine or to any other drugs.

Because delavirdine acts on liver enzymes, side effects associated with use of this drug can be life-threatening. Therefore, you should have your liver enzyme levels monitored regularly. If you have liver disease, use this drug with extreme caution.

If you develop a severe rash alone or accompanied by fever, blisters, eye irritation, swelling, muscle or joint aches, or mouth sores, stop taking delavirdine and contact your health-care practitioner.

DRUG INTERACTIONS

Tell your health-care practitioner and pharmacist if you are taking any prescription or nonprescription drugs, as well as any vitamins, herbs, or other supplements. Possible drug interactions include the following:

- Anticonvulsants (e.g., phenobarbital, carbamazepine), rifabutin, and rifampin may reduce blood levels of delavirdine.
- Clarithromycin and delavirdine, when combined, may double the blood levels of either drug.

- Antacids and didanosine may reduce the level of delavirdine in the blood. These drugs should be taken at least one hour before or after your delavirdine dose.
- Cimetidine, ranitidine, and similar drugs may reduce the amount of delavirdine your body absorbs.
- Antimicrobials (e.g., clarithromycin, dapsone), benzodiazepine tranquilizers and sleeping pills (e.g., diazepam, clonazepam), ergot drugs (e.g., ergotamine, pergolide), quinidine, and warfarin should not be taken if you have been prescribed delavirdine.
- Fluoxetine and ketoconazole increase the blood levels of delavirdine by about 50%.
- Delavirdine effects the breakdown of protease inhibitors, which may cause your health-care practitioner to adjust your inhibitor dosage.

FOOD, VITAMIN, AND HERBAL INTERACTIONS

No food, vitamin, or herbal interactions have been noted.

RECOMMENDED DOSAGE

Delavirdine is available as tablets and oral solution. The dosage given here is typical. However, your health-care practitioner will determine the most appropriate dose and schedule for your needs.

- *Children Up to 16 Years:* dose to be determined by your health-care practitioner
- *Adults 16 Years and Older:* 400 mg 3 times daily

The tablets can be taken with or without food. The oral suspension should be swallowed with liquid.

If you miss a dose, take it as soon as you remember. If it is nearly time for your next dose, do not take the missed dose. Continue with your regular dosing schedule. Never take a double dose.

SYMPTOMS OF OVERDOSE AND WHAT TO DO

Symptoms of overdose are unknown. If overdose occurs, seek immediate medical attention and bring the prescription container with you to the hospital.

SPECIAL INFORMATION FOR PREGNANT OR NURSING WOMEN

No adequate studies have been done of the effects of delavirdine on pregnant or nursing women. The drug has caused birth defects in laboratory animals. If you are pregnant or plan to become pregnant and this drug is crucial for your health, you and your health-care practitioner must weigh the potential benefits against the potential risks to the fetus.

Delavirdine passes into breast milk in concentrations that are higher than those found in the mother's blood. If you are breast-feeding, you should switch to bottle feeding while taking this drug.

SPECIAL INFORMATION FOR SENIORS

No special precautions have been noted for seniors.

GENERIC NAME

Demeclocycline

see Tetracycline Antibiotics, page 1013

GENERIC NAME

Desipramine

see Tricyclic Antidepressants, page 1076

GENERIC NAME

Desloratadine

BRAND NAME

Clarinex

No generic available

ABOUT THIS DRUG

Desloratadine is a tricyclic antihistamine antagonist used to treat symptoms of seasonal and perennial allergy rhinitis, which include runny nose, sneezing, scratchy throat, and itchy, runny eyes.

This drug inhibits the release of histamine, chemicals normally released by the body in response to allergens (substances that cause an allergic reaction).

SIDE EFFECTS

Be sure to tell your health-care practitioner if you experience any side effects while taking desloratadine. Only your health-care practitioner can determine whether it is safe for you to continue taking this drug.

- *Common:* pharyngitis (inflamed pharynx), muscle pain, dry mouth, insomnia, headache, menstrual problems, fatigue
- *Rare:* drowsiness (unlike other antihistamines, in which it is common)

IMPORTANT PRECAUTIONS

Tell your health-care practitioner if you are sensitive or allergic to desloratadine or to any other drugs, especially loratadine.

If you have a liver or kidney condition, your health-care practitioner may need to adjust your dosage.

DRUG INTERACTIONS

Tell your health-care practitioner and pharmacist if you are taking any prescription or nonprescription drugs, as well as any vitamins, herbs, or other supplements. Desloratadine is relatively new to the market (approved December 2001), and no drug-drug interactions have been reported. There may be yet unknown interactions because of limited clinical experience with this drug.

FOOD, VITAMIN, AND HERBAL INTERACTIONS

No food, vitamin, or herbal interactions have been noted.

RECOMMENDED DOSAGE

Desloratadine is available in 5-mg tablets. The dosages given here are typical. However, your health-care practitioner will determine the most appropriate dose and schedule for your needs.

- *Children Up to Age 12:* not recommended
- *Children 12 to 18 Years and Adults:* 5 mg once daily. If you have a kidney disorder, the usual dose is 5 mg every other day

Desloratadine can be taken with or without food.

If you miss a dose, take it as soon as you remember. If it is nearly time for your next dose, do not take the missed dose. Continue with your regular dosing schedule. Never take a double dose.

SYMPTOMS OF OVERDOSE AND WHAT TO DO

Little is known about desloratadine overdose, although prolonged drowsiness is likely. If overdose occurs, seek immediate medical assistance and bring the prescription container with you to the hospital.

SPECIAL INFORMATION FOR PREGNANT OR NURSING WOMEN

No adequate studies of the effects of desloratadine on pregnant or nursing women have been done. If you are pregnant or plan to become pregnant and this drug is crucial for your health, you and your health-care practitioner must weigh the potential benefits against the potential risks to the fetus.

Desloratadine passes into breast milk. If you are breastfeeding, your health-care practitioner will likely advise you to bottle feed until your treatment is done.

SPECIAL INFORMATION FOR SENIORS

No special precautions have been noted for older adults.

GENERIC NAME

Desmopressin

BRAND NAMES

DDAVP, Stimate

No generic available

ABOUT THIS DRUG

Desmopressin is an antidiuretic used to prevent and control symptoms associated with diabetes insipidus.

This drug increases the amount of water that is reabsorbed by the kidney, resulting in less urine output.

SIDE EFFECTS

Be sure to tell your health-care practitioner if you experience any side effects while taking desmopressin. Only your health-care practitioner can determine whether it is safe for you to continue taking this drug.

- *Less Common:* flushed or red skin, headache, nausea, nasal congestion
- *Rare:* water intoxication, characterized by confusion, headache, seizures, drowsiness, rapid weight gain, and decreased urination

IMPORTANT PRECAUTIONS

Tell your health-care practitioner if you are sensitive or allergic to desmopressin or to any other drugs.

While taking desmopressin, drink only enough fluid to satisfy your thirst. Too high an intake of liquids can result in water intoxication.

During your treatment, your health-care practitioner should periodically monitor your urine.

Before taking desmopressin, talk to your health-care practitioner if you have allergic rhinitis, nasal congestion, a cold or other upper respiratory infection, heart disease, high blood pressure, or cystic fibrosis.

DRUG INTERACTIONS

Tell your health-care practitioner and pharmacist if you are taking any prescription or nonprescription drugs, as well as any vitamins, herbs, or other supplements. Possible interactions include the following:

- Carbamazepine, chlorpropamide, and clofibrate may increase the effect of desmopressin.
- Demeclocycline, lithium, and norepinephrine may decrease the effect of desmopressin.

FOOD, VITAMIN, AND HERBAL INTERACTIONS

No interactions with food, vitamins, or herbs have been noted.

RECOMMENDED DOSAGE

Desmopressin is available as a nasal spray and in tablets. The dosages given here are typical. However, your health-care practitioner will determine the most appropriate dose and schedule for your needs.

- *Children 3 Months to 12 Years:* 0.05 to 0.3 ml nasal spray daily in 1 to 2 doses. For tablets: start with 0.05 mg, to be adjusted by your health-care practitioner
- *Adults:* 0.1 to 0.4 ml daily for nasal solution. For tablets: start with 0.05 mg twice daily, increased gradually by your health-care practitioner up to 1.2 mg daily in 2 to 3 doses

If you miss a dose, take it as soon as you remember if it is less than 2 hours past your scheduled dose. If it is more than 2 hours, do not take the missed dose. Continue with your regular dosing schedule. Never take a double dose.

SYMPTOMS OF OVERDOSE AND WHAT TO DO

Symptoms of overdose include headache, confusion, coma, seizures, breathing problems, abdominal cramps, nausea, and facial flushing. If an overdose occurs, seek immediate medical attention and bring the prescription container with you to the hospital.

SPECIAL INFORMATION FOR PREGNANT OR NURSING WOMEN

No adequate studies of desmopressin have been done on pregnant or nursing women. However, animal studies have not revealed any birth defects or development problems, and the drug has been given to pregnant women to treat diabetes insipidus without harming the infant. If you are pregnant or plan to become pregnant and your health-care practitioner believes desmopressin is necessary for your health, you and your health-care practitioner must weigh the potential benefits against the potential risks to the fetus.

Desmopressin may pass into breast milk. If you are breastfeeding, your health-care practitioner will likely advise you to bottle feed until you are done with treatment.

SPECIAL INFORMATION FOR SENIORS

No special precautions are needed for older adults. Fluid consumption should be watched carefully.

GENERIC NAME

Desonide

see Corticosteroids, Topical, page 337

GENERIC NAME

Desoximetasone

see Corticosteroids, Topical, page 337

GENERIC NAME

Dexamethasone

see Corticosteroids, Oral, page 330

GENERIC NAME

Dexbrompheniramine

see Antihistamine-Decongestant Combination, page 132

GENERIC NAMES

(1) Dextroamphetamine; (2) dextroamphetamine + amphetamine

BRAND NAMES

(1) Dexedrine, Dextrostat; (2) Adderall, Adderall XR
No generic available

ABOUT THIS DRUG

Dextroamphetamine and the dextroamphetamine/amphetamine combination are central nervous system stimulants (amphetamines) used to treat attention-deficit hyperactivity disorder (ADHD) and narcolepsy (an uncontrollable desire to sleep), and to control weight.

Dextroamphetamine/amphetamine and dextroamphetamine alone activate nerve cells in the spinal cord and brain, which increases alertness and reduces fatigue and drowsiness. When used to treat ADHD and narcolepsy, they improve mental concentration.

SIDE EFFECTS

Be sure to tell your health-care practitioner if you experience any side effects while taking these amphetamines. Only your health-care practitioner can determine whether it is safe for you to continue taking these drugs.

- *Most Common:* palpitations, restlessness, overstimulation, dizziness, sleeplessness, high blood pressure
- *Less Common:* hallucinations, muscle spasms, headache, dry mouth, diarrhea, constipation, itching, diminished sex drive, euphoria, taste changes
- *Rare:* psychotic drug reactions

IMPORTANT PRECAUTIONS

Tell your health-care practitioner if you are sensitive or allergic to dextroamphetamine, amphetamines, or to any other drugs.

Dextroamphetamine and amphetamine have a high potential for abuse and addiction. Your health-care practitioner should monitor your use carefully.

Because these drugs can cause dizziness and sleeplessness, you should be certain of your response to them before you drive or operate dangerous equipment.

Do not use dextroamphetamine or amphetamine if you have

hardening of the arteries, heart disease, high blood pressure, glaucoma, or an overactive thyroid gland.

There are no adequate studies of the effects of long-term treatment of ADHD in children using dextroamphetamine/ amphetamine medications.

Amphetamine-based medications can stunt growth of children. Your health-care practitioner should conduct an extensive evaluation before prescribing these drugs.

To help prevent their interference with sleep, take these drugs at least 6 to 8 hours before bedtime.

Dextroamphetamine/amphetamine and dextroamphetamine alone should not be used for longer than a few months for weight control, and their use for ADHD is a topic of controversy (see "Open Questions or Controversies").

If you take dextroamphetamine/amphetamine for weight control, it may gradually lose its effectiveness. Do not increase your dose; discontinue taking the drug.

DRUG INTERACTIONS

Tell your health-care practitioner and pharmacist if you are taking any prescription or nonprescription drugs, as well as any vitamins, herbs, or other supplements. Possible interactions include the following:

- Tricyclic antidepressants (e.g., amitriptyline, imipramine), chlorpromazine, guanethidine, haloperidol, lithium, methenamine, reserpine, and sodium acid phosphate may reduce the effects of dextroamphetamine.
- Acetazolamide, MAOI inhibitors (e.g., phenelzine), propoxyphene, and thiazide diuretics (e.g., chlorothiazide, hydrochlorothiazide) may increase the effects of dextroamphetamine.
- Dextroamphetamine may decrease the effects of antihistamines (e.g., doxylamine, loratadine), blood-pressure medications (e.g., clonidine, prazosin), ethosuximide, and veratrum alkaloids (found in some blood-pressure medications).
- Dextroamphetamine can increase the effects of antidepressants (Norpramin, Vivactil), meperidine, norepinephrine, phenobarbital, and phenytoin.
- Monoamine oxidase inhibitors (MAOIs; e.g., phenelzine) may cause a severe rise in blood pressure and bleeding inside the brain. You should stop taking an MAOI at least 2 weeks before starting treatment with dextroamphetamines/amphetamines.

FOOD, VITAMIN, AND HERBAL INTERACTIONS

Vitamin C supplements can reduce the absorption of amphetamines. Take such supplements at least 1 hour before or 2 hours after taking your dextroamphetamine/ amphetamine dose. Fruit juices also can reduce the absorption of amphetamines by acidifying the intestinal contents. Drink these beverages at least 1 hour before or 2 hours after taking your medication.

RECOMMENDED DOSAGE

Dextroamphetamine/amphetamine is available in tablets; dextroamphetamine is available in tablets and capsules. The dosages given here are typical and are for both dextroamphetamine/amphetamine and dextroamphetamine alone. Your health-care practitioner will determine the most appropriate dose and schedule for your needs.

- *Children 3 to 6 Years:* for ADHD, 2.5 mg daily to start
- *Children 6 Years and Older:* for ADHD, 5 mg, 1 to 2 times daily, to start. For narcolepsy, 5 mg once daily
- *Children 12 to 18 Years:* for narcolepsy, 10 mg once daily
- *Adults:* for ADHD or narcolepsy: 5 to 60 mg daily, taken in 1 to 3 doses, but not to exceed 60 mg daily. For weight control, 5 to 30 mg daily in divided doses 30 to 60 minutes before meals

Dextroamphetamines and amphetamines can be taken with food to help prevent stomach irritation.

If you miss a dose, take it as soon as you remember unless it is within 6 hours of bedtime. If it is nearly time for your next dose, do not take the missed dose. Continue with your regular dosing schedule. Never take a double dose.

SYMPTOMS OF OVERDOSE AND WHAT TO DO

An overdose of dextroamphetamine/amphetamine or dextroamphetamine can be fatal. Symptoms of overdose include tremors, restlessness, muscle spasms, rapid breathing, hallucinations, confusion, panic, high fever, seizures, coma, and overaggressive behavior. If overdose occurs, seek immediate medical assistance and bring the prescription container with you to the hospital.

SPECIAL INFORMATION FOR PREGNANT OR NURSING WOMEN

Dextroamphetamine/amphetamine and dextroamphetamine can cause birth defects when used during the early stages of pregnancy.

Use of amphetamines also increases the risk of low-birth-weight infants, premature delivery, and symptoms of drug withdrawal in newborns. If you are pregnant or plan to become pregnant, and either of these drugs is crucial for your health, you and your health-care practitioner must weigh the potential benefits against the potential risks to the fetus.

These drugs pass into breast milk. If you are breastfeeding, your health-care practitioner will likely advise you to bottle feed until your treatment is complete.

SPECIAL INFORMATION FOR SENIORS

Side effects are more likely to occur and to be more severe in older adults.

OPEN QUESTIONS OR CONTROVERSIES

Some controversy surrounds the use of dextroamphetamines/amphetamines (Adderall) for treatment of ADHD in children because of the drug's high potential for dependence and the lack of information about long-term effects. One question is whether treatment with Adderall sensitizes the brain to future use of this and other stimulants and thus increases the risk of substance abuse and addiction. Animal studies indicate that repeated use of amphetamines make the animals more sensitive to future administration of these drugs. Whether this is true in humans is not known.

For now, parents are advised to use these drugs cautiously and to enroll their children in other behavior modification methods, including counseling, to deal with ADHD.

GENERIC NAME

Dextromethorphan hydrobromide

see Promethazine, page 879

GENERIC NAME

Diazepam

BRAND NAMES

Di-Tran, Diastat, Diazepam Intensol, Valium, Valrelease, Vazepam X-O'Spaz, Zetran

Generic available

ABOUT THIS DRUG

Diazepam is a benzodiazepine tranquilizer used primarily to treat anxiety, panic attacks, and muscle spasms.

This drug produces mild sedation by enhancing the effect of a chemical (gamma-aminobutyric acid, or GABA), which in turn dampens the transmission of nerve signals and reduces nerve excitation.

SIDE EFFECTS

Be sure to tell your health-care practitioner if you experience any side effects while taking diazepam. Only your health-care practitioner can determine whether it is safe for you to continue taking this drug.

- *Most Common:* drowsiness (especially during the first few days of treatment), loss of coordination, dizziness, lightheadedness, slurred speech, unsteady gait
- *Less Common or Rare:* constipation, nausea, vomiting, urinary difficulties, unusual fatigue, change in sexual desire or ability, salivation changes, hallucinations, headache, rage, rash, slow heartbeat, vertigo, yellowing of eyes and skin (jaundice)

IMPORTANT PRECAUTIONS

Tell your health-care practitioner if you are sensitive or allergic to diazepam or to any other drugs, especially other benzodiazepines (e.g., clonazepam, temazepam).

If you have liver or kidney problems, use this drug with caution.

Because diazepam can cause drowsiness, make sure you know how you react to it before you drive or operate hazardous equipment.

Diazepam can be addictive, even after only 4 weeks of treatment, and you can experience withdrawal symptoms if you suddenly stop taking it. Follow your health-care practitioner's use instructions carefully.

Do not take diazepam if you have narrow-angle glaucoma (but it is safe if you have open-angle glaucoma), severe depression, severe lung disease, sleep apnea, psychotic problems, alcoholism, or kidney disease. Diazepam can worsen these conditions, and the depressive effects of the drug may be enhanced as well.

DRUG INTERACTIONS

Tell your health-care practitioner and pharmacist if you are taking any prescription or nonprescription drugs, as well as any vitamins, herbs, or other supplements. Possible drug interactions with diazepam may include the following:

- Diazepam can increase the effects of alcohol. Do not drink alcohol while taking this drug.
- Narcotics (e.g., codeine, oxycodone), barbiturates (e.g., phenobarbital), monoamine oxidase inhibitors (e.g., phenelzine), antihistamines (e.g., cetirizine, loratadine), and antidepressants (e.g., amitriptyline, doxepin) may lead to excessive drowsiness, difficulty breathing, and extreme depression.
- Cimetidine, oral contraceptives, disulfiram, fluoxetine, isoniazid, ketoconazole, rifampin, metoprolol, probenecid, propoxyphene, propranolol, and valproic acid may prolong the effects of diazepam.
- Diazepam may raise the blood levels of digoxin and increase the risk of digoxin toxicity.
- Diazepam may decrease the effects of levodopa.
- Smoking may reduce how quickly diazepam is broken down by the body, thus reducing its effectiveness.
- Diazepam along with phenytoin may elevate phenytoin levels and increase the risk of phenytoin toxicity.

FOOD, VITAMIN, AND HERBAL INTERACTIONS

Herbs that produce a sedative effect may cause significantly depressant interactions when used with diazepam. Some of those herbs include calendula, capsicum, catnip, goldenseal, gotu kola, hops, kava, lady's slipper, passionflower, sage, Siberian ginseng, skullcap, St. John's wort, and valerian, among others.

Because grapefruit juice does slow the breakdown of some benzodiazepines, it is best to avoid this beverage while being treated with diazepam.

RECOMMENDED DOSAGE

Diazepam is available in tablets, capsules, injection, and rectal gel; however, the injection and gel dosages are not discussed here. The dosages given here are typical. Your health-care practitioner will determine the most appropriate dose and schedule for your needs.

- *Children 6 Months and Older*: 1 to 2.5 mg 3 or 4 times daily.
- *Adults:* 2 to 10 mg, 4 times daily

If you miss a dose, take it as soon as you remember. If it is nearly time for your next dose, do not take the missed dose. Continue with your regular dosing schedule. Never take a double dose.

SYMPTOMS OF OVERDOSE AND WHAT TO DO

Symptoms of overdose include extreme drowsiness, confusion, slurred speech, poor coordination, staggering, tremor, slowed breathing, and loss of consciousness. If overdose occurs, seek immediate medical attention and bring the prescription container with you to the hospital.

SPECIAL INFORMATION FOR PREGNANT OR NURSING WOMEN

Diazepam crosses the placenta, and it may cause birth defects if taken during the first 3 months of pregnancy. This drug should not be used during pregnancy unless it is considered to be crucial by your health-care practitioner. Then you and your health-care practitioner must weigh the potential benefits against the potential risks.

Diazepam passes into breast milk. If you are breastfeeding, your health-care practitioner may advise you to switch to bottle feeding.

SPECIAL INFORMATION FOR SENIORS

Older adults, especially those who have kidney or liver disease, are more likely to experience side effects, and perhaps more severe ones. Seniors may require lower doses.

GENERIC NAME

Diclofenac

BRAND NAMES

Cataflam, Voltaren, Voltaren-XR
Generic available

ABOUT THIS DRUG

Diclofenac is a nonsteroidal anti-inflammatory drug (NSAID) used to treat the pain and inflammation associated with rheumatoid arthritis, osteoarthritis, and arthritis of the spine, as well as menstrual pain and cramps.

Diclofenac blocks the body's production of prostaglandins, substances that cause inflammation and make nerves more sensitive to pain signals.

SIDE EFFECTS

Be sure to tell your health-care practitioner if you experience any side effects while taking diclofenac. Only your health-care practi-

tioner can determine whether it is safe for you to continue taking this drug.

- *Most Common:* nausea, vomiting, constipation, stomach gas, diarrhea, loss of appetite, especially during the first few days of treatment
- *Less Common:* gastrointestinal bleeding, stomach ulcers, hepatitis, gallbladder attacks, painful urination, kidney inflammation or poor function, bloody urine, hallucinations, dizziness, fainting, nervousness, depression, disorientation, tingling in the feet or hands, itching, increased sweating, dry nose, palpitations, chest pain, muscle cramps
- *Rare:* severe allergic reactions (fever, chills, closing of the throat, jaundice), kidney failure

IMPORTANT PRECAUTIONS

Tell your health-care practitioner if you are sensitive or allergic to diclofenac or to any other drugs, especially other NSAIDs.

Do not take diclofenac if you have a history of asthma associated with the use of NSAIDs, iodides, or aspirin; or if you have clotting problems and are taking warfarin.

Diclofenac may cause swelling of the arms, legs, or feet if you have heart problems.

Prolonged use of diclofenac may lead to gastrointestinal problems, including bleeding stomach, stomach ulcers, kidney problems, and an inflamed liver.

When taking diclofenac, you may be extremely sensitive to the effects of the sun. Protect yourself against sunlight by wearing protective clothing and sunscreen.

DRUG INTERACTIONS

Tell your health-care practitioner and pharmacist if you are taking any prescription or nonprescription drugs, as well as any vitamins, herbs, or other supplements. Possible interactions include the following:

- Aspirin and other salicylates should never be taken along with diclofenac.
- Probenecid may increase the risk of side effects from diclofenac.
- Diclofenac may increase the effects of oral anticoagulants (blood-thinning drugs; e.g., warfarin). Your health-care practitioner may alter your anticoagulant dosage.
- Diclofenac may increase the side effects of methotrexate and the kidney-related side effects of cyclosporine.

- Cimetidine may affect the blood levels of diclofenac.
- Diclofenac may reduce the blood-pressure-lowering effect of loop diuretics (e.g., bendroflumethiazide, furosemide) and beta-blockers (e.g., acebutolol, nadolol).
- Diclofenac may increase the side effects of phenytoin.
- Diclofenac may increase the blood levels of lithium.

FOOD, VITAMIN, AND HERBAL INTERACTIONS

Alfalfa, clove oil, cinchona bark, feverfew, garlic, ginseng, and ginkgo may affect blood clotting, so use of these herbs along with diclofenac is not recommended.

St. John's wort and dong quai are associated with an increased sensitivity to the sun. Be sure to wear protective clothing and use sunscreen if you take these herbs while taking diclofenac.

RECOMMENDED DOSAGE

Diclofenac is available in tablets. The dosages given here are typical. However, your health-care practitioner will determine the most appropriate dose and schedule for your needs.

- *Children:* not recommended
- *Adults:* for osteoarthritis, 100 to 150 mg daily, divided into 2 or 3 doses. For rheumatoid arthritis, 100 to 200 mg daily, divided into 2 to 4 doses. For menstrual discomfort and pain, 100 mg for the starting dose, followed by 50 mg 3 times daily

Diclofenac can be taken with food to help avoid stomach irritation.

If you miss a dose, take it as soon as you remember. If it is nearly time for your next dose, do not take the missed dose. Continue with your regular dosing schedule. Never take a double dose.

SYMPTOMS OF OVERDOSE AND WHAT TO DO

An overdose of NSAIDs can be fatal. Symptoms of overdose include drowsiness, nausea, vomiting, diarrhea, rapid breathing, rapid heartbeat, increased sweating, ringing in the ears, confusion, disorientation, stupor, and coma. If overdose occurs, seek immediate medical attention and bring the prescription container with you to the hospital.

SPECIAL INFORMATION FOR PREGNANT OR NURSING WOMEN

Diclofenac may affect heart development of the fetus during the second half of pregnancy. If you are pregnant or plan to become pregnant and diclofenac is crucial for your health, you and your health-care practitioner must weigh the potential benefits against the potential risks to the fetus.

This drug passes into breast milk. If you are breastfeeding, your health-care practitioner will likely advise you to switch to bottle feeding.

SPECIAL INFORMATION FOR SENIORS

Older adults may be more susceptible to side effects, especially stomach ulcers.

GENERIC NAME

Dicloxacillin sodium

see Penicillin Antibiotics, page 812

GENERIC NAME

Dicyclomine

BRAND NAMES

Bemote, Bentyl, Byclomine, Di-Spaz
Generic available

ABOUT THIS DRUG

Dicyclomine is an antispasmodic and anticholinergic drug used to treat irritable bowel syndrome and similar digestive conditions.

This drug blocks the effects of acetylcholine, a neurohormone in the gastrointestinal tract, which in turn reduces production of enzymes and other stomach secretions.

SIDE EFFECTS

Be sure to tell your health-care practitioner if you experience any side effects while taking dicyclomine. Only your health-care practitioner can determine whether it is safe for you to continue taking this drug.

- *Most Common:* constipation, dry mouth, throat, or skin, decreased sweating
- *Less Common:* blurred vision, sensitivity to bright light, difficulty swallowing

- *Rare:* allergic reactions (rash, itching, breathing problems), confusion, eye pain, dizziness when rising from a lying or sitting position, urination problems, drowsiness, unusual tiredness, headache, memory loss, nausea, vomiting

IMPORTANT PRECAUTIONS

Tell your health-care practitioner if you are sensitive or allergic to dicyclomine or to any other drugs.

Use dicyclomine with caution if you have heart disease, Down's syndrome, fever, stomach obstruction, glaucoma, acute bleeding hiatal hernia, intestinal paralysis, myasthenia gravis, overactive thyroid, prostate problems, urinary problems, kidney or liver disease, rapid heartbeat, high blood pressure, ulcerative colitis, or reduced mobility of the lower esophagus or stomach.

Exercise caution if using dicyclomine during hot weather or strenuous exercise, or if taking hot baths or using a sauna, because this drug can reduce your ability to sweat.

Because this drug can cause blurred vision, be sure you know how you react to dicyclomine before you drive or operate dangerous equipment.

DRUG INTERACTIONS

Tell your health-care practitioner and pharmacist if you are taking any prescription or nonprescription drugs, as well as any vitamins, herbs, or other supplements. Possible interactions include the following:

- Antacids that contain calcium or magnesium, citrates, and sodium bicarbonate may decrease the therapeutic effect and side effects of dicyclomine.
- Combining other anticholinergic drugs (e.g., atropine, hyoscyamine) with dicyclomine may increase the side effects.
- Tricyclic antidepressants (e.g., amitriptyline, imipramine), antihistamines (e.g., clemastine, doxylamine), meperidine, methylphenidate, orphenadrine, phenothiazines (e.g., chlorpromazine, promazine), and quinidine may increase the effect of dicyclomine.
- Digitalis may not be absorbed as well if taken along with dicyclomine.
- Narcotic pain relievers (e.g., codeine, oxycodone) may cause severe constipation.
- Metoclopramide may be less effective in reducing nausea and vomiting.
- Dicyclomine may reduce the blood levels of oral ketoconazole and stomach acidity.

FOOD, VITAMIN, AND HERBAL INTERACTIONS

Large doses of vitamin C can reduce the effects of dicyclomine. Supplements of potassium can increase the risk of intestinal ulcers.

RECOMMENDED DOSAGE

Dicyclomine is available in tablets, capsules, and syrup. The dosages given here are typical. However, your health-care practitioner will determine the most appropriate dose and schedule for your needs.

- *Children Younger than 6 Months:* not recommended
- *Children 6 Months to 2 Years:* 5 to 10 mg syrup 3 to 4 times daily
- *Children Older than 2 Years:* 10 mg 3 to 4 times daily
- *Adults:* starting dose, 20 mg taken 4 times daily, increased by your health-care practitioner to 40 mg taken 4 times daily

You can take dicyclomine with food to help prevent stomach irritation.

If you miss a dose, take it as soon as you remember. If it is nearly time for your next dose, do not take the missed dose. Continue with your regular dosing schedule. Never take a double dose.

SYMPTOMS OF OVERDOSE AND WHAT TO DO

Symptoms of overdose include blurred vision, swallowing difficulties, dilated pupils, dizziness, dry mouth, headache, nausea, nerve blockage causing weakness and possibly paralysis, and vomiting. If an overdose occurs, seek immediate medical attention and bring the prescription container with you to the hospital.

SPECIAL INFORMATION FOR PREGNANT OR NURSING WOMEN

No adequate studies of the effects of dicyclomine on pregnant or nursing women have been done. If you are pregnant or plan to become pregnant and this drug is crucial for your health, you and your health-care practitioner must weigh the potential benefits against the potential risks to the fetus.

Dicyclomine passes into breast milk. If you are breastfeeding, your health-care practitioner will likely advise you to switch to bottle feeding until your treatment is done.

SPECIAL INFORMATION FOR SENIORS

Older adults are more likely to experience side effects and more severe ones.

GENERIC NAME

Didanosine

BRAND NAME

Videx

No generic available

ABOUT THIS DRUG

Didanosine is an antiviral medication used to treat HIV (human immunodeficiency virus) infection.

Didanosine hinders the activity of the enzymes that are required for the reproduction of DNA in viral cells, which in turn can delay the progression of the disease. This drug is typically used along with another anti-HIV medication as part of a "drug cocktail."

SIDE EFFECTS

Be sure to tell your health-care practitioner if you experience any side effects while taking didanosine. It can be difficult to discern side effects associated with the drug from a symptom of the disease. Only your health-care practitioner can make that determination and tell you whether it is safe for you to continue taking this drug.

- ➤ *Most Common:* abdominal pain, chills, headache, itching, nausea, vomiting, diarrhea, pain, tingling or numbness in the feet and hands, weakness
- ➤ *Less Common:* allergic reactions (hives, breathing difficulties), dry mouth, dry eyes, gas, indigestion, joint pain, loss of appetite, muscle disorders, swollen glands, vision problems

IMPORTANT PRECAUTIONS

Tell your health-care practitioner if you are sensitive or allergic to didanosine or to any other drugs.

Didanosine does not prevent the spread of HIV through sexual relations or contact with infected blood.

The powdered form of didanosine contains 1,380 mg of sodium per packet. If you are on a sodium (salt)-restricted diet, or if you have the hereditary disease phenylketonuria, talk to your health-care practitioner before taking this drug.

About half of all patients who take didanosine experience nervous system inflammation, characterized by numbness, tingling, or pain in the hand and feet. Reducing the dosage can control these symptoms. If you already have signs of nerve damage, do not take didanosine.

About 3 percent of people who take didanosine experience an inflamed pancreas, which is potentially fatal. Symptoms include nausea, vomiting, abdominal pain, changes in blood-sugar levels, an increase in triglyceride blood levels, and a decline in blood calcium levels. If you develop these symptoms, stop taking didanosine and contact your health-care practitioner immediately.

Between 15 and 20 percent of people who take didanosine develop liver failure. Therefore, liver function should be checked regularly by your health-care practitioner.

If you have liver or kidney disease, you may need lower dosages of this drug.

DRUG INTERACTIONS

Tell your health-care practitioner and pharmacist if you are taking any prescription or nonprescription drugs, as well as any vitamins, herbs, or other supplements. Possible drug interactions with didanosine include the following:

- Alcohol increases your chance of developing serious side effects, such as pancreatitis.
- Do not take zalcitabine or drugs that may cause inflammation of the pancreas, such as intravenous pentamidine.
- Quinolone anti-infectives (e.g., fleroxacin, ofloxacin), tetracycline antibiotics (e.g., doxycycline, minocycline), and other drugs whose absorption can be affected by antacids should not be taken within 2 hours of taking didanosine.
- Drugs that may cause inflammation of the nervous system (e.g., chloramphenicol, cisplatin, dapsone, disulfiram, ethionamide, glutethamide, gold, hydralazine, isoniazid, metronidazole, nitrofurantoin, ribavirin, and vincristine) should not be taken with didanosine.

FOOD, VITAMIN, AND HERBAL INTERACTIONS

Food can prevent absorption of didanosine by up to 50 percent. Therefore, take this drug on an empty stomach.

RECOMMENDED DOSAGE

Didanosine is available as a chewable tablet and as a powder for solution. The dosages given here are typical. However, your health-care practitioner will determine the most appropriate dose and schedule for your needs.

Tablets

- *Children Up to Age 12 Years:* dose can range from 25 to 100 mg every 8 to 12 hours.
- *Children 12 Years and Older and Adults:* if you weigh 132 pounds or more, take 200 mg every 12 hours. If you weigh less than 132 pounds, take 125 mg every 12 hours.

Powder

- *Children Up to Age 12 Years:* a special pediatric form is available. Dose can range from 31 to 125 mg every 8 to 12 hours
- *Adults and Teens:* if you weigh 132 pound or more, take 250 mg every 12 hours. If you weigh less than 132 pounds, take 167 mg every 12 hours

Take didanosine on an empty stomach: at least 1 hour before or 2 hours after eating.

If you take the tablets, chew them thoroughly, or crush them and dissolve them in about ¼ cup water. Do not mix them with juice or any other acidic drink. If you take the powder, mix it into ½ cup water and stir until completely dissolved. Drink it immediately. Do not mix the powder with juice or any other acidic beverage.

If you miss a dose, take it as soon as you remember. If it is nearly time for your next dose, do not take the missed dose. Continue with your regular dosing schedule. Never take a double dose.

SYMPTOMS OF OVERDOSE AND WHAT TO DO

Symptoms of overdose include abdominal pain, diarrhea, numbness, and burning and tingling in the hands and feet. If overdose occurs, seek immediate medical attention and bring the prescription container with you to the hospital.

SPECIAL INFORMATION FOR PREGNANT OR NURSING WOMEN

No adequate studies of the effects of didanosine have been done on pregnant or nursing women. If you are pregnant or plan to become pregnant and this drug is crucial for your health, you and your health-care practitioner must weigh the potential benefits against the potential risks to the fetus.

It is not known whether didanosine passes into breast milk. However, because HIV can be passed to an infant through breast milk, do not breastfeed while taking this drug.

SPECIAL INFORMATION FOR SENIORS

Older adults and others who have diminished kidney or liver function should take lower dosages of didanosine.

GENERIC NAME

Dienestrol *see Estrogens, page 436*

GENERIC NAME

Diethylpropion

BRAND NAMES

Tenuate, Tepanil
Generic available

ABOUT THIS DRUG

Diethylpropion is a sympathomimetic (central nervous system stimulant) taken to suppress the appetite of obese individuals. It should be used in conjunction with a strict diet and exercise.

This drug appears to affect the appetite-control center in the brain, located in the hypothalamus, and suppress the nerve impulses in that region.

SIDE EFFECTS

Be sure to tell your health-care practitioner if you experience any side effects while taking diethylpropion. Only your health-care practitioner can determine whether it is safe for you to continue taking this drug.

- ➤ *Most Common:* lightheadedness, irritability, nervousness, difficulty falling asleep, euphoria, increased heartbeat, palpitations, increased blood pressure
- ➤ *Less Common or Rare:* unusual fever, chills, sore throat, cough, unusual bruising or bleeding, gastrointestinal problems, chest pain, extreme dizziness, headache along with nausea or vomiting, convulsions, rash

IMPORTANT PRECAUTIONS

Tell your health-care practitioner if you are sensitive or allergic to diethylpropion or to any other drugs.

This drug should be taken for only a few weeks, typically 8 to 12. Prolonged use may lead to mental or physical dependence.

Do not take diethylpropion if you have an overactive thyroid, glaucoma, severe high blood pressure, or severe hardening of the arteries, or if you are agitated, have a history of drug or alcohol abuse, or are taking or have taken a monoamine oxidase inhibitor (MAOI; e.g., phenelzine) within the last 14 days.

This drug should be used with caution if you have heart disease, high blood pressure, epilepsy, or kidney disease.

DRUG INTERACTIONS

Tell your health-care practitioner and pharmacist if you are taking any prescription or nonprescription drugs, as well as any vitamins, herbs, or other supplements. Possible interactions include the following:

- Antihypertensive drugs (e.g., enalapril, guanfacine), rauwolfia alkaloids, methyldopa, and guanethidine may be less effective.
- Insulin and antidiabetic drug (e.g., glipizide, glyburide) dosages may need to be adjusted.
- Other appetite suppressants may cause dangerous overstimulation.
- Central nervous system depressants (e.g., amitriptyline, temazepam) may increase the depressive effects of both drugs.
- Central nervous system stimulants (e.g., amphetamine, caffeine) may increase the stimulant effects of both drugs.

FOOD, VITAMIN, AND HERBAL INTERACTIONS

Avoid all beverages and foods that contain caffeine, such as colas, coffee, tea, and chocolate, as they may lead to overstimulation.

RECOMMENDED DOSAGE

Diethylpropion is available in 25-mg immediate release tablets and 75-mg sustained release tablets. The dosages given here are typical. However, your health-care practitioner will determine the most appropriate dose and schedule for your needs.

- *Children Up to Age 12*: not recommended
- *Children 12 Years and Older and Adults:* one 25-mg tablet one hour before meals and another midevening if needed to control nighttime hunger. This bedtime dose may interfere with sleep, however. If taking the sustained release tablet, take one midmorning.

If you miss a dose, take it as soon as you remember. If it is nearly time for your next dose, do not take the missed dose. Continue with your regular dosing schedule. Never take a double dose.

SYMPTOMS OF OVERDOSE AND WHAT TO DO

Symptoms of overdose include abdominal cramps, confusion, depression, diarrhea, elevated blood pressure, hallucinations, irregular heartbeat, nausea, panic, rapid breathing, restlessness, tremors, and vomiting. If overdose occurs, seek immediate medical assistance and bring the prescription container with you to the hospital.

SPECIAL INFORMATION FOR PREGNANT OR NURSING WOMEN

No adequate studies of the impact of diethylpropion on pregnant or nursing women have been done. If you are pregnant or plan to become pregnant, you and your health-care practitioner must weigh the potential benefits against the potential risks to the fetus.

This drug passes into breast milk. If you are breastfeeding, your health-care practitioner will likely advise you to switch to bottle feeding until your treatment is done.

SPECIAL INFORMATION FOR SENIORS

No special instructions are available for older adults.

GENERIC NAME

Difenoxin-atropine combination

BRAND NAME

Motofen

No generic available

ABOUT THIS DRUG

The combination of difenoxin and atropine is an antidiarrheal used to treat severe diarrhea in adults. Because difenoxin is related chemically to some narcotics and thus has the potential to be habit-forming, atropine (an anticholinergic) has been added as a safety mechanism. If you try to take high doses of the combination drug, the atropine portion causes unpleasant side effects, which discourages abuse.

Difenoxin/atropine slows down the movement (peristalsis) of the intestinal tract.

SIDE EFFECTS

Be sure to tell your health-care practitioner if you experience any side effects while taking difenoxin/atropine. Only your health-care practitioner can determine whether it is safe for you to continue taking this drug.

- *Most Common:* drowsiness, dizziness
- *Less Common:* bloating, constipation, appetite loss, blurred vision, flushed skin, fast heartbeat, dry mouth, frequent urination, dry skin, headache, insomnia
- *Rare:* weakness, confusion, fever

IMPORTANT PRECAUTIONS

Tell your health-care practitioner if you are sensitive or allergic to difenoxin or atropine or to any other drugs.

This drug combination should not be given to children, as they are more sensitive to the drugs' side effects.

If you have a history of alcohol or drug abuse, taking difenoxin/atropine increases your risk of becoming addicted to the drug.

If you have colitis, chronic respiratory problems (e.g., asthma, emphysema), dysentery, gallbladder problems, enlarged prostate, urinary tract problems, hiatal hernia, glaucoma, heart disease, high blood pressure, intestinal blockage, liver or kidney disease, myasthenia gravis, peptic ulcer, or overactive or underactive thyroid, consult your health-care practitioner before taking this drug combination, because it can make these conditions worse.

Because difenoxin/atropine can cause drowsiness and dizziness, make sure you know how you react to this drug before you drive or operate dangerous equipment.

Before undergoing any type of surgery (including dental surgery) or emergency treatment, make sure you tell the health-care practitioner you are taking this medication.

DRUG INTERACTIONS

Tell your health-care practitioner and pharmacist if you are taking any prescription or nonprescription drugs, as well as any vitamins, herbs, or other supplements. Possible interactions include the following:

- Antibiotics (e.g., cefaclor, clindamycin) cause diarrhea and when taken with difenoxin/atropine can make the condition worse.
- Central nervous system depressants (e.g., antidepressants, antipsychotics) can make drowsiness and other central nervous system effects more pronounced.

- Monoamine oxidase inhibitors (MAOIs) (e.g., procarbazine, furazolidone) should not be taken within 2 weeks of taking difenoxin/atropine.
- Naltrexone makes difenoxin less effective and can also lead to withdrawal effects among people who have become addicted to the difenoxin in the combination drug.
- Methyprylon can cause dangerous sedation. Do not take this drug when using difenoxin/atropine.
- Antihypertensive drugs (e.g., amlodipine, methyldopa) can increase sedation.
- Amantadine, meperidine, methylphenidate, orphenadrine, phenothiazines (e.g., chlorpromazine, promazine), and procainamide can cause increased atropine effect.

FOOD, VITAMIN, AND HERBAL INTERACTIONS

High doses of vitamin C can decrease the effect of atropine. Potassium supplements can lead to intestinal ulcers.

RECOMMENDED DOSAGE

Difenoxin/atropine is available in tablets. The dosages given here are typical. However, your health-care practitioner will determine the most appropriate dose and schedule for your needs.

- *Children Up to 12 Years:* not recommended
- *Children 12 Years and Older and Adults:* 2 mg starting dose, then 1 mg every 3 to 4 hours as needed, or after every loose stool. Do not exceed 8 mg within any 24-hour period

You can take difenoxin/atropine with food to reduce stomach irritation.

If you miss a dose, take it as soon as you remember. If it is nearly time for your next dose, do not take the missed dose. Continue with your regular dosing schedule. Never take a double dose.

SYMPTOMS OF OVERDOSE AND WHAT TO DO

Symptoms of overdose include dilated pupils, rapid pulse, rapid breathing, dizziness, fever, hallucinations, confusion, slurred speech, convulsions, flushed face, and coma. If an overdose occurs, seek immediate medical attention and bring the prescription container with you to the hospital.

SPECIAL INFORMATION FOR PREGNANT OR NURSING WOMEN

No adequate studies of the effects of difenoxin/atropine have been done in pregnant or nursing women. This combination, when given to lab animals in high doses, does increase delivery time and can result in death. If you are pregnant or plan to become pregnant, you and your health-care practitioner must weigh the potential benefits against the potential risks to the fetus.

Both difenoxin and atropine pass into breast milk. If you are breastfeeding, your health-care practitioner will likely advise you to switch to bottle feeding.

SPECIAL INFORMATION FOR SENIORS

Older adults are more likely to experience breathing difficulties when taking this drug combination. Seniors should also be extremely careful about maintaining their fluid levels by drinking lots of water and diluted juices to replace fluids lost to diarrhea.

GENERIC NAME

Diflorasone diacetate *see Corticosteroids, Topical, page 337*

GENERIC NAME

Diflunisal

BRAND NAME

Dolobid

Generic available

ABOUT THIS DRUG

Diflunisal is a nonsteroidal anti-inflammatory drug (NSAID) used to treat mild-to-moderate pain and inflammation associated with arthritis, bursitis, tendinitis, migraine, headaches, menstrual cramps, and other conditions.

Diflunisal, like other NSAIDs, interferes with the formation of natural substances called prostaglandins, which cause inflammation and make nerves more sensitive to pain signals.

SIDE EFFECTS

Be sure to tell your health-care practitioner if you experience any side effects while taking diflunisal. Only your health-care practitioner can determine whether it is safe for you to continue taking this drug.

- *Most Common:* nausea, vomiting, heartburn, diarrhea, constipation, headache, dizziness, sleepiness
- *Less Common or Rare:* mouth sores, depression, rash, ringing in the ears, tingling or numbness of the feet or hands, seizures, blurred vision, decreased blood counts, abdominal bleeding, dry mouth, fluid retention, vertigo, jaundice, painful urination, nervousness, shortness of breath, chest pain, black stools

IMPORTANT PRECAUTIONS

Tell your health-care practitioner if you are sensitive or allergic to diflunisal, other NSAIDs, or any other drugs.

Prolonged use of diflunisal can cause gastrointestinal problems, including stomach bleeding, stomach ulcers, kidney dysfunction, and inflamed liver.

Use diflunisal with caution if you have liver or kidney disease, heart disease, diabetes, epilepsy, lupus, anemia, asthma, Parkinson's disease, kidney stones, high blood pressure, or a history of alcohol abuse.

Because diflunisal may cause dizziness and sleepiness, make sure you know how you react to this drug before you drive or operate dangerous equipment.

DRUG INTERACTIONS

Tell your health-care practitioner and pharmacist if you are taking any prescription or nonprescription drugs, as well as any vitamins, herbs, or other supplements. Possible interactions may include the following:

- Adrenocorticoids (e.g., betamethasone, cortisone) increase the risk of ulcers.
- Angiotensin-converting enzyme (ACE) inhibitors may reduce the ACE inhibitor effects.
- Antacids may decrease the pain relief effects of diflunisal.
- Oral anticoagulants (e.g., warfarin), other NSAIDs, and cephalosporins (e.g., cefadroxil, cefotaxime) increase your risk of bleeding.
- Anticonvulsants (e.g., carbamazepine, clonazepam) may cause an increased anticonvulsant effect.
- Beta-blockers (e.g., acebutolol, metoprolol) and carteolol may be less effective in lowering high blood pressure.
- Diflunisal may decrease the effects of diuretics (e.g., amiloride, indapamide), losartan, terazosin, minoxidil, and triamterene.
- Diflunisal may increase the effects of lithium.

- Gold compounds and tiopronin may increase the risk of kidney toxicity.
- Thyroid hormones may result in rapid heartbeat and a rise in blood pressure.

FOOD, VITAMIN, AND HERBAL INTERACTIONS

Alfalfa, clove oil, cinchona bark, feverfew, garlic, ginseng, and ginkgo may affect blood clotting, so use of these herbs along with diflunisal is not recommended.

St. John's wort and dong quai are associated with an increased sensitivity to the sun. Be sure to wear protective clothing and use sunscreen if you take these herbs while taking diflunisal.

RECOMMENDED DOSAGE

Diflunisal is available in tablets. The dosages given here are typical. However, your health-care practitioner will determine the most appropriate dose and schedule for your needs.

- *Children Up to 12 Years:* not recommended
- *Children 12 Years and Older and Adults:* 500 to 1,000 mg daily in 2 divided doses
- *Adults Older than 65*: 250 to 500 mg a day in 2 divided doses

Always take diflunisal with food.

If you miss a dose, take it as soon as you remember. If it is nearly time for your next dose, do not take the missed dose. Continue with your regular dosing schedule. Never take a double dose.

SYMPTOMS OF OVERDOSE AND WHAT TO DO

An overdose of NSAIDs can be fatal. Symptoms of overdose include drowsiness, nausea, vomiting, diarrhea, rapid breathing and heartbeat, increased sweating, ringing in the ears, confusion, disorientation, stupor, and coma. If overdose occurs, seek immediate medical attention and bring the prescription container with you to the hospital.

SPECIAL INFORMATION FOR PREGNANT OR NURSING WOMEN

No adequate studies of the effects of diflunisal have been done on pregnant or nursing women. If you are pregnant or plan to become pregnant, you and your health-care practitioner must weigh the potential benefits against the potential risks to the fetus.

Diflunisal passes into breast milk. If you are breastfeeding, your health-care practitioner will likely advise you to stop until your treatment is done.

SPECIAL INFORMATION FOR SENIORS

The dosage for seniors is usually half that of the adult dosage because they have a greater risk of gastrointestinal problems.

GENERIC NAMES

Class: Digitalis preparations

Generics: (1) digitoxin; (2) digoxin

BRAND NAMES

(1) Crystodigin; (2) Lanoxicaps, Lanoxin, Novodigoxin
Generic available

ABOUT THIS DRUG

Digitalis preparations are used to strengthen weak heart muscle contractions with the goal of preventing congestive heart failure. They are also used to correct irregular heartbeat.

These drugs enhance the force of the heart's contractions, which then helps regulate the rate and rhythm of the heartbeat and improve heart function in congestive heart failure.

SIDE EFFECTS

Be sure to tell your health-care practitioner if you experience any side effects while taking digitoxin or digoxin. Only your health-care practitioner can determine whether it is safe for you to continue taking these drugs.

- *Most Common:* loss of appetite, diarrhea
- *Less Common:* extreme drowsiness, lethargy, fainting, headache, disorientation
- *Rare:* rash, cardiac arrhythmias, hallucinations, double vision, enlarged, sensitive male breasts, tiredness, weakness, depression, decreased sex drive

IMPORTANT PRECAUTIONS

Tell your health-care practitioner if you are sensitive or allergic to digitoxin or digoxin or to any other drugs.

Do not take digitoxin or digoxin if your heartbeat is lower than 50 beats per minute.

Before taking digitoxin or digoxin, consult with your health-care practitioner if you have taken another digitalis preparation or diuretics within the past 2 weeks, or if you have kidney disease or a thyroid disorder, or if you will have surgery or dental surgery within the next 2 months.

Some digitalis medications contain tartrazine dye. Do not use these products, especially if you are allergic to aspirin.

Never suddenly stop taking these medications because it could cause a serious change in heart function.

DRUG INTERACTIONS

Tell your health-care practitioner and pharmacist if you are taking any prescription or nonprescription drugs, as well as any vitamins, herbs, or other supplements. Possible drug interactions include the following:

- Amiodarone, beta-blockers (e.g., acebutolol, propranolol), anticholinergics (e.g., atropine, mepenzolate), hydroxychloroquine, nefazodone, nicardipine, nizatidine, quinidine, rauwolfia alkaloids, verapamil, and spironolactone may increase the effect of digitalis.
- Antacids (e.g., Maalox, Mylanta), cholestyramine, colestipol, dextrothyroxine, laxatives, oxyphenbutazone, phenobarbital, phenylbutazone, metronidazole, rifampin, and triamterene may decrease the effect of digitalis.
- Tetracycline, propafenone, and erythromycins may increase the absorption of digitalis.
- Sulfasalazine and metoclopramide may decrease digitalis absorption.
- Sotalol may either increase or decrease heart rate.
- Diuretics (e.g., amiloride, indapamide) may cause digitalis toxicity.
- Ephedrine and epinephrine may cause disturbed heart rhythm. Do not take these drugs when using digitalis.
- Fluoxetine may cause agitation, convulsions, high blood pressure, and confusion. Do not use this drug while taking digitalis.

FOOD, VITAMIN, AND HERBAL INTERACTIONS

Avoid foods and beverages that contain caffeine, as they may cause irregular heartbeat. Foods high in fiber, such as bran cereals and prune juice, can decrease the effect of digitalis. Calcium supplements also can decrease the effects of digitalis. St. John's wort lowers blood levels of digoxin and may reduce its effectiveness. Avoid using St. John's wort while taking digoxin. Low blood potassium levels may increase the risk of side effects with digoxin; your health-care practitioner should monitor your potassium levels during treatment with digoxin.

RECOMMENDED DOSAGE

Digitoxin is available in tablets; digoxin is available in tablets, capsules, and elixir. The dosages given here are typical. However, your health-care practitioner will determine the most appropriate dose and schedule for your needs.

- *Children Up to Age 10*: your health-care practitioner will determine the appropriate dosage.
- *Adults:* starting dose is 0.2 mg, twice daily for 4 days. Maintenance dosage ranges from 0.05 to 0.3 mg once daily. Individual requirements vary widely.

Digitalis should be taken on an empty stomach at the same time each day. It can be taken with food if you experience stomach irritation; however, taking digitoxin or digoxin with food can decrease the drugs' absorption rate.

If you miss a dose, take it as soon as you remember. If it is nearly time for your next dose, do not take the missed dose. Continue with your regular dosing schedule. Never take a double dose.

SYMPTOMS OF OVERDOSE AND WHAT TO DO

Symptoms of overdose include abdominal pain, irregular heartbeat, loss of appetite, nausea, very slow pulse, vomiting, and diarrhea. If overdose occurs, seek immediate medical assistance and bring the prescription container with you to the hospital.

SPECIAL INFORMATION FOR PREGNANT OR NURSING WOMEN

No adequate studies have been done of the effects of digitoxin and digoxin on pregnant or nursing women. If you are pregnant or plan to become pregnant, and either of these drugs is crucial for your health, you and your health-care practitioner must weigh the potential benefits against the potential risks to the fetus.

Both of these drugs pass into breast milk. If you are breastfeeding, your health-care practitioner may advise you to stop until your treatment is done.

SPECIAL INFORMATION FOR SENIORS

Frail or underweight older adults may need a lower maintenance dose.

GENERIC NAME
Diltiazem

BRAND NAMES
Cardizem, Cardizem CD, Cardizem SR, Dilacor XR, Tiazac
Generic available

ABOUT THIS DRUG
Diltiazem is a calcium channel blocker that is used to treat angina and reduce high blood pressure.

This drug interferes with the transport of calcium into heart muscle cells and smooth muscles. The result is relaxation of the blood vessels, which increases the supply of blood to the heart and reduces blood pressure.

SIDE EFFECTS
Be sure to tell your health-care practitioner if you experience any side effects while taking diltiazem. Only your health-care practitioner can determine whether it is safe for you to continue taking this drug.

- *Most Common:* headache, drowsiness, swelling of ankles and feet, constipation, fatigue, nausea
- *Less Common or Rare:* dizziness, confusion, diarrhea, weakness, depression, nervousness, insomnia, excessive urination, jaundice rash, overgrowth of the gums, dry mouth, hair loss, heart attack, muscle cramps, nosebleed, rapid or pounding heartbeat, sexual difficulties, taste changes, thirst, tremor, vision changes, weight gain

IMPORTANT PRECAUTIONS
Tell your health-care practitioner if you are sensitive or allergic to diltiazem, other calcium channel blockers, or any other drugs.

Because diltiazem can cause drowsiness and dizziness, make sure you know how you react to this drug before you drive or operate dangerous equipment.

If you are taking diltiazem for angina, do not stop suddenly because it can cause an increase in attacks.

Do not take diltiazem if you have sick sinus syndrome or second- or third-degree heart block, unless you also have a ventricular pacemaker. Avoid use of diltiazem if you have a recent history of heart attack or if you have lung congestion or low blood pressure.

Before starting diltiazem, talk to your health-care practitioner if you have kidney disease, liver disease, or any kind of heart or blood vessel disease.

DRUG INTERACTIONS

Tell your health-care practitioner and pharmacist if you are taking any prescription or nonprescription drugs, as well as any vitamins, herbs, or other supplements. Possible drug interactions include the following:

- Cimetidine, fluoxetine, fluvoxamine, quinupristin, ranitidine, and sertraline may increase the effects of diltiazem.
- Toxicity of the following drugs may occur when they are taken along with diltiazem: carbamazepine, cilostazol, cyclosporine, digoxin, dofetilide, midazolam, nifedipine, quinidine, theophylline, tretinoin, and triazolam.
- Cisapride may cause heart toxicity.
- Amiodarone and beta-blockers, such as atenolol and carteolol, may result in abnormal heart rhythm.
- Aspirin may result in prolonged bleeding time or hemorrhage, and NSAIDs (e.g., diclofenac, sulindac) may cause gastrointestinal bleeding.
- Diltiazem may increase anticoagulation when taken with oral anticoagulants, such as warfarin.
- Diltiazem may cause abnormally low blood sugar when taken with oral antidiabetic drugs, such as glipizide.

FOOD, VITAMIN, AND HERBAL INTERACTIONS

Avoid excessive intake of salt or salty foods.

Herbs that can raise blood pressure, including goldenseal, ephedra (ma huang), ginseng, licorice, and saw palmetto, may reduce the benefits of diltiazem. St. John's wort may reduce the drug's levels in the body.

RECOMMENDED DOSAGE

Diltiazem is available in tablets and capsules. The dosages given here are typical. However, your health-care practitioner will determine the most appropriate dose and schedule for your needs.

- *Children:* safety and effectiveness have not been determined
- *Adults:* dosage depends on the brand taken. Daily doses are as follows:
- Cardizem, for angina, 180 to 360 mg divided into 3 or 4 doses
- Cardizem SR, for angina, 60 to 120 mg twice daily, which can be increased to 240 to 360 mg daily

- Cardizem CD, 180 to 240 mg once daily for high blood pressure, and 120 to 180 mg for angina
- Dilacor XR, 180 to 240 mg daily, which can be increased to up to 540 mg. For angina, starting dose is 120 mg and may be increased to 480 mg
- Tiazac, starting dose for high blood pressure is 120 to 240 mg daily, which can eventually be increased up to 540 mg daily. For angina, 120 to 180 mg daily, increased to 540 mg if needed

Diltiazem should be taken before meals or at bedtime.

If you miss a dose, take it as soon as you remember. If it is nearly time for your next dose, do not take the missed dose. Continue with your regular dosing schedule. Never take a double dose.

SYMPTOMS OF OVERDOSE AND WHAT TO DO

Symptoms of overdose include fainting, dizziness, irregular pulse, heart failure, very slow heartbeat, and low blood pressure. If an overdose occurs, seek immediate medical attention and bring the prescription container with you to the hospital.

SPECIAL INFORMATION FOR PREGNANT OR NURSING WOMEN

No adequate studies have been done on the effects of diltiazem on pregnant or nursing women. Animal studies have shown that this drug causes birth defects in animals. If you are pregnant or plan to become pregnant, and either of these drugs is crucial for your health, you and your health-care practitioner must weigh the potential benefits against the potential risks to the fetus. Diltiazem should not be taken at all during the first trimester.

Diltiazem passes into breast milk. If you are breastfeeding, your health-care practitioner will likely advise you to stop until your treatment is done.

SPECIAL INFORMATION FOR SENIORS

Older adults are more likely to experience weakness, dizziness, and fainting.

GENERIC NAME
Diphenhydramine

BRAND NAMES
Benadryl, Benahist, Benylin Cough, Compoz, Diphenhist, Nytol, Phendry, Sleep-Eze 3, Sominex Formula 2, Unisom SleepGels Maximum Strength
Generic available

ABOUT THIS DRUG
Diphenhydramine is an antihistamine that is available both by prescription and over-the-counter (depending on the strength). Its primary uses are to relieve symptoms of hay fever (allergic rhinitis) and other allergic reactions (e.g., swelling, itching, hives), motion sickness, and symptoms of Parkinson's disease.

This drug blocks the release of histamine (a chemical released by the body during an allergic reaction). Histamine is responsible for the symptoms associated with seasonal allergies, as well as itching, rash, and hives. In patients with Parkinson's disease, it decreases muscle stiffness and tremors.

SIDE EFFECTS
Be sure to tell your health-care practitioner if you experience any side effects while taking diphenhydramine. Only your health-care practitioner can determine whether it is safe for you to continue taking this drug.

- *Most Common:* drowsiness, dry mouth, nausea, thickening of mucus
- *Less Common or Rare:* confusion, difficult urination, blurred vision, diarrhea, excessive perspiration, fluttery heartbeat, fatigue, headache, hives, irritability, loss of appetite, low blood pressure, ringing in the ears, tight chest, tremor, euphoria, vertigo

IMPORTANT PRECAUTIONS
Tell your health-care practitioner if you are sensitive or allergic to diphenhydramine, other antihistamines, or any other drugs.

Use diphenhydramine cautiously if you have narrow-angle glaucoma, peptic ulcer or other stomach problems, intestinal blockage, enlarged prostate, or obstructed bladder, or if you have a history of asthma or other chronic lung disease, high blood pressure, heart disease, or overactive thyroid.

Because this drug can cause drowsiness, make sure you know how it affects you before you drive or operate dangerous equipment.

DRUG INTERACTIONS

Tell your health-care practitioner and pharmacist if you are taking any prescription or nonprescription drugs, as well as any vitamins, herbs, or other supplements. Possible interactions include the following:

- Alcohol, tranquilizers, sleeping pills, or other central nervous system depressants may increase the sedative effects of diphenhydramine. These drugs should not be combined.
- Tricyclic antidepressants may increase the risk of urinary retention.
- Phenothiazines (e.g., chlorpromazine, promazine) may result in increased urinary difficulties, intestinal obstruction, or glaucoma, especially if you are older than 70.
- Monoamine oxidase inhibitor (MAOI) antidepressants and anticholinergics (e.g., atropine, scopolamine) may increase the side effects of diphenhydramine.

FOOD, VITAMIN, AND HERBAL INTERACTIONS

Herbs that produce a sedative effect may cause significant depressant interactions when used with diphenhydramine. Some of those herbs include calendula, capsicum, catnip, goldenseal, gotu kola, hops, kava, lady's slipper, passionflower, sage, Siberian ginseng, skullcap, St. John's wort, and valerian, among others.

RECOMMENDED DOSAGE

Diphenhydramine is available in capsules, tablets, elixir, and syrup. The dosages given here are typical. However, your health-care practitioner will determine the most appropriate dose and schedule for your needs.

For Hay Fever

- *Children Up to Age 6 Years:* 6.25 to 12.5 mg every 4 to 6 hours
- *Children 6 to 12 Years:* 12.5 to 25 mg every 4 to 6 hours
- *Children 12 Years and Older and Adults:* 25 to 50 mg every 4 to 6 hours

For Motion Sickness, Nausea, Vomiting

- *Children Up to Age 12:* 1 to 1.5 mg per 2.2 lbs every 4 to 6 hours
- *Children 12 Years and Older and Adults:* 25 to 50 mg every 4 to 6 hours

For Parkinsonian Symptoms

- *Children:* to be determined by your health-care practitioner
- *Adults:* 25 mg three times daily. Your health-care practitioner may gradually increase the dose as needed

Diphenhydramine should be taken with food to reduce stomach irritation.

If you miss a dose, take it as soon as you remember. If it is nearly time for your next dose, do not take the missed dose. Continue with your regular dosing schedule. Never take a double dose.

SYMPTOMS OF OVERDOSE AND WHAT TO DO

Symptoms of overdose include severe drowsiness, dilated pupils, fever, excitability, interrupted breathing, aggression, confusion, loss of coordination, seizures, and loss of consciousness. If overdose occurs, seek immediate medical attention and bring the prescription container with you to the hospital.

SPECIAL INFORMATION FOR PREGNANT OR NURSING WOMEN

No adequate studies of the effects of diphenhydramine on pregnant or nursing women have been done. No birth defects have been noted in animal studies. If you are pregnant or plan to become pregnant, you and your health-care practitioner must weigh the potential benefits against the potential risks to the fetus.

Diphenhydramine passes into breast milk. If you are breastfeeding, your health-care practitioner will likely advise you to stop until your treatment is done.

SPECIAL INFORMATION FOR SENIORS

Older adults are more likely to experience side effects, which may be more severe as well.

GENERIC NAME

Dipivefrin

BRAND NAMES

AKPro, Propine

Generic available

ABOUT THIS DRUG

Dipivefrin is an antiglaucoma medication used to treat chronic open-angle glaucoma, the most common form of this eye disease characterized by abnormal pressure in the eye (intraocular pressure), which can cause vision problems or blindness.

Once dipivefrin is placed into the eye, it converts to epinephrine, which lowers the production of fluid in the eye and increases its outflow, thus reducing intraocular pressure.

SIDE EFFECTS

Be sure to tell your health-care practitioner if you experience any side effects while taking dipivefrin. Only your health-care practitioner can determine whether it is safe for you to continue taking this drug.

- *Most Common:* if you have had prior cataract surgery, dipivefrin may cause swelling of the retina, which is usually reversible
- *Less Common or Rare:* increased sensitivity to light, burning, stinging, or other eye irritation, change in heart rhythm, increased blood pressure

IMPORTANT PRECAUTIONS

Tell your health-care practitioner if you are sensitive or allergic to dipivefrin or to any other drugs.

Dipivefrin controls glaucoma, but it does not cure it. You will likely need to be treated for life.

Dipivefrin is dispensed in an eye dropper. To avoid contamination, do not allow the dropper to touch any surface, including the eye.

Do not use this drug for narrow-angle glaucoma unless instructed to do so by your health-care practitioner.

Because dipivefrin can cause blurred vision or other temporary vision changes, do not drive or operate dangerous equipment until you know how you react to this drug.

DRUG INTERACTIONS

Tell your health-care practitioner and pharmacist if you are taking any prescription or nonprescription drugs, as well as any vitamins, herbs, or other supplements. Possible interactions include the following:

- Other eye drugs may reduce the antiglaucoma effect of dipivefrin.

- Tricyclic antidepressants (e.g., amitriptyline, imipramine), maprotiline, nomifensine, ophthalmic beta-blockers (e.g., betaxolol, timolol), digitalis drugs, and systemic sympathomimetics (e.g., ephedrine, guaifenesin) may interact with dipivefrin. Consult with your health-care practitioner.

FOOD, VITAMIN, AND HERBAL INTERACTIONS

No food, vitamin, or herbal interactions have been noted.

RECOMMENDED DOSAGE

Dipivefrin is available as an ophthalmic solution. The dosage given here is typical. However, your health-care practitioner will determine the most appropriate dose and schedule for your needs.

- *Children and Adults:* 1 drop in each eye every 12 hours. Your health-care practitioner may adjust this dose depending on your response.

To use the drops, first wash your hands. Tilt your head back and gently pull downward on the lower eyelid. Administer a drop into this space, close your eye, and apply pressure for 1 to 2 minutes.

If you miss a dose, take it as soon as you remember. If it is nearly time for your next dose, do not take the missed dose. Continue with your regular dosing schedule. Never take a double dose.

SYMPTOMS OF OVERDOSE AND WHAT TO DO

A rapid or irregular heartbeat is the symptom of an overdose in the eye. If an overdose occurs, flush the eye with water and call your health-care practitioner or emergency department. If someone accidentally ingests dipivefrin, seek immediate medical assistance and bring the prescription container with you to the hospital.

SPECIAL INFORMATION FOR PREGNANT OR NURSING WOMEN

No adequate studies of the effects of dipivefrin on pregnant or nursing women have been done. Animal studies have not revealed any birth defects. If you are pregnant or plan to become pregnant, you and your health-care practitioner must weigh the potential benefits against the potential risks to the fetus.

Dipivefrin may pass into breast milk. If you are breastfeeding, your health-care practitioner may advise you to switch to bottle feeding.

SPECIAL INFORMATION FOR SENIORS

No special instructions are noted for older adults.

GENERIC NAME
Dipyridamole

BRAND NAMES

Dipridacot, Persantine
Generic available

ABOUT THIS DRUG

Dipyridamole is an antiplatelet drug used to prevent blood clots while you are recovering from heart surgery and to reduce the intensity and frequency of angina attacks.

This drug appears to increase the blood levels of adenosine, a substance that causes blood vessels to expand, and to prevent platelets from sticking together and forming clots.

SIDE EFFECTS

Be sure to tell your health-care practitioner if you experience any side effects while taking dipyridamole. Only your health-care practitioner can determine whether it is safe for you to continue taking this drug.

- *Most Common:* headache, nausea, rash
- *Less Common or Rare:* chest pain, itching, dizziness and weakness related to low blood pressure, flushing, liver problems that result in nausea, vomiting, yellowish skin and eyes, bloating

IMPORTANT PRECAUTIONS

Tell your health-care practitioner if you are sensitive or allergic to dipyridamole or to any other drugs.

Before taking dipyridamole, tell your health-care practitioner if you have low blood pressure or liver disease, or if you are recovering from a heart attack.

Aspirin is sometimes prescribed along with dipyridamole to better protect against clot formation. Because aspirin increases the risk of bleeding, be sure to take only the amount of aspirin prescribed by your health-care practitioner.

Before you have surgery or dental treatment or if there's a medical emergency, tell the health-care practitioner or dentist that you are taking dipyridamole.

DRUG INTERACTIONS

Tell your health-care practitioner and pharmacist if you are taking any prescription or nonprescription drugs, as well as any vitamins,

herbs, or other supplements. Possible drug interactions with dipyridamole may include the following:

- Alcohol may lower blood pressure excessively.
- Anticoagulants may result in an increased tendency to bleed.
- Aspirin and drugs containing aspirin may cause an increased dipyridamole effect.

FOOD, VITAMIN, AND HERBAL INTERACTIONS

Taking dipyridamole with food can reduce absorption.

RECOMMENDED DOSAGE

Dipyridamole is available in tablets. The dosages given here are typical. However, your health-care practitioner will determine the most appropriate dose and schedule for your needs.

- *Children Up to Age 12:* safety and effectiveness have not been determined
- *Children 12 Years and Older and Adults:* 75 to 100 mg, 4 times daily

Dipyridamole should be taken on an empty stomach, as food decreases absorption. However, if it causes stomach irritation, take it with food.

If you miss a dose, take it as soon as you remember. If it is nearly time for your next dose, do not take the missed dose. Continue with your regular dosing schedule. Never take a double dose.

SYMPTOMS OF OVERDOSE AND WHAT TO DO

Symptoms of an overdose include dizziness and weakness caused by extremely low blood pressure. If an overdose occurs, seek immediate medical attention and bring the prescription container with you to the hospital.

SPECIAL INFORMATION FOR PREGNANT OR NURSING WOMEN

No adequate studies of the effects of dipyridamole on pregnant or nursing women have been done. If you are pregnant or plan to become pregnant, you and your health-care practitioner must weigh the potential benefits against the potential risks to the fetus.

Dipyridamole passes into breast milk. If you are breastfeeding, your health-care practitioner may advise you to stop until your treatment is done.

SPECIAL INFORMATION FOR SENIORS
Older adults may require a lower starting dose.

GENERIC NAME
Dirithromycin

BRAND NAME
Dynabac
No generic available

ABOUT THIS DRUG
Dirithromycin is a macrolide antibiotic that is used to treat bronchitis, certain types of pneumonia, skin infections, and throat infections. It is only effective against infections caused by bacteria.

This drug prevents the bacteria cells from producing certain proteins that they need to survive.

SIDE EFFECTS
Be sure to tell your health-care practitioner if you experience any side effects while taking dirithromycin. Only your health-care practitioner can determine whether it is safe for you to continue taking this drug.

- *Most Common:* abdominal pain, diarrhea, headache, nausea
- *Less Common:* dizziness, vomiting, unusual fatigue, stomach upset
- *Rare:* colitis (inflammation of the lower intestinal tract, symptoms that can include severe abdominal pain, cramps, bloody stools, and severe diarrhea), liver toxicity (fever, nausea, vomiting, yellowish skin or eyes), allergic reaction (swelling of the tongue, face, lips, and throat, breathing problems, rash or hives), unusual bleeding or bruising

IMPORTANT PRECAUTIONS
Tell your health-care practitioner if you are sensitive or allergic to dirithromycin, other macrolide antibiotics, erythromycins, or any other drugs.

Before taking dirithromycin, talk to your health-care practitioner if you have a blood or liver disorder.

DRUG INTERACTIONS
Tell your health-care practitioner and pharmacist if you are taking any prescription or nonprescription drugs, as well as any vitamins,

herbs, or other supplements. Possible drug interactions include the following:

- Antacids that contain magnesium or aluminum should be taken at least one hour apart from your dirithromycin dose.
- Astemizole and dofetilide may increase your risk of heart problems.
- Dirithromycin may increase the effects of benzodiazipines (e.g., diazepam, clonazepam), bromocriptine, carbamazepine, cyclosporine, digoxin, tacrolimus, and theophylline.
- Dirithromycin may decrease the effects of zidovudine.
- Rifabutin and rifampin may reduce the effects of dirithromycin.
- Erythromycin reacts with the following drugs, although it is not certain that dirithromycin reacts as well. Caution should be used when combining these drugs with dirithromycin: digoxin, ergotamine, cyclosporine, carbamazepine, disopyramide, phenytoin, lovastatin, valproate acid, and anticoagulants (e.g., warfarin).

FOOD, VITAMIN, AND HERBAL INTERACTIONS

No food, vitamin, or herbal interactions have been noted.

RECOMMENDED DOSAGE

Dirithromycin is available in tablets. The dosage given here is typical. However, your health-care practitioner will determine the most appropriate dose and schedule for your needs.

- *Children Up to Age 12:* use to be determined by your health-care practitioner
- *Children 12 Years and Older and Adults:* 500 mg once daily for 5 to 14 days, depending on the condition being treated

Dirithromycin should be taken at the same time each day, with or without food.

If you miss a dose, take it as soon as you remember. If it is nearly time for your next dose, do not take the missed dose. Continue with your regular dosing schedule. Never take a double dose.

SYMPTOMS OF OVERDOSE AND WHAT TO DO

Symptoms of an overdose include diarrhea, nausea, vomiting, and abdominal pain. If an overdose occurs, seek immediate medical attention and bring the prescription container with you to the hospital.

SPECIAL INFORMATION FOR PREGNANT OR NURSING WOMEN

No adequate studies of the effects of dirithromycin on pregnant or nursing women have been done. If you are pregnant or plan to become pregnant, you and your health-care practitioner must weigh the potential benefits against the potential risks to the fetus.

Dirithromycin may pass into breast milk. If you are breastfeeding, your health-care practitioner will probably advise you to stop until you finish your treatment course.

SPECIAL INFORMATION FOR SENIORS

No special precautions have been noted.

GENERIC NAME

Disopyramide

BRAND NAMES

Norpace, Norpace CR

Generic available

ABOUT THIS DRUG

Disopyramide is an antiarrhythmic drug used to control abnormal or irregular heart rhythms, also referred to as cardiac arrhythmias.

The heart has a natural pacemaker, and disopyramide slows its activity, while it also delays the transmission of electrical impulses through the heart, which then stabilizes the heartbeat.

SIDE EFFECTS

Be sure to tell your health-care practitioner if you experience any side effects while taking disopyramide. Only your health-care practitioner can determine whether it is safe for you to continue taking this drug.

- *Common:* dizziness, constipation, blurred vision, dry eyes, dry nose, dry mouth, weakness caused by low blood pressure, hypoglycemia (cold sweats, rapid heartbeat, extreme hunger, shakiness, nervousness, drowsiness), difficulty urinating

- *Less Common or Rare:* depression, agitation, fatigue, muscle weakness, nausea, vomiting, abdominal pain, diarrhea, congestive heart failure, shortness of breath, rash, sore throat, fever, headache, yellowish skin and eyes, eye pain, diminished sex drive, psychosis

IMPORTANT PRECAUTIONS

Tell your health-care practitioner if you are sensitive or allergic to disopyramide or to any other drugs.

Use disopyramide with extreme caution if you have structural heart disease, inflamed heart muscle, or other heart conditions, or if you have glaucoma, myasthenia gravis, or urination difficulties.

If you have liver or kidney disease, you will likely need lower doses of this drug.

Before starting disopyramide, your health-care practitioner should check your potassium levels, because high levels can increase its toxicity.

Disopyramide can cause or worsen congestive heart failure and can cause severe low blood pressure.

Do not suddenly stop taking this drug, because it can cause serious changes in your heart function.

DRUG INTERACTIONS

Tell your health-care practitioner and pharmacist if you are taking any prescription or nonprescription drugs, as well as any vitamins, herbs, or other supplements. Possible interactions include the following:

- Alcohol should be avoided, because it can decrease blood pressure and blood sugar.
- Other antiarrthymic drugs (e.g., amiodarone, mexiletine) can increase the effects and toxicity of each drug.
- Anticholinergics (e.g., atropine, pirenzepine) and anticoagulants (e.g., warfarin) may have increased effects.
- Astemizole, chloroquine, clarithromycin, diphenhydramine, erythromycin, fludrocortisone, haloperidol, indapamide, maprotiline, beta-blockers (e.g., propranolol, sotalol), amiodarone, bepridil, diltiazem, flecainide, procainamide, propafenone, phenothiazines (e.g., chlorpromazine, promazine), pimozide, risperidone, tamoxifen, nicardipine, and nimodipine may have adverse effects on the heart.
- Phenobarbital, phenytoin, and rifampin may increase metabolism and decrease the effects of disopyramide.
- Propafenone may increase the effect and toxicity of both drugs.
- Tocainide may increase the adverse reactions of either drug.

FOOD, VITAMIN, AND HERBAL INTERACTIONS

The herbs ephedra (ma huang), kola, and St. John's wort may overstimulate the heart and should be avoided.

RECOMMENDED DOSAGE

Disopyramide is available in tablets and capsules. The dosages given here are typical. However, your health-care practitioner will determine the most appropriate dose and schedule for you.

- *Children:* 2.75 to 13.64 mg per pound of body weight per day, taken in divided doses every 6 hours
- *Adults:* if you weigh more than 110 pounds, take 150 mg every 6 hours. Adults who weigh less than 110 pounds must have their dose determined by their health-care practitioner

Disopyramide should be taken with liquid.

If you miss a dose, take it as soon as you remember. If it is nearly time for your next dose, do not take the missed dose. Continue with your regular dosing schedule. Never take a double dose.

SYMPTOMS OF OVERDOSE AND WHAT TO DO

Symptoms of an overdose include stopping breathing, irregular heartbeat, loss of consciousness, low blood pressure, and worsening congestive heart failure. If an overdose occurs, seek immediate medical assistance and bring the prescription container with you to the hospital.

SPECIAL INFORMATION FOR PREGNANT OR NURSING WOMEN

No adequate studies of the effects of disopyramide on pregnant or nursing women have been done. If you are pregnant or plan to become pregnant, and this drug is crucial for your health, you and your health-care practitioner must weigh the potential benefits against the potential risks to the fetus.

Disopyramide passes into breast milk. If you are breastfeeding, your health-care practitioner may advise you to switch to bottle feeding until your treatment is done.

SPECIAL INFORMATION FOR SENIORS

Older adults are more likely to require lower dosing and to experience difficulty urinating, to be constipated, or to have a decline in blood pressure.

GENERIC NAME

Divalproex sodium

see Valproic Acid, page 1096

GENERIC NAME
Dolasetron

see Antiemetics, page 128

GENERIC NAME
Donepezil

BRAND NAME
Aricept
No generic available

ABOUT THIS DRUG
Donepezil is an acetylcholinesterase inhibitor used to treat mild-to-moderate Alzheimer's disease.

This drug inhibits the breakdown of acetylcholine, a chemical in the brain that is needed for memory. A deficiency of this chemical may result in the memory loss associated with Alzheimer's disease.

SIDE EFFECTS
Be sure to tell your health-care practitioner if you experience any side effects while taking donepezil. Only your health-care practitioner can determine whether it is safe for you to continue taking this drug.

- *Most Common:* nausea, vomiting, diarrhea, headache, dizziness, fatigue, insomnia
- *Less Common:* drowsiness, depression, loss of appetite, unusual bleeding, fainting, muscle cramps, joint pain, vivid dreams

IMPORTANT PRECAUTIONS
Tell your health-care practitioner if you are sensitive or allergic to donepezil, biperiden, bupivacaine, methylphenidate, paroxetine, rifabutin, trihexyphenidyl, or any other drugs.

Because donepezil can make you drowsy and dizzy, make sure you know how the drug affects you before you drive or operate dangerous equipment.

Consult with your health-care practitioner before taking donepezil if you have any of the following conditions: asthma, chronic obstructive pulmonary disease, urinary problems, heart disease, liver disease, seizure disorder, stomach ulcers, and urinary tract blockage.

DRUG INTERACTIONS

Tell your health-care practitioner and pharmacist if you are taking any prescription or nonprescription drugs, as well as any vitamins, herbs, or other supplements. Possible drug interactions include the following:

- Ketoconazole and quinidine may decrease the metabolism of donepezil.
- Carbamazepine, dexamethasone, phenobarbital, phenytoin, and rifampin may increase the rate at which donepezil is eliminated from the body.

FOOD, VITAMIN, AND HERBAL INTERACTIONS

No food, vitamin, or herbal interactions have been noted.

RECOMMENDED DOSAGE

Donepezil is available in 5- and 10-mg tablets. The dosage given here is typical. However, your health-care practitioner will determine the most appropriate dose and schedule for your needs.

- *Children:* not intended for children
- *Adults:* staring dose of 5 mg at bedtime. Your health-care practitioner may increase the dose to 10 mg after 4 to 6 weeks

If you miss a dose, take it as soon as you remember. If it is nearly time for your next dose, do not take the missed dose. Continue with your regular dosing schedule. Never take a double dose.

SYMPTOMS OF OVERDOSE AND WHAT TO DO

Symptoms of an overdose include seizures, severe nausea, slowed heartbeat, muscle weakness, vomiting, excessive sweating, excessive salivation, irregular breathing, enlarged pupils, and weak pulse. If overdose occurs, seek immediate medical assistance and bring the prescription container with you to the hospital.

SPECIAL INFORMATION FOR PREGNANT OR NURSING WOMEN

No adequate studies of the effects of donepezil on pregnant or nursing women have been done. Animal studies show, however, that high doses can cause adverse effects. If you are pregnant or plan to become pregnant, and this drug is crucial for your health, you and your health-care practitioner must weigh the potential benefits against the potential risks to the fetus.

Donepezil may pass into breast milk. If you are breastfeeding, your health-care practitioner may advise you to switch to bottle feeding.

SPECIAL INFORMATION FOR SENIORS

No special precautions have been noted.

OPEN QUESTIONS OR CONTROVERSIES

Will donepezil be helpful for people who have a type of dementia other than Alzheimer's disease? That question may be answered in the near future. A unique clinical study presented at the American Association for Geriatric Psychiatry's 15th Annual meeting in February 2002 stated that donepezil significantly improved the cognitive and overall functioning of patients who had vascular dementia, which is caused by stroke. Vascular dementia is second only to Alzheimer's disease as a cause of dementia. About one-third of people who are diagnosed with dementia have the vascular type.

GENERIC NAME

Dorzolamide

BRAND NAME

Trusopt

No generic available

ABOUT THIS DRUG

Dorzolamide is an antiglaucoma (ophthalmic) medication used to treat open-angle glaucoma and ocular hypertension.

Dorzolamide helps reduce production of fluid in the eye, which lowers the pressure inside the eye.

SIDE EFFECTS

Be sure to tell your health-care practitioner if you experience any side effects while using dorzolamide. Only your health-care practitioner can determine whether it is safe for you to continue using this drug.

- *Most Common:* burning, stinging, or discomfort in the eye after the drug is given, bitter taste in the mouth
- *Less Common or Rare:* severe tearing, nausea, vomiting, bloody urine, eye pain, allergic reaction (red, itchy, swollen eyelid), severe sensitivity to light

IMPORTANT PRECAUTIONS

Tell your health-care practitioner if you are sensitive or allergic to dorzolamide, sulfonamides (e.g., sulfadiazine, sulfamethizole), furosemide, thiazide diuretics (e.g., bendroflumethiazide, hydrochlorothiazide), oral antidiabetics (e.g., glipizide, glyburide), oral carbonic anhydrase inhibitor glaucoma drugs (e.g., acetazolamide, methazolamide), substances such as benzalkonium chloride or other preservatives, or any other drugs.

To avoid contamination, make sure the eye dropper does not touch your eye or any other surface.

Because dorzolamide can cause temporary vision problems, do not drive or operate dangerous equipment until you know how you react to the drug.

DRUG INTERACTIONS

Tell your health-care practitioner and pharmacist if you are taking any prescription or nonprescription drugs, as well as any vitamins, herbs, or other supplements. Dorzolamide should not be used along with eye medications that contain silver, such as silver nitrate.

FOOD, VITAMIN, AND HERBAL INTERACTIONS

No food, vitamin, or herbal interactions have been noted.

RECOMMENDED DOSAGE

Dorzolamide is available as an ophthalmic solution. The dosage given here is typical. However, your health-care practitioner will determine the most appropriate dose and schedule for your needs.

- *Children Up to Age 12:* safety and dosage for children have not been established
- *Children 12 Years and Older and Adults:* 1 drop in each eye 3 times daily

If you miss a dose, take it as soon as you remember. If it is nearly time for your next dose, do not take the missed dose. Continue with your regular dosing schedule. Never take a double dose.

SYMPTOMS OF OVERDOSE AND WHAT TO DO

No specific symptoms of an overdose have been reported. If a large amount of the drug enters the eye, flush the eye with water. If someone accidentally ingests the drug, seek immediate medical attention and bring the prescription container with you to the hospital.

SPECIAL INFORMATION FOR PREGNANT OR NURSING WOMEN

No adequate studies of the effects of dorzolamide on pregnant or nursing women have been done. One animal study showed birth defects when very large doses were given. If you are pregnant or plan to become pregnant, you and your health-care practitioner must weigh the potential benefits against the potential risks to the fetus.

Dorzolamide may pass into breast milk. If you are breastfeeding, your health-care practitioner may advise you to stop until your treatment is done.

SPECIAL INFORMATION FOR SENIORS

No special precautions have been reported for older adults.

GENERIC NAME

Doxazosin

BRAND NAME

Cardura
Generic available

ABOUT THIS DRUG

Doxazosin is an antihypertensive drug, as well as an agent for benign prostatic hyperplasia (BPH, noncancerous enlargement of the prostate gland). It is given to individuals to treat mild-to-moderate high blood pressure and to relieve the urinary tract symptoms associated with BPH.

SIDE EFFECTS

Be sure to tell your health-care practitioner if you experience any side effects while taking doxazosin. Only your health-care practitioner can determine whether it is safe for you to continue taking this drug.

- ➤ *Most Common:* drowsiness, dizziness
- ➤ *Less Common or Rare:* weakness, palpitations, rapid pulse, headache, diarrhea, constipation, runny nose, rash, hives, itchy skin, depression, muscle or joint pain, irregular heartbeat. Priapism (prolonged or painful erection lasting more than 4 hours) is a very rare occurrence and requires medical attention

IMPORTANT PRECAUTIONS

Tell your health-care practitioner if you are sensitive or allergic to doxazosin, prazosin, terazosin, or any other drugs.

Use this drug with extreme caution if you have liver disease.

Consult with your health-care practitioner before taking doxazosin if you have experienced orthostatic hypotension (lightheadedness and dizziness when rising from a lying or seated position) when taking other antihypertensive drugs, if you have a history of depression or of low white blood cell count, or if you have impaired circulation, coronary artery disease, stroke and high blood pressure, or kidney problems. Also talk to your health-care practitioner first if you have angina and you are not treating it with a beta-blocker (e.g., acebutolol, nadolol).

Your first dose of this drug is likely to cause dizziness and lightheadedness. Take the drug at bedtime and be careful if you get up during the night and when you get up in the morning.

DRUG INTERACTIONS

Tell your health-care practitioner and pharmacist if you are taking any prescription or nonprescription drugs, as well as any vitamins, herbs, or other supplements. Possible drug interactions with doxazosin may include the following:

- Estrogen, amphetamines (e.g., amphetamine, dextroamphetamine), nonsteroidal anti-inflammatory drugs (e.g., naproxen, ibuprofen), and sympathomimetics (e.g., guaifenesin, phenylephrine) may decrease the effect of doxazosin.
- Other antihypertensives (e.g., clonidine, methyldopa) may increase the antihypertensive effect. Your health-care practitioner will need to adjust your dosages.

FOOD, VITAMIN, AND HERBAL INTERACTIONS

Herbs that produce a sedative effect may cause significant depressant interactions when used with doxazosin. Some of those herbs include calendula, capsicum, catnip, goldenseal, gotu kola, hops, kava, lady's slipper, passionflower, sage, Siberian ginseng, skullcap, St. John's wort, and valerian, among others.

RECOMMENDED DOSAGE

Doxazosin is available in tablets. The dosages given here are typical. However, your health-care practitioner will determine the most appropriate dose and schedule for your needs.

- *Children:* for hypertension, dose to be determined by your health-care practitioner
- *Adults:* for hypertension, start with 1 mg once daily. Your health-care practitioner may increase your dose up to a maximum of 16 mg daily. For BPH, start with 1 mg once daily, which your health-care practitioner may increase up to a maximum of 8 mg daily.

Take your doxazosin dose at the same time each day. Swallow the tablet with liquid, or you can crush the tablet and take it with food or liquid.

If you miss a dose, take it as soon as you remember. If it is nearly time for your next dose, do not take the missed dose. Continue with your regular dosing schedule. Never take a double dose.

SYMPTOMS OF OVERDOSE AND WHAT TO DO

Symptoms of overdose include extreme weakness, rapid or irregular heartbeat, cold sweaty skin, loss of consciousness, weak, rapid pulse, and coma. If overdose occurs, seek immediate medical attention and bring the prescription container with you to the hospital.

SPECIAL INFORMATION FOR PREGNANT OR NURSING WOMEN

No adequate studies of the effects of doxazosin on pregnant or nursing women have been done. Very high doses of the drug given to lab animals have damaged the fetus. If you are pregnant or plan to become pregnant, you and your health-care practitioner must weigh the potential benefits against the potential risks to the fetus.

Doxazosin may pass into breast milk. If you are breastfeeding, your health-care practitioner may advise you to stop until your treatment is done.

SPECIAL INFORMATION FOR SENIORS

Older adults are more likely to experience dizziness, lightheadedness, and fainting than younger patients.

GENERIC NAME

Doxepin *see Tricyclic Antidepressants, page 1076*

GENERIC NAME

Doxycycline *see Tetracycline Antibiotics, page 1013*

GENERIC NAME

Dronabinol

BRAND NAME
Marinol
No generic available

ABOUT THIS DRUG
Dronabinol is an antiemetic (antinausea) used to prevent nausea and vomiting caused by cancer medications. It is also given to patients who have AIDS (acquired immunodeficiency syndrome) to stimulate their appetite.

This drug appears to inhibit the areas of the brain that control the vomiting reflex. The exact mechanism, however, is unknown.

SIDE EFFECTS
Be sure to tell your health-care practitioner if you experience any side effects while taking dronabinol. Only your health-care practitioner can determine whether it is safe for you to continue taking this drug.

- *Most Common:* drowsiness, poor coordination, trouble thinking, dizziness
- *Less Common or Rare:* anxiety, blurred vision, convulsions, dry mouth, hallucinations, nervousness, headache, severe mood changes, difficult urination, rapid heartbeat

IMPORTANT PRECAUTIONS
Tell your health-care practitioner if you are sensitive or allergic to dronabinol or to any other drugs.

Do not take dronabinol if your nausea and vomiting are caused by factors other than cancer treatment, if you are sensitive or allergic to sesame oil or any form of marijuana, or if your chemotherapy cycle is longer than 7 consecutive days.

Consult your health-care practitioner before taking dronabinol if you have heart disease, high blood pressure, schizophrenia, or manic-depressive disorder, or if you are an alcoholic or drug addict.

Dronabinol is habit forming if used for a prolonged period. Withdrawal symptoms, including insomnia, restlessness, sweating, diarrhea, hiccups, loss of appetite, and irritability, may occur if you stop abruptly.

Dronabinol is not recommended for children younger than 12 years or for children who have AIDS cachexia.

DRUG INTERACTIONS

Tell your health-care practitioner and pharmacist if you are taking any prescription or nonprescription drugs, as well as any vitamins, herbs, or other supplements. Possible drug interactions include the following:

- Drugs that cause central nervous system depression or sedation, including alcohol, anticonvulsants, barbiturates, tricyclic antidepressants, antihistamines, tranquilizers, muscle relaxants, narcotics, and sedatives, may result in oversedation.
- Clozapine may have a toxic effect on the central nervous system.
- Molindone may cause dangerous increased effects of both drugs. Do not take this drug.
- Sertraline and guanfacine may increase the depressant effects of both drugs.
- Leucovorin has a high alcohol content and may cause adverse reactions.
- Fluoxetine may increase the depressant effects of both drugs.

FOOD, VITAMIN, AND HERBAL INTERACTIONS

No food, vitamin, or herbal interactions have been noted.

RECOMMENDED DOSAGE

Dronabinol is available in capsules. The dosages given here are typical. However, your health-care practitioner will determine the most appropriate dose and schedule for you.

- *Children Up to Age 12:* not recommended
- *Children 12 Years and Older and Adults:* for nausea and vomiting, 5 mg per square meter of body surface, 1 to 3 hours before chemotherapy and before meals. The dose can be repeated every 2 to 4 hours after therapy for 4 to 6 doses daily. To stimulate appetite, 2.5 mg twice daily, before lunch and dinner. If needed, the maximum dose is up to 20 mg daily.

If you miss a dose, take it as soon as you remember. If it is nearly time for your next dose, do not take the missed dose. Continue with your regular dosing schedule. Never take a double dose.

SYMPTOMS OF OVERDOSE AND WHAT TO DO

Symptoms of overdose include confusion, slurred speech, hallucinations, changes in taste, sound, touch, smell, or sight, drastic mood changes, rapid heartbeat, urination difficulties, nervousness, dry mouth, loss of coordination, fainting, and dizziness. If overdose occurs, seek immediate medical assistance and bring the prescription container with you to the hospital.

SPECIAL INFORMATION FOR PREGNANT OR NURSING WOMEN

No adequate studies of the effects of dronabinol on pregnant or nursing women have been completed. If you are pregnant or plan to become pregnant, you and your health-care practitioner must weigh the potential benefits against the potential risks to the fetus.

Dronabinol passes into breast milk. Your health-care practitioner will likely advise you to stop breastfeeding until you have completed treatment.

SPECIAL INFORMATION FOR SENIORS

Older adults are more likely to experience side effects, and they may be more severe. In particular, changes in mental functioning should be noted and not mistaken for other conditions, such as Alzheimer's disease or other dementias.

GENERIC NAME

Duloxetine

BRAND NAME

Cymbalta
No generic available

ABOUT THIS DRUG

Duloxetine is approved for treatment of major depressive disorder and for physical pain associated with depression. Symptoms of major depressive disorder include sleep and appetite changes, recurrent thoughts of death or suicide, decrease in sex drive, unusual difficulty concentrating or thinking, irritability, feelings of hopelessness, worthlessness, or inappropriate guilt, for more than two weeks.

Duloxetine is a type of drug known as a serotonin norepinephrine reuptake inhibitor (SNRI). It works by making more serotonin and norepinephrine available in the brain.

SIDE EFFECTS

Be sure to tell your health-care practitioner if you experience any side effects while taking duloxetine. Only your health-care practitioner can determine whether it is safe for you to continue taking this drug. The following side effects are those associated with the use of duloxetine.

- *Most Common:* nausea, constipation, dizziness, drowsiness, dry mouth, decreased appetite, fatigue, increased sweating, insomnia
- *Less Common:* abdominal pain, palpitations, back pain, headache, cough, pharyngitis, upper respiratory infection, sexual difficulties, urinary retention

IMPORTANT PRECAUTIONS

Tell your health-care practitioner if you are sensitive or allergic to duloxetine or to any other drugs.

Duloxetine should not be taken along with MAO inhibitors (e.g., phenelzine, furazolidone, linezolid) or within at least 14 days of stopping treatment with an MAOI. Serious reactions can occur if MAOIs are mixed with duloxetine.

Duloxetine should be prescribed with caution if you have a history of seizures.

Talk to your health-care practitioner before taking duloxetine if you have liver or kidney disease.

You should not take this drug if you have uncontrolled narrow-angle glaucoma or if you are taking thioridazine.

Your health-care practitioner may check your blood pressure periodically while you are being treated with duloxetine.

Do not discontinue duloxetine abruptly without consulting your physician; if the drug needs to be stopped, the dose should be decreased gradually.

DRUG INTERACTIONS

Tell your health-care practitioner and pharmacist if you are taking any prescription or nonprescription drugs, as well as any vitamins, herbs, or other supplements. Possible drug interactions include the following:

- MAOIs should not be used with duloxetine, and this SNRI should not be used within at least 14 days of discontinuing an MAOI.
- Thioridazine should not be used with duloxetine, as it can cause serious ventricular arrhythmias or sudden death.
- Use of cimetidine, ciprofloxacin, enoxacin, fluvoxamine, or paroxetine can increase the blood levels of duloxetine.
- Amitriptyline, flecainide, imipramine, nortriptyline, phenothiazines, and propafenone should be used with caution if taking duloxetine.

FOOD, VITAMIN, AND HERBAL INTERACTIONS

No food, vitamin, or herbal interactions have been documented.

RECOMMENDED DOSAGE

Duloxetine is available in 20-, 30-, and 60-mg enteric-coated capsules. The dosages given here are typical. However, your health-care practitioner will determine the most appropriate dose and schedule for your needs.

- *Children*: Not indicated for use in children
- *Adults*: 40 mg per day in divided doses. Your health-care practitioner may increase your dose to 60 mg as needed.

Duloxetine can be taken with or without food and should be swallowed whole. If you miss a dose, take it as soon as you remember. If it is nearly time for your next dose, skip the missed dose and return to your normal dosing schedule. Never take a double dose.

SYMPTOMS OF OVERDOSE AND WHAT TO DO

Symptoms of overdose have not been recorded. If overdose occurs, seek immediate medical attention and bring the prescription container with you to the hospital.

SPECIAL INFORMATION FOR PREGNANT OR NURSING WOMEN

No adequate studies of the effects of duloxetine on pregnant or breastfeeding women have been done. It's been shown that neonates who are exposed to SSRIs and SNRIs during the third trimester can develop respiratory distress, seizures, vomiting, apnea, and other problems. If you are pregnant or plan to become pregnant and this drug is crucial for your health, you and your health-care practitioner must weigh the potential benefits against the potential risks to the fetus.

It is not known whether duloxetine appears in breast milk. If you are breastfeeding, your health-care practitioner will likely advise you to switch to bottle feeding until your treatment is complete.

SPECIAL INFORMATION FOR SENIORS

Although no studies have indicated such, older adults may experience more side effects and more serious ones.

GENERIC NAME
Econazole

BRAND NAME
Spectazole
No generic available

ABOUT THIS DRUG
Econazole is an antifungal medication used to treat athlete's foot, jock itch, and other fungal infections of the skin.

This drug prevents fungal organisms from making substances they need to grow and function.

SIDE EFFECTS
Be sure to tell your health-care practitioner if you experience any side effects while taking econazole. Only your health-care practitioner can determine whether it is safe for you to continue taking this drug.

➤ *Less Common:* itching, stinging, redness, burning, or other irritation symptoms not present before treatment

IMPORTANT PRECAUTIONS
Tell your health-care practitioner if you are sensitive or allergic to econazole or to any other drugs, especially other antifungal medications.

Econazole should not be used in or near the eyes.

Do not apply tight coverings or bandages to the treated areas, and do not wear tight clothing over the treated skin.

Use econazole for the prescribed treatment period, even if you feel better before treatment is scheduled to end. Stopping too soon may allow the infection to return.

DRUG INTERACTIONS
Tell your health-care practitioner and pharmacist if you are taking any prescription or nonprescription drugs, as well as any vitamins, herbs, or other supplements. No drug interactions have been noted. However, talk to your health-care practitioner if you are also using a topical corticosteroid, because it may inhibit the effectiveness of econazole.

FOOD, VITAMIN, AND HERBAL INTERACTIONS
No food, vitamin, or herbal interactions have been noted.

RECOMMENDED DOSAGE

Econazole is available as a cream. The dosages given here are typical. However, your health-care practitioner will determine the most appropriate dose and schedule for you.

- *Children and Adults:* Apply an even, thin layer to the affected area 1 to 2 times daily. For athlete's foot, treatment typically lasts 1 month; for jock itch and other fungal infections, 2 weeks.

If you miss a dose, apply it as soon as you remember. If it is nearly time for your next dose, do not apply the missed dose. Continue with your regular dosing schedule. Never take a double dose.

SYMPTOMS OF OVERDOSE AND WHAT TO DO

An overdose of econazole is unlikely. If someone accidentally ingests the cream, seek immediate medical attention and bring the prescription container with you to the hospital.

SPECIAL INFORMATION FOR PREGNANT OR NURSING WOMEN

Before you use econazole, tell your health-care practitioner if you are pregnant or plan to become pregnant. This drug should not be used during the first trimester unless your health-care practitioner says it is crucial for your health, and should be used during the last two trimesters only if your health-care practitioner feels it is needed.

Econazole may pass into breast milk. If you are breastfeeding, your health-care practitioner may advise you to stop until treatment is complete.

SPECIAL INFORMATION FOR SENIORS

No special precautions are noted for older adults.

GENERIC NAME

Efavirenz

BRAND NAME

Sustiva
No generic available

ABOUT THIS DRUG

Efavirenz is an antiviral drug used to treat human immunodeficiency virus (HIV) infection. It is combined with other drugs as part of a "drug cocktail."

This drug helps prevent HIV by inhibiting the activity of an enzyme the virus needs to replicate its DNA, and by stopping the formation of the complete DNA.

SIDE EFFECTS

Be sure to tell your health-care practitioner if you experience any side effects while taking efavirenz. Only your health-care practitioner can determine whether it is safe for you to continue taking this drug.

- *Most Common:* dizziness, sleeping difficulties, fatigue, impaired concentration, abnormal dreams, fever, cough, vomiting, diarrhea, stomach upset. If you develop a rash, contact your health-care practitioner immediately.
- *Less Common or Rare:* severe depression, mood changes, confusion

IMPORTANT PRECAUTIONS

Tell your health-care practitioner if you are sensitive or allergic to efavirenz or to any other drugs.

It is especially important to take efavirenz on schedule to help ensure a constant level of the drug in the bloodstream.

Because efavirenz can cause dizziness and compromised concentration, make sure you know how you react to the drug before you drive or operate dangerous equipment.

Use of efavirenz does not prevent the risk of transmitting the AIDS virus to others. Appropriate preventive measures need to be taken.

DRUG INTERACTIONS

Tell your health-care practitioner and pharmacist if you are taking any prescription or nonprescription drugs, as well as any vitamins, herbs, or other supplements. Drugs that may interact with efavirenz include the following:

- Efavirenz may reduce the blood levels of amprenavir, clarithromycin, indinavir, methadone, and sildenafil.
- Amprenavir, fluconazole, and ritonavir may raise blood levels of efavirenz.
- Efavirenz may raise blood levels of ethinyl estradiol.
- Nevirapine and rifampin may reduce blood levels of efavirenz.

FOOD, VITAMIN, AND HERBAL INTERACTIONS

Efavirenz should not be taken with high-fat foods.

Avoid taking St. John's wort, as it may reduce blood levels of efavirenz.

RECOMMENDED DOSAGE

Efavirenz is available in capsules. The dosages given here are typical. However, your health-care practitioner will determine the most appropriate dose and schedule for you.

- *Children:* use and dose to be determined by your health-care practitioner
- *Adults:* Starting dose is 500 mg once daily. Efavirenz is always taken as part of a drug cocktail. During the first 2 to 4 weeks of treatment, take the dose at bedtime to help alleviate dizziness, drowsiness, and impaired concentration.

Efavirenz should be taken with a low-fat meal and with lots of water or other liquid.

If you miss a dose, take it as soon as you remember. If it is nearly time for your next dose, do not take the missed dose. Continue with your regular dosing schedule. Never take a double dose.

SYMPTOMS OF OVERDOSE AND WHAT TO DO

An increased severity of side effects is the most common indication of an overdose. If an overdose occurs, seek immediate medical assistance and bring the prescription container with you to the hospital.

SPECIAL INFORMATION FOR PREGNANT OR NURSING WOMEN

No adequate studies of the effects of efavirenz on pregnant or nursing women have been done. Animal studies have shown birth defects. If you are pregnant or plan to become pregnant and this drug is crucial for your health, you and your health-care practitioner must weigh the potential benefits against the potential risks to the fetus.

Women who have HIV should not breastfeed because they can pass the infection on to their infant.

SPECIAL INFORMATION FOR SENIORS

No special precautions are noted for older adults.

GENERIC NAME

Eflornithine (topical)

BRAND NAME

Vaniqa
No generic available

ABOUT THIS DRUG

Eflornithine is an enzyme inhibitor used to slow the growth of unwanted facial hair on women.

This drug appears to block an enzyme that is necessary for hair growth. It does not remove facial hair; it significantly slows its growth.

SIDE EFFECTS

Be sure to tell your health-care practitioner if you experience any side effects while taking eflornithine. Only your health-care practitioner can determine whether it is safe for you to continue taking this drug.

- *Most Common:* acne, stinging skin
- *Less Common:* burning or bleeding skin, chapped red lips, hair bumps, numbness, rash, tingling skin, swollen lips

IMPORTANT PRECAUTIONS

Tell your health-care practitioner if you are sensitive or allergic to eflornithine or to any other drugs.

If you do not have improvement after six months of treatment, stop using eflornithine and call your health-care practitioner.

If irritation occurs, reduce the number of treatments. If the irritation continues, stop using eflornithine and call your health-care practitioner.

Wait until eflornithine dries before you apply makeup or sunscreen.

Do not wash the treated areas for at least four hours after you apply the medication.

Because eflornithine does not remove hair, you must continue to use hair removal products or methods while using eflornithine.

DRUG INTERACTIONS

Tell your health-care practitioner and pharmacist if you are taking any prescription or nonprescription drugs, as well as any vitamins, herbs, or other supplements. No drug interactions have been noted to date.

FOOD, VITAMIN, AND HERBAL INTERACTIONS

No food, vitamin, or herbal interactions have been noted.

RECOMMENDED DOSAGE

Eflornithine is available as a cream. The dosage given here is typical. However, your health-care practitioner will determine the most appropriate dose and schedule for you.

- *Children Up to Age 12 Years:* not recommended
- *Children 12 Years and Older and Adults:* coat the problem areas around the lips and chin twice daily. The second daily application should be done at least eight hours after the first one.

If you miss a dose, apply it as soon as you remember. If it is nearly time for your next dose, do not apply the missed dose. Continue with your regular dosing schedule. Never apply a double dose.

SYMPTOMS OF OVERDOSE AND WHAT TO DO

Overdose with eflornithine is unlikely. If someone accidentally ingests the drug, seek immediate medical attention and bring the prescription container with you to the hospital.

SPECIAL INFORMATION FOR PREGNANT OR NURSING WOMEN

No adequate studies of the effects of eflornithine on pregnant or nursing women have been done. If you are pregnant or plan to become pregnant and this drug is crucial for your health, you and your health-care practitioner must weigh the potential benefits against the potential risks to the fetus.

Eflornithine may pass into breast milk. If you are breastfeeding, your health-care practitioner will likely advise you to stop until treatment is complete.

SPECIAL INFORMATION FOR SENIORS

Older adults may experience more severe skin irritation problems.

GENERIC NAME

Emedastine

BRAND NAME

Emadine
No generic available

ABOUT THIS DRUG

Emedastine is an ophthalmic solution prescribed as short-term treatment of itchy eyes associated with seasonal allergic conjunctivitis (inflamed inner surface of the eyelids and whites of the eyes).

This drug blocks the effects of histamine, a substance the body produces that causes sneezing, watery eyes, itching, swelling, and other symptoms.

SIDE EFFECTS

Be sure to tell your health-care practitioner if you experience any side effects while taking emedastine. Only your health-care practitioner can determine whether it is safe for you to continue taking this drug.

- *Most Common:* headache
- *Less Common:* abnormal dreams, dry eyes, blurry vision, rash, weakness, runny nose, bad taste in the mouth, burning or stinging eyes

IMPORTANT PRECAUTIONS

Tell your health-care practitioner if you are sensitive or allergic to emedastine or to any other drugs.

To avoid contamination, do not allow the tip of the dropper to touch your eye or any other surface.

Make sure you know how you react to this drug before you drive or operate dangerous equipment, as it may temporarily affect your vision.

Before you use emedastine, tell your health-care practitioner if you wear soft contact lenses.

DRUG INTERACTIONS

Tell your health-care practitioner and pharmacist if you are taking any prescription or nonprescription drugs, as well as any vitamins, herbs, or other supplements. No significant drug interactions have been noted.

FOOD, VITAMIN, AND HERBAL INTERACTIONS

No food, vitamin, or herbal interactions have been noted.

RECOMMENDED DOSAGE

Emedastine is available as an ophthalmic solution. The dosages given here are typical. However, your health-care practitioner will determine the most appropriate dose and schedule for you.

- *Children up to Age 3:* not recommended
- *Children Age 3 and Older and Adults:* 1 drop in the affected eyes up to 4 times daily

If you miss a dose, take it as soon as you remember. If it is nearly time for your next dose, do not take the missed dose. Continue with your regular dosing schedule. Never take a double dose.

SYMPTOMS OF OVERDOSE AND WHAT TO DO

An overdose of emedastine is unlikely. If someone accidentally ingests the solution, seek immediate medical assistance and bring the prescription container with you to the hospital.

SPECIAL INFORMATION FOR PREGNANT OR NURSING WOMEN

No adequate studies of the effects of emedastine on pregnant or nursing women have been done. If you are pregnant or plan to become pregnant and emedastine is crucial to your health, you and your health-care practitioner must weigh the potential benefits against the potential risks to the fetus.

Emedastine may pass into breast milk. If you are breastfeeding, your health-care practitioner may advise you to stop until your treatment is complete.

SPECIAL INFORMATION FOR SENIORS

No special precautions are needed for older adults.

GENERIC NAME

Enalapril

BRAND NAME

Vasotec

Generic available

ABOUT THIS DRUG

Enalapril is an angiotensin-converting enzyme (ACE) inhibitor prescribed primarily to control high blood pressure and to treat congestive heart failure.

Like other ACE inhibitors, enalapril blocks an enzyme that produces angiotensin, a substance that causes blood vessels to constrict and promotes production of aldosterone, which causes the body to retain sodium. Thus ACE inhibitors cause blood vessels to relax and reduce sodium retention, which lowers blood pressure.

SIDE EFFECTS

Be sure to tell your health-care practitioner if you experience any side effects while taking enalapril. Only your health-care practitioner can determine whether it is safe for you to continue taking this drug.

➤ *Most Common:* persistent dry cough

- *Less Common or Rare:* dizziness, fainting, rash, tingling or numbness in the feet, lips, or hands, unusual fatigue, muscle weakness, nausea, abnormal dreams, drowsiness, loss of taste, fever and chills, sudden breathing difficulties, swelling

IMPORTANT PRECAUTIONS

Tell your health-care practitioner if you are sensitive or allergic to enalapril or to any other drugs, especially other ACE inhibitors.

It's important that you continue to take enalapril as prescribed, even if you feel better. Stopping without your health-care practitioner's knowledge may result in serious health problems.

If you develop swelling of your tongue, throat, face, arms, or legs while taking enalapril, stop taking the drug and contact your health-care practitioner immediately.

Before starting enalapril, tell your health-care practitioner if you have kidney disease or dysfunction, scleroderma, lupus, heart or liver disease, diabetes, or renal artery stenosis.

Do not take enalapril if you have an abnormally high blood potassium level or if you have a blood cell or bone marrow disorder.

DRUG INTERACTIONS

Tell your health-care practitioner and pharmacist if you are taking any prescription or nonprescription drugs, as well as any vitamins, herbs, or other supplements. Possible drug interactions include the following:

- Azathioprine may cause severe anemia.
- Cyclosporine may cause kidney failure.
- Lithium may result in toxic lithium levels.
- Loop diuretics (e.g., bendroflumethiazide, furosemide) and phenothiazines (e.g., chlorpromazine, promazine) may cause excessively low blood pressure when standing from a seated or lying position.
- Oral hypoglycemic drugs (e.g., glyburide, glipizide) may cause decreased insulin resistance and the need to lower the dose of the hypoglycemic drugs.
- Thiazide diuretics (e.g., hydrochlorothiazide, bendroflumethiazide) may cause an increased reduction in blood pressure.
- Potassium preparations, potassium-sparing diuretics, and co-trimoxazole may cause blood potassium levels to rise and risk serious heart rhythm problems.
- COX-2 inhibitors (e.g., celecoxib, rofecoxib) may decrease the effects of enalapril.
- Alcohol can further reduce blood pressure. Use it with caution.

FOOD, VITAMIN, AND HERBAL INTERACTIONS

Discuss your salt intake with your health-care practitioner when taking enalapril. Avoid using salt substitutes or drinking low-salt milk, as these substances can cause abnormally high potassium levels, which can lead to heart problems. Also avoid foods high in potassium, such as bananas and citrus, unless you are also taking medications that reduce potassium levels. Do not take potassium supplements while taking enalapril unless directed to do so by your health-care practitioner.

If you are taking or plan to take any herbs or supplements, talk with your health-care practitioner before starting enalapril. Ginseng, goldenseal, licorice, ephedra (ma huang), and saw palmetto may raise your blood pressure; garlic and calcium may help lower it.

RECOMMENDED DOSAGE

Enalapril is available in tablets. The dosages given here are typical. However, your health-care practitioner will determine the most appropriate dose and schedule for you.

- *Children:* safety and effectiveness have not been established
- *Adults:* for high blood pressure (if not taking a diuretic), 5 mg once daily, with a gradual increase up to 40 mg daily in a single dose or divided doses as determined by your health-care practitioner. For congestive heart failure, 2.5 to 10 mg once or twice daily to a maximum of 40 mg daily.

Enalapril can be taken with or without food. Doses should be taken at the same time each day.

If you miss a dose, take it as soon as you remember. If it is nearly time for your next dose, do not take the missed dose. Continue with your regular dosing schedule. Never take a double dose.

SYMPTOMS OF OVERDOSE AND WHAT TO DO

The main symptom of overdose is a sudden drop in blood pressure, characterized by lightheadedness, dizziness, and fainting. If overdose occurs, seek immediate medical attention and bring the prescription container with you to the hospital.

SPECIAL INFORMATION FOR PREGNANT OR NURSING WOMEN

Enalapril can cause birth defects, premature delivery, and death to a developing or newborn infant. If you are pregnant or plan to become pregnant, talk to your health-care practitioner immediately.

Enalapril passes into breast milk. If you are breastfeeding, your health-care practitioner will advise you to switch to bottle feeding until your treatment is complete.

SPECIAL INFORMATION FOR SENIORS

Older adults usually have lower starting doses. Some seniors may be more susceptible to side effects.

GENERIC NAME

Enoxacin

see Fluoroquinolone Antibiotics, page 468

GENERIC NAME

Eplerenone

BRAND NAME

Inspra
No generic available

ABOUT THIS DRUG

Eplerenone is an antihypertensive used to treat high blood pressure, either alone or in combination with other medications designed to treat hypertension.

Eplerenone works by blocking the action of aldosterone, a substance produced in the body that raises blood pressure.

SIDE EFFECTS

Be sure to tell your health-care practitioner if you experience any side effects while taking eplerenone. Only your health-care practitioner can determine whether it is safe for you to continue taking this drug.

- *Most Common:* cough, dizziness, fatigue, flu-like symptoms, headache, stomach pain, increased blood potassium concentration
- *Rare:* allergic reaction (closing of the throat, difficulty breathing, hives, swelling of the tongue, lips, or face)

IMPORTANT PRECAUTIONS

Tell your health-care practitioner if you are sensitive or allergic to eplerenone or to any other drugs.

Do not take eplerenone if you have any of the following: high levels of potassium in your blood, type II diabetes with protein in your urine, or kidney disease. Use of eplerenone is also not recommended if you are using a salt substitute or taking a potassium supplement or a potassium-sparing diuretic.

If you have liver disease, talk to your health-care practitioner before taking eplerenone. You may need special dosing or to be monitored during treatment.

DRUG INTERACTIONS

Tell your health-care practitioner and pharmacist if you are taking any prescription or nonprescription drugs, as well as any vitamins, herbs, or other supplements. If you are taking any of the following drugs, your health-care practitioner may need to modify your dose or monitor your drug levels. Possible interactions may occur with the following drugs:

- Potassium supplements or salt substitutes that contain potassium
- Potassium-sparing diuretics, such as triamterene, spironolactone, and amiloride
- Angiotensin converting enzyme inhibitors such as benazepril, captopril, enalapril, fosinopril, lisinopril, moexipril, perindopril, quinapril, ramipril, and trandolapril.
- Angiotensin II receptor inhibitors such as candesartan, eprosartan, irbesartan, losartan, olmesartan, telmisartan, and valsartan
- Aspirin and other nonsteroidal anti-inflammatory drugs such as ibuprofen and naproxen
- Cimetidine, clarithromycin, danazol, delavirdine, erythromycin, fluconazole, fluoxetine, fluvoxamine, itraconazole, ketoconazole, lithium, nefazodone, protease inhibitors (e.g., amprenavir, nelfinavir, ritonavir, saquinavir), verpamil, and zafirlukast.

FOOD, VITAMIN, AND HERBAL INTERACTIONS

Talk to your health-care practitioner before drinking grapefruit juice or before using St. John's wort while taking eplerenone.

RECOMMENDED DOSAGE

Eplerenone is available in 25-, 50-, and 100-mg tablets. The dosages given here are typical. However, your health-care practitioner will determine the most appropriate dose and schedule for your needs.

- *Children:* Not recommended for children
- *Adults:* 1 tablet one to two times per day, as prescribed by your health-care practitioner

Eplerenone should be taken with an 8-ounce glass of water, with or without food. You should take your dose(s) at the same time each day for maximum benefit. If you miss a dose, take it as soon as you remember. However, if it is nearly time for your next dose, skip the missed dose and take your next scheduled dose. Never take a double dose. Do not stop taking this drug without first discussing it with your health-care practitioner. Suddenly stopping this drug can cause your condition to worsen.

SYMPTOMS OF OVERDOSE AND WHAT TO DO
Symptoms of overdose may include fainting, dizziness, blurred vision, upset stomach, loss of muscle tone, heaviness or weakness in legs, tingling in legs and arms, confusion, lack of energy, cold skin, and slow or irregular heartbeat. If overdose occurs, seek immediate medical attention and bring the prescription container with you to the hospital.

SPECIAL INFORMATION FOR PREGNANT OR NURSING WOMEN
No adequate studies of the effects of eplerenone on pregnant or nursing women have been done. If you are pregnant or plan to become pregnant, talk to your health-care practitioner. Eplerenone should be used during pregnancy only if the potential benefit justifies the potential risk to the fetus.

If you are breastfeeding, your health-care practitioner may advise you to stop while you use eplerenone, as this drug may appear in breast milk.

SPECIAL INFORMATION FOR SENIORS
No special instructions are needed for seniors.

GENERIC NAME

Eprosartan mesylate/hydrochlorothiazide

see Angiotensin II Blockers, page 123

GENERIC NAME

Ergoloid mesylates

BRAND NAMES

Gerimal, Hydergine, Hydergine LC
Generic available

ABOUT THIS DRUG

Ergoloid mesylates are ergot preparations prescribed for elderly individuals who have reduced alertness, poor memory, confusion, and other age-related declines in mental capability.

These drugs stimulate the metabolism of brain cells to promote use of oxygen and nutrients.

SIDE EFFECTS

Be sure to tell your health-care practitioner if you experience any side effects while taking ergoloid mesylates. Only your health-care practitioner can determine whether it is safe for you to continue taking this drug.

➤ *Most Common:* runny nose, flushed skin, headache

➤ *Less Common or Rare:* slow heartbeat, tingling in fingers, blurred vision, fainting, rash, nausea, vomiting, stomach cramps, dizziness when rising from a seated or lying position, soreness under tongue, appetite loss

IMPORTANT PRECAUTIONS

Tell your health-care practitioner if you are sensitive or allergic to ergoloid mesylates or to any other drugs.

Do not take ergoloid mesylates if you have a heart rate of less than 60 beats per minute, or if your systolic blood pressure is consistently lower than 100.

Before starting ergoloid mesylates, tell your health-care practitioner if you have had low blood pressure, liver disease, or a severe mental illness.

Ergoloid mesylates may reduce your body's ability to adjust to cold temperatures.

DRUG INTERACTIONS

Tell your health-care practitioner and pharmacist if you are taking any prescription or nonprescription drugs, as well as any vitamins, herbs, or other supplements. Drug interactions with ergoloid mesylates may include the following:

- Ergoloid mesylates should not be taken with other ergot preparations or with sympathomimetics (e.g., albuterol, ephedrine) because the combination may cause decreased circulation to the extremities.
- Alcohol and medications that contain alcohol (e.g., cough remedies, elixirs) should be avoided.

FOOD, VITAMIN, AND HERBAL INTERACTIONS
No food, vitamin, or herbal interactions have been noted.

RECOMMENDED DOSAGE
Ergoloid mesylates are available in capsules, oral solution, and sublingual tablets. The dosages given here are typical. However, your health-care practitioner will determine the most appropriate dose and schedule for you.

- *Children:* this drug is primarily for people 60 and older
- *Adults:* 1 mg three times daily

If you miss a dose, take it as soon as you remember. If it is nearly time for your next dose, do not take the missed dose. Continue with your regular dosing schedule. Never take a double dose.

SYMPTOMS OF OVERDOSE AND WHAT TO DO
Symptoms of overdose include headache, flushed face, nasal congestion, nausea, vomiting, drop in blood pressure, blurred vision, weakness, collapse, and coma. If overdose occurs, seek immediate medical attention and bring the prescription container with you to the hospital.

SPECIAL INFORMATION FOR PREGNANT OR NURSING WOMEN
This drug is not intended for women of childbearing age.

SPECIAL INFORMATION FOR SENIORS
No special precautions are noted for older adults.

OPEN QUESTIONS OR CONTROVERSIES
Whether ergoloid mesylates are helpful in treating dementia is debatable. Some experts say there is some benefit; others say there is not. An attempt to settle the debate was made by the National Institutes of Health, which published the Cochrane

(continued from page 422)
Database System Review of 2000. The study reviewed 19 studies in which ergoloid mesylates were used in people with dementia. Unfortunately, the researchers concluded that the effectiveness of these drugs is still uncertain. Newer drugs to treat dementia (e.g., rivastigmine) should also be considered if you are looking for treatment for Alzheimer's disease and other types of dementia.

GENERIC NAME
Ergotamine

BRAND NAMES
Cafergot, Cafergot-PB, Cafetrate, Ercaf, Ergomar, Ergostat, Medihaler Ergotamine, Wigraine
No generic available

ABOUT THIS DRUG
Ergotamine is an antimigraine medication used for the prevention and relief of vascular headache, especially migraine and cluster headache. The drug is often combined with caffeine, which increases its absorption, and/or with atropine (belladonna) and barbiturates to relieve premenstrual tension, nausea, and hot flashes.

Ergotamine causes the blood vessels in the head to constrict, which prevents their dilation and thus the pain associated with migraine.

SIDE EFFECTS
Be sure to tell your health-care practitioner if you experience any side effects while taking ergotamine. Only your health-care practitioner can determine whether it is safe for you to continue taking this drug.

- *Most Common:* cold hands and feet with mild tingling and numbness
- *Less Common or Rare:* nausea, diarrhea, vomiting, headache, drowsiness, dizziness, confusion, chest pain, abdominal pain, gangrene of the extremities, gangrene of the intestines

IMPORTANT PRECAUTIONS
Tell your health-care practitioner if you are sensitive or allergic to ergotamine or to any other drugs.

Do not take ergotamine if you have a severe infection, angina,

Buerger's disease, arteriosclerosis (hardening of the arteries), high blood pressure, ischemic heart disease, peptic ulcer malnutrition, liver or kidney disease, Raynaud's phenomenon, thrombophlebitis, or glaucoma.

If you experience numbness in your fingers or toes, or you have chest pain or muscle cramping, contact your health-care practitioner immediately.

The safety and effectiveness of ergotamine has not been determined for children younger than 12 years.

Excessive use of ergotamine may increase the frequency of migraines.

This drug may cause drowsiness or dizziness; therefore be sure you know how you react to ergotamine before you drive or operate dangerous equipment.

DRUG INTERACTIONS

Tell your health-care practitioner and pharmacist if you are taking any prescription or nonprescription drugs, as well as any vitamins, herbs, or other supplements. Possible drug interactions include the following:

- Amprenavir, indinavir, and ritonavir should not be taken with ergotamine.
- Ergotamine may decrease the effects of nitroglycerin.
- Beta-blockers (e.g., atenolol, carvedilol), dopamine, erythromycins, and sumatriptan may increase the effects of ergotamine.

FOOD, VITAMIN, AND HERBAL INTERACTIONS

Use of ephedra may cause additional constriction of the blood vessels and should be avoided. Talk to your health-care practitioner if you are taking St. John's wort, because this herb can change how your body eliminates the drug.

RECOMMENDED DOSAGE

Ergotamine is available as an aerosol and in sublingual tablets. The dosages given here are typical. However, your health-care practitioner will determine the most appropriate dose and schedule for you.

- *Children:* not recommended for children younger than 12 years
- *Adults:* for the aerosol, one spray when the headache starts, with repeat sprays 30 to 60 minutes later as needed, up to a maximum of six sprays every 24 hours. Tablets, one 2-mg tablet under the tongue

when the pain begins, followed by 2 mg in 30 to 60 minutes as needed, up to a maximum of 6 mg per attack

Follow the dosing instructions set forth by your health-care practitioner.

SYMPTOMS OF OVERDOSE AND WHAT TO DO

Symptoms of overdose include nausea, vomiting, diarrhea, numbness in the hands and feet, cold skin, confusion, seizures, and coma. If overdose occurs, seek immediate medical assistance and bring the prescription container with you to the hospital.

SPECIAL INFORMATION FOR PREGNANT OR NURSING WOMEN

Studies in both animals and humans have shown that ergotamine can cause fetal deaths. Ergotamine should never be used during pregnancy.

Ergotamine passes into breast milk. If you are breastfeeding, your health-care practitioner will advise you to switch to bottle feeding.

SPECIAL INFORMATION FOR SENIORS

Older adults have a greater risk of experiencing more severe side effects.

GENERIC NAME

Erythromycins

Generics: erythromycin estolate, erythromycin ethylsuccinate, erythromycin gluceptate, erythromycin lactobionate, erythromycin stearate, erythromycin-base

BRAND NAMES

Eryzole, Ilosone Sulfa, Pediazole, Sulfimycin (for ear infections); Ilotycin (for eye infections); E-Base, E-Mycin, EES, Ery-Tab, ERYC, EryPed, Erythro, Erythrocin, Erythrocot, Ilosone, Ilotycin, My-E, PCE, Wintrocin (for other infections)
Generics available

ABOUT THIS DRUG

Erythromycins belong to a class of antibiotics (macrolide antibiotics) that are used to treat various bacterial infections, including those that afflict the throat, ears, eyes, respiratory tract, urinary tract, intestinal tract, and heart.

Erythromycins prevent bacteria from producing specific proteins that they need to survive.

SIDE EFFECTS

Be sure to tell your health-care practitioner if you experience any side effects while taking erythromycins. Only your health-care practitioner can determine whether it is safe for you to continue taking this drug.

- *Most Common:* stomach or abdominal cramps and discomfort, diarrhea, loss of appetite, nausea, vomiting, blurred vision for up to 30 minutes after treatment (ophthalmic product only)
- *Less Common or Rare:* sore tongue or mouth, vaginal discharge or itching, rash, itching, aching joints and muscles, swallowing difficulty, pale, red, blistered, peeling, or loose skin, sore throat, fever, unusual bleeding or bruising, unusual fatigue, jaundice, blood in urine, lower back pain, painful urination, swollen neck, increased sensitivity to light. For ophthalmic solution only: eye irritation, redness, itching, or swelling that was not present before therapy began.

IMPORTANT PRECAUTIONS

Tell your health-care practitioner if you are sensitive or allergic to erythromycins or to any other drugs.

Prolonged use of erythromycins may result in your becoming more susceptible to infections caused by organisms that do not respond to erythromycins.

Before starting erythromycins, tell your health-care practitioner if you have liver disease, myasthenia gravis, a history of heart rhythm problems, or hearing loss.

Erythromycins may cause a severe form of intestinal inflammation. If diarrhea develops, call your health-care practitioner immediately.

The oral suspension form of erythromycins, which is for treatment of ear infections in children, is not intended for children younger than 2 months of age.

DRUG INTERACTIONS

Tell your health-care practitioner and pharmacist if you are taking any prescription or nonprescription drugs, as well as any vitamins, herbs, or other supplements. Possible drug interactions include the following:

- Erythromycins may increase the effects of benzodiazepines (e.g., diazepam, clonazepam), buspirone, carbamazepine, clozapine, digoxin, ergotamine, methylprednisolone, quetiapine, quinidine, sibutramine, sildenafil, tacrolimus, theophylline, tretinoin, valproic acid, vinblastine, and warfarin.

- Erythromycins may decrease the effects of clindamycin, lincomycin, and penicillins.
- Astemizole may cause serious arrhythmias.
- Atorvastatin and similar drugs (e.g., fluvastatin, lovastatin) may increase the risk of myopathy (serious muscle damage).
- Oral contraceptives may lose their effectiveness.
- Cyclosporine, corticosteroids (e.g., prednisone, hydrocortisone), ergot derivatives (e.g., dihydroergotamine), fluoxetinenevirapine, delavirdine, efavirenz, ritonavir, triazolam, and trimexate may result in toxicity of each of these individual drugs.
- Disopyramide may cause heart arrhythmias.
- Grepafloxacin may cause heartbeat changes.
- Midazolam (and perhaps other benzodiazepines) may cause excessive central nervous system depression.
- Zidovudine levels may decrease and be less effective.
- Valproic acid may lead to toxic blood levels.

FOOD, VITAMIN, AND HERBAL INTERACTIONS

Do not drink carbonated beverages or fruit juices for at least 1 hour after you take a nonenteric-coated form of erythromycin.

Avoid using St. John's wort because extreme reactions to sunlight may occur.

RECOMMENDED DOSAGE

Erythromycins are available in capsules, tablets, and oral suspension, and as an ophthalmic ointment. The dosages for each brand name of erythromycin differ, and the dosages vary widely depending on the condition being treated. The dosages given here are examples only. Your health-care practitioner will determine the most appropriate dose and schedule for you.

For Streptococcal Infections of Respiratory Tract

- *Children:* 30 to 50 mg daily for each 2.2 pounds of body weight, divided into equal doses. Children who weigh more than 44 pounds can take the recommended adult dose
- *Adults:* 333 mg every 8 hours or 500 mg every 12 hours for at least 10 days. The dose may be increased up to 4 g daily

For Urinary, Reproductive, or Rectal Infections

- *Children:* 30 to 50 mg daily for each 2.2 pounds of body weight, divided into equal doses. Children who weigh more than 44 pounds can take the recommended adult dose
- *Adults:* 500 mg 4 times daily or 666 mg every 8 hours for at least 7 days

For Intestinal Infections

- *Children:* 30 to 50 mg daily for each 2.2 pounds of body weight, divided into equal doses. Children who weigh more than 44 pounds can take the recommended adult dose
- *Adults:* 500 mg every 12 hours or 333 mg every 8 hours, for 10 to 14 days

For Ear Infections (Oral Suspension)

- *Children (less than 18 Pounds):* to be determined by your health-care practitioner
- *Children (18 to 35 Pounds):* ½ teaspoon 4 times daily for 10 days
- *Children (35 to 53 Pounds):* 1 teaspoon 4 times daily for 10 days
- *Children (53 to 100 Pounds):* 1½ teaspoons 4 times daily for 10 days
- *Children (more than 100 Pounds):* 2 teaspoons 4 times daily for 10 days

The oral forms are best taken on an empty stomach. However, they can be taken with food to help prevent stomach irritation.

If you miss a dose, take it as soon as you remember. If it is nearly time for your next dose, do not take the missed dose. Continue with your regular dosing schedule. Never take a double dose.

SYMPTOMS OF OVERDOSE AND WHAT TO DO

Symptoms of overdose include diarrhea, nausea, vomiting, and stomach cramps. If overdose occurs, seek immediate medical assistance and bring the prescription container with you to the hospital.

SPECIAL INFORMATION FOR PREGNANT OR NURSING WOMEN

No adequate studies of the effects of most of the erythromycins on pregnant or nursing women have been done. Erythromycin estolate can cause toxic liver reactions during pregnancy and should not be used during that time. If you are pregnant or plan to become pregnant, and any of these drugs are crucial for your health, you and your health-care practitioner must weigh the potential benefits against the potential risks to the fetus.

Erythromycins pass into breast milk. If you are breastfeeding, your health-care practitioner will likely advise you to switch to bottle feeding until your treatment is complete.

SPECIAL INFORMATION FOR SENIORS

Older adults have a greater risk of hearing loss when taking the oral forms.

GENERIC NAME

Escitalopram

BRAND NAME

Lexapro
No generic available

ABOUT THIS DRUG

Escitalopram is a selective serotonin reuptake inhibitor (SSRI) antidepressant that is prescribed for treatment of depression and generalized anxiety disorder.

This drug impacts the level of serotonin, a chemical in the brain that is believed to be associated with mood, mental state, and emotions.

SIDE EFFECTS

Be sure to tell your health-care practitioner if you experience any side effects while taking escitalopram oxalate. Only your health-care practitioner can determine whether it is safe for you to continue taking this drug.

- *Most Common:* agitation, blurred vision, changes in taste, difficulty sleeping, drowsiness, dry mouth, fever, frequent urination, headache, indigestion, nausea, increased or decreased appetite, increased sweating, sexual difficulties (decreased sexual desire, ejaculatory delay), tremor, weight changes
- *Less Common:* abdominal pain, chills, diarrhea, fever, joint pain, runny nose
- *Rare:* shortness of breath, increased thirst, headache, confusion, muscle pain or cramps, coma

IMPORTANT PRECAUTIONS

Tell your health-care practitioner if you are sensitive or allergic to escitalopram oxalate, citalopram, or to any other drugs.

Escitalopram should not be taken along with MAO inhibitors (e.g., phenelzine, furazolidone), and do not take escitalopram within at least 14 days of stopping treatment with an MAOI. If you want to take an MAOI after discontinuing escitalopram, wait at least 14 days before starting the MAOI.

Because this medication can cause drowsiness and blurred vision, you should make sure you know how you react to it before you drive or operate dangerous equipment.

Escitalopram should be used with caution if you have severe kidney disease, diabetes, or a history of seizures or mania.

Rarely, a condition known as serotonin syndrome occurs in patients who take SSRIs. A combination of symptoms, including agitation, confusion, tremor, twitching, and hyperthermia, may indicate this condition.

Do not discontinue escitalopram abruptly without consulting your physician; if the drug needs to be stopped, the dose should be decreased gradually.

DRUG INTERACTIONS

Tell your health-care practitioner and pharmacist if you are taking any prescription or nonprescription drugs, as well as any vitamins, herbs, or other supplements. Possible drug interactions include the following:

- Alcohol should be avoided while taking escitalopram.
- Monoamine oxidase inhibitors (MAOIs; e.g., phenelzine, selegiline, furazolidone, linezolid) should not be taken along with escitalopram (see "Important Precautions").
- Citalopram should not be taken at the same time as escitalopram.
- Lithium may enhance the effects of escitalopram, so caution should be used if these two drugs are taken together.
- Sumatriptan taken along with escitalopram can, in rare cases, cause weakness, hyperreflexia, and incoordination.
- Carbamazepine may reduce levels of escitalopram in the body.
- Before starting escitalopram, inform your health-care practitioner if you are taking any of the following medications: other antidepressants (e.g, citalopram, fluoxetine, fluvoxamine, sertraline, paroxetine, trazodone, nefazodone, amitriptyline, imipramine, doxepin, nortriptyline, and others), stomach medications (e.g., cimetidine, ranitidine), antibiotics (e.g., erythromycin, clarithromycin), antifungals (e.g., fluconzaole, itraconazole, ketoconazole), asthma medications (e.g., zafirlukast), and NSAIDs (e.g., naproxen, ibuprofen), aspirin, or drugs that affect blood coagulation.

FOOD, VITAMIN, AND HERBAL INTERACTIONS

Herbs that produce a sedative effect may cause significant depressant interactions when used with escitalopram. Some of those herbs include calendula capsicum, catnip, goldenseal, gotu kola, kava, lady's slipper, passionflower, sage, Siberian ginseng, skullcap, St. John's wort, and valerian, among others.

Do not take this drug with grapefruit or grapefruit juice, as dangerous interactions may occur.

RECOMMENDED DOSAGE

Escitalopram is available in 5-, 10-, and 20-mg tablets. The dosages given here are typical. However, your health-care practitioner will determine the most appropriate dose and schedule for your needs.

- *Children:* Not recommended for use in children
- *Adults:* Starting dose is 10 mg once daily; can be increased to 20 mg once daily after one week by a health-care practitioner, as needed

Escitalopram should be taken with water, and can be taken with or without food either in the morning or evening.

If you miss a dose, take it as soon as you remember. If it is nearly time for your next dose, do not take the missed dose. Continue with your regular dosing schedule. Never take a double dose.

SYMPTOMS OF OVERDOSE AND WHAT TO DO

Symptoms of overdose include dizziness, sweating, nausea, vomiting, tremor, and severe drowsiness. In some cases, individuals experience confusion, convulsions, coma, hyperventilation, and rapid heartbeat. If overdose occurs, seek immediate medical attention and bring the prescription container with you to the hospital.

SPECIAL INFORMATION FOR PREGNANT OR NURSING WOMEN

Adequate studies of the effects of escitalopram on pregnant or nursing women have not been done. If you are pregnant or plan to become pregnant, talk to your health-care practitioner. If this drug is crucial for your health, you and your health-care practitioner must weigh the potential benefits against the potential risks to the fetus.

Escitalopram appears in breast milk. If you are breastfeeding, your health-care practitioner will likely advise you to switch to bottle feeding until your treatment is complete.

SPECIAL INFORMATION FOR SENIORS

Most seniors should take no more than 10 mg daily.

GENERIC NAME
Esomeprazole

BRAND NAME
Nexium
No generic available

ABOUT THIS DRUG
Esomeprazole is a gastric acid pump inhibitor prescribed to treat and prevent gastroesophageal reflux disease (GERD).

This drug inhibits the secretion of gastric acid.

SIDE EFFECTS
Be sure to tell your health-care practitioner if you experience any side effects while taking esomeprazole. Only your health-care practitioner can determine whether it is safe for you to continue taking this drug.

➤ *Most Common:* abdominal pain, diarrhea, headache

➤ *Less Common:* constipation, dry mouth, gas, nausea

IMPORTANT PRECAUTIONS
Tell your health-care practitioner if you are sensitive or allergic to esomeprazole or to any other drugs.

Take the full course of treatment as prescribed by your health-care practitioner, even if you feel better before you've completed it.

Liver disease or a history of liver disease may cause esomeprazole to build up in the body.

DRUG INTERACTIONS
Tell your health-care practitioner and pharmacist if you are taking any prescription or nonprescription drugs, as well as any vitamins, herbs, or other supplements. No drug interactions have been noted.

FOOD, VITAMIN, AND HERBAL INTERACTIONS
No food, vitamin, or herbal interactions have been noted.

RECOMMENDED DOSAGE
Esomeprazole is available in delayed-release capsules. The dosages given here are typical. However, your health-care practitioner will determine the most appropriate dose and schedule for you.

- *Children Up to 18 Years:* safety and dose to be determined by your health-care practitioner
- *Adults:* to treat GERD, 20 to 40 mg once daily for 4 to 8 weeks. To prevent GERD, 20 mg once daily.

Take esomeprazole at least one hour before meals.

If you cannot swallow the capsule, open it up and add the granules to one tablespoon yogurt or applesauce or a small amount of water and swallow immediately.

If you miss a dose, take it as soon as you remember. If it is nearly time for your next dose, do not take the missed dose. Continue with your regular dosing schedule. Never take a double dose.

SYMPTOMS OF OVERDOSE AND WHAT TO DO

No reports of overdose have been made. However, symptoms of overdose of a similar drug, omeprazole, include confusion, drowsiness, blurred vision, slow heartbeat, nausea, flushing, and headache. If an overdose with esomeprazole occurs, seek immediate medical attention and bring the prescription container with you to the hospital.

SPECIAL INFORMATION FOR PREGNANT OR NURSING WOMEN

No adequate studies of the effects of esomeprazole on pregnant or nursing women have been done. No birth defects or abnormalities have been noted in animal studies. If you are pregnant or plan to become pregnant and this drug is crucial for your health, you and your health-care practitioner must weigh the potential benefits against the potential risks to the fetus.

Esomeprazole may pass into breast milk. If you are breastfeeding, your health-care practitioner may advise you to stop until treatment is complete.

SPECIAL INFORMATION FOR SENIORS

No special precautions have been noted for older adults.

GENERIC NAME

Estazolam

BRAND NAME

ProSom
Generic available

ABOUT THIS DRUG

Estazolam is a benzodiazepine tranquilizer that is prescribed for short-term treatment of insomnia.

This drug produces mild sedation by enhancing the effect of a chemical (gamma-aminobutyric acid, or GABA), which in turn dampens the transmission of nerve signals and reduces nerve excitation.

SIDE EFFECTS

Be sure to tell your health-care practitioner if you experience any side effects while taking estazolam. Only your health-care practitioner can determine whether it is safe for you to continue taking this drug.

➤ *Most Common:* dizziness, drowsiness, lightheadedness, slurred speech, loss of coordination, unsteady gait, headache

➤ *Less Common or Rare:* constipation, euphoria, nausea, vomiting, urinary difficulties, unusual fatigue, change in sexual desire or ability, abnormal dreams, acne, agitation, arthritis, asthma, back pain, double vision, dry mouth, gas, hallucinations, indigestion, loss of memory, muscle stiffness, neck pain, nosebleed, rapid, heavy breathing, rash, ringing in the ears, seizure, sore throat, stupor, swollen breast, thirst, tremor, vomiting, weight gain or loss

IMPORTANT PRECAUTIONS

Tell your health-care practitioner if you are sensitive or allergic to estazolam or to any other drugs, especially other benzodiazepines.

Estazolam is potentially addictive, even after only a few weeks' use. If the drug is taken for too long, withdrawal symptoms can occur when the drug is stopped suddenly. Symptoms of withdrawal include tremors, insomnia, agitation, diarrhea, vomiting, muscle cramps, sweating, and convulsions.

Because estazolam can cause dizziness, drowsiness, and other symptoms that can affect vision and alertness, make sure you know how you react to this drug before you drive or operate dangerous equipment.

If you have liver or kidney problems, have breathing difficulties, or are physically run down, use estazolam with caution.

If you have a respiratory disease, taking estazolam may cause sleep apnea (intermittent cessation of breathing during sleep).

DRUG INTERACTIONS

Tell your health-care practitioner and pharmacist if you are taking any prescription or nonprescription drugs, as well as any vitamins, herbs, or other supplements. Possible drug interactions include the following:

- Central nervous system depressants (e.g., alcohol, antiseizure drugs, antihistamines, tranquilizers, narcotics, barbiturates, and MAO inhibitors) may slow down functioning of your central nervous system and make you comatose.
- Cimetidine, disulfiram, isoniazid, probenecid, and oral contraceptives may increase the effect of estazolam.
- Cigarette smoking, rifampin, and theophylline may reduce the effects of estazolam.
- Estazolam may reduce the effectiveness of levodopa.
- Estazolam may increase the amount of zidovudine, digoxin, or phenytoin in the blood, which in turn increases the risk of side effects.

FOOD, VITAMIN, AND HERBAL INTERACTIONS

Herbs that produce a sedative effect may cause significant depressant interactions when used with estazolam. Some of those herbs include calendula, capsicum, catnip, goldenseal, gotu kola, hops, kava, lady's slipper, passionflower, sage, Siberian ginseng, skullcap, St. John's wort, and valerian, among others.

Because grapefruit juice does slow the breakdown of some benzodiazepines, it is best to avoid this beverage while being treated with estazolam.

RECOMMENDED DOSAGE

Estazolam is available in tablets. The dosages given here are typical. However, your health-care practitioner will determine the most appropriate dose and schedule for you.

- *Children Up to 18 Years:* safety and effectiveness information is not available
- *Adults:* 1 mg 60 minutes before bedtime; may be increased to 2 mg by your health-care practitioner
- *Adults 60 and Older:* 0.5 to 1 mg 60 minutes before bedtime

Estazolam may be taken with food to help minimize stomach irritation.

If you miss a dose, take it as soon as you remember. If it is nearly time for your next dose, do not take the missed dose. Continue with your regular dosing schedule. Never take a double dose.

SYMPTOMS OF OVERDOSE AND WHAT TO DO

Symptoms of overdose include confusion, depression, loss of muscle coordination, slurred speech, and sleepiness. If overdose occurs, call your local poison control center, health-care practitioner, or emergency room. You may be told to induce vomiting using ipecac syrup (available at any pharmacy) and then to seek immediate medical assistance. Bring the prescription container with you to the hospital.

SPECIAL INFORMATION FOR PREGNANT OR NURSING WOMEN

Estazolam may cause birth defects in your child. If you are pregnant or plan to become pregnant, you must not take estazolam. Infants born to women who take this drug shortly before giving birth are likely to experience drug withdrawal symptoms or to have poor muscle tone.

Estazolam passes into breast milk. If you are breastfeeding, your health-care practitioner will advise you to switch to bottle feeding until your treatment is complete.

SPECIAL INFORMATION FOR SENIORS

Like many other benzodiazepines and sleeping pills, estazolam is especially dangerous when used by older adults, because these drugs often cause dizziness, unsteady gait, and loss of coordination.

GENERIC NAME

Esterified estrogens *see Estrogens, page 436*

GENERIC NAME

Estradiol *see Estrogens, page 436*

GENERIC NAME

Estrogens (female hormones)

Generics: (1) esterified estrogens; (2) estradiol; (3) conjugated estrogens; (4) conjugated estrogen (synthetic); (5) ethinyl estradiol; (6) estropipate; (7) conjugated estrogens/medroxyprogesterone acetate

BRAND NAMES

(1) Estratab, Menest; (2) Alora, Climara, Depo-Estradiol, Dioval, Dura-Estrin, Duragen, Estrace, Estraderm, EstroGel, Estro-Span, Femi-

nate, Femogex, Menaval, Vagifem, Vivelle, Vivelle-Dot; (3) Premarin; (4) Cenestin; (5) Estinyl; (6) Ogen, Ortho-Est; (7) Premphase, Prempro
Generics available for all except (7)

ABOUT THIS DRUG

Estrogens are female hormones which, in their various forms, are prescribed primarily to relieve symptoms of menopause (e.g., hot flashes, vaginal dryness, sleep disturbances) and to help prevent heart disease and osteoporosis in postmenopausal women.

Estrogens play a major role in the growth and maintenance of the female sex characteristics and the reproductive system. They promote the release of essential hormones from the pituitary gland, hormones that are involved in the functioning of capillaries (tiny blood vessels), the development of bone, fluid retention, and ovulation, among other tasks.

SIDE EFFECTS

Be sure to tell your health-care practitioner if you experience any side effects while taking estrogen. Only your health-care practitioner can determine whether it is safe for you to continue taking this drug.

- *Most Common:* abdominal bloating, stomach cramps, loss of appetite, skin irritation (with patches), breast tenderness, headache, nausea
- *Less Common or Rare:* dizziness, diarrhea, unusual increase in sexual desire, vomiting, breast pain, swelling of feet and lower legs, rapid weight gain, vaginal bleeding changes, lumps in or discharge from the breast, vision problems, jaundice, discomfort when wearing contact lenses

IMPORTANT PRECAUTIONS

Tell your health-care practitioner if you are sensitive or allergic to estrogens or to any other drugs.

Prolonged use (5 years or longer) may increase your risk of endometrial cancer and breast cancer. The combination of conjugated estrogens and medroxyprogesterone nearly eliminates the increased risk of endometrial cancer, because of the protective power of medroxyprogesterone.

You should not take estrogens if you have a blood clot disorder, breast cancer, abnormal genital bleeding, or any type of hormone-dependent cancer.

Before taking any type of estrogen, talk to your health-care practitioner if you have a history of liver disease, heart attack, stroke, a blood clotting disorder, gallbladder disease, or gallstones, or if you are a heavy smoker.

Estrogens can raise blood pressure. Once treatment stops, blood pressure usually returns to normal.

Swollen or bleeding gums may occur with use of the estradiol, estropipate, and ethinyl estradiol. The latter also may cause excessive gum growth.

DRUG INTERACTIONS

Tell your health-care practitioner and pharmacist if you are taking any prescription or nonprescription drugs, as well as any vitamins, herbs, or other supplements. Possible drug interactions with estrogen may include the following:

- Ethotoin, mephenytoin, and phenytoin may interfere with the effects of estrogen.
- Estrogens may increase the side effects of antidepressants (e.g., amitriptyline, imipramine) and phenothiazine tranquilizers (e.g., chlorpromazine, promazine).
- Estrogens may reduce the effect of oral anticoagulants (e.g., warfarin), thyroid hormones, guanfacine, dextrothyroxine, and clofibrate.
- Estrogens may interfere with the effects of bromocriptine and tamoxifen.
- Anticonvulsants (e.g., clonazepam, felbamate), carbamazepine, primidone, and rifampin may decrease the effect of estrogen.
- Estrogens may decrease the effect of insulin and require dosage adjustments.
- Estrogens and oral antidiabetic drugs may cause sudden increases or decreases in blood sugar.
- Meprobamate may increase the effect of estrogens.

FOOD, VITAMIN, AND HERBAL INTERACTIONS

Grapefruit juice should be avoided while you are taking estrogen because it slows the body's normal breakdown of the drug, allowing it to accumulate to excessive levels in the blood and cause increased effects.

Vitamin C may increase the effect of estrogens, while estrogens may decrease the effects of vitamin B_6.

RECOMMENDED DOSAGE

Estrogens are available in tablets, skin patch, and vaginal cream. The dosages given here are typical. However, your health-care practitioner will determine the most appropriate dose and schedule for you.

Estradiol

- *Children:* not recommended
- *Adults:* for postmenopausal vaginal dryness or prevention of osteoporosis, take 1 to 2 mg daily, or apply 1 or 2 patches weekly, depending on the brand. For women who have not had a hysterectomy, progestin should be added to the treatment course for 10 to 14 days.

Conjugated Estrogens

- *Children:* not recommended
- *Adults:* dosing is in cycles, with progestin added 10 to 14 days, except for women who have had a hysterectomy. To prevent bone loss, 0.3 to 1.25 mg daily. To relieve menopausal symptoms, 0.625 to 1.25 mg daily

Ethinyl Estradiol

- *Children:* not recommended
- *Adults:* for menopausal symptoms, 0.02 to 0.05 mg daily. EstroGel is applied once daily, 1.25 g delivered in a metered dose pump.

Esterified Estrogens

- *Children:* not recommended
- *Adults:* for menopausal symptoms, 0.3 to 1.25 mg daily

Estropipate

- *Children:* not recommended
- *Adults:* for menopausal symptoms, 1.25 to 2.5 mg daily of the tablets; take for 3 weeks and then stop for 1 week.

Conjugated Estrogens/Medroxyprogesterone

- *Children:* not recommended
- *Adults:* 1 tablet daily

All forms of estrogen can be taken with food to help reduce stomach irritation.

If you miss a dose, take it as soon as you remember. If it is nearly time for your next dose, do not take the missed dose. Continue with your regular dosing schedule. Never take a double dose.

SYMPTOMS OF OVERDOSE AND WHAT TO DO

Symptoms of overdose may include nausea, unexpected vaginal bleeding, and vomiting. If overdose occurs, seek immediate medical assistance and bring the prescription container with you to the hospital.

SPECIAL INFORMATION FOR PREGNANT OR NURSING WOMEN

Estrogens used during pregnancy can cause birth defects. If you are pregnant or plan to become pregnant, talk to your health-care practitioner.

Estrogens should not be used while you are breastfeeding.

SPECIAL INFORMATION FOR SENIORS

No special precautions are needed for older adults.

GENERIC NAME

Estropipate *see Estrogens, page 436*

GENERIC NAME

Etanercept

BRAND NAME

Enbrel

No generic available

ABOUT THIS DRUG

Etanercept is a disease-modifying antirheumatic drug (DMARD) prescribed to reduce the signs and symptoms of moderate to severe rheumatoid arthritis. It is generally reserved for individuals who have not responded well to other antirheumatic drugs.

This drug is a tumor necrosis factor (TNF) antagonist, a substance that blocks the action of TNF, which is a naturally occurring protein that helps cause inflammation. Etanercept absorbs TNF and thus hinders its activity. It can be given along with methotrexate.

SIDE EFFECTS

Be sure to tell your health-care practitioner if you experience any side effects while taking etanercept. Only your health-care practitioner can determine whether it is safe for you to continue taking this drug.

- *Most Common:* itching, redness, swelling, or pain at the injection site, upper respiratory infection. About one-third of patients experience injection site reactions or infection
- *Less Common:* headache, dizziness, sore throat, cough, nasal congestion, general weakness, abdominal discomfort, rash, runny nose
- *Rare:* heart failure, myocardial infarction, high blood pressure, low blood pressure, gastrointestinal bleeding, depression, inflamed gallbladder, pancreatitis

IMPORTANT PRECAUTIONS

Tell your health-care practitioner if you are sensitive or allergic to etanercept or to any other drugs.

Etanercept has been associated with serious and fatal infections. Do not take etanercept if you have an active infection.

The needle cover of the syringe contains latex. People who are allergic to this substance should not handle the needle cover.

DRUG INTERACTIONS

Tell your health-care practitioner and pharmacist if you are taking any prescription or nonprescription drugs, as well as any vitamins, herbs, or other supplements. No specific drug interactions have been noted (see "Open Questions or Controversies").

FOOD, VITAMIN, AND HERBAL INTERACTIONS

No food, vitamin, or herbal interactions have been noted.

RECOMMENDED DOSAGE

Etanercept is available in injectable form only. The dosages given here are typical. However, your health-care practitioner will determine the most appropriate dose and schedule for you.

- *Children:* dose to be determined by your health-care practitioner
- *Adults:* 25 mg given by injection twice weekly. You can do self-injections once you have been properly instructed by a health professional.

If you miss a dose, take it as soon as you remember. If it is nearly time for your next dose, do not take the missed dose. Continue with your regular dosing schedule. Never take a double dose.

SYMPTOMS OF OVERDOSE AND WHAT TO DO

No cases of overdose with etanercept have been reported. If an overdose occurs, seek immediate medical attention and bring the prescription container with you to the hospital.

SPECIAL INFORMATION FOR PREGNANT OR NURSING WOMEN

No adequate studies of the effects of etanercept on pregnant or nursing women have been done. If you are pregnant or plan to become pregnant and this drug is crucial for your health, you and your health-care practitioner must weigh the potential benefits against the potential risks to the fetus.

Etanercept may pass into breast milk. If you are breastfeeding, your health-care practitioner may advise you to stop until your treatment is complete.

SPECIAL INFORMATION FOR SENIORS

No special precautions have been noted for older adults.

OPEN QUESTIONS OR CONTROVERSIES

Some studies suggest that people who take etanercept are at higher risk of developing autoantibodies, substances characteristic of autoimmune disease (e.g., lupus, scleroderma, multiple sclerosis). In October 2000, Immunex Corporation (makers of Enbrel) warned health-care practitioners and pharmacists about prescribing the drug to patients with rheumatoid arthritis who also had multiple sclerosis (MS), and to look for signs of serious anemia as well. This warning came after 11 cases of MS and MS-like diseases and 10 cases of serious anemia (five patients died) occurred within two years of Enbrel's release to market.

Postmarketing studies have revealed many cases of serious infections, some resulting in death (at least six), from etanercept. Many of these cases involved people who had underlying conditions, in addition to rheumatoid arthritis, that predisposed them to infection. In addition, a report in *Lancet* (2002; 359:579-80) found that use of etanercept may induce symptoms of lupus. The researchers report on four cases of lupus that appeared in women who had been taking etanercept for rheumatoid arthritis.

Because little postmarketing information about additional side effects and drug interactions associated with the use of etanercept was available at press time, you can stay abreast of any new information about the drug by contacting the FDA at 1-888-FDA-INFO or visiting their website: *www.fda.gov/default.htm*

GENERIC NAME
Ethinyl estradiol
see Estrogens, page 436

GENERIC NAME
Ethotoin
see Phenytoin, page 840

GENERIC NAME
Etidronate
see Bisphosphonates, page 200

GENERIC NAME
Etodolac

BRAND NAMES
Lodine, Lodine XL
Generic available

ABOUT THIS DRUG
Etodolac is a nonsteroidal anti-inflammatory drug (NSAID) prescribed primarily for treatment of mild-to-moderate pain and inflammation associated with osteoarthritis and rheumatoid arthritis, as well as bursitis, gout, migraine, menstrual cramps, soft tissue injuries, tendinitis, and other conditions.

SIDE EFFECTS
Be sure to tell your health-care practitioner if you experience any side effects while taking etodolac. Only your health-care practitioner can determine whether it is safe for you to continue taking this drug.

- ➤ *Most Common:* abdominal pain, black stools, blurred vision, chills, constipation, depression, diarrhea, dizziness, fever, gas, heartburn, itching, nausea, nervousness, rash, ringing in the ears, urinary difficulties, vomiting, weakness
- ➤ *Less Common or Rare:* anemia, blood disorders, congestive heart failure, dry mouth, fainting, hypersensitivity to light, flushing, hepatitis, high blood pressure, inflamed blood vessels, sleep disturbances, inflamed mouth or upper intestinal tract, kidney problems, peptic ulcer, stomach bleeding, rapid heartbeat, rash, skin disorders, peeling skin, sweating, fluid retention, thirst, visual problems, jaundice

IMPORTANT PRECAUTIONS

Tell your health-care practitioner if you are sensitive or allergic to etodolac or to any other drugs, or if you have ever had an allergic reaction (e.g., hives, asthma attacks, breathing difficulties) caused by aspirin or other nonsteroidal anti-inflammatory drugs.

Before using this drug, tell your health-care practitioner if you have liver or kidney problems, as this drug can cause serious liver inflammation, or if you have Parkinson's disease, diabetes, lupus, anemia, or epilepsy.

If you have heart disease or high blood pressure, this drug should be used with caution as it can cause fluid retention.

Avoid use of etodolac if you have active peptic ulcer disease, any other type of gastrointestinal bleeding or ulceration, severely impaired kidney function, or a bleeding disorder.

The safety and effectiveness of etodolac have not been determined for children.

DRUG INTERACTIONS

Tell your health-care practitioner and pharmacist if you are taking any prescription or nonprescription drugs, as well as any vitamins, herbs, or other supplements. Possible drug interactions with etodolac include the following:

- Aspirin and other NSAIDs pose a greater risk of stomach bleeding and stomach ulcers.
- Etodolac may decrease the effects of angiotensin-converting enzyme (ACE) inhibitors (e.g., captopril, enalapril), carteolol, diuretics (e.g., amiloride, indapamide), losartan, minoxidil, terazosin, and triamterene.
- Thyroid hormones may result in rapid heartbeat and a rise in blood pressure.
- Etodolac may increase the effects of lithium.
- Adrenocorticoids (e.g., cortisone, hydrocortisone) may result in an increased risk of ulcers and increased effects of adrenocorticoids.
- Cephalosporins (e.g., cefaclor, cefixime) and warfarin may cause an increased risk of bleeding.
- Etodolac may increase the side effects of methotrexate and meloxicam.
- Etodolac may increase the levels of cyclosporine and digoxin. Cyclosporine also increases the risk of cyclosporine-induced kidney toxicity.

FOOD, VITAMIN, AND HERBAL INTERACTIONS

Alfalfa, clove oil, cinchona bark, feverfew, garlic, ginseng, and ginkgo may affect blood clotting, so use of these herbs along with etodolac is not recommended.

RECOMMENDED DOSAGE

Etodolac is available in capsules (regular and extended-release) and tablets. The dosages given here are typical. However, your health-care practitioner will determine the most appropriate dose and schedule for you.

- *Children:* not recommended
- *Adults:* for osteoarthritis, starting dose is 400 mg 2 or 3 times daily, or 300 mg 3 or 4 times daily. For pain, starting dose is 400 mg, then 200 to 400 mg every 6 to 8 hours as needed.

Take etodolac with food to help reduce stomach irritation.

If you miss a dose, take it as soon as you remember. If it is nearly time for your next dose, do not take the missed dose. Continue with your regular dosing schedule. Never take a double dose.

SYMPTOMS OF OVERDOSE AND WHAT TO DO

Symptoms of overdose include drowsiness, lethargy, nausea, stomach pain, and vomiting. If overdose occurs, seek immediate medical attention and bring the prescription container with you to the hospital.

SPECIAL INFORMATION FOR PREGNANT OR NURSING WOMEN

No adequate studies of the effects of etodolac on pregnant or nursing women have been done; however, it should not be taken during the latter part of pregnancy because of possible damage to the fetus. If you are pregnant or plan to become pregnant and this drug is crucial for your health, you and your health-care practitioner must weigh the potential benefits against the potential risks to the fetus.

Etodolac may pass into breast milk. If you are breastfeeding, your health-care practitioner may advise you to stop until treatment is complete.

SPECIAL INFORMATION FOR SENIORS

Older adults often are prescribed lower doses because of the increased risk of gastrointestinal side effects.

GENERIC NAME

Exemestane

BRAND NAME

Aromasin

No generic available

ABOUT THIS DRUG

Exemestane is an antineoplastic (anticancer) drug prescribed for postmenopausal women who have advanced breast cancer that does not respond to tamoxifen.

This drug prevents the natural synthesis of estrogen, which stimulates breast cancer in many cases, by inactivating the enzyme aromatase, a key player in postmenopausal breast cancer.

SIDE EFFECTS

Be sure to tell your health-care practitioner if you experience any side effects while taking exemestane. Only your health-care practitioner can determine whether it is safe for you to continue taking this drug.

➤ *Most Common:* anxiety, insomnia, hot flashes, fatigue, depression, pain, shortness of breath

➤ *Less Common:* changes in appetite, cough, dizziness, diarrhea, abdominal pain, sweating, flulike symptoms, headache, vomiting, constipation, weight gain, cough, swollen feet, ankles, lower legs, and hands

IMPORTANT PRECAUTIONS

Tell your health-care practitioner if you are sensitive or allergic to exemestane or to any other drugs.

Exemestane can lower your white-blood-cell levels (the cells that fight infections), although no increase in infections have been seen in studies.

Before taking exemestane, tell your health-care practitioner if you have liver or kidney disease.

DRUG INTERACTIONS

Tell your health-care practitioner and pharmacist if you are taking any prescription or nonprescription drugs, as well as any vitamins, herbs, or other supplements. To date, the only significant drug interaction with exemestane is with estrogens, which may reduce the effect of exemestane.

FOOD, VITAMIN, AND HERBAL INTERACTIONS

No food, vitamin, or herbal interactions have been noted.

RECOMMENDED DOSAGE

Exemestane is available in tablets. The dosages given here are typical. However, your health-care practitioner will determine the most appropriate dose and schedule for you.

- *Children:* not applicable
- *Adults:* one 25-mg tablet daily

Exemestane should be taken after a meal.

Because exemestane is taken once daily, if you miss a dose, simply resume your regular dosing schedule the next day. Never take a double dose.

SYMPTOMS OF OVERDOSE AND WHAT TO DO

No overdose cases have been noted. If an overdose occurs, seek immediate medical attention and bring the prescription container with you to the hospital.

SPECIAL INFORMATION FOR PREGNANT OR NURSING WOMEN

Exemestane is for postmenopausal women, so use during pregnancy does not apply. However, it should be noted that this drug should not be used by pregnant women.

Use during breastfeeding does not apply.

SPECIAL INFORMATION FOR SENIORS

No special precautions are noted for older adults.

GENERIC NAME

Famciclovir

BRAND NAME

Famvir

No generic available

ABOUT THIS DRUG

Famciclovir is an antiviral medication prescribed to treat shingles (herpes zoster) and recurrent genital herpes. It treats the symptoms but does not cure these conditions.

This drug hinders the activity of certain enzymes that the viral cells need to reproduce DNA.

SIDE EFFECTS

Be sure to tell your health-care practitioner if you experience any side effects while taking famciclovir. Only your health-care practitioner can determine whether it is safe for you to continue taking this drug.

- *Most Common:* headache, nausea
- *Less Common:* confusion, diarrhea, vomiting, itching, rash, hallucinations, sore throat, joint or back pain, sinus infection, fever, chills

IMPORTANT PRECAUTIONS

Tell your health-care practitioner if you are sensitive or allergic to famciclovir or to any other drugs.

Famciclovir is most effective if used within 48 hours of the appearance of symptoms (pain, blisters, burning) of shingles, or within 6 hours of the appearance of symptoms (pain, blisters) of genital herpes. It may not be helpful if it is taken more than 72 hours after the first shingles symptoms appear, or more than 6 hours after symptoms of genital herpes appear.

Make sure you take the entire course of treatment even if you feel better before it is done.

The safety and effectiveness of famciclovir has not been determined for children younger than 18 years.

This drug should not be used if you have had a bone marrow transplant or a kidney transplant. If your immune system is compromised, talk to your health-care practitioner before taking famciclovir.

DRUG INTERACTIONS

Tell your health-care practitioner and pharmacist if you are taking any prescription or nonprescription drugs, as well as any vitamins, herbs, or other supplements. Possible drug interactions include the following:

- Digoxin blood levels may rise slightly.
- Probenecid may cause famciclovir blood levels to increase.

FOOD, VITAMIN, AND HERBAL INTERACTIONS

No food, vitamin, or herbal interactions have been noted.

RECOMMENDED DOSAGE

Famciclovir is available in tablets. The dosages given here are typical. However, your health-care practitioner will determine the most appropriate dose and schedule for you.

- *Children:* safety and effectiveness not determined for those younger than 18 years
- *Adults:* for shingles, 500 mg every 8 hours for 7 days. For recurrent genital herpes, 250 mg twice daily for up to 1 year.

If you miss a dose, take it as soon as you remember. If it is nearly time for your next dose, do not take the missed dose. Continue with your regular dosing schedule. Never take a double dose.

SYMPTOMS OF OVERDOSE AND WHAT TO DO

An overdose of famciclovir is unlikely. If an overdose occurs, seek immediate medical attention and bring the prescription container with you to the hospital.

SPECIAL INFORMATION FOR PREGNANT OR NURSING WOMEN

No adequate studies of the effects of famciclovir on pregnant or nursing women have been done. If you are pregnant or plan to become pregnant, you and your health-care practitioner must weigh the potential benefits against the potential risks to the fetus.

Famciclovir may pass into breast milk. If you are breastfeeding, your health-care practitioner may advise you to stop until your treatment is done.

SPECIAL INFORMATION FOR SENIORS

Older adults infrequently experience hallucinations, confusion, delirium, and disorientation.

GENERIC NAME

Famotidine

BRAND NAME

Pepcid

No generic available

ABOUT THIS DRUG

Famotidine is a histamine (H_2) blocker prescribed primarily for the short-term treatment of active peptic ulcers for 4 to 8 weeks, and for active gastric ulcers for 6 to 8 weeks. It is also prescribed for short-term treatment of gastroesophageal reflux disease (GERD), which is the backwash of stomach acid into the esophagus.

This drug blocks the action of histamine (which the body produces naturally), which in turn reduces the secretion of hydrochloric acid by the stomach. The reduction of stomach acid allows the body to better heal itself.

SIDE EFFECTS

Be sure to tell your health-care practitioner if you experience any side effects while taking famotidine. Only your health-care practitioner can determine whether it is safe for you to continue taking this drug.

- *Most Common:* abdominal pain, diarrhea, constipation, drowsiness, dizziness, fatigue, headache, nausea, vomiting
- *Less Common or Rare:* blurred vision, temporary hair loss, hallucinations, depression, insomnia, rash, hives, reduced sexual desire or function, palpitations, slowed heartbeat, unusual bleeding, fever, chills, increased susceptibility to infection

IMPORTANT PRECAUTIONS

Tell your health-care practitioner if you are sensitive or allergic to famotidine, other histamine blockers, or any other drugs.

You must take this drug for the entire treatment course, even if you feel better before it is done.

Before starting famotidine, tell your health-care practitioner if you have stomach cancer or severe kidney disease.

If you have phenylketonuria (a hereditary disease in which brain damage may occur), note that the orally disintegrating tablets contain phenylalanine.

Because famotidine can cause dizziness and drowsiness, make sure you know how you react to the drug before you drive or operate dangerous equipment.

Do not take this drug for more than 8 weeks unless your health-care practitioner prescribes it.

DRUG INTERACTIONS

Tell your health-care practitioner and pharmacist if you are taking any prescription or nonprescription drugs, as well as any vitamins, herbs, or other supplements.

FOOD, VITAMIN, AND HERBAL INTERACTIONS

Foods and beverages that may interfere with the effectiveness of famotidine include caffeine, carbonated drinks, citrus fruits and juices, and any acidic foods or liquids that irritate the stomach (e.g., tomatoes, tomato juice).

RECOMMENDED DOSAGE

Famotidine is available in tablets, powder for suspension, and orally disintegrating and chewable tablets. The dosages given here are typical. However, your health-care practitioner will determine the most appropriate dose and schedule for you.

- *Children 1 to 16 Years:* for peptic ulcer, 0.5 mg per 2.2 pounds of body weight. It can be taken as one dose at bedtime or two smaller doses. Do not exceed 40 mg daily. For GERD, 1 mg per 2.2 pounds of body weight, given in 2 doses. Do not exceed 40 mg daily
- *Adults:* for duodenal ulcer, starting dose is 40 mg or 5 ml once daily at bedtime. Your health-care practitioner may change your dose to 20 mg or 2.5 ml twice a day. For benign gastric ulcer, 40 mg or 5 ml once at bedtime. For GERD, 20 mg or 2.5 ml twice daily for up to 5 weeks.

If you are using the oral suspension, shake it well for 10 seconds before use. The disintegrating tablets do not require water; they dissolve immediately on your tongue. The chewable tablets can be taken with water. All forms can be taken with food to help minimize stomach irritation.

If you miss a dose, take it as soon as you remember. If it is nearly time for your next dose, do not take the missed dose. Continue with your regular dosing schedule. Never take a double dose.

SYMPTOMS OF OVERDOSE AND WHAT TO DO

Symptoms of overdose include confusion, slurred speech, difficulty breathing, delirium, and rapid heartbeat. If overdose occurs, seek immediate medical attention and bring the prescription container with you to the hospital.

SPECIAL INFORMATION FOR PREGNANT OR NURSING WOMEN

No adequate studies of the effects of famotidine on pregnant or nursing women have been done. If you are pregnant or plan to become pregnant, you and your health-care practitioner must weigh the potential benefits against the potential risks to the fetus.

Famotidine may pass into breast milk. If you are breastfeeding, your health-care practitioner may advise you to stop until you complete treatment.

SPECIAL INFORMATION FOR SENIORS

Older adults are more likely to experience side effects, and they may be more severe.

GENERIC NAME

Felbamate

BRAND NAME

Felbatol
No generic available

ABOUT THIS DRUG

Felbamate is an anticonvulsant prescribed to control certain types of seizures associated with epilepsy or other seizure disorders. Because it has a high rate of potentially deadly side effects, it is used only for individuals who do not respond to other seizure control medications.

This drug suppresses the activity of specific parts of the brain and the abnormal firing of neurons that cause seizures.

SIDE EFFECTS

Be sure to tell your health-care practitioner if you experience any side effects while taking felbamate. Only your health-care practitioner can determine whether it is safe for you to continue taking this drug.

- *Most Common:* loss of appetite, headache, nausea, vomiting, stomach upset, constipation, insomnia, dizziness, drowsiness, anxiety, nervousness, tremor, muscle incoordination, runny nose, upper respiratory tract infections
- *Less Common:* cough, diarrhea, abdominal pain, dry mouth, blurred or double vision
- *Rare:* fever, weakness, sore throat, swollen glands, unusual bruising, blisters, jaundice, and tiny purple or red spots on the skin may indicate liver problems, aplastic anemia, or other potentially life-threatening conditions. Call your health-care practitioner immediately.

IMPORTANT PRECAUTIONS

Tell your health-care practitioner if you are sensitive or allergic to felbamate or to any other drugs.

Because this drug causes drowsiness and dizziness, make sure you know how you react to it before you drive or operate dangerous equipment.

Before taking felbamate, tell your health-care practitioner if you have a history of any blood condition, bone marrow depression (which causes anemia), or liver disease.

DRUG INTERACTIONS

Tell your health-care practitioner and pharmacist if you are taking any prescription or nonprescription drugs, as well as any vitamins, herbs, or other supplements. Possible drug interactions include the following:

- Carbamazepine, phenytoin, and valproic acid may cause increased side effects.
- Check with your health-care practitioner before combining felbamate with other anticonvulsant drugs (e.g., phenobarbital, clonazepam).

FOOD, VITAMIN, AND HERBAL INTERACTIONS

Herbs that produce a sedative effect may cause significant depressant interactions when used with felbamate. Some of those herbs include calendula, capsicum, catnip, goldenseal, gotu kola, hops, kava, lady's slipper, passionflower, sage, Siberian ginseng, skullcap, St. John's wort, and valerian, among others.

RECOMMENDED DOSAGE

Felbamate is available in tablets and oral suspension. The dosages given here are typical. However, your health-care practitioner will determine the most appropriate dose and schedule for you.

- *Children 2 to 14 Years:* 15 mg per 2.2 pounds of body weight daily in divided smaller does (3 to 4 times daily). Your health-care practitioner may gradually increase the dose to 45 mg per 2.2 pounds of body weight daily.
- *Children 14 Years and Older and Adults:* starting dose is 1,200 mg daily, divided into 3 to 4 doses. Your health-care practitioner may gradually increase the dose up to 3,600 mg daily.

Take felbamate with food to reduce stomach irritation.

If you miss a dose, take it as soon as you remember. If it is nearly time for your next dose, do not take the missed dose. Continue with your regular dosing schedule. Never take a double dose.

SYMPTOMS OF OVERDOSE AND WHAT TO DO

Symptoms of overdose include gastric upset and increased heart rate. If an overdose occurs, seek immediate medical attention and bring the prescription container with you to the hospital.

SPECIAL INFORMATION FOR PREGNANT OR NURSING WOMEN

No adequate studies of the effects of felbamate on pregnant or nursing women have been done. If you are pregnant or plan to become pregnant, you and your health-care practitioner must weigh the potential benefits against the potential risks to the fetus.

Felbamate passes into breast milk. If you are breastfeeding, your health-care practitioner may advise you to stop breastfeeding until your treatment is complete.

SPECIAL INFORMATION FOR SENIORS

Older adults may need lower doses to help minimize side effects.

GENERIC NAME

Felodipine

BRAND NAME

Plendil

No generic available

ABOUT THIS DRUG

Felodipine is a calcium channel blocker that is prescribed to treat high blood pressure. It can be used alone or along with other medications for high blood pressure. It is also prescribed to help prevent angina (chest pain).

Like other calcium channel blockers, felodipine interferes with the movement of calcium into heart muscle, which in turn relaxes the blood vessels and reduces heart rate. It also results in a lowering of blood pressure and reduced chest pain.

SIDE EFFECTS

Be sure to tell your health-care practitioner if you experience any side effects while taking felodipine. Only your health-care practitioner can determine whether it is safe for you to continue taking this drug.

➤ *Most Common:* headache, flushing, swelling of the feet and legs

- *Less Common or Rare:* chest pain, palpitations, dizziness, numbness or tingling sensation, rapid pulse, sore throat, abdominal discomfort, nausea, constipation, diarrhea, cough, muscle cramps, back pain, overgrowth of the gums, low blood pressure, irregular heartbeat, weakness

IMPORTANT PRECAUTIONS

Tell your health-care practitioner if you are sensitive or allergic to felodipine, other calcium channel blockers, or any other drugs.

When taking felodipine for high blood pressure, it is only effective if you take it regularly. Do not stop taking it when you feel better: this drug controls high blood pressure but does not cure it.

Before taking felodipine, tell your health-care practitioner if you have congestive heart failure, a history of heart attack or stroke, heart rhythm disturbances, or liver or kidney impairment, or if you are taking any drugs that lower blood pressure.

Felodipine may cause your blood pressure to drop too low. If you feel faint or lightheaded, your heart begins to race, or you have chest pain, contact your health-care practitioner immediately.

Do not take felodipine if you have active liver disease, uncorrected congestive heart failure, severe dysfunction in the left side of your heart, atrioventricular blockage, or sick sinus syndrome.

DRUG INTERACTIONS

Tell your health-care practitioner and pharmacist if you are taking any prescription or nonprescription drugs, as well as any vitamins, herbs, or other supplements. Possible drug interactions include the following:

- Nonsteroidal anti-inflammatory drugs (NSAIDs; e.g., ibuprofen, etodolac) and anticoagulants (e.g., warfarin) may increase the risk of gastrointestinal bleeding.
- Beta-blockers (e.g., nadolol, propranolol) and digitalis preparations may cause heart rate and heart rhythm problems.
- Delavirdine, itraconazole, fluconazole, or ketoconazole may lead to felodipine toxicity.
- Phenobarbital, rifampin, and carbamazepine may decrease felodipine's benefits.
- Cyclosporine may change the blood levels of either drug.
- Digoxin may result in digoxin toxicity.
- Phenytoin and theophylline may cause decreased levels of each of these drugs.
- Cimetidine and erythromycin may increase the effects of felodipine.

FOOD, VITAMIN, AND HERBAL INTERACTIONS

Avoid herbs that can increase blood pressure, including ginseng, goldenseal, ephedra (ma huang), licorice, and saw palmetto. Calcium and garlic can be beneficial as they help lower blood pressure. Be sure to talk to your health-care practitioner before taking these supplements.

Do not take felodipine with grapefruit juice because the effects of the drug can double.

RECOMMENDED DOSAGE

Felodipine is available in tablets. The dosages given here are typical. However, your health-care practitioner will determine the most appropriate dose and schedule for you.

- *Children:* not recommended
- *Adults:* starting dose is 5 to 10 mg once daily. Your health-care practitioner may increase the dose to a maximum of 20 mg once daily.
- *Adults Older than 65:* starting dose is 2.5 mg daily, to a maximum of 10 mg daily

Felodipine can be taken on an empty stomach or with a light meal.

If you miss a dose, take it as soon as you remember. If it is nearly time for your next dose, do not take the missed dose. Continue with your regular dosing schedule. Never take a double dose.

SYMPTOMS OF OVERDOSE AND WHAT TO DO

Symptoms of overdose include very low blood pressure, shortness of breath, weakness, lightheadedness, rapid pulse, fainting, slurred speech, tremors, and flushed skin. If overdose occurs, seek immediate medical attention and bring the prescription container with you to the hospital.

SPECIAL INFORMATION FOR PREGNANT OR NURSING WOMEN

No adequate studies of the effects of felodipine on pregnant or nursing women have been done, although animal studies have shown birth defects. If you are pregnant or plan to become pregnant, you and your health-care practitioner must weigh the potential benefits against the potential risks to the fetus.

Felodipine may pass into breast milk. If you are breastfeeding, your health-care practitioner may advise you to stop until your treatment is complete.

SPECIAL INFORMATION FOR SENIORS
Older adults are given lower doses, and their blood pressure should be monitored regularly by their health-care practitioner.

GENERIC NAME
Fenofibrate

BRAND NAME
Tricor
No generic available

ABOUT THIS DRUG
Fenofibrate is an antilipidemic (triglyceride-lowering drug) that is prescribed to treat high levels of triglycerides, fatty substances in the blood. Triglycerides play a significant role in causing heart disease.

Fenofibrate inhibits the formation of triglycerides, which helps prevent heart disease and high blood pressure.

SIDE EFFECTS
Be sure to tell your health-care practitioner if you experience any side effects while taking fenofibrate. Only your health-care practitioner can determine whether it is safe for you to continue taking this drug.

- *Most Common:* rash, flulike symptoms, infection
- *Less Common or Rare:* belching, flatulence, nausea, vomiting, constipation, dizziness, nasal congestion, itching, irritated eyes, visual problems, headache, fatigue, decreased libido, fever, unusual muscle aches and tenderness, irregular heartbeat, angina

IMPORTANT PRECAUTIONS
Tell your health-care practitioner if you are sensitive or allergic to fenofibrate or to any other drugs.

Do not take fenofibrate if you have serious liver disease.

Before taking fenofibrate, talk to your health-care practitioner if you have had liver or kidney disease, peptic ulcer disease, diabetes, or gallbladder disease or gallstones.

Prolonged use of fenofibrate may cause gallbladder infection or possibly stomach cancer.

Fenofibrate may make you hypersensitive to sunlight. Protect yourself by wearing sunscreen and protective clothing.

DRUG INTERACTIONS

Tell your health-care practitioner and pharmacist if you are taking any prescription or nonprescription drugs, as well as any vitamins, herbs, or other supplements. Possible drug interactions include the following:

- Fenofibrate may increase the effects of anticoagulants (e.g., warfarin), oral antidiabetic drugs (e.g., glyburide, glipizide), and insulin.
- Oral contraceptives and estrogens may decrease the effect of fenofibrate.
- Cyclosporine may cause kidney problems or make them worse.
- Fenofibrate may reduce the effect of desmopressin and ursodiol.
- Probenecid may lead to an increased effect and toxicity of fenofibrate.
- Thyroid hormones may increase the effect of fenofibrate.

FOOD, VITAMIN, AND HERBAL INTERACTIONS

Fatty foods may decrease the effect of fenofibrate.

RECOMMENDED DOSAGE

Fenofibrate is available in 67-mg capsules. The dosages given here are typical. However, your health-care practitioner will determine the most appropriate dose and schedule for you.

- *Children:* Safety and effectiveness have not been established for children younger than 18 years.
- *Adults:* 67 mg once daily. Your health-care practitioner may increase your dose; daily maximum is 201 mg.

If you miss a dose one day, do not double up the next day. Return to your regular dosing schedule.

SYMPTOMS OF OVERDOSE AND WHAT TO DO

Symptoms of overdose include diarrhea, muscle pain, and headache. If overdose occurs, seek immediate medical attention and bring the prescription container with you to the hospital.

SPECIAL INFORMATION FOR PREGNANT OR NURSING WOMEN

No adequate studies of the effects of fenofibrate on pregnant or nursing women have been done. If you are pregnant or plan to become pregnant, and this drug is crucial for your health, you and your health-care practitioner must weigh the potential benefits against the potential risks to the fetus.

Fenofibrate may harm the nursing child. If you are breastfeeding, your health-care practitioner will advise you to stop until your treatment is complete.

SPECIAL INFORMATION FOR SENIORS

Older individuals are more likely to experience side effects, and they may be more severe. They also may develop flulike symptoms.

GENERIC NAME

Fenoprofen *see Propionic Acid (NSAID) Family, page 880*

GENERIC NAME

Fexofenadine *see Antihistamine-Decongestant Combination, page 132*

GENERIC NAME

Finasteride

BRAND NAMES

Propecia, Proscar

No generic available

ABOUT THIS DRUG

Finasteride is prescribed for the treatment of benign prostatic hyperplasia, a noncancerous enlargement of the prostate gland in men. It is also taken to treat male pattern baldness. This drug belongs to a class known as dihydrotestosterone inhibitors.

Finasteride inhibits the activity of an enzyme that is required for the conversion of testosterone to dihydrotestosterone, a compound that is needed for the development of benign prostatic hyperplasia.

SIDE EFFECTS

Be sure to tell your health-care practitioner if you experience any side effects while taking finasteride. Only your health-care practitioner can determine whether it is safe for you to continue taking this drug.

- *Less Common:* back or stomach pain, headache, decreased volume of ejaculation
- *Rare:* impotence, breast enlargement and tenderness, allergic reaction (rash, swollen lips)

IMPORTANT PRECAUTIONS

Tell your health-care practitioner if you are sensitive or allergic to finasteride or any other drugs.

Before taking finasteride, tell your health-care practitioner if you have a liver disorder or reduced urinary flow, or if your sexual partner is pregnant or may become pregnant.

Finasteride is not intended for women or children.

Before taking finasteride, men should undergo a digital rectal examination and other screening tests for prostate cancer. This drug may alter the results of the prostate-specific antigen (PSA) test for prostate cancer.

DRUG INTERACTIONS

Tell your health-care practitioner and pharmacist if you are taking any prescription or nonprescription drugs, as well as any vitamins, herbs, or other supplements. No significant drug interactions have been reported.

FOOD, VITAMIN, AND HERBAL INTERACTIONS

The herb saw palmetto has anti-inflammatory and anti-androgenic (male hormones, such as testosterone) actions and is used by some men to treat benign prostatic hyperplasia and maintain prostate health. Although saw palmetto and finasteride have not been studied together, you should talk to your health-care practitioner before you decide to take both the herb and the drug.

RECOMMENDED DOSAGE

Finasteride is available in tablets. The dosages given here are typical. However, your health-care practitioner will determine the most appropriate dose and schedule for you.

- *Children:* not indicated
- *Adults:* for benign prostatic hyperplasia, 5 mg once daily; for hair loss, 1 mg once daily.

Finasteride can be taken with or without food. If you cannot swallow the tablet, it can be crushed and taken with liquid or food.

If you miss a dose, take it as soon as you remember. If it is nearly time for your next dose, do not take the missed dose. Continue with your regular dosing schedule. Never take a double dose.

SYMPTOMS OF OVERDOSE AND WHAT TO DO

No symptoms of overdose have been reported. If overdose occurs, seek immediate medical assistance and bring the prescription container with you to the hospital.

SPECIAL INFORMATION FOR PREGNANT OR NURSING WOMEN

Finasteride is not intended for women. However, women who are pregnant or plan to become pregnant should not touch the medication, especially if it has been crushed, because it can be absorbed by the skin and can affect the fetus. Men who are taking finasteride should wear a condom to prevent the small amount of the drug found in the semen from making contact with their sexual partner.

Women who are breastfeeding should avoid touching finasteride and avoid exposure to the semen of men who are taking the drug.

SPECIAL INFORMATION FOR SENIORS

No special precautions are needed for older adults.

GENERIC NAME

Flecainide

BRAND NAME

Tambocor
No generic available

ABOUT THIS DRUG

Flecainide is an antiarrhythmic drug prescribed for individuals who have an irregular heartbeat (cardiac arrhythmia).

This drug slows nerve signals in the heart and makes the heart less sensitive to those signals.

SIDE EFFECTS

Be sure to tell your health-care practitioner if you experience any side effects while taking flecainide. Only your health-care practitioner can determine whether it is safe for you to continue taking this drug.

➤ *Most Common:* headache, blurred vision or other visual disturbances, dizziness, lightheadedness

- *Less Common:* nausea, constipation, tremor, fatigue, abdominal pain, swollen hands, rash, anxiety, depression

IMPORTANT PRECAUTIONS

Tell your health-care practitioner if you are sensitive or allergic to flecainide or to any other drugs.

Before you take flecainide, tell your health-care practitioner if you have heart disease, heart block, a slow heart rate, or liver or kidney disease.

Because flecainide causes dizziness and blurred vision, make sure you know how you react to this drug before you drive or operate dangerous equipment.

Take flecainide for the entire treatment course, even if you feel better before it is complete.

DRUG INTERACTIONS

Tell your health-care practitioner and pharmacist if you are taking any prescription or nonprescription drugs, as well as any vitamins, herbs, or other supplements. Possible drug interactions include the following:

- Alcohol can further suppress heart function.
- Antacids (e.g., Maalox, Mylanta), cimetidine, and sodium bicarbonate may increase the effect of flecainide.
- Other antiarrhythmic drugs may cause irregular heartbeat.
- Flecainide may increase the effect of digitalis.
- Verapamil may cause decreased efficiency of heart muscle contraction, which may lead to congestive heart failure.
- Propafenone may cause an increased effect of both drugs and a greater risk of toxicity.
- Paroxetine may cause an increased effect of both drugs.

FOOD, VITAMIN, AND HERBAL INTERACTIONS

Beverages containing caffeine should be avoided because they may decrease the effect of flecainide.

RECOMMENDED DOSAGE

Flecainide is available in tablets. The dosages given here are typical. However, your health-care practitioner will determine the most appropriate dose and schedule for you.

- *Children:* not recommended for children younger than 18 years
- *Adults:* for potentially fatal arrhythmias, starting dose is 100 mg every 12 hours, increased by 50 mg every 4 days if necessary. The maximum is 200 mg every 12 hours.

Flecainide tablets should be taken with liquid, and can also be taken with or between meals.

If you miss a dose, take it as soon as you remember. If it is nearly time for your next dose, do not take the missed dose. Continue with your regular dosing schedule. Never take a double dose.

SYMPTOMS OF OVERDOSE AND WHAT TO DO

Symptoms of overdose include dizziness, fainting, rapid or irregular heartbeat, unusual sweating, drowsiness, tremor, and loss of consciousness. If overdose occurs, seek immediate medical attention and bring the prescription container with you to the hospital.

SPECIAL INFORMATION FOR PREGNANT OR NURSING WOMEN

No adequate studies of the effects of flecainide on pregnant or nursing women have been done. In animal studies, however, large doses have caused birth defects. If you are pregnant or plan to become pregnant and this drug is crucial for your health, you and your health-care practitioner must weigh the potential benefits against the potential risks to the fetus.

Flecainide passes into breast milk and may harm your infant. If you are breastfeeding, your health-care practitioner will advise you to stop until your treatment is complete.

SPECIAL INFORMATION FOR SENIORS

Older adults are more likely to experience side effects, especially heartbeat irregularities.

GENERIC NAME

Fluconazole

BRAND NAME

Diflucan

No generic available

ABOUT THIS DRUG

Fluconazole is an antifungal medication prescribed to treat fungal infections of the throat (thrush), mouth, vagina (yeast infection), or elsewhere in the body.

This drug prevents fungal organisms from producing substances they need to grow and reproduce. This medication is effective against fungi only; bacteria and viruses are not effected.

SIDE EFFECTS

Be sure to tell your health-care practitioner if you experience any side effects while taking fluconazole. Only your health-care practitioner can determine whether it is safe for you to continue taking this drug.

- *Less Common:* constipation, dizziness, diarrhea, nausea, vomiting, headache, red or flushed skin, fever, chills, rash

IMPORTANT PRECAUTIONS

Tell your health-care practitioner if you are sensitive or allergic to fluconazole or to any other drugs.

Take fluconazole for the entire course of treatment, even if you feel better before you are done.

If your condition does not improve within a few weeks, or it becomes worse, contact your health-care practitioner.

Before starting fluconazole, tell your health-care practitioner if you have a history of alcohol abuse or any type of liver or kidney disease.

DRUG INTERACTIONS

Tell your health-care practitioner and pharmacist if you are taking any prescription or nonprescription drugs, as well as any vitamins, herbs, or other supplements. Possible drug interactions include the following:

- Fluconazole may increase the effects of benzodiazepines (e.g., diazepam, clonazepam), oral antidiabetic drugs (e.g., glyburide, glipizide), cyclosporine, phenytoin, triazolam, tricyclic antidepressants (e.g., amitriptyline, imipramine), trimetrexate, warfarin, and zidovudine.
- Cimetidine and rifampin may decrease the effects of fluconazole.
- Amphotericin B may decrease this drug's benefits.
- Atorvastatin and possibly other similar drugs (e.g., fluvastatin, lovastatin) may increase muscle toxicity.

- Hydrochlorothiazide may increase potassium loss.
- Loratadine may result in elevated levels of loratadine. Dose adjustments of loratadine may be needed.
- Losartan may suppress blood pressure control.
- Oral contraceptives may not be effective and pregnancy may result.

FOOD, VITAMIN, AND HERBAL INTERACTIONS

Do not eat grapefruit for an hour after taking fluconazole, and do not take this medication with grapefruit juice.

RECOMMENDED DOSAGE

Fluconazole is available in tablets and oral suspension. The dosages given here are typical. However, your health-care practitioner will determine the most appropriate dose and schedule for you.

- *Children Younger than 14 Years:* not usually prescribed for those younger than 14 years
- *Children 14 Years and Older and Adults:* for fungal infection, 200 to 400 mg on day 1, then 100 to 400 mg once daily. For vaginal infection, 150 mg taken once

Tablets should be taken with liquid. The oral suspension should be shaken before use.

If you miss a dose, take it as soon as you remember. If it is nearly time for your next dose, do not take the missed dose. Continue with your regular dosing schedule. Never take a double dose.

SYMPTOMS OF OVERDOSE AND WHAT TO DO

Symptoms of overdose include nausea, vomiting, and diarrhea. If overdose occurs, seek immediate medical attention and bring the prescription container with you to the hospital.

SPECIAL INFORMATION FOR PREGNANT OR NURSING WOMEN

No adequate studies of the effects of fluconazole on pregnant or nursing women have been done. Abnormalities in bone growth have been seen in animal studies. If you are pregnant or plan to become pregnant, you and your health-care practitioner must weigh the potential benefits against the potential risks to the fetus.

Fluconazole may pass into breast milk. If you are breastfeeding, your health-care practitioner may advise you to stop until your treatment is complete.

SPECIAL INFORMATION FOR SENIORS

Older adults who have reduced kidney function may need a dose adjustment.

GENERIC NAME

Flucytosine

BRAND NAME

Ancobon

No generic available

ABOUT THIS DRUG

Flucytosine is an antifungal drug prescribed to treat general fungal infection as well as severe infections of the bone and bone marrow, the protective covering of the brain (meningitis), the blood (septicemia), the respiratory tract (pneumonia), and the genitourinary tract.

This drug prevents the synthesis of genetic material by infectious organisms, which thus prevents the cells from reproducing.

SIDE EFFECTS

Be sure to tell your health-care practitioner if you experience any side effects while taking flucytosine. Only your health-care practitioner can determine whether it is safe for you to continue taking this drug.

- *Most Common:* abdominal pain, nausea, vomiting, diarrhea, loss of appetite
- *Less Common or Rare:* dizziness, headache, unusual drowsiness, unusual fatigue, jaundice, unusual bleeding or bruising, rash, sore throat, fever, hypersensitivity to light, confusion, hallucinations

IMPORTANT PRECAUTIONS

Tell your health-care practitioner if you are sensitive or allergic to flucytosine or to any other drugs.

Flucytosine make you hypersensitive to sunlight, so protect yourself by wearing sunscreen and protective clothing.

Take this drug for the entire treatment course, even if you feel better before treatment is scheduled to end.

Do not take flucytosine if you have an active blood cell or bone marrow disorder or active liver disease.

Before taking flucytosine, tell your health-care practitioner if you have impaired liver or kidney function, a history of peripheral neuritis (nerve inflammation), a blood disease, or drug-induced bone marrow depression.

Flucytosine may cause blood problems, which can lead to an increased risk of infection, bleeding gums, and slow healing.

DRUG INTERACTIONS

Tell your health-care practitioner and pharmacist if you are taking any prescription or nonprescription drugs, as well as any vitamins, herbs, or other supplements. Possible drug interactions include the following:

- Amphotericin B, antineoplastics (e.g., cyclophosphamide, methotrexate), antithyroid drugs, azathioprine, chloramphenicol, colchicine, ganciclovir, interferon, plicamycin, and zidovudine may increase the chance of side effects in the blood.

FOOD, VITAMIN, AND HERBAL INTERACTIONS

Avoid the herb St. John's wort, because it, along with flucytosine, can cause increased sensitivity to sunlight.

RECOMMENDED DOSAGE

Flucytosine is available in capsules. The dosages given here are typical. However, your health-care practitioner will determine the most appropriate dose and schedule for you.

- *Children and Adults:* 12.5 to 37.5 mg per 2.2 pounds of body weight every 6 hours

If you miss a dose, take it as soon as you remember. If it is nearly time for your next dose, do not take the missed dose. Continue with your regular dosing schedule. Never take a double dose.

SYMPTOMS OF OVERDOSE AND WHAT TO DO

Symptoms of overdose include severe nausea, vomiting, abdominal pain, confusion, and diarrhea. If overdose occurs, seek immediate medical attention and bring the prescription container with you to the hospital.

SPECIAL INFORMATION FOR PREGNANT OR NURSING WOMEN

No adequate studies of the effects of flucytosine on pregnant or nursing women have been done. If you are pregnant or plan to become pregnant, you and your health-care practitioner must weigh the potential benefits against the potential risks to the fetus.

Flucytosine may pass into breast milk. If you are breastfeeding, your health-care practitioner will likely advise you to stop until your treatment is complete.

SPECIAL INFORMATION FOR SENIORS

Older adults who have impaired kidney function may need a reduced dosage.

GENERIC NAME

Flunisolide

see Corticosteroids, Nasal Inhalation, page 327; Corticosteroids, Oral Inhalers, page 334

GENERIC NAME

Fluocinolone acetonide

see Corticosteroids, Topical, page 337

GENERIC NAME

Fluocinonide

see Corticosteroids, Topical, page 337

GENERIC NAME

Class: Fluoroquinolone antibiotics

Generics: (1) ciprofloxacin; (2) enoxacin; (3) gatifloxacin; (4) levofloxacin; (5) lomefloxacin; (6) moxifloxacin; (7) norfloxacin; (8) ofloxacin; (9) sparfloxacin

BRAND NAMES

(1) Cipro; (2) Penetrex; (3) Tequin; (4) Levaquin; (5) Maxaquin; (6) Avelox; (7) Noroxin; (8) Floxin; (9) Zagam

No generic available

ABOUT THIS DRUG

Fluoroquinolone antibiotics are prescribed to treat bacterial infections, including those that affect the urinary tract, upper respiratory tract, skin, bones, and joints.

The fluoroquinolone antibiotics inhibit the activity of gyrase, an enzyme that is necessary for DNA formation and reproduction. Thus these drugs prevent the bacteria cells from reproducing.

SIDE EFFECTS

Be sure to tell your health-care practitioner if you experience any side effects while taking fluoroquinolone antibiotics. Only your health-care practitioner can determine whether it is safe for you to continue taking this drug.

- *Most Common:* blisters, burning, sunburn, and itching skin when exposed to the sun
- *Less Common:* dizziness, lightheadedness, headache, nervousness, drowsiness, stomach pain, nausea, vomiting, taste changes, vaginal itching, diarrhea
- *Rare:* agitation, confusion, shortness of breath, neck or face swelling, bloody or cloudy urine, swollen legs or feet, seizures

IMPORTANT PRECAUTIONS

Tell your health-care practitioner if you are sensitive or allergic to fluoroquinolones or quinolone derivatives, or to any other drugs.

Before you take any of the fluoroquinolone antibiotics, tell your health-care practitioner if you have liver or kidney disease or any disorder of the central nervous system (e.g., stroke, epilepsy).

If you have kidney problems, your health-care practitioner will need to adjust your dosage.

Levofloxacin can cause changes in blood sugar levels in people who have diabetes.

Gatifloxacin, moxifloxacin, and sparfloxacin may make heart conditions worse.

Fluoroquinolones may increase the risk of tendon injury.

Some fluoroquinolones cause rash or intense sunburn in some individuals. When taking any of these drugs, avoid overexposure to the sun and protect yourself with sunscreen and protective clothing.

Fluoroquinolones are not recommended for people younger than 18 years because they can interfere with bone development.

DRUG INTERACTIONS

Tell your health-care practitioner and pharmacist if you are taking any prescription or nonprescription drugs, as well as any vitamins, herbs, or other supplements. Possible drug interactions include the following:

- Ciprofloxacin, enoxacin, and norfloxacin may increase the chance of side effects of aminophylline, oxtriphylline, and theophylline.
- Gatifloxacin, levofloxacin, moxifloxacin, and sparfloxacin may cause heart problems if taken with amiodarone, astemizole, bepridil, disopyramide, erythromycin, pentamidine, phenothiazines (e.g., chlorpromazine, perphenazine), procainamide, quinidine, sotalol, and tricyclic antidepressants (e.g., amitriptyline, doxepin).
- Antacids, didanosine, and sucralfate may prevent fluoroquinolones from working effectively.
- Ciprofloxacin may prevent phenytoin from working effectively.
- Ciprofloxacin and norfloxacin may increase the effect of warfarin and increase bleeding.

FOOD, VITAMIN, AND HERBAL INTERACTIONS

Dairy foods may reduce the effect of fluoroquinolones. To prevent this reaction, consume dairy products as far apart as possible from your drug dose, or avoid them altogether. Consumption of caffeine-containing beverages may result in an increased effect of caffeine.

The herb fennel can reduce blood levels of ciprofloxacin and may make the drug less effective. Fennel may also interact with other fluoroquinolones in the same way.

The minerals calcium, iron, and zinc may interfere with the absorption of some fluoroquinolones. To avoid this situation, take these supplements as far before or after your drug dose as possible.

RECOMMENDED DOSAGE

Fluoroquinolones are available as tablets, eye drops, and oral suspension. The dosages given here are typical. However, your health-care practitioner will determine the most appropriate dose and schedule for you. Some fluoroquinolones are prescribed to treat more specific conditions than are others.

Ciprofloxacin

- *Children:* not recommended for persons younger than 18 years
- *Adults:* 250 to 750 mg every 12 hours for 5 to 14 days, depending on the infection being treated

Enoxacin

- *Children:* not recommended for persons younger than 18 years
- *Adults:* 200 to 400 mg every 12 hours for 7 to 14 days, depending on the severity of the urinary tract infection. For gonorrhea, 400 mg in one dose

Gatifloxacin

- *Children:* not recommended for persons younger than 18 years
- *Adults:* for most infections, 400 mg once daily for 7 to 10 days. For uncomplicated urinary tract infections, 400 mg as a single dose or 200 mg once daily for 3 days

Levofloxacin

- *Children:* not recommended for persons younger than 18 years
- *Adults:* 250 to 500 mg once daily for 7 to 14 days

Lomefloxacin

- *Children:* not recommended for persons younger than 18 years
- *Adults:* 400 mg once daily for 10 to 14 days, depending on the infection. To help prevent infections presurgically, 400 mg 2 to 6 hours before surgery

Moxifloxacin

- *Children:* not recommended for persons younger than 18 years
- *Adults:* for acute sinusitis or community-acquired pneumonia, 400 mg once daily for 10 days. For acute bacterial complications associated with chronic bronchitis, 400 mg once daily for 5 days

Norfloxacin

- *Children:* not recommended for persons younger than 18 years
- *Adults:* for urinary tract infections, 400 mg twice daily for 3 to 21 days. For sexually transmitted diseases, 800 mg as a single dose. For eye infections, 1 drop in each affected eye 4 times daily for 7 days

Ofloxacin

- *Children:* not recommended for persons younger than 18 years
- *Adults:* for most infections, 200 to 400 mg twice daily for 3 to 10 days. For gonorrhea, 400 mg in a single dose

Sparfloxacin

- *Children:* not recommended for persons younger than 18 years
- *Adults:* 400 mg on day one, then 200 mg once daily for 9 days

Enoxacin and norfloxacin should be taken on an empty stomach. All others may be taken on an empty stomach or with food to help reduce stomach irritation. All fluoroquinolones should be taken with a full glass of water.

If you miss a dose, take it as soon as you remember. If it is nearly time for your next dose, do not take the missed dose. Continue with your regular dosing schedule. Never take a double dose.

SYMPTOMS OF OVERDOSE AND WHAT TO DO

Symptoms of overdose include confusion, hallucinations, headache, abdominal pain, and convulsions. If overdose occurs, seek immediate medical attention and bring the prescription container with you to the hospital.

SPECIAL INFORMATION FOR PREGNANT OR NURSING WOMEN

No adequate studies of the effects of fluoroquinolone antibiotics on pregnant or nursing women have been done. However, animal studies have shown that these drugs cause birth defects. If you are pregnant or plan to become pregnant, and any of these drugs are crucial for your health, you and your health-care practitioner must weigh the potential benefits against the potential risks to the fetus.

Fluoroquinolones pass into breast milk. If you are breastfeeding, your health-care practitioner will advise you to switch to bottle feeding until your treatment is complete.

SPECIAL INFORMATION FOR SENIORS

Older adults usually need lower doses and shorter treatment periods. They also may experience more frequent and more severe side effects than younger patients.

GENERIC NAME

Fluoxetine

BRAND NAME

Prozac
Generic *available*

ABOUT THIS DRUG

Fluoxetine is a selective serotonin reuptake inhibitor (SSRI) antidepressant that is prescribed for individuals who have major depression (continuing depression that interferes with daily activities), obsessive-compulsive disorder, and panic disorder.

This drug affects the level of serotonin, a chemical in the brain that is believed to affect mood, mental state, and emotions.

SIDE EFFECTS

Be sure to tell your health-care practitioner if you experience any side effects while taking fluoxetine. Only your health-care practitioner can determine whether it is safe for you to continue taking this drug.

- *Most Common:* abnormal dreams, amnesia, anxiety, bronchitis, mood swings, chills, confusion, conjunctivitis, cough, diarrhea, dilated pupils, dizziness, drowsiness, fatigue, dry eyes, dry mouth, ear pain, high blood pressure, impotence, light intolerability, insomnia, headache, nervousness, excessive sweating, nausea, decreased appetite, rash, ringing in the ears, sore throat, tremors, vomiting, weakness, yawning
- *Less Common:* abnormal gain, abnormal cessation of menstrual flow, acne, apathy, arthritis, asthma, bone pain, breast pain, bursitis, convulsions, dark stool, euphoria, facial swelling, fever, hair loss, hallucinations, hiccups, hives, hostility, infection, inflamed esophagus, inflamed stomach lining, involuntary movements, irregular heartbeat, lack of muscle coordination, low blood pressure when standing from a seated or lying position, migraine, inflamed mouth, muscle spasm, nosebleed, swallowing difficulties, pelvic pain, rapid breathing, inflamed skin, thirst, twitching, urinary problems, vertigo, vision problems
- *Rare:* antisocial behavior, belching, bleeding gums, bloody urine, bloody diarrhea, breast enlargement, dehydration, deafness, coma, delusions, diabetes, double vision, duodenal ulcer, enlarged liver, enlarged thyroid gland, eye bleeding, female milk production, gallstones, glaucoma, gout, heart attack, heart failure, hepatitis, high blood sugar, increased salivation, inflamed eyes, inflamed intestinal tract, breathing difficulties, muscle spasms, weakness, psoriasis, rash, rheumatoid arthritis, skin discoloration, slurred speech, gastrointestinal bleeding, loss of taste, tongue swelling, vomiting blood

NOTE: Studies of the use of fluoxetine in children ages 7 to 18 years found that its use was associated with the following side effects: unusual excitement, restlessness, sleeping problems. More studies are needed to investigate these side effects.

IMPORTANT PRECAUTIONS

Tell your health-care practitioner if you are sensitive or allergic to fluoxetine or to any other drugs.

Fluoxetine should not be taken along with MAO inhibitors (e.g., phenelzine, furazolidone), and do not take fluoxetine within at least 14 days of stopping treatment with an MAOI. If you want to start taking an MAOI after stopping fluoxetine, wait at least five weeks to start the MAOI. Serious and even fatal reactions can occur if these two drugs are used together.

If you are recovering from a heart attack or if you have diabetes, liver disease, Parkinson's disease, or a history of seizures, talk to your health-care practitioner before taking this drug.

The safety and effectiveness of this drug has not been determined for children.

If you develop a rash or hives while taking fluoxetine, stop taking the drug and call your health-care practitioner immediately.

Because fluoxetine can make you dizzy and drowsy, make sure you know how you react to the drug before you drive or operate dangerous equipment.

DRUG INTERACTIONS

Tell your health-care practitioner and pharmacist if you are taking any prescription or nonprescription drugs, as well as any vitamins, herbs, or other supplements. Possible drug interactions include the following:

- Alcohol should be avoided while taking fluoxetine.
- Monoamine oxidase inhibitors (MAOIs; e.g., phenelzine, furazolidone) can cause dangerous reactions; see "Important Precautions."
- Alprazolam may raise the levels of this drug in the blood and side effects may be increased.
- Anticoagulants (e.g., warfarin) and digitalis may raise or lower levels of these drugs or of fluoxetine. Dose adjustments may be necessary.
- Astemizole may result in higher levels of astemizole and an increased chance of very serious arrhythmias.
- Buspirone, bromocriptine, levodopa, dextromethorphan, lithium, meperidine, nefazodone, pentazocine, sumatriptan, tramadol, trazodone, tryptophan, venlafaxine, and SSRIs (e.g., paroxetine, sertraline): using any of these drugs with fluoxetine or within five weeks of stopping fluoxetine may increase the chance of developing a condition called serotonin syndrome, characterized by restlessness, confusion, diarrhea, shivering, sweating, uncontrolled excitement, shaking, and twitching. Tramadol with fluoxetine increases your chance of seizures.
- Moclobemide along with fluoxetine is not recommended. The recommendation is to let seven days pass between stopping moclobemide and starting fluoxetine, and let five weeks pass between stopping fluoxetine and starting moclobemide.
- Higher levels of phenytoin and tricyclic antidepressants (e.g., amitriptyline, imipramine) may occur and increase your chance of side effects.

FOOD, VITAMIN, AND HERBAL INTERACTIONS

Herbs that produce a sedative effect may cause significant depressant interactions when used with fluoxetine. Some of those herbs include calendula, capsicum, catnip, goldenseal, gotu kola, hops, kava, lady's slipper, passionflower, sage, Siberian ginseng, skullcap, St. John's wort, and valerian, among others. St. John's wort can cause delirium and mild serotonin syndrome when taken with fluoxetine; avoid St. John's wort when using this medication.

Do not take fluoxetine with grapefruit juice because it may cause increased blood levels of the drug.

RECOMMENDED DOSAGE

Fluoxetine is available in capsules and oral solution. The dosages given here are typical. However, your health-care practitioner will determine the most appropriate dose and schedule for you.

- *Children:* not recommended for children younger than 12 years
- *Adults:* starting dose is 20 mg daily taken in the morning. Your health-care practitioner may increase your dose as needed. The typical dose for depression and obsessive-compulsive disorder is 20 to 60 mg daily. Once your depression is under control, your health-care practitioner may switch you to once-weekly fluoxetine, which is a 90-mg capsule taken the same day each week.

If you miss a dose, take it as soon as you remember. If it is nearly time for your next dose, do not take the missed dose. Continue with your regular dosing schedule. Never take a double dose.

SYMPTOMS OF OVERDOSE AND WHAT TO DO

Symptoms of overdose include agitation, nausea, vomiting, seizures, and restlessness. If overdose occurs, seek immediate medical attention and bring the prescription container with you to the hospital.

SPECIAL INFORMATION FOR PREGNANT OR NURSING WOMEN

No adequate studies of the effects of fluoxetine on pregnant or nursing women have been done. One study found that some children born to mothers who took fluoxetine were born prematurely, had breathing problems or nursing difficulties, or experienced jitteriness. Four other studies, however, did not have these findings. If you are pregnant or plan to become pregnant, and this drug is crucial for your health, you and your health-care practitioner must weigh the potential benefits against the potential risks to the fetus.

Fluoxetine appears in breast milk. If you are breastfeeding, your health-care practitioner will likely advise you to switch to bottle feeding until your treatment is complete.

SPECIAL INFORMATION FOR SENIORS
Older adults may experience more side effects and more severe ones. Dosages also may need to be reduced.

OPEN QUESTIONS OR CONTROVERSIES

In June 2004, the Food and Drug Administration asked manufacturers of fluoxetine to include in their labeling a warning statement that recommends close observation of adult and pediatric patients for clinical worsening of depression or the emergence of suicidality when being treated with this drug, especially when beginning the drug, or at the time of dose changes, either increases or decreases.

GENERIC NAME

Fluoxymesterone

BRAND NAMES
Android-F, Halotestin
Generic available

ABOUT THIS DRUG
Fluoxymesterone is a hormone (androgen) treatment and an antineoplastic (anticancer) agent given to treat certain types of breast cancer in women, as a hormone replacement in men, and to treat delayed sexual development in boys. Androgens are male hormones that are responsible for the normal growth and development of male sexual organs and characteristics.

This drug replaces natural testosterone in men and boys who have abnormally low levels of the hormone, and it also blocks the activity of certain hormones that promote the growth of some types of breast cancers.

SIDE EFFECTS
Be sure to tell your health-care practitioner if you experience any side effects while taking fluoxymesterone. Only your health-care

practitioner can determine whether it is safe for you to continue taking this drug.

- *Most Common:* Women may experience acne, oily skin, decreased breast size, hoarseness or deepening of the voice, male-type baldness, or excessive hair growth. Men may experience frequent urination, frequent or prolonged erections, sore or enlarged breasts, or temporary infertility.
- *Less Common:* changes in skin color, confusion, constipation, dizziness, headaches (frequent), depression, nausea, vomiting, swollen feet or lower legs, unusual bleeding, unusual fatigue, rapid weight gain, diarrhea, insomnia, change in sexual desire, increased thirst and urination. Men only: erectile dysfunction, irritated scrotum, testicular shrinkage. Boys only: acne, premature growth of pubic hair, enlarged penis, increased frequency of erections

IMPORTANT PRECAUTIONS

Tell your health-care practitioner if you are sensitive or allergic to fluoxymesterone or to any other drugs. This drug contains tartrazine, a dye that causes allergic reactions in some people.

Long-term, high-dose use of this drug may increase your risk of hepatitis, liver disease, and liver cancer, as well as cause a reduced sperm count or water retention.

In some cases, fluoxymesterone can be transmitted to a sexual partner and cause side effects. Therefore, a nonhormonal contraceptive (barrier type, such as a condom or an IUD) is recommended during therapy.

Men who have prostate cancer, prostate damage, breast cancer, or abnormally high blood levels of calcium should not take fluoxymesterone.

Anyone who has heart, liver, or kidney disease should not take fluoxymesterone.

Fluoxymesterone can raise blood cholesterol levels, which can be a serious problem for people who have heart disease.

Because the effects of fluoxymesterone can vary widely, your health-care practitioner should regularly monitor your use of and response to this drug.

DRUG INTERACTIONS

Tell your health-care practitioner and pharmacist if you are taking any prescription or nonprescription drugs, as well as any vitamins, herbs, or other supplements. Possible drug interactions include the following:

- Tricyclic antidepressants may result in severe paranoid reactions.

- Fluoxymesterone may increase the effect of oral anticoagulants (e.g., warfarin), requiring an adjustment of your anticoagulant dose. It can also increase the effects of antidiabetic drugs (e.g., glyburide, glipizide), cyclosporine, and insulin.
- Chlorzoxazone, oxyphenbutazone, phenobarbital, and phenylbutazone may decrease the effects of fluoxymesterone.

FOOD, VITAMIN, AND HERBAL INTERACTIONS

Fluoxymesterone can cause excessive fluid retention, so reduce your intake of salt and salty foods while using this medication.

RECOMMENDED DOSAGE

Fluoxymesterone is available in tablets. The dosages given here are typical. However, your health-care practitioner will determine the most appropriate dose and schedule for you.

- *Boys:* for delayed sexual development, 2.5 to 10 mg daily for 4 to 6 months, under strict supervision of your health-care practitioner
- *Men:* for hormone replacement, 5 to 20 mg daily in divided doses
- *Women:* for treatment of breast cancer, 10 to 40 mg daily in divided doses

Fluoxymesterone can be taken with food to help prevent stomach irritation.

If you miss a dose, take it as soon as you remember. If it is nearly time for your next dose, do not take the missed dose. Continue with your regular dosing schedule. Never take a double dose.

SYMPTOMS OF OVERDOSE AND WHAT TO DO

No specific symptoms of a fluoxymesterone overdose have been reported, and an overdose is unlikely to be life-threatening. However, if overdose occurs, seek immediate medical assistance and bring the prescription container with you to the hospital.

SPECIAL INFORMATION FOR PREGNANT OR NURSING WOMEN

Fluoxymesterone should not be used during pregnancy because it can damage the fetus. If you are pregnant or plan to become pregnant, tell your health-care practitioner immediately.

This drug passes into breast milk. If you are breastfeeding, your health-care practitioner will advise you to switch to bottle feeding until your treatment is complete.

SPECIAL INFORMATION FOR SENIORS

Older men may experience prostate enlargement or urinary retention. The drug may also heighten sexual activity or worsen high blood pressure or heart disease in both men and women.

GENERIC NAME

Fluphenazine hydrochloride *see Chlorpromazine, page 267*

GENERIC NAME

Flurandrenolide *see Corticosteroids, Topical, page 337*

GENERIC NAME

Flurazepam

BRAND NAME

Dalmane
Generic available

ABOUT THIS DRUG

Flurazepam is a benzodiazepine tranquilizer prescribed for the short-term treatment of insomnia.

This drug produces mild sedation by enhancing the effect of a chemical (gamma-aminobutyric acid, or GABA), which in turn dampens the transmission of nerve signals and reduces nerve excitation.

SIDE EFFECTS

Be sure to tell your health-care practitioner if you experience any side effects while taking flurazepam. Only your health-care practitioner can determine whether it is safe for you to continue taking this drug.

- *Most Common:* dizziness, falling, lack of muscle coordination, lightheadedness, staggering, drowsiness
- *Less Common or Rare:* abnormal salivation, apprehension, bad taste in the mouth, blurred vision, body pain, breathing difficulties, chest pains, confusion, constipation, depression, diarrhea, dry mouth, euphoria, faintness, flushes, genitourinary tract disorders, hallucina-

tions, headache, heartburn, irritability, itching, loss of appetite, low blood pressure, nausea, nervousness, fluttering heartbeat, restlessness, rash, slurred speech, gastrointestinal pain, sweating, vomiting, weakness

IMPORTANT PRECAUTIONS

Tell your health-care practitioner if you are sensitive or allergic to flurazepam or to any other drugs, especially other benzodiazepines.

Because this drug can cause dizziness and drowsiness, make sure you know how you react to it before you drive or operate dangerous equipment.

You may experience withdrawal symptoms (e.g., abdominal cramps, convulsions, sweating, tremors, vomiting) if you suddenly stop taking flurazepam. Your health-care practitioner will help you slowly taper off this drug.

If you are severely depressed or have suffered with severe depression in the past, or if you have reduced liver or kidney function, a chronic respiratory or lung disease, sleep apnea, myasthenia gravis, or a history of alcohol or drug abuse, talk to your health-care practitioner before taking flurazepam.

DRUG INTERACTIONS

Tell your health-care practitioner and pharmacist if you are taking any prescription or nonprescription drugs, as well as any vitamins, herbs, or other supplements. Possible drug interactions include the following:

- ➤ Drugs that depress the central nervous system, such as antihistamines (e.g., astemizole, cetirizine), antidepressants (e.g., imipramine, fluoxetine), barbiturates (e.g., amobarbital, phenobarbital), sedatives (e.g., temazepam, zolpidem), pain killers (e.g., codeine, oxycodone), cough medicine, and decongestants may cause additional suppression of the nervous system. Talk to your health-care practitioner before taking any of these drugs when taking flurazepam.

FOOD, VITAMIN, AND HERBAL INTERACTIONS

Herbs that produce a sedative effect may cause significant depressant interactions when used with flurazepam. Some of those herbs include calendula, capsicum, catnip, goldenseal, gotu kola, hops, kava, lady's slipper, passionflower, sage, Siberian ginseng, skullcap, St. John's wort, and valerian, among others.

Because grapefruit juice does slow the breakdown of some benzodiazepines, it is best to avoid this beverage while being treated with flurazepam. Also limit your intake of caffeine-containing beverages and foods while taking flurazepam.

RECOMMENDED DOSAGE

Flurazepam is available in capsules. The dosages given here are typical. However, your health-care practitioner will determine the most appropriate dose and schedule for you.

- *Children:* should not be taken by children younger than 6 months and is generally not prescribed for children younger than 15 years. Dosing will be determined by your health-care practitioner.
- *Adults:* 15 or 30 mg at bedtime

If you miss a dose, take it as soon as you remember, unless it is late at night. You should not take a dose unless the time remaining allows you a full night's sleep. Never take a double dose.

SYMPTOMS OF OVERDOSE AND WHAT TO DO

Symptoms of overdose include extreme drowsiness, confusion, slow reflexes, poor coordination, staggering, tremor, slowed breathing, and loss of consciousness. If an overdose occurs, seek immediate medical assistance and bring the prescription container with you to the hospital.

SPECIAL INFORMATION FOR PREGNANT OR NURSING WOMEN

Flurazepam should not be taken during pregnancy, because it is associated with an increased risk of birth defects. If you are pregnant or plan to become pregnant, tell your health-care practitioner immediately.

This drug may pass into breast milk and could injure a nursing infant. If you are breastfeeding, your health-care practitioner will likely advise you to switch to bottle feeding until you have completed treatment with flurazepam.

SPECIAL INFORMATION FOR SENIORS

Older adults usually require a lower dose to help prevent dizziness, confusion, oversedation, and poor muscle coordination.

GENERIC NAME

Flurbiprofen

see Propionic Acid (NSAID) Family, page 880

GENERIC NAME
Flutamide

BRAND NAME
Eulexin
No generic available

ABOUT THIS DRUG
Flutamide is an antiandrogen (male hormone) and antineoplastic (anticancer) medication prescribed to treat prostate cancer.

Some types of prostate tumors are stimulated by the male hormone testosterone. Flutamide interferes with the activity of the hormone, which then slows or stops the growth of the tumor.

SIDE EFFECTS
Be sure to tell your health-care practitioner if you experience any side effects while taking flutamide. Only your health-care practitioner can determine whether it is safe for you to continue taking this drug.

➤ *Most Common:* diarrhea, impotence, loss of sexual desire, sudden sweating and feeling warm

➤ *Less Common or Rare:* loss of appetite, swollen and tender breasts, swollen feet or lower legs, tingling or numbness of hands or feet, jaundice, pain or tenderness in the upper right abdomen

IMPORTANT PRECAUTIONS
Tell your health-care practitioner if you are sensitive or allergic to flutamide or to any other drugs.

DRUG INTERACTIONS
Tell your health-care practitioner and pharmacist if you are taking any prescription or nonprescription drugs, as well as any vitamins, herbs, or other supplements. Possible drug interactions include the following:

➤ Anticoagulants (e.g., warfarin) may result in changes in clotting time. The dose of your anticoagulant may need to be adjusted.

FOOD, VITAMIN, AND HERBAL INTERACTIONS
No food, vitamin, or herbal interactions have been noted.

RECOMMENDED DOSAGE

Flutamide is available in capsules. The dosages given here are typical. However, your health-care practitioner will determine the most appropriate dose and schedule for you.

- *Children*: not indicated for children
- *Adults*: 2 capsules 3 times daily, at 8-hour intervals

If you miss a dose, take it as soon as you remember. If it is nearly time for your next dose, do not take the missed dose. Continue with your regular dosing schedule. Never take a double dose.

SYMPTOMS OF OVERDOSE AND WHAT TO DO

Symptoms of overdose include dramatically slowed movements, excessive tearing, slowed breathing, loss of appetite, loss of muscle coordination, breast tenderness, and vomiting. If overdose occurs, seek immediate medical assistance and bring the prescription container with you to the hospital.

SPECIAL INFORMATION FOR PREGNANT OR NURSING WOMEN

Flutamide is for men only, but it can affect pregnancy because it can lower sperm count. The medication that is typically taken along with flutamide can cause permanent sterility. If you plan to have children, talk to your health-care practitioner before you start this medication.

SPECIAL INFORMATION FOR SENIORS

The dosage may be reduced, because the drug takes longer to be eliminated from the body than do some other drugs.

GENERIC NAME

Fluticasone propionate

see Corticosteroids, Nasal Inhalation, page 327; Corticosteroids, Oral Inhalers, page 334; Corticosteroids, Topical, page 337

GENERIC NAME

Fluvastatin

see Statin Cholesterol-Lowering Drugs, page 959

GENERIC NAME
Fluvoxamine

BRAND NAME
Luvox
Generic available

ABOUT THIS DRUG
Fluvoxamine is a selective serotonin reuptake inhibitor (SSRI) antidepressant that is prescribed for treatment of obsessive-compulsive disorder.

This drug impacts the levels of serotonin, a chemical in the brain that is believed to be associated with mood, mental state, and emotions.

SIDE EFFECTS
Be sure to tell your health-care practitioner if you experience any side effects while taking fluvoxamine. Only your health-care practitioner can determine whether it is safe for you to continue taking this drug.

- *Most Common:* decreased appetite, constipation, dry mouth, drowsiness, heartburn, insomnia, runny nose, weight loss, headache, frequent urination, sweating, taste changes, yawning
- *Less Common or Rare:* swollen feet or lower legs, chills, gas, weight gain, decreased libido, diarrhea, dizziness, rapid heartbeat, breathing difficulties, trembling, vomiting, swallowing difficulties, fainting, psychotic reactions

IMPORTANT PRECAUTIONS
Tell your health-care practitioner if you are sensitive or allergic to fluvoxamine or to any other drugs.

Take fluvoxamine for the entire treatment course as prescribed, even if you begin to feel better. Suddenly stopping this drug may result in withdrawal symptoms (e.g., tremors, seizures, blurred vision, breathing and swallowing difficulties). Your health-care practitioner will help you gradually reduce your dose.

Before taking fluvoxamine, tell your health-care practitioner if you have ever had suicidal thoughts, if you suffer from seizures, if you have a history of mania, if you have liver disease, or if you smoke.

Because fluvoxamine can cause drowsiness and dizziness, make sure you know how you react to this drug before you drive or operate dangerous equipment.

DRUG INTERACTIONS

Tell your health-care practitioner and pharmacist if you are taking any prescription or nonprescription drugs, as well as any vitamins, herbs, or other supplements. Possible drug interactions include the following:

- ➤ Monoamine oxidase inhibitors (MAOIs; e.g., phenelzine, procarbazine) should not be taken at least 2 weeks before starting or 2 weeks after stopping fluvoxamine.
- ➤ Astemizole should not be taken with fluvoxamine because of potentially serious reactions.
- ➤ Benzodiazepines (e.g., diazepam, clonazepam) should be used with caution because some may accumulate in the blood and cause more serious side effects.
- ➤ Theophylline and warfarin doses may need to be adjusted lower when taken with fluvoxamine.

FOOD, VITAMIN, AND HERBAL INTERACTIONS

Herbs that produce a sedative effect may cause significant depressant interactions when used with fluvoxamine. Some of those herbs include calendula, capsicum, catnip, goldenseal, gotu kola, hops, kava, lady's slipper, passionflower, sage, Siberian ginseng, skullcap, St. John's wort, and valerian, among others.

RECOMMENDED DOSAGE

Fluvoxamine is available in tablets. The dosages given here are typical. However, your health-care practitioner will determine the most appropriate dose and schedule for you.

- ➤ *Children 8 to 17 Years:* starting dose is 25 mg as a single dose at bedtime. Your health-care practitioner may increase it by 25 mg every 4 to 7 days as needed. The maximum daily dosage is 200 mg in divided doses.
- ➤ *Adults:* starting dose is 50 mg as a single dose at bedtime. Your health-care practitioner may increase it by 50 mg every 4 to 7 days as needed. Maximum daily dosage is 300 mg in divided doses.

Fluvoxamine can be taken with or without food. If you miss a dose, and you are taking one dose daily, skip the missed dose and return to your regular schedule. If you are taking two doses daily, take the missed dose as soon as you remember, then return to your regular dosing schedule. Never take a double dose.

SYMPTOMS OF OVERDOSE AND WHAT TO DO

Symptoms of overdose may include severe diarrhea, dizziness, drowsiness, low blood pressure, rapid or slow heartbeat, seizures, and severe vomiting. If overdose occurs, seek immediate medical attention and bring the prescription container with you to the hospital.

SPECIAL INFORMATION FOR PREGNANT OR NURSING WOMEN

No adequate studies of the effects of fluvoxamine on pregnant or nursing women have been done. If you are pregnant or plan to become pregnant, you and your health-care practitioner must weigh the potential benefits against the potential risks to the fetus.

Fluvoxamine passes into breast milk. If you are breastfeeding, your health-care practitioner may advise you to stop until your treatment is complete.

SPECIAL INFORMATION FOR SENIORS

Older adults may experience more side effects, and they may be more severe. Lower doses may be required.

OPEN QUESTIONS OR CONTROVERSIES

In June 2004, the Food and Drug Administration asked manufacturers of fluvoxamine to include in their labeling a warning statement that recommends close observation of adult and pediatric patients for clinical worsening of depression or the emergence of suicidality when being treated with this drug, especially when beginning the drug, or at the time of dose changes, either increases or decreases.

GENERIC NAME

Formoterol

BRAND NAME

Foradil

No generic available

ABOUT THIS DRUG

Formoterol is a bronchodilator and beta-2 agonist that is prescribed to prevent the symptoms of asthma. It is typically taken along with other medications known as corticosteroids (e.g., cortisone, flunisolide).

Formoterol is inhaled into the lungs, where it helps prevent certain cells from releasing substances that cause asthma symptoms.

SIDE EFFECTS

Be sure to tell your health-care practitioner if you experience any side effects while taking formoterol. Only your health-care practitioner can determine whether it is safe for you to continue taking this drug.

- *Most Common:* headache, cough, flulike symptoms, sore throat, sneezing, hoarseness
- *Less Common:* agitation, anxiety, back pain, cramps, dizziness, hives, mucous in the lungs and throat, red skin, itching, shaky legs, arms, hands, or feet, sleeplessness, body aches, chest pain, congestion, difficulty breathing, dry throat, tenderness around the eyes, swollen neck glands, trouble swallowing, wheezing

IMPORTANT PRECAUTIONS

Tell your health-care practitioner if you are sensitive or allergic to formoterol or to any other drugs.

Before taking formoterol, tell your health-care practitioner if you have any type of heart problems, acutely deteriorating asthma, high blood pressure, diabetes, overactive thyroid, or a seizure disorder.

Formoterol is used to help prevent asthma attacks. It is not effective against an attack that has already started. Other medications are needed for that situation.

If you are using formoterol for a prolonged period, you should be checked regularly by your health-care practitioner for blood or heart problems that may be caused by the drug.

Formoterol comes with a special inhaler. Do not wash your inhaler, and use a new inhaler with each drug refill.

DRUG INTERACTIONS

Tell your health-care practitioner and pharmacist if you are taking any prescription or nonprescription drugs, as well as any vitamins, herbs, or other supplements. Possible drug interactions include the following:

- Tricyclic antidepressants (e.g., imipramine, amitriptyline), monoamine oxidase inhibitors (e.g., phenelzine, procarbazine), phenothiazines (e.g., chlorpromazine, promazine), disopyramide, quinidine, procainamide, and beta-receptor blockers (e.g., acebutolol, nadolol)—tell your health-care practitioner if you are taking any of these medications before you begin to take formoterol.
- Other beta-agonists (e.g., albuterol, terbutaline) may increase the risk of heart-related side effects.

FOOD, VITAMIN, AND HERBAL INTERACTIONS

No food, vitamin, or herbal interactions have been noted.

RECOMMENDED DOSAGE

Formoterol is available in capsules for inhalation. The dosages given here are typical. However, your health-care practitioner will determine the most appropriate dose and schedule for you.

- *Children Younger than 6 Years:* dose and schedule to be determined by your health-care practitioner
- *Children 6 Years and Older and Adults:* 12 mcg by oral inhalation every 12 hours

If you miss a dose, take it as soon as you remember. If it is nearly time for your next dose, do not take the missed dose. Continue with your regular dosing schedule. Never take a double dose.

SYMPTOMS OF OVERDOSE AND WHAT TO DO

Symptoms of overdose may include blurred vision, chest tightness, convulsions, dizziness, fainting, irregular heartbeat, increased urination, muscle pain or cramps, muscle spasms or jerking, nausea, vomiting, pounding heartbeat, shortness of breath, stopping of heart, sudden loss of consciousness, or unconsciousness. If overdose occurs, seek immediate medical attention and bring the prescription container with you to the hospital.

SPECIAL INFORMATION FOR PREGNANT OR NURSING WOMEN

No adequate studies of the effects of formoterol on pregnant or nursing women have been done. However, animal studies have shown birth defects and other negative effects on the fetus. If you are pregnant or plan to become pregnant and this drug is crucial for your health, you and your health-care practitioner must weigh the potential benefits against the potential risks to the fetus.

Formoterol may pass into breast milk. If you are breastfeeding, your health-care practitioner may advise you to stop until you have completed your treatment.

SPECIAL INFORMATION FOR SENIORS

No special precautions have been noted for older adults.

GENERIC NAME

Fosfomycin

BRAND NAME

Monurol
No generic available

ABOUT THIS DRUG

Fosfomycin is an antibiotic that is specifically used to treat uncomplicated urinary tract infections (acute cystitis) in women.

This drug prevents the disease-causing bacteria from forming cell walls, which makes them unable to reproduce and spread.

SIDE EFFECTS

Be sure to tell your health-care practitioner if you experience any side effects while taking fosfomycin. Only your health-care practitioner can determine whether it is safe for you to continue taking this drug.

- *Most Common:* diarrhea, vaginal itching, nausea, headache, runny nose, back pain, irritated throat, dizziness, abdominal pain, weakness, rash, indigestion, painful menstruation
- *Less Common:* loss of appetite, constipation, dry mouth, ear disorders, fever, gas, flulike symptoms, bloody urine, insomnia, swollen lymph glands, nerve pain, nervousness, sleepiness, vomiting, failure to urinate

IMPORTANT PRECAUTIONS

Tell your health-care practitioner if you are sensitive or allergic to fosfomycin or to any other drugs.

If you do not notice an improvement within 2 to 3 days, call your health-care practitioner. You will need a different prescription.

Because fosfomycin can cause dizziness, be cautious about driving or operating potentially dangerous equipment after you take your dose.

DRUG INTERACTIONS

Tell your health-care practitioner and pharmacist if you are taking any prescription or nonprescription drugs, as well as any vitamins, herbs, or other supplements.

- Metoclopramide and similar drugs that increase the contractions of the stomach and small intestine may reduce the effectiveness of fosfomycin.

FOOD, VITAMIN, AND HERBAL INTERACTIONS

No food, vitamin, or herbal interactions have been noted.

RECOMMENDED DOSAGE

Fosfomycin is available as a powder for solution. The dosages given here are typical. However, your health-care practitioner will determine the most appropriate dose and schedule for you.

- ➤ *Children 12 Years and Younger:* safety and effectiveness have not been established
- ➤ *Children 13 Years and Older and Adults:* 1 packet (3 grams) dissolved in water. Only one dose is needed. Do not take a second dose.

SYMPTOMS OF OVERDOSE AND WHAT TO DO

No overdoses have been reported. However, if an overdose occurs, seek immediate medical assistance and bring the prescription container with you to the hospital.

SPECIAL INFORMATION FOR PREGNANT OR NURSING WOMEN

No adequate studies of the effects of fosfomycin on pregnant or nursing women have been done. If you are pregnant or plan to become pregnant, you and your health-care practitioner must weigh the potential benefits against the potential risks to the fetus.

Fosfomycin may pass into breast milk. If you are breastfeeding, talk to your health-care practitioner about stopping temporarily while you take your one dose of fosfomycin.

SPECIAL INFORMATION FOR SENIORS

No special precautions are noted for older adults.

GENERIC NAME

Fosinopril

BRAND NAME

Monopril
Generic available

ABOUT THIS DRUG

Fosinopril is an ACE (angiotensin-converting enzyme) inhibitor that is prescribed as treatment for high blood pressure. It can be used alone or in combination with other drugs for hypertension. It is also used to treat heart failure.

Like other ACE inhibitors, fosinopril blocks an enzyme that produces angiotensin, a substance that causes blood vessels to constrict, and promotes production of aldosterone, which causes the body to retain sodium. Thus ACE inhibitors cause blood vessels to relax and reduce sodium retention, which lowers blood pressure.

SIDE EFFECTS

Be sure to tell your health-care practitioner if you experience any side effects while taking fosinopril. Only your health-care practitioner can determine whether it is safe for you to continue taking this drug.

When Taken to Treat Hypertension

➤ *Most Common:* cough, dizziness, nausea, vomiting

➤ *Less Common:* abdominal pain, severe allergic reaction, appetite and weight changes, confusion, constipation, decreased sex drive, diarrhea, drowsiness, dry mouth, sweating, irritated eyes, fatigue, gas, headache, heartburn, itching, kidney failure, liver failure, muscle cramps, rash, skin sensitivity to sunlight, sleep problems, tremors, vertigo, vision problems, weakness, jaundice

When Taken for Heart Failure

➤ *Most Common:* cough, dizziness, low blood pressure, muscle and bone pain

➤ *Less Common or Rare:* breathing difficulties, arm or leg weakness, behavior changes, bronchitis, chest pain, constipation, decreased appetite, depression, diarrhea, distended abdomen, dry mouth, sweating, fainting, fever, flu, fluid retention, gas, gout, heart rhythm disturbances, high blood pressure, itching, kidney pain, muscle aches, inflamed nasal passages, nausea, numbness, pins and needles, rapid or slow heartbeat, sexual problems, change in taste, tremors, stroke, swollen arms or legs, upper respiratory infection, urinary problems, vertigo, vision problems, vomiting, lightheadedness when standing from a lying or seated position

IMPORTANT PRECAUTIONS

Tell your health-care practitioner if you are sensitive or allergic to fosinopril or to any other drugs, especially other ACE inhibitors.

Fosinopril must be used regularly if it is to be effective, and you must continue to take it even when you feel better. Suddenly stopping fosinopril can result in a rise in blood pressure.

If you develop a sore throat, fever, or swollen legs, arms, tongue, lips, throat, or face, or if you have trouble swallowing, contact your health-care practitioner immediately.

Before starting fosinopril, tell your health-care practitioner if you have kidney or liver problems.

This drug should be used with extreme caution if you are on dialysis, or if you have received bee or wasp venom to protect against stings. Dangerous allergic reactions have been known to occur.

DRUG INTERACTIONS

Tell your health-care practitioner and pharmacist if you are taking any prescription or nonprescription drugs, as well as any vitamins, herbs, or other supplements. Possible drug interactions include the following:

- Potassium preparations, potassium-sparing diuretics, and cotrimoxazole may cause blood potassium levels to rise and cause serious heart rhythm problems.
- Allopurinol may increase the risk of serious skin reactions.
- Azathioprine may cause severe anemia.
- Cyclosporine may cause kidney failure.
- Lithium may result in toxic levels of lithium.
- Loop diuretics (e.g., furosemide, bumetanide) and phenothiazines (e.g., chlorpromazine, promazine) may cause very low blood pressure when standing from a seated or lying position.
- Oral antidiabetes drugs (e.g., glyburide, glipizide) may require you to decrease your dose of these drugs.
- Cotrimoxazole may raise blood potassium levels, which increases the risk of serious heart rhythm disturbances.
- Antacids (e.g., Maalox, Mylanta), COX-2 inhibitors (e.g., celecoxib, rofecoxib), naloxone, and salicylates (e.g., aspirin) and other NSAIDs (e.g., naproxen, ibuprofen) may reduce the effects of fosinopril.
- Alcohol can further reduce blood pressure. Use it with caution.

FOOD, VITAMIN, AND HERBAL INTERACTIONS

Discuss your salt intake with your health-care practitioner when taking fosinopril. Avoid using salt substitutes or drinking low-salt milk, as these substances can cause abnormally high potassium levels, which can lead to heart problems. Also avoid foods high in potassium, such as bananas and citrus, unless you are also taking medications that reduce potassium levels. Do not take potassium supplements while taking fosinopril unless directed to do so by your health-care practitioner.

If you plan to or are taking any herbs or supplements, talk with your health-care practitioner before starting fosinopril. Ginseng, goldenseal, licorice, ephedra (ma huang), and saw palmetto may raise your blood pressure; garlic and calcium may help lower it.

RECOMMENDED DOSAGE

Fosinopril is available in tablets. The dosages given here are typical. However, your health-care practitioner will determine the most appropriate dose and schedule for you.

- *Children:* not recommended for children
- *Adults:* for high blood pressure, starting dose is 10 mg taken once daily, either alone or with a diuretic. Once your blood pressure is adjusted, your health-care practitioner may change your dosage to 20 to 40 mg daily, perhaps in divided doses. For heart failure, starting dose is 10 mg once daily. Your health-care practitioner will gradually increase the dose to fit your needs. The typical maintenance dose is 20 to 40 mg daily.

It is best to take fosinopril one hour before meals, but you can take it with food if it causes stomach irritation.

If you miss a dose, take it as soon as you remember. If it is nearly time for your next dose, do not take the missed dose. Continue with your regular dosing schedule. Never take a double dose.

SYMPTOMS OF OVERDOSE AND WHAT TO DO

The main symptom of an overdose of fosinopril is a sudden drop in blood pressure, characterized by lightheadedness, dizziness, and fainting. If overdose occurs, seek immediate medical attention and bring the prescription container with you to the hospital.

SPECIAL INFORMATION FOR PREGNANT OR NURSING WOMEN

ACE inhibitors such as fosinopril can cause injury and death to the developing fetus. If you are pregnant, your health-care practitioner should have you stop this drug immediately.

Fosinopril passes into breast milk and may affect a nursing infant. If you are breastfeeding, your health-care practitioner will advise you to stop until your treatment is complete.

SPECIAL INFORMATION FOR SENIORS

Older adults may encounter more side effects, and they may be more severe.

GENERIC NAME

Fosphenytoin *see Phenytoin, page 840*

GENERIC NAME

Frovatriptan succinate *see Triptan-Type Antimigraine Drugs, page 1083*

GENERIC NAME

Furosemide *see Loop Diuretics, page 622*

GENERIC NAME

Gabapentin

BRAND NAME

Neurontin
No generic available

ABOUT THIS DRUG

Gabapentin is an anticonvulsant used to control specific types of seizures associated with epilepsy. It is often given along with another anticonvulsant drug.

This drug appears to suppress the abnormal firing of neurons in the brain that cause seizures.

SIDE EFFECTS

Be sure to tell your health-care practitioner if you experience any side effects while taking gabapentin. Only your health-care practitioner can determine whether it is safe for you to continue taking this drug.

- *Most Common:* fatigue, dizziness, blurred or altered vision, nausea, vomiting, tremor, clumsiness, unusual eye movements, sedation. Among children 3 to 12 years, common side effects include aggressiveness, anxiety, crying, euphoria, hyperactivity, restlessness, and other behavior problems.

- *Less Common:* dry mouth, sleep problems, irritability, slurred speech, headache, diarrhea, muscle aches or weakness
- *Rare:* fever, sore throat, swollen glands, rash, blistering or peeling skin lesions, confusion, lethargy, and seizures may indicate a potentially fatal blood condition called aplastic anemia or other complications. Contact your health-care practitioner immediately.

IMPORTANT PRECAUTIONS

Tell your health-care practitioner if you are sensitive or allergic to gabapentin or to any other drugs.

Do not suddenly stop taking this drug, as seizures can occur. Only your health-care practitioner can advise you on how to gradually reduce your dosage.

Do not take gabapentin if you have pancreatitis.

Before taking gabapentin, consult with your health-care practitioner if you have low blood pressure, or if you have a history of kidney disease or impaired kidney function.

Because gabapentin can cause dizziness and sleepiness, make sure you know how you react to the drug before you drive or operate dangerous equipment.

DRUG INTERACTIONS

Tell your health-care practitioner and pharmacist if you are taking any prescription or nonprescription drugs, as well as any vitamins, herbs, or other supplements. Possible drug interactions include the following:

- Antacids (e.g., Maalox, Mylanta) can reduce the effectiveness of gabapentin and should be taken at least 2 hours after taking gabapentin.
- Drugs that have depressive effects on the central nervous system, including antihistamines, sedatives, tranquilizers, narcotics, barbiturates, muscle relaxants, anesthetics (including dental anesthetics), and other anticonvulsants may add to the depressive effect.

FOOD, VITAMIN, AND HERBAL INTERACTIONS

No food, vitamin, or herbal interactions have been noted.

RECOMMENDED DOSAGE

Gabapentin is available in tablets, capsules, and oral solution. The dosages given here are typical. However, your health-care practitioner will determine the most appropriate dose and schedule for you.

- *Children Up to Age 3 Years:* dose and schedule to be determined by your health-care practitioner
- *Children 3 to 12 Years:* 4.5 to 6.8 mg per pound of body weight, divided into 3 doses. This dosage may be increased by your health-care practitioner as needed.
- *Children 12 Years and Older and Adults:* 300 mg three times daily, which can be increased by your health-care practitioner as needed. Maximum daily dose is 3,600 mg.
- *Adults 60 and Older:* your health-care practitioner will determine the dose. The typical dose is no more than 400 mg three times daily.

Gabapentin can be taken with or after eating food to help reduce stomach irritation. The capsules can be opened and the contents mixed with food if desired. Only mix one dose at a time.

If you miss a dose, take it as soon as you remember. If it is nearly time for your next dose, do not take the missed dose. Continue with your regular dosing schedule. Never take a double dose.

SYMPTOMS OF OVERDOSE AND WHAT TO DO

Symptoms of overdose include double vision, slurred speech, lethargy, diarrhea, and drowsiness. If an overdose occurs, seek immediate medical attention. Bring the prescription container with you to the hospital.

SPECIAL INFORMATION FOR PREGNANT OR NURSING WOMEN

Adequate studies of the effects of gabapentin on pregnant or nursing women have not been done. However, other anticonvulsants have been linked with an increased risk of birth defects. Because seizures during pregnancy also pose risks to unborn children, use of gabapentin during pregnancy must be discussed with your health-care practitioner and the potential benefits weighed against the potential risks.

Gabapentin may pass into breast milk. If you are breastfeeding, your health-care practitioner may advise you to switch to bottle feeding until your treatment is complete.

SPECIAL INFORMATION FOR SENIORS

Older adults typically need lower doses.

GENERIC NAME
Galantamine

BRAND NAME
Reminyl
No generic available

ABOUT THIS DRUG
Galantamine is a dementia symptom treatment adjunct used to treat the symptoms of mild-to-moderate Alzheimer's disease. It is not a cure for the disease, nor can it change the course of the disease.

This drug blocks the action of acetylcholinesterase, an enzyme that helps break down a substance called acetylcholine. A loss of acetylcholine has been associated with a decline in cognitive functioning.

SIDE EFFECTS
Be sure to tell your health-care practitioner if you experience any side effects while taking galantamine. Only your health-care practitioner can determine whether it is safe for you to continue taking this drug. Approximately 80 percent of patients who take galantamine experience some adverse reactions.

- *Most Common:* nausea, vomiting, diarrhea, loss of appetite, weight loss
- *Less Common:* abdominal pain, dizziness, confusion, sleepiness or sleeplessness

IMPORTANT PRECAUTIONS
Tell your health-care practitioner if you are sensitive or allergic to galantamine or to any other drugs. The 12-mg galantamine tablets contain a dye called E110, which causes an asthma-like reaction in some people, especially those who are allergic to aspirin.

Galantamine should not be used if you have severe liver or kidney conditions.

Before talking galantamine, consult with your health-care practitioner if you have liver or kidney problems, a heart condition, galactose intolerance, lactase deficiency, glucose-galactose malabsorption, recent gut or bladder surgery, urinary difficulties, stomach or duodenal ulcer, acute abdominal pain, or epilepsy.

DRUG INTERACTIONS

Tell your health-care practitioner and pharmacist if you are taking any prescription or nonprescription drugs, as well as any vitamins, herbs, or other supplements. Possible drug interactions include the following:

- Ketoconazole, erythromycin, and cimetidine cause galantamine blood levels to be high and thus increase the risk of side effects.
- Galantamine may increase the effects of cholinomimetics (e.g., bethanechol, succinylcholine).
- Amitriptyline, fluvoxamine, and quinidine reduce the elimination of galantamine from the body by up to 33%.
- Paroxetine increases the bioavailability of galantamine by 40%.

FOOD, VITAMIN, AND HERBAL INTERACTIONS

No food, vitamin, or herbal interactions have been noted.

RECOMMENDED DOSAGE

Galantamine is available in 4-, 8-, and 12-mg tablets. The dosage given here is typical. However, your health-care practitioner will determine the most appropriate dose and schedule for you.

- *Children:* not indicated
- *Adults:* starting dose is usually 4 mg taken twice daily, with morning and evening meals. Your health-care practitioner may increase the dose gradually up to 8 to 12 mg twice daily.

If you miss a dose, take it as soon as you remember. If it is nearly time for your next dose, do not take the missed dose. Continue with your regular dosing schedule. Never take a double dose.

SYMPTOMS OF OVERDOSE AND WHAT TO DO

Symptoms of overdose include convulsions, rapid, weak pulse, increased salivation, nausea, vomiting, breathing difficulties, increased sweating, dilated pupils, and increased muscle weakness. If overdose occurs, seek immediate medical assistance and bring the prescription container with you to the hospital.

SPECIAL INFORMATION FOR PREGNANT OR NURSING WOMEN

No adequate studies of the effects of galantamine on pregnant or nursing women have been done. Animal studies have shown that the drug can cause birth defects and other problems with the fetus. If you are pregnant or plan to become pregnant, you and your health-care practitioner should weigh the potential benefits against the potential risks.

Galantamine may pass into breast milk. If you are breastfeeding, your health-care practitioner will likely advise you to switch to bottle feeding.

SPECIAL INFORMATION FOR SENIORS

No special precautions have been noted.

GENERIC NAME

Ganciclovir

BRAND NAMES

Cytovene, Vitrasert
Generic available

ABOUT THIS DRUG

Ganciclovir is an antiviral used to treat or prevent infections caused by cytomegalovirus (CMV). This infection is common in people who have a weakened immune system, especially among those with AIDS (acquired immunodeficiency syndrome).

This drug prevents the CMV virus from replicating by interfering with the functioning of enzymes that are necessary for the reproduction of viral DNA in cells.

SIDE EFFECTS

Be sure to tell your health-care practitioner if you experience any side effects while taking ganciclovir. Only your health-care practitioner can determine whether it is safe for you to continue taking this drug.

- *Less Common:* abdominal discomfort, nausea, vomiting, sweating, decreased appetite
- *Rare:* serious anemia (signs include unusual fever, chills, fatigue, sore throat, bruising or bleeding), rash, tremor, eye pain, sudden vision changes

IMPORTANT PRECAUTIONS

Tell your health-care practitioner if you are sensitive or allergic to ganciclovir or to any other drugs.

Ganciclovir may cause cancer and reproductive toxicity. It is used in children only with extreme caution.

Before taking ganciclovir, talk to your health-care practitioner if you have a sore throat or fever, you have a history of blood cell disorders, or you think you are dehydrated.

Males who are planning pregnancy should avoid attempted conception for at least 3 months after stopping ganciclovir treatment.

The oral form of this drug should be given only when a health-care practitioner has determined the patient is not a candidate for the intravenous form.

DRUG INTERACTIONS

Tell your health-care practitioner and pharmacist if you are taking any prescription or nonprescription drugs, as well as any vitamins, herbs, or other supplements. Possible drug interactions include the following:

- Amphotericin B, cotrimoxazole, pentamidine, zidovudine, and cancer chemotherapy may increase bone marrow suppression.
- Cyclosporine may result in increased kidney toxicity.
- Flucytosine may cause additive bone marrow toxicity.
- Probenecid may interfere with the elimination of ganciclovir by the kidneys and thus increase the effects of ganciclovir.

FOOD, VITAMIN, AND HERBAL INTERACTIONS

Do not take echinacea while undergoing treatment with ganciclovir because it may weaken your immune system if you take the herb for too long or too often. Also avoid St. John's wort, as both this herb and ganciclovir can cause photosensitivity.

RECOMMENDED DOSAGE

Ganciclovir is available in capsules (also by injection and intraocular implant, both not discussed here). The dosages given here are typical. However, your health-care practitioner will determine the most appropriate dose and schedule for you.

- *Adults:* once the intravenous dosing has been completed, 1,000 mg three times daily is taken orally. An alternative is 500 mg taken 6 times daily, every three hours

Ganciclovir should be taken with food and at the same time each day.

If you miss a dose, take it as soon as you remember. If it is nearly time for your next dose, do not take the missed dose. Continue with your regular dosing schedule. Never take a double dose.

SYMPTOMS OF OVERDOSE AND WHAT TO DO

Symptoms of overdose include extreme weakness, dizziness, severe diarrhea, kidney failure, nausea, and vomiting. If overdose occurs, seek immediate medical attention and bring the prescription container with you to the hospital.

SPECIAL INFORMATION FOR PREGNANT OR NURSING WOMEN

No adequate studies of the effects of ganciclovir on pregnant or nursing women have been done. Animal studies have shown birth defects and fetal death. If you are pregnant or plan to become pregnant, talk to your health-care practitioner. Ganciclovir should not be used by pregnant women, and a reliable birth control method should be used by both men and women both during treatment and for three months after treatment ends.

Ganciclovir passes into breast milk and may harm a nursing infant. If you are breastfeeding, your health-care practitioner will advise you to stop until your treatment is done.

SPECIAL INFORMATION FOR SENIORS

Older adults are more likely to experience side effects, and they may be more severe.

GENERIC NAME

Gatifloxacin

see Fluoroquinolone Antibiotics, page 468

GENERIC NAME

Gefitinib

BRAND NAME

Iressa

No generic available

ABOUT THIS DRUG

Gefitinib is an anticancer drug used for the treatment of non-small cell lung cancer that has progressed after or failed to respond to use of two other types of anticancer medications.

This drug works by inhibiting the activity of an enzyme (tyrosine kinase) that is associated with epidermal growth factor receptor, a protein that is present on cancer cells and normal cells. Abnormal activity of this receptor appears to play a significant role in the growth of cancer cells.

SIDE EFFECTS

Be sure to tell your health-care practitioner if you experience any side effects while taking gefitinib. Only your health-care practitioner can determine whether it is safe for you to continue taking this drug.

- *Most Common:* acne, diarrhea, dry mouth, dry skin, nausea, vomiting
- *Less Common:* anorexia, itching, weakness, weight loss
- *Rare:* corneal erosion, eye pain, interstitial lung disease (indications include sudden onset or worsening of pulmonary symptoms such as cough, shortness of breath, and fever), pancreatitis

IMPORTANT PRECAUTIONS

Tell your health-care practitioner if you are sensitive or allergic to gefitinib or to any other drugs.

Seek immediate medical help if you develop severe or persistent diarrhea, nausea, anorexia, or vomiting while taking this drug.

Interstitial lung disease has been observed in about one percent of patients who receive gefitinib, and one-third of cases are fatal. If you experience sudden onset or worsening of pulmonary symptoms (cough, fever, shortness of breath), you should notify your health-care practitioner immediately.

Your health-care practitioner may periodically conduct liver function tests while you are using this drug to monitor you for toxicity.

DRUG INTERACTIONS

Tell your health-care practitioner and pharmacist if you are taking any prescription or nonprescription drugs, as well as any vitamins, herbs, or other supplements. Possible drug interactions include the following:

- Itraconazole, ketoconazole, and similar drugs may increase the concentration of gefitinib.
- Rifampicin, phenytoin, and similar drugs may reduce the concentration of gefitinib, and an increase in dosage may be necessary.
- Ranitidine, cimetidine, and similar drugs may reduce the absorption of gefitinib.
- Metoprolol concentrations may increase when taken with gefitinib.
- Use of warfarin along with gefitinib may increase bleeding events.

FOOD, VITAMIN, AND HERBAL INTERACTIONS

No food, vitamin, or herbal interactions have been reported.

RECOMMENDED DOSAGE

Gefitinib is available in 250-mg tablets. The dosages given here are typical. However, your health-care practitioner will determine the most appropriate dose and schedule for your needs.

- *Children:* Not recommended for children
- *Adults:* 250 mg once daily

Gefitinib can be taken with or without food. If you forget a dose, take it as soon as you remember. If it is almost time for the next dose, skip the missed dose and resume your normal schedule. Never take a double dose.

SYMPTOMS OF OVERDOSE AND WHAT TO DO

Symptoms of overdose include diarrhea and rash. If overdose occurs, seek immediate medical attention and bring the prescription container with you to the hospital.

SPECIAL INFORMATION FOR PREGNANT OR NURSING WOMEN

No studies have adequately investigated the effects of gefitinib during pregnancy or breastfeeding. However, animal studies suggest this drug may harm the fetus. If you are pregnant or plan to become pregnant, talk with your health-care practitioner before starting this drug. Only a health-care practitioner can determine whether the potential benefits outweigh the potential dangers.

It is not known whether gefitinib can be found in breast milk, but you should not breastfeed while taking gefitinib. Your health-care practitioner will likely advise you to switch to bottle feeding until your treatment is complete.

SPECIAL INFORMATION FOR SENIORS

There are no special instructions for seniors.

GENERIC NAME

Gemfibrozil

BRAND NAMES

Gemcor, Lopid
Generic available

ABOUT THIS DRUG

Gemfibrozil is an anticholesterol drug used to help reduce abnormally high blood levels of triglycerides in people who have not responded well to diet, weight loss, and exercise. It is also given to decrease the risk for developing coronary artery disease.

This drug lowers triglyceride levels by interfering with the liver's ability to make them.

SIDE EFFECTS

Be sure to tell your health-care practitioner if you experience any side effects while taking gemfibrozil. Only your health-care practitioner can determine whether it is safe for you to continue taking this drug.

- *Most Common:* diarrhea, gas, acute appendicitis, constipation, eczema, headache, nausea, vomiting, rash, vertigo
- *Less Common:* anemia, dizziness, blurred vision, confusion, convulsions, inflamed colon, itching, joint pain, laryngeal swelling, reduced sexual ability, flu-like symptoms, weakness, unusual tiredness, inflamed mouth and lips, heartburn, sleepiness

IMPORTANT PRECAUTIONS

Tell your health-care practitioner if you are sensitive or allergic to gemfibrozil or to any other drugs.

If you want to get the full benefit of gemfibrozil, you must follow the exercise and diet programs prescribed by your health-care practitioner.

Unless directed to do so by your health-care practitioner, do not take gemfibrozil if you are being treated for severe liver or kidney disorders or gallbladder disease.

There is a slight risk associated with use of gemfibrozil and getting malignancy, gallbladder disease and gallstones, myositis (a muscle disease characterized by muscle tenderness, pain, and weakness), abdominal pain that results in appendectomy, or other serious or even deadly abdominal conditions.

If your cholesterol levels are not significantly lower after three months of treatment, your health-care practitioner will likely discontinue your treatment.

DRUG INTERACTIONS

Tell your health-care practitioner and pharmacist if you are taking any prescription or nonprescription drugs, as well as any vitamins, herbs, or other supplements. Possible drug interactions include the following:

- Ritonavir may lead to gemfibrozil toxicity.
- Gemfibrozil may increase the effects of oral antidiabetes drugs (e.g., glyburide, glipizide).
- Statin-lowering drugs (e.g., lovastatin, fluvastatin) may increase the risk of muscle damage.
- Warfarin may increase the risk of bleeding.
- Gemfibrozil may decrease the effects of colestipol. Take these two drugs at least two hours apart.

FOOD, VITAMIN, AND HERBAL INTERACTIONS

Garlic may increase the risk of rhabdomyolysis (a sometimes fatal muscle disease) or myopathy (a general term for muscle disease). Avoid taking garlic and gemfibrozil.

RECOMMENDED DOSAGE

Gemfibrozil is available in 600-mg tablets. The dosages given here are typical. However, your health-care practitioner will determine the most appropriate dose and schedule for you.

- *Children:* safety and effectiveness have not been established for children. It should not be used in children younger than 2 years.
- *Adults:* 600 mg twice daily, taken 30 minutes before your morning and evening meals

If you miss a dose, take it as soon as you remember. If it is nearly time for your next dose, do not take the missed dose. Continue with your regular dosing schedule. Never take a double dose.

SYMPTOMS OF OVERDOSE AND WHAT TO DO

Symptoms of overdose may include abdominal pain, nausea, vomiting, and diarrhea. If overdose occurs, seek immediate medical attention and bring the prescription container with you to the hospital.

SPECIAL INFORMATION FOR PREGNANT OR NURSING WOMEN

No adequate studies of the effects of gemfibrozil on pregnant or nursing women have been done. In animal studies, this drug causes tumors. If you are pregnant or plan to become pregnant, you and your health-care practitioner should weigh the potential benefits against the potential risks.

Gemfibrozil passes into breast milk. If you are breastfeeding, your health-care practitioner will likely advise you to stop until your treatment is done.

SPECIAL INFORMATION FOR SENIORS

Older adults have an increased tendency to get infections when taking gemfibrozil.

GENERIC NAME

Glatiramer

BRAND NAME

Copaxone
No generic available

ABOUT THIS DRUG

Glatiramer is an immunomodulator that is prescribed to prevent or reduce the frequency of relapses in people who have relapsing-remitting multiple sclerosis (MS), the most common form of this disease. In this form of MS, periods of active disease alternate with periods of reduced symptoms or remission.

In MS, the myelin sheath, a fatty insulation material that protects the nerves, is damaged in various places throughout the body by the body's own immune system. Glatiramer blocks the body's attack on myelin, which slows the progression of the disease.

SIDE EFFECTS

Be sure to tell your health-care practitioner if you experience any side effects while taking glatiramer. Only your health-care practitioner can determine whether it is safe for you to continue taking this drug.

- *Most Common:* flushed skin, dizziness, depression, palpitations, anxiety, breathing difficulties, tremor, hives, chest pain, loss of appetite, gastrointestinal problems, joint pain, bronchitis, ear pain; lump, hives, itching, redness, pain, or swelling at the injection site
- *Less Common:* agitation, bloating, chills, confusion, fainting, fever, swelling in arms, fingers, legs, and feet, constricted throat, migraine, muscle aches

IMPORTANT PRECAUTIONS

Tell your health-care practitioner if you are sensitive or allergic to glatiramer or to any other drugs.

Glatiramer should be injected at a different site every day during the week.

Because glatiramer can cause dizziness, make sure you know how you react to the drug before you drive or operate dangerous equipment.

DRUG INTERACTIONS

Tell your health-care practitioner and pharmacist if you are taking any prescription or nonprescription drugs, as well as any vitamins, herbs, or other supplements. Glatiramer has not been shown to interact negatively with other drugs.

FOOD, VITAMIN, AND HERBAL INTERACTIONS

No food, vitamin, or herbal interactions have been noted.

RECOMMENDED DOSAGE

Glatiramer is available as an injection. The dosage given here is typical. However, your health-care practitioner will determine the most appropriate dose and schedule for you.

- *Children:* dose and use to be determined by your health-care practitioner
- *Adults:* 20 mg once daily

If you miss a dose, take it as soon as you remember. If it is nearly time for your next dose, do not take the missed dose. Continue with your regular dosing schedule. Never take a double dose.

SYMPTOMS OF OVERDOSE AND WHAT TO DO

No specific symptoms of overdose have been reported. If you or someone else takes too large a dose or if the drug is accidentally ingested, seek immediately medical assistance and bring the prescription container with you to the hospital.

SPECIAL INFORMATION FOR PREGNANT OR NURSING WOMEN

No adequate studies of the effects of glatiramer on pregnant or nursing women have been done. If you are pregnant or plan to become pregnant, and this drug is crucial for your health, you and your health-care practitioner must weigh the potential benefits against the potential risks to the fetus.

Glatiramer may pass into breast milk. If you are breastfeeding, your health-care practitioner may advise you to switch to bottle feeding.

SPECIAL INFORMATION FOR SENIORS
No special precautions are noted for older adults.

GENERIC NAME
Glimepiride
see Sulfonylurea Antidiabetes Drugs, page 971

GENERIC NAME
Glipizide
see Sulfonylurea Antidiabetes Drugs, page 971

GENERIC NAME
Glipizide/metformin

BRAND NAME
Metaglip
No generic available

ABOUT THIS DRUG
The glipizide/metformin combination drug is used to treat the form of diabetes mellitus known as type 2. Type 2 diabetes was formerly known as adult-onset, and is also referred to as non-insulin-dependent. Diet and exercise play a key role in the management of this disease.

Glipizide is a sulfonylurea drug, which helps the body regulate the amount of glucose (sugar) in blood. This drug lowers blood sugar by stimulating the pancreas to secret insulin and make insulin work more efficiently. The pancreas must produce insulin in order for glipizide to work. Metformin also helps the body regulate the amount of glucose, but it does so by decreasing glucose production and increasing the body's sensitivity to insulin.

SIDE EFFECTS
Be sure to tell your health-care practitioner if you experience any side effects while taking glipizide/metformin. Only your health-care practitioner can determine whether it is safe for you to continue taking this drug.

People with diabetes need to learn to recognize the symptoms of low blood sugar and high blood sugar and what to do when they occur. It is essential to control these symptoms before they progress to more serious conditions.

Rarely, people who have taken metformin have developed a life-threatening condition called lactic acidosis, an accumulation of lactic acid in the blood. In most cases, this condition occurs in people who have kidney or liver problems, and it is fatal in about 50 percent of cases. (See symptoms of lactic acidosis below.)

- *Most Common:* nausea, vomiting, abdominal pain, diarrhea, all of which begin at the start of treatment; headache
- *Hypoglycemia (Low Blood Sugar):* "drunken" behavior, drowsiness, unusual tiredness or weakness, slurred speech, shakiness, dizziness, difficulty concentrating, headache, confusion, anxiety, nervousness, blurred vision, cold sweats, cool pale skin, excessive hunger, restless sleep, nightmares, nausea, fast heartbeat
- *Hyperglycemia (High Blood Sugar):* dry mouth, thirst, frequent urination, dry skin, flushing, appetite loss, difficulty breathing, tiredness
- *Lactic Acidosis:* diarrhea, stomach discomfort, unusual tiredness or sleepiness, feeling cold, dizziness, lightheadedness, weakness, muscle pain and cramping, fast shallow breathing, slow or irregular heartbeat

IMPORTANT PRECAUTIONS

Tell your health-care practitioner if you are sensitive or allergic to glipizide, metformin, or any other drugs.

This drug combination should not be taken if you have kidney or liver disease, heart or lung disease, or chronic metabolic acidosis or diabetic ketoacidosis (see symptoms under "Side Effects"). Tell your health-care practitioner if you have pituitary or thyroid disease, adrenal insufficiency, or hormone problems. Do not take this drug if you are an alcoholic.

Do not take this drug 2 days before or after having an X-ray using an injectable iodinated contrast agent (e.g., Omnipaque). Your health-care practitioner will also most likely advise you to stop taking this drug for a short time before and after having any type of surgery or dental procedure.

Hyperglycemia is a possible side effect of this drug combination (see symptoms above). If this condition is not treated, it can lead to diabetic coma and death. Another possible side effect is lactic acidosis (see symptoms above). In order to prevent these types of complications, carefully follow all diet and exercise recommendations made by your health-care practitioner and nutritionist. In fact, many people with type 2 diabetes are able to successfully control this disease by making healthy lifestyle changes, cutting back on the need for medication.

DRUG INTERACTIONS

Tell your health-care practitioner and pharmacist if you are taking any prescription or nonprescription drugs, as well as any vitamins, herbs, or other supplements. Possible drug interactions include the following:

- Alcohol should be avoided when using this drug combination.
- Prescription and over-the-counter medications for cold, cough, pain, and weight loss should not be taken without first talking with your health-care practitioner.
- Metformin increases the blood-sugar-lowering effects of insulin.
- ACE inhibitors, amiloride, beta-blockers, cimetidine, clotrimazole, digoxin, furosemide, morphine, procainamide, quinidine, quinine, ranitidine, triamterene, trimethoprim, and vancomycin may increase the risk of side effects of metformin.
- Consult your health-care practitioner if you are taking any of the following drugs: estrogens, niacin, nifedipine, phenytoin, predisone, sulfonamides, thyroid hormones, warfarin, and water pills (diuretics).

FOOD, VITAMIN, AND HERBAL INTERACTIONS

Supplements such as chromium, garlic, ginger, ginseng, hawthorn, and nettle may affect blood sugar levels. Check with your health-care practitioner before using any dietary supplements.

Metformin is associated with malabsorption of vitamin B12. Supplementation with vitamin B12 and calcium (which helps your body absorb B12) may be helpful.

RECOMMENDED DOSAGE

The combination of glipizide/metformin is available in various formulations: 2.5 mg/250 mg, 5 mg/500 mg, and 5 mg/500 mg tablets. The dosages given here are typical. However, your health-care practitioner will determine the most appropriate dose and schedule for your needs.

- *Children:* Not recommended for children
- *Adults not previously treated with diabetes medications:* starting dose is 2.5 mg glipizide with 250 mg metformin once daily. Your health-care practitioner may increase the dose to twice daily if needed. Maximum daily dose is 10 mg glipizide with 2,000 mg metformin.

➤ *Adults previously treated with glipizide (or similar drug) or metformin:* starting dose is 2.5 or 5 mg of glipizide with 500 mg of metformin twice daily. Your health-care practitioner may increase this dose in increments of up to 5 mg (glipizide)/500 mg (metformin). Maximum daily dose is 20 mg glipizide and 2,000 mg metformin.

This drug combination should be taken with a meal to avoid stomach distress, such as nausea, diarrhea, and upset stomach. These symptoms are more likely to occur during the first few weeks of therapy.

If you forget a dose, take it as soon as you remember. If it is almost time for the next dose, skip the missed dose and resume your normal schedule. Never take a double dose.

SYMPTOMS OF OVERDOSE AND WHAT TO DO

Symptoms of overdose include nausea, anxiety, cold sweats, weakness, unconsciousness, and coma. If overdose occurs, seek immediate medical attention and bring the prescription container with you to the hospital.

SPECIAL INFORMATION FOR PREGNANT OR NURSING WOMEN

This drug should not be used during pregnancy. It is critically important to monitor and control blood sugar during pregnancy. However, it is safer to accomplish this through diet or a combination of diet and insulin. Consult your health-care practitioner as soon as you think you may be pregnant or if you are planning to become pregnant.

The combination of glipizide/metformin passes into breast milk. If you are breastfeeding or plan to do so, talk with your health-care practitioner before starting this drug. Only a health-care practitioner can determine whether the potential benefits outweigh the potential dangers.

SPECIAL INFORMATION FOR SENIORS

Adults 65 years and older are at increased risk of developing lactic acidosis when taking this drug because of a natural decline in kidney function. Your health-care practitioner should assess kidney function before prescribing this drug.

GENERIC NAME

Glyburide *see Sulfonylurea Antidiabetes Drugs, page 971*

GENERIC NAME
Granisetron *see Antiemetics, page 128*

GENERIC NAME
Grepafloxacin *see Fluoroquinolone Antibiotics, page 468*

GENERIC NAME
Griseofulvin

BRAND NAMES
Fulvicin P/G, Fulvicin U/F, Grifulvin V, Grisactin, Grisactin Ultra, Grisovin-FP, Gris-PEG
Generic available

ABOUT THIS DRUG
Griseofulvin is an antifungal used to treat a variety of fungal infections that are susceptible to this drug.

Griseofulvin prevents certain fungi from growing and reproducing.

SIDE EFFECTS
Be sure to tell your health-care practitioner if you experience any side effects while taking griseofulvin. Only your health-care practitioner can determine whether it is safe for you to continue taking this drug.

➤ *Most Common:* headache

➤ *Less Common:* confusion, rash, itch, mouth or tongue irritation, soreness, nausea, vomiting, diarrhea, stomach pain, insomnia, tiredness

➤ *Rare:* sore throat, fever, numbness or tingling in feet or hands, cloudy urine, sensitivity to sunlight, jaundice. All these side effects are more likely to occur if you take high doses for long periods

IMPORTANT PRECAUTIONS
Tell your health-care practitioner if you are sensitive or allergic to griseofulvin or to any other drugs, especially other antifungal medications and penicillin.

Do not take griseofulvin if you have liver disease or porphyria (a rare inherited disease characterized by abdominal pain and depression, among other symptoms), or if your infection is minor and will respond to other, less potent drugs. Griseofulvin should be used with caution if you have lupus.

Prolonged use of griseofulvin may make you susceptible to infections that do not respond to griseofulvin.

Griseofulvin may make you more likely to burn in sunlight. Protect yourself against excessive exposure by wearing protective clothing and sunscreen.

DRUG INTERACTIONS

Tell your health-care practitioner and pharmacist if you are taking any prescription or nonprescription drugs, as well as any vitamins, herbs, or other supplements. Possible drug interactions include the following:

- Griseofulvin may reduce the effect of oral anticoagulants (e.g., warfarin) and oral contraceptives.
- Barbiturates (e.g., pentobarbital, phenobarbital) may decrease the effect of griseofulvin.

FOOD, VITAMIN, AND HERBAL INTERACTIONS

No food, vitamin, or herbal interactions have been noted.

RECOMMENDED DOSAGE

Griseofulvin is available in tablets, capsules, and oral suspension. The dosages given here are typical. However, your health-care practitioner will determine the most appropriate dose and schedule for you.

- *Children Up to Age 12:* for feet, nails, scalp, and groin, 5 mg per 2.2 pounds of body weight every 12 hours, or 10 mg per 2.2 pounds of body weight once daily
- *Children 12 Years and Older and Adults:* for feet and nails, 500 mg every 12 hours. For scalp, skin, and groin, 250 mg every 12 hours or 500 mg once daily

Griseofulvin should be taken either with or after meals or milk. Fatty foods, such as milk, peanut butter, and avocados, increase the amount of the drug your body absorbs. Talk to your health-care practitioner if you are on a low-fat diet.

If you miss a dose, take it as soon as you remember. If it is nearly time for your next dose, do not take the missed dose. Continue with your regular dosing schedule. Never take a double dose.

SYMPTOMS OF OVERDOSE AND WHAT TO DO

Symptoms of overdose include nausea, vomiting, and diarrhea. If overdose occurs, seek immediate medical assistance and bring the prescription container with you to the hospital.

SPECIAL INFORMATION FOR PREGNANT OR NURSING WOMEN

Griseofulvin causes birth defects in both humans and animals. If you are pregnant or plan to become pregnant, talk to your health-care practitioner immediately. This drug should not be taken during pregnancy because the risks outweigh the benefits.

Griseofulvin may pass into breast milk. If you are breastfeeding, your health-care practitioner may advise you to switch to bottle feeding until your treatment is done.

SPECIAL INFORMATION FOR SENIORS

Older adults may experience more side effects, and they may be more severe.

GENERIC NAME

Guanabenz

BRAND NAME

Wytensin
Generic available

ABOUT THIS DRUG

Guanabenz is an antihypertensive used to treat high blood pressure.

This drug affects certain areas of the brain and spinal cord that regulate the activity of the heart and the muscles that surround the arteries. Guanabenz causes the blood vessels to relax, which then lowers blood pressure.

SIDE EFFECTS

Be sure to tell your health-care practitioner if you experience any side effects while taking guanabenz. Only your health-care practitioner can determine whether it is safe for you to continue taking this drug.

- *Most Common:* dizziness or lightheadedness, drowsiness, dry mouth, weakness, faintness
- *Less Common:* headache, nausea, decreased sexual ability

IMPORTANT PRECAUTIONS

Tell your health-care practitioner if you are sensitive or allergic to guanabenz or to any other drugs, especially any sympathomimetic drugs (e.g., ephedrine, guaifenesin).

Consult your health-care practitioner before stopping guanabenz. Do not stop taking guanabenz suddenly, because you may experience serious health problems, including a sudden rise in blood pressure to dangerous levels (known as rebound effect). Symptoms include severe headache, nausea, vomiting, abdominal pain, confusion, blurred vision, chest pain, anxiety, heartbeat irregularities, and breathing difficulties. Contact your health-care practitioner immediately if these symptoms occur.

Because guanabenz can cause dizziness, drowsiness, and faintness, make sure you know how you react to the drug before you drive or operate dangerous equipment.

Before taking guanabenz, talk to your health-care practitioner if you have a blood disease, heart disease, stroke, kidney or liver disease, diabetes, or an overactive thyroid, or if you will be having surgery requiring general or spinal anesthesia (including dental surgery) within the next 2 months.

DRUG INTERACTIONS

Tell your health-care practitioner and pharmacist if you are taking any prescription or nonprescription drugs, as well as any vitamins, herbs, or other supplements. Possible drug interactions include the following:

- Alcohol can cause oversedation and should be avoided while taking guanabenz.
- Other antihypertensive drugs (e.g., clonidine, enalapril) and diuretics (e.g., amiloride, furosemide) may decrease blood pressure more than either drug alone. Dosage adjustments may be needed.
- Fluoxetine and sertraline may cause an increased depressive effect of both drugs.
- Central nervous system depressants (e.g., sedatives, tranquilizers, antidepressants, narcotics) may increase brain depression. Do not use these drugs when taking guanabenz.
- Clozapine may result in toxic effects on the central nervous system.
- Angiotensin-converting enzyme (ACE) inhibitors (e.g., captopril, enalapril) may result in excessive blood potassium levels.
- Methyprylon may cause a dangerous sedative effect. Do not use along with guanabenz.

- Nimodipine may result in a dangerous drop in blood pressure. Do not use along with guanabenz.

FOOD, VITAMIN, AND HERBAL INTERACTIONS

It is best to avoid excessive salt intake if you have high blood pressure. Foods and beverages that contain caffeine (e.g., colas, coffee, tea, chocolate) should be avoided as well because they can cause overstimulation.

If you plan to or are taking any herbs or supplements, talk with your health-care practitioner before starting guanabenz. Ginseng, goldenseal, licorice, ephedra (ma huang), and saw palmetto may raise your blood pressure; garlic and calcium may help lower it.

RECOMMENDED DOSAGE

Guanabenz is available in tablets. The dosages given here are typical. However, your health-care practitioner will determine the most appropriate dose and schedule for you.

- *Children Up to 12 Years:* safety and effectiveness have not been established for children younger than 12 years
- *Children 12 Years and Older and Adults:* 4 mg twice daily. Your health-care practitioner will gradually increase the dose as needed. The daily maximum dose is 32 mg in divided doses.

Guanabenz can be taken with food to reduce stomach irritation. The tablet can be crushed and taken with liquid or food if swallowing the tablet is difficult.

If you miss a dose, take it as soon as you remember. If it is nearly time for your next dose, do not take the missed dose. Continue with your regular dosing schedule. Never take a double dose. If you miss two or more doses in a row, contact your health-care practitioner.

SYMPTOMS OF OVERDOSE AND WHAT TO DO

Symptoms of overdose include severe dizziness, slow heartbeat, pinpoint pupils, fainting, unusual weakness, and coma. If overdose occurs, seek immediate medical assistance and bring the prescription container with you to the hospital.

SPECIAL INFORMATION FOR PREGNANT OR NURSING WOMEN

No adequate studies of the effects of guanabenz on pregnant or nursing women have been done. If you are pregnant or plan to become pregnant, talk to your health-care practitioner. You and your health-care practitioner must weigh the potential benefits against the potential risks to the fetus.

Guanabenz may pass into breast milk. If you are breastfeeding, your health-care practitioner will likely advise you to stop until treatment is done.

SPECIAL INFORMATION FOR SENIORS

Older adults may experience more side effects, and they may be more severe.

GENERIC NAME

Halazepam

BRAND NAME

Paxipam
No generic available

ABOUT THIS DRUG

Halazepam is a benzodiazepine tranquilizer used primarily to treat anxiety, panic attacks, and muscle spasms.

This drug produces mild sedation by enhancing the effect of a chemical (gamma-aminobutyric acid, or GABA), which in turn dampens the transmission of nerve signals and reduces nerve excitation.

SIDE EFFECTS

Be sure to tell your health-care practitioner if you experience any side effects while taking halazepam. Only your health-care practitioner can determine whether it is safe for you to continue taking this drug.

- *Most Common:* dizziness, drowsiness, clumsiness
- *Less Common:* constipation, diarrhea, nausea, vomiting, urinary difficulties, vivid dreams, behavior changes, abdominal pain, dry mouth, headache, confusion, depression, rash, itch, vision changes, sore throat, fever, chills
- *Rare:* breathing difficulties, slow heartbeat, mouth ulcers, jaundice, decreased sex drive

IMPORTANT PRECAUTIONS

Tell your health-care practitioner if you are sensitive or allergic to halazepam or to any other drugs, especially other benzodiazepines (e.g., diazepam, clonazepam).

If you have liver or kidney problems, use this drug with caution.

Because halazepam can cause drowsiness, make sure you know how you react to it before you drive or operate hazardous equipment.

Halazepam can be addictive, and you can experience withdrawal symptoms if you suddenly stop taking it. Follow your health-care practitioner's use instructions carefully.

Do not take halazepam if you have narrow-angle glaucoma (but it is safe if you have open-angle glaucoma), severe depression, severe lung disease, sleep apnea, psychotic problems, alcoholism, or kidney disease. Halazepam can worsen these conditions, and the depressive effects of the drug may be enhanced as well.

DRUG INTERACTIONS

Tell your health-care practitioner and pharmacist if you are taking any prescription or nonprescription drugs, as well as any vitamins, herbs, or other supplements. Possible drug interactions include the following:

- Halazepam can increase the effects of alcohol. Do not drink alcohol while taking this drug.
- Narcotics (e.g., codeine, oxycodone), barbiturates (e.g., phenobarbital), monoamine oxidase inhibitors (e.g., phenelzine), antihistamines (e.g., cetirizine, loratadine), and antidepressants (e.g., amitriptyline, doxepin) may lead to excessive drowsiness, difficulty breathing, and extreme depression.
- Cimetidine, oral contraceptives, disulfiram, fluoxetine, isoniazid, ketoconazole, rifampin, metoprolol, probenecid, propoxyphene, propranolol, and valproic acid may prolong the effects of halazepam.
- Halazepam may raise the blood levels of digoxin and increase the risk of digoxin toxicity.
- Halazepam may decrease the effects of levodopa.
- Smoking may reduce how quickly halazepam is broken down by the body, thus reducing its effectiveness.
- Halazepam along with phenytoin may elevate phenytoin levels and increase the risk of phenytoin toxicity.
- Anticonvulsants (e.g., phenobarbital, felbamate) may result in a change in seizure pattern.

FOOD, VITAMIN, AND HERBAL INTERACTIONS

Herbs that produce a sedative effect may cause significant depressant interactions when used with halazepam. Some of those herbs include calendula, capsicum, catnip, goldenseal, gotu kola, hops, kava, lady's slipper, passionflower, sage, Siberian ginseng, skullcap, St. John's wort, and valerian, among others.

Because grapefruit juice does slow the breakdown of some benzodiazepines, it is best to avoid this beverage while being treated with halazepam.

RECOMMENDED DOSAGE

Halazepam is available in tablets. The dosages given here are typical. However, your health-care practitioner will determine the most appropriate dose and schedule for you.

- *Children Up to 18 Years:* use and dose to be determined by your health-care practitioner
- *Adults:* 20 to 40 mg 3 to 4 times daily
- *Adults Older than 60:* 20 mg 1 to 2 times daily

If you miss a dose, take it as soon as you remember. If it is nearly time for your next dose, do not take the missed dose. Continue with your regular dosing schedule. Never take a double dose.

SYMPTOMS OF OVERDOSE AND WHAT TO DO

Symptoms of overdose include extreme drowsiness, confusion, slurred speech, poor coordination, staggering, tremor, slowed breathing, and loss of consciousness. If overdose occurs, seek immediate medical attention and bring the prescription container with you to the hospital.

SPECIAL INFORMATION FOR PREGNANT OR NURSING WOMEN

No adequate studies of the effects of halazepam on pregnant or nursing women have been done, but animal studies have shown some fetal deaths. If you are pregnant or plan to become pregnant and this drug is necessary for your health, you and your health-care practitioner must weigh the potential benefits against the potential risks to the fetus.

Halazepam may pass into breast milk. If you are breastfeeding, your health-care practitioner may advise you to switch to bottle feeding.

SPECIAL INFORMATION FOR SENIORS

Older adults, especially those who have kidney or liver disease, are more likely to experience side effects, and perhaps more severe ones. Seniors may require lower doses.

GENERIC NAME
Halcinonide *see Corticosteroids, Topical, page 337*

GENERIC NAME
Halobetasol propionate
see Corticosteroids, Topical, page 337

GENERIC NAME
Halofantrine

BRAND NAME
Halfan
No generic available

ABOUT THIS DRUG
Halofantrine is an antimalarial drug used to treat victims of mild-to-moderate infections of malaria, a red blood cell infection carried by mosquitoes. More severe cases require more potent drugs.

This drug kills malaria organisms in the blood; it does not affect immature forms of the organism or those that may be in the liver.

SIDE EFFECTS
Be sure to tell your health-care practitioner if you experience any side effects while taking halofantrine. Only your health-care practitioner can determine whether it is safe for you to continue taking this drug.

- *Most Common:* diarrhea, abdominal pain
- *Less Common:* nausea, vomiting, dizziness, cough, headache, muscle ache, chills
- *Rare:* rare side effects may occur anywhere throughout the body

IMPORTANT PRECAUTIONS
Tell your health-care practitioner if you are sensitive or allergic to halofantrine or to any other drugs.

Halofantrine can cause fatal changes in heart ventricle rhythm. Do not take this drug if you have a ventricular disorder.

Before starting this drug, tell your health-care practitioner if you have any heart problems, a thiamine deficiency, or unexplained fainting.

This drug is associated with more frequent relapse than other malaria drugs.

Because halofantrine can cause dizziness, make sure you know how the drug affects you before you drive or operate hazardous equipment.

If you develop anxiety, reduced urine volume, chest or lower back pain, black urine, rapid and irregular heartbeat, restlessness, flushing, or rapid breathing, call your health-care practitioner immediately.

DRUG INTERACTIONS

Tell your health-care practitioner and pharmacist if you are taking any prescription or nonprescription drugs, as well as any vitamins, herbs, or other supplements. Possible drug interactions include the following:

- Mefloquine may have a fatal effect on heart ventricular rhythm. Do not take halofantrine if you have been treated with mefloquine.

FOOD, VITAMIN, AND HERBAL INTERACTIONS

No food, vitamin, or herbal interactions have been noted.

RECOMMENDED DOSAGE

Halofantrine is available in tablets. The dosages given here are typical. However, your health-care practitioner will determine the most appropriate dose and schedule for you.

- *Children (less than 50 pounds):* dosage has not been established
- *Children (50 to 68 pounds):* 250 mg every 6 hours for 3 doses
- *Children (68 to 82 pounds):* 375 mg every 6 hours for 3 doses
- *Adults and Children (more than 82 pounds):* 500 mg every 5 hours for 3 doses

Take halofantrine on an empty stomach to reduce the risk of side effects.

If you miss a dose, take it as soon as you remember. If it is nearly time for your next dose, do not take the missed dose. Continue with your regular dosing schedule. Never take a double dose.

SYMPTOMS OF OVERDOSE AND WHAT TO DO

Symptoms of overdose include abdominal pain, gastrointestinal problems, cramping, diarrhea, vomiting, and palpitations. If overdose occurs, you can induce vomiting using ipecac syrup and then seek treatment, or you can seek immediate medical assistance. Always bring the prescription container with you to the hospital.

SPECIAL INFORMATION FOR PREGNANT OR NURSING WOMEN

No adequate studies of the effects of halofantrine on pregnant or nursing women have been done. Animal studies show that halofantrine may harm the fetus. If you are pregnant or plan to become pregnant, and this drug is crucial for your health, you and your health-care practitioner must weigh the potential benefits against the potential risks to the fetus.

Halofantrine may pass into breast milk. If you are breastfeeding, your health-care practitioner may advise you to stop until your treatment is done.

SPECIAL INFORMATION FOR SENIORS

No special precautions are needed for older adults.

GENERIC NAME

Haloperidol

BRAND NAMES

Haldol, Haldol Decanoate
Generic available

ABOUT THIS DRUG

Haloperidol is an antipsychotic drug used primarily to reduce severe anxiety, agitation, and psychotic behavior, including schizophrenia, manic states, and drug-induced psychosis. It is also used to treat behavior problems in children, including infantile autism, and to reduce the symptoms of Tourette's syndrome.

This drug blocks the effects of dopamine, a chemical that aids in the transmission of nerve impulses in the brain. The blockage results in a tranquilizing effect.

SIDE EFFECTS

Be sure to tell your health-care practitioner if you experience any side effects while taking haloperidol. Only your health-care practitioner can determine whether it is safe for you to continue taking this drug.

- *Most Common:* involuntary or jerky movements (especially in the face, lips, or tongue), slow-frequency tremor of the head or limbs, lack of facial expression, slow inflexible movements, restlessness, intermittent spasms of the facial muscles or muscles of the body or limbs
- *Less Common:* dry mouth, blurred vision, constipation, urination difficulties, sedation, low blood pressure, dizziness

People taking antipsychotic drugs may experience a rare but life-threatening set of side effects known as neuroleptic malignant syndrome (NMS). Symptoms include fever, difficulty breathing, rapid heartbeat, rigid muscles, mental changes, increased sweating, irregular blood pressure, and convulsions. Immediate medical attention is required.

Side effects such as lip smacking, wormlike movements of the tongue, and slow, rhythmical, involuntary movements are characteristic of a disorder known as tardive dyskinesia. Older adults (especially women) are more susceptible to this condition, which may become permanent. If you experience tardive dyskinesia, your health-care practitioner will probably advise you to stop taking this drug.

IMPORTANT PRECAUTIONS

Tell your health-care practitioner if you are sensitive or allergic to haloperidol or to any other drugs.

Do not take haloperidol if you are depressed or if you have Parkinson's disease. It also should not be given to children younger than 3 years old.

Prolonged use of haloperidol may cause tardive dyskinesia (involuntary movements of the tongue, lips, and jaw).

Haloperidol may cause rash or a serious sunburn in skin areas exposed to the sun. Protect yourself by wearing protective clothing and applying sunscreen.

Because haloperidol may cause involuntary movements, make sure you know how you react to this drug before you drive or operate dangerous equipment.

DRUG INTERACTIONS

Tell your health-care practitioner and pharmacist if you are taking any prescription or nonprescription drugs, as well as any vitamins, herbs, or other supplements. Possible drug interactions include the following:

- Haloperidol may increase the effects of anticholinergics (e.g., atropine, scopolamine) and also result in elevated pressure within the eye.
- Antidepressants (e.g., amitriptyline, fluoxetine), antihistamines (e.g., clemastine, cetirizine), barbiturates (e.g., amobarbital, secobarbital), narcotics (e.g., codeine, oxycodone), and procarbazine may result in increased sedation.
- Antihypertensives (e.g., clonidine, guanfacine) may cause a severe drop in blood pressure.
- Clozapine may cause toxic effects on the nervous system.
- Haloperidol may decrease the effects of levodopa, pergolide, and guanethidine.
- Lithium may result in increased toxicity.
- Methyldopa may cause psychosis.
- Fluoxetine and sertraline may result in an increased depressive effect of both drugs.
- Bupropion use increases your risk of seizures.

FOOD, VITAMIN, AND HERBAL INTERACTIONS

No food, vitamin, or herbal interactions have been noted.

RECOMMENDED DOSAGE

Haloperidol is available in tablets and liquid. The dosages given here are typical. However, your health-care practitioner will determine the most appropriate dose and schedule for you.

For Psychotic Disorders

- *Children 3 to 12 Years:* 0.05 to 0.15 mg per 2.2 pounds of body weight.
- *Adults:* 0.5 to 5 mg, 2 or 3 times daily, depending on the severity of symptoms. The maximum dose is 100 mg a day.

For Tourette's Syndrome

- *Children 3 to 12 Years:* 0.075 mg per 2.2 pounds of body weight
- *Adults:* 0.5 to 5 mg, 2 or 3 times daily, depending on the severity of symptoms

Haloperidol should be taken with food or a full glass of milk or water. If you are taking the oral solution, you can prevent stomach irritation if you dilute the solution in beverages such as apple or orange juice.

If you miss a dose, take it as soon as you remember. Then take the remaining doses for the day at equally spaced intervals. Continue with your regular dosing schedule. Never take a double dose.

SYMPTOMS OF OVERDOSE AND WHAT TO DO

Symptoms of overdose include slow, shallow breathing, weak or rapid pulse, dizziness, confusion, seizures, deep sleep leading to coma, and muscle weakness or tremor. If overdose occurs, seek immediate medical attention and bring the prescription container with you to the hospital.

SPECIAL INFORMATION FOR PREGNANT OR NURSING WOMEN

No adequate studies of the effects of haloperidol on pregnant or nursing women have been done. If you are pregnant or plan to become pregnant, and haloperidol is crucial for your health, you and your health-care practitioner must weigh the potential benefits against the potential risks to the fetus.

Haloperidol passes into breast milk and may harm the infant. If you are breastfeeding, your health-care practitioner will advise you to stop until your treatment is done.

SPECIAL INFORMATION FOR SENIORS

Generally, older adults take lower dosages. Seniors, especially older women, may be more susceptible to tardive dyskinesia, a condition marked by involuntary muscle spasms and twitches.

GENERIC NAME

Hydralazine

BRAND NAMES

Apresoline, Alazine
Generic available

ABOUT THIS DRUG

Hydralazine is an antihypertensive used for treatment of high blood pressure and congestive heart failure.

This drug causes the blood vessels to relax and expand, which then lowers blood pressure.

SIDE EFFECTS

Be sure to tell your health-care practitioner if you experience any side effects while taking hydralazine. Only your health-care practitioner can determine whether it is safe for you to continue taking this drug.

- *Most Common:* nausea, vomiting, headache, diarrhea, loss of appetite, difficult or painful urination, irregular or rapid heartbeat
- *Less Common:* rash, facial flush, sore throat, fever, chest pain, swelling of lymph glands, skin blisters, swollen feet or legs, joint pain, confusion, dizziness, anxiety, depression, muscle pain, watery eyes, constipation
- *Rare:* jaundice, weakness and faintness when rising from a lying or seated position, numbness or tingling in the feet or hands, nasal congestion, impotence

IMPORTANT PRECAUTIONS

Tell your health-care practitioner if you are sensitive or allergic to hydralazine or to any other drugs, or to tartrazine dye, which is used in making this drug.

Do not take hydralazine if you have a history of coronary artery disease or rheumatic heart disease.

Before starting hydralazine, consult with your health-care practitioner if you have chest, neck, or arm pain upon physical exertion, or if you have lupus, stroke, or kidney disease or impaired function.

Prolonged use may cause lupus, psychosis, or numbness or tingling in the hands or feet (peripheral neuropathy).

Take hydralazine for the entire treatment course as prescribed by your health-care practitioner, even if you begin to feel better.

DRUG INTERACTIONS

Tell your health-care practitioner and pharmacist if you are taking any prescription or nonprescription drugs, as well as any vitamins, herbs, or other supplements. Possible drug interactions include the following:

- Amphetamines (dextroamphetamine, amphetamine) and nonsteroidal anti-inflammatory drugs (e.g., ibuprofen, naproxen) may decrease the effect of hydralazine.
- Hydralazine may decrease the effectiveness of terazosin.
- Hydralazine may increase the effects of beta-blockers (e.g., metoprolol, propranolol).
- Other antihypertensives (e.g., clonidine, guanabenz), carteolol, diazoxide, lisinopril, and sotalol may increase the antihypertensive effect.

- Oral diuretics (e.g., amiloride, indapamide) may increase the effects of both drugs. If monitored carefully, this combination can be used successfully to control hypertension.
- Guanfacine may increase the effects of both drugs.
- Nicardipine may cause blood pressure to drop.

FOOD, VITAMIN, AND HERBAL INTERACTIONS

It is best to avoid excessive salt intake if you have high blood pressure. Foods and beverages that contain caffeine (e.g., colas, coffee, tea, chocolate) should be avoided as weli because they can cause overstimulation.

If you plan to or are taking any herbs or supplements, talk with your health-care practitioner before starting guanabenz. Ginseng, goldenseal, licorice, ephedra (ma huang), and saw palmetto may raise your blood pressure; garlic and calcium may help lower it.

Because of a risk of peripheral neuropathy associated with hydralazine, ask your health-care practitioner about taking pyridoxine (vitamin B_6).

RECOMMENDED DOSAGE

Hydralazine is available in tablets. The dosages given here are typical. However, your health-care practitioner will determine the most appropriate dose and schedule for you.

- *Children:* dose and safety to be determined by your health-care practitioner
- *Adults:* starting dose is 10 mg, four times daily for 2 to 4 days. Your health-care practitioner may increase the dose to 25 mg or higher, four times daily. The total daily dose usually should not exceed 200 mg.

Hydralazine should be taken with food and at the same time each day. The tablet can be crushed and taken with liquid or food if swallowing the tablet is difficult.

If you miss a dose, take it as soon as you remember. If it is nearly time for your next dose, do not take the missed dose. Continue with your regular dosing schedule. Never take a double dose.

SYMPTOMS OF OVERDOSE AND WHAT TO DO

Symptoms of overdose include dizziness, headache, flushed skin, nausea, vomiting, loss of consciousness, cold and sweaty skin, weak and rapid pulse, and irregular heart rhythm. If overdose occurs, seek immediate medical attention and bring the prescription container with you to the hospital.

SPECIAL INFORMATION FOR PREGNANT OR NURSING WOMEN

No adequate studies of the effects of hydralazine on pregnant or nursing women have been done. In animal studies, birth defects have been noted. If you are pregnant or plan to become pregnant and this drug is crucial for your health, you and your health-care practitioner must weigh the potential benefits against the potential risks to the fetus.

Hydralazine passes into breast milk. If you are breastfeeding, your health-care practitioner will likely advise you to stop until treatment is done.

SPECIAL INFORMATION FOR SENIORS

Side effects may be more likely to occur, and to be more severe, in older adults. Headache, palpitations, and rapid heart rates are more common in seniors.

GENERIC NAME

Hydrochlorothiazide

see Thiazide Diuretics, page 1020

GENERIC NAME

Hydrocodone + chlorpheniramine

BRAND NAME

Tussionex

No generic available

ABOUT THIS DRUG

Hydrocodone plus chlorpheniramine is a narcotic-based cough suppressant and antihistamine combination drug prescribed for coughs and upper respiratory symptoms of allergies and colds.

Hydrocodone is a narcotic that works directly on the cough center in the brain. Chlorpheniramine, an antihistamine, reduces swelling and itching and also dries up secretions released from the nose, throat, and eyes.

SIDE EFFECTS

Be sure to tell your health-care practitioner if you experience any side effects while taking hydrocodone and chlorpheniramine. Only your health-care practitioner can determine whether it is safe for you to continue taking this drug combination.

- *Most Common:* lightheadedness, dizziness, sleepiness, nausea, vomiting, increased sweating, itching rash, dry mouth, throat, and nose, sensitivity to bright light, chills
- *Less Common:* euphoria, weakness, agitation, uncoordinated muscle movement, disorientation, hallucinations, palpitations, urinary difficulties, low blood sugar, anemia, jaundice, blurred or double vision, ringing in the ears, wheezing

IMPORTANT PRECAUTIONS

Tell your health-care practitioner if you are sensitive or allergic to hydrocodone, chlorpheniramine, other narcotics, or any other drugs.

Use this drug combination with caution if you have a history of glaucoma, stomach ulcer, alcoholism, drug abuse, lung disease, narrow-angle glaucoma, asthma, hypertension, heart disease, diabetes, thyroid or adrenal gland disorders, urinary difficulties, an intestinal disorder, liver or kidney disease, or convulsions.

Because this drug combination can cause dizziness, lightheadedness, and sleepiness, make sure you know how you react to the drug before you drive or operate dangerous equipment.

This drug combination contains a mild narcotic that can cause dependence and tolerance if it is taken for several weeks. Dependence is unlikely, however, with short-term treatment of cough.

DRUG INTERACTIONS

Tell your health-care practitioner and pharmacist if you are taking any prescription or nonprescription drugs, as well as any vitamins, herbs, or other supplements. Possible drug interactions include the following:

- Antidepressants (e.g., amitriptyline, fluoxetine), antihistamines (e.g., clemastine, loratadine), methyprylon, phenothiazines (e.g., chlorpromazine, promazine), sedatives, tranquilizers, sleeping pills, and tramadol may increase the sedative effect.
- Alcohol increases the intoxicating effect of alcohol. Do not take alcohol and hydrocodone/chlorpheniramine.
- Sertraline may increase the depressive effects of both drugs.
- Selegiline may cause severe toxicity, marked by breathing problems, seizures, and coma.
- Phenytoin and rifampin may decrease the narcotic effect.

- Other narcotics (e.g., codeine, oxycodone), sotalol, nonsteroidal anti-inflammatory drugs (NSAIDs; e.g., naproxen, aspirin), and molindone may increase the narcotic effect.
- Naltrexone may cause respiratory arrest, coma, and death.
- Carteolol may cause increased narcotic effect and dangerous sedation.

FOOD, VITAMIN, AND HERBAL INTERACTIONS

Herbs that produce a sedative effect may cause potentially serious depressant interactions when used with hydrocodone. Some of those herbs include calendula, capsicum, catnip, goldenseal, gotu kola, hops, kava, lady's slipper, passionflower, sage, Siberian ginseng, skullcap, St. John's wort, and valerian, among others.

RECOMMENDED DOSAGE

Hydrocodone/chlorpheniramine is available as syrup. The dosages given here are typical. However, your health-care practitioner will determine the most appropriate dose and schedule for you.

- *Children Up to 6 Years:* not recommended
- *Children 6 Years and Older:* one-half teaspoon every 12 hours. Do not take more than 1 teaspoon in 24 hours.
- *Adults:* 1 teaspoon every 12 hours. Do not exceed 2 teaspoons in 24 hours.

You can take this drug combination with food to help prevent stomach upset.

If you miss a dose, take it as soon as you remember. If it is nearly time for your next dose, do not take the missed dose. Continue with your regular dosing schedule. Never take a double dose.

SYMPTOMS OF OVERDOSE AND WHAT TO DO

Symptoms of overdose include bluish skin due to lack of oxygen, cardiac arrest, cold and clammy skin, extreme sleepiness leading to stupor or coma, low blood pressure, slow heartbeat, temporary cessation of breathing, and breathing difficulties. If overdose occurs, seek immediate medical attention and bring the prescription container with you to the hospital.

SPECIAL INFORMATION FOR PREGNANT OR NURSING WOMEN

Although no adequate studies of the effects of hydrocodone and chlorpheniramine on pregnant or nursing women have been done, infants born to mothers who have been taking narcotics regularly before they deliver are born addicted. If you are pregnant or plan to become pregnant, talk to your health-care practitioner immediately.

Hydrocodone/chlorpheniramine may pass into breast milk. If you are breastfeeding, your health-care practitioner will likely advise you to stop until your treatment is done.

SPECIAL INFORMATION FOR SENIORS

Older adults are more likely to experience side effects, especially dizziness, fainting when rising from a lying or seated position, confusion, nervousness, dry mouth, difficult urination, restlessness, irritability, and nightmares.

GENERIC NAME

Hydrocodone + ibuprofen

BRAND NAME

Vicoprofen

No generic available

ABOUT THIS DRUG

Hydrocodone + ibuprofen is an opioid (narcotic) painkiller used to relieve mild-to-moderate pain and to control cough. The combination of drugs may provide better pain relief at lower doses than taking either drug alone.

Hydrocodone acts on certain areas in the brain and spinal cord that process pain messages from the nerves in the body. Ibuprofen (a nonsteroidal anti-inflammatory drug, or NSAID) interferes with the production of prostaglandins, natural substances that cause inflammation and make nerves more sensitive to pain signals.

SIDE EFFECTS

Be sure to tell your health-care practitioner if you experience any side effects while taking hydrocodone plus ibuprofen. Only your health-care practitioner can determine whether it is safe for you to continue taking this drug.

- ➤ *Most Common:* dizziness, nausea, stomach upset, drowsiness, constipation, headache, lightheadedness, abdominal pain, anxiety, diarrhea, dry mouth, unusual sweating, insomnia, itching, swollen limbs
- ➤ *Less Common:* confusion, breathing difficulties, tarry stool, fever, frequent urination, hiccups, inflamed throat and nasal passages,

mouth ulcers, ringing in the ears, loss of appetite, tension, thinking abnormalities, thirst, throbbing heartbeat

- *Rare:* abnormal dreams, allergic reaction, vision problems, asthma, bad taste, bronchitis, decreased sex drive, depression, dry eyes, hives, hoarseness, inflamed sinuses or tongue, joint pain, low blood pressure, lung congestion, mood changes, irregular heartbeat, slurred speech, tremor, vertigo, weight loss

IMPORTANT PRECAUTIONS

Tell your health-care practitioner if you are sensitive or allergic to hydrocodone, ibuprofen, or any other drugs, especially other narcotic painkillers (e.g., codeine, oxycodone) or NSAIDs (e.g., aspirin, naproxen).

Because hydrocodone plus ibuprofen can make you drowsy, dizzy, and lightheaded, make sure you know how you react to the drug before you drive or operate dangerous equipment.

Do not take this drug combination if you have had a head injury, because hydrocodone can increase the pressure of the fluid inside the skull.

Before taking hydrocodone plus ibuprofen, talk to your health-care practitioner if you have severe liver or kidney disease, gallbladder disease, a seizure disorder, urinary difficulties, heart failure, lupus, underactive adrenal or thyroid glands, an enlarged prostate, a history of drug abuse or alcoholism, or any type of bladder obstruction.

Hydrocodone suppresses the cough reflex. If you have had surgery recently or if you have a lung condition, use this drug with caution.

This drug combination can be habit forming. Prolonged use can lead to mental and physical dependence, with a need for higher and higher doses to get the same results.

DRUG INTERACTIONS

Tell your health-care practitioner and pharmacist if you are taking any prescription or nonprescription drugs, as well as any vitamins, herbs, or other supplements. Possible drug interactions include the following:

- Hydrocodone may increase the effects of atropine and similar drugs and increase the risk of urinary retention and constipation.
- Hydrocodone may increase the effects of drugs with sedative effects, including tranquilizers, barbiturates, antidepressants, and sleeping pills.

- Cimetidine and tramadol may increase the risk of breathing difficulties and central nervous system suppression.
- Ritonavir and perhaps other protease inhibitors (e.g., amprenavir, indinavir) may result in toxicity.
- Monoamine oxidase inhibitors (MAOIs; e.g., phenelzine, furazolidone) may cause an increased effect and the need to reduce the hydrocodone dose.

FOOD, VITAMIN, AND HERBAL INTERACTIONS

Herbs that produce a sedative effect may cause potentially serious depressant interactions when used with hydrocodone. Some of those herbs include calendula, capsicum, catnip, goldenseal, gotu kola, hops, kava, lady's slipper, passionflower, sage, Siberian ginseng, skullcap, St. John's wort, and valerian, among others.

RECOMMENDED DOSAGE

Hydrocodone and ibuprofen is available in tablets. The dosages given here are typical. However, your health-care practitioner will determine the most appropriate dose and schedule for you.

- *Children Up to 16 Years:* not recommended
- *Adults:* 1 tablets every 4 to 6 hours as needed. The maximum 24-hour dose is 5 tablets.

Hydrocodone and ibuprofen should be taken with food.

If you miss a dose, take it as soon as you remember. If it is nearly time for your next dose, do not take the missed dose. Continue with your regular dosing schedule. Never take a double dose.

SYMPTOMS OF OVERDOSE AND WHAT TO DO

Symptoms of overdose include severe nausea, vomiting, breathing difficulties, severe dizziness or drowsiness, cold clammy skin, irregular or slow heartbeat, severe weakness, confusion, and loss of consciousness. If overdose occurs, seek immediately medical attention and bring the prescription container with you to the hospital.

SPECIAL INFORMATION FOR PREGNANT OR NURSING WOMEN

Hydrocodone and ibuprofen should not be taken during pregnancy unless your health-care practitioner determines that it is crucial for your health and the benefits of therapy clearly outweigh the potential risks to the fetus. Infants born to mothers who take this drug combination regularly during pregnancy can be born with a drug dependency.

This drug combination may pass into breast milk. If you are breastfeeding, your health-care practitioner will likely advise you to stop until your treatment is done.

SPECIAL INFORMATION FOR SENIORS

Older adults should be given a lower dose. Side effects are more likely to occur and to be more severe.

GENERIC NAME

Hydrocortisone

see Corticosteroids, Oral, page 330; Corticosteroids, Topical, page 337

GENERIC NAME

Hydroflumethiazide

see Thiazide Diuretics, page 1020

GENERIC NAME

Hydroxyzine

BRAND NAMES

Anxanil, Atarax, E-Vista, Hydroxacen, Hyzine-50, Vistaject-25, Vistaject-50, Vistaril, Vistazine 50
Generic available

ABOUT THIS DRUG

Hydroxyzine is a tranquilizer (sedative) and antihistamine used to treat anxiety, agitation, insomnia, and tension, and to relieve itching associated with allergic reactions.

This drug blocks the action of histamines, substances that cause itching, sneezing, watery eyes, runny nose, and other typical allergy symptoms.

SIDE EFFECTS

Be sure to tell your health-care practitioner if you experience any side effects while taking hydroxyzine. Only your health-care practitioner can determine whether it is safe for you to continue taking this drug.

- *Most Common:* drowsiness, dizziness, dry mouth, nose, or throat, nausea
- *Less Common:* vision changes, clumsiness, rash, difficult or painful urination, loss of appetite

- *Rare:* nightmares, agitation, sore throat, fever, rapid heartbeat, unusual bleeding or bruising, fatigue, fainting, seizures, confusion

IMPORTANT PRECAUTIONS

Tell your health-care practitioner if you are sensitive or allergic to hydroxyzine, any other antihistamines, or any other drugs.

Before you take hydroxyzine, tell your health-care practitioner if you have asthma or kidney disease, or if you will be having surgery (including dental surgery) within the next 2 months that will require general or spinal anesthesia.

Prolonged use of this drug results in tolerance and reduced effectiveness.

DRUG INTERACTIONS

Tell your health-care practitioner and pharmacist if you are taking any prescription or nonprescription drugs, as well as any vitamins, herbs, or other supplements. Possible drug interactions include the following:

- Tricyclic antidepressants (e.g., imipramine, clomipramine) and narcotics (e.g., codeine, oxycodone) may increase the effects of both drugs.
- Antihistamines (e.g., cetirizine, loratadine) may increase the effect of hydroxyzine.
- Central nervous system depressants (e.g., sedatives, antidepressants, barbiturates) may result in greater depression of the central nervous system.
- Clozapine may cause a toxic effect on the central nervous system.
- Fluoxetine and sertraline may cause increased depressant effects of both drugs.
- Guanfacine may increase the depressant effects of either drug.
- Alcohol may result in increased sedation and intoxication. Exercise caution if using alcohol when taking hydroxyzine.

FOOD, VITAMIN, AND HERBAL INTERACTIONS

Beverages and foods that contain caffeine (e.g., colas, coffee, tea, chocolate) may decrease the tranquilizer effect of hydroxyzine.

RECOMMENDED DOSAGE

Hydroxyzine is available in tablets, syrup, and capsules. The dosages given here are typical. However, your health-care practitioner will determine the most appropriate dose and schedule for you.

For Allergy Symptoms

- *Children Up to 6 Years:* 12.5 mg every 6 hours as needed
- *Children 6 Years and Older:* 12.5 to 25 mg every 6 hours as needed
- *Adults:* 25 to 100 mg, 3 or 4 times daily as needed

For Sedation

- *Children:* to be determined by your health-care practitioner
- *Adults:* 50 to 100 mg daily

If you have difficulty swallowing the tablet, you can crush it and mix it with liquid or food. The syrup can be diluted in liquid.

If you miss a dose, take it as soon as you remember. If it is nearly time for your next dose, do not take the missed dose. Continue with your regular dosing schedule. Never take a double dose.

SYMPTOMS OF OVERDOSE AND WHAT TO DO

Symptoms of overdose include severe dry mouth, nose, and throat, extreme drowsiness, loss of coordination, flushing, tremors, faintness, hallucinations, and difficulty breathing. If overdose occurs, seek immediate medical attention and bring the prescription container with you to the hospital.

SPECIAL INFORMATION FOR PREGNANT OR NURSING WOMEN

No adequate studies of the effects of hydroxyzine on pregnant or nursing women have been done. If you are pregnant or plan to become pregnant, you and your health-care practitioner must weigh the potential benefits against the potential risks to the fetus.

Hydroxyzine may pass into breast milk. If you are breastfeeding, your health-care practitioner may advise you to stop until your treatment is done.

SPECIAL INFORMATION FOR SENIORS

Older adults are more likely to experience side effects, and those reactions may be more severe.

GENERIC NAME

Hyoscyamine

BRAND NAMES

Anaspaz, A-Spas S/L, Donnamar, Gastroseda, Levbid, Levsin, Levsinex

Generic available

ABOUT THIS DRUG

Hyoscyamine is prescribed to help prevent painful spasms of the urinary bladder and the gut, and can be helpful in treating irritable or spastic bowel and diverticulosis (a painful inflammatory disease of the bowel). It is a belladonna alkaloid in a class of drugs called anticholinergic antispasmodics.

This drug relaxes the muscles and helps prevent spasms from occurring. It also reduces the production of gastric acid.

SIDE EFFECTS

Be sure to tell your health-care practitioner if you experience any side effects while taking hyoscyamine. Only your health-care practitioner can determine whether it is safe for you to continue taking this drug.

- *Most Common:* dizziness, sleepiness, faintness, lightheadedness, dry mouth, constipation, urinary difficulties, headache, blurred vision, decreased sweating, bloating
- *Less Common or Rare:* tight chest, irregular or fast heartbeat, eye pain, fever, itching, bad cough, blue skin color, swelling of the lips, tongue, throat, or face

IMPORTANT PRECAUTIONS

Tell your health-care practitioner if you are sensitive or allergic to hyoscyamine, other belladonna alkaloids, or any other drugs.

Do not take hyoscyamine if you have glaucoma, blockage of the urinary tract, myasthenia gravis, kidney disease, or severe ulcerative colitis.

Before taking hyoscyamine, tell your health-care practitioner if you have high blood pressure, congestive heart failure, asthma, hiatal hernia or reflux disease, an enlarged prostate, allergies, chronic lung problems, tingling in your hands or feet, or urinary difficulties.

Men older than 65 who have urinary problems should not take hyoscyamine.

Avoid becoming overheated while taking hyoscyamine. This drug reduces your ability to sweat, thus increasing your risk for heatstroke.

Severe mental changes have been reported in people who are sensitive to belladonna alkaloids. Symptoms may include agitation, confusion, hallucinations, and short-term memory loss, all of which usually disappear within 12 to 48 hours after stopping the drug.

DRUG INTERACTIONS

Tell your health-care practitioner and pharmacist if you are taking any prescription or nonprescription drugs, as well as any vitamins, herbs, or other supplements. Possible drug interactions with hyoscyamine include the following:

- Antimuscarinics (e.g., atropine, scopolamine), amantadine, haloperidol, phenothiazines (chlorpromazine, promazine), monoamine oxidase inhibitors (e.g., phenelzine, procarbazine), tricyclic antidepressants (e.g., clomipramine, imipramine), decongestants and appetite suppressants (e.g., phenylephrine, pseudoephedrine), and some antihistamines may increase adverse effects.
- Antacids should be taken after meals (hyoscyamine is taken before) because they may interfere with the absorption of hyoscyamine.
- Hyoscyamine may increase levels of digoxin.

FOOD, VITAMIN, AND HERBAL INTERACTIONS

Hyoscyamine reduces the absorption of ferrous citrate, an iron supplement, and so the two substances should be taken at least several hours apart.

The herb *Anisodus tanguticus* (used to vitalize blood flow) contains a chemical that causes effects similar to those of atropine, which is related to hyoscyamine. Although no human studies have investigated a possible interaction between hyoscyamine and this herb, it is best to avoid using them together until further research is done.

RECOMMENDED DOSAGE

Hyoscyamine is available in tablets. The dosages given here are typical. However, your health-care practitioner will determine the most appropriate dose and schedule for you.

- *Children Up to 2 Years:* not recommended
- *Children 2 to 11 Years:* 1/2 to 1 tablet every 4 hours as needed. Do not exceed 6 tablets in 24 hours.

- *Children 12 Years and Older and Adults:* 1 to 2 tablets every 4 hours as needed.

For best results, take hyoscyamine 30 to 60 minutes before eating.

If you miss a dose, take it as soon as you remember. If it is nearly time for your next dose, do not take the missed dose. Continue with your regular dosing schedule. Never take a double dose.

SYMPTOMS OF OVERDOSE AND WHAT TO DO

Symptoms of overdose include nausea, vomiting, headache, blurred vision, dilated pupils, hot dry skin, dizziness, dry mouth, swallowing difficulties, and central nervous system stimulation. If overdose occurs, seek immediate medical attention and bring the prescription container with you to the hospital.

SPECIAL INFORMATION FOR PREGNANT OR NURSING WOMEN

No adequate studies of the effects of hyoscyamine on pregnant or nursing women have been done. If you are pregnant or plan to become pregnant, and this drug is crucial for your health, you and your health-care practitioner must weigh the potential benefits against the potential risks to the fetus.

Hyoscyamine may pass into breast milk. If you are breastfeeding, your health-care practitioner may advise you to switch to bottle feeding until your treatment is complete.

SPECIAL INFORMATION FOR SENIORS

Older adults often experience more side effects, and more severe ones.

GENERIC NAME

Ibuprofen *see Propionic Acid (NSAID) Family, page 880*

GENERIC NAME

Imipramine *see Tricyclic Antidepressants, page 1076*

GENERIC NAME

Imiquimod

BRAND NAME

Aldara

No generic available

ABOUT THIS DRUG

Imiquimod is an immunomodulator prescribed to treat genital and perianal warts in adults. It is not a cure for these conditions.

Exactly how imiquimod eliminates genital and perianal warts is unknown. One theory is that it stimulates the skin to produce chemicals called cytokines that attack the warts.

SIDE EFFECTS

Be sure to tell your health-care practitioner if you experience any side effects while using imiquimod. Only your health-care practitioner can determine whether it is safe for you to continue using this drug.

- *Most Common:* at treated areas only, you may see redness, thinning of the skin, swelling, flaking
- *Less Common:* at treated areas only, you may see hardening or stiffening of the skin, sores, scabbing, blisters
- *Rare*: swollen eyelids, face, or lips, rash, wheezing, all of which are symptoms of an allergic reaction. Contact your health-care practitioner immediately.

IMPORTANT PRECAUTIONS

Tell your health-care practitioner if you are sensitive or allergic to imiquimod or to any other drugs.

Do not apply imiquimod to any areas that have not healed from previous medical treatment or surgery.

Before using imiquimod, tell your health-care practitioner if you have a history of any type of inflammatory skin disease.

Imiquimod may reduce the effectiveness of condoms and vaginal diaphragms. Sexual contact should be avoided while the cream is on your skin.

Do not apply bandages to the treated area or wear tight clothing during treatment.

Always wash your hands before and after applying imiquimod, and do not get the drug into your eyes.

DRUG INTERACTIONS

Tell your health-care practitioner and pharmacist if you are taking any prescription or nonprescription drugs, as well as any vitamins, herbs, or other supplements. Imiquimod should not be used along with any other medications that may cause skin irritation.

FOOD, VITAMIN, AND HERBAL INTERACTIONS

No food, vitamin, or herbal interactions have been noted.

RECOMMENDED DOSAGE

Imiquimod is available as a cream. The dosages given here are typical. However, your health-care practitioner will determine the most appropriate dose and schedule for you.

- *Children Up to 18 Years:* not recommended
- *Adults:* apply a thin layer to external warts and rub it in until the cream disappears. Imiquimod should be left on the skin for 6 to 10 hours, then removed with mild soap and water. This treatment process should be repeated three times a week (e.g., Monday, Wednesday, and Friday) for up to 16 weeks or until the warts disappear.

If you miss a dose, skip it and stay on your regular schedule. You should never apply imiquimod two days in a row.

SYMPTOMS OF OVERDOSE AND WHAT TO DO

Symptoms of topical overdose are unlikely because only a small amount of the drug is absorbed through the skin. If someone accidentally ingests imiquimod, low blood pressure may occur. Seek medical attention at an emergency room and bring the prescription container with you.

SPECIAL INFORMATION FOR PREGNANT OR NURSING WOMEN

No adequate studies of the effects of imiquimod on pregnant or nursing women have been done. If you are pregnant or plan to become pregnant, and this drug is crucial for your health, you and your health-care practitioner must weigh the potential benefits against the potential risks to the fetus.

Imiquimod may pass into breast milk. If you are breastfeeding, your health-care practitioner may advise you to switch to bottle feeding until treatment is done.

SPECIAL INFORMATION FOR SENIORS

No special precautions have been noted for older adults.

GENERIC NAME

Indapamide *see Thiazide Diuretics, page 1020*

GENERIC NAME

Indinavir

BRAND NAME

Crixivan
No generic available

ABOUT THIS DRUG

Indinavir is a protease inhibitor used to treat HIV (human immunodeficiency virus) infection. It is used as part of a multidrug "cocktail" that includes nucleoside antiviral drugs (e.g., AZT, ddI [didanosine]) in the fight against HIV and AIDS (acquired immunodeficiency syndrome).

Indinavir, when taken as part of a multidrug "cocktail," helps reduce the amount of HIV virus in the blood, and helps prevent the mature HIV virus from forming.

SIDE EFFECTS

Be sure to tell your health-care practitioner if you experience any side effects while taking indinavir. Only your health-care practitioner can determine whether it is safe for you to continue taking this drug.

➤ *Most Common:* headache, nausea, abdominal pain

➤ *Common:* weakness or fatigue, diarrhea, vomiting, taste changes, pain in the side, acid regurgitation, sleeplessness

➤ *Less Common:* back pain, dizziness, drowsiness

IMPORTANT PRECAUTIONS

Tell your health-care practitioner if you are sensitive or allergic to indinavir or to any other drugs.

If you have mild or moderate liver disease or cirrhosis, you are more likely to develop side effects, and your dosage may need to be adjusted.

About 4 percent of people who take indinavir develop a kidney stone or painful urination. To help avoid these complications, drink at least 48 ounces of liquid daily.

Indinavir may worsen diabetes, awaken latent diabetes, or raise your blood sugar levels. Your health-care practitioner may need to adjust your antidiabetes medication.

DRUG INTERACTIONS

Tell your health-care practitioner and pharmacist if you are taking any prescription or nonprescription drugs, as well as any vitamins, herbs, or other supplements. Possible drug interactions include the following:

- Terfenadine, astemizole, triazolam, and midazolam are not properly broken down when taken with indinavir. Do not use these drugs when taking indinavir.
- Rifampin reduces the amount of indinavir in the blood.
- Indinavir along with either clarithromycin or zidovudine increases the amount of both drugs in the blood.
- Combining indinavir with isoniazid increases the amount of the latter in the blood.
- Didanosine (ddI) interferes with the absorption of indinavir. If you must take both of these drugs, take them at least one hour apart.
- Fluconazole reduces the amount of indinavir in the blood.
- Ketoconazole increases the amount of indinavir in the blood.
- Quinidine increases indinavir levels.
- Indinavir raises the amounts of zidovudine, stavudine, and trimethoprim in the blood.
- Oral contraceptives may result in higher blood hormone levels, which can cause hormone-related side effects.

FOOD, VITAMIN, AND HERBAL INTERACTIONS

Do not drink grapefruit juice while you are taking indinavir because it reduces the drug's effectiveness.

Do not eat meals high in fat, calories, or protein 1 hour before or 2 hours after taking indinavir. St. John's wort lowers blood concentrations of indinavir and can reduce its effectiveness; avoid using St. John's wort while taking indinavir.

RECOMMENDED DOSAGE

Indinavir is available in capsules. The dosages given here are typical. However, your health-care practitioner will determine the most appropriate dose and schedule for you.

- *Children Up to Age 16*: safety and effectiveness not established

➤ *Adults:* 800 mg every 8 hours, either alone or as part of a drug "cocktail"

Indinavir should be taken with water, juice, milk, or another nonalcoholic beverage at least 1 hour before or 2 hours after eating. It also can be taken with a light meal.

If you miss a dose, take it as soon as you remember. If it is nearly time for your next dose, do not take the missed dose. Continue with your regular dosing schedule. Never take a double dose.

SYMPTOMS OF OVERDOSE AND WHAT TO DO

Symptoms of overdose include lower back pain, blood in the urine, nausea, vomiting, and diarrhea. If an overdose occurs, seek immediate medical attention and bring the prescription container with you to the hospital.

SPECIAL INFORMATION FOR PREGNANT OR NURSING WOMEN

No adequate studies of the effects of indinavir on pregnant or nursing women have been done, but the drug does cause birth defects in animals. If you are pregnant or plan to become pregnant, and this drug is crucial for your health, you and your health-care practitioner must weigh the potential benefits against the potential risks to the fetus.

Women with HIV should not breastfeed, because they can transmit the virus to an uninfected infant.

SPECIAL INFORMATION FOR SENIORS

No special precautions have been noted for older adults.

GENERIC NAME

Indomethacin

BRAND NAMES

Indocin, Indocin SR, Novo-Methacin
Generic available

ABOUT THIS DRUG

Indomethacin is a nonsteroidal anti-inflammatory drug (NSAID) taken to treat mild-to-moderate pain and inflammation associated with arthritis, bursitis, gout, tendinitis, migraine, menstrual cramps, and other painful conditions. It should be prescribed only if other NSAIDs have proven to be ineffective.

Indomethacin, like other NSAIDs, interferes with the production of prostaglandins, substances that cause inflammation and make nerves more sensitive to pain signals.

SIDE EFFECTS

Be sure to tell your health-care practitioner if you experience any side effects while taking indomethacin. Only your health-care practitioner can determine whether it is safe for you to continue taking this drug.

➤ *Most Common:* nausea, vomiting, diarrhea, constipation, headache, dizziness, drowsiness, heartburn, ringing in the ears, vertigo

➤ *Less Common or Rare:* anemia, anxiety, asthma, behavior disturbances, blurred vision, heart rate changes, chest pain, coma, congestive heart failure, convulsions, fluid retention, decrease in white blood cells, fever, flushing, hair loss, hepatitis, hives, itching, rise in blood sugar levels, kidney failure, breathing difficulties, muscle weakness, nosebleed, peptic ulcer, rectal bleeding, skin peeling, gastrointestinal bleeding, sweating, twitching, vaginal bleeding, jaundice

IMPORTANT PRECAUTIONS

Tell your health-care practitioner if you are sensitive or allergic to indomethacin, other NSAIDs, or any other drugs.

While you take indomethacin, frequent checkups with your health-care practitioner are recommended, because internal bleeding or ulcers can appear suddenly.

Before you take indomethacin, tell your health-care practitioner if you have a history of alcohol abuse, anemia, asthma, bleeding problems, epilepsy, gastrointestinal inflammation or ulcers, diabetes, heart, liver, or kidney disease, kidney stones, lupus, or Parkinson's disease.

DRUG INTERACTIONS

Tell your health-care practitioner and pharmacist if you are taking any prescription or nonprescription drugs, as well as any vitamins, herbs, or other supplements. Possible drug interactions include the following:

➤ Aspirin and other nonsteroidal anti-inflammatory drugs should never be taken along with indomethacin.

➤ Probenecid may increase the risk of side effects from indomethacin.

- Indomethacin may increase the effects of oral anticoagulants (blood-thinning drugs; e.g., warfarin). Your health-care practitioner may alter your anticoagulant dosage.
- Indomethacin may increase the side effects of methotrexate and the kidney-related side effects of cyclosporine.
- Cimetidine may affect the blood levels of indomethacin.
- Indomethacin may reduce the blood-pressure-lowering effect of loop diuretics (e.g., bendroflumethiazide, furosemide) and beta-blockers (e.g., acebutolol, nadolol).
- Indomethacin may increase the risk of side effects of methotrexate and meloxicam.
- Indomethacin may increase the blood levels of lithium.

FOOD, VITAMIN, AND HERBAL INTERACTIONS

Alfalfa, clove oil, cinchona bark, feverfew, garlic, ginseng, and ginkgo may affect blood clotting, so use of these herbs along with indomethacin is not recommended. Combining feverfew and indomethacin may result in stomach problems.

St. John's wort and dong quai are associated with an increased sensitivity to the sun. Be sure to wear protective clothing and use sunscreen if you take these herbs while taking indomethacin.

RECOMMENDED DOSAGE

Indomethacin is available in capsules and liquid. The dosages given here are typical. However, your health-care practitioner will determine the most appropriate dose and schedule for you.

- *Children Up to 14 Years:* safety and effectiveness have not been established
- *Children 14 Years and Older and Adults:* for moderate to severe osteoarthritis and rheumatoid arthritis, 25 mg 2 or 3 times daily. Dosage can be increased up to 250 mg by your health-care practitioner. For bursitis or tendinitis, 75 to 150 mg daily taken in 3 to 4 equal doses for 1 to 2 weeks until symptoms go away. Consult your health-care practitioner for liquid dosages.

Indomethacin should be taken with food.

If you miss a dose, take it as soon as you remember. If it is nearly time for your next dose, do not take the missed dose. Continue with your regular dosing schedule. Never take a double dose.

SYMPTOMS OF OVERDOSE AND WHAT TO DO

Symptoms of overdose include severe nausea, vomiting, headache, seizures, and confusion. If an overdose occurs, seek immediate medical attention and bring the prescription container with you to the hospital.

SPECIAL INFORMATION FOR PREGNANT OR NURSING WOMEN

No adequate studies of the effects of indomethacin on pregnant or nursing women have been done. If you are pregnant or plan to become pregnant and this drug is crucial for your health, you and your health-care practitioner must weigh the potential benefits against the potential risks to the fetus.

Indomethacin passes into breast milk. If you are breastfeeding, your health-care practitioner will advise you to switch to bottle feeding while you are being treated.

SPECIAL INFORMATION FOR SENIORS

Older adults typically are prescribed a lower dose because they have a greater risk of gastrointestinal side effects.

GENERIC NAME

Infliximab

BRAND NAME

Remicade
No generic available

ABOUT THIS DRUG

Infliximab is a monoclonal antibody prescribed for the treatment of Crohn's disease, an inflammatory intestinal disorder, and for rheumatoid arthritis. It is typically classified as a disease-modifying antirheumatic drug (DMARD).

High levels of tumor necrosis factor, a substance involved in the inflammatory process associated with Crohn's disease and rheumatoid arthritis, play a role in the worsening of these diseases. Infliximab interferes with tumor necrosis factor so that it cannot increase disease severity.

SIDE EFFECTS

Be sure to tell your health-care practitioner if you experience any side effects while taking infliximab. Eighty percent of people experience at least two side effects, and 16 percent have a drug reaction (e.g., chills, fever, itching, rash, chest pain, breathing problems, or low blood pressure). Only your health-care practitioner can determine whether it is safe for you to continue taking this drug.

- *Most Common:* abdominal pain, headache, nausea, upper respiratory infection, fatigue, fever
- *Common:* bronchitis, dizziness, rash, runny nose, chest pain, cough, itching, sore throat, vomiting, muscle aches, back pain, fungal infection
- *Less Common:* bloody or cloudy urine, cracked skin at the corners of the mouth, diarrhea, painful urination, high or low blood pressure, tenderness or pain around the eyes and cheekbones, redness and soreness around toenails and fingernails, vaginal burning or itching and discharge
- *Rare:* abscess, black tarry stools, bone or joint pain, constipation, hernia, infection, irregular heartbeat, rectal pain, severe stomach pain, swollen or painful glands, unusual bleeding or bruising, jaundice, feeling of fullness

IMPORTANT PRECAUTIONS

Tell your health-care practitioner if you are sensitive or allergic to infliximab or to any other drugs, or if you have a reaction to rodents, because mouse cells are used in the preparation of this injectable drug.

The safety and effectiveness of receiving more than three infusions of infliximab are not known.

Lupus erythematosus develops in some patients but disappears once treatment is stopped.

Because infliximab suppresses the immune system, it should be used cautiously by anyone who has a compromised immune system.

Infliximab is not recommended for people who have congestive heart failure or an active infection. If you have tuberculosis, it should be treated before you take infliximab.

DRUG INTERACTIONS

Tell your health-care practitioner and pharmacist if you are taking any prescription or nonprescription drugs, as well as any vitamins, herbs, or other supplements. Infliximab should not be used along with any drug that is infused into the bloodstream.

FOOD, VITAMIN, AND HERBAL INTERACTIONS

No food, vitamin, or herbal interactions have been noted.

RECOMMENDED DOSAGE

Infliximab is available as an injection, given by a medical professional. The dosages given here are typical. However, your health-care practitioner will determine the most appropriate dose and schedule for you.

For Crohn's Disease

- *Children:* use and dose to be determined by your health-care practitioner
- *Adults:* 2.27 mg per pound of body weight

For Rheumatoid Arthritis

- *Children:* use and dose to be determined by your health-care practitioner
- *Adults:* 1.36 mg per pound of body weight

SYMPTOMS OF OVERDOSE AND WHAT TO DO

Symptoms of overdose include those associated with a drug reaction (e.g., chills, fever, itching, rash, chest pains, breathing problems, or low blood pressure). If overdose occurs, seek immediate medical assistance.

SPECIAL INFORMATION FOR PREGNANT OR NURSING WOMEN

No adequate studies of the effects of infliximab on pregnant or nursing women have been done; nor have studies been done in animals. If you are pregnant or plan to become pregnant, you and your health-care practitioner must weigh the potential benefits against the potential risks to the fetus.

Infliximab may pass into breast milk. If you are breastfeeding, your health-care practitioner may advise you to switch to bottle feeding until your treatment is done.

SPECIAL INFORMATION FOR SENIORS

There is no specific information on the effects of infliximab in older adults. It is possible that seniors may experience more infections as a side effect of this drug, because older people generally get more infections.

GENERIC NAME

Influenza vaccine, live, intranasal

BRAND NAME

FluMist

No generic available

ABOUT THIS DRUG

This live trivalent vaccine is given to prevent influenza illness due to influenza A and B in healthy children ages 5 to 17 and healthy adults ages 18 to 49.

This medication induces immunity in the body by producing specific antibodies against influenza A and B.

SIDE EFFECTS

Be sure to tell your health-care practitioner if you experience any side effects after you have received a dose of the vaccine. Only your health-care practitioner can determine whether it is safe for you to receive a subsequent dose.

- *Common:* cough, decreased activity, headache, irritability, muscle ache, nasal congestion, runny nose, sore throat
- *Rare:* allergic reaction (closed throat, difficulty breathing, hives, swelling of the lips, tongue, or face)

IMPORTANT PRECAUTIONS

Tell your health-care practitioner if you are sensitive or allergic to eggs or egg products or if you have had a reaction to previous vaccinations.

The safety of this vaccine in people who have asthma has not been established and so should not be used if you have asthma.

Do not get this vaccine if you have a chronic underlying medical condition that could predispose you to severe flu infection, or if you have health problems associated with heart, kidney, lung, or metabolic diseases, anemia and blood disorders, diseases that are known to affect the immune system, or if you have a history of Guillain-Barre syndrome.

This vaccine does not protect 100 percent of individuals vaccinated or protect against strains not in the vaccine.

Administration of the vaccine should be withheld for at least 72 hours from experiencing a fever or respiratory illness.

DRUG INTERACTIONS

Tell your health-care practitioner and pharmacist if you are taking any prescription or nonprescription drugs, as well as any vitamins, herbs, or other supplements. Possible drug interactions include the following:

- Children ages 5 to 17 who are taking aspirin or aspirin-therapy should not receive this vaccine.

- This vaccine should not be administered to anyone who is on immunosuppression therapy.
- This vaccine should not be administered until 48 hours after stopping antiviral therapy, and antiviral agents should not be used until two weeks after receiving this vaccine.
- This vaccine should not be taken along with any other vaccines.

FOOD, VITAMIN, AND HERBAL INTERACTIONS
No food, vitamin, or herbal interactions have been noted.

RECOMMENDED DOSAGE
This vaccine is available as a nasal spray and is administered by a health-care practitioner. The dosages given here are typical. However, your health-care practitioner will determine the most appropriate dose and schedule for your needs.

- *Children 5 to 8 Years:* two doses at least 6 weeks apart during the first year of vaccination
- *Children 9 to 17 Years and Adults 18 to 49 Years:* one dose yearly

SYMPTOMS OF OVERDOSE AND WHAT TO DO
There is no information on symptoms of an overdose.

SPECIAL INFORMATION FOR PREGNANT OR NURSING WOMEN
Do not get this vaccine if you are pregnant. If you plan to become pregnant, talk to your health-care practitioner before getting this vaccine.

Shedding of the virus into breast milk may occur. If you are breastfeeding, your health-care practitioner will likely advise you to switch to bottle feeding.

SPECIAL INFORMATION FOR SENIORS
The safe use of this vaccine in seniors has not been established.

GENERIC NAME

Insulin

BRAND NAMES
Humalog, Humulin, Humulin N, Novolin N, Novolin R, Humulin BR&R, Velosulin Human, Humulin 70/30, Novolin 70/30, Humulin L&U, Novolin L, NPH Iletin I, NPH Insulin, Iletin I Regular, Regular In-

sulin, Iletin I Lente, Protamine Ainc and Iletin, Iletin I Semilente, Iletin I, Lente Insulin, Ultralente Insulin
Generic available

ABOUT THIS DRUG

Insulin is an antidiabetic agent prescribed for diabetes mellitus when the disease cannot be controlled through diet and oral antidiabetic drugs. Insulin drugs are derived from either animals or humans, or are genetically engineered, and vary in the amount of time until they take effect and how long they remain effective.

The insulin produced naturally by the body is a hormone that the body needs to utilize food correctly. Insulin helps sugar (glucose) enter cells, where it is used by the cells to produce energy. The drug insulin is designed to mimic natural insulin.

SIDE EFFECTS

Be sure to tell your health-care practitioner if you experience any side effects while taking insulin. Side effects are rare, although symptoms of low blood sugar and allergic reactions are more common. Contact your health-care practitioner if you experience any of the following symptoms:

- ➤ *Most Common:* redness, itching, or swelling at the injection site
- ➤ *Less Common:* low blood pressure, perspiration, body rash, shortness of breath, shallow breathing, fast pulse, wheezing

IMPORTANT PRECAUTIONS

Tell your health-care practitioner if you are sensitive or allergic to insulin or to any other drugs.

It is important that you follow your health-care practitioner's exercise and dietary guidelines and to take your insulin exactly as prescribed.

Do not change the type of insulin or the brand or model of syringe or needle without first consulting your health-care practitioner.

Smoking can decrease the amount of insulin absorbed. If you smoke, you should stop.

Various diseases and symptoms can increase your insulin requirements, including but not limited to infections, stress, an uncontrolled overactive thyroid gland, and surgical procedures. Conditions that may reduce your insulin needs include an underactive adrenal or pituitary gland and kidney disease. Eating a large number of calories or lots of simple carbohydrates and sugars also increases your insulin needs.

DRUG INTERACTIONS

Tell your health-care practitioner and pharmacist if you are taking any prescription or nonprescription drugs, as well as any vitamins, herbs, or other supplements. Possible drug interactions include the following:

- Excessive alcohol can cause severe hypoglycemia and result in brain damage.
- Acarbose, aspirin and other salicylates, some beta-blockers, clofibrate, disopyramide, fenfluramine, monoamine oxidase inhibitors, and other oral antidiabetic drugs (e.g., glipizide, glyburide) may increase the effects of insulin.
- Oral contraceptives, chlorthalidone, cortisone-like drugs (e.g., betamethasone, cortisone), furosemide, phenytoin, thiazide diuretics (e.g., chlorothiazide, hydrochlorothiazide), and thyroid preparations may decrease the effects of insulin.

FOOD, VITAMIN, AND HERBAL INTERACTIONS

Before using any of the following herbs, talk to your health-care practitioner, as they change blood sugar levels: garlic, ginger, ginseng, hawthorn, licorice, and nettle.

Chromium supplements may improve your ability to use glucose and increase your risk of abnormally low blood sugar. The hormone DHEA may alter your sensitivity to insulin or insulin resistance. Talk to your health-care practitioner before using any of these supplements.

RECOMMENDED DOSAGE

Insulin is available in injectable form. Dosages of insulin are highly individual, and your health-care practitioner will determine the most appropriate dose and schedule for you.

Your health-care practitioner should tell you what to do if you miss a dose.

SYMPTOMS OF OVERDOSE AND WHAT TO DO

An overdose of insulin can cause hypoglycemia (low blood sugar), with symptoms that include abnormal behavior and personality changes, blurred vision, cold sweat, confusion, depressed mood, dizziness, drowsiness, headache, hunger, lightheadedness, nausea, nervousness, rapid heartbeat, sleep problems, slurred speech, tingling in the tongue, lips, hands, or feet, and tremor. Severe low blood sugar may result in disorientation and coma. Eating sugar or a food that is high in sugar often corrects the situation. If overdose occurs, seek medical attention immediately.

SPECIAL INFORMATION FOR PREGNANT OR NURSING WOMEN

Insulin is safe for pregnant women. Its use should be carefully monitored, because properly controlled diabetes is crucial for the health of both the mother and fetus.

Insulin does not pass into breast milk; therefore it is safe to use during breastfeeding. The genetically engineered insulin lispro may appear in breast milk. If you are taking this form of insulin, talk to your health-care practitioner about breastfeeding.

SPECIAL INFORMATION FOR SENIORS

Insulin requirements may change with age; thus periodic adjustments may be needed. Older adults often adapt well to higher blood sugar levels.

GENERIC NAME

Interferon alfa

Generics: (1) Interferon alfa-2A; (2) Interferon alfa-2B; (3) Interferon alfa-3N

BRAND NAMES

(1) Roferon-A; (2) Intron A; (3) Alferon N
No generic available

ABOUT THIS DRUG

The interferon alfa drugs are immunomodulators prescribed primarily to treat hairy-cell leukemia, Kaposi's sarcoma (associated with acquired immunodeficiency syndrome [AIDS]), genital warts, and types of chronic hepatitis.

This drug imitates the action of the body's natural interferons, proteins released by the immune system cells to fight viruses and cancer cells.

SIDE EFFECTS

Be sure to tell your health-care practitioner if you experience any side effects while taking interferon alfa drugs. Only your health-care practitioner can determine whether it is safe for you to continue taking them.

- *Most Common:* flulike symptoms, fever, chills (usually during the first few weeks of treatment), general ill feeling, fatigue, muscle aches, loss of appetite, headache, nausea, vomiting, altered taste, rash, temporary hair loss

- *Less Common:* back pain, blurred vision, dizziness, dry mouth, itching skin, unusual sweating, joint pain, leg cramps, mouth or lip sores, weight loss

IMPORTANT PRECAUTIONS

Tell your health-care practitioner if you are sensitive or allergic to interferon alfa drugs or to any other drugs. Also tell your health-care practitioner if you have had a severe allergic reaction to bovine or ovine immunoglobulins, egg protein, polymyxin B, or neomycin sulfate.

Use interferon alfa drugs with caution if you have preexisting cardiac disease, a clinically significant depressive disorder, any severe preexisting autoimmune, renal, or liver disease (including decompensated liver disease and autoimmune hepatitis), seizure disorders, bleeding or clotting disorders, pulmonary problems (including asthma), compromised central nervous system function, leukopenia, or thrombocytopenia.

Among adolescent females, interferon alfa drugs have the potential to cause changes in the menstrual cycle.

It is important to drink plenty of liquids during treatment with interferon alfa drugs to help prevent low blood pressure caused by a loss of water.

Do not switch to another brand of interferon alfa drug without first consulting your health-care practitioner. Each of the brands has a different dose and schedule.

Avoid individuals who have infections because interferon alfa drugs increase your susceptibility to disease.

DRUG INTERACTIONS

Tell your health-care practitioner and pharmacist if you are taking any prescription or nonprescription drugs, as well as any vitamins, herbs, or other supplements. Interferon alfa drugs may interact with the following medications:

- Acyclovir increases antiviral activity in test tubes.
- Antineoplastics (e.g., vincristine, vinblastine), flucytosine, ganciclovir, AZT, pentamidine, and pyrimethamine may increase the risk of bone marrow toxicity.
- Talk to your health-care practitioner if you are taking antihistamines, tranquilizers, or psychiatric medications.

FOOD, VITAMIN, AND HERBAL INTERACTIONS

No food, vitamin, or herbal interactions have been noted.

RECOMMENDED DOSAGE

Interferon alfa drugs are available by injection and can be self-administered. The dosages vary widely and depend on the condition being treated, the person's weight, whether other drugs are being used, and the brand used. Your health-care practitioner will determine the most appropriate dose and schedule for you.

If you miss a dose, take it as soon as you remember. If it is nearly time for your next dose, do not take the missed dose. Continue with your regular dosing schedule. Never take a double dose.

SYMPTOMS OF OVERDOSE AND WHAT TO DO

No specific symptoms of overdose with interferon alfa drugs have been noted. If an overdose occurs, seek immediate medical attention and bring the prescription container with you to the hospital.

SPECIAL INFORMATION FOR PREGNANT OR NURSING WOMEN

No adequate studies of the effects of interferon alfa drugs on pregnant or nursing women have been done. High doses have caused the death of the fetus in animals. If you are pregnant or plan to become pregnant, and any of these drugs is crucial for your health, you and your health-care practitioner must weigh the potential benefits against the potential risks to the fetus.

Interferon alfa drugs may pass into breast milk. If you are breastfeeding, your health-care practitioner will likely advise you to stop until your treatment is done.

SPECIAL INFORMATION FOR SENIORS

Some side effects of interferon alfa drugs are more common among older adults, including confusion, unusual tiredness, loss of concentration, depression, chest pain, and irregular heartbeat.

GENERIC NAME

Interferon beta

Generics: (1) Interferon beta 1a; (2) Interferon beta 1b

BRAND NAMES

(1) Avonex, Rebif; (2) Betaseron

No generic available

ABOUT THIS DRUG

Interferon beta is an immunomodulator prescribed for relapsing-remitting multiple sclerosis, which is the most common form of the disease. This form of multiple sclerosis is characterized by periods of active disease alternating with periods of remission or less severe symptoms.

The drug interferon beta was designed to mimic the body's natural interferons, which are proteins released by the immune system to fight against viruses, cancer, and other diseases.

SIDE EFFECTS

Be sure to tell your health-care practitioner if you experience any side effects while taking interferon beta. Only your health-care practitioner can determine whether it is safe for you to continue taking this drug.

- *Most Common:* inflammation, pain, or allergic reaction at the injection site; headache, fever, muscle aches, fatigue, general weakness, insomnia, increased susceptibility to infection, nausea, vomiting, diarrhea, abdominal pain
- *Less Common or Rare:* dizziness, dry mouth, dry or itchy skin, increased sweating, joint pain, hearing difficulties, vision changes, thyroid goiter, palpitations, laryngitis, uncontrolled movements, breast pain, cystitis, urinary urgency, seizures, swelling and fluid retention, anxiety, confusion, depression

IMPORTANT PRECAUTIONS

Tell your health-care practitioner if you are sensitive or allergic to interferon beta, human albumin, or any other drugs.

The safety and effectiveness of interferon beta in chronic progressive multiple sclerosis is not known.

Up to three-quarters of people who take interferon beta develop flulike symptoms (e.g., fever, chills, muscle aches, sweating). If you have heart disease, these symptoms may be especially stressful.

If you have a seizure disorder, you are more likely to develop seizures while taking this drug.

Interferon beta can increase your sensitivity to sunlight. To protect yourself, wear sunscreen and protective clothing.

Some studies suggest that in people with a history of depression, interferon beta may lead to suicidal impulses.

Before taking interferon beta, tell your health-care practitioner if you have a history of clotting or bleeding disorders, chicken pox, shingles, psychological problems, diabetes, autoimmune disorders, heart disease, kidney disease, lung disease, liver disease, or thyroid disease.

DRUG INTERACTIONS

Tell your health-care practitioner and pharmacist if you are taking any prescription or nonprescription drugs, as well as any vitamins, herbs, or other supplements. No significant drug interactions have been noted for interferon beta.

FOOD, VITAMIN, AND HERBAL INTERACTIONS

No food, vitamin, or herbal interactions have been noted.

RECOMMENDED DOSAGE

Interferon beta is available as an injection, which can be self-administered. The dosages given here are typical. However, your health-care practitioner will determine the most appropriate dose and schedule for you.

- *Children:* use and dosage to be determined by your health-care practitioner
- *Adults:* injectable dose varies depending on the brand name used, and may be given once a week, three times a week, or every other day by intramuscular or subcutaneous injection

If you miss a dose, do not take the missed dose and do not double a dose. Call your health-care practitioner for instructions.

SYMPTOMS OF OVERDOSE AND WHAT TO DO

Little is known about overdosing with interferon beta, but symptoms would probably include exaggerated side effects. If an overdose occurs, call your local poison control center or emergency department for more information. If you seek treatment, bring the prescription container with you.

SPECIAL INFORMATION FOR PREGNANT OR NURSING WOMEN

No adequate studies of the effects of interferon beta on pregnant or nursing women have been done. Animal studies show that interferon beta may cause abortion. If you are pregnant or plan to become pregnant and this drug is crucial for your health, you and your health-care practitioner must weigh the potential benefits against the potential risks to the fetus.

Interferon beta may pass into breast milk. If you are breastfeeding, your health-care practitioner may advise you to switch to bottle feeding until your treatment is done.

SPECIAL INFORMATION FOR SENIORS

Older adults are more likely to experience side effects, which may be more severe.

GENERIC NAME

Ipratropium

BRAND NAMES

Atrovent, Atrovent Nasal Spray
Generic available

ABOUT THIS DRUG

Ipratropium is an anticholinergic/bronchodilator prescribed for treatment of bronchitis, chronic obstructive pulmonary disease, and emphysema.

This drug, when inhaled, opens the air passages and allows more oxygen to reach the lungs. It also decreases production and secretion of mucus.

SIDE EFFECTS

Be sure to tell your health-care practitioner if you experience any side effects while taking ipratropium. Only your health-care practitioner can determine whether it is safe for you to continue taking this drug.

- *Most Common (for inhalation aerosol and inhalation solution):* blurred vision, cough, dizziness, dry mouth, headache, nausea, nervousness, rash, gastrointestinal upset, worsening of symptoms, fluttering heartbeat
- *Most Common (for nasal spray):* blurred vision, taste changes, conjunctivitis, cough, dizziness, dry mouth, dry throat, eye irritation, headache, hoarseness, inflamed nasal ulcers, nasal congestion, nasal irritation, nausea, nosebleed, nasal drip, pounding heartbeat, ringing in the ears, rash, sore throat, swollen nose, thirst, upper respiratory infection
- *Less Common (for inhalation aerosol and inhalation solution):* allergic reaction, constipation, problems with coordination, urinary difficulties, drowsiness, fatigue, flushing, hives, hoarseness, sleep problems, hair loss, itching, low blood pressure, mouth sores, eye pain, swollen tongue, lips, and face, tight throat, tingling sensation, tremors

IMPORTANT PRECAUTIONS

Tell your health-care practitioner if you are sensitive or allergic to ipratropium, atropine, aerosol propellants (fluorocarbons; in inhalational form), benzalkonium chloride, edetate disodium (in nasal form), or any other drugs.

Do not take ipratropium if you are allergic to peanuts (if using the inhalational form), soy lecithin, or soybeans.

Avoid use of ipratropium if you have narrow-angle glaucoma, an enlarged prostate, or bladder neck obstruction unless your health-care practitioner advises you to do so.

Because ipratropium can cause blurred vision, make sure you know how you react to this drug before you drive or operate dangerous equipment.

Before taking ipratropium, talk to your health-care practitioner if you have had an adverse reaction to any belladonna derivative in the past, if you have a history of glaucoma, or if you have urinary retention or prostate problems.

DRUG INTERACTIONS

Tell your health-care practitioner and pharmacist if you are taking any prescription or nonprescription drugs, as well as any vitamins, herbs, or other supplements. No significant drug interactions have been reported. Use of anticholinergics (e.g., atropine, scopolamine) may result in an increased anticholinergic effect.

FOOD, VITAMIN, AND HERBAL INTERACTIONS

Do not inhale a dose of ipratropium if you have food in your mouth.

Do not use fir or pine needle oil when taking this drug.

RECOMMENDED DOSAGE

Ipratropium is available as an inhalation aerosol, an inhalation solution, and a nasal spray. The dosages given here are typical. However, your health-care practitioner will determine the most appropriate dose and schedule for you.

Aerosol and Solution

- *Children Up to 12 Years:* not recommended
- *Children Older than 12 Years and Adults:* starting dose is 2 inhalations, 4 times daily. Total daily inhalations should not exceed 12.

Nasal Spray 0.03%

- *Children Up to 6 Years:* not recommended
- *Children 6 Years and Older and Adults:* 2 sprays in each nostril 2 or 3 times daily

Nasal Spray 0.06%

- *Children Up to 6 Years:* not recommended
- *Children 6 to 11 Years:* 2 sprays in each nostril 3 times daily
- *Children 12 Years and Older and Adults:* 2 sprays in each nostril 3 or 4 times daily

If you miss a dose, take it as soon as you remember. If it is nearly time for your next dose, do not take the missed dose. Continue with your regular dosing schedule. Never take a double dose.

SYMPTOMS OF OVERDOSE AND WHAT TO DO

No specific symptoms of overdose have been reported, but it is unlikely that they would be life-threatening. If an overdose occurs, contact your health-care practitioner, local poison control center, or emergency department for instructions.

SPECIAL INFORMATION FOR PREGNANT OR NURSING WOMEN

No adequate studies of the effects of ipratropium on pregnant or nursing women have been done. If you are pregnant or plan to become pregnant, you and your health-care practitioner must weigh the potential benefits against the potential risks to the fetus.

Ipratropium may pass into breast milk. If you are breastfeeding, your health-care practitioner may advise you to switch to bottle feeding until your treatment is done.

SPECIAL INFORMATION FOR SENIORS

No special precautions have been noted for older adults.

GENERIC NAME

Irbesartan *see Angiotensin II Blockers, page 123*

GENERIC NAME
Isocarboxazid

BRAND NAME
Marplan
No generic available

ABOUT THIS DRUG
Isocarboxazid is an antidepressant used to treat depression and panic. It should be administered only after other antidepressants have not been successful. Isocarboxazid belongs to the monoamine oxidase inhibitor class of drugs.

Like other MAO inhibitors, isocarboxazid increases the levels of neurotransmitters in the brain and interferes with their normal breakdown in the body.

SIDE EFFECTS
Contact your health-care practitioner if you experience any side effects while taking isocarboxazid. Only he or she can determine whether you should continue to take this drug.

- *Common*: lightheadedness, reduced sexual ability, blurred vision, drowsiness, weakness, slow or fast heartbeat, dry mouth
- *Rare*: constipation, diarrhea, chills, allergies, rash, chest pain, severe headache, jaundice

IMPORTANT PRECAUTIONS
Always inform your physician about any other medical conditions you may have, especially congestive heart failure, hyperthyroid, high blood pressure, any seizure disorder, a history of heart attack or stroke, diabetes, kidney or liver impairment, severe or frequent headaches, or an adrenal gland tumor. Tell your doctor if you have ever had an allergic reaction to this or another MAOI antidepressant.

If you plan to undergo surgery or a dental procedure, tell your doctor or dentist that you are taking isocarboxazid. You should stop taking this drug at least 10 days before such procedures.

Isocarboxazid is not indicated for children younger than 16 years.

This drug can make you drowsy and less alert than usual. Until you know how isocarboxazid affects you, do not drive a car, operate machinery, or perform other tasks that require concentration.

When you first start taking this drug or when the dosage is increased, you may experience dizziness or faintness when you rise quickly from a sitting or reclining position (postural hypotension). Try to get up slowly, and consult your doctor if the problem continues.

If this drug causes mouth dryness, use sugarless gum or candy, ice chips, or artificial saliva. If the problem continues, consult your doctor or dentist.

DRUG INTERACTIONS

Inform your health-care practitioner if you are taking any other prescription or over-the-counter drugs, as well as any vitamins, herbs, or other supplements. Possible drug interactions include the following:

- Isocarboxazid should not be taken along with any other MAO inhibitors or debenzazepine derivatives.
- Fluoxetine and other selective serotonin reuptake inhibitors should not be taken in combination with isocarboxazid or within 14 days of stopping therapy with isocarboxazid. At least five weeks should be allowed after stopping fluoxetine and starting isocarboxazid.
- Sympathomimetics, including amphetamines and over-the-counter medications (for colds, weight reduction, or hay fever), as well as guanethidine, methyldopa, reserpine, dopamine, levodopa, and tyrosine should not be taken along with isocarboxazid.
- Buproprion and buspirone should not be taken along with isocarboxazid. Wait at least 14 days after stopping isocarboxazid and starting buproprion and 10 days after stopping isocarboxazid and starting buspirone.
- Wait at least 14 days after stopping sertraline or paroxetine before starting isocarboxazid.
- Do not take meperidine along with isocarboxazid or within two to three weeks after stopping isocarboxazid.
- Use of dextromethorphan and isocarboxazid together can cause psychosis or bizarre behavior.
- Antihypertensive drugs (e.g., rauwolfia alkaloids and thiazide diuretics) should not be taken with isocarboxazid.
- Anti-parkinsonism drugs may cause severe reactions.

FOOD, VITAMIN, AND HERBAL INTERACTIONS

It is essential to avoid foods that are rich in the amino acid tyramine while taking and for 2 weeks after taking isocarboxazid. This combination may result in an excessive and potentially fatal rise in blood pressure. Tyramine-rich foods include (but are not limited to) aged cheeses, bologna, chicken liver, chocolate, figs, pickled herring, pepperoni, raisins, salami, soy sauce, and yeast extracts. Also avoid beverages that contain meat or meat tenderizers, and alcoholic beverages that may contain tyramine, which include some beers, vermouth, and Chianti wines.

Herbs that affect the central nervous system—including St. John's wort, guarana, ephedra (ma huang), ginseng, scotch broom, and kola—must also be avoided when taking isocarboxazid. In addition, avoid caffeinated beverages, such as coffee, tea, and cola.

RECOMMENDED DOSAGE

Isocarboxazid comes as a tablet. The doses given below are typical, but dosage is always carefully individualized according to a person's particular needs and reactions to therapy.

- *Children Younger than 16 Years:* not indicated for this age group
- *Adults:* starting dose of 10 mg twice daily. Your health-care practitioner may then increase your dosage by 10 mg every two to four days. Maximum recommended dosage is 60 mg, taken in two to four doses. Benefit may not be apparent for up to six weeks.

If you miss a dose and you're no more than one hour late, take the dose. However, if it is within two hours of your next dose, do not take the missed dose and continue with your regular dosing schedule. Never take a double dose.

Do not suddenly stop taking isocarboxazid, because you can experience withdrawal symptoms if you have been taking the drug for more than three weeks. Your doctor will gradually reduce your dose for you.

SYMPTOMS OF OVERDOSE AND WHAT TO DO

Symptoms of overdose include drowsiness, rapid heartbeat, hypotension, breathing difficulties, convulsions, and coma. If an overdose occurs, seek immediately medical attention and bring the prescription container to the hospital with you.

SPECIAL INFORMATION FOR PREGNANT AND NURSING WOMEN

No studies have adequately investigated the effects of isocarboxazid during pregnancy or breastfeeding. If you are pregnant or plan to become pregnant, or if you are breastfeeding or plan to do so, talk with your doctor before starting this drug. Only a physician can determine whether the potential benefits outweigh the potential dangers.

SPECIAL INFORMATION FOR SENIORS

Seniors are at higher risk of side effects and usually require a lower dose.

GENERIC NAME

Isosorbide

Generics: (1) Isosorbide dinitrate; (2) isosorbide mononitrate

BRAND NAMES

(1) Dilatrate-SR, Isonate, Isordil Tembids, Isordil Titradose, Sorbitrate; (2) Imdur, ISMO, Monoket
Generic available

ABOUT THIS DRUG

Isosorbide is an antianginal drug prescribed for treatment of the pain associated with angina, and to prevent the recurrence of heart and chest pain in other heart conditions.

Isosorbide dinitrate, isosorbide mononitrate, and other nitrates relax the muscles in blood vessels, allowing for freer blood flow and less stress on the heart muscle.

SIDE EFFECTS

Be sure to tell your health-care practitioner if you experience any side effects while taking isosorbide. Only your health-care practitioner can determine whether it is safe for you to continue taking this drug.

- ➤ *Most Common:* headache, flushing, dizziness, weakness, blurred vision, dry mouth
- ➤ *Less Common:* nausea, vomiting, sweating, rash with itching, redness, and peeling skin

IMPORTANT PRECAUTIONS

Tell your health-care practitioner if you are sensitive or allergic to isosorbide, other nitrates, or any other drugs.

If you have a recent history of head injury, use this drug with caution.

This drug is not recommended if you have had a recent heart attack or if you have glaucoma, severe liver disease, overactive thyroid, cardiomyopathy, low blood pressure, severe kidney problems, an overactive gastrointestinal tract, or severe anemia.

Because isosorbide can cause dizziness and compromised vision, make sure you know how you react to this drug before you drive or operate dangerous equipment.

DRUG INTERACTIONS

Tell your health-care practitioner and pharmacist if you are taking any prescription or nonprescription drugs, as well as any vitamins, herbs, or other supplements. Possible drug interactions include the following:

- Avoid over-the-counter cold and cough medicines, because many of them contain ingredients that may aggravate heart disease.
- Large amounts of alcohol may significantly lower blood pressure.
- Nitrates raise the blood levels of dihydroergotamine, which may raise blood pressure or block the effects of isosorbide.
- Aspirin and calcium channel blockers (e.g., amlodipine, verapamil) may increase the blood levels of isosorbide and the risk of side effects.
- Sildenafil can enhance the action of isosorbide and other nitrates. Do not take isosorbide within 24 hours of taking sildenafil.

FOOD, VITAMIN, AND HERBAL INTERACTIONS

Talk to your health-care practitioner before taking the herb hawthorn or using the supplement coenzyme Q10, as both have an effect on the heart.

RECOMMENDED DOSAGE

Isosorbide is available in tablets, capsules, chewable tablets, and sublingual forms. The dosages given here are typical. However, your health-care practitioner will determine the most appropriate dose and schedule for you.

- *Children:* use and dose to be determined by your health-care practitioner
- *Adults:* to prevent angina attacks, 20 to 80 mg every 8 to 12 hours of extended release capsules or tablets; 5 to 40 mg 4 times daily of short-acting capsules or tablets. If you feel an angina attack coming, place a sublingual tablet in your mouth or chew a chewable tablet. If the pain remains after 5 minutes, take another tablet. After another 5 minutes, take a third tablet if the pain continues. If the pain persists, seek immediate medical attention.

If you miss a dose, take it as soon as you remember. If it is nearly time for your next dose, do not take the missed dose. Continue with your regular dosing schedule. Never take a double dose.

SYMPTOMS OF OVERDOSE AND WHAT TO DO

Symptoms of overdose include extreme dizziness or fainting, unusual weakness, fever, weak and fast heartbeat, seizures, and bluish fingernails, lips, or palms. If overdose occurs, seek immediate medical attention and bring the prescription container with you to the hospital.

SPECIAL INFORMATION FOR PREGNANT OR NURSING WOMEN

No adequate studies of the effects of isosorbide on pregnant or nursing women have been done. Animal studies have shown adverse effects on the fetus. If you are pregnant or plan to become pregnant, and either of these drugs is crucial for your health, you and your health-care practitioner must weigh the potential benefits against the potential risks to the fetus.

Isosorbide may pass into breast milk. If you are breastfeeding, your health-care practitioner may advise you to switch to bottle feeding until treatment is done.

SPECIAL INFORMATION FOR SENIORS

Older adults are more likely to experience adverse reactions, which may be more severe.

GENERIC NAME

Isotretinoin

BRAND NAME

Accutane
No generic available

ABOUT THIS DRUG

Isotretinoin is an antiacne drug that is related to vitamin A (retinol). It is used primarily to treat severe nodular and cystic acne and some less common skin conditions caused by disorders of keratin (skin cell) production, such as keratinization (hardening of skin cells) and mycosis fungoides.

This drug reduces the size of the oil (sebaceous) glands, inhibits production of skin oils (sebum), and reduces keratinization.

SIDE EFFECTS

Be sure to tell your health-care practitioner if you experience any side effects while taking isotretinoin. Only your health-care practi-

tioner can determine whether it is safe for you to continue taking this drug.

- *Most Common:* dry mouth, dry nose, inflamed lips, peeling of the palms and soles, extreme increase in triglyceride levels (seen in 25% of users), liver inflammation (15% of users), dry, itchy skin
- *Less Common:* rash, thinning hair, decreased night vision, muscle and joint ache, headache, fatigue, indigestion, conjunctivitis
- *Rare*: depression and suicide (see "Open Questions or Controversies"), skin infections, inflammatory bowel disorders, opacities in the cornea of the eye, reduced red and white blood cell counts, increased blood platelet count, abnormal acceleration of bone development (in children), seizures, myopathy, tendonitis, kidney and liver toxicity, abnormal blood glucose control, increased pressure in the head (causing headache, visual disturbances, nausea, vomiting), decreased sex drive, pancreatitis

IMPORTANT PRECAUTIONS

Tell your health-care practitioner if you are sensitive or allergic to isotretinoin or to any other drugs.

Do not take isotretinoin if you have mild acne (this drug is for severe acne only), if you are allergic to parabens (preservatives used in this drug), if you are unable or unwilling to take adequate birth control precautions (see "Special Information for Pregnant or Nursing Women"), or if you have not had a negative serum or urine pregnancy test one week before you start this medication.

Before starting isotretinoin, tell your health-care practitioner if you have diabetes, a cholesterol or triglyceride disorder, a history of depression, liver disease, or kidney disease; if you have had an allergic reaction to vitamin A in the past; or if you regularly take a vitamin A supplement or a multivitamin supplement that contains vitamin A.

Inform your health-care practitioner if plan to donate blood. You must not donate blood during treatment and for at least 30 days after you stop because of the risk of passing the drug along to a pregnant woman.

If you wear contact lenses, you may have less tolerance for them while taking isotretinoin.

Sudden difficulty seeing at night (night blindness) can develop while taking isotretinoin.

DRUG INTERACTIONS

Tell your health-care practitioner and pharmacist if you are taking any prescription or nonprescription drugs, as well as any vitamins,

herbs, or other supplements. Possible drug interactions include the following:

- Isotretinoin may reduce the amount of carbamazepine in the blood.
- Minocycline may cause severe headache, visual problems, and papilledema.
- Tetracyclines may increase your risk of pseudotumor cerebri (increased pressure in the brain).
- Alcohol can severely raise blood triglyceride levels.
- More than one hundred drugs that can cause photosensitivity can significantly increase sun sensitivity if taken with isotretinoin. Consult with your health-care practitioner or pharmacist about this possible reaction if you are taking other medications.

FOOD, VITAMIN, AND HERBAL INTERACTIONS

Because isotretinoin is related to vitamin A, avoid eating liver because of its high vitamin A content, and limit your intake of foods (e.g., carrots) and supplements that have moderate to large amounts of the vitamin. Taking St. John's wort while being treated with isotretinoin can cause extreme photosensitivity to the sun.

RECOMMENDED DOSAGE

Isotretinoin is available in 10-, 20-, and 40-mg capsules. The dosages given here are typical. However, your health-care practitioner will determine the most appropriate dose and schedule for you.

- *Children Up to 12 Years:* not recommended
- *Children 12 Years and Older and Adults:* 0.5 to 1 mg per 2.2 pounds of body weight in 1 or 2 doses daily. Average length of treatment is 20 weeks. If treatment needs to be repeated, you should wait at least two months before taking the drug again. Any use of this drug needs to be monitored by your health-care practitioner.

If you are a female who has begun menstruation, treatment must be coordinated with your menstrual cycle. The first dose should be taken only on the second or third day of your next normal menstrual period.

Isotretinoin should always be taken with food. If you miss a dose, take it as soon as you remember. However, if it is nearly time for your next dose, skip the one you missed and continue with your regular schedule. Never take a double dose.

SYMPTOMS OF OVERDOSE AND WHAT TO DO

Symptoms of overdose can include a rise in blood pressure, lethargy, mild gastrointestinal bleeding, elevated calcium levels in the blood, nausea and vomiting, hallucinations, and psychosis. If overdose occurs, seek immediate medical attention and bring the prescription container with you. You may be instructed to take ipecac syrup to help remove the drug from your stomach, then to seek medical help immediately thereafter.

SPECIAL INFORMATION FOR PREGNANT OR NURSING WOMEN
Isotretinoin should never be used by females who are pregnant. Many serious birth defects, including major abnormalities of the brain, heart, blood vessels, head, and hormone-producing glands, have been reported, even if the drug is used only for a short time. This drug should never be used if you are breastfeeding.

SPECIAL INFORMATION FOR SENIORS
There are no special restrictions for seniors.

OPEN QUESTIONS AND CONTROVERSIES

Isotretinoin has received media attention because of its apparent link with depression and suicide in some users. One of the most profiled cases came to light in October 2000, when Rep. Bart Stupak (D-Mich) announced on national television that he believed isotretinoin was responsible for the suicide death of his 17-year-old son.

In 2000, Rep. Dan Burton (R-Ind), chairman of the Government Reform Committee, reported that 66 suicides and 1,373 other psychiatric incidents associated with use of isotretinoin had been reported to the FDA since the drug's introduction in 1982. Rep. Henry Laxman (D-Calif) said that the FDA numbers represented only 1 to 10 percent of all adverse cases. Given the seriousness of these reactions, the FDA now requires that all patients sign a consent form which explains the potential psychiatric effects associated with the drug.

The FDA has also taken strong measures to ensure that female patients are sufficiently warned about the risk of severe birth defects associated with use of isotretinoin. If you are a female of childbearing age, before you can be prescribed isotretinoin, you must receive a medication guide, which tells you about the serious adverse effects. You also must produce monthly documentation of negative pregnancy tests in order to continue taking the drug.

GENERIC NAME
Isradipine

BRAND NAME
DynaCirc
No generic available

ABOUT THIS DRUG
Isradipine is a calcium channel blocker used primarily to treat high blood pressure. It can be used alone or along with a thiazide-type diuretic (e.g., bendroflumethiazide, chlorothiazide).

Like other calcium channel blockers, isradipine interferes with the movement of calcium into heart muscle, which in turn relaxes the blood vessels and reduces heart rate. It also results in a lowering of blood pressure and reduced chest pain.

SIDE EFFECTS
Be sure to tell your health-care practitioner if you experience any side effects while taking isradipine. Only your health-care practitioner can determine whether it is safe for you to continue taking this drug.

- *Most Common:* headache, dizziness, swelling of the feet, ankles, or calves, palpitations, feeling warm and skin flushing
- *Less Common:* diarrhea, chest pain, fatigue, nausea, rapid heartbeat, rash, shortness of breath, abnormally frequent urination, vomiting, weakness, stomach upset
- *Rare*: constipation, cough, depression, sleeping problems, drowsiness, dry mouth, heart attack or heart failure, hives, reduced sex drive, low blood pressure, nervousness, numbness, severe dizziness, stroke, tingling or pins and needles, vision changes

IMPORTANT PRECAUTIONS
Tell your health-care practitioner if you are sensitive or allergic to isradipine or to any other drugs, especially other calcium channel blockers.

Before taking isradipine, tell your health-care practitioner if you have a history of congestive heart failure, heart attack, or stroke, if you have a tendency to experience heart rhythm disturbances, if you have muscular dystrophy or myasthenia gravis, or if you have impaired liver or kidney function.

Do not take isradipine if you have left ventricular dysfunction (severe problem in the left side of your heart), advanced narrowing of the aorta, or symptomatic low blood pressure.

Be sure to take isradipine exactly as prescribed by your health-care practitioner, even if your symptoms disappear. Your condition may worsen if you miss doses.

Isradipine can cause dizziness; therefore make sure you know how you react to it before you drive or operate dangerous equipment.

The safety and effectiveness of isradipine has not been determined for children up to age 18.

DRUG INTERACTIONS

Tell your health-care practitioner and pharmacist if you are taking any prescription or nonprescription drugs, as well as any vitamins, herbs, or other supplements. Possible drug interactions include the following:

- Beta-blockers (e.g., acebutolol, metoprolol) or digitalis may cause heart rate and rhythm problems or very low blood pressure.
- Isradipine may increase the effects of anticonvulsants (e.g., carbamazepine), anticoagulants (e.g., warfarin), digitalis, metformin, quinidine, salicylates (e.g., aspirin), and theophylline.
- Fentanyl can result in very low blood pressure.
- Some antifungals (e.g., fluconazole, itraconazole) may result in toxic levels of isradipine.
- Delavirdine may cause increased isradipine levels and toxicity.
- Nonsteroidal anti-inflammatory drugs (NSAIDs; e.g., etodolac, naproxen) may suppress the benefits of isradipine.
- Isradipine may reduce blood levels of carbamazepine.
- Phenytoin may cause isradipine to lose its effectiveness.
- Rifampin may reduce the therapeutic effect of isradipine.
- Ritonavir and probably other protease inhibitors (e.g., nelfinavir) may cause isradipine toxicity.

FOOD, VITAMIN, AND HERBAL INTERACTIONS

Do not take this medication with grapefruit or grapefruit juice, and do not ingest either of these foods for at least one hour after taking your dose. Also avoid excessive salt intake.

Avoid herbs that can increase blood pressure, including ginseng, goldenseal, ephedra (ma huang), licorice, and saw palmetto. Calcium and garlic can be beneficial as they help lower blood pressure. Be sure to talk to your health-care practitioner before taking these supplements.

RECOMMENDED DOSAGE

Isradipine is available in 2.5- and 5-mg capsules. The dosages given here are typical. However, your health-care practitioner will determine the most appropriate dose and schedule for you.

- *Children:* not recommended
- *Adults:* starting dose for hypertension is 2.5 mg twice daily for 2 to 4 weeks. Your health-care practitioner may increase the dose by 5 mg per day at monthly intervals. Maximum daily dose is 20 mg. The timed released tablets are started at 5 mg once daily and increased as determined by your health-care practitioner.

Isradipine can be taken with or following food to help reduce stomach irritation. The capsules may be opened and mixed with food if needed. The tablets must not be crushed.

If you miss a dose, take it as soon as you remember. If it is nearly time for your next dose, do not take the missed dose. Continue with your regular dosing schedule. Never take a double dose.

SYMPTOMS OF OVERDOSE AND WHAT TO DO

Symptoms of overdose include weakness, lightheadedness, fainting, low blood pressure, shortness of breath, tremors, abnormal heartbeats, and fast pulse. If an overdose occurs, seek immediate medical attention, and bring the prescription container with you.

SPECIAL INFORMATION FOR PREGNANT OR NURSING WOMEN

No adequate studies of the effects of isradipine on pregnant or nursing women have been done. Isradipine should not be used during the first trimester, and only during the second and third trimester if essential for your health. You and your health-care practitioner need to weigh the potential benefits against the potential risks to the fetus.

Isradipine may pass into breast milk. If you are breastfeeding, your health-care practitioner will likely advise you to switch to bottle feeding until your treatment is complete.

SPECIAL INFORMATION FOR SENIORS

Older adults typically start with 2.5 mg twice daily but should have their dosage monitored carefully.

GENERIC NAME
Itraconazole

BRAND NAME
Sporanox
Generic available

ABOUT THIS DRUG
Itraconazole is an antifungal medication prescribed to treat various serious fungal infections, including those that affect the lungs, bones, and skin (blastomycosis); heart, blood, and lungs (histoplasmosis); lungs, kidneys, and other organs (aspergillosis); nails (onychomycosis); and mouth, throat, and esophagus (candidiasis). Such infections frequently occur in people who have a weakened immune system.

This drug prevents fungal organisms from producing substances they need to grow and function.

SIDE EFFECTS
Be sure to tell your health-care practitioner if you experience any side effects while taking itraconazole. Only your health-care practitioner can determine whether it is safe for you to continue taking this drug.

- *Most Common:* anxiety, bursitis, diarrhea, fatigue, fever, gas, headache, high blood pressure, indigestion, nausea and vomiting, respiratory infection, inflamed sinuses, fluid retention, urinary infection
- *Less Common:* abdominal pain, low sex drive, dizziness, extreme sleepiness, gum inflammation, hives, increased or loss of appetite, inflamed gastrointestinal tract, itching, sore throat, tremor, weakness
- *Rare:* constipation, depression, hepatitis, breast development (in males), menstrual disorders, ringing in the ears, severe allergic reaction, sleeplessness
- *Additional Side Effects Associated with the Oral Solution:* back pain, blood in the urine, breathing problems, chest pain, cough, dehydration, swallowing difficulties, hemorrhoids, insomnia, pneumonia, sweating, vision problems, weight loss

IMPORTANT PRECAUTIONS
Tell your health-care practitioner if you are sensitive or allergic to itraconazole, any other antifungal medication, or any other drugs.

Itraconazole treatment often takes months to complete, and prolonged use may increase the risk of side effects.

This drug is not recommended for children younger than 16.

Be sure to take itraconazole exactly as prescribed by your health-care practitioner. If you stop treatment before completing the entire course, the infection may return.

Before starting itraconazole, tell your health-care practitioner if you have liver or kidney disease, a history of alcohol abuse, or low or no stomach acid.

DRUG INTERACTIONS

Tell your health-care practitioner and pharmacist if you are taking any prescription or nonprescription drugs, as well as any vitamins, herbs, or other supplements. Possible drug interactions include the following:

- Adrenocorticoids (e.g., cortisone, prednisone), carbamazepine, hyoscyamine, isoniazid, nizatidine, omeprazole, propantheline, ranitidine, rifampin, and sodium bicarbonate can lead to decreased effect of itraconazole.
- Antacids, anticholinergics (e.g., atropine, scopolamine), belladonna, clininium, glycopyrrolate, and histamine H_2 receptor antagonists (e.g., cimetidine, ranitidine) may cause decreased absorption of itraconazole. Antacids should be taken at least 2 hours after taking itraconazole.
- Itraconazole may reduce the effect of losartan, mifepristone, and oral contraceptives.
- Astemizole may cause serious heart problems. Do not combine these drugs.
- Itraconazole may increase the effects of oral hypoglycemics, sibutramine, and warfarin.

FOOD, VITAMIN, AND HERBAL INTERACTIONS

Avoid grapefruit juice while taking itraconazole, as it can either significantly increase or decrease the absorption of the drug.

RECOMMENDED DOSAGE

Itraconazole is available in capsules and as an oral solution. The dosages given here are typical. However, your health-care practitioner will determine the most appropriate dose and schedule for you.

Blastomycosis and Histoplasmosis

- *Children:* not recommended

- *Adults:* two 100-mg capsules once daily after a full meal. If necessary, your health-care practitioner may increase the dose 100 mg at a time to a maximum of 400 mg daily, taken in divided doses.

Aspergillosis

- *Children:* not recommended
- *Adults:* 200 to 400 mg daily, usually for a minimum of 3 months

Onychomycosis

- *Children:* not recommended
- *Adults:* 200 mg once daily for 12 weeks for toenail infections (with or without fingernail involvement). If only the fingernails are infected, treatment is given as follows: seven days of taking 200 mg twice daily, followed by three weeks without treatment, followed by seven days of taking 200 mg twice daily.

Candidiasis

- *Children:* not recommended
- *Adults:* 20 ml of oral solution daily for 1 to 2 weeks for mouth and throat candidiasis. For infection of the esophagus, 10 ml of oral solution daily for at least 3 weeks

Capsules should be taken with a full meal; the oral solution should be taken without food. Some people find that taking the capsules with cola improves absorption of the drug.

If you miss a dose, take it as soon as you remember. If it is nearly time for your next dose, do not take the missed dose. Continue with your regular dosing schedule. Never take a double dose.

SYMPTOMS OF OVERDOSE AND WHAT TO DO

An overdose with itraconazole is unlikely. If one occurs, seek immediate medical assistance and bring the prescription container with you to the hospital.

SPECIAL INFORMATION FOR PREGNANT OR NURSING WOMEN

No adequate studies of the effects of itraconazole on pregnant or nursing women have been done. Itraconazole should not be used during pregnancy to treat nail infections. In other cases, consult with your health-care practitioner. You and your health-care practitioner must weigh the potential benefits against the potential risks to the fetus.

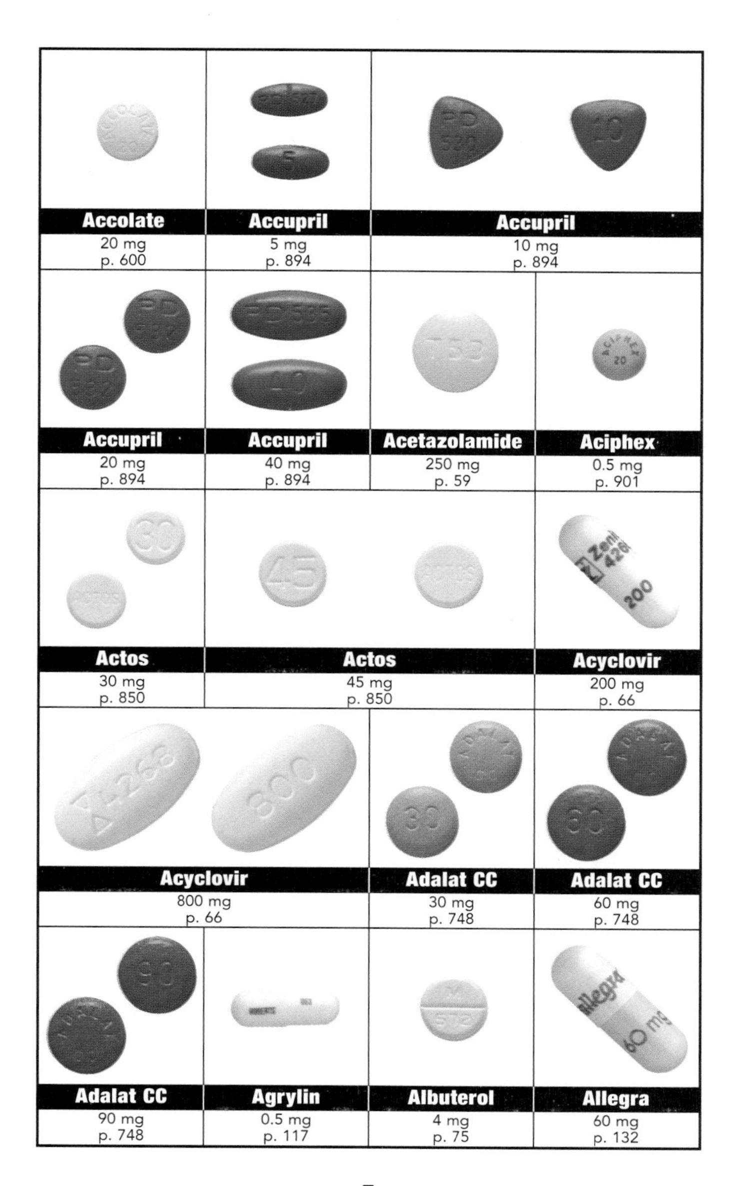
Accolate
20 mg
p. 600
Accupril
5 mg
p. 894
Accupril
10 mg
p. 894
Accupril
20 mg
p. 894
Accupril
40 mg
p. 894
Acetazolamide
250 mg
p. 59
Aciphex
0.5 mg
p. 901
Actos
30 mg
p. 850
Actos
45 mg
p. 850
Acyclovir
200 mg
p. 66
Acyclovir
800 mg
p. 66
Adalat CC
30 mg
p. 748
Adalat CC
60 mg
p. 748
Adalat CC
90 mg
p. 748
Agrylin
0.5 mg
p. 117
Albuterol
4 mg
p. 75
Allegra
60 mg
p. 132

A

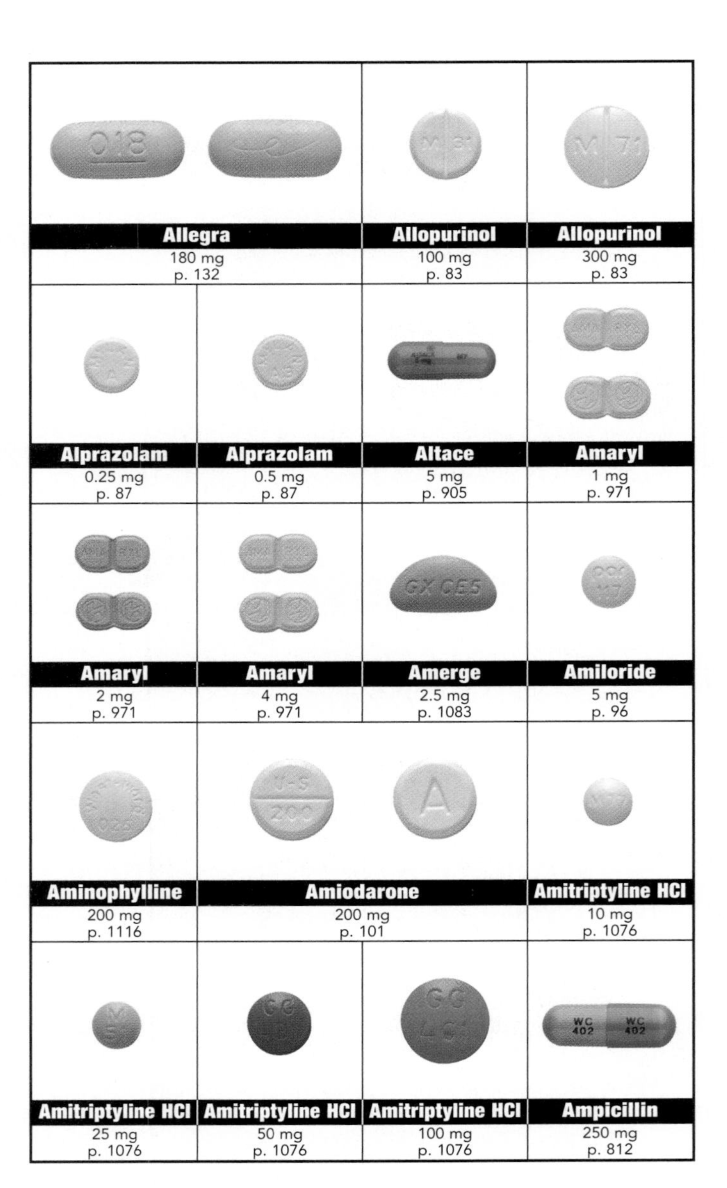
Allegra
180 mg
p. 132
Allopurinol
100 mg
p. 83
Allopurinol
300 mg
p. 83
Alprazolam
0.25 mg
p. 87
Alprazolam
0.5 mg
p. 87
Altace
5 mg
p. 905
Amaryl
1 mg
p. 971
Amaryl
2 mg
p. 971
Amaryl
4 mg
p. 971
Amerge
2.5 mg
p. 1083
Amiloride
5 mg
p. 96
Aminophylline
200 mg
p. 1116
Amiodarone
200 mg
p. 101
Amitriptyline HCl
10 mg
p. 1076
Amitriptyline HCl
25 mg
p. 1076
Amitriptyline HCl
50 mg
p. 1076
Amitriptyline HCl
100 mg
p. 1076
Ampicillin
250 mg
p. 812

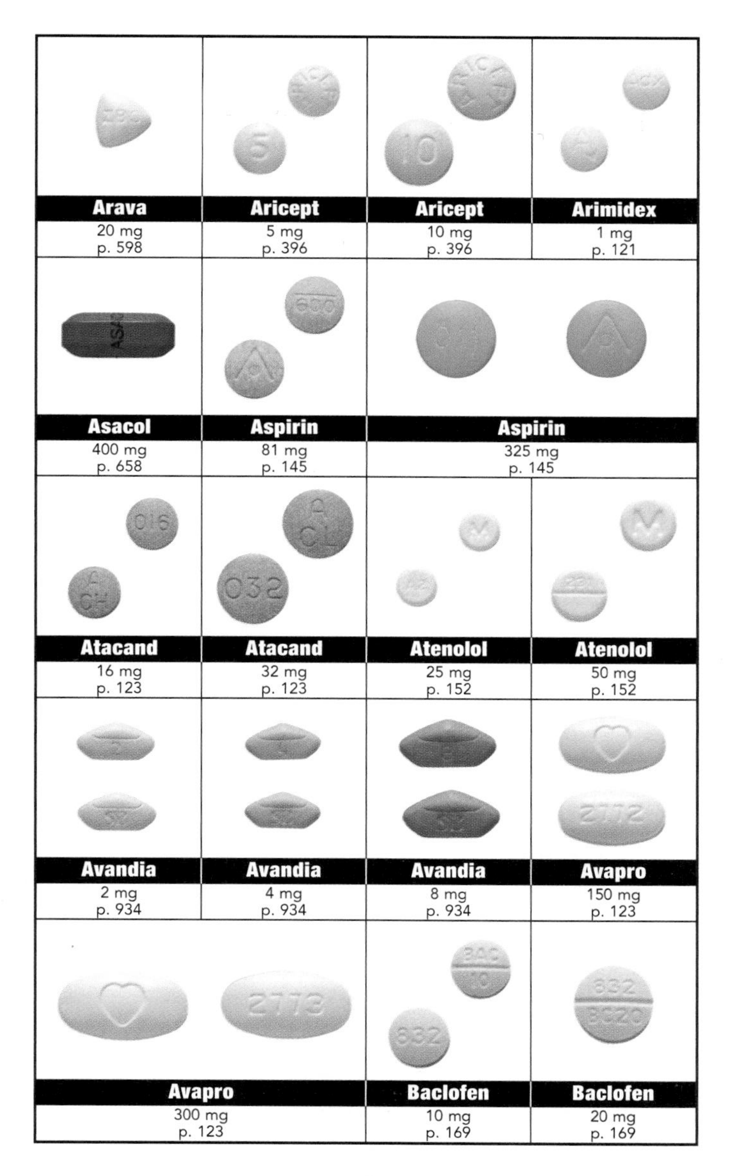
Arava
20 mg
p. 598
Aricept
5 mg
p. 396
Aricept
10 mg
p. 396
Arimidex
1 mg
p. 121
Asacol
400 mg
p. 658
Aspirin
81 mg
p. 145
Aspirin
325 mg
p. 145
Atacand
16 mg
p. 123
Atacand
32 mg
p. 123
Atenolol
25 mg
p. 152
Atenolol
50 mg
p. 152
Avandia
2 mg
p. 934
Avandia
4 mg
p. 934
Avandia
8 mg
p. 934
Avapro
150 mg
p. 123
Avapro
300 mg
p. 123
Baclofen
10 mg
p. 169
Baclofen
20 mg
p. 169

Drug	Strength	Page
Benztropine	1 mg	p. 180
Benztropine	2 mg	p. 180
Biaxin	500 mg	p. 286
Bumetanide	2 mg	p. 622
Bupropion	75 mg	p. 214
Bupropion	100 mg	p. 214
BuSpar	5 mg	p. 217
BuSpar	10 mg	p. 217
Butalbital/aspirin/caffeine	50/325/40 mg	p. 222
Captopril	12.5 mg	p. 234
Captopril	25 mg	p. 234
Captopril	50 mg	p. 234
Carbidopa/Levodopa	10/100 mg	p. 240
Carbidopa/Levodopa	25/100 mg	p. 240
Casodex	50 mg	p. 193

D

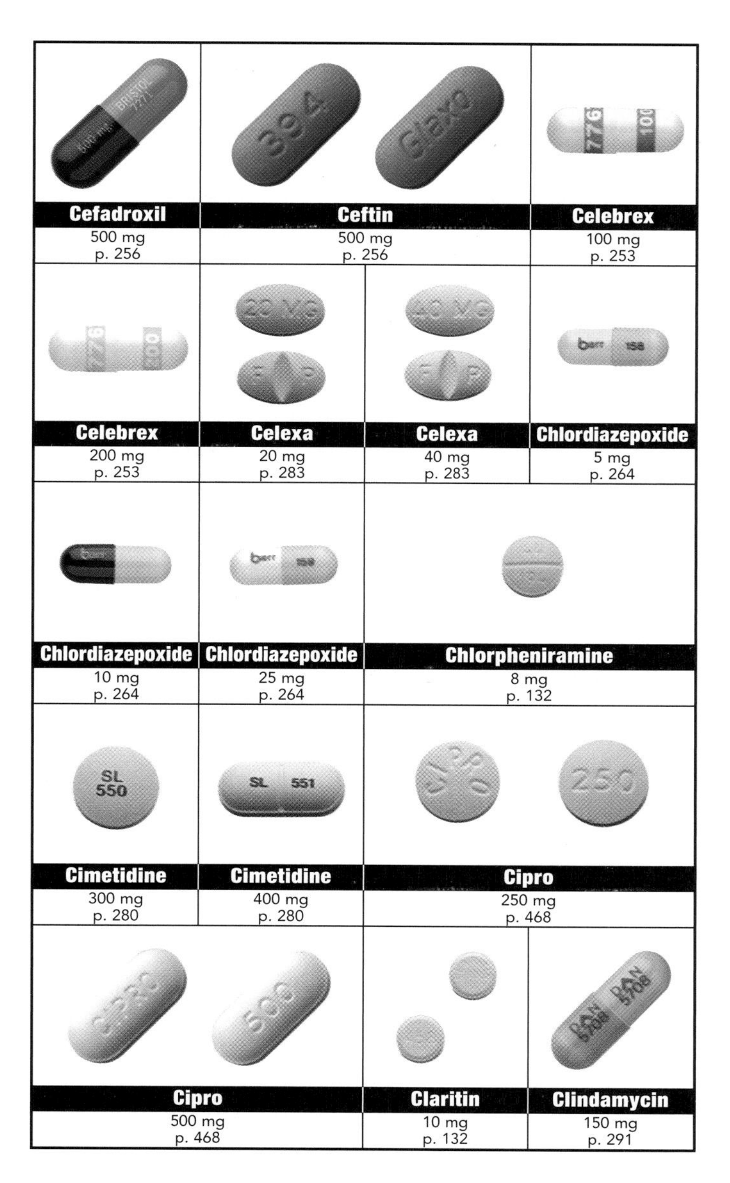
Cefadroxil
500 mg
p. 256
Ceftin
500 mg
p. 256
Celebrex
100 mg
p. 253
Celebrex
200 mg
p. 253
Celexa
20 mg
p. 283
Celexa
40 mg
p. 283
Chlordiazepoxide
5 mg
p. 264
Chlordiazepoxide
10 mg
p. 264
Chlordiazepoxide
25 mg
p. 264
Chlorpheniramine
8 mg
p. 132
Cimetidine
300 mg
p. 280
Cimetidine
400 mg
p. 280
Cipro
250 mg
p. 468
Cipro
500 mg
p. 468
Claritin
10 mg
p. 132
Clindamycin
150 mg
p. 291

E

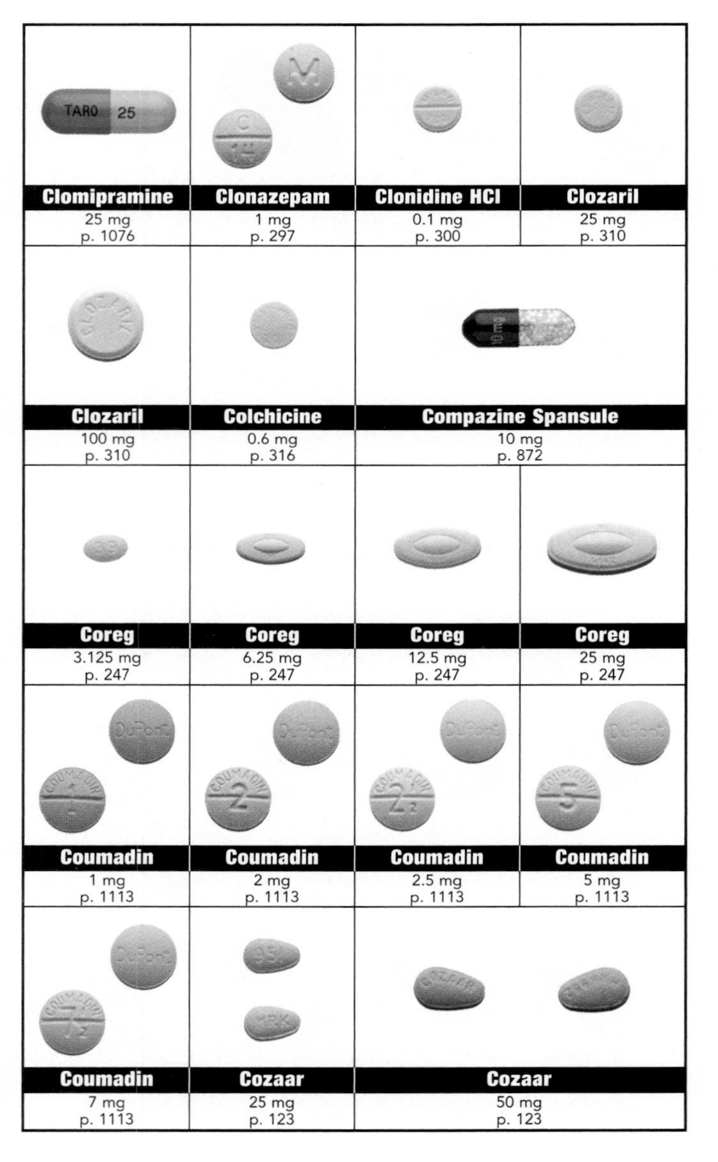
TARO 25
Clomipramine
25 mg
p. 1076
Clonazepam
1 mg
p. 297
Clonidine HCl
0.1 mg
p. 300
Clozaril
25 mg
p. 310
Clozaril
100 mg
p. 310
Colchicine
0.6 mg
p. 316
Compazine Spansule
10 mg
p. 872
Coreg
3.125 mg
p. 247
Coreg
6.25 mg
p. 247
Coreg
12.5 mg
p. 247
Coreg
25 mg
p. 247
Coumadin
1 mg
p. 1113
Coumadin
2 mg
p. 1113
Coumadin
2.5 mg
p. 1113
Coumadin
5 mg
p. 1113
Coumadin
7 mg
p. 1113
Cozaar
25 mg
p. 123
Cozaar
50 mg
p. 123

F

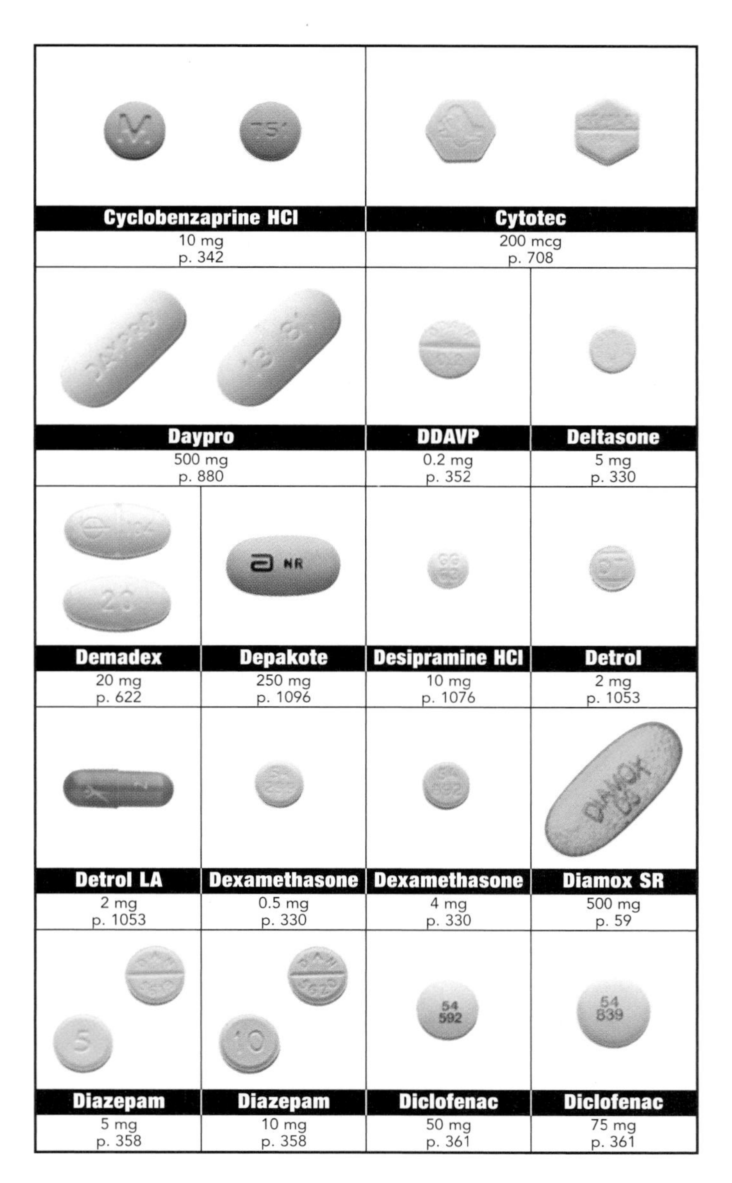
Cyclobenzaprine HCl
10 mg
p. 342
Cytotec
200 mcg
p. 708
Daypro
500 mg
p. 880
DDAVP
0.2 mg
p. 352
Deltasone
5 mg
p. 330
Demadex
20 mg
p. 622
Depakote
250 mg
p. 1096
Desipramine HCl
10 mg
p. 1076
Detrol
2 mg
p. 1053
Detrol LA
2 mg
p. 1053
Dexamethasone
0.5 mg
p. 330
Dexamethasone
4 mg
p. 330
Diamox SR
500 mg
p. 59
Diazepam
5 mg
p. 358
Diazepam
10 mg
p. 358
Diclofenac
50 mg
p. 361
Diclofenac
75 mg
p. 361

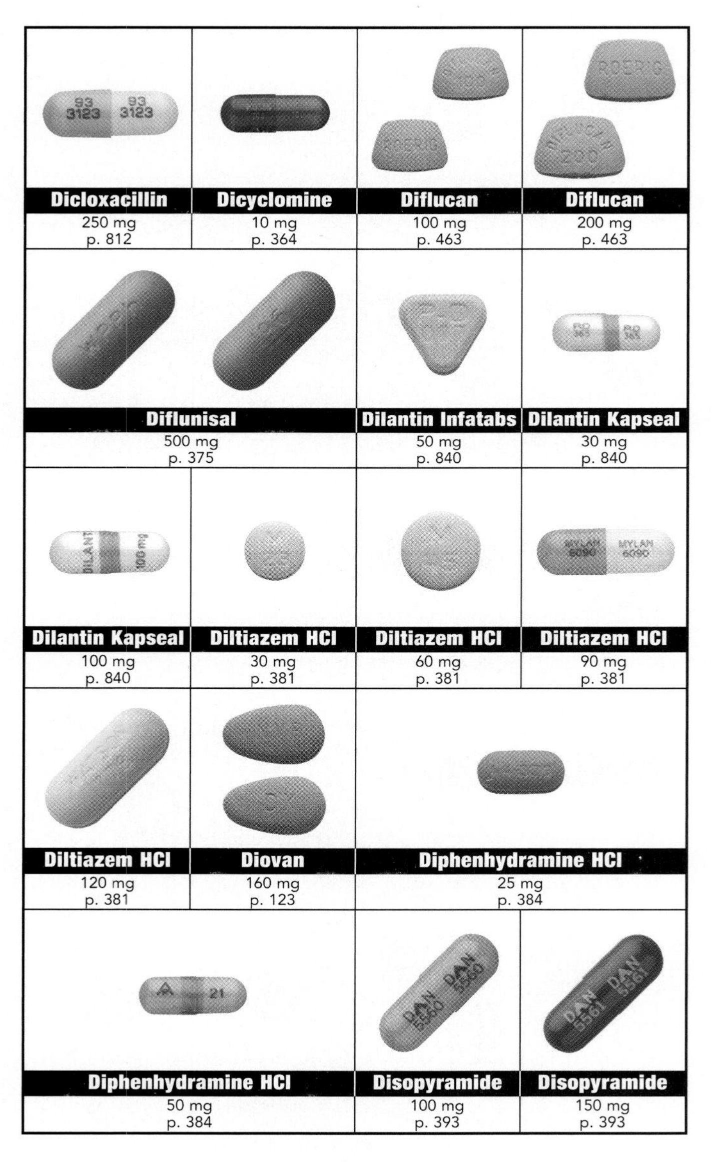
Dicloxacillin
250 mg
p. 812
Dicyclomine
10 mg
p. 364
Diflucan
100 mg
p. 463
Diflucan
200 mg
p. 463
Diflunisal
500 mg
p. 375
Dilantin Infatabs
50 mg
p. 840
Dilantin Kapseal
30 mg
p. 840
Dilantin Kapseal
100 mg
p. 840
Diltiazem HCl
30 mg
p. 381
Diltiazem HCl
60 mg
p. 381
Diltiazem HCl
90 mg
p. 381
Diltiazem HCl
120 mg
p. 381
Diovan
160 mg
p. 123
Diphenhydramine HCl
25 mg
p. 384
Diphenhydramine HCl
50 mg
p. 384
Disopyramide
100 mg
p. 393
Disopyramide
150 mg
p. 393

Doxepin HCl 10 mg p. 1076	**Doxepin HCl** 50 mg p. 1076	**Doxepin HCl** 75 mg p. 1076	**Doxycycline** 100 mg p. 1013
Effexor 37.5 mg p. 1102	**Effexor** 75 mg p. 1102	**Effexor XR** 75 mg p. 1102	**Elmiron** 100 mg p. 816
Enalapril maleate 10 mg p. 415		**Endocet** 5/325 mg p. 56	**Epivir** 150 mg p. 587
Erythrocin Stearate Filmtab 250 mg p. 425		**Etodolac** 300 mg p. 443	**Evista** 60 mg p. 903
Exelon 1.5 mg p. 929	**Exelon** 3 mg p. 929	**Exelon** 6 mg p. 929	**Famvir** 125 mg p. 447

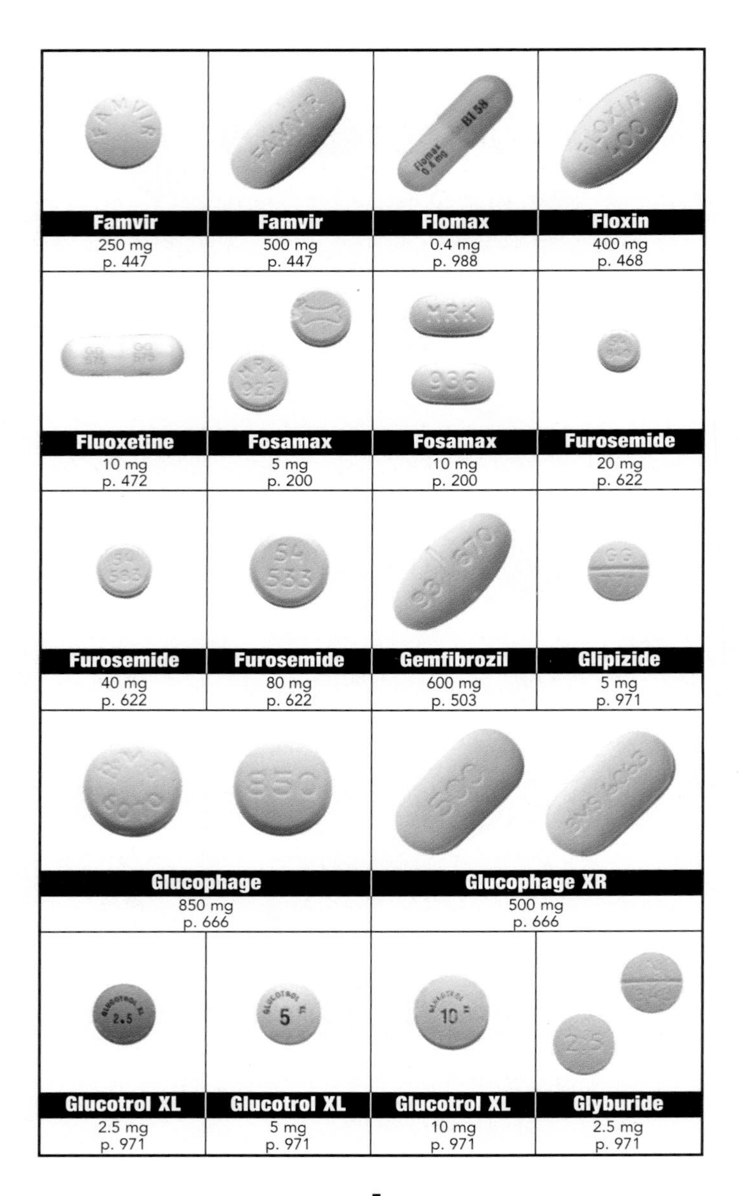
Famvir
250 mg
p. 447
Famvir
500 mg
p. 447
Flomax
0.4 mg
p. 988
Floxin
400 mg
p. 468
Fluoxetine
10 mg
p. 472
Fosamax
5 mg
p. 200
Fosamax
10 mg
p. 200
Furosemide
20 mg
p. 622
Furosemide
40 mg
p. 622
Furosemide
80 mg
p. 622
Gemfibrozil
600 mg
p. 503
Glipizide
5 mg
p. 971
Glucophage
850 mg
p. 666
Glucophage XR
500 mg
p. 666
Glucotrol XL
2.5 mg
p. 971
Glucotrol XL
5 mg
p. 971
Glucotrol XL
10 mg
p. 971
Glyburide
2.5 mg
p. 971

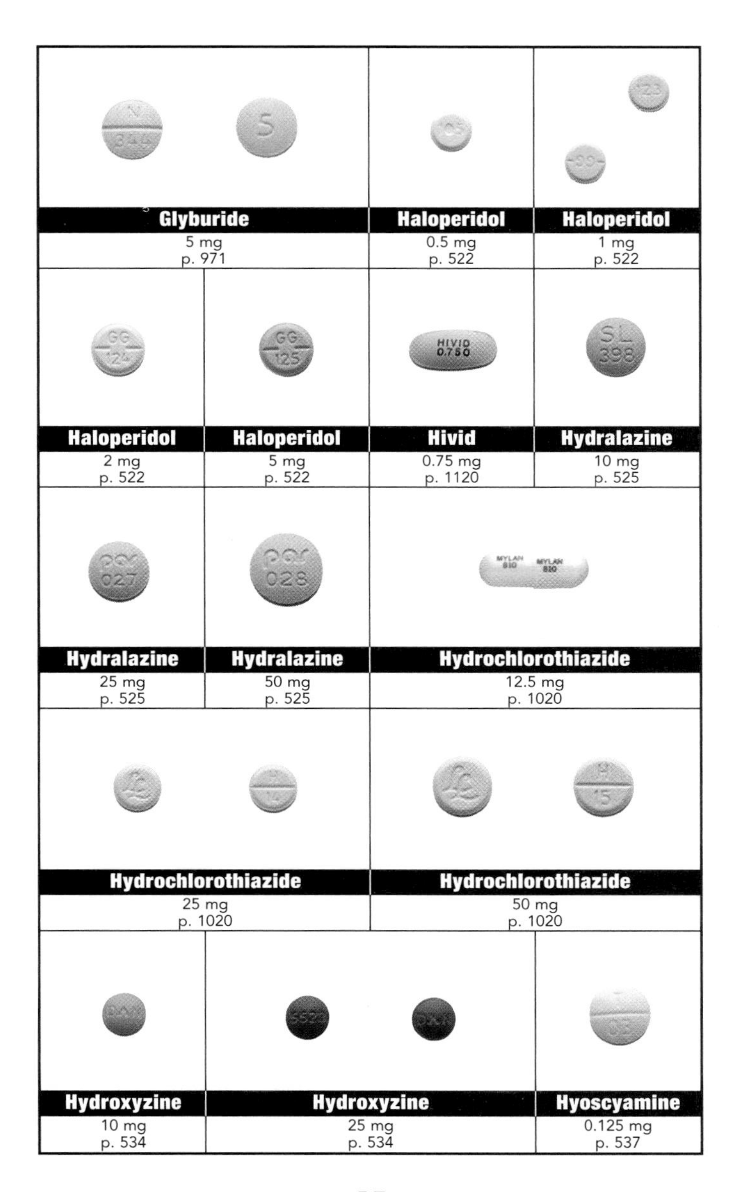

Glyburide
5 mg
p. 971
Haloperidol
0.5 mg
p. 522
Haloperidol
1 mg
p. 522
Haloperidol
2 mg
p. 522
Haloperidol
5 mg
p. 522
Hivid
0.75 mg
p. 1120
Hydralazine
10 mg
p. 525
Hydralazine
25 mg
p. 525
Hydralazine
50 mg
p. 525
Hydrochlorothiazide
12.5 mg
p. 1020
Hydrochlorothiazide
25 mg
p. 1020
Hydrochlorothiazide
50 mg
p. 1020
Hydroxyzine
10 mg
p. 534
Hydroxyzine
25 mg
p. 534
Hyoscyamine
0.125 mg
p. 537

K

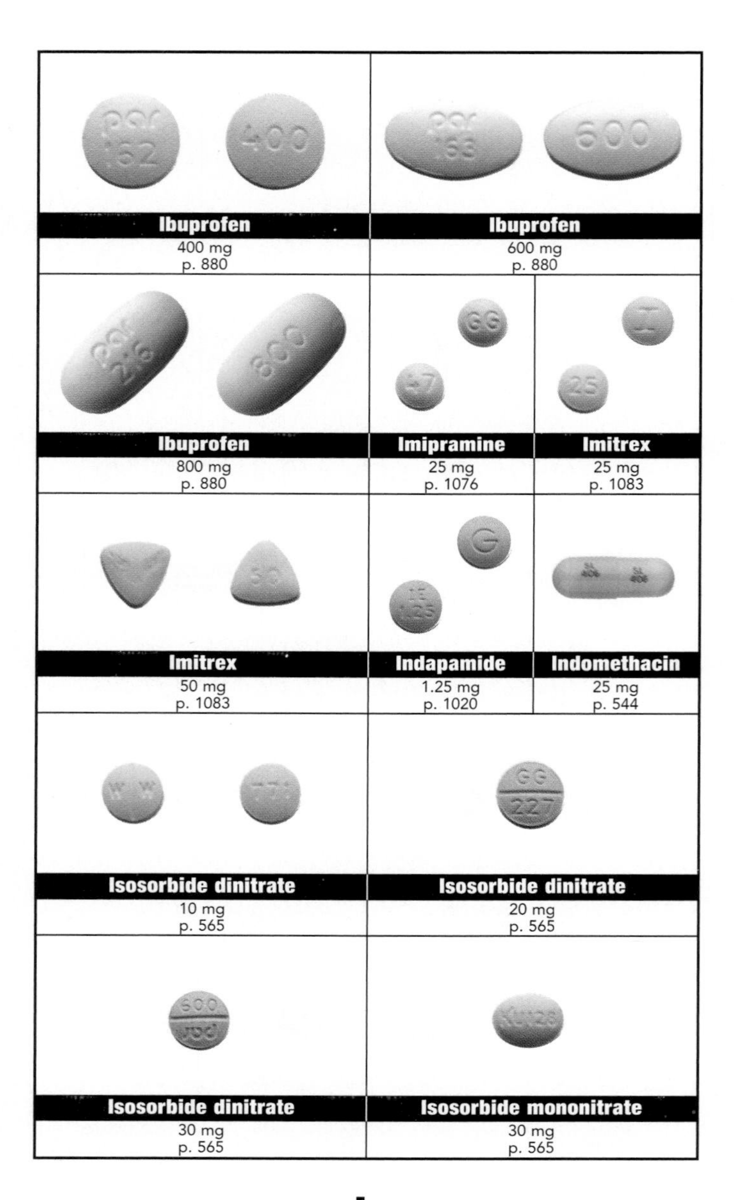
Ibuprofen
400 mg
p. 880
Ibuprofen
600 mg
p. 880
Ibuprofen
800 mg
p. 880
Imipramine
25 mg
p. 1076
Imitrex
25 mg
p. 1083
Imitrex
50 mg
p. 1083
Indapamide
1.25 mg
p. 1020
Indomethacin
25 mg
p. 544
Isosorbide dinitrate
10 mg
p. 565
Isosorbide dinitrate
20 mg
p. 565
Isosorbide dinitrate
30 mg
p. 565
Isosorbide mononitrate
30 mg
p. 565

L

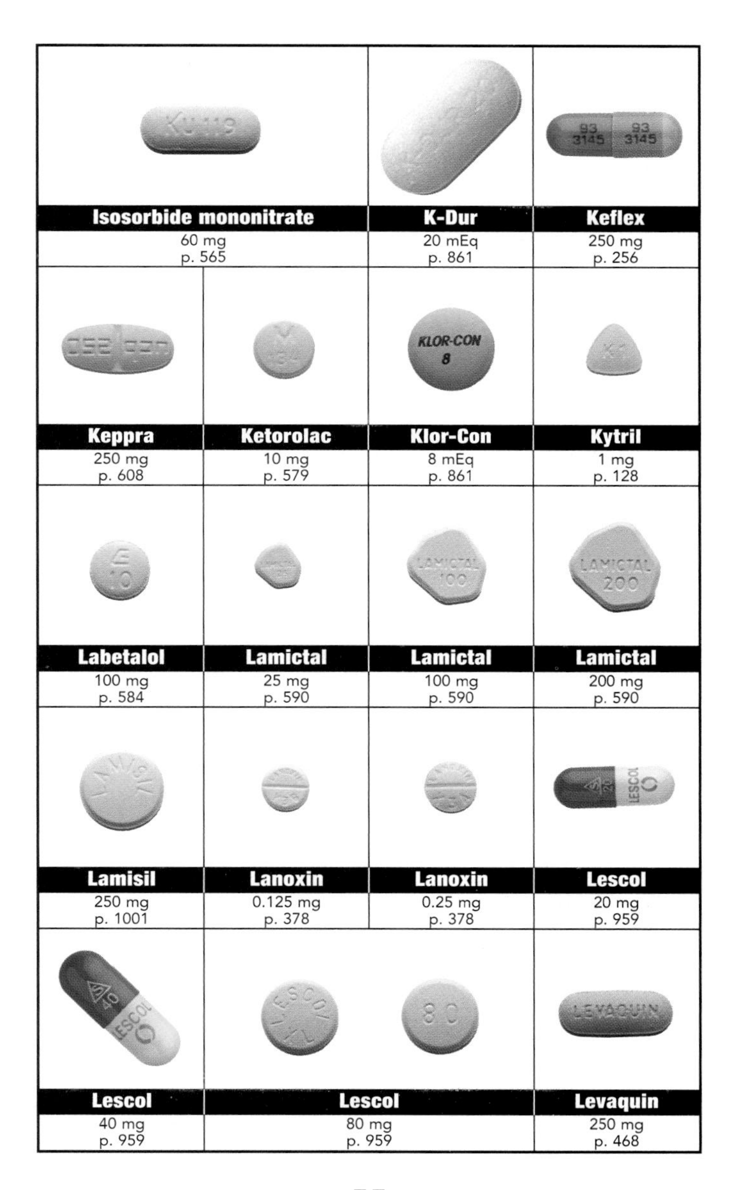

Drug	Strength	Page
Isosorbide mononitrate	60 mg	p. 565
K-Dur	20 mEq	p. 861
Keflex	250 mg	p. 256
Keppra	250 mg	p. 608
Ketorolac	10 mg	p. 579
Klor-Con	8 mEq	p. 861
Kytril	1 mg	p. 128
Labetalol	100 mg	p. 584
Lamictal	25 mg	p. 590
Lamictal	100 mg	p. 590
Lamictal	200 mg	p. 590
Lamisil	250 mg	p. 1001
Lanoxin	0.125 mg	p. 378
Lanoxin	0.25 mg	p. 378
Lescol	20 mg	p. 959
Lescol	40 mg	p. 959
Lescol	80 mg	p. 959
Levaquin	250 mg	p. 468

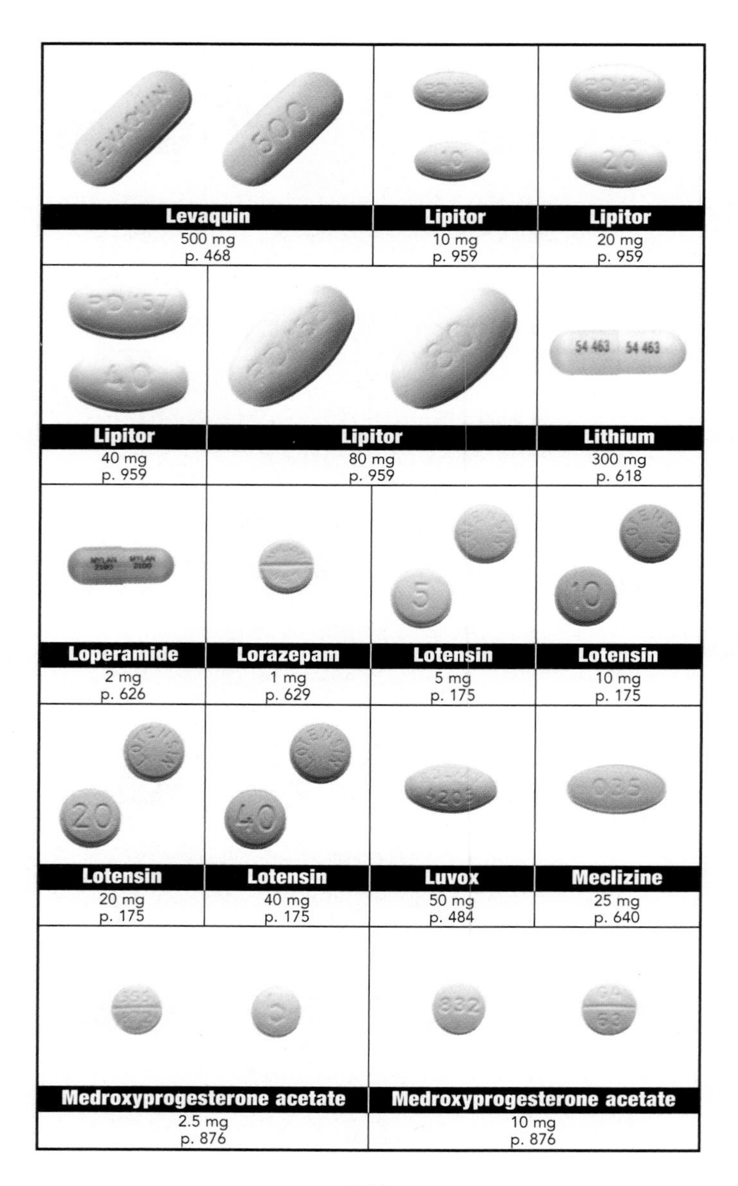

Levaquin
500 mg
p. 468
Lipitor
10 mg
p. 959
Lipitor
20 mg
p. 959
Lipitor
40 mg
p. 959
Lipitor
80 mg
p. 959
Lithium
300 mg
p. 618
Loperamide
2 mg
p. 626
Lorazepam
1 mg
p. 629
Lotensin
5 mg
p. 175
Lotensin
10 mg
p. 175
Lotensin
20 mg
p. 175
Lotensin
40 mg
p. 175
Luvox
50 mg
p. 484
Meclizine
25 mg
p. 640
Medroxyprogesterone acetate
2.5 mg
p. 876
Medroxyprogesterone acetate
10 mg
p. 876

N

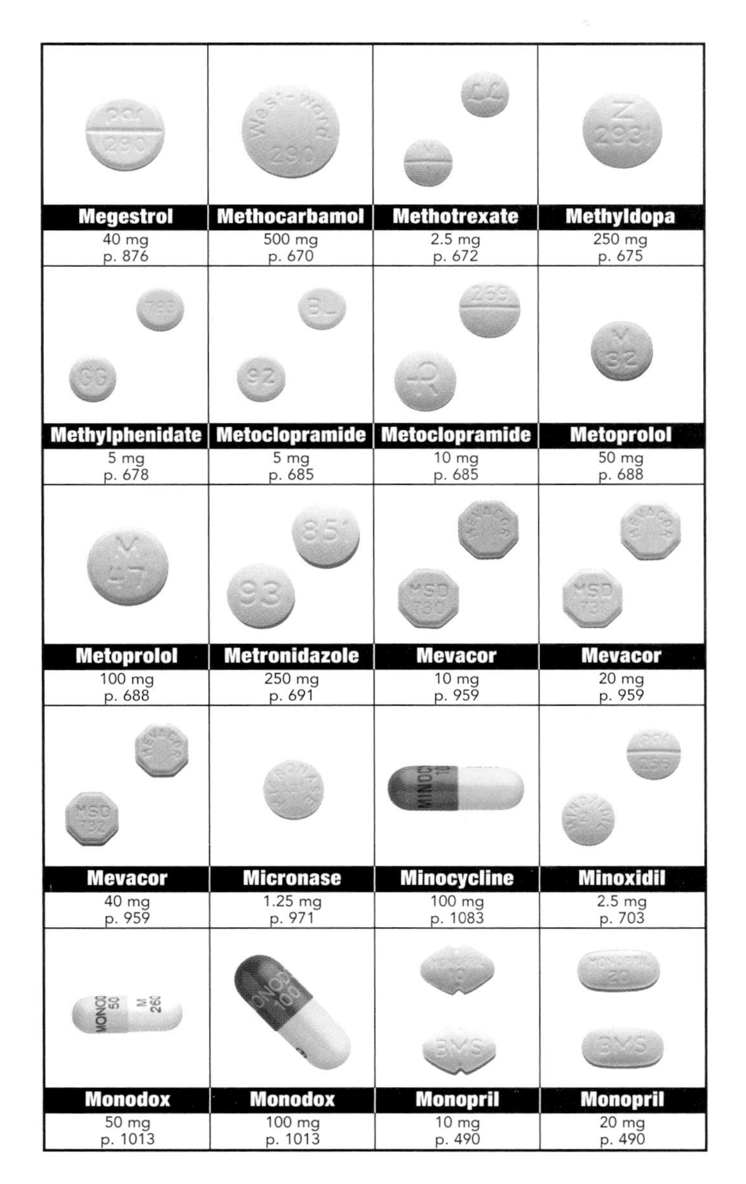

Megestrol 40 mg p. 876	Methocarbamol 500 mg p. 670	Methotrexate 2.5 mg p. 672	Methyldopa 250 mg p. 675
Methylphenidate 5 mg p. 678	Metoclopramide 5 mg p. 685	Metoclopramide 10 mg p. 685	Metoprolol 50 mg p. 688
Metoprolol 100 mg p. 688	Metronidazole 250 mg p. 691	Mevacor 10 mg p. 959	Mevacor 20 mg p. 959
Mevacor 40 mg p. 959	Micronase 1.25 mg p. 971	Minocycline 100 mg p. 1083	Minoxidil 2.5 mg p. 703
Monodox 50 mg p. 1013	Monodox 100 mg p. 1013	Monopril 10 mg p. 490	Monopril 20 mg p. 490

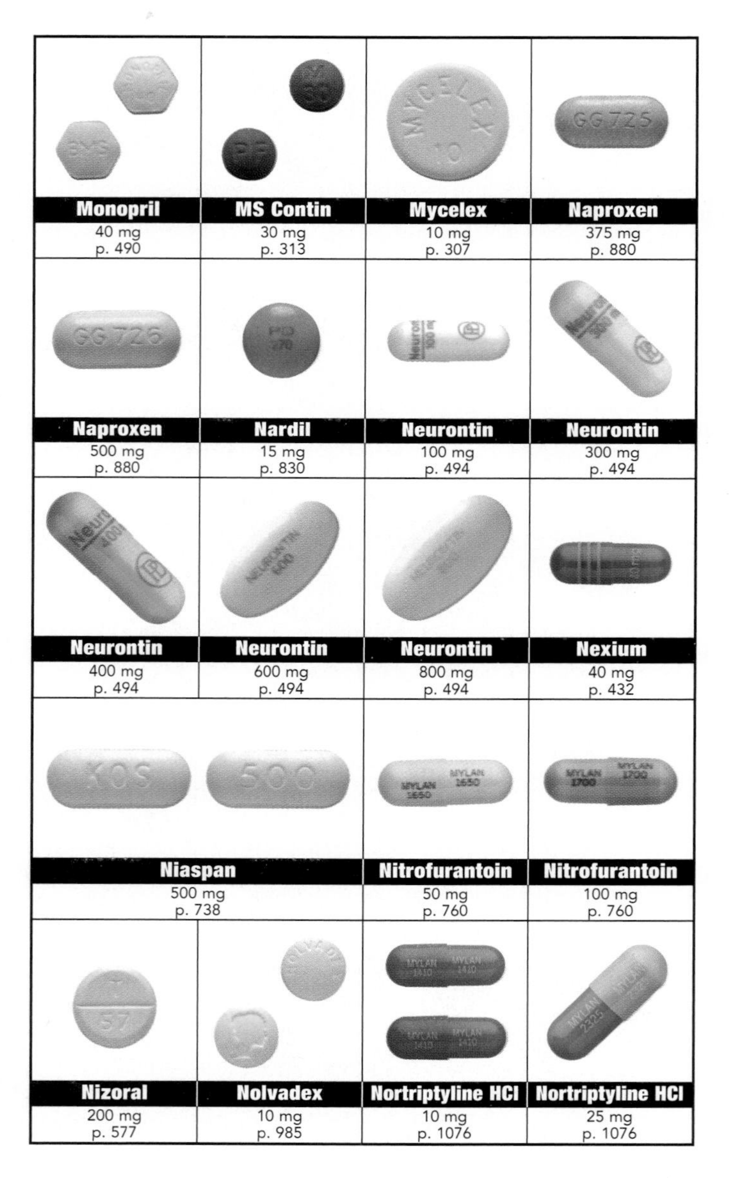
Monopril
40 mg
p. 490
MS Contin
30 mg
p. 313
Mycelex
10 mg
p. 307
Naproxen
375 mg
p. 880
Naproxen
500 mg
p. 880
Nardil
15 mg
p. 830
Neurontin
100 mg
p. 494
Neurontin
300 mg
p. 494
Neurontin
400 mg
p. 494
Neurontin
600 mg
p. 494
Neurontin
800 mg
p. 494
Nexium
40 mg
p. 432
Niaspan
500 mg
p. 738
Nitrofurantoin
50 mg
p. 760
Nitrofurantoin
100 mg
p. 760
Nizoral
200 mg
p. 577
Nolvadex
10 mg
p. 985
Nortriptyline HCl
10 mg
p. 1076
Nortriptyline HCl
25 mg
p. 1076

P

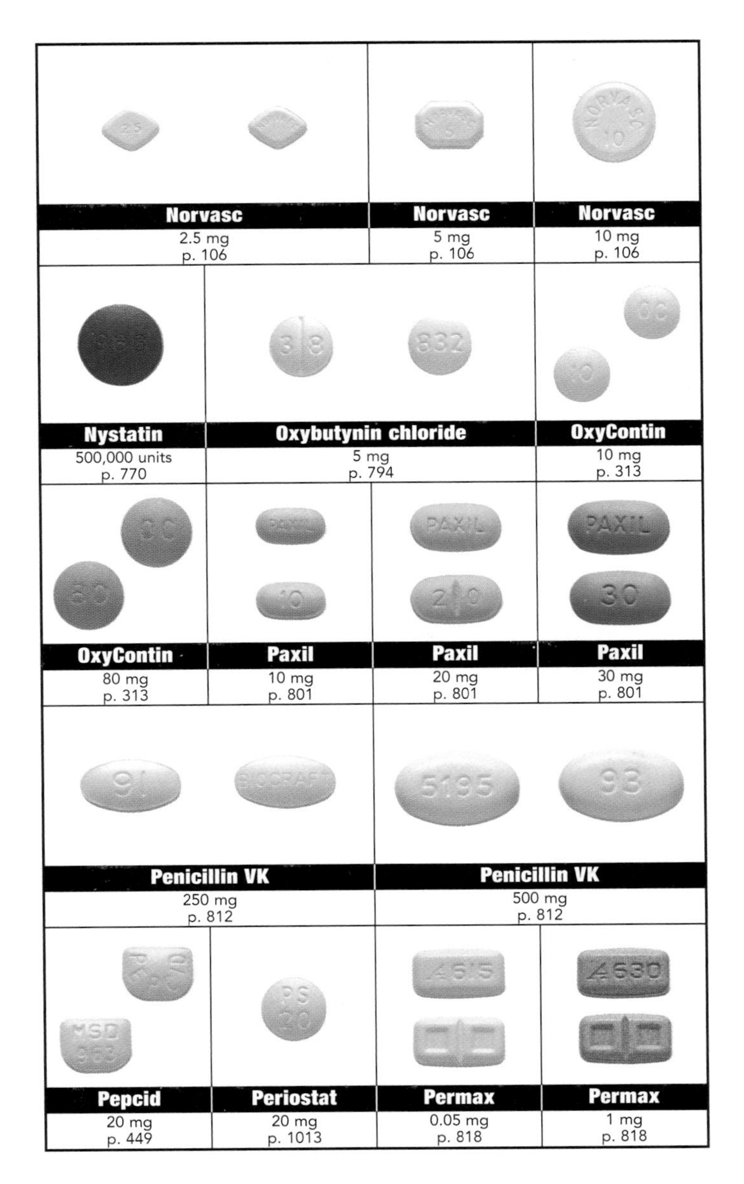

Norvasc
2.5 mg
p. 106
Norvasc
5 mg
p. 106
Norvasc
10 mg
p. 106
Nystatin
500,000 units
p. 770
Oxybutynin chloride
5 mg
p. 794
OxyContin
10 mg
p. 313
OxyContin
80 mg
p. 313
Paxil
10 mg
p. 801
Paxil
20 mg
p. 801
Paxil
30 mg
p. 801
Penicillin VK
250 mg
p. 812
Penicillin VK
500 mg
p. 812
Pepcid
20 mg
p. 449
Periostat
20 mg
p. 1013
Permax
0.05 mg
p. 818
Permax
1 mg
p. 818

Q

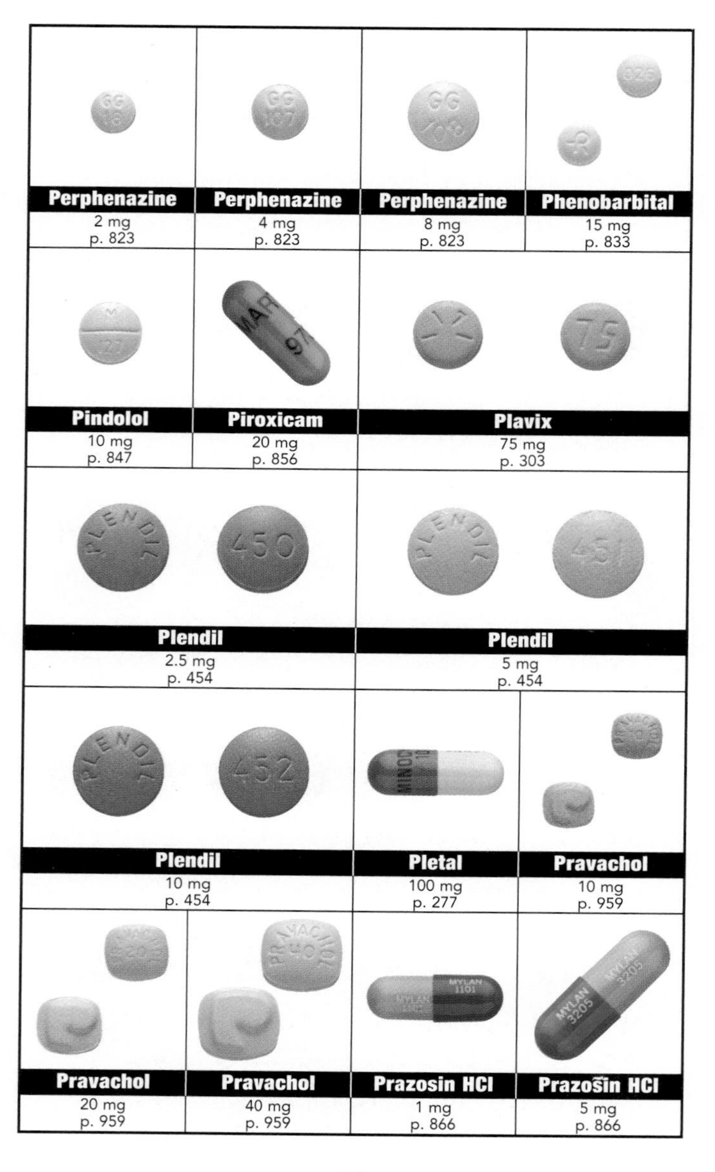
Perphenazine
2 mg
p. 823
Perphenazine
4 mg
p. 823
Perphenazine
8 mg
p. 823
Phenobarbital
15 mg
p. 833
Pindolol
10 mg
p. 847
Piroxicam
20 mg
p. 856
Plavix
75 mg
p. 303
Plendil
2.5 mg
p. 454
Plendil
5 mg
p. 454
Plendil
10 mg
p. 454
Pletal
100 mg
p. 277
Pravachol
10 mg
p. 959
Pravachol
20 mg
p. 959
Pravachol
40 mg
p. 959
Prazosin HCl
1 mg
p. 866
Prazosin HCl
5 mg
p. 866

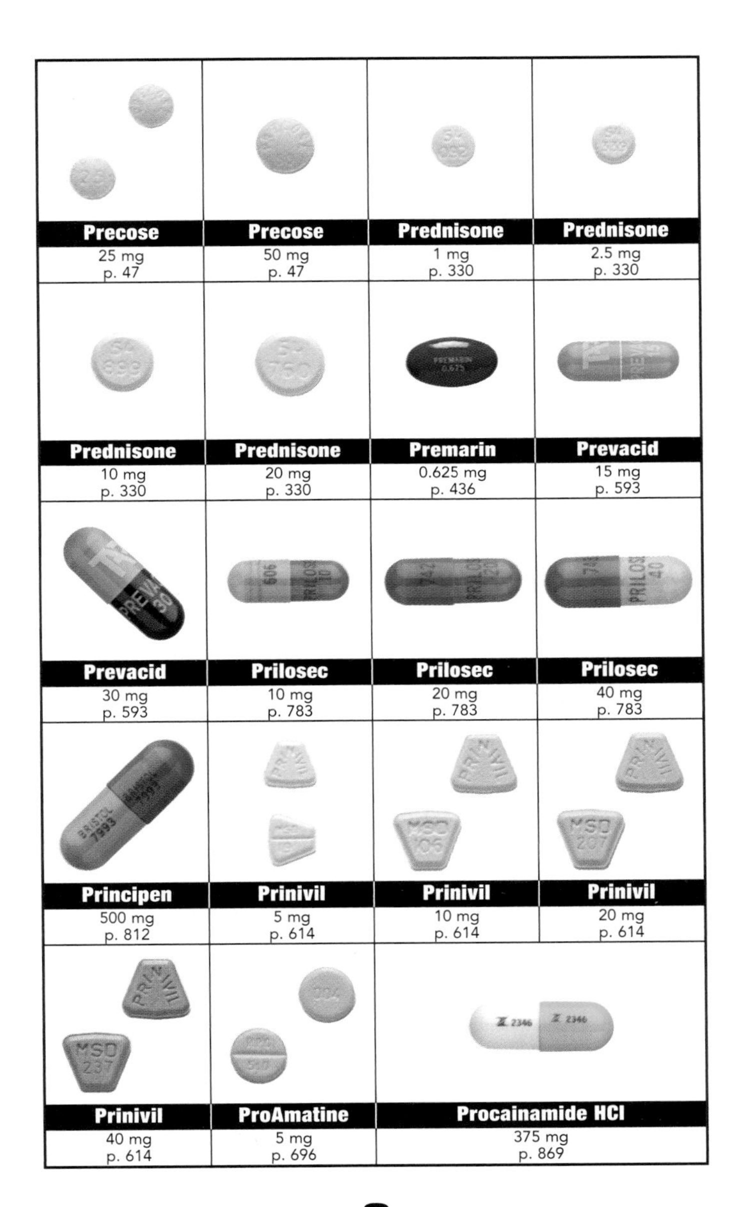
Precose
25 mg
p. 47
Precose
50 mg
p. 47
Prednisone
1 mg
p. 330
Prednisone
2.5 mg
p. 330
Prednisone
10 mg
p. 330
Prednisone
20 mg
p. 330
Premarin
0.625 mg
p. 436
Prevacid
15 mg
p. 593
Prevacid
30 mg
p. 593
Prilosec
10 mg
p. 783
Prilosec
20 mg
p. 783
Prilosec
40 mg
p. 783
Principen
500 mg
p. 812
Prinivil
5 mg
p. 614
Prinivil
10 mg
p. 614
Prinivil
20 mg
p. 614
Prinivil
40 mg
p. 614
ProAmatine
5 mg
p. 696
Procainamide HCl
375 mg
p. 869

S

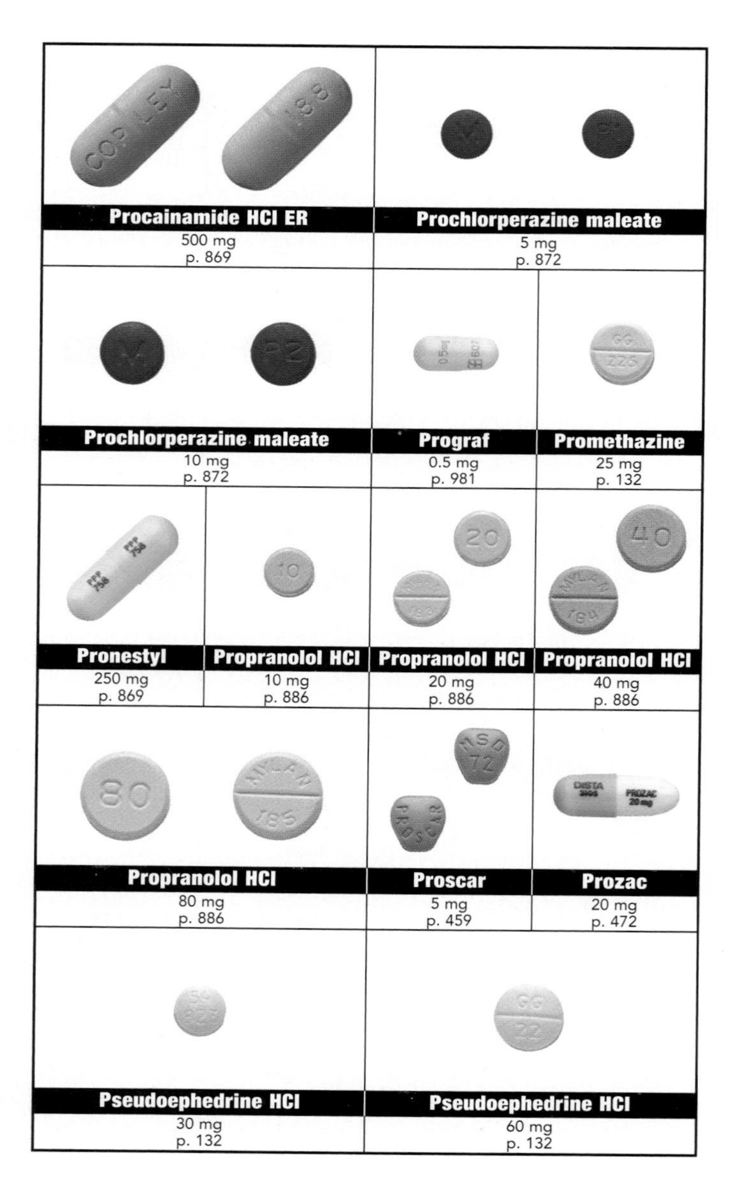

Procainamide HCl ER
500 mg
p. 869
Prochlorperazine maleate
5 mg
p. 872
Prochlorperazine maleate
10 mg
p. 872
Prograf
0.5 mg
p. 981
Promethazine
25 mg
p. 132
Pronestyl
250 mg
p. 869
Propranolol HCl
10 mg
p. 886
Propranolol HCl
20 mg
p. 886
Propranolol HCl
40 mg
p. 886
Propranolol HCl
80 mg
p. 886
Proscar
5 mg
p. 459
Prozac
20 mg
p. 472
Pseudoephedrine HCl
30 mg
p. 132
Pseudoephedrine HCl
60 mg
p. 132

T

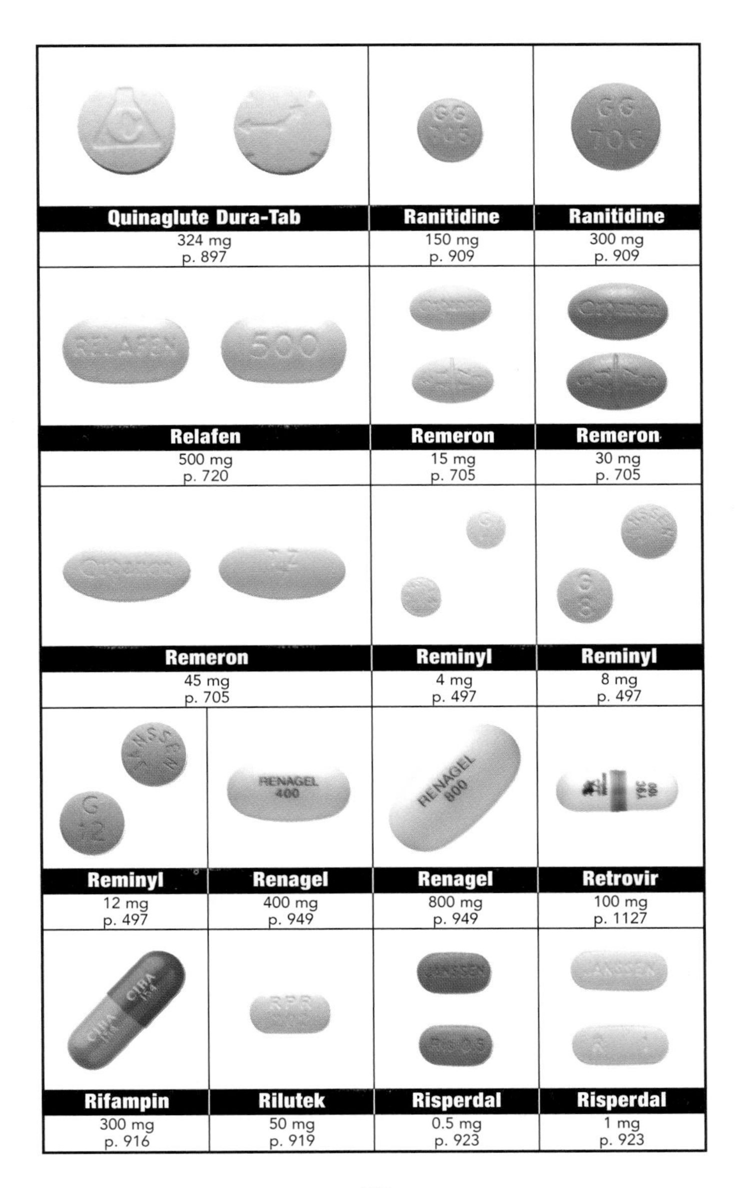
Quinaglute Dura-Tab
324 mg
p. 897
Ranitidine
150 mg
p. 909
Ranitidine
300 mg
p. 909
Relafen
500 mg
p. 720
Remeron
15 mg
p. 705
Remeron
30 mg
p. 705
Remeron
45 mg
p. 705
Reminyl
4 mg
p. 497
Reminyl
8 mg
p. 497
Reminyl
12 mg
p. 497
Renagel
400 mg
p. 949
Renagel
800 mg
p. 949
Retrovir
100 mg
p. 1127
Rifampin
300 mg
p. 916
Rilutek
50 mg
p. 919
Risperdal
0.5 mg
p. 923
Risperdal
1 mg
p. 923

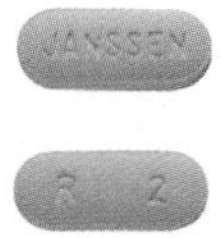

Drug	Strength	Page
Risperdal	2 mg	p. 923
Risperdal	3 mg	p. 923
Sansert	2 mg	p. 682
Serentil	25 mg	p. 267
Seroquel	25 mg	p. 891
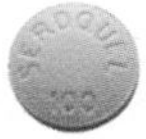 Seroquel	100 mg	p. 891
Serzone	100 mg	p. 728
Serzone	200 mg	p. 728
Serzone	250 mg	p. 728
Sinemet	25/250 mg	p. 610
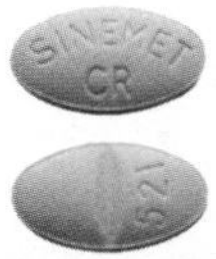 Sinemet	50/200 mg	p. 610
Singulair	10 mg	p. 600
Skelaxin	400 mg	p. 664
Soriatane	25 mg	p. 63
Spironolactone	25 mg	p. 956
Sporanox	100 mg	p. 574

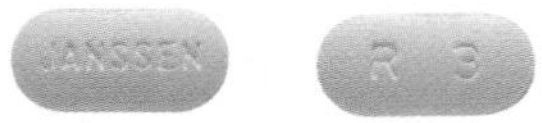

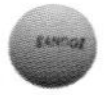

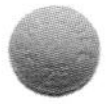

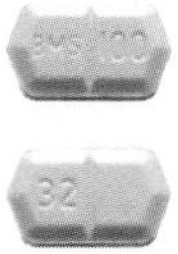

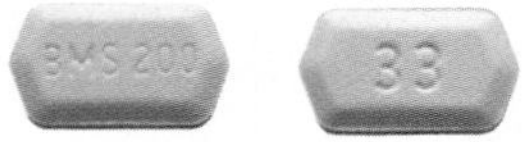

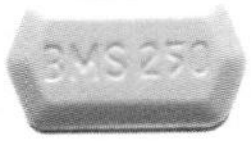

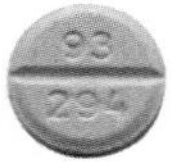

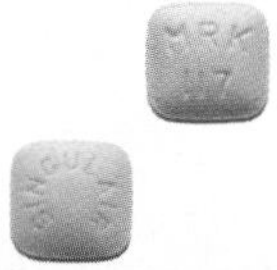

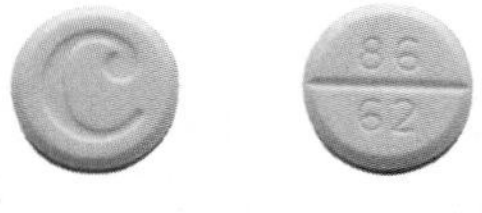

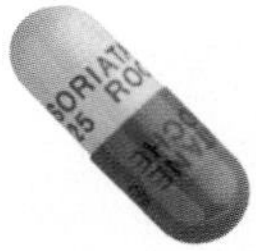

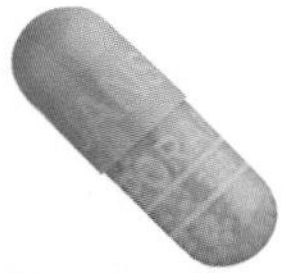

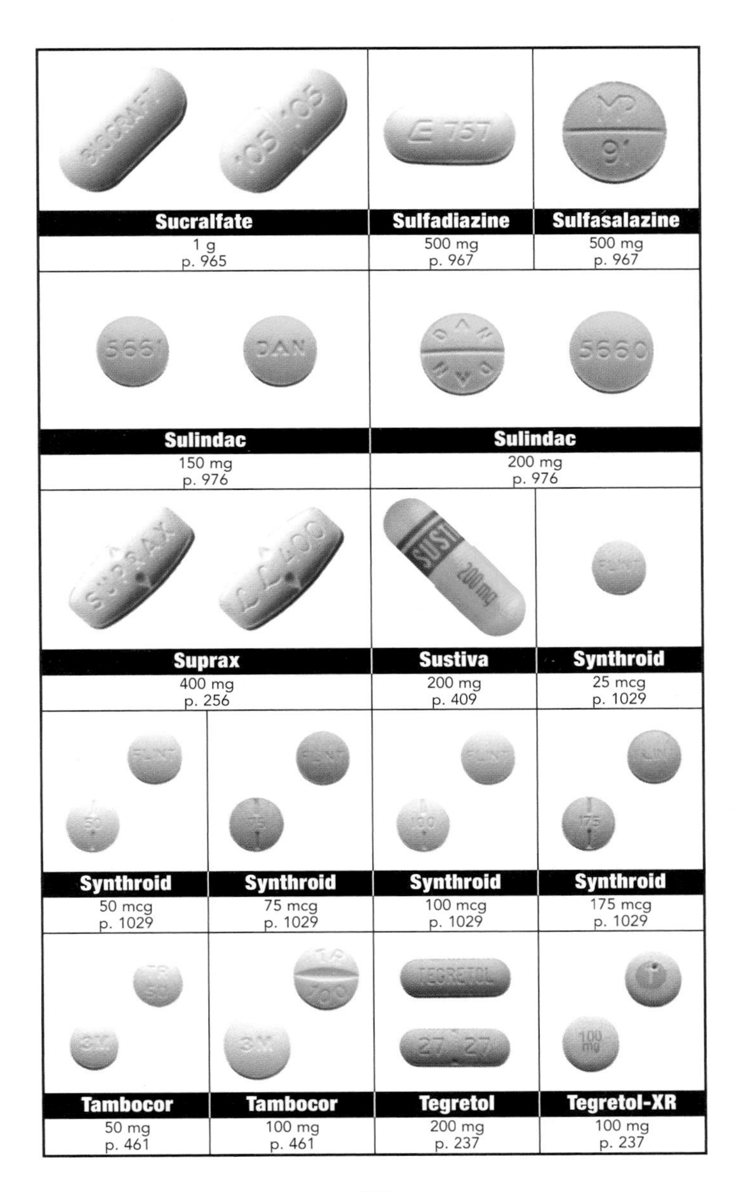
Sucralfate
1 g
p. 965
Sulfadiazine
500 mg
p. 967
Sulfasalazine
500 mg
p. 967
Sulindac
150 mg
p. 976
Sulindac
200 mg
p. 976
Suprax
400 mg
p. 256
Sustiva
200 mg
p. 409
Synthroid
25 mcg
p. 1029
Synthroid
50 mcg
p. 1029
Synthroid
75 mcg
p. 1029
Synthroid
100 mcg
p. 1029
Synthroid
175 mcg
p. 1029
Tambocor
50 mg
p. 461
Tambocor
100 mg
p. 461
Tegretol
200 mg
p. 237
Tegretol-XR
100 mg
p. 237

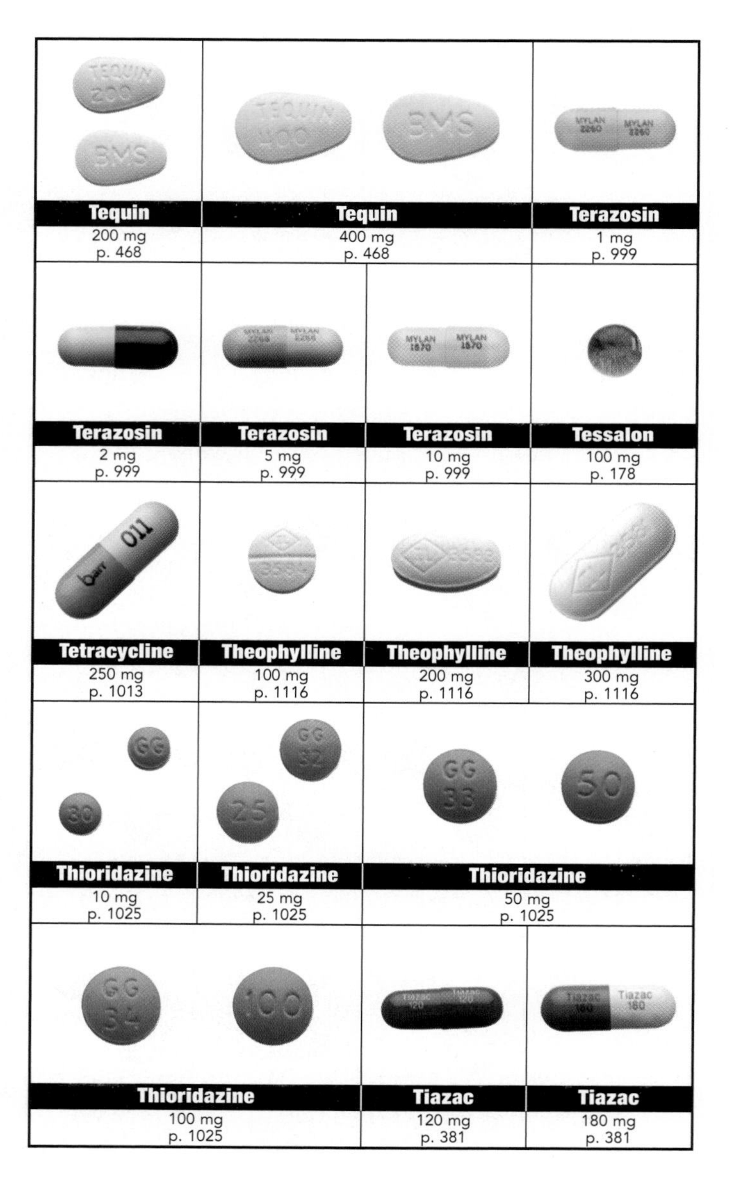
Tequin
200 mg
p. 468
Tequin
400 mg
p. 468
Terazosin
1 mg
p. 999
Terazosin
2 mg
p. 999
Terazosin
5 mg
p. 999
Terazosin
10 mg
p. 999
Tessalon
100 mg
p. 178
Tetracycline
250 mg
p. 1013
Theophylline
100 mg
p. 1116
Theophylline
200 mg
p. 1116
Theophylline
300 mg
p. 1116
Thioridazine
10 mg
p. 1025
Thioridazine
25 mg
p. 1025
Thioridazine
50 mg
p. 1025
Thioridazine
100 mg
p. 1025
Tiazac
120 mg
p. 381
Tiazac
180 mg
p. 381

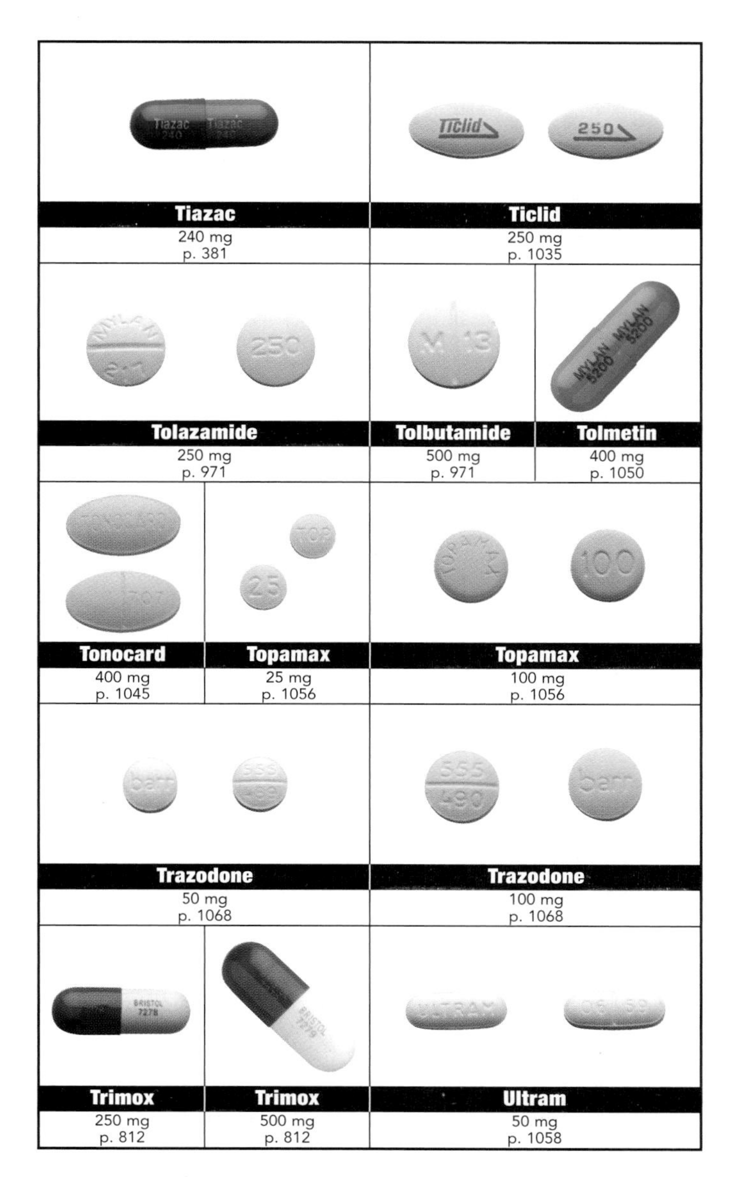

Tiazac
240 mg
p. 381
Ticlid
250 mg
p. 1035
Tolazamide
250 mg
p. 971
Tolbutamide
500 mg
p. 971
Tolmetin
400 mg
p. 1050
Tonocard
400 mg
p. 1045
Topamax
25 mg
p. 1056
Topamax
100 mg
p. 1056
Trazodone
50 mg
p. 1068
Trazodone
100 mg
p. 1068
Trimox
250 mg
p. 812
Trimox
500 mg
p. 812
Ultram
50 mg
p. 1058

Y

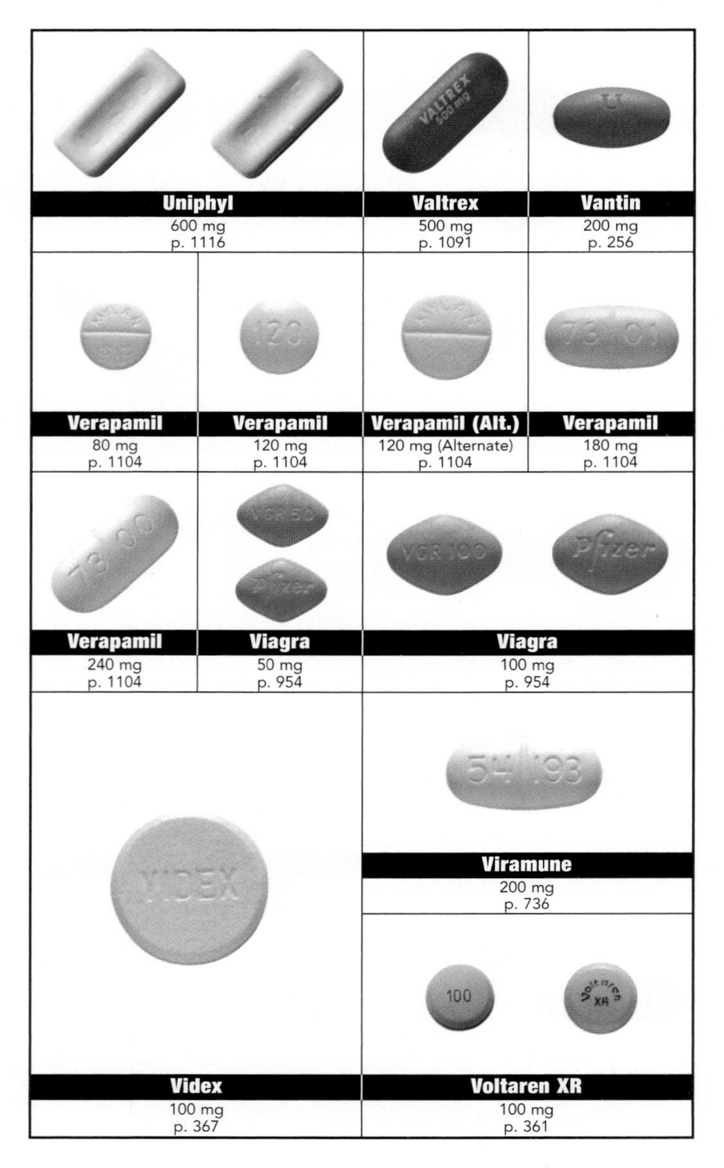
VALTREX 500 mg
Uniphyl
600 mg
p. 1116
Valtrex
500 mg
p. 1091
Vantin
200 mg
p. 256
120
73 01
Verapamil
80 mg
p. 1104
Verapamil
120 mg
p. 1104
Verapamil (Alt.)
120 mg (Alternate)
p. 1104
Verapamil
180 mg
p. 1104
73 00
VGR 50
Pfizer
VGR 100
Pfizer
Verapamil
240 mg
p. 1104
Viagra
50 mg
p. 954
Viagra
100 mg
p. 954
54 193
VIDEX
Viramune
200 mg
p. 736
100
Voltaren XR
Videx
100 mg
p. 367
Voltaren XR
100 mg
p. 361

Z

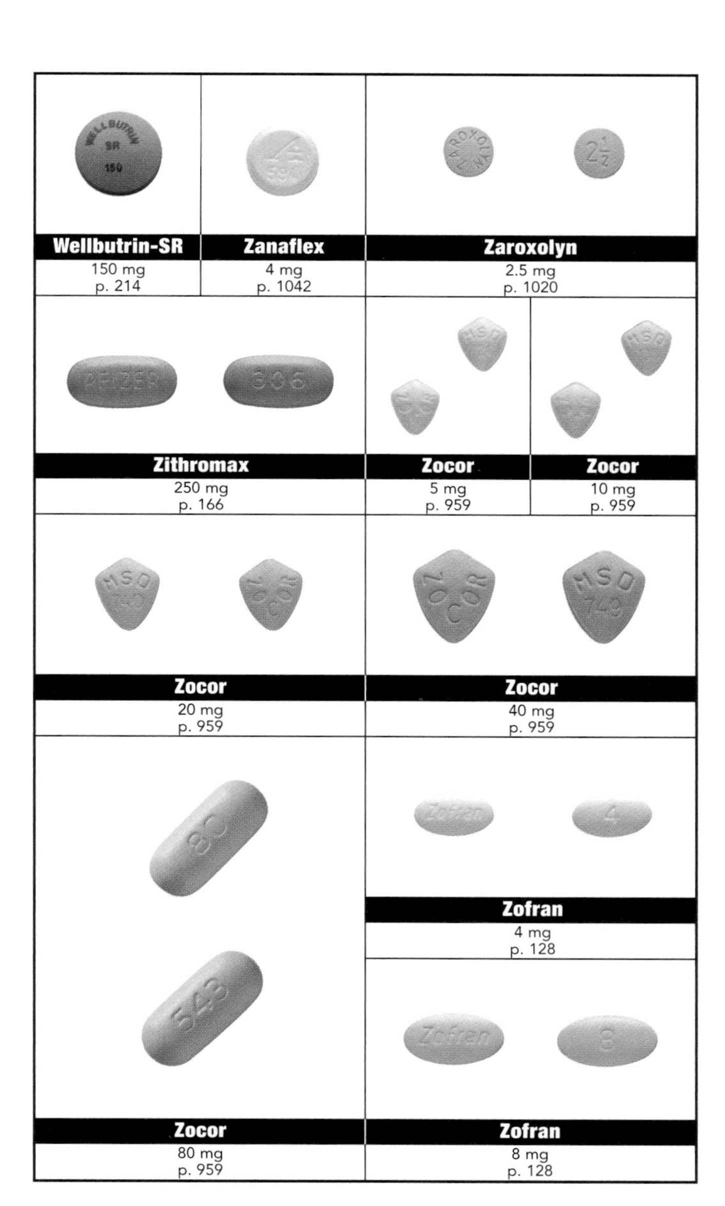
Wellbutrin-SR
150 mg
p. 214
Zanaflex
4 mg
p. 1042
Zaroxolyn
2.5 mg
p. 1020
Zithromax
250 mg
p. 166
Zocor
5 mg
p. 959
Zocor
10 mg
p. 959
Zocor
20 mg
p. 959
Zocor
40 mg
p. 959
Zofran
4 mg
p. 128
Zocor
80 mg
p. 959
Zofran
8 mg
p. 128

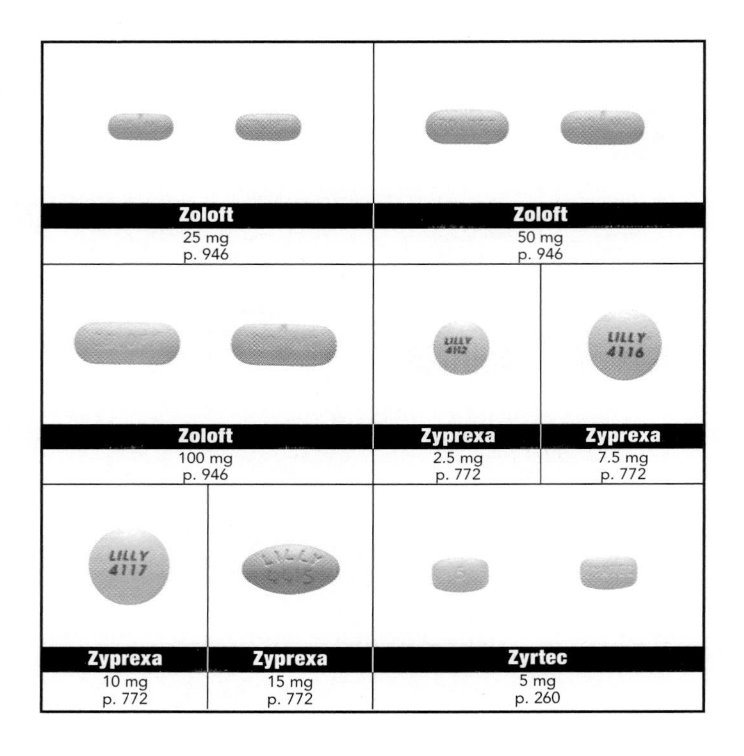

Zoloft
25 mg
p. 946
Zoloft
50 mg
p. 946
Zoloft
100 mg
p. 946
LILLY 4112
Zyprexa
2.5 mg
p. 772
LILLY 4116
Zyprexa
7.5 mg
p. 772
LILLY 4117
Zyprexa
10 mg
p. 772
Zyprexa
15 mg
p. 772
5
Zyrtec
5 mg
p. 260

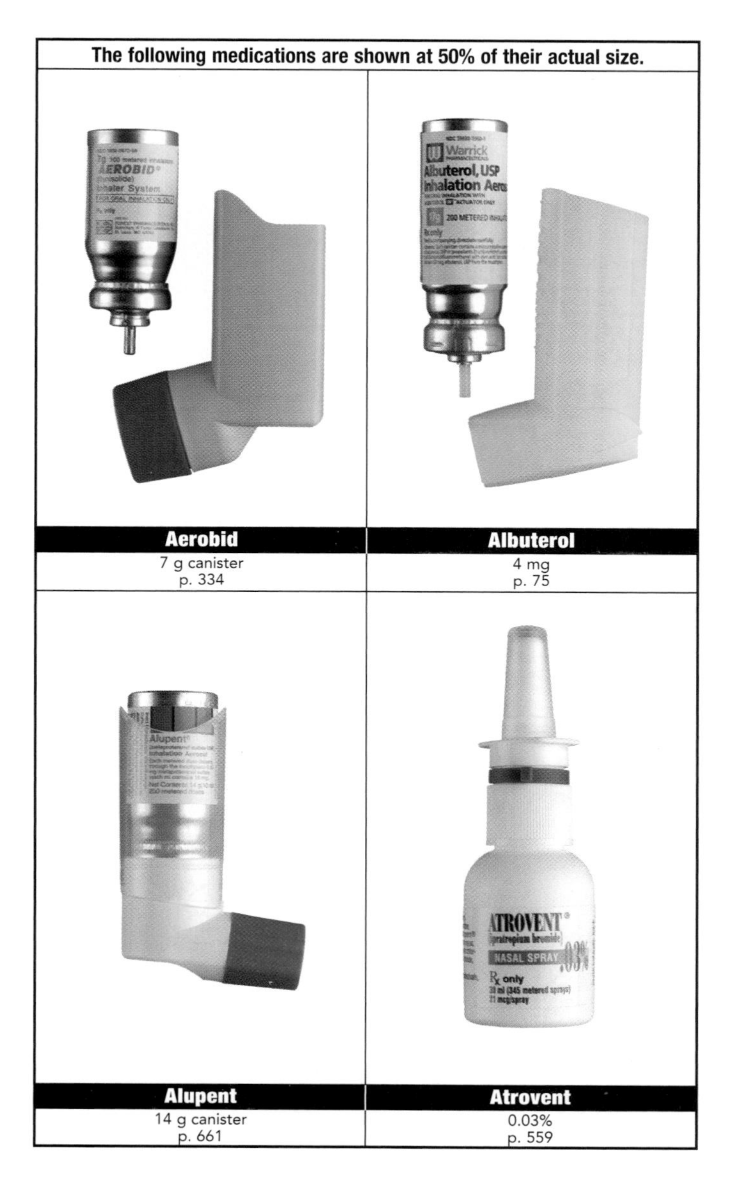

The following medications are shown at 50% of their actual size.

Aerobid	Albuterol
7 g canister p. 334	4 mg p. 75

Alupent	Atrovent
14 g canister p. 661	0.03% p. 559

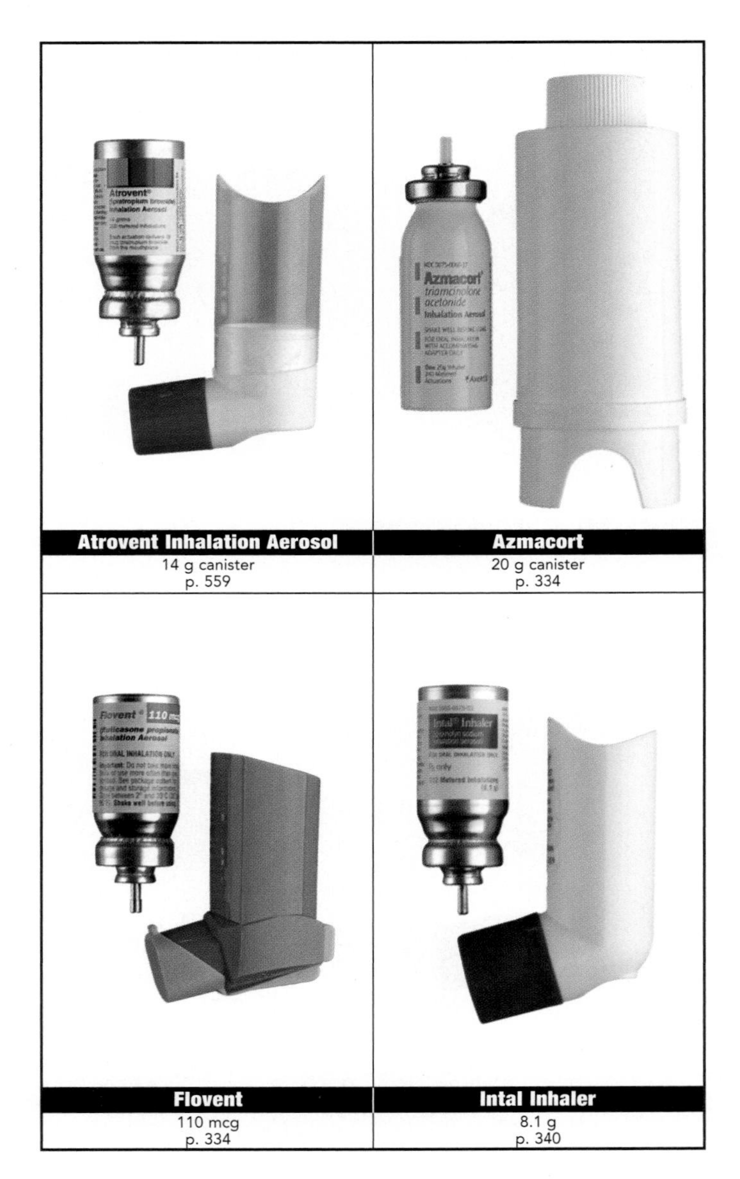

Atrovent Inhalation Aerosol
14 g canister
p. 559

Azmacort
20 g canister
p. 334

Flovent
110 mcg
p. 334

Intal Inhaler
8.1 g
p. 340

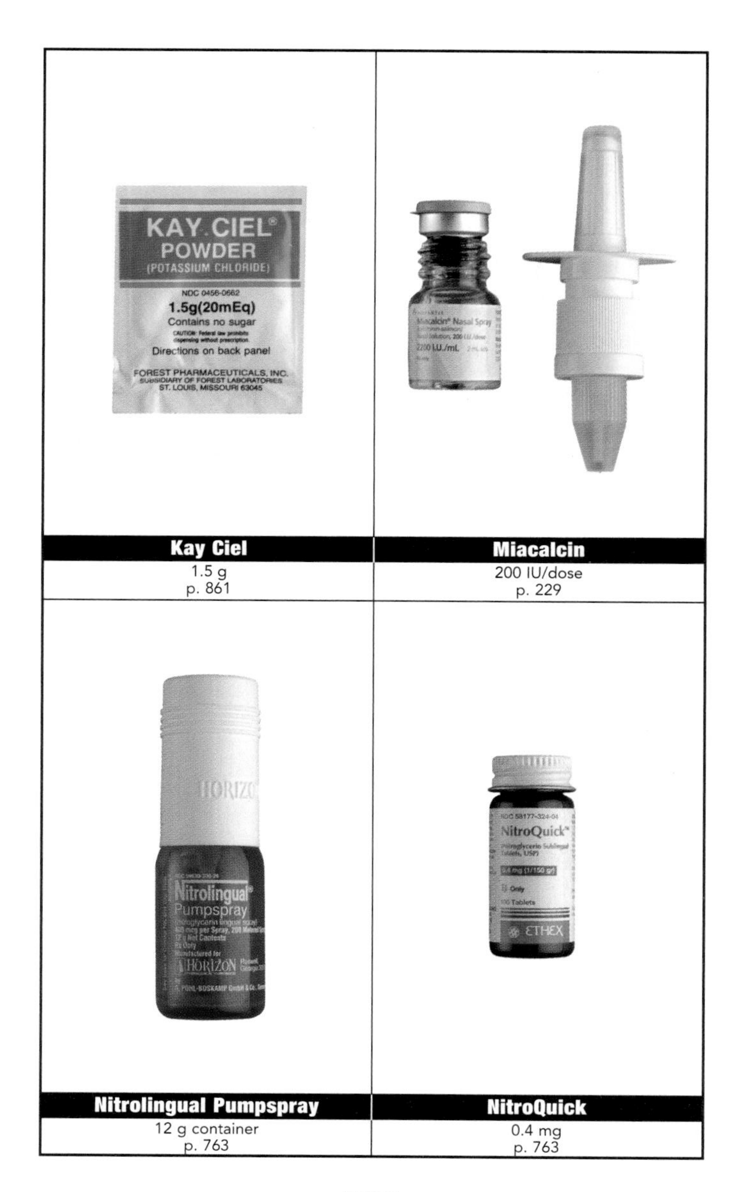

Kay Ciel
1.5 g
p. 861

Miacalcin
200 IU/dose
p. 229

Nitrolingual Pumpspray
12 g container
p. 763

NitroQuick
0.4 mg
p. 763

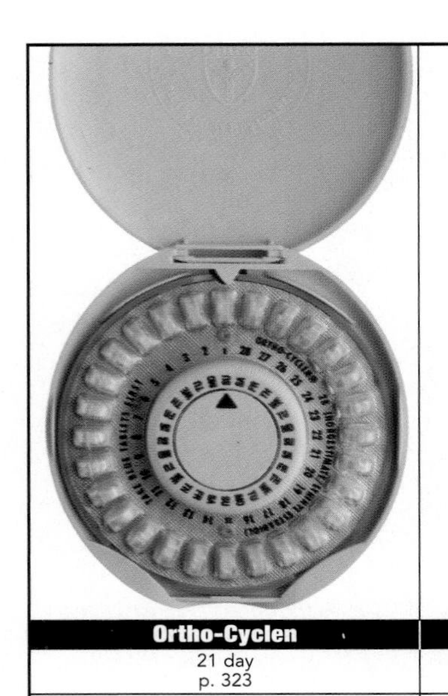

Ortho-Cyclen

21 day
p. 323

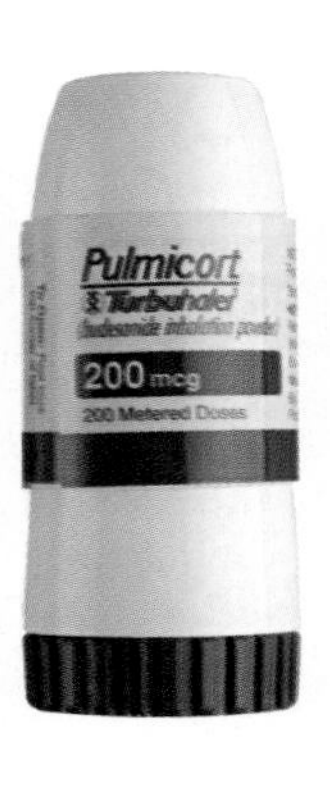

Pulmicort Turbuhaler

200 mcg
p. 334

Serevent

13 g canister
p. 940

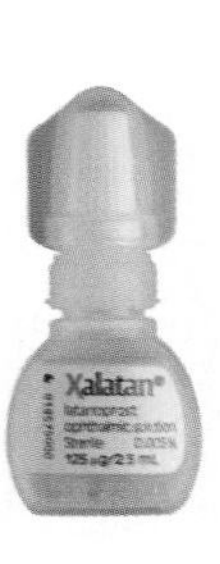

Xalatan

0.005%
p. 596

Itraconazole passes into breast milk. If you are breastfeeding, your health-care practitioner will likely advise you to switch to bottle feeding until your treatment is complete.

SPECIAL INFORMATION FOR SENIORS

Adverse reactions are more likely and are more severe in older adults.

GENERIC NAME

Ketoconazole

BRAND NAME

Nizoral
No generic available

ABOUT THIS DRUG

Ketoconazole is an antifungal medication used to treat serious fungal infections that affect the lungs and other parts of the body, especially the skin. Common skin infections include athlete's foot and jock itch.

This drug prevents fungal organisms from producing the essential elements they need to grow and reproduce.

SIDE EFFECTS

Be sure to tell your health-care practitioner if you experience any side effects while taking ketoconazole. Only your health-care practitioner can determine whether it is safe for you to continue taking this drug.

- *Less Common:* diarrhea, nausea, vomiting, dizziness, headache, flushed or red skin, constipation

IMPORTANT PRECAUTIONS

Tell your health-care practitioner if you are sensitive or allergic to ketoconazole or to any other drugs, especially antifungal medications.

Take ketoconazole for the entire treatment period, even if you feel better before the end of treatment. If you stop too early, the infection may return.

Sometimes treatment takes several months, which increases the risk of adverse effects. Prolonged use also may interfere with the body's steroid hormone functioning, which can lead to erectile dysfunction in men and cessation of menstruation in women.

Ketoconazole is not recommended for children younger than 2 years.

Ketoconazole may make your eyes more sensitive to sunlight. You may need to avoid exposure to bright light and to wear sunglasses.

Before taking ketoconazole, talk to your health-care practitioner if you have a history of alcohol abuse, liver or kidney disease, or a low amount of stomach acid.

DRUG INTERACTIONS

Tell your health-care practitioner and pharmacist if you are taking any prescription or nonprescription drugs, as well as any vitamins, herbs, or other supplements. Possible drug interactions include the following:

- Antacids (e.g, Maalox, Mylanta), anticholinergics (e.g., atropine, scopolamine), histamine H_2 blockers (e.g., cimetidine, ranitidine), omeprazole, and sucralfate should be taken at least 2 hours after taking ketoconazole.
- Astemizole and terfenadine may cause serious side effects involving the heart.
- Alcohol and medications that contain alcohol, such as cough syrups, elixirs, and tonics, should be avoided.
- Ketoconazole may increase the effects of benzodiazepines (e.g., alprazolam, diazepam), carbamazepine, cortisone-like drugs (e.g., cortisone, prednisone), cyclosporine, delavirdine, some calcium channel blockers (e.g., nifedipine, amlodipine), oral antidiabetic drugs (e.g., glyburide, glipizide), quinidine, ritonavir, sildenafil, tretinoin, warfarin, and trimexate.
- Ketoconazole may decrease the effects of amphotericin B, didanosine, and theophyllines.
- Phenytoin taken with ketoconazole may change the levels of both drugs.

FOOD, VITAMIN, AND HERBAL INTERACTIONS

St. John's wort may change the way ketoconazole is eliminated from the body, as well as cause sun sensitivity.

RECOMMENDED DOSAGE

Ketoconazole is available in tablets. The dosages given here are typical. However, your health-care practitioner will determine the most appropriate dose and schedule for you.

- *Children 2 Years to 12 Years:* 3.3 to 6.6 mg per 2.2 pounds of body weight once daily. Your health-care practitioner will determine the exact dosage.
- *Children 12 Years and Older and Adults:* 200 to 400 mg once daily.

Take ketoconazole with food or after eating to aid absorption and to help prevent stomach irritation.

If you miss a dose, take it as soon as you remember. If it is nearly time for your next dose, do not take the missed dose. Continue with your regular dosing schedule. Never take a double dose.

SYMPTOMS OF OVERDOSE AND WHAT TO DO
Symptoms of overdose include nausea, vomiting, and diarrhea. If an overdose occurs, seek immediate medical assistance and bring the prescription container with you to the hospital.

SPECIAL INFORMATION FOR PREGNANT OR NURSING WOMEN
No adequate studies of the effects of ketoconazole on pregnant or nursing women have been done. Animal studies have shown significant toxicity and birth defects. If you are pregnant or plan to become pregnant and this drug is crucial for your health, you and your health-care practitioner must weigh the potential benefits against the potential risks to the fetus.

Ketoconazole passes into breast milk. If you are breastfeeding, your health-care practitioner will likely advise you to stop until your treatment is complete.

SPECIAL INFORMATION FOR SENIORS
Adverse reactions are more likely and can be more severe in older adults. Ketoconazole requires an acidic environment in the stomach to be effective. Make sure you have not been diagnosed with achlorhydria (lack of stomach acid).

GENERIC NAME

Ketoprofen *see Propionic Acid (NSAID) Family, page 880*

GENERIC NAME

Ketorolac

BRAND NAME
Toradol
Generic available

ABOUT THIS DRUG

Ketorolac is a nonsteroidal anti-inflammatory drug (NSAID) prescribed to relieve moderately severe, acute pain. Typically it is taken for no longer than 5 days because it can cause serious side effects.

This drug interferes with the action of prostaglandins, naturally produced substances that cause inflammation and cause nerves to be more sensitive to pain signals.

SIDE EFFECTS

Be sure to tell your health-care practitioner if you experience any side effects while taking ketorolac. Only your health-care practitioner can determine whether it is safe for you to continue taking this drug.

- *Most Common:* stomach distress, diarrhea, dizziness, headache, drowsiness, nausea, fluid retention, ringing in the ears
- *Less Common:* abdominal fullness, constipation, gas, high blood pressure, inflammation of the mouth, itching, rash, sweating purple or red spots on the skin, vomiting, sensitivity to sunlight
- *Rare:* abnormal dreams, allergic reactions, asthma, belching, black stools, breathing problems, euphoria, fainting, fever, hallucinations, hearing problems, kidney inflammation or failure, loss of appetite, low blood pressure, nosebleeds, pallor, peptic ulcer, rapid heartbeat, skin inflammation, peeling, or flaking, swollen throat or tongue, thirst, dry mouth, tremors, urinary difficulties, vertigo, vision problems, jaundice

IMPORTANT PRECAUTIONS

Tell your health-care practitioner if you are sensitive or allergic to ketorolac, other NSAIDs, or any other drugs. Also tell your health-care practitioner if you have ever had an allergic reaction (e.g., swelling of the face, limbs, and throat, hives, wheezing, lightheadedness) after taking aspirin or other NSAIDs.

Avoid ketorolac if you have a history of peptic ulcer or gastrointestinal bleeding, or if you have severe kidney disease or bleeding problems.

This drug should not be taken for longer than 5 days because of a high risk of adverse reactions.

Ketorolac can cause water retention, which can be dangerous if you have heart disease or high blood pressure.

Before you take ketorolac, tell your health-care practitioner if you have a history of alcohol abuse, anemia, asthma, bleeding problems, epilepsy, gastrointestinal inflammation or ulcers, diabetes, heart, liver, or kidney disease, kidney stones, lupus, or Parkinson's disease.

DRUG INTERACTIONS

Tell your health-care practitioner and pharmacist if you are taking any prescription or nonprescription drugs, as well as any vitamins, herbs, or other supplements. Possible drug interactions include the following:

- Aspirin, NSAIDs (e.g., ibuprofen, naproxen), and probenecid should not be combined with ketorolac.
- Anticoagulants (e.g., warfarin) may prolong bleeding time.
- Ketorolac may increase the effects of cyclosporine, lithium, methotrexate, phenytoin, and zidovudine.
- Ketorolac may decrease the effects of angiotensin-converting enzyme (ACE) inhibitors (e.g., captopril, enalapril), bumetanide, and loop and thiazide diuretics (e.g., amiloride, furosemide).

FOOD, VITAMIN, AND HERBAL INTERACTIONS

Alfalfa, clove oil, cinchona bark, feverfew, garlic, ginseng, and ginkgo may change blood clotting; therefore do not take these herbs with ketorolac. Also avoid St. John's wort, because it can increase your sensitivity to sunlight.

RECOMMENDED DOSAGE

Ketorolac is available in tablets and by injection. The dosages given here are typical. However, your health-care practitioner will determine the most appropriate dose and schedule for you.

- *Children:* safety and effectiveness have not been established for children younger than age 3; for all others, dose to be determined by your health-care practitioner
- *Adults:* your health-care practitioner will give you your first dose by injection, then you will take tablets: 20 mg for your first oral dose, followed by 10 mg every 4 to 6 hours. Do not exceed 40 mg daily or take this drug for longer than 5 days.
- *Adults 65 and Older:* your health-care practitioner will determine your dose, which is typically lower than the normal adult dose.

Ketorolac works fastest when taken on an empty stomach, but it can be taken with food to help prevent stomach irritation.

If you miss a dose, take it as soon as you remember. If it is nearly time for your next dose, do not take the missed dose. Continue with your regular dosing schedule. Never take a double dose.

SYMPTOMS OF OVERDOSE AND WHAT TO DO

Symptoms of overdose include nausea, vomiting, severe headache, confusion, and seizures. If an overdose occurs, seek immediate medical attention and bring the prescription container with you to the hospital.

SPECIAL INFORMATION FOR PREGNANT OR NURSING WOMEN

No adequate studies of the effects of ketorolac on pregnant or nursing women have been done. If you are pregnant or plan to become pregnant, and ketorolac is crucial for your health, you and your health-care practitioner must weigh the potential benefits against the potential risks to the fetus.

Ketorolac passes into breast milk. If you are breastfeeding, your health-care practitioner will likely advise you to switch to bottle feeding until your treatment is complete.

SPECIAL INFORMATION FOR SENIORS

Doses are typically lower for older adults.

GENERIC NAME

Ketotifen

BRAND NAME

Zaditor

No generic available

ABOUT THIS DRUG

Ketotifen is a histamine (H_1) blocker prescribed for short-term treatment of itchy eyes associated with seasonal allergic conjunctivitis (inflamed mucous membranes that line the whites of the eyes and the inner surface of the eyelids).

This drug blocks the action of histamine, a substance produced by the body that causes itching, sneezing, swelling, hives, watery eyes, and other symptoms associated with an allergic reaction.

SIDE EFFECTS

Be sure to tell your health-care practitioner if you experience any side effects while using ketotifen. Only your health-care practitioner can determine whether it is safe for you to continue using this drug.

- *Most Common:* headache, runny nose
- *Less Common or Rare:* allergic reaction, blurred vision, eye irritation not present before treatment, eye tearing or discharge, dry eyes or

nose, drowsiness, feeling of heat in the eye or body, nausea, stomach discomfort, eye pain, sensitivity to light, dizziness, rash

IMPORTANT PRECAUTIONS

Tell your health-care practitioner if you are sensitive or allergic to ketotifen or to any other drugs.

Before you use ketotifen, tell your health-care practitioner if you wear soft contact lenses.

To avoid contamination, do not allow the tip of the dropper to touch your eye or any other surface.

Make sure you know how you react to this medication before you drive or operate any dangerous equipment.

DRUG INTERACTIONS

Tell your health-care practitioner and pharmacist if you are taking any prescription or nonprescription drugs, as well as any vitamins, herbs, or other supplements. No significant drug interactions have been noted.

FOOD, VITAMIN, AND HERBAL INTERACTIONS

No food, vitamin, or herbal interactions have been noted.

RECOMMENDED DOSAGE

Ketotifen is available as an ophthalmic solution. The dosages given here are typical. However, your health-care practitioner will determine the most appropriate dose and schedule for you.

- *Children Up to 3 Years:* not recommended
- *Children 3 Years and Older and Adults:* 1 drop in the affected eye every 8 to 12 hours

If you miss a dose, take it as soon as you remember. If it is nearly time for your next dose, do not take the missed dose. Continue with your regular dosing schedule. Never take a double dose.

SYMPTOMS OF OVERDOSE AND WHAT TO DO

No specific symptoms of overdose have been reported. If someone accidentally ingests the solution, seek immediate medical attention and bring the prescription container with you to the hospital.

SPECIAL INFORMATION FOR PREGNANT OR NURSING WOMEN

No adequate studies of the effects of ketotifen on pregnant or nursing women have been done. If you are pregnant or plan to become pregnant and ketotifen is crucial for your health, you and your health-care practitioner must weigh the potential benefits against the potential risks to the fetus.

Ketotifen may pass into breast milk. If you are breastfeeding, your health-care practitioner may advise you to stop until treatment is done.

SPECIAL INFORMATION FOR SENIORS

No special precautions are noted for older adults.

GENERIC NAME

Labetalol

BRAND NAMES

Normodyne, Trandate
Generic available

ABOUT THIS DRUG

Labetalol is a beta-adrenergic blocking agent (beta-blocker) prescribed to treat mild-to-moderate high blood pressure (hypertension) and pregnancy-related high blood pressure. It is also used to limit the damage caused by heart attacks, and to reduce the risk of repeat heart attacks. This drug is sometimes combined with other high blood pressure medications, such as thiazide diuretics.

Labetalol works by interfering with alpha- and beta-adrenergic nerve impulses. This combination action reduces blood pressure. An advantage of labetalol over other beta-blockers is that it rarely affects your heart rate.

SIDE EFFECTS

Speak to your health-care practitioner if you develop side effects while taking this drug. Only he or she can determine whether it is safe for you to continue taking labetalol.

- *Common:* scalp tingling, dizziness, lightheadedness, fainting, nausea, upset stomach, indigestion, vomiting, diarrhea, cramps, sweating, fatigue, urinary difficulties, impotence, muscle weakness, blurred vision, dry eyes, rash, hair loss, bronchial spasm, stuffy nose
- *Less Common or Rare:* disorientation, confusion, anxiety, depression, short-term memory loss, insomnia, vivid dreams, hallucinations, excessive tiredness or weakness, slow heartbeat, constipation, cold hands and feet, breathing difficulties, fever with sore throat, heart failure

IMPORTANT PRECAUTIONS

Always inform your health-care practitioner about any other medical conditions you suffer from, especially a slow heart rate or serious heart block, congestive heart failure, angina, asthma or other lung ailments, liver or kidney problems, diabetes or hypoglycemia, or a thyroid condition. Tell your health-care practitioner if you have ever experienced an allergic reaction to labetalol or other beta-blockers.

Before having any type of surgery or dental procedure, inform your surgeon or dentist that you are taking labetalol.

This drug may make you more sensitive to the cold. Beta-blockers including labetalol can decrease blood circulation in the fingers, toes, and skin. Be sure to dress warmly in low temperatures, especially if you already have blood circulation problems.

This drug may make you drowsy. Until you know how labetalol affects you, do not drive a car, operate machinery, or perform other tasks that demand concentration.

When you first start taking this drug or when the dosage is increased, you may experience dizziness or faintness when you rise quickly from a sitting or reclining position (postural hypotension). Try to get up slowly, and consult your health-care practitioner if the problem continues.

Treatment of high blood pressure also entails certain lifestyle changes, such as weight control, smoking cessation, and close attention to diet.

Be extremely careful when you exercise in hot weather. Heavy sweating can lead to dizziness, lightheadedness, fainting, vomiting, dehydration, and low blood pressure.

DRUG INTERACTIONS

Tell your health-care practitioner and pharmacist if you are taking any other prescription or over-the-counter drugs, as well as any vitamins, herbs, or other supplements. Possible drug interactions include the following:

- Drugs that contain aspirin can lessen the blood pressure lowering effects of labetalol.
- Taking other blood pressure medications (including clonidine, reserpine, and calcium channel blockers) can increase the effects of labetalol.
- Medications such as cimetidine may increase the effects of labetalol.
- Labetalol can interfere with the action of oral antidiabetes medications. It may also change blood glucose levels.

- Labetalol may interfere with the effectiveness of certain asthma medications, including aminophylline, epinephrine, isoproterenol, and theophylline.
- Labetalol can increase the effect of antianxiety benzodiazepine drugs.
- If you are also taking ergot alkaloids for migraines, labetalol may worsen side effects such as cold hands and feet. In rare cases, this drug combination can lead to gangrene.
- Monoamine oxidase inhibitor (MAOI) antidepressants should not be taken at the same time or within 14 days of labetalol.
- Labetalol may interact with anesthetics during surgery, increasing the risk of heart problems. As a result, your health-care practitioner will instruct you how to stop taking this drug two days before surgery.
- Alcohol intensifies the drowsiness caused by this drug.
- Cocaine and cigarette smoking may reduce the effectiveness of labetalol.
- Ask your health-care practitioner about taking over-the-counter cough, cold, allergy, and weight loss remedies. Many of these can raise blood pressure.

FOOD, VITAMIN, AND HERBAL INTERACTIONS

Do not take herbs that increase blood pressure, including ephedra (ma huang), ginseng, goldenseal, licorice, and saw palmetto. Consult your health-care practitioner before taking substances that may lower blood pressure, such as calcium, soy, or garlic. Your health-care practitioner will probably recommend a low-sodium diet.

RECOMMENDED DOSAGE

Labetalol is available in oral form as tablets. Although the doses given below are typical, only your health-care practitioner can determine the dose and schedule that are most appropriate for you.

- *Children:* This drug is not recommended for children under the age of 12.
- *Adults:* 100 to 400 mg 2 times a day

If labetalol upsets your stomach, take it with food. If you forget to take a dose, take it as soon as you remember. If it is almost time for the next dose, skip the forgotten one, and resume your normal schedule. Never take double doses.

Continue to take this drug even if you feel well. Do not discontinue use without consulting your health-care practitioner. Abrupt withdrawal can cause chest pain, breathing difficulties, increased sweating, irregular heartbeat, and even heart attack in some people. To end treatment, in most cases your health-care practitioner will reduce dosage gradually over a 2-week period.

SYMPTOMS OF OVERDOSE AND WHAT TO DO

The symptoms of labetalol overdose include slow heart rate, low blood pressure, dizziness, fainting, difficulty breathing, bluish fingernails and palms, and seizures. If overdose occurs, seek immediate medical attention and take the bottle of labetalol to the hospital with you.

SPECIAL INFORMATION FOR PREGNANT OR NURSING WOMEN

Some studies have shown that women who take beta-blockers during pregnancy give birth to babies with lower birth weight, heart rate, and blood pressure. As a result, labetalol should be avoided if you are pregnant.

Small amounts of labetalol can pass into breast milk and cause problems such as slow heart rate, low blood pressure, and trouble breathing. If you must take labetalol, your health-care practitioner may recommend bottle-feeding.

SPECIAL INFORMATION FOR SENIORS

Seniors usually require lower doses of labetalol. Older people are more apt to experience side effects such as heightened sensitivity to the cold, a general feeling of unwellness, chest pain, breathing difficulties, sweating, and variations in heartbeat.

GENERIC NAME

Lamivudine

BRAND NAMES

Epivir, Epivir-HBV

No generic available

ABOUT THIS DRUG

Lamivudine is an antiviral drug prescribed to treat HIV, the human immunodeficiency virus that causes acquired immune deficiency syndrome (AIDS). It is used in combination with zidovudine (AZT) and other antiretroviral drugs. Lower doses are used to treat hepatitis B (HBV) infection.

Lamivudine is known as a transcriptase inhibitor. This drug interferes with the reproduction of HIV and HBV, which slows the progression of these viruses.

SIDE EFFECTS

Contact your health-care practitioner if you develop side effects while taking this drug. Only he or she can determine if you should continue to take lamivudine.

➤ *Common:* an overall feeling of unwellness, abdominal discomfort, nausea, appetite loss, feeling of fullness, vomiting, headache, stuffy or runny nose, canker sores, tingling, pins and needles, numbness, and burning in the extremities

➤ *Less Common or Rare:* diarrhea, fever, chills, cough, dizziness, sore throat, muscle pain and cramps, shallow breathing, shortness of breath, hair loss, rash, unusual fatigue, trouble sleeping, pancreas irritation

IMPORTANT PRECAUTIONS

Tell your health-care practitioner about any other medical conditions you suffer from, such as nerve damage or kidney disease. Nerve damage may develop or worsen when taking lamivudine. If you have kidney disease, your health-care practitioner will prescribe a lower dosage.

Children with advanced AIDS may be more susceptible to pancreatitis (inflammation of the pancreas) when taking this drug. Call your health-care practitioner immediately if your child develops symptoms such as severe abdominal pain, tense abdominal muscles, fever, sweating, shallow breathing, nausea, and vomiting.

If your health-care practitioner recommends lamivudine for hepatitis B and you do not know your HIV status, get tested. Health-care practitioners prescribe a lower dosage for HBV, and if you later learn that you are HIV-positive, the lower dosage may be less effective in slowing the progression of HIV.

Lamivudine does not cure AIDS or HBV, nor does it prevent you from passing on these infectious viruses to others. Therefore it is important to always practice safe sex while taking this drug.

DRUG INTERACTIONS

Tell your health-care practitioner and pharmacist if you are taking any other prescription or over-the-counter drugs, as well as any vitamins, herbs, or other supplements. Possible drug interactions include the following:

- Lamivudine increases the absorption of AZT, making it more effective.
- Nelfinavir may increase the level of lamivudine.
- The combination of sulfamethoxazole and trimethoprim (Bactrim or Septra) increases the absorption of lamivudine.

FOOD, VITAMIN, AND HERBAL INTERACTIONS

Consult your health-care practitioner if you want to use the herb milk thistle (an antioxidant and liver tonic) along with lamivudine in the treatment of hepatitis B.

RECOMMENDED DOSAGE

Oral dosage forms of lamivudine include solution and tablets. Although the doses given below are typical, only your health-care practitioner can determine the dose and schedule that are most appropriate for you. Dosage is reduced for people who weigh less than 110 pounds.

HIV and AIDS

- *Children 3 Months to 12 Years:* 2 mg per pound of body weight twice a day; the maximum is 150 mg per dose
- *Children Older than 12 and Adults:* 150 mg twice a day

Hepatitis B

- *Children 16 Years and Younger:* Dosage must be determined by your health-care practitioner.
- *Adults:* 100 mg once a day

Lamivudine can be taken with or without food. It is absorbed more slowly with food. It is essential to take lamivudine exactly as prescribed. If you miss a dose, take it as soon as you remember. However, if it is nearly time for your next scheduled dose, do not take the missed dose. Follow your regular dosing schedule. Never take a double dose. Call your health-care practitioner if you forget 2 doses in a row.

SYMPTOMS OF OVERDOSE AND WHAT TO DO

No specific information on overdosing with lamivudine is available. However, symptoms that may occur include nausea, vomiting, diarrhea, and bone marrow depression. If overdose does occur, seek medical attention immediately, and bring the prescription bottle with you to the hospital so that health-care practitioners will know exactly what drug was used.

SPECIAL INFORMATION FOR PREGNANT OR NURSING WOMEN

Lamivudine is known to cross the placenta, and high doses have caused birth defects in animals. Do not use this drug unless the benefits of therapy clearly outweigh the potential risks to the fetus.

Lamivudine may pass into breast milk, and HIV and HBV can be transferred by breast milk. Bottle-feeding is preferable.

SPECIAL INFORMATION FOR SENIORS

Smaller doses of lamivudine are usually appropriate for seniors, due to their lower levels of kidney function.

GENERIC NAME

Lamotrigine

BRAND NAME

Lamictal

No generic available

ABOUT THIS DRUG

Lamotrigine is an anticonvulsant prescribed to treat adult epilepsy. It is used to control absence, myoclonic, partial, and tonic-clonic seizures. In some cases, lamotrigine is prescribed for children who fail to respond to other treatments. This drug is taken in combination with other antiepileptic medications. It has also been approved for treatment of bipolar disorder.

Lamotrigine works by blocking voltage-dependent sodium channels in the brain. This prevents the release of chemicals such as glutamate and aspartate transmitters, which decreases the likelihood of seizures.

SIDE EFFECTS

Consult your health-care practitioner if you develop side effects while taking this drug. Only he or she can determine whether it is safe for you to continue taking lamotrigine.

- *Common:* dizziness, drowsiness, headache, nausea, vomiting, rash, clumsiness, uncoordinated movements, vision changes such as blurred or double vision, weight gain

- *Less Common or Rare:* anxiety, confusion, depression, irritability, memory loss, poor concentration, sleep disorders, heart palpitations, tremors, constipation, diarrhea, dry mouth, sore throat, fever, ear pain, cough, chills, muscle weakness or spasm, ringing in the ears, vaginal inflammation, hot flashes, painful menstruation, absence of periods

If you develop a rash, swollen lymph nodes, and fever while taking lamotrigine, call your health-care practitioner immediately. Rashes associated with this drug can be life-threatening, particularly in children. The risk of this reaction is greatest in the first 2 to 8 weeks that you take lamotrigine. A slight risk remains for 6 months after initiation of therapy.

IMPORTANT PRECAUTIONS

Inform your health-care practitioner about any other medical conditions you suffer from. Lamotrigine must be used with caution if you have heart problems or liver or kidney disease.

Because lamotrigine may cause side effects such as dizziness, clumsiness, and blurred vision, do not drive a car, operate machinery, or perform other tasks that require concentration until you know how this drug affects you.

Lamotrigine may cause unusual sensitivity to the sun. Wear protective clothing and apply sunscreen when using this drug.

DRUG INTERACTIONS

Tell your health-care practitioner and pharmacist if you are taking any other prescription or over-the-counter drugs, as well as any vitamins, herbs, or other supplements. Possible drug interactions include the following:

- Lamotrigine is often prescribed in combination with other medications for epilepsy, including carbamazepine, phenobarbital, phenytoin, primidone, and valproic acid. Your health-care practitioner will make dosage adjustments as required.
- Regular use of acetaminophen may decrease blood levels of lamotrigine and increase the risk of seizures. However, occasional use of acetaminophen is not a problem.
- Lamotrigine may inhibit the action of sulfa drugs such Bactrim or Septra.
- Ritonavir may decrease lamotrigine levels and lead to seizures.
- Sertraline may increase the concentration of lamotrigine to toxic levels.

- Lamotrigine may increase the effects of alcohol and other central nervous system depressants (such as tranquilizers, sedatives, sleeping pills, barbiturates, narcotics, muscle relaxants, antihistamines, and anesthetics). Check with your health-care practitioner before using any of these substances in combination with lamotrigine.

FOOD, VITAMIN, AND HERBAL INTERACTIONS

Combining the herbs kola or St. John's wort with this drug may cause nervousness.

RECOMMENDED DOSAGE

Oral dosage forms of lamotrigine include tablets and chewable tablets. Although the doses given below are typical, only your health-care practitioner can determine the dose and schedule that are most appropriate for you. The dosage will be adjusted according to what other epilepsy medications are prescribed in combination with lamotrigine, and how effectively seizures are controlled.

- *Children:* This drug is not recommended for children under the age of 16.
- *Adults:* 25 to 50 mg to start, which may be gradually increased as needed to a maximum daily dosage of 500 mg, divided into 2 equal doses

Lamotrigine can be taken with or without food. It is essential to take this drug exactly as prescribed. If you miss a dose, take it as soon as you remember. However, if it is nearly time for your next scheduled dose, do not take the missed dose. Follow your regular dosing schedule. Never take a double dose. Do not stop taking this drug suddenly, as seizures may occur.

SYMPTOMS OF OVERDOSE AND WHAT TO DO

No specific information on overdosing with lamotrigine is available. However, symptoms that may occur include dizziness, headache, changes in muscle reflexes, and coma. If overdose does occur, seek medical attention immediately, and bring the prescription bottle with you to the hospital so that health-care practitioners will know exactly what drug was used.

SPECIAL INFORMATION FOR PREGNANT OR NURSING WOMEN

Lamotrigine is known to cross the placenta, and high doses have caused birth defects in animals. Do not use this drug unless the benefits of therapy clearly outweigh the potential risks to the fetus. If you do take lamotrigine while pregnant, your health-care practitioner will probably recommend folic acid supplements. Because lamotrigine may pass into breast milk, bottle-feeding is preferable.

SPECIAL INFORMATION FOR SENIORS

Smaller doses of lamotrigine are usually recommended for seniors.

GENERIC NAME

Lansoprazole

BRAND NAMES

Prevacid, Prevpac
No generic available

ABOUT THIS DRUG

Lansoprazole is used to treat conditions in which there is too much acid in the stomach. It is prescribed for duodenal and gastric ulcers, erosive esophagitis, gastroesophageal reflux disease (GERD), and other excess acid conditions (such as Zollinger-Ellison syndrome, mastocytosis, and endocrine adenoma). In some cases, lansoprazole is used in combination with antibiotics to treat ulcers associated with *H. pylori* bacteria.

This drug is one of the most powerful medications for reducing acid levels in the stomach. It works by blocking the stomach's ability to produce acid.

SIDE EFFECTS

Contact your health-care practitioner if you experience side effects while taking lansoprazole. Only he or she can determine whether or not you should continue to take this drug.

- *Common:* diarrhea, rash, itching
- *Less Common or Rare:* abdominal or stomach pain, changes in appetite, joint or muscle pain, cold or flu-like symptoms, nausea, vomiting, headache, dizziness, fatigue, anxiety, depression, constipation, cough, ringing in the ears, unusual bleeding or bruising, mouth inflammation, black tongue

IMPORTANT PRECAUTIONS

This drug should be taken with caution if you suffer from liver problems. Tell your health-care practitioner if you have ever experienced an allergic reaction to this or similar medications.

Lansoprazole may cause drowsiness, so limit activities such as driving as necessary.

DRUG INTERACTIONS

Inform your health-care practitioner and pharmacist if you are taking any other prescription or over-the-counter drugs, as well as any vitamins, herbs, or other supplements. Possible drug interactions include the following:

- Antacids may reduce the effects of lansoprazole.
- Ritonavir may change levels of lansoprazole in the blood.
- Sucralfate may decrease the absorption and effects of lansoprazole.
- Lansoprazole may decrease the effects of itraconazole, ketoconazole, and theophylline.
- If lansoprazole is taken with an antibiotic, also be certain to refer to the drugs that interact with that particular antibiotic.
- Do not smoke cigarettes. This can worsen acid secretion.

FOOD, VITAMIN, AND HERBAL INTERACTIONS

Lansoprazole may interfere with the absorption of iron, zinc, and B vitamins such as folate. Taking a daily multivitamin-multimineral supplement is recommended. Do not use the herb St. John's wort while taking lansoprazole.

RECOMMENDED DOSAGE

Lansoprazole is available in capsule form. Although the doses given below are typical, only your health-care practitioner can determine the dose and schedule that are most appropriate for you.

Gastroesophageal Reflux Disease (GERD)

- *Children:* This drug is not recommended for children.
- *Adults:* 15 to 30 mg once a day for up to 8 weeks

Duodenal Ulcers

- *Children:* This drug is not recommended for children.
- *Adults:* 15 to 30 mg once a day for 4 weeks

Prevention of Duodenal Ulcer Relapse

- *Children:* This drug is not recommended for children.
- *Adults:* 15 mg once a day

Duodenal Ulcers Associated with *H. pylori* Bacteria

- ➤ *Children:* This drug is not recommended for children.
- ➤ *Adults:* 30 mg lansoprazole, 1,000 mg amoxicillin, and 500 mg clarithromycin twice daily for 7 to 14 days

Gastric Ulcers

- ➤ *Children:* This drug is not recommended for children.
- ➤ *Adults:* 15 mg once a day for up to 8 weeks

Erosive Esophagitis

- ➤ *Children:* This drug is not recommended for children.
- ➤ *Adults:* 30 mg once a day for up to 8 weeks

Other Excess Acid Conditions

- ➤ *Children:* This drug is not recommended for children.
- ➤ *Adults:* 60 to 180 mg a day, with daily doses larger than 120 mg divided into 2 doses

Lansoprazole should be taken on an empty stomach, preferably in the morning. If you cannot swallow the capsule whole, open it and sprinkle the grains on a spoonful of applesauce. However, do not crush or chew the grains.

If you miss a dose, take it as soon as you remember. However, if it is nearly time for your next scheduled dose, do not take the missed dose. Follow your regular dosing schedule. Never take a double dose.

SYMPTOMS OF OVERDOSE AND WHAT TO DO

Possible symptoms of overdose include nausea, vomiting, abdominal pain, dizziness, and lethargy. If you suspect an overdose, seek immediate medical attention, and bring the prescription bottle to the hospital with you.

SPECIAL INFORMATION FOR PREGNANT OR NURSING WOMEN

No studies have adequately investigated the effects of lansoprazole during pregnancy or breastfeeding. If you are pregnant or plan to become pregnant, or if you are breastfeeding or plan to do so, talk with your health-care practitioner before starting this drug. Only a

health-care practitioner can determine whether the potential benefits outweigh the potential dangers.

SPECIAL INFORMATION FOR SENIORS

No special instructions are provided for seniors.

GENERIC NAME

Latanoprost

BRAND NAME

Xalatan
No generic available

ABOUT THIS DRUG

Latanoprost ophthalmic eye solution is used to treat open-angle glaucoma and ocular hypertension (high blood pressure within the eye). This drug lowers pressure in the eye by increasing the outflow of eye fluid.

SIDE EFFECTS

Consult your health-care practitioner if you experience side effects while using latanoprost. Only he or she can determine whether or not you should continue to use this drug.

- *Common:* blurred vision, eye burning and irritation, stinging, tearing, bloodshot eyes, itchy eyes or eyelids, foreign body sensation, darkening of eyelid skin color, increased pigmentation of the iris, lengthening and darkening of eyelashes, inflammatory disease of the cornea, upper respiratory infection
- *Less Common or Rare:* eyelid crusting, eye discomfort or pain, dry eye, eye swelling, excessive tearing, redness of eye or inside of eyelid, eyelid crusting or swelling, double vision, pinkeye, eye discharge, allergic reactions, back pain, chest pain, muscle or joint pain, cough, difficulty breathing, wheezing, rash

IMPORTANT PRECAUTIONS

Before using this drug, tell your health-care practitioner if you wear contact lenses; have had an eye infection in the last 3 months; or have sudden (acute) angle closure of the eye.

Latanoprost may cause blurred vision. Until you know how this medication affects you, do not drive a car, operate machinery, or perform other tasks that demand concentration.

DRUG INTERACTIONS

Tell your health-care practitioner and pharmacist if you are taking any other prescription or over-the-counter drugs, as well as any vitamins, herbs, or other supplements. Possible interactions may include the following:

- ➤ Taking latanoprost with eye drops that contain thiomersal may cause solid substances to form in the eye. To avoid this effect, use the drops at least 5 minutes apart.

FOOD, VITAMIN, AND HERBAL INTERACTIONS

Do not take the herb scopolia root, which has glaucoma as a possible side effect.

RECOMMENDED DOSAGE

Latanoprost comes as an eyedrop solution. Although the dosage below is typical, consult your health-care practitioner for exact instructions.

- ➤ *Children:* This drug is not recommended for children.
- ➤ *Adults:* Apply 1 drop of latanoprost daily in the evening.

Remove contact lenses before using latanoprost, and do not reinsert them for at least 15 minutes. Be careful not to touch the dropper to the eye. To limit absorption into the body, press your finger to the inner corner of the eye during and for one minute after administration.

If you miss a dose of latanoprost, administer it as soon as you remember. However, if it is nearly time for your next scheduled dose, do not administer the missed dose. Follow your regular dosing schedule. Never use a double dose.

SYMPTOMS OF OVERDOSE AND WHAT TO DO

Symptoms of overdose may include bloodshot eyes and eye irritation, which can progress to abdominal pain, nausea, sweating, flushing, dizziness, and fatigue. Seek immediate medical attention, and bring the prescription bottle to the hospital with you.

SPECIAL INFORMATION FOR PREGNANT OR NURSING WOMEN

No studies have adequately investigated the effects of latanoprost during pregnancy or breastfeeding. If you are pregnant or plan to become pregnant, or if you are breastfeeding or plan to do so, talk with your health-care practitioner before starting this drug. Only a

health-care practitioner can determine whether the potential benefits outweigh the potential dangers.

SPECIAL INFORMATION FOR SENIORS

No special instructions are provided for seniors.

GENERIC NAME

Leflunomide

BRAND NAME

Arava
No generic available

ABOUT THIS DRUG

Leflunomide is prescribed for the treatment of rheumatoid arthritis in adults. It relieves symptoms such as inflammation, swelling, stiffness, and pain. Leflunomide works by stopping the immune system from producing too many of the immune cells that are responsible for inflammation.

SIDE EFFECTS

Speak to your health-care practitioner if you develop side effects while taking this drug. Only he or she can determine whether it is safe for you to continue taking leflunomide.

- *Common:* diarrhea, nausea, appetite loss, abdominal or stomach pain, stomach upset, indigestion, rash, high blood pressure, respiratory infection, difficulty breathing, sore throat, fever, headache, weakness, back pain, urinary infection, abnormal liver function
- *Less Common or Rare:* anxiety, constipation, chest pain, fast or pounding heartbeat, dizziness, tingling in the hands and feet, dry mouth, mouth ulcer, dry skin, eczema, itching, hair loss, unexplained weight loss, vomiting, bloody or cloudy urine, joint or muscle pain, severe stomach pain, tender stomach, shortness of breath, unusual tiredness or weakness, immune suppression, liver toxicity

IMPORTANT PRECAUTIONS

Do not take leflunomide if you are or plan to become pregnant. This drug may cause birth defects. Men who take this drug should wear condoms, and when possible stop taking it when they plan to start a family.

Inform your health-care practitioner about any other medical conditions you suffer from. Leflunomide must be used with caution if you have liver or kidney disease, an immune system disease, or a severe infection. Leflunomide suppresses the immune system, and may decrease the body's ability to combat infection.

Because leflunomide may cause blurred vision, do not drive a car, operate machinery, or perform other tasks that require concentration until you know how this drug affects you.

DRUG INTERACTIONS

Inform your health-care practitioner and pharmacist if you are taking any other prescription or over-the-counter drugs, as well as any vitamins, herbs, or other supplements. Possible drug interactions include the following:

- Charcoal and cholestyramine reduce leflunomide blood levels. When you stop taking leflunomide, cholestyramine is usually prescribed to help your body eliminate this drug from your body.
- Rifampin increases the effects of leflunomide.
- Leflunomide increases the blood levels of tolbutamide and NSAIDs.
- Leflunomide may increase the liver toxicity of drugs (such as methotrexate) that are toxic to the liver.
- Do not drink alcohol while taking leflunomide. This increases the risk of liver problems.
- Do not have any immunizations without your health-care practitioner's approval.

FOOD, VITAMIN, AND HERBAL INTERACTIONS

Do not use the herb echinacea while taking leflunomide.

RECOMMENDED DOSAGE

Leflunomide comes in tablet form. Although the doses given below are typical, only your health-care practitioner can determine the dose and schedule that are most appropriate for you.

- *Children:* This drug is not recommended for children.
- *Adults:* Recommended starting dose is one 100-mg tablet daily for 3 days. This will be reduced to 20 mg daily, or to 10 mg daily if side effects are troublesome.

Leflunomide can be taken with or without food. It is essential to take this drug exactly as prescribed, especially during the first days of therapy. If you miss a dose, take it as soon as you remember. However, if it is nearly time for your next scheduled dose, do not take the missed dose. Follow your regular dosing schedule. Never take a double dose.

SYMPTOMS OF OVERDOSE AND WHAT TO DO
No specific information on overdosing with leflunomide is available. However, if you experience severe side effects, you may have taken too much medication. Seek immediate medical attention, and bring the prescription bottle with you to the hospital so that health-care practitioners will know exactly what drug was taken.

SPECIAL INFORMATION FOR PREGNANT OR NURSING WOMEN
Do not take leflunomide during pregnancy. This drug may cause birth defects. It is not known whether leflunomide passes into breast milk. However, because of possible unwanted effects to nursing infants, breastfeeding is not recommended while you take this drug.

SPECIAL INFORMATION FOR SENIORS
No special instructions are provided for seniors.

GENERIC NAME

Letrozole *see Anastrozole, page 121*

GENERIC NAME

Class: Leukotriene antagonist/inhibitors

Generics: (1) montelukast; (2) zafirlukast; (3) zileuton

BRAND NAMES
(1) Singulair; (2) Accolate; (3) Zyflo Filmtab
No generic available

ABOUT THIS DRUG
Leukotriene antagonists and inhibitors are prescribed to treat asthma. Montelukast is also used to prevent exercise-induced asthma. However, these medications are not used to treat sudden asthma attacks.

Leukotrienes are substances involved in the body's allergic responses. Zafirlukast and montelukast work by blocking leukotrienes from binding to receptors in the body. Zileuton inhibits the formation of leukotrienes.

SIDE EFFECTS
Consult your health-care practitioner if you develop side effects while taking one of these drugs. Only he or she can determine

whether it is safe for you to continue taking a leukotriene antagonist or inhibitor.

Montelukast

- *Common:* headache
- *Less Common or Rare:* abdominal or stomach pain, cough, dental pain, dizziness, fatigue, fever, heartburn, rash, stuffy nose, weakness

Zafirlukast

- *Common:* headache
- *Less Common or Rare:* nausea, diarrhea, infections, stomach upset, abdominal pain, vomiting, dizziness, muscle aches, back pain, overall pain, weakness, liver inflammation

Zileuton

- *Common:* headache, pain, upset stomach, nausea, liver inflammation
- *Less Common or Rare:* abdominal pain, weakness, flu-like symptoms, itching, unusual tiredness or weakness, yellow eyes or skin, muscle or joint pain, chest pain, dizziness, vomiting, fever, gas, constipation, insomnia, swollen lymph glands, neck pain, general feeling of unwellness, urinary infections, vaginal inflammation

IMPORTANT PRECAUTIONS

Always tell your health-care practitioner about any other medical conditions you suffer from. If you have elevated liver enzymes or liver disease, this group of drugs may not be appropriate for you. Zileuton should not be taken if you have active liver disease. Use these drugs with caution if you have impaired kidney function or if you are a heavy drinker.

Side effects of leukotriene antagonist/inhibitors may include dizziness and confusion. Do not drive a car, operate machinery, or perform other tasks that require concentration until you know how the drug you are taking affects you.

DRUG INTERACTIONS

Tell your health-care practitioner and pharmacist if you are taking any other prescription or over-the-counter drugs, as well as any vitamins, herbs, or other supplements. If your need for other asthma medication increases while taking one of these drugs, inform your health-care practitioner at once. Possible drug interactions include the following:

Montelukast

- Phenobarbital or rifampin may lower montelukast blood levels, so you may require a higher dosage.

Zafirlukast

- Because aspirin significantly increases zafirlukast blood levels, consult your health-care practitioner before taking aspirin remedies along with this drug.
- Erythromycin, terfenadine, and theophylline reduce zafirlukast blood levels. You may require a higher dosage.
- Zafirlukast may increase the effects of a number of other drugs, including carbamazepine, cisapride, cyclosporine, felodipine, isradipine, nicardipine, nifedipine, nimodipine, phenytoin, tolbutamide, and warfarin.

Zileuton

- Zileuton may increase the effects of a number of other drugs, including beta-blockers such as propranolol, cisapride, cyclosporine, felodipine, isradipine, nicardipine, nifedipine, nimodipine, theophylline, and warfarin.

FOOD, VITAMIN, AND HERBAL INTERACTIONS

Do not use herbal remedies for asthma—such as ephedra (ma huang)—in conjunction with leukotriene antagonist/inhibitors.

RECOMMENDED DOSAGE

These drugs come in tablet form. Although the doses given below are typical, only your health-care practitioner can determine the dose and schedule that are most appropriate for you.

Montelukast

- *Children 6 to 14 Years:* one 5-mg tablet daily
- *Children 15 Years and Older and Adults:* one 10-mg tablet daily

Zafirlukast

- *Children Younger than 12 Years:* This drug is not recommended for children under 12.
- *Children 12 Years and Older and Adults:* 20 mg twice daily

Zileuton

- *Children Younger than 12 Years:* This drug is not recommended for children under 12.
- *Children 12 Years and Older and Adults:* 600 mg 4 times a day

Take montelukast in the evening. Zafirlukast should be taken on an empty stomach, 1 hour before or 2 hours after meals. Zileuton can be taken with or without food.

These drugs must be taken on a regular basis to prevent asthma attacks. If you miss a dose, take it as soon as you remember. However, if it is nearly time for your next scheduled dose, do not take the missed dose. Follow your regular dosing schedule. Never take a double dose.

SYMPTOMS OF OVERDOSE AND WHAT TO DO

No specific information on overdosing with these drugs is available. If you suspect an overdose, seek immediate medical attention, and bring the prescription bottle with you to the hospital so that health-care practitioners will know exactly what drug was used.

SPECIAL INFORMATION FOR PREGNANT OR NURSING WOMEN

No studies have adequately investigated the effects of these drugs during pregnancy or breastfeeding. If you are pregnant or plan to become pregnant, or if you are breastfeeding or plan to do so, talk with your health-care practitioner before starting one of these medications. Only a health-care practitioner can determine whether the potential benefits outweigh the risks.

SPECIAL INFORMATION FOR SENIORS

Studies have shown that people over 55 who take zafirlukast have more respiratory infections. Seniors may benefit from a reduced dosage.

GENERIC NAME

Leuprolide

BRAND NAME

Eligard
No generic available

ABOUT THIS DRUG

Leuprolide is a synthetic form of gonadotropin releasing hormone that, when given continuously, suppresses formation of testosterone (from the testes) in men and estrogen (from the ovaries) in women. Leuprolide is used to treat prostate cancer in men and endometriosis in women.

This drug works by stopping testosterone production in men, and because testosterone promotes growth of prostate cancer, leuprolide helps slow cancer growth. In women, estrogen promotes growth of fibroids and endometriosis; leuprolide stops estrogen production and thus reduces growth of fibroids and endometriosis.

SIDE EFFECTS

Be sure to tell your health-care practitioner if you experience any side effects while taking leuprolide. Only your health-care practitioner can determine whether it is safe for you to continue taking this drug.

➤ *Most Common:* aches and pains, headache, hot flashes, irritation at injection site

➤ *Less Common:* anxiety, blurred vision, breast enlargement in men, constipation, decreased sexual desire, impotence, nausea, shrinking of testes

➤ *Rare:* allergic reaction (closing of throat, difficulty breathing, hives, swelling of lips, mouth, or face)

IMPORTANT PRECAUTIONS

Tell your health-care practitioner if you are sensitive or allergic to leuprolide or to any other drugs.

Leuprolide may stop sperm production in men and interfere with normal menstrual cycles in women. Women who have not reached menopause and who take 10 weeks or more of leuprolide therapy may experience cessation of their monthly menstrual cycle and/or vaginal bleeding or discharge. The presence of any of these symptoms does not mean you cannot get pregnant or that you cannot get someone pregnant.

Before taking leuprolide, tell your health-care practitioner if you have or have ever had liver disease or abnormal vaginal bleeding.

Leuprolide causes an initial increase in testosterone levels before causing them to decline. This causes some men to experience increased bone pain and increased difficulty in urinating during the first few weeks of treatment. Contact your health-care practitioner if these symptoms occur.

Prolonged periods of use can decrease bone density, thereby increasing risk of bone fractures in men and women. Your physician may recommend calcium supplements and weight-bearing exercise to reduce these effects.

DRUG INTERACTIONS

No drug-drug interactions have been documented. However, you should still tell your health-care practitioner and pharmacist if you are taking any prescription or nonprescription drugs, as well as any vitamins, herbs, or other supplements.

FOOD, VITAMIN, AND HERBAL INTERACTIONS

No food, vitamin, or herbal interactions have been reported.

RECOMMENDED DOSAGE

Leuprolide is available as an injectable, either under the skin (subcutaneously) or into the muscle (intramuscularly; this form is called Lupron Depot and is administered by a health-care practitioner). Viadur is an implant that is administered by subcutaneous injection in the upper arm once every 12 months. The dosages given here are typical. However, your health-care practitioner will determine the most appropriate dose and schedule for your needs.

For Prostate Cancer

- Leuprolide can be administered daily at a dose of 1 mg.
- Lupron Depot can be administered monthly or at 3- to 4-month intervals: 3.5- and 7.5-mg doses of Lupron Depot are given monthly; 11.25- and 22.5-mg doses are given every 3 months; the 30-mg dose is given every 4 months.
- Eligard is given intramuscularly as 7.5 mg every month.

For Endometriosis and Fibroids

- For endometriosis, Lupron Depot is administered 3.75 mg monthly or 11.5 mg every 3 months.
- For fibroids, a single 11.5-mg dose of Lupron Depot or 3.75-mg doses given monthly

Leuprolide should be taken exactly as prescribed by your health-care practitioner. If you miss a dose, take it as soon as you remember. If it is nearly time for your next dose, do not take the missed dose, and resume your normal schedule. Do not take a double dose.

SYMPTOMS OF OVERDOSE AND WHAT TO DO

Symptoms of overdose are not known, but may include difficulty breathing and reduced activity. If overdose occurs, seek immediate medical attention and bring the prescription container with you to the hospital.

SPECIAL INFORMATION FOR PREGNANT OR NURSING WOMEN

Leuprolide may harm the fetus and should not be used if you are pregnant. Talk to your health-care practitioner before using this drug about using a reliable method of birth control to prevent pregnancy. You should not plan to become pregnant while you receive hormone therapy or for some time after stopping treatment.

It is not known whether leuprolide passes into breast milk. Your health-care practitioner will likely recommend you switch to bottle feeding while you are taking this medication.

SPECIAL INFORMATION FOR SENIORS

No special precautions have been noted for older adults.

GENERIC NAME

Levamisole

BRAND NAME

Ergamisol

No generic available

ABOUT THIS DRUG

Levamisole is prescribed along with fluorouracil for the treatment of colon cancer.

This drug works by stimulating the immune system and restoring depressed immune function. It is not known exactly how it makes fluorouracil more effective.

SIDE EFFECTS

Side effects are extremely common. Consult your health-care practitioner if they are persistent or severe. Only he or she can determine whether it is safe for you to continue taking levamisole.

- *Common:* nausea, vomiting, diarrhea, constipation, metallic taste, appetite loss, mouth sores, abdominal pain, muscle and joint aches, dizziness, headache, tingling in the hands and feet, hair loss, rash, fatigue, fever, chills, drop in white blood cells, infection

- *Less Common or Rare:* anxiety, depression, nervousness, confusion, insomnia, paranoia, trembling or shaking, tingling in the hands and feet, gas, stomach upset, blurred vision, eye redness or swelling, rash, intense itching, painful urination, trouble walking, unusual bleeding or bruising, black, tarry stools, hallucinations, convulsions, kidney failure

Some people develop a sudden and dangerous drop in their white blood cells while taking levamisole. This is known as agranulocytosis. Symptoms include fever, chills, and flu-like symptoms. Your health-care practitioner will monitor your blood while you take this drug, but also report these types of symptoms at once.

IMPORTANT PRECAUTIONS

Inform your health-care practitioner about any other medical conditions you suffer from. Levamisole must be used with caution if you have an infection, because this drug impedes your body's ability to fight infection.

DRUG INTERACTIONS

Inform your health-care practitioner and pharmacist if you are taking any other prescription or over-the-counter drugs, as well as any vitamins, herbs, or other supplements. Possible drug interactions include the following:

- Combining alcohol with levamisole can result in severe side effects.
- If you take phenytoin along with levamisole and fluorouracil, you may experience an increased risk of phenytoin's side effects.

FOOD, VITAMIN, AND HERBAL INTERACTIONS

No food, vitamin, or herbal interactions have been noted.

RECOMMENDED DOSAGE

Levamisole comes in tablet form. Although the doses given below are typical, only your health-care practitioner can determine the dose and schedule that are most appropriate for you.

Colon Cancer

- *Children:* Consult your health-care practitioner.
- *Adults:* Recommended dosage 7 to 30 days after surgery is 50 mg every 8 hours for 3 days; followed by 50 mg every 8 hours for 3 days every 2 weeks

Malignant Melanoma

- *Children:* Consult your health-care practitioner.
- *Adults:* 2.5 mg once daily for 2 consecutive days each week

It is very important to take levamisole exactly as directed by your health-care practitioner. Taking more than the recommended dosage can result in serious side effects. If you vomit shortly after taking levamisole, call your health-care practitioner to see whether you should take another dose. If you miss a dose of this medication, *do not* take the missed dose or double the next one. Check with your health-care practitioner for instructions.

SYMPTOMS OF OVERDOSE AND WHAT TO DO

An overdose of levamisole can be potentially fatal. Symptoms include severe side effects such as those that involve the blood, stomach, kidneys, or intestines. If overdose occurs, seek immediate medical attention, and bring the prescription bottle with you to the hospital so that health-care practitioners will know exactly what drug was used.

SPECIAL INFORMATION FOR PREGNANT OR NURSING WOMEN

Levamisole may cause fetal damage. Use effective contraception to make sure that you do not become pregnant while taking this drug. If you are already pregnant, talk with your health-care practitioner before taking levamisole. Only a health-care practitioner can determine whether the potential benefits of treatment outweigh its dangers. Because levamisole passes into breast milk, it is probably best to stop breastfeeding during the periods that you must take this drug.

SPECIAL INFORMATION FOR SENIORS

No special instructions are provided for seniors.

GENERIC NAME

Levetiracetam

BRAND NAME

Keppra
No generic available

ABOUT THIS DRUG

Levetiracetam is an anticonvulsant used to control epileptic seizures in adults. It is always prescribed in combination with other antiepileptic drugs.

Although levetiracetam can help prevent seizures, it works in a different manner from other antiepileptic drugs. That is, it does not directly affect the pathways that block or stimulate nerve transmissions.

SIDE EFFECTS

Consult your health-care practitioner if you develop side effects while taking this drug. Only he or she can determine whether it is safe for you to continue taking levetiracetam.

- *Common:* dizziness, weakness, tiredness, infection, pain, sore throat
- *Less Common or Rare:* tingling or "pins and needles" sensations, sensation of spinning, cough, sinus irritation, swollen gums, double vision, appetite loss, memory loss, anxiety, depression, hostility, nervousness, poor muscle coordination, muscle aches, fever, flu-like symptoms, diarrhea, constipation, bruising, rash, insomnia, weight gain, middle ear infections, tremors, convulsions

IMPORTANT PRECAUTIONS

Inform your health-care practitioner about any other medical conditions you suffer from. Levetiracetam must be used with caution if you have kidney disease, which may increase the risk of unwanted side effects. A lower dosage will probably be prescribed.

Because levetiracetam may cause side effects such as dizziness, drowsiness, and fatigue, do not drive a car, operate machinery, or perform other tasks that require concentration until you know how this drug affects you.

DRUG INTERACTIONS

Although there are no specific drug interactions associated with levetiracetam, always inform your health-care practitioner and pharmacist about all other prescription and over-the-counter drugs that you take, as well as any vitamins, herbs, or other supplements.

FOOD, VITAMIN, AND HERBAL INTERACTIONS

No food, vitamin, or herbal interactions have been noted.

RECOMMENDED DOSAGE

Levetiracetam is available in tablet form. Although the doses given below are typical, only your health-care practitioner can determine the dose and schedule that are most appropriate for you. The dosage will be adjusted according to which other epilepsy medications are prescribed in combination with levetiracetam, and how effectively seizures are controlled.

- *Children:* This drug is not recommended for children.
- *Adults:* 1,000 to 3,000 mg daily, divided into 2 doses

Levetiracetam can be taken with or without food. If you miss a dose, take it as soon as you remember. However, if it is almost time for the next dose, skip the one you missed and go back to your regular dosing schedule. Never take a double dose. Do not stop taking this drug suddenly, as seizures may occur.

SYMPTOMS OF OVERDOSE AND WHAT TO DO

Drowsiness is the primary symptom of overdose. If overdose occurs, seek medical attention immediately, and bring the prescription bottle with you to the hospital so that health-care practitioners will know exactly what drug was used.

SPECIAL INFORMATION FOR PREGNANT OR NURSING WOMEN

Levetiracetam may cause birth defects. Do not use this drug while pregnant unless the benefits of therapy clearly outweigh the potential risks to the fetus. Because levetiracetam may pass into breast milk, bottle-feeding is preferable.

SPECIAL INFORMATION FOR SENIORS

Smaller doses of levetiracetam are usually recommended for seniors.

GENERIC NAME

Levodopa *see also Carbidopa, page 240*

BRAND NAMES

Bendopa, Dopar, Larodopa; Sinemet (Carbidopa/Levodopa combination)
Generic available

ABOUT THIS DRUG

Levodopa—also known as L-dopa—is an antiparkinsonian drug prescribed for Parkinson's disease, restless leg syndrome, and herpes zoster (shingles). When levodopa enters the brain, it is converted to dopamine, an important neurotransmitter (a chemical messenger in the brain). Levodopa is often prescribed with a similar drug known as carbidopa, resulting in fewer side effects.

Levodopa works by correcting the dopamine deficiency that is believed to be the cause of Parkinson's disease and related problems. Yet an important aspect of treatment is the "on-off" phenomenon—that is, after 2 to 3 years of taking levodopa, many people find that this drug temporarily loses its effect, only to regain it later. This effect becomes more pronounced after 5 years of treatment.

SIDE EFFECTS

Side effects from levodopa are common. Call your health-care practitioner if symptoms become severe or do not go away. Contact your health-care practitioner immediately if you experience fainting, dizziness, and lightheadedness; severe nausea and vomiting; palpitations; mood changes; uncontrollable movements; abnormal results in urine tests for sugar and ketones; or difficulty urinating. Only your health-care practitioner can determine if you should continue to take this drug.

- *Common:* abdominal pain, dry mouth, appetite loss, nightmares, gas, muscle spasms, inability to control muscles, nausea, vomiting, drooling, difficulty eating, headache, fatigue, weakness, faint feeling, dizziness, numbness, hand tremors, agitation, anxiety, delusions, hallucinations, a general feeling of unwellness
- *Less Common or Rare:* diarrhea, constipation, flushing, hiccups, increased sweating, muscle twitching, trouble sleeping, blurred or double vision, difficulty urinating, changes in mental state (which may include paranoia and suicidal tendencies), loss of intellectual function, heart palpitations, hot flashes, weight changes, darkening of urine, dizziness upon rising, high blood pressure, ulcer, stomach bleeding, loss of eye muscle control, hair loss, fluid retention, convulsions

IMPORTANT PRECAUTIONS

You should not take this drug if you have a history of gastric or stomach ulcers. If you have heart or lung disease, a history of heart attacks, glaucoma, kidney or liver disease, a hormonal disorder, asthma, or a family history of malignant melanoma, use levodopa with caution. Because this drug is associated with hallucinations and suicidal tendencies, extreme caution must be exercised when using this drug in people with a history of psychosis. Also inform your health-care practitioner of any other medical conditions you have, especially diabetes, emphysema, or seizure disorders such as epilepsy.

Because levodopa may cause side effects such as dizziness and fatigue, do not drive a car, operate machinery, or perform other tasks that require concentration until you know how this drug affects you.

DRUG INTERACTIONS

Tell your health-care practitioner and pharmacist if you are taking any other prescription or over-the-counter drugs, as well as any vitamins, herbs, or other supplements. Possible drug interactions include the following:

- Levodopa has fewer side effects when prescribed with carbidopa.
- Do not take levodopa while you are taking or within 2 weeks of taking monoamine oxidase inhibitors. This can cause extremely high blood pressure.
- Antacids may increase levodopa's effects.
- Metoclopramide may increase levodopa's effects, while levodopa may reduce metoclopramide's effects.
- Anticholinergic drugs decrease levodopa's effects.
- Levodopa may interact with high blood pressure medications by further reducing pressure. The antihypertensive medication methyldopa may reduce levodopa's effects.
- Other drugs that may interact with levodopa include tranquilizers, medications for depression, antipsychotic medications, and phenytoin.
- Using cocaine while taking levodopa can cause an irregular heartbeat.

FOOD, VITAMIN, AND HERBAL INTERACTIONS

High doses of vitamin B_6 (pyroxidine) may interfere with levodopa's action in the body, especially when this drug is taken by itself (without carbidopa). Also keep in mind that pyroxidine is present in many foods such as bananas, egg yolks, peanuts, lima beans, whole grain cereals, and meats. If you take levodopa alone, ask your health-care practitioner how many of these foods it is safe to include in your diet.

The herb kava may also interfere with the absorption of levodopa. Avoid combining levodopa with dietary supplements such as 5-HTP (5-hydroxytryptophan) and BCCAs (branched chain amino acids). Because iron may inhibit the absorption of levodopa, if you use an iron supplement be sure to take it at a different time of day.

RECOMMENDED DOSAGE

Levodopa is available in tablet form. Although the doses given below are typical, only your health-care practitioner can determine the dose and schedule that are most appropriate for you.

- *Children:* This drug is not recommended for children.
- *Adults:* 500 mg to 8,000 mg daily

At the start of treatment, in order to prevent stomach upset, take levodopa with food. As time goes on and your body grows used to this drug, your health-care practitioner may prefer you to take it on an empty stomach, so that it will be more effective. If you miss a dose of levodopa, take it as soon as you remember. However, if it is almost time for the next dose, skip the one you missed and go back to your regular dosing schedule. Never take a double dose.

SYMPTOMS OF OVERDOSE AND WHAT TO DO

Symptoms of levodopa overdose may include nausea, vomiting, diarrhea, muscle twitching, spastic closure of the eyelids, fainting, agitation, confusion, and hallucinations. If overdose does occur, seek medical attention immediately, and bring the prescription bottle with you to the hospital so that health-care practitioners will know exactly what drug was used.

SPECIAL INFORMATION FOR PREGNANT OR NURSING WOMEN

Levodopa may cause birth defects. Do not use this drug while pregnant unless the benefits of therapy clearly outweigh the potential risks to the fetus. Because levodopa may pass into breast milk, bottle-feeding is preferable.

SPECIAL INFORMATION FOR SENIORS

Significantly smaller doses of levodopa are usually prescribed for seniors, who are more susceptible to side effects. Older people with heart disease are more apt to experience cardiac effects such as abnormal heart rhythms.

GENERIC NAME

Levofloxacin

see Fluoroquinolone Antibiotics, page 468

GENERIC NAME
Levothyroxine sodium *see Thyroid Hormone Replacements, page 1029*

GENERIC NAME
Liothyronine sodium *see Thyroid Hormone Replacements, page 1029*

GENERIC NAME
Liotrix *see Thyroid Hormone Replacements, page 1029*

GENERIC NAME
Lisinopril

BRAND NAMES
Prinivil, Zestril
Generic available

ABOUT THIS DRUG
Lisinopril is an angiotensin-converting enzyme (ACE) inhibitor used to treat mild to severe high blood pressure (hypertension). It is also used to reduce the risk of death after heart attacks, and for congestive heart failure. Lisinopril may be prescribed alone or with other high blood pressure medications. This drug works by blocking an enzyme in the body, which relaxes blood vessels and lowers blood pressure.

SIDE EFFECTS
Speak to your health-care practitioner if you develop side effects while taking lisinopril. Only he or she can determine whether you should continue taking this drug.

- *Common:* dizziness, headache, tiredness, diarrhea, nausea, cough
- *Less Common or Rare:* chest pain, low blood pressure, upset stomach, vomiting, rash, breathing difficulties, muscle weakness, joint pain, changes in mental status or sex drive, respiratory difficulties, kidney or liver problems, heart rhythm disturbances, increased susceptibility to infection

IMPORTANT PRECAUTIONS

Always inform your health-care practitioner about any other medical conditions you suffer from, especially heart, kidney, or liver disease, diabetes, an elevated potassium level, a blood cell disorder, lupus, or scleroderma.

Lisinopril can affect your kidneys, especially if you have congestive heart failure. If you already have kidney disease, your dosage should be lower than usual.

Before having any type of surgery or dental procedure, tell your surgeon or dentist that you are taking lisinopril.

When you first start taking this drug or when the dosage is increased, you may experience dizziness or faintness when you rise quickly from a sitting or reclining position (postural hypotension). Try to get up slowly, and consult your health-care practitioner if the problem continues.

Treatment of high blood pressure also entails certain lifestyle changes, such as weight control, smoking cessation, and close attention to diet.

Be extremely careful when you exercise in hot weather. Heavy sweating can lead to dizziness, lightheadedness, fainting, vomiting, dehydration, and low blood pressure.

Do not take this drug if you have ever experienced an allergic reaction to it or to other ACE inhibitors. If you have an allergic reaction such as swelling of the face and mouth and a sudden problem with breathing, seek immediate medical attention.

DRUG INTERACTIONS

Tell your health-care practitioner and pharmacist if you are taking any other prescription or over-the-counter drugs, as well as any vitamins, herbs, or other supplements. Possible drug interactions include the following:

- Taking other blood pressure medications can increase the blood pressure lowering effects of lisinopril. It is best to stop taking all other antihypertensive drugs (especially diuretics) 1 week before beginning treatment with lisinopril. Otherwise, if you are already taking a diuretic, you may experience a rapid and dangerous drop in blood pressure when you begin taking this drug. After your health-care practitioner sees how you react to lisinopril, other high blood pressure medications can be restarted as needed.
- Lisinopril increases blood levels of potassium, particularly when taken with potassium-sparing diuretics. Too much potassium can cause heart rhythm disturbances.

- Combining lisinopril with loop diuretics increases the risk of postural hypotension (low blood pressure and dizziness when you stand up).
- Do not combine lisinopril with potassium medications, such as K-Lyte or Slow-K.
- Bactrim and Septra may also increase blood potassium, increasing the risk of heart rhythm disturbances.
- Do not combine lisinopril with interferons. This combination is associated with an increased risk of blood problems.
- Combining lisinopril with allopurinal increases the risk of serious skin reactions.
- Taking lisinopril with lithium can result in toxic levels of lithium in the blood.
- Phenothiazine tranquilizers and antiemetics may increase the effects of lisinopril.
- Aspirin and other NSAIDs (such as ibuprofen and indomethacin) can reduce the blood pressure lowering effects of lisinopril.
- Separate doses of antacids and lisinopril by 2 hours.
- Lisinopril increases blood levels of digoxin.
- Alcohol may further lower blood pressure. Use with caution.
- Consult your health-care practitioner before taking over-the-counter cough, cold, sinus, allergy, or weight loss medications. Many of these can raise blood pressure.

FOOD, VITAMIN, AND HERBAL INTERACTIONS

Do not take herbs that increase blood pressure, such as ephedra (ma huang), ginseng, goldenseal, licorice, and saw palmetto. Consult your health-care practitioner before taking substances that may lower blood pressure, such as calcium, soy, or garlic. To minimize possible interactions, take lisinopril and iron supplements 2 or 3 hours apart. Because ACE inhibitors such as lisinopril raise potassium levels in the body, *do not* take potassium supplements or use salt substitutes containing potassium, and ask your health-care practitioner how many potassium-rich foods (such as bananas, prunes, raisins, melons, tomatoes, citrus fruit, and orange juice) you can safely include in your diet. Also talk to your health-care practitioner about salt intake.

RECOMMENDED DOSAGE

Lisinopril is available in oral form as tablets. Although the doses given below are typical, only your health-care practitioner can determine the dose and schedule that best fit your needs.

High Blood Pressure

- *Children:* This drug is not recommended for children.
- *Adults:* 5 to 40 mg once daily

Heart Failure

- *Children:* This drug is not recommended for children.
- *Adults:* 5 to 40 mg once daily

Heart Attack

- *Children:* This drug is not recommended for children.
- *Adults:* 5 mg in the first 24 hours after a heart attack, followed by 5 mg 24 hours later, and then 10 mg daily for 6 weeks

Take lisinopril with food or milk to prevent stomach upset. Continue to take this drug even if you feel well. Do not discontinue use without consulting your health-care practitioner. If you miss a dose, take it as soon as you remember. If it is almost time for the next dose, skip the forgotten one, and resume your normal schedule. Never take a double dose.

SYMPTOMS OF OVERDOSE AND WHAT TO DO

The symptoms of lisinopril overdose include dizziness and fainting caused by a severe drop in blood pressure. If overdose occurs, seek immediate medical attention and take the bottle of lisinopril to the hospital with you.

SPECIAL INFORMATION FOR PREGNANT OR NURSING WOMEN

Do not take lisinopril if you are pregnant (especially during the final six months). This drug can cause fetal injury and death. If you become pregnant while taking lisinopril, call your health-care practitioner immediately.

Small amounts of lisinopril may pass into breast milk. If you are breastfeeding, your health-care practitioner will likely advise you to stop until your treatment is done.

SPECIAL INFORMATION FOR SENIORS

Seniors usually require lower doses of lisinopril.

GENERIC NAME
Lithium carbonate

BRAND NAMES
Cibalith-S, Eskalith, Eskalith CR, Lithane, Lithobid, Lithonate, Lithotabs
Generic available
NOTE: The information in this profile also applies to lithium citrate, which is available only in generic form.

ABOUT THIS DRUG
Lithium is an antipsychotic drug used to treat bipolar disorder (manic-depressive illness). People with this disorder experience extreme mood changes from depression or anger to excitement and elation. Lithium can be used on a short-term basis to control an acute manic episode, or on a long-term basis to reduce the frequency and severity of manic states. This drug works by changing the way nerve signals are sent and interpreted.

SIDE EFFECTS
Talk to your health-care practitioner if you develop side effects while taking lithium. Only he or she can determine whether it is safe for you to continue taking this drug and whether it is necessary to readjust your dosage.

- *Common:* slight tremor in the hands, increased thirst, increased urination, nausea, discomfort
- *Less Common or Rare:* drowsiness, diarrhea, vomiting, weakness, unsteady gait, tremor, slurred speech, muscle weakness, poor coordination, stiffness of arms and legs, ringing in the ears, blurred vision, giddiness, fainting, confusion, impaired memory, weight gain, dry skin, hair loss, hoarseness, sensitivity to cold, swelling of feet or lower legs, unusual tiredness, trouble breathing, change in heartbeat, loss of bladder control, and goiter, thyroid, and kidney problems

Stop taking lithium and contact your health-care practitioner immediately if you experience side effects such as vomiting, diarrhea, drowsiness, weakness, unsteady gait, and tremor. These may be signs of severe toxic reactions that can occur at close to therapeutic doses.

IMPORTANT PRECAUTIONS
You should not take lithium if you have uncontrolled diabetes, poorly managed hypothyroidism, or severe kidney failure. Also do

not use this drug if you are breastfeeding. Lithium should be used with caution if you have brain or spinal cord disease; epilepsy; schizophrenia; diabetes; heart disease; thyroid problems; difficulty urinating; impaired kidney function; Parkinson's disease; psoriasis; or a history of leukemia; or if you are in a weak and dehydrated condition, or on a low-sodium diet.

When you take lithium, it is essential to comply with frequent testing of its level in your blood. This is because the level at which you derive benefit from lithium is very close to the level of drug toxicity. Blood tests are particularly frequent when you first start therapy.

Long-term use of lithium is associated with thyroid and kidney problems. Thyroid and kidney function should thus be routinely monitored during treatment. Frequent thirst and urination may be signs of diabetes mellitus.

Before having any type of surgery or dental procedure, tell your surgeon or dentist that you are taking lithium.

This drug may impair your physical coordination and mental alertness. Until you know how lithium affects you, do not drive a car, operate machinery, or perform other tasks that demand concentration.

Be careful when you exercise in hot weather or take a hot bath or sauna. Heavy sweating can lead to dizziness, lightheadedness, fainting, vomiting, and dehydration. The loss of too much water and salt from your body can lead to serious side effects.

Alert your health-care practitioner if you experience an illness accompanied by diarrhea, vomiting, and sweating. You may need to stop taking lithium until you get better.

DRUG INTERACTIONS

Inform your health-care practitioner and pharmacist if you are taking any other prescription or over-the-counter drugs, as well as any vitamins, herbs, or other supplements. Possible drug interactions include the following:

- Taking lithium with other antipsychotic drugs may alter the levels of both medications, increasing the risk of side effects.
- Combining lithium with haloperidol can cause symptoms such as tiredness, weakness, confusion, and fever. In some cases, this has led to permanent brain damage.
- Taking lithium with chlorpromazine can reduce chlorpromazine's effects and increase lithium's effects.
- Concurrent use of diuretics can lead to serious side effects.
- Avoid over-the-counter medications that contain iodides. These add to lithium's antithyroid effect.

- Lithium may increase blood levels of insulin. If you are diabetic, ask your health-care practitioner whether it is necessary to adjust your medication.
- Lithium may affect the absorption of estrogen-containing drugs such as birth control pills and hormone replacement therapy. Ask your health-care practitioner whether your dosage should be adjusted.
- Lithium may increase your absorption of warfarin, leading to an increased risk of bleeding.
- Lithium may increase the effects of tricyclic antidepressants.
- Lithium may decrease the effects of digoxin, resulting in the need for a higher dosage.
- Drugs that reduce the absorption of lithium include acetazolamide, mannitol, sodium bicarbonate, theophylline drugs, urea, and verapamil.
- Drugs that increase the absorption of lithium include carbamazepine, methyldopa, NSAIDs (such as aspirin and ibuprofen), loop and thiazide diuretics, and the SSRIs (such as fluoxetine).

FOOD, VITAMIN, AND HERBAL INTERACTIONS

While taking this drug, drink 10 to 12 glasses of water a day. Do not drink large amounts of caffeinated beverages such as coffee, tea, or soft drinks, and use a normal amount of salt in your diet. Do not go on a weight loss plan or make other drastic changes in your diet without consulting your health-care practitioner. The loss of too much water and salt from your body can lead to serious side effects.

Do not combine lithium with herbs that produce sedative effects, such as catnip, elecampane, goldenseal, gotu kola, hops, kava, lemon balm, skullcap, St. John's wort, and valerian.

RECOMMENDED DOSAGE

Lithium comes as a tablet, capsule, extended-release tablet, and liquid. The doses given below are typical, but each lithium dosage is always carefully individualized according to a person's particular needs and reactions to therapy.

Acute Manic Episodes

- *Children:* This drug is not recommended for children under the age of 12.
- *Adults:* 1,800 mg daily, in divided doses

Long-Term Control

- *Children:* This drug is not recommended for children under the age of 12.
- *Adults:* 900 to 1,200 mg daily, in divided doses

Take lithium with food or milk to prevent stomach upset. Extended-release tablets must be swallowed whole. If you forget a dose, *do not* take it as soon as you remember. Skip it, and take your next dose at the normal time. Never take a double dose.

SYMPTOMS OF OVERDOSE AND WHAT TO DO

The symptoms of lithium overdose include drowsiness, dizziness, nausea, vomiting, diarrhea, lack of coordination, muscle spasms, staggering gait, blurred vision, slurred speech, confusion, stupor, seizures, and coma. If overdose occurs, seek immediate medical attention and take the bottle of lithium to the hospital with you.

SPECIAL INFORMATION FOR PREGNANT OR NURSING WOMEN

Lithium is not recommended during pregnancy, especially during the first three months. Studies have also shown that lithium causes muscle weakness and extreme drowsiness in newborns of mothers who take this drug around the time of childbirth. If you become pregnant while taking lithium, call your health-care practitioner immediately.

Lithium passes into breast milk and causes effects such as muscle weakness, heart problems, and lowered body temperature in nursing babies. If you must take this drug, bottle-feeding is preferable.

SPECIAL INFORMATION FOR SENIORS

Seniors require lower doses of lithium. This age group is more likely to experience effects such as unusual thirst, an increase in urine output, trembling, muscle weakness, drowsiness, slurred speech, nausea, vomiting, loss of appetite, diarrhea, and goiter.

GENERIC NAME

Lomefloxacin

see Fluoroquinolone Antibiotics, page 468

GENERIC NAME

Class: Loop diuretics

Generics: (1) bumetanide; (2) furosemide; (3) torsemide

BRAND NAMES

(1) Bumex; (2) Lasix; (3) Demadex

Only (1) and (2) available in generic

ABOUT THIS DRUG

Loop diuretics are used to reduce the amount of water in the body. Also known as "water pills," these drugs are prescribed for congestive heart failure, high blood pressure, cirrhosis, kidney problems, fluid accumulation in the lungs, and other conditions that require the removal of excess fluid from the body.

Loop diuretics, which are stronger than thiazide diuretics, cause the kidneys to get rid of unneeded water and salt from the body into the urine. They impact the same part of the kidneys as thiazide diuretics, but also another part of the kidneys known as the "loop of Henle."

SIDE EFFECTS

Consult your health-care practitioner if you develop side effects while taking one of these drugs. Only he or she can determine whether it is safe for you to continue taking a loop diuretic.

- *Common:* frequent urination (up to 6 hours after a dose), dizziness or lightheadedness when getting up from a sitting or lying down position, changes in blood levels of potassium and possibly other electrolytes, a decrease in magnesium, an increase in blood sugar or blood uric acid levels
- *Less Common or Rare:* appetite loss, abdominal discomfort, diarrhea, nausea, vomiting, fatigue, rash, weakness, dizziness, lightheadedness, blurred vision, confusion, tingling in the arms and legs, rash, temporary hearing loss, jaundice, acute gout attacks

Beware of symptoms of low blood potassium (hypokalemia), which may include excessive thirst, dry mouth, decreased urination, drowsiness, weakness, lethargy, muscle pain or cramps, abnormal heart rate, upset stomach, nausea, vomiting, and low blood pressure.

IMPORTANT PRECAUTIONS

Tell your health-care practitioner if you have or have ever had a medical condition such as diabetes, gout, history of a recent heart attack, hearing problems, lupus, kidney or liver disease, or low blood potassium or other electrolytes.

Loop diuretics may affect blood sugar levels. If you have diabetes, be careful when testing your glucose levels, and closely monitor your diet.

Before having any type of surgery or dental procedure, tell your surgeon or dentist that you are taking a loop diuretic.

Treatment of high blood pressure also entails certain lifestyle changes, such as weight control, smoking cessation, and close attention to diet.

When you first start taking this drug or when the dosage is increased, you may experience dizziness or faintness when you rise quickly from a sitting or reclining position (postural hypotension). Try to get up slowly, and consult your health-care practitioner if the problem continues.

Loop diuretics may cause side effects such as dizziness and confusion. Do not drive a car, operate machinery, or perform other tasks that require concentration until you know how the drug you are taking affects you.

Alert your health-care practitioner if you experience an illness accompanied by diarrhea, vomiting, and sweating. This may cause the loss of too much water and potassium.

Be careful when you exercise in hot weather or take a hot bath or sauna. Heavy sweating can lead to dizziness, lightheadedness, fainting, vomiting, dehydration, and low blood pressure.

Furosemide may cause increased sensitivity to sunlight. When you take this drug, avoid direct sunlight and wear sunscreen.

DRUG INTERACTIONS

Tell your health-care practitioner and pharmacist if you are taking any other prescription or over-the-counter drugs, as well as any vitamins, herbs, or other supplements. Possible drug interactions include the following:

- Loop diuretics enhance the effectiveness of other blood pressure medications.
- Loop diuretics increase the risk of lithium side effects.
- NSAIDs (such as aspirin and ibuprofen) may lessen the effectiveness of loop diuretics.
- Other drugs that may reduce the effects of loop diuretics are charcoal tablets, phenytoin, and probenecid.
- Thiazide diuretics and clofibrate increase the effects of loop diuretics.

- Combining a loop diuretic with adrenal corticosteroids or digitalis drugs increases the risk of electrolyte imbalances. In addition, loop diuretic–induced potassium loss can increase digitalis toxicity.
- Loop diuretics may increase the absorption of blood thinners such as warfarin, leading to an increased risk of bleeding.
- In rare cases, taking chloral hydrate with a loop diuretic may cause high blood pressure, hot flashes, sweating, abnormal heart rhythms, nausea, and weakness.
- Loop diuretics may alter theophylline levels.
- Combining a loop diuretic with cisplatin or an aminoglycoside antibiotic may cause ringing or buzzing in the ears and periodic hearing loss.
- Consult your health-care practitioner before taking over-the-counter cough, cold, sinus, allergy, or weight loss medications. Many of these can raise blood pressure.
- It may be necessary to adjust the dosages of oral diabetes drugs taken along with loop diuretics.
- Your health-care practitioner may recommend medication to prevent potassium loss.
- Limit your alcohol intake. You are more likely to experience effects such as dizziness, lightheadedness, and fainting if you use alcohol.

FOOD, VITAMIN, AND HERBAL INTERACTIONS

Do not take herbs that increase blood pressure, such as ephedra (ma huang), ginseng, goldenseal, licorice, and saw palmetto. Consult your health-care practitioner before taking substances that may lower blood pressure, such as calcium, soy, or garlic. Do not combine furosemide with St. John's wort, since both cause heightened sensitivity to the sun.

Because loop diuretics may deplete your body's supply of potassium, consult your health-care practitioner about possible dietary changes. However, do not change your diet on your own (especially if you have other health issues such as diabetes). Your health-care practitioner may recommend a higher intake of potassium-rich foods such as bananas, prunes, raisins, citrus fruits, orange juice, melons, and tomatoes. Magnesium levels may also be affected, so inquire about a daily nutritional supplement. A low-sodium diet may be advised.

RECOMMENDED DOSAGE

Loop diuretics come primarily in tablet form. (Furosemide is also available as a liquid medication.) Ask your health-care practitioner to help you plan the best way to take this medication. If you are prescribed a single dose, it is best to take it in the morning to avoid nighttime urination. If you take more than one dose a day, take the last dose before 6 p.m. Although the doses given below are typical, only your health-care practitioner can determine the dose and schedule that are most appropriate for you.

Bumetanide

- *Children:* This drug is not recommended for children.
- *Adults:* 0.5 to 2 mg a day on an intermittent schedule, such as every other day

Furosemide

- *Children:* 2 mg per 2.2 pounds of body weight once daily, which may be slowly increased
- *Adults:* 20 to 80 mg daily, in either 1 or 2 doses; total daily dosages of 600 mg or more can be prescribed

Torsemide

- *Children:* This drug is not recommended for children.
- *Adults:* 5 to 20 mg once daily; total daily dosages of up to 200 mg can be prescribed

Take furosemide 1 hour before or 2 hours after meals. If they cause stomach upset, other loop diuretics can be taken with food or milk. If you miss a dose of a loop diuretic, take it as soon as you remember. However, if it is nearly time for your next scheduled dose, do not take the missed dose. Follow your regular dosing schedule. Never take a double dose.

SYMPTOMS OF OVERDOSE AND WHAT TO DO

Symptoms of overdose may include nausea, vomiting, weakness, lethargy, dizziness, confusion, thirst, muscle cramps, weak and rapid pulse, electrolyte disturbances, and drowsiness progressing to coma. If overdose occurs, seek immediate medical attention, and bring the prescription bottle with you to the hospital so that health-care practitioners will know exactly what drug was used.

SPECIAL INFORMATION FOR PREGNANT OR NURSING WOMEN

No studies have adequately investigated the effects of these drugs during pregnancy or breastfeeding. If you are pregnant or plan to become pregnant, or if you are breastfeeding or plan to do so, talk with your health-care practitioner before starting one of these medications. Only a health-care practitioner can determine whether the potential benefits outweigh the risks.

SPECIAL INFORMATION FOR SENIORS

Because seniors are more sensitive to the effects of these drugs, lower doses are usually prescribed. Smaller starting doses are crucial.

GENERIC NAME

Loperamide

BRAND NAME

Imodium
Generic available

ABOUT THIS DRUG

Loperamide is used to control cramping and diarrhea. It is available with or without a prescription. This drug should only be used for short periods, and is not an appropriate remedy in every case of diarrhea. Loperamide works by acting on the nerve supply of the gastrointestinal tract, slowing intestinal movement, and decreasing secretions.

SIDE EFFECTS

Side effects are generally mild. However, if they become persistent or severe, call your health-care practitioner to determine whether you should continue taking this drug.

- *Common:* drowsiness, constipation
- *Less Common or Rare:* dry mouth, dehydration, dizziness, fever, loss of appetite, cramps, stomach pain, nausea, vomiting, bloating, rash

Tell your health-care practitioner at once if you develop bloating, swelling (distention) of the abdomen, abdominal pain, nausea, and vomiting. These may be signs of a serious bowel problem.

IMPORTANT PRECAUTIONS

Tell your health-care practitioner if you suffer from any other medical conditions, especially colitis, dysentery, or liver disease. Loperamide may worsen gastrointestinal problems such as severe colitis and dysentery, while the chance of side effects is greater in people with liver disease.

Loperamide may cause drowsiness. Do not drive a car, operate machinery, or perform other tasks that require concentration until you know how this drug affects you.

Loperamide is for short-term use only (up to 2 days for sudden or acute diarrhea, and 10 days for chronic, long-lasting diarrhea). If diarrhea continues or you develop a fever or bloody stools, consult your health-care practitioner.

DRUG INTERACTIONS

Inform your health-care practitioner and pharmacist if you are taking any other prescription or over-the-counter drugs, as well as any vitamins, herbs, or other supplements. Possible drug interactions include the following:

- Do not combine loperamide with tranquilizers, sleeping pills, or alcohol. This increases loperamide's sedative effect and also the risk of constipation.
- Antibiotics such as clindamycin and lincomycin must not be taken with loperamide. This combination can result in severe and life-threatening colitis.

FOOD, VITAMIN, AND HERBAL INTERACTIONS

Drink plenty of clear fluids to help prevent dry mouth and dehydration, which may accompany diarrhea. Speak to your health-care practitioner about dietary measures to help control diarrhea, such as eliminating fried and fatty foods and adding more fiber to your diet. St. John's wort may cause delirium when taken with loperamide.

RECOMMENDED DOSAGE

Loperamide is available by prescription in capsule form. (Tablets and liquid are sold over-the-counter.) It can be taken for either acute (sudden) or chronic (long-lasting) diarrhea. Acute diarrhea is generally treated for 2 days, and chronic diarrhea for up to 10 days. The following doses are typical, but only your health-care practitioner can determine the dose and schedule that are most appropriate for you.

Acute Diarrhea

- ➤ *Children 2 to 5 Years:* 1 mg 3 times a day as needed
- ➤ *Children 6 to 8 Years:* 2 mg twice daily as needed on the first day; on the second day, 1 mg after each loose bowel movement, for a maximum of 4 mg
- ➤ *Children 9 to 12 Years:* 2 mg 3 times daily as needed on the first day; on the second day, 1 mg after each loose bowel movement, for a maximum of 6 mg
- ➤ *Children Older than 12 Years and Adults:* 4 mg after the first loose bowel movement, followed by 2 mg after each subsequent loose stool, up to a maximum daily dosage of 16 mg for 2 days; no more than 16 mg should be taken in any 24-hour period

Chronic Diarrhea

- ➤ *Children Older than 12 and Adults:* 4 to 8 mg daily as needed for up to 10 days

Diarrhea with Irinotecan Chemotherapy

- ➤ *Adults:* 4 mg after the first loose bowel movement, followed by 2 mg every 2 hours until diarrhea-free for 12 hours. At night, 4 mg can be taken every 4 hours. If diarrhea cannot be controlled within 24 hours, contact your health-care practitioner immediately.

Take loperamide on an empty stomach. If you are taking scheduled doses of loperamide, take a missed dose as soon as you remember it. If it is almost time for the next dose, skip the forgotten one and resume your normal schedule. Never take a double dose.

SYMPTOMS OF OVERDOSE AND WHAT TO DO

The symptoms of loperamide overdose include drowsiness, lethargy, depression, dry mouth, and vomiting. If you suspect an overdose, seek immediate medical attention and take the bottle of loperamide to the hospital with you.

SPECIAL INFORMATION FOR PREGNANT OR NURSING WOMEN

No studies have adequately investigated the effects of loperamide during pregnancy or breastfeeding. If you are pregnant or plan to become pregnant, or if you are breastfeeding or plan to do so, ask your health-care practitioner about taking loperamide. Only a health-care practitioner can determine whether its potential benefits outweigh the risks.

SPECIAL INFORMATION FOR SENIORS
Seniors are more susceptible to side effects such as constipation and dehydration. Lower doses are generally recommended.

GENERIC NAME
Loracarbef
see Cephalosporin Antibiotics, page 256

GENERIC NAME
Loratadine
see Antihistamine-Decongestant Combinations, page 132

GENERIC NAME
Lorazepam

BRAND NAME
Ativan
Generic available

ABOUT THIS DRUG
Lorazepam is used to treat anxiety. It belongs to a class of central nervous system depressant drugs known as benzodiazepines. Lorazepam works by attaching to a site in the brain that results in decreased activity of nervous tissue.

SIDE EFFECTS
Although side effects from lorazepam are fairly common, they occur less frequently than with some other benzodiazepines. If symptoms are severe or prolonged, ask your health-care practitioner whether your dosage requires adjustment, and whether it is safe for you to continue taking this drug.

- *Common:* sedation, dizziness, weakness, unsteadiness, a hangover sensation on the day after bedtime use
- *Less Common or Rare:* sleep disturbances, agitation, disorientation, depression, appetite loss, headache, nausea, skin problems, eye problems, stomach and intestinal disorders

IMPORTANT PRECAUTIONS
Lorazepam should not be taken if you have narrow-angle glaucoma, excessively low blood pressure, primary depression or psychosis, or

kidney or liver failure. If you have mild-to-moderate kidney or liver impairment, the lowest effective dose of lorazepam is recommended. Also inform your health-care practitioner if you have asthma, emphysema, epilepsy, myasthenia gravis, or a low white blood cell count, or if you have ever experienced an allergic reaction to this drug or another benzodiazepine.

Lorazepam is recommended for short-term use (up to 4 months). Longer use can lead to physical and/or psychological addiction. This drug should be used with caution in anyone with a history of drug or alcohol abuse or depression.

Lorazepam can make you drowsy and less alert than usual. Until you know how this drug affects you, do not drive a car, operate machinery, or perform other tasks that require concentration.

DRUG INTERACTIONS

Tell your health-care practitioner and pharmacist if you are taking any other prescription or over-the-counter drugs, as well as any vitamins, herbs, or other supplements. Dosage adjustments may be necessary when you begin taking lorazepam. Possible drug interactions include the following:

- Macrolide antibiotics, heparin, probenecid, quetiapine, and valproic acid may increase the effects of lorazepam.
- Taking other central nervous system depressants along with lorazepam can result in respiratory depression.
- Combining lorazepam and clozapine may cause increased sedation and loss of muscle coordination.
- Birth control pills, theophylline, caffeine, and other stimulants reduce the effects of lorazepam.
- Combining lorazepam and phenytoin may result in altered levels of both drugs in the body.
- Taking lithium with lorazepam may cause a drop in body temperature.
- Do not drink alcohol while taking lorazepam. This combination worsens coordination and impairs mental function.
- Marijuana causes increased drowsiness and impaired physical function.

FOOD, VITAMIN, AND HERBAL INTERACTIONS

Do not drink grapefruit juice while taking lorazepam. Grapefruit juice slows the body's breakdown of benzodiazepine drugs, which can lead to their potentially dangerous concentration in the blood.

Do not take lorazepam with hops, kava, passionflower, and valerian. These can increase its sedative effects. Lorazepam should not be combined with hawthorn.

Avoid caffeinated beverages such as coffee, tea, and cola.

RECOMMENDED DOSAGE

Lorazepam comes as a tablet or liquid. Although the doses given below are typical, only your health-care practitioner can determine the dose and schedule that best fit your needs.

- *Children:* Lorazepam is not recommended for children under the age of 12.
- *Adults:* 1 to 2 mg daily in divided doses to start. Over time this can be increased as needed to a maximum daily dose of 10 mg in divided doses. If anxiety is accompanied by insomnia, your health-care practitioner may prescribe a single daily dose of 2 to 4 mg at bedtime.

Lorazepam can be taken with or without food. If you forget a dose, take it as soon as you remember. If it is almost time for the next dose, skip the missed one and resume your normal schedule. Never take a double dose. If you have been taking lorazepam for more than 4 weeks, do not stop taking it suddenly. Abrupt withdrawal can lead to symptoms such as cramps, vomiting, sweating, tremor, ringing in the ears, sleep disturbances, depression, and convulsions. Speak to your health-care practitioner about gradually reducing dosage.

SYMPTOMS OF OVERDOSE AND WHAT TO DO

The symptoms of lorazepam overdose include drowsiness, sluggishness, confusion, lack of coordination, low blood pressure, and coma. If overdose occurs, seek immediate medical attention and take the prescription bottle to the hospital with you.

SPECIAL INFORMATION FOR PREGNANT OR NURSING WOMEN

Do not take lorazepam if you are pregnant or planning to become pregnant. This drug is associated with an increased risk of birth effects. Since lorazepam may pass into breast milk, breastfeeding is not advisable while taking this medication.

SPECIAL INFORMATION FOR SENIORS

Side effects such as lethargy, fatigue, and weakness are more likely to occur in older people. Smaller doses are generally recommended, especially at the beginning of therapy.

OPEN QUESTIONS OR CONTROVERSIES
Lorazepam can cause psychological and/or physical dependence. Tolerance may develop with long-term use, making it less effective. Do not take a larger dose of lorazepam, take it more often, or use it for a longer period that your health-care practitioner recommends. This is not an appropriate remedy for anxiety related to everyday stress.

GENERIC NAME

Losartan potassium

see Angiotensin II Blockers, page 123

GENERIC NAME

Lovastatin

see Statin Cholesterol-Lowering Drugs, page 959

GENERIC NAME

Malathion

BRAND NAME

Ovide
No generic available

ABOUT THIS DRUG

Malathion is a lotion applied to the scalp to treat head lice and their eggs. This drug is an extremely toxic substance once used as an agricultural insecticide. Because the potential for absorption through the skin is not known, extreme care must be exercised when using this drug.

Malathion works by inhibiting cholinesterase activity.

SIDE EFFECTS

Consult your health-care practitioner if you experience side effects when using malathion. If stinging or skin irritation are severe, you will probably be advised to discontinue use.

- *Common:* slight stinging sensation, irritation to the skin and scalp, conjunctivitis due to accidental eye contact

- *Less Common or Rare:* If too much malathion is absorbed through the skin, symptoms of overdose may occur. (See "Symptoms of Overdose and What to Do.")

IMPORTANT PRECAUTIONS

Malathion is for external use only. If it is accidentally swallowed, induce vomiting and proceed to the nearest hospital. Bring the malathion container with you.

If lotion accidentally gets in the eyes, flush them immediately with plenty of water. Call your health-care practitioner if eye irritation persists or if you experience vision changes.

Malathion lotion is flammable. Do not use a hair dryer, electric curlers, or any other electric heat source on wet hair. Stay away from lit cigarettes, candles, or any other open flame.

Do not apply malathion if you have broken skin or open sores on your scalp or neck.

Always inform your health-care practitioner about any other medical conditions you suffer from. Malathion should be used with caution if you have asthma, severe anemia, a history of a recent heart attack or brain surgery, low blood pressure, slow heartbeat, stomach ulcer, dehydration, liver disease, malnutrition, or a seizure disorder.

Head lice are easily transferred from one person to another via direct contact or by touching the clothing, hats, hairbrushes, or other items of infected people. To prevent infection or reinfection, wash clothing, bedding, and towels in very hot water; soak hairbrushes and combs in hot water and do not share them with others; and thoroughly vacuum your home (including upholstered furniture).

DRUG INTERACTIONS

Inform your health-care practitioner and pharmacist if you are taking any other prescription or over-the-counter drugs, as well as any vitamins, herbs, or other supplements. Possible drug interactions include the following:

- Avoid exposure to other insecticides during treatment with malathion.
- Combining malathion with glaucoma eyedrops or local anesthetics may lead to increased side effects.

FOOD, VITAMIN, AND HERBAL INTERACTIONS

No food, vitamin, or herbal interactions have been noted.

RECOMMENDED DOSAGE

Malathion comes as a lotion. Follow dosage instructions exactly. Using too much of this toxic substance may cause serious adverse reactions. Safety has not been established in children under the age of six. To use malathion lotion, follow these instructions:

- Malathion lotion should be used on children only under the direct supervision of an adult.
- Apply a small amount of lotion to *dry* hair. Use just enough to thoroughly wet the hair and scalp. Pay special attention to the back of the head and neck.
- Immediately wash hands after application.
- Allow hair to dry naturally and remain uncovered.
- Because malathion lotion is flammable, do not use a hair dryer or other electric heat source on wet hair, and stay away from any open flame.
- A slight stinging sensation is natural. But if skin irritation occurs, wash scalp and hair immediately.
- After 8 to 12 hours, shampoo hair.
- Rinse and use a fine-toothed comb to remove any nits (lice eggs).
- If lice are still detected after 7 to 9 days, repeat the process.

SYMPTOMS OF OVERDOSE AND WHAT TO DO

No specific information on overdosing with malathion lotion is available. However, symptoms that may occur include severe respiratory distress, cramps, sweating, depression, drowsiness, dizziness, confusion, trembling, weakness, restlessness, anxiety, slow heartbeat, and seizures. If you suspect an overdose, seek immediate medical attention and take the prescription container to the hospital with you.

SPECIAL INFORMATION FOR PREGNANT OR NURSING WOMEN

No studies have adequately investigated the effects of malathion during pregnancy or breastfeeding. However, if you are or think you may be pregnant, or if you are breastfeeding, consult your health-care practitioner before using this extremely toxic drug (either on yourself or applying it to another person's scalp). Only your health-care practitioner can determine if the benefits outweigh the potential dangers.

SPECIAL INFORMATION FOR SENIORS

There are no special guidelines for seniors.

GENERIC NAME

Maprotiline

BRAND NAME

Ludiomil
Generic available

ABOUT THIS DRUG

Maprotiline is used to relieve symptoms of major depression. It belongs to the drug class of tetracyclic antidepressants.

Maprotiline works by affecting the neurotransmitter norepinephrine, which is believed to impact mood, emotions, and mental state.

SIDE EFFECTS

Contact your health-care practitioner if you experience any side effects while taking maprotiline. Only he or she can determine whether you should continue to take this drug.

- ➤ *Common:* dizziness, drowsiness, visual problems, dry mouth, headache, sexual dysfunction, fatigue
- ➤ *Less Common and Rare:* diarrhea, constipation, heartburn, increased sensitivity to light, insomnia, weight loss, weight gain, increased sweating, fever, palpitations, breast enlargement, confusion, hallucinations, jaundice, skin swelling, redness, itching

IMPORTANT PRECAUTIONS

Tell your health-care practitioner if you have ever had any unusual or allergic reactions to maprotiline or to tricyclic antidepressants.

Consult your health-care practitioner before taking maprotiline if you have any of the following medical conditions: seizure disorder, asthma, difficulty urinating, enlarged prostate, glaucoma, mental illness, gastrointestinal problems, history of alcohol abuse, heart or blood vessel disease, hyperactive thyroid, or liver disease.

Because maprotiline can cause drowsiness, dizziness, and blurred vision, do not drive a car, operate machinery, or perform other tasks that require concentration until you know how the drug affects you.

Before you undergo any type of dental or medical surgery or

emergency treatment, tell the health-care practitioner that you are taking maprotiline.

Maprotiline can cause dry mouth, which can be alleviated by chewing sugarless gum, melting ice in your mouth, or using a saliva substitute. If dry mouth continues for more than two weeks despite your efforts to eliminate it, consult with your health-care practitioner.

DRUG INTERACTIONS

Inform your health-care practitioner if you are taking any other prescription or over-the-counter drugs, as well as any vitamins, herbs, or other supplements. Possible drug interactions include the following:

- Taking amphetamines, appetite suppressants, asthma medications, and any prescription or over-the-counter medications for colds, sinus problems, allergies, or hay fever may cause serious effects on your heart and blood pressure.
- Central nervous system depressants (e.g., sedatives) may increase the central nervous system effects.
- MAO inhibitors (e.g., isocarboxazid, phenelzine) should not be taken along with or within 14 days of maprotiline. At least 14 days should pass between stopping treatment with one medication and starting another.

FOOD, VITAMIN, AND HERBAL INTERACTIONS

Do not combine maprotiline with dietary supplements such as dong quai, hops, kava, passionflower, St. John's wort, valerian, SAMe, or 5-HTP. Consult your physician before taking this drug with grapefruit juice.

RECOMMENDED DOSAGE

Maprotiline comes as a tablet. Although the doses given below are typical, only your doctor can determine the dose and schedule that best fit your needs.

- *Children:* to be determined by your health-care practitioner
- *Adults:* starting dose is 25 mg one to three times daily. Your health-care practitioner may increase your dose as needed. Maximum dosage is 150 mg daily.

If you miss a dose and you normally take only one dose at bedtime, do not take the forgotten dose in the morning. Call your health-care practitioner for advice. If you take maprotiline more than once daily and you miss a dose, take it as soon as you remember. However, if it is nearly time for the next dose, skip the missed dose and resume your regular dosing schedule. Never take a double dose.

SYMPTOMS OF OVERDOSE AND WHAT TO DO

Symptoms of overdose can include severe dizziness or drowsiness, nausea, vomiting, irregular heartbeat, seizures, breathing difficulties, fever, muscle stiffness, or fatigue. If an overdose occurs, seek immediate medical assistance and bring the prescription container with you to the hospital.

SPECIAL PRECAUTIONS FOR PREGNANT OR NURSING WOMEN

No studies have adequately investigated the effects of maprotiline during pregnancy. If you are pregnant or plan to become pregnant, talk with your health-care practitioner before starting this drug so the potential benefits and dangers can be weighed.

Maprotiline passes into breast milk. Your health-care practitioner will likely advise you to bottle feed until your treatment is complete.

SPECIAL PRECAUTIONS FOR SENIORS

Seniors are more likely to experience adverse reactions, and they may be more severe.

GENERIC NAME

Mazindol

BRAND NAMES

Mazanor, Sanorex

No generic available

ABOUT THIS DRUG

Mazindol is an appetite suppressant used in the treatment of obesity. This drug should be used on a short-term basis only and under a health-care practitioner's close supervision. Appetite suppressants are not a substitute for a sensible, healthy, overall weight loss program. Although not an amphetamine, mazindol works by affecting similar parts of the brain.

SIDE EFFECTS

If you develop side effects while taking mazindol, ask your health-care practitioner whether it is safe for you to continue taking this drug.

- *Common:* overstimulation, nervousness, restlessness, difficulty sleeping, a sense of euphoria, false sense of well-being, "feeling high"
- *Less Common or Rare:* high blood pressure, palpitations, dizziness, blurred vision, tremors, headache, sweating, chills, fever, weakness, changes in sex drive, nausea, vomiting, diarrhea, dry mouth, difficulty urinating, rash, itching, hair loss, muscle pain

IMPORTANT PRECAUTIONS

This drug is not an appropriate remedy for people who have heart disease, high blood pressure, glaucoma, or thyroid disease. Do not use mazindol if you have experienced an allergic reaction to this or other appetite suppressants. Because appetite suppressants have habit-forming potential, inform your health-care practitioner if you have a history of mental illness or substance abuse. If you have diabetes, mazindol may alter the amount of medication you require.

In order to lose weight, follow a reduced calorie diet while taking mazindol. To keep weight off, continue to follow a sensible program of diet and exercise under the supervision of your health-care practitioner.

Mazindol makes some people dizzy, lightheaded, and less alert than usual. Until you know how this drug affects you, do not drive a car, operate machinery, or engage in other actions that require concentration.

Because mazindol may cause dryness in the mouth, use sugarless candy or gum, ice chips, or a saliva substitute. If the problem continues, consult your health-care practitioner or dentist.

Before having surgery or a dental procedure, tell your health-care practitioner or dentist that you take mazindol.

If you have a urine test while taking mazindol, you may test positive for amphetamines.

DRUG INTERACTIONS

Tell your health-care practitioner and pharmacist if you are taking any other prescription or over-the-counter drugs, as well as any vitamins, herbs, or other supplements. Possible drug interactions include the following:

- Do not take mazindol with or within 14 days of taking a monoamine oxidase (MAO) inhibitor. This combination can cause very high blood pressure.
- Diabetes and asthma medications may require adjustment when you take mazindol.

- Mazindol may reduce the effects of high blood pressure medications.
- Combining mazindol with other stimulants (such as other appetite suppressants, amphetamines, methylphenidate, caffeine, or cocaine) can result in unwanted effects ranging from overstimulation to heart problems.
- Taking tricyclic antidepressants with mazindol may cause high blood pressure or an irregular heartbeat.
- Be careful when you use over-the-counter remedies while taking mazindol. Many cough, cold, sinus, and allergy remedies raise blood pressure.

FOOD, VITAMIN, AND HERBAL INTERACTIONS

Do not take mazindol with herbs that raise blood pressure, such as ephedra (ma huang), ginseng, goldenseal, or saw palmetto.

Moderate your consumption of caffeinated beverages such as coffee, tea, and cola.

RECOMMENDED DOSAGE

Mazindol comes in tablet form. The doses given below are typical, but only your health-care practitioner can determine the dose and schedule that best fit your particular needs.

- *Children:* This drug is not recommended for children under the age of 16.
- *Adults:* 1 to 2 mg once daily

Take mazindol with food or milk to prevent stomach upset. To prevent trouble sleeping, take medication 10 to 14 hours before bedtime. Swallow tablets whole; do not break, crush, or chew them. If you find that several weeks of therapy do not affect your appetite, do not increase the dose. Consult your health-care practitioner. If you miss a dose, skip it. Never take double doses.

SYMPTOMS OF OVERDOSE AND WHAT TO DO

The symptoms of mazindol overdose include nausea, vomiting, diarrhea, blood pressure changes, confusion, restlessness, clammy skin, tremors, hallucinations, and fever. If overdose occurs, seek immediate medical attention and take the bottle of mazindol to the hospital with you.

SPECIAL INFORMATION FOR PREGNANT OR NURSING WOMEN

Large doses of mazindol may cause birth defects. If you are or think you may be pregnant, consult your health-care practitioner before using this drug. Only your health-care practitioner can determine if the benefits outweigh the potential dangers. It is not known whether mazindol passes into breast milk. However, if you are breastfeeding, your health-care practitioner will likely advise you to stop until your treatment is done.

SPECIAL INFORMATION FOR SENIORS

Mazindol aggravates many diseases associated with old age, including heart disease, high blood pressure, and diabetes.

OPEN QUESTIONS OR CONTROVERSIES

Appetite suppressants can cause dependence. They should be used on a short-term basis only, and should be avoided by those with a history of mental illness or drug or alcohol abuse. Signs of dependence include a strong need for medication, a desire to increase the dosage, and withdrawal symptoms (such as depression, cramps, nausea, and fatigue) when you stop taking mazindol.

GENERIC NAME

Meclizine

BRAND NAMES

Antivert, Bonine
Generic available

ABOUT THIS DRUG

Meclizine is an antihistamine used for the treatment of nausea, vomiting, and dizziness associated with motion sickness. This drug works by countering the effects of histamine, a chemical released by your body that can cause irritating effects.

SIDE EFFECTS

If you develop side effects while taking meclizine, ask your health-care practitioner whether it is safe for you to continue taking this drug.

- *Common:* drowsiness, dry mouth
- *Less Common or Rare:* blurred vision

IMPORTANT PRECAUTIONS

Meclizine should be used with caution in people who suffer from asthma, glaucoma, and enlargement of the prostate gland.

This drug can make you drowsy. Until you know how meclizine affects you, do not drive a car, operate machinery, or perform other tasks that require concentration.

DRUG INTERACTIONS

Tell your health-care practitioner and pharmacist if you are taking any other prescription or over-the-counter drugs, as well as any vitamins, herbs, or other supplements. Possible drug interactions include the following:

- Do not drink alcohol while you are taking meclizine.

FOOD, VITAMIN, AND HERBAL INTERACTIONS

No food, vitamin, or herbal interactions have been noted.

RECOMMENDED DOSAGE

Meclizine comes in tablet form. Although the doses given below are typical, only your health-care practitioner can determine the dose and schedule that best fit your individual needs.

- *Children:* This drug is not recommended for children under the age of 12.
- *Adults:* Take 25 to 50 mg one hour before traveling. This dose may be repeated every 24 hours for the duration of your trip.

Pay close attention to correct dosage, and take only on an as-needed basis.

SYMPTOMS OF OVERDOSE AND WHAT TO DO

No specific information is available regarding meclizine overdose. However, if you suspect that an overdose has occurred, seek immediate medical attention and take the bottle of meclizine to the hospital with you so the health-care practitioner will know exactly what medication was taken.

SPECIAL INFORMATION FOR PREGNANT OR NURSING WOMEN

No studies have adequately investigated the effects of meclizine during pregnancy. If you are pregnant or planning to become pregnant, or if you are breastfeeding, consult your health-care practitioner about taking this medication. Only a health-care practitioner can determine whether the potential benefits outweigh the risks.

SPECIAL INFORMATION FOR SENIORS

There are no special instructions for seniors.

GENERIC NAME

Meclocycline sulfosalicylate

see Tetracycline Antibiotics, page 1013

GENERIC NAME

Meclofenamate

BRAND NAME

Meclomen
Generic available

ABOUT THIS DRUG

Meclofenamate is a nonsteroidal anti-inflammatory drug (NSAID) prescribed for the relief of pain associated with osteoarthritis, rheumatoid arthritis, and menorrhagia (excessive menstrual bleeding). Pain relief usually comes shortly after taking your first dose, while the full anti-inflammatory impact occurs 2 to 3 weeks into therapy. This drug works by reducing the level of prostaglandins, chemicals in the body that produce inflammation and pain.

SIDE EFFECTS

Consult your health-care practitioner if you experience side effects while taking meclofenamate. Only he or she can determine whether it is safe for you to continue taking this drug.

- ➤ *Common:* diarrhea, constipation, stomach upset, gas, nausea, vomiting, drowsiness, fluid retention, ringing in the ears, appetite loss
- ➤ *Less Common or Rare:* headache, dizziness, blurred vision, confusion, fainting, tingling in the hands or feet, mouth sores, rash, hives,

itching, heart palpitations, difficulty breathing, gastrointestinal bleeding, ulcers, painful urination, kidney damage

IMPORTANT PRECAUTIONS

Like all NSAIDs, meclofenamate can cause gastrointestinal bleeding, ulcers, and stomach perforation. If you take this drug on a regular basis, these types of side effects can occur at any time, with or without warning. People with a history of gastrointestinal disorders such as ulcers, colitis, or bleeding should be extremely careful when taking this drug.

Do not take meclofenamate if you have a bleeding disorder (such as hemophilia) or asthma or nasal polyps associated with aspirin use. Use this drug with caution if you have high blood pressure or other heart problems or impaired liver or kidney function. Tell your health-care practitioner if you have ever experienced an allergic reaction to aspirin or related drugs.

Meclofenamate may cause dizziness or altered vision. Until you know how this drug affects you, do not drive a car, operate machinery, or perform other tasks that require concentration.

Meclofenamate may cause increased sun sensitivity. Wear protective clothing and apply sunscreen when using this drug.

DRUG INTERACTIONS

Inform your health-care practitioner and pharmacist if you are taking any other prescription or over-the-counter drugs, as well as any vitamins, herbs, or other supplements. Possible drug interactions include the following:

- Do not combine aspirin, ibuprofen, or other prescription or over-the-counter NSAIDs with meclofenamate. This increases the risk of bleeding.
- Other drugs that may increase the risk of bleeding include dipyridamole, sulfinpyrazone, valproic acid, and blood thinners such as warfarin.
- Taking meclofenamate with antihypertensive medications such as ACE inhibitors, beta-blockers, and diuretics decreases their blood pressure lowering effects.
- The combination of meclofenamate and ofloxacin can result in an increased risk of seizures.
- Taking meclofenamate with lithium or methotrexate can lead to toxic levels of lithium or methotrexate in the body.
- The combination of sulfonylureas and meclofenamate may increase the risk of hypoglycemia.

- Do not use alcohol while you are taking meclofenamate. Both are stomach irritants, and using them together can increase the risk of stomach bleeding and ulcers.

FOOD, VITAMIN, AND HERBAL INTERACTIONS

Do not combine meclofenamate with the herbal remedies clove oil, feverfew, garlic, ginkgo, and ginseng. These herbs affect clotting.

RECOMMENDED DOSAGE

Meclofenamate comes in capsule form. Low starting doses and smallest effective doses are recommended. Although the doses given below are typical, only your health-care practitioner can determine the dose and schedule that best fit your individual needs.

Osteoarthritis and Rheumatoid Arthritis

- *Children:* This drug is not recommended for children under the age of 14.
- *Adults:* 200 to 400 mg daily in divided doses

Menorrhagia

- *Children:* This drug is not recommended for children under the age of 14.
- *Adults:* 300 mg daily in divided doses, for up to 6 days

Take meclofenamate after meals to prevent stomach upset. Take medication with an 8-ounce glass of water and remain sitting upright or standing (do not lie down) for 30 minutes. If you forget to take a dose, take it as soon as you remember. But if it is almost time for the next dose, skip the one you missed and resume your normal schedule. Never take a double dose.

SYMPTOMS OF OVERDOSE AND WHAT TO DO

Symptoms of meclofenamate overdose include nausea, vomiting, diarrhea, abdominal pain, drowsiness, rapid breathing, rapid heartbeat, agitation, confusion, disorientation, sweating, ringing in the ears, stupor, and seizures. If an overdose occurs, seek immediate medical attention and take the prescription bottle to the hospital with you so the health-care practitioner will know exactly what medication was taken.

SPECIAL INFORMATION FOR PREGNANT OR NURSING WOMEN

No studies have adequately investigated the effects of meclofenamate during pregnancy. If you are pregnant or planning to become pregnant, consult your health-care practitioner about taking this medication. Only a health-care practitioner can determine whether the potential benefits outweigh the risks. Because meclofenamate may pass into breast milk, it is best to stop breastfeeding while you take this drug.

SPECIAL INFORMATION FOR SENIORS

Smaller doses are recommended for seniors, who are more susceptible to side effects such as diarrhea, dizziness, confusion, fluid retention, stomach ulcers, and kidney or liver effects.

GENERIC NAME

Medroxyprogesterone acetate

see Progestins, page 876

GENERIC NAME

Mefenamic acid

BRAND NAME

Ponstel

Generic available

ABOUT THIS DRUG

Mefenamic acid is a nonsteroidal anti-inflammatory drug (NSAID) used to treat pain, such as menstrual and postoperative pain. Taking this drug for more than seven days is not recommended. Mefenamic acid works by reducing the level of prostaglandins, chemicals in the body that produce inflammation and pain.

SIDE EFFECTS

If you develop side effects while taking mefenamic acid, ask your health-care practitioner whether it is safe for you to continue taking this drug.

➤ *Common:* diarrhea, constipation, stomach upset, gas, nausea, vomiting, drowsiness, fluid retention, ringing in the ears, appetite loss

- *Less Common or Rare:* headache, dizziness, blurred vision, confusion, fainting, tingling in the hands or feet, mouth sores, fatigue, weakness, abnormal bleeding or bruising, rash, hives, itching, heart palpitations, difficulty breathing, gastrointestinal bleeding, ulcers, painful urination, kidney damage

IMPORTANT PRECAUTIONS

Like all NSAIDs, mefenamic acid can cause gastrointestinal bleeding, ulcers, and stomach perforation. If you take this drug on a regular basis, these types of side effects can occur at any time, with or without warning. People with a history of ulcers, colitis, or any type of gastrointestinal bleeding should be extremely careful when taking mefenamic acid.

Do not take mefenamic acid if you have a bleeding disorder or asthma or nasal polyps associated with aspirin use. Use this drug with caution if you have high blood pressure or other heart problems or impaired liver or kidney function. Tell your health-care practitioner if you have ever experienced an allergic reaction to aspirin or related drugs.

Mefenamic acid may make you drowsy. Until you know how this drug affects you, do not drive a car, operate machinery, or perform other tasks that require concentration.

Mefenamic acid may cause increased sun sensitivity. Wear protective clothing and apply sunscreen when using this drug.

DRUG INTERACTIONS

Tell your health-care practitioner and pharmacist if you are taking any other prescription or over-the-counter drugs, as well as any vitamins, herbs, or other supplements. Possible drug interactions include the following:

- Do not combine aspirin, ibuprofen, or other prescription or over-the-counter NSAIDs with mefenamic acid. This increases the risk of bleeding.
- Other drugs that may increase the risk of bleeding include dipyridamole, sulfinpyrazone, valproic acid, and blood thinners such as warfarin.
- Taking mefenamic acid with antihypertensive medications such as ACE inhibitors, beta-blockers, and diuretics decreases their blood pressure lowering effects.
- The combination of mefenamic acid and ofloxacin can result in an increased risk of seizures.
- Taking mefenamic acid with lithium or methotrexate can lead to toxic levels of lithium or methotrexate in the body.

- The combination of sulfonylurea drugs and mefenamic acid may increase the risk of hypoglycemia.
- Do not use alcohol when you are taking mefenamic acid. Both are stomach irritants, and using them together can increase the risk of stomach bleeding and ulcers.

FOOD, VITAMIN, AND HERBAL INTERACTIONS

Do not combine mefenamic acid with the herbal remedies clove oil, feverfew, garlic, ginkgo, and ginseng. These herbs may affect clotting.

RECOMMENDED DOSAGE

Mefenamic acid comes in capsule form. Low starting doses and smallest effective doses are recommended. The doses given below are typical. However, only your health-care practitioner can determine the dose and schedule that best fit your individual needs.

- *Children:* This drug is not recommended for children under the age of 14.
- *Adults:* 500 mg to start, followed by 250 mg every 6 hours as needed for up to 7 days

Mefenamic acid can be taken with food or milk to prevent stomach upset. Take medication with an 8-ounce glass of water and remain sitting upright or standing (do not lie down) for 30 minutes. If you forget to take a dose, take it as soon as you remember. But if it is almost time for the next dose, skip the one you missed and resume your normal schedule. Never take a double dose.

SYMPTOMS OF OVERDOSE AND WHAT TO DO

Symptoms of mefenamic acid overdose include nausea, vomiting, diarrhea, abdominal pain, drowsiness, rapid breathing, rapid heartbeat, agitation, confusion, disorientation, sweating, ringing in the ears, stupor, and seizures. If an overdose occurs, seek immediate medical attention and take the bottle of mefenamic acid to the hospital with you so the health-care practitioner will know exactly what medication was taken.

SPECIAL INFORMATION FOR PREGNANT OR NURSING WOMEN

Use of mefenamic acid should be avoided in late pregnancy. If you want to take this drug in early pregnancy, ask your health-care practitioner whether the potential benefits outweigh the risks. Because mefenamic acid may pass into breast milk, it is best to stop breastfeeding while you take this drug.

SPECIAL INFORMATION FOR SENIORS

Smaller doses are recommended for seniors, who are more susceptible to side effects such as diarrhea, dizziness, confusion, fluid retention, stomach ulcers, and kidney or liver effects.

GENERIC NAME

Megestrol

see Progestins, page 876

GENERIC NAME

Meloxicam

BRAND NAME

Mobic
No generic available

ABOUT THIS DRUG

Meloxicam is a nonsteroidal anti-inflammatory drug (NSAID) used to relieve the pain and inflammation of arthritis. Like all NSAIDs, meloxicam can cause gastrointestinal bleeding and ulcers. This drug works by reducing the level of prostaglandins, chemicals in the body that produce inflammation and pain.

SIDE EFFECTS

Tell your health-care practitioner if you develop side effects while taking meloxicam. Only he or she can determine whether it is safe for you to continue taking this drug.

➤ *Common:* diarrhea, stomach upset, indigestion, gas, heartburn

➤ *Less Common or Rare:* abdominal pain, anxiety, confusion, constipation, nausea, vomiting, dry mouth, sun sensitivity, headache, dizziness, blurred vision, fainting, tingling in the hands or feet, fatigue, weakness, skin eruptions, hives, heart problems, difficulty breathing, gastrointestinal bleeding, ulcers, painful urination, kidney damage, bloody or black, tarry stools

Certain effects associated with meloxicam can be life-threatening. Seek immediate medical attention if you experience symptoms such as fast or irregular breathing, wheezing, fainting, change in skin color, swelling of the eyelids or face, swelling of the extremities, hives, severe stomach pain, black, tarry stools, or vomiting material that looks like coffee grounds.

IMPORTANT PRECAUTIONS

Like all NSAIDs, meloxicam can cause gastrointestinal bleeding, ulcers, and stomach perforation. If you take this drug on a regular basis, these types of side effects can occur at any time, with or without warning.

Do not take meloxicam if you have asthma or nasal polyps associated with aspirin use, ulcers, colitis, gastrointestinal bleeding, or a bleeding or blood cell disorder. Use this drug with caution if you have high blood pressure or other heart problems, dehydration or fluid retention, impaired liver or kidney function, or a bleeding disorder. Tell your health-care practitioner if you have ever experienced an allergic reaction to aspirin or related drugs.

Meloxicam may make you drowsy. Until you know how this drug affects you, do not drive a car, operate machinery, or perform other tasks that require concentration.

Meloxicam may cause increased sun sensitivity. Wear protective clothing and apply sunscreen when using this drug.

DRUG INTERACTIONS

Tell your health-care practitioner and pharmacist if you are taking any other prescription or over-the-counter drugs, as well as any vitamins, herbs, or other supplements. Possible drug interactions include the following:

- Do not combine aspirin, ibuprofen, or other prescription or over-the-counter NSAIDs with meloxicam. This increases the risk of bleeding.
- Other drugs that may increase the risk of bleeding include blood thinners such as warfarin.
- Taking meloxicam with antihypertensive medications such as ACE inhibitors may decrease their blood pressure lowering effects.
- Taking meloxicam with lithium can lead to toxic levels of lithium in the body.
- Combining meloxicam with alcohol increases the risk of stomach bleeding and ulcers.

FOOD, VITAMIN, AND HERBAL INTERACTIONS

Do not combine meloxicam with the herbal remedies clove oil, feverfew, garlic, ginkgo, and ginseng. Like meloxicam, these herbs may affect clotting.

RECOMMENDED DOSAGE

Meloxicam comes in capsule form. Low starting doses and smallest effective doses are recommended. Although the doses given below are typical, only your health-care practitioner can determine the dose and schedule that best fit your individual needs.

- *Children:* This drug is not recommended for children.
- *Adults:* 7.5 to 15 mg once daily

Take meloxicam with food or milk to prevent stomach upset. If you forget to take a dose, take it as soon as you remember. But if it is almost time for the next dose, skip the one you missed and resume your normal schedule. Never take double doses.

SYMPTOMS OF OVERDOSE AND WHAT TO DO

Symptoms of meloxicam overdose include fast or irregular breathing, wheezing, unusual fatigue, fainting, heartbeat changes, tight chest, blurred vision, confusion, fever, chills, swelling of the eyelids or face, rash, severe stomach pain, black, tarry stools, vomiting material that looks like coffee grounds, pounding in the ears, yellow eyes or skin, blue lips, fingernails, or skin, and convulsions. If an overdose occurs, seek immediate medical attention and take the bottle of meloxicam to the hospital with you so the health-care practitioner will know exactly what medication was taken.

SPECIAL INFORMATION FOR PREGNANT OR NURSING WOMEN

No studies have adequately investigated the effects of meloxicam during pregnancy. If you are pregnant or plan to become pregnant, talk with your health-care practitioner before starting this drug. Only a health-care practitioner can determine whether the potential benefits outweigh the risks. Because meloxicam may pass into breast milk, it is best to stop breastfeeding while you take this drug.

SPECIAL INFORMATION FOR SENIORS

There are no special instructions for seniors.

GENERIC NAME

Memantine

BRAND NAME

Namenda
No generic available

ABOUT THIS DRUG

Memantine is an NMDA (N-methyl-d-aspartate) receptor antagonist used to treat moderate to severe Alzheimer's disease. It can help slow progression of the disease; it is not a cure.

Memantine appears to protect the brain cells against high levels of glutamate, a chemical that is released at high levels by cells that have been damaged by Alzheimer's disease. This drug regulates the release of glutamate.

SIDE EFFECTS

Be sure to tell your health-care practitioner if you experience any side effects while taking memantine. Only your health-care practitioner can determine whether it is safe for you to continue taking this drug.

- *Most Common:* confusion, constipation, dizziness, headache
- *Less Common/Rare:* back pain, cough, fatigue, hallucinations, vomiting

IMPORTANT PRECAUTIONS

Tell your health-care practitioner if you are sensitive or allergic to memantine or to any other drugs.

Do not take memantine if you have severe kidney failure.

Because memantine can cause dizziness, you should make sure you know how you react to the drug before you drive or operate hazardous equipment.

DRUG INTERACTIONS

Tell your health-care practitioner and pharmacist if you are taking any prescription or nonprescription drugs, as well as any vitamins, herbs, or other supplements. Possible drug interactions include the following:

- Use of memantine with other NMDA antagonists (e.g., amantadine, ketamine) has not been evaluated and should be approached with caution.
- Side effects may occur if you take memantine with cimetidine, hydrochlorothiazide, nicotine, quinidine, ranitidine, triamterene, sodium bicarbonate, or acetazolamide.

FOOD, VITAMIN, AND HERBAL INTERACTIONS

No food, vitamin, or herbal interactions have been noted.

RECOMMENDED DOSAGE

Memantine is available in 5- and 10-mg tablets. The dosages given here are typical. However, your health-care practitioner will determine the most appropriate dose and schedule for your needs.

- *Children*: Not indicated for use in children
- *Adults*: 5 mg once daily as a starting dose. Your health-care practitioner may increase your dose in 5-mg increments weekly until 20 mg daily is reached. Doses greater than 5 mg are taken twice daily.

Memantine can be taken with or without food. If you miss a dose, take it as soon as you remember. If it is nearly time for your next dose, skip the missed dose and return to your normal dosing schedule. Never take a double dose.

SYMPTOMS OF OVERDOSE AND WHAT TO DO

Symptoms of overdose may include restlessness, abnormal psychologic behavior, visual hallucinations, somnolence, and loss of consciousness. If overdose occurs, seek immediate medical attention and bring the prescription container with you to the hospital.

SPECIAL INFORMATION FOR PREGNANT OR NURSING WOMEN

Adequate studies of the effects of memantine on pregnant or nursing women have not been done. If you are pregnant or plan to become pregnant, talk to your health-care practitioner.

SPECIAL INFORMATION FOR SENIORS

Side effects are more likely to occur and are more severe in older adults.

GENERIC NAME

Meperidine

BRAND NAME

Demerol

Generic available

ABOUT THIS DRUG

Meperidine is a narcotic analgesic prescribed to relieve moderate to severe pain. This medication is best limited to short-term use. If narcotics are used for a long time, physical and/or psychological dependence may develop.

Meperidine acts on the central nervous system. It works by depressing select brain functions and suppressing the perception of pain.

SIDE EFFECTS

Inform your health-care practitioner if you develop side effects while taking meperidine. If symptoms are severe or prolonged, ask your health-care practitioner whether your dosage requires adjustment, and whether it is safe for you to continue taking this drug.

- *Common:* drowsiness, weakness, feeling faint, lightheadedness, euphoria, dry mouth, constipation, urinary retention
- *Less Common or Rare:* nausea, vomiting, headache, dizziness, agitation, confusion, mental sluggishness, disorientation, depression, blurred or double vision, impaired concentration, sensation of drunkenness, slow heartbeat, heart palpitations, flushing, sweating, hallucinations, restlessness, muscle twitching, uncoordinated muscle movements, hives, seizures

IMPORTANT PRECAUTIONS

Always inform your health-care practitioner about any other medical conditions you may have. Meperidine should not be taken if you have an abnormal heart rhythm, a head injury, respiratory depression, kidney failure, or a history of convulsions or seizures. Use this drug with caution if you have mild-to-moderate kidney or liver impairment, asthma, chronic bronchitis, emphysema, epilepsy, glaucoma, lung or thyroid disease, urinary problems, chronic constipation, or an enlarged prostate. Do not take meperidine during an asthma attack.

Meperidine can lead to physical and/or psychological dependence. This drug should be used with caution in anyone with a history of drug or alcohol abuse.

If you plan to undergo surgery or a dental procedure, tell your health-care practitioner or dentist that you are taking meperidine.

This drug can make you drowsy and less alert than usual. Until you know how meperidine affects you, do not drive a car, operate machinery, or perform other tasks that require concentration.

DRUG INTERACTIONS

Tell your health-care practitioner and pharmacist if you are taking any other prescription or over-the-counter drugs, as well as any vitamins, herbs, or other supplements. Possible drug interactions include the following:

- Do not take monoamine oxidase inhibitor (MAOI) antidepressants at the same time as or within 14 days of meperidine.
- Tricyclic antidepressants increase the risk of respiratory depression.
- Combining tramadol with meperidine increases seizure risk.
- Taking other central nervous system depressants along with meperidine can result in more drowsiness.
- Combining acyclovir with meperidine boosts the risk of nerve toxicity.
- Drugs such as cimetidine, famotidine, ranitidine, and omeprazole increase blood levels and thus the effects of meperidine.
- Combining meperidine with atropinelike drugs raises the risks of urinary retention and impaired intestinal function.
- Other drugs that may cause difficulties when taken with meperidine include phenothiazines, phenytoin, sibutramine, and ritonavir.
- Narcotics such as meperidine are not effective if you take naltrexone.
- Do not drink alcohol while taking meperidine.
- Marijuana causes increased drowsiness and pain relief, while impairing mental and physical function.

FOOD, VITAMIN, AND HERBAL INTERACTIONS

Do not take meperidine with herbs such as hops, kava, passionflower, and valerian. These can increase its sedative effects. Meperidine should not be combined with ginseng.

RECOMMENDED DOSAGE

Meperidine comes as a tablet or syrup. This drug is not recommended for children under age one. Although the doses given below are typical, only your health-care practitioner can determine the dose and schedule that best fit your needs.

- *Children 1 Year and Older:* 0.5 to 0.8 mg per pound of body weight every 3 to 4 hours
- *Adults:* 50 to 150 mg every 3 to 4 hours, with a maximum daily dose of 900 mg

To prevent stomach upset, the tablet can be crushed and taken with food. The syrup is usually mixed with a half glass of water (4 ounces) to reduce meperidine's numbing effect on your mouth and throat.

Meperidine must be taken exactly as directed. Too much medication can be habit-forming and can possibly lead to overdose. If you forget a dose, take it as soon as you remember. If it is almost time for the next dose, skip the missed one and resume your normal schedule. Never take a double dose. If you have been taking meperidine for several weeks and you feel it is not working, do not take a higher dose. Consult your health-care practitioner.

SYMPTOMS OF OVERDOSE AND WHAT TO DO

The symptoms of meperidine overdose may include drowsiness, sluggishness, confusion, tremors, low blood pressure, breathing problems, stupor, and coma. If overdose occurs, seek immediate medical attention and take the prescription bottle to the hospital with you.

SPECIAL INFORMATION FOR PREGNANT OR NURSING WOMEN

If you are pregnant or planning to become pregnant, discuss the potential risks versus the benefits of meperidine with your health-care practitioner. Narcotic use during pregnancy may cause the fetus to become drug-dependent, potentially leading to withdrawal effects after birth. Because this drug may pass into breast milk, breastfeeding is not advisable while taking it.

SPECIAL INFORMATION FOR SENIORS

Seniors are at higher risk of side effects such as drowsiness, dizziness, falling, constipation, and urinary retention. Smaller doses and short-term therapy are preferable.

OPEN QUESTIONS OR CONTROVERSIES

Meperidine can cause psychological and/or physical dependence. Tolerance may develop with long-term use, making it less effective. Do not take a larger dose of meperidine, take it more often, or use it for a longer period than your health-care practitioner recommends.

GENERIC NAME

Mephenytoin *see Phenytoin, page 840*

GENERIC NAME
Meprobamate

BRAND NAMES
Equanil, Meprospan, Miltown, Neuramate, Probate, Trancot
Generic available

ABOUT THIS DRUG
Meprobamate is used for the short-term relief of anxiety. Because it can be habit-forming, check with your health-care practitioner at least every 4 months to make sure that you still need to take this medication. Meprobamate should not be used to relieve nervousness and anxiety related to ordinary, everyday stress.

This drug works by acting on the central nervous system.

SIDE EFFECTS
Consult your health-care practitioner if you develop side effects from meprobamate. Only he or she can determine whether your dosage requires adjustment, and whether it is safe for you to continue taking this drug.

- *Common:* drowsiness, clumsiness, unsteadiness
- *Less Common or Rare:* nausea, vomiting, diarrhea, headache, dizziness, lightheadedness, false sense of well-being, tiredness, weakness, confusion, pounding heartbeat, inappropriate excitement, difficulty breathing, slurred speech, staggering, tingling sensations or numbness, fluid retention, vision problems, itchy rash, allergic reactions, breathing difficulty, chills, fever, blood disorders

Seek immediate medical attention if you experience allergic reactions such as shortness of breath, sore throat, fever, and rash.

IMPORTANT PRECAUTIONS
Always inform your health-care practitioner about all other disorders you may have, especially kidney or liver disease, porphyria, or epilepsy. If you have mild-to-moderate kidney or liver impairment, the lowest effective dose of meprobamate is recommended.

Meprobamate is recommended for short-term use only (up to 4 months). Longer use can lead to physical and/or psychological addiction. This may not be an appropriate remedy if you have a history of drug or alcohol abuse.

Meprobamate can make you drowsy and less alert than usual. Until you know how this drug affects you, do not drive a car, operate machinery, or perform other tasks that require concentration.

Meprobamate may cause dryness of the mouth. Use sugarless candy or gum, ice chips, or a saliva substitute. If the problem persists, consult your health-care practitioner or dentist.

DRUG INTERACTIONS

Tell your health-care practitioner and pharmacist if you are taking any other prescription or over-the-counter drugs, as well as any vitamins, herbs, or other supplements. Dosage adjustments may be necessary when you begin taking meprobamate. Possible drug interactions include the following:

- Consult your health-care practitioner before combining meprobamate with other central nervous system depressants, such as antihistamines, sedatives, tranquilizers, sleeping pills, barbiturates, muscle relaxants, seizure medications, cough and cold remedies, pain medication, and narcotics.
- Do not drink alcohol while taking meprobamate. This combination worsens coordination and impairs mental function.

FOOD, VITAMIN, AND HERBAL INTERACTIONS

Do not take meprobamate with hops, kava, passionflower, and valerian. These can increase its sedative effects. Avoid caffeinated beverages such as coffee, tea, and cola.

RECOMMENDED DOSAGE

Meprobamate comes in tablet form. The doses given below are typical. However, only your health-care practitioner can determine the dose and schedule that best match your particular needs. This drug is not recommended for children under age six.

- *Children 6 to 12 Years:* 100 to 200 mg 2 to 3 times daily
- *Children Older than 12 Years and Adults:* 400 mg 3 to 4 times daily, or 600 mg twice a day; maximum daily dose is 2,400 mg

Meprobamate can be taken with or without food. If you forget a dose, take it as soon as you remember. If it is almost time for the next dose, skip the missed one and resume your normal schedule. Never take a double dose. If you have been taking this drug for more than 4 weeks, do not stop taking it suddenly. Abrupt withdrawal can lead to symptoms such as anxiety, confusion, hallucinations, appetite loss, vomiting, tremor, sleep disturbances, loss of coordination, muscle twitching, and convulsions. Speak to your health-care practitioner about gradually reducing dosage.

SYMPTOMS OF OVERDOSE AND WHAT TO DO

The symptoms of meprobamate overdose include drowsiness, sluggishness, slurred speech, staggering, confusion, dizziness, lightheadedness, difficulty breathing, wheezing, slow heartbeat, shock, unresponsiveness, and coma. If overdose occurs, seek immediate medical attention and take the prescription bottle to the hospital with you.

SPECIAL INFORMATION FOR PREGNANT OR NURSING WOMEN

Do not take meprobamate if you are pregnant or planning to become pregnant. This drug is associated with an increased risk of birth effects. Since meprobamate may pass into breast milk, breastfeeding is not advisable while taking this medication.

SPECIAL INFORMATION FOR SENIORS

Smaller doses are generally recommended for seniors in order to avoid oversedation.

OPEN QUESTIONS OR CONTROVERSIES

Meprobamate can cause psychological and/or physical dependence. Tolerance may develop with long-term use, making it less effective. Do not take a larger dose of meprobamate, take it more often, or use it for a longer period than your health-care practitioner recommends. This is not an appropriate remedy for anxiety related to everyday stress.

GENERIC NAME

Mesalamine

BRAND NAMES

Asacol, Pentasa, Rowasa, 5-ASA
No generic available

ABOUT THIS DRUG

Mesalamine is an anti-inflammatory medicine used to treat inflammatory bowel disease such as ulcerative colitis. Enemas may also be used for inflammation of the lower colon and rectum, and suppositories for inflammation of the rectum.

This drug reduces diarrhea, rectal bleeding, and stomach pain. It works by reducing inflammation in the bowel.

SIDE EFFECTS

Consult your health-care practitioner if you experience side effects while taking this drug. Only he or she can determine whether it is safe for you to continue taking mesalamine.

- *Common:* flu-like symptoms, stomach cramps, abdominal pain, diarrhea, headache, dizziness, runny nose, sneezing, anal irritation (with enemas and suppositories)
- *Less Common or Rare:* gas, bloody diarrhea, indigestion, appetite loss, unusual tiredness, back or joint pain, hair loss, acne, rash, itching, severe headache, sudden, severe stomach pain, anxiety, blurred vision, ringing in the ears, chest pain, pale or blue skin, nausea, vomiting, fever, chills, shortness of breath, fast heartbeat, swollen stomach, yellow eyes or skin

IMPORTANT PRECAUTIONS

Tell your health-care practitioner about any other medical conditions you may have, especially allergies, a blood clotting disorder, a low white blood cell count, and liver or kidney impairment. If you have kidney disease, taking mesalamine may cause further kidney damage. Some people using this drug have experienced flare-ups of colitis. Rare cases of swelling of the membrane around the heart have also been reported; tell your health-care practitioner if you experience chest pain while taking this medication.

Inform your health-care practitioner if you have experienced any previous allergic reactions to this drug or to aspirin (or other salicylates), olsalazine, or sulfasalazine. Several mesalamine preparations contain sulfites, which can cause life-threatening allergic reactions in susceptible individuals. Some people with asthma are also sensitive to sulfites.

Enemas may stain clothes and fabrics.

DRUG INTERACTIONS

Inform your health-care practitioner if you are taking any other prescription or over-the-counter drugs, as well as any vitamins, herbs, or supplements. Possible drug interactions include the following:

- Mesalamine, like aspirin, is a type of drug known as a salicylate. Do not take mesalamine with other medications or in other conditions in which aspirin is not recommended.
- Tell your health-care practitioner if you are taking sulfasalazine or medications that affect the bone marrow.

FOOD, VITAMIN, AND HERBAL INTERACTIONS

Do not take mesalamine with supplements such as arginine, dong quai, feverfew, garlic, ginkgo, policosanol, potassium citrate, St. John's wort, white willow, and vitamin E.

RECOMMENDED DOSAGE

Mesalamine comes as a tablet and capsule to take by mouth and suppositories and an enema to use in the rectum. The doses given below are typical, but only your health-care practitioner can determine the best dose and schedule for you. This drug is not recommended for children.

Tablets and Capsules

- The number and schedule of tablets or capsules recommended depends on the brand and strength of the medication. Swallow the tablets or capsules whole. Do not cut, crush, or chew them.

Enemas

- 1 rectal enema (60 milliliters) per day at bedtime
- The enema—a liquid to be given directly into the rectum—comes in a disposable bottle with an applicator. Each bottle contains one dose. Remove the bottle from the protective foil pouch by tearing it or cutting it with a scissors. Be careful not to puncture the bottle. Carefully read the instructions before using.

Suppositories

- 1 rectal suppository (500 mg) 2 times a day
- When inserting a suppository, follow the directions on your prescription label carefully. Ask your health-care practitioner or pharmacist to explain any part you do not understand.

Mesalamine must be used regularly to be effective. You may need to use it for up to 6 weeks before your symptoms improve. If you forget a dose, take it as soon as you remember. If it is almost time for the next dose, skip the missed one and resume your normal schedule. Never take a double dose.

SYMPTOMS OF OVERDOSE AND WHAT TO DO

No specific information on overdosing with mesalamine is available. But if you suspect an overdose, seek immediate medical attention and take the prescription bottle to the hospital with you.

SPECIAL INFORMATION FOR PREGNANT OR NURSING WOMEN

No studies have adequately investigated the effects of mesalamine during pregnancy or breastfeeding. If you are pregnant or plan to become pregnant, or if you are breastfeeding or plan to do so, talk with your health-care practitioner before starting this drug. Only a health-care practitioner can determine whether the potential benefits outweigh the potential dangers.

SPECIAL INFORMATION FOR SENIORS

There are no special instructions for seniors.

GENERIC NAME

Mesoridazine besylate

see Chlorpromazine, page 267

GENERIC NAME

Metaproterenol

BRAND NAMES

Alupent, Arm-a-Med, Dey-Dose, Dey-Lute, Metaprel, Metaprel Nasal Inhaler, Prometa
Generic available

ABOUT THIS DRUG

Metaproterenol is a bronchodilator medication used to prevent and treat wheezing, shortness of breath, and troubled breathing caused by asthma, chronic bronchitis, emphysema, and other lung diseases. This drug works by dilating bronchial tubes that are in constriction. It relaxes and opens air passages in the lungs, making it easier to breathe.

SIDE EFFECTS

Speak to your health-care practitioner if you develop side effects while taking this drug. Only he or she can determine whether you should continue taking metaproterenol.

- *Common:* dry mouth, throat irritation, changes in taste, nervousness, fast or irregular heartbeat, heart palpitations, trembling
- *Less Common or Rare:* bad taste in mouth, cough, dizziness, tiredness, headache, stomach upset, nausea, vomiting, diarrhea, tremors, insomnia, heart rhythm disturbances, high blood pressure, worsening of asthma

IMPORTANT PRECAUTIONS

Tell your health-care practitioner about any other medical conditions you may have, especially heart disease, an irregular heartbeat, increased heart rate, high blood pressure, an overactive thyroid, glaucoma, diabetes, or seizures.

Inform your health-care practitioner if you have experienced allergies to this or similar medications in the past.

Because metaproterenol may cause side effects such as nervousness and dizziness, do not drive a car, operate machinery, or perform other tasks that require concentration until you know how this drug affects you.

To relieve dry mouth or throat irritation, use sugarless gum or hard candy, or rinse your mouth with water.

DRUG INTERACTIONS

Tell your health-care practitioner if you are taking any other prescription or over-the-counter drugs, as well as any vitamins, herbs, or supplements. Possible drug interactions include the following:

- Taking metaproterenol at the same time as or within 14 days of monoamine oxidase inhibitor (MAOI) antidepressants can cause a dangerous increase in blood pressure.
- Do not use other inhaled medications without consulting your health-care practitioner. This can result in increased cardiovascular side effects.
- Do not take metaproterenol at the same time as epinephrine. Take at least 4 hours apart.
- Medications such as beta-blockers and phenothiazines may decrease the effects of metaproterenol.
- Use tricyclic antidepressants with caution.
- Check with your health-care practitioner before using over-the-counter drugs. Many cold, cough, allergy, sinus, and weight loss remedies can raise blood pressure.

FOOD, VITAMIN, AND HERBAL INTERACTIONS

Do not take herbs that increase blood pressure, such as ephedra (ma huang), ginseng, goldenseal, licorice, and saw palmetto. Combining metaproterenol with kola can cause nervousness. Avoid caffeinated beverages such as coffee, tea, and cola while you are taking this drug.

RECOMMENDED DOSAGE

Metaproterenol comes as a tablet and syrup to take by mouth and as a solution and an aerosol to inhale by mouth. Although the doses given below are typical, only your health-care practitioner can determine the dose and schedule that best fit your individual needs.

Syrup

➤ *Children 6 to 9 Years (Less than 60 Pounds):* 1 teaspoon 3 to 4 times daily

➤ *Children 10 Years and Older (and More than 60 Pounds) and Adults:* 2 teaspoons 3 to 4 times daily

Tablets

➤ *Children 6 to 9 Years (Less than 60 Pounds):* 10 mg 3 to 4 times daily

➤ *Children 10 Years and Older (and More than 60 Pounds) and Adults:* 20 mg 3 to 4 times daily

Inhalation Aerosol

➤ *Children:* Inhalation aerosol is not recommended for children under the age of 12.

➤ *Adults:* 2 to 3 inhalations every 3 to 4 hours, for a maximum daily dosage of 12 inhalations

Inhalation Solution

➤ This medication is used in a nebulizer and taken by inhalation. The amount recommended depends on the brand and strength ordered by your health-care practitioner. Doses should be taken at least 4 hours apart 3 to 4 times daily. Inhalation solution is not recommended for children under the age of six.

It is important to take metaproterenol exactly as prescribed. Taking it more often than recommended can result in a loss in effectiveness and heart rhythm disturbances, possibly even cardiac arrest. Oral medication can be taken with or without food. If you forget a dose, take it as soon as you remember. Take the rest of the day's doses at evenly spaced intervals, and resume your normal schedule the next day. Never take a double dose.

SYMPTOMS OF OVERDOSE AND WHAT TO DO

Symptoms of metaproterenol overdose include chest pain, rapid heart rate, heart palpitations, nervousness, tremor, sweating, vomiting, and headache. If overdose occurs, seek immediate medical attention and take the prescription bottle to the hospital with you.

SPECIAL INFORMATION FOR PREGNANT OR NURSING WOMEN

No studies have adequately investigated the effects of metaproterenol during pregnancy or breastfeeding. If you are pregnant or plan to become pregnant, or if you are breastfeeding or plan to do so, talk with your health-care practitioner before starting this drug. Only a health-care practitioner can determine whether the potential benefits outweigh the potential dangers.

SPECIAL INFORMATION FOR SENIORS

Seniors are more susceptible to side effects such as nervousness, heart rhythm disturbances, heart palpitations, and muscle tremors. Metaproterenol should be used with extreme caution in older people who have heart problems or high blood pressure.

GENERIC NAME

Metaxalone

BRAND NAME

Skelaxin
No generic available

ABOUT THIS DRUG

Metaxalone is a muscle relaxant prescribed to relax muscles in the body and thus relieve the pain and stiffness of sprains, strains, and other injuries. This drug is used along with rest, physical therapy, and other treatment. Muscle relaxants work by acting on the central nervous system.

SIDE EFFECTS

Inform your health-care practitioner if you develop side effects while taking metaxalone. If symptoms are severe or prolonged, ask your health-care practitioner whether your dosage requires adjustment, and whether it is safe for you to continue taking this drug.

- *Common:* drowsiness, weakness, blurred or double vision, headache, dizziness, lightheadedness, nausea, vomiting, upset stomach, stomach cramps, nervousness, irritability
- *Less Common or Rare:* fast heartbeat, fainting, depression, fever, stinging or burning eyes, stuffy nose, red or bloodshot eyes, swollen glands, tight chest, abdominal cramps, clumsiness, unsteadiness, confusion, excitement, nervousness, constipation, flushing, heartburn, hiccups, muscle weakness

Seek immediate medical attention if you experience symptoms such as painful urination, blood in urine, convulsions, yellow skin or eyes, breathing difficulties, hives, pinpoint red spots on the skin, swelling around the eyes, severe stomach pain, lower back or side pain, unusual bleeding or bruising, extreme fatigue, fever, chills, cough, hoarseness, black, tarry stools, or vomiting material that looks like coffee grounds.

IMPORTANT PRECAUTIONS

Always inform your health-care practitioner about any other medical conditions you may have. Metaxalone should not be taken if you have kidney or liver impairment, seizures, or a blood disorder such as anemia. Long-term use can cause liver damage.

This drug can make you drowsy and less alert than usual. Until you know how metaxalone affects you, do not drive a car, operate machinery, or perform other tasks that require concentration.

DRUG INTERACTIONS

Tell your health-care practitioner and pharmacist if you are taking any other prescription or over-the-counter drugs, as well as any vitamins, herbs, or other supplements. Possible drug interactions include the following:

- Consult your health-care practitioner before combining metaxalone with other central nervous system depressants, including tranquilizers, sedatives, sleep aids, antihistamines, narcotics or other pain medication, barbiturates, seizure medications, and anesthesia. These can result in increased effects such as drowsiness and dizziness.
- Do not drink alcohol while taking metaxalone. This combination can also add to drowsiness.

FOOD, VITAMIN, AND HERBAL INTERACTIONS

Do not take metaxalone with herbs such as hops, kava, passionflower, and valerian. These can increase effects such as drowsiness.

RECOMMENDED DOSAGE

Metaxalone comes in tablet form. Although the doses given below are typical, only your health-care practitioner can determine the dose and schedule that best fit your needs.

- *Children:* This drug is not recommended for children under the age of 12.
- *Adults:* 800 mg 3 or 4 times daily

If the tablets are hard to swallow, they can be crushed and mixed with a small amount of food or liquid. If you forget a dose, take it as soon as you remember. If it is almost time for the next dose, skip the missed one and resume your normal schedule. Never take a double dose.

SYMPTOMS OF OVERDOSE AND WHAT TO DO

No specific information on overdosing with metaxalone is available. However, symptoms that may occur include exaggerated side effects. If you suspect that an overdose has occurred, seek immediate medical attention and take the prescription bottle to the hospital with you.

SPECIAL INFORMATION FOR PREGNANT OR NURSING WOMEN

No studies have adequately investigated the effects of metaxalone during pregnancy or breastfeeding. If you are pregnant or plan to become pregnant, or if you are breastfeeding or plan to do so, talk with your health-care practitioner before starting this drug. Only a health-care practitioner can determine whether the potential benefits outweigh the potential dangers.

SPECIAL INFORMATION FOR SENIORS

Lower doses may be prescribed for seniors with impaired liver or kidney function.

GENERIC NAME

Metformin

BRAND NAMES

Apo-Metformin, Glucophage
No generic available

ABOUT THIS DRUG

Metformin is used to treat the form of diabetes mellitus known as type 2. Type 2 diabetes was formerly known as adult-onset, and is also referred to as noninsulin-dependent. Diet and exercise play a key role in the management of this disease, and often metformin is used along with other antidiabetes drugs called sulfonylureas.

Metformin may also moderately lower blood fats.

This drug helps your body regulate the amount of glucose (sugar) in blood. It works by decreasing glucose production and increasing the body's sensitivity to insulin.

SIDE EFFECTS

Side effects are most common at the start of treatment. As your body gets used to metformin, in several weeks there should be few problems. Get emergency help at once if you experience the symptoms of lactic acidosis, a rare but life-threatening condition. Also learn to recognize the symptoms of low blood sugar and high blood sugar and know what to do when you experience them. It is essential to control these symptoms before they progress to more serious conditions.

- *Common:* nausea, vomiting, diarrhea, abdominal bloating, gas, appetite loss, a metallic or unpleasant taste
- *Hypoglycemia (Low Blood Sugar):* "drunken" behavior, drowsiness, unusual tiredness or weakness, slurred speech, shakiness, dizziness, difficulty concentrating, headache, confusion, anxiety, nervousness, blurred vision, cold sweats, cool pale skin, excessive hunger, restless sleep, nightmares, nausea, fast heartbeat
- *Hyperglycemia (High Blood Sugar):* dry mouth, thirst, frequent urination, dry skin, flushing, appetite loss, difficulty breathing, tiredness
- *Lactic Acidosis:* diarrhea, stomach discomfort, unusual tiredness or sleepiness, feeling cold, dizziness, lightheadedness, weakness, muscle pain and cramping, fast shallow breathing, slow or irregular heartbeat

IMPORTANT PRECAUTIONS

Metformin should not be taken if you have kidney or liver impairment, heart or lung disease, or chronic metabolic acidosis or diabetic ketoacidosis (a life-threatening condition caused by insufficient insulin, with symptoms such as nausea, fatigue, excessive thirst, lower chest pain, and fruity breath).

Also inform your health-care practitioner if you have other medical conditions such as pituitary or thyroid disease, adrenal insufficiency, or hormone problems. Do not take this drug if you are an alcoholic.

Serious infection increases the risk of lactic acidosis, especially if you experience nausea, vomiting, or diarrhea. Call your health-care practitioner for instructions. You may need to switch from metformin to insulin for the duration of your illness.

Do not take metformin 2 days before or after having an X ray using an injectable contrast agent (such as radioactive iodide). Your health-care practitioner will also most likely advise you to stop taking this drug for a short time before and after having any type of surgery or dental procedure.

Unlike other oral antidiabetes medications, metformin does not usually cause low blood sugar (hypoglycemia). However, this condition can occur. The people most susceptible to hypoglycemia are older, weak, or malnourished, or have kidney, liver, adrenal, or hormone problems. Symptoms vary from person to person, so it is essential to learn which symptoms you usually have. As soon as you experience the characteristic signs, address and control them quickly by taking a fast-acting sugar, such as a glucose tablet, glass of fruit juice or nondiet soft drink, tablespoon of corn syrup or honey, or tablespoon of table sugar dissolved in water.

People with uncontrolled diabetes may also experience high blood sugar, or hyperglycemia. (See symptoms above.) If this condition is not treated, it can lead to diabetic coma and death. Another problem associated with metformin is a rare but life-threatening condition called lactic acidosis, a buildup of lactic acid in the blood. At the highest risk of this effect are people who take multiple medications and those who have kidney or liver damage, congestive heart failure, or multiple medical problems. Older individuals and alcoholics also face increased risk.

In order to prevent these types of complications, carefully follow all diet and exercise recommendations made by your health-care practitioner and nutritionist. In fact, many people with type 2 diabetes are able to successfully control this disease by making healthy lifestyle changes, cutting back on the need for medication.

To monitor the effectiveness of metformin, measure the amount of glucose in your urine or blood on a regular basis. Your health-care practitioner may also tell you to test your urine for ketones (substances that appear in urine when diabetes is not properly controlled). Carefully follow the instructions of your health-care practitioner and pharmacist when conducting these tests at home. If blood sugar is high or sugar or ketones are present in urine, call your health-care practitioner.

DRUG INTERACTIONS

Inform your health-care practitioner and pharmacist if you are taking any other prescription or over-the-counter drugs, as well as any vitamins, herbs, or other supplements. Possible drug interactions include the following:

- Metformin increases the blood-sugar-lowering effects of insulin.
- ACE inhibitors, amiloride, beta-blockers, cimetidine, clotrimazole, digoxin, furosemide, morphine, procainamide, quinidine, quinine, ranitidine, triamterene, trimethoprim, and vancomycin may increase the risk of side effects of metformin.
- Metformin may reduce the effect of glyburide, a sulfonylurea.

- Do not drink alcohol while taking metformin. Alcohol alters blood sugar.

FOOD, VITAMIN, AND HERBAL INTERACTIONS

Metformin is associated with malabsorption of vitamin B_{12}. Supplementation with vitamin B_{12} and calcium (which helps your body absorb B_{12}) may be helpful.

Herbs such as garlic, ginger, ginseng, hawthorn, and nettle may affect blood sugar levels. Check with your health-care practitioner before using any herbal remedy.

RECOMMENDED DOSAGE

Metformin comes in tablet form. Although the doses given below are typical, only your health-care practitioner can determine the dose and schedule that best fit your needs.

- *Children:* This drug is not recommended for children.
- *Adults:* The starting dose is 500 mg twice a day before morning and evening meals, or 850 mg once a day before breakfast. This may be increased by 500 to 850 mg a week, to a daily total of 2,000 to 2,550 mg.

To reduce side effects such as nausea and diarrhea, take metformin with food. If you forget a dose, take it as soon as you remember. If it is almost time for the next dose, skip the missed one and resume your normal schedule. Never take a double dose.

SYMPTOMS OF OVERDOSE AND WHAT TO DO

An overdose of metformin may cause lactic acidosis. (See symptoms under Side Effects.) If you suspect that an overdose has occurred, seek immediate medical attention and take the prescription bottle to the hospital with you.

SPECIAL INFORMATION FOR PREGNANT OR NURSING WOMEN

Metformin should not be used during pregnancy. It is critically important to monitor and control blood sugar during pregnancy. However, it is safer to accomplish this through diet or a combination of diet and insulin. Consult your health-care practitioner as soon as you think you may be pregnant or if you are planning to become pregnant.

If you are breastfeeding or plan to do so, talk with your health-care practitioner before starting this drug. Only a health-care practitioner can determine whether the potential benefits outweigh the potential dangers.

SPECIAL INFORMATION FOR SENIORS

Seniors may require lower doses. Metformin is also used to treat hyperglycemia (high blood sugar) in older people.

GENERIC NAME

Methocarbamol

BRAND NAME

Robaxin
Generic available

ABOUT THIS DRUG

Methocarbamol is a muscle relaxant prescribed to relax muscles in the body and thus relieve the pain and stiffness of sprains, strains, and other injuries. This drug is used along with rest, physical therapy, and other treatment. Muscle relaxants work by acting on the central nervous system.

SIDE EFFECTS

Tell your health-care practitioner if you experience side effects while taking methocarbamol. If symptoms are severe or prolonged, ask your health-care practitioner whether your dosage requires adjustment, and whether it is safe for you to continue taking this drug.

- *Common:* drowsiness, weakness, blurred or double vision, headache, dizziness, lightheadedness, nausea, vomiting, upset stomach, stomach cramps, nervousness, irritability
- *Less Common or Rare:* fast heartbeat, fainting, depression, fever, stinging or burning eyes, stuffy nose, red or bloodshot eyes, swollen glands, tight chest, abdominal cramps, clumsiness, unsteadiness, confusion, excitement, nervousness, constipation, flushing, heartburn, hiccups, muscle weakness

Seek immediate medical attention if you experience symptoms such as painful urination, blood in urine, convulsions, yellow skin or eyes, breathing difficulties, hives, pinpoint red spots on the skin, swelling around the eyes, severe stomach pain, lower back or side pain, unusual bleeding or bruising, extreme fatigue, fever, chills, cough, hoarseness, black, tarry stools, or vomiting material that looks like coffee grounds.

IMPORTANT PRECAUTIONS

Always tell your health-care practitioner about any other medical conditions you may have. Methocarbamol should not be taken if you have kidney or liver impairment, seizures, or a blood disorder such as anemia. Long-term use can cause liver damage.

This drug can make you drowsy and less alert than usual. Until you know how methocarbamol affects you, do not drive a car, operate machinery, or perform other tasks that require concentration.

DRUG INTERACTIONS

Inform your health-care practitioner and pharmacist if you are taking any other prescription or over-the-counter drugs, as well as any vitamins, herbs, or other supplements. Possible drug interactions include the following:

- Consult your health-care practitioner before combining methocarbamol with other central nervous system depressants, including tranquilizers, sedatives, sleep aids, antihistamines, narcotics or other pain medication, barbiturates, seizure medications, and anesthesia. This can result in increased effects such as drowsiness and dizziness.
- Do not drink alcohol while taking methocarbamol. This combination can also add to drowsiness.

FOOD, VITAMIN, AND HERBAL INTERACTIONS

Do not take methocarbamol with herbs such as hops, kava, passionflower, and valerian. These can increase effects such as drowsiness.

RECOMMENDED DOSAGE

Methocarbamol comes in tablet form. Although the doses given below are typical, only your health-care practitioner can determine the dose and schedule that best fit your needs.

- *Children:* This drug is not recommended for children under the age of 12.
- *Adults:* Starting dose is 1,500 mg 4 times daily; your health-care practitioner will then reduce your dose to 500 mg 3 to 4 times daily.

If the tablets are hard to swallow, they can be crushed and mixed with a small amount of food or liquid. If you forget a dose, take it as soon as you remember. If it is almost time for the next dose, skip the missed one and resume your normal schedule. Never take a double dose.

SYMPTOMS OF OVERDOSE AND WHAT TO DO

No specific information on overdosing with methocarbamol is available. However, symptoms that may occur include exaggerated side effects. If you suspect that an overdose has occurred, seek immediate medical attention and take the prescription bottle to the hospital with you.

SPECIAL INFORMATION FOR PREGNANT OR NURSING WOMEN

No studies have adequately investigated the effects of methocarbamol during pregnancy or breastfeeding. If you are pregnant or plan to become pregnant, or if you are breastfeeding or plan to do so, talk with your health-care practitioner before starting this drug. Only a health-care practitioner can determine whether the potential benefits outweigh the potential dangers.

SPECIAL INFORMATION FOR SENIORS

Lower doses may be prescribed for seniors with impaired liver or kidney function.

GENERIC NAME

Methotrexate

BRAND NAMES

Abitrexate, Amethopterin, Folex, Mexate, Rheumatrex
Generic available

ABOUT THIS DRUG

Methotrexate is an antimetabolite drug used in the treatment of lymph, blood, bone, breast, uterine, head, neck, and other kinds of cancer. It is prescribed for cancer in children as well as adults. This drug is also recommended for rheumatoid arthritis and severe psoriasis. Even low doses of methotrexate can prove toxic, so this drug is prescribed with extreme care.

Methotrexate works by suppressing the immune system. It blocks an enzyme required by abnormal cells to live, thus slowing the growth of abnormal tissue. Unfortunately, at the same time this medication also affects normal cells, accounting for the great number of side effects.

SIDE EFFECTS

Side effects of methotrexate can be extremely serious, and must be promptly reported to your health-care practitioner. Some effects, such as hair loss, are distressing but pose no physical danger. On the other hand, a dangerous form of lung disease can develop at any point during therapy. Some effects develop months or even years after treatment.

- *Common:* nausea, vomiting, diarrhea, stomach upset, appetite loss, hair loss, dizziness, reduced platelet count, rash, itchiness, mouth and lip sores, increased risk of infection, liver and kidney problems
- *Less Common or Rare:* increased sensitivity to the sun, headache, fatigue, sore throat, inflammation of the gums and mouth, peeling skin, vision problems, bruises, changes in skin color, muscle or joint pain, infertility, birth defects, miscarriage, lung disease, stomach ulcers and bleeding, inability to speak, boils, infection, black or tarry stools, diabetes, kidney failure, osteoporosis, paralysis, convulsions

Methotrexate may cause serious lung problems. Contact your health-care practitioner immediately if you experience symptoms such as breathing difficulties, dry cough, and fever.

IMPORTANT PRECAUTIONS

Always tell your health-care practitioner about any other medical conditions you may have, especially alcohol abuse, active infection, chicken pox, colitis, gout, intestinal blockage, kidney or liver disease, mouth sores, shingles, ulcers, or immune system diseases. Methotrexate is prescribed with extreme caution in such cases.

Methotrexate can cause birth defects if either a man or woman is taking it at the time of conception. It is also associated with miscarriage, impaired fertility, menstrual irregularities, and loss of sexual desire.

Methotrexate suppresses the immune system, and may decrease the body's ability to combat infection.

This drug may cause drowsiness, dizziness, and blurred vision. Until you know how methotrexate affects you, do not drive a car, operate machinery, or perform other tasks that require concentration. Prolonged treatment with methotrexate increases risk of opportunistic infections.

People taking methotrexate for psoriasis may experience a burning sensation in patches of psoriasis and increased sensitivity to the sun. Wear protective clothing and apply sunscreen when using this drug.

High doses of this drug may cause confusion, paralysis, seizures, and coma. People taking any dose of methotrexate must be closely monitored with regular complete blood counts and other tests.

DRUG INTERACTIONS

Inform your health-care practitioner and pharmacist if you are taking any other prescription or over-the-counter drugs, as well as any vitamins, herbs, or other supplements. Possible drug interactions include the following:

- If you are taking methotrexate for cancer or psoriasis, do not take aspirin, ibuprofen, ketoprofen, naproxen, or other NSAIDs. This increases the toxic effects of methotrexate. (People with rheumatoid arthritis who continue to take NSAIDs will be very closely monitored.)
- Other drugs that increase the effects of methotrexate include cisplatin, etretinate, leflunomide, penicillin drugs, phenylbutazone, phenytoin, probenecid, and sulfa drugs.
- Some antibiotics reduce the effectiveness of methotrexate.
- Do not have live-virus immunizations while taking this drug without your health-care practitioner's approval. You are at risk of infection from the virus.
- Methotrexate may alter the absorption of theophylline.
- Do not drink alcohol while taking methotrexate. This increases the possibility of undesirable liver effects.

FOOD, VITAMIN, AND HERBAL INTERACTIONS

Do not take methotrexate with supplements such as potassium citrate, dong quai, echinacea, St. John's wort, or white willow. Drink extra fluids while taking this drug, so it will pass through your body more quickly and prevent kidney problems. Avoid spicy foods. Ask your health-care practitioner about taking folic acid supplements, which alter the absorption of methotrexate.

RECOMMENDED DOSAGE

Methotrexate comes in tablet form. Dosage is highly individualized and must be determined by your health-care practitioner. In some cases, medication is taken once a week rather than once a day, and it is essential to adhere to this schedule in order to prevent dangerous side effects.

Tablets can be crushed and mixed with food to prevent stomach upset. If you miss a dose, skip it and resume your regular schedule. Never take a double dose.

SYMPTOMS OF OVERDOSE AND WHAT TO DO

Symptoms of methotrexate overdose include breathing difficulties, mouth ulcers, and diarrhea. If you suspect that an overdose has occurred, seek immediate medical attention and take the prescription bottle to the hospital with you.

SPECIAL INFORMATION FOR PREGNANT OR NURSING WOMEN

Do not take this drug if you are pregnant or think you may be pregnant. Methotrexate may cause birth defects and miscarriage. Because of the possibility of serious side effects, breastfeeding is not recommended while you take this drug.

SPECIAL INFORMATION FOR SENIORS

Side effects are more likely to occur in seniors. Kidney function must be closely monitored throughout treatment.

GENERIC NAME

Methyclothiazide

see Thiazide Diuretics, page 1020

GENERIC NAME

Methyldopa

BRAND NAMES

Aldoclor, Aldomet
Generic available

ABOUT THIS DRUG

Methyldopa is used to treat high blood pressure (hypertension). It may be prescribed alone or with other antihypertensive medications. This drug must be taken regularly in order to be effective.

Methyldopa works by controlling impulses along select nerve pathways in the body. This action relaxes blood vessels and lowers blood pressure.

SIDE EFFECTS

Speak to your health-care practitioner if you develop side effects while taking methyldopa. Only he or she can determine whether you should continue taking this drug.

- *Common:* drowsiness (especially at the start of treatment), dry mouth, headache, weakness, fluid retention, swelling of feet or lower legs, weight gain

- *Less Common or Rare:* increased angina or chest pain, rash, joint pain, muscle spasms, depression, decreased mental acuity, anxiety, nightmares, loss of interest or ability in sex, swollen breasts, unusual milk production, stuffy nose, nausea, vomiting, diarrhea, constipation, dizziness, lightheadedness, numbness, tingling, yellow eyes and skin, fever, chills, difficulty breathing, fast heartbeat, fatigue, dark or amber urine, pale stools, liver problems, involuntary movements

IMPORTANT PRECAUTIONS

Always inform your health-care practitioner about any other medical conditions you suffer from, especially angina, depression, Parkinson's disease, and kidney or liver disease.

Methyldopa can cause liver problems. Your health-care practitioner will monitor your liver function before and during treatment with this drug. If you already have liver disease, your health-care practitioner may advise you not to take methyldopa, or to take a lower dosage than usual. Immediately report symptoms such as a fever shortly after starting this medication. Also consult your health-care practitioner if you develop yellow eyes and skin anytime in the course of treatment.

Before having any type of surgery or dental procedure, tell your surgeon or dentist that you are taking methyldopa.

This drug may make you dizzy or drowsy. Until you know how methyldopa affects you, do not drive a car, operate machinery, or perform other tasks that demand concentration.

Treatment of high blood pressure also entails certain lifestyle changes, such as weight control, smoking cessation, and close attention to diet.

When you first start taking this drug or when the dosage is increased, you may experience dizziness or faintness when you rise quickly from a sitting or reclining position (postural hypotension). Try to get up slowly, and consult your health-care practitioner if the problem continues.

Be extremely careful when you exercise in hot weather. Heavy sweating can lead to dizziness, lightheadedness, fainting, vomiting, dehydration, and low blood pressure.

Methyldopa may cause mouth dryness. To counteract this effect, use sugarless gum or candy, ice chips, or a saliva substitute. If the problem continues, consult your health-care practitioner or dentist.

If you have ever experienced an allergic reaction to methyldopa or to sulfa drugs, do not take this medication. If you experience an allergic reaction such as swelling of the face and mouth and a sudden problem with breathing, seek immediate medical attention.

DRUG INTERACTIONS

Tell your health-care practitioner and pharmacist if you are taking any other prescription or over-the-counter drugs, as well as any vitamins, herbs, or other supplements. Possible drug interactions include the following:

- Other blood pressure medications are commonly prescribed in combination with methyldopa. Your health-care practitioner will carefully adjust the dosages of these medications in the first months of treatment.
- Do not take methyldopa at the same time or within 14 days of monoamine oxidase inhibitor (MAOI) antidepressants. This combination can lead to severe high blood pressure.
- Alcohol may further lower blood pressure. Use with caution.
- Consult your health-care practitioner before taking over-the-counter cough, cold, sinus, allergy, or weight loss medications. Many of these can raise blood pressure.

FOOD, VITAMIN, AND HERBAL INTERACTIONS

Do not take herbs that increase blood pressure, such as ephedra (ma huang), ginseng, goldenseal, licorice, and saw palmetto. Consult your health-care practitioner before taking substances that may lower blood pressure, such as calcium, soy, or garlic. Because iron supplements may affect your body's absorption of methyldopa, take at different times of day. Talk to your health-care practitioner about diet and salt intake.

RECOMMENDED DOSAGE

Methyldopa is available in tablet or suspension form. Although the doses given below are typical, only your health-care practitioner can determine the dose and schedule that best fit your needs. During the first few months of treatment, your health-care practitioner may adjust your dosage and add other antihypertensive drugs to your treatment.

- *Children:* 10 mg per 2.2 pounds of body weight daily in divided doses, to be adjusted as necessary
- *Adults:* 250 mg to 2 grams daily in divided doses

Methyldopa is best taken on an empty stomach. However, if you experience stomach upset, take it with food or milk. Continue to take this drug even if you feel well. Do not discontinue use without consulting your health-care practitioner. If you miss a dose, take it as soon as you remember. If it is almost time for the next dose, skip the forgotten one, and resume your normal schedule. Never take a double dose.

SYMPTOMS OF OVERDOSE AND WHAT TO DO

The symptoms of methyldopa overdose include drowsiness, weakness, dizziness, and lightheadedness brought on by a severe drop in blood pressure. There may also be gas, bloating, nausea, vomiting, and constipation. If overdose occurs, seek immediate medical attention and take the prescription bottle to the hospital with you.

SPECIAL INFORMATION FOR PREGNANT OR NURSING WOMEN

No studies have adequately investigated the effects of methyldopa during pregnancy or breastfeeding. If you are pregnant or plan to become pregnant, or if you are breastfeeding or plan to do so, talk with your health-care practitioner before starting this drug. Only a health-care practitioner can determine whether the potential benefits outweigh the potential dangers.

SPECIAL INFORMATION FOR SENIORS

Seniors are more susceptible to side effects such as drowsiness and dizziness, and usually require lower doses.

GENERIC NAME

Methylphenidate

BRAND NAMES

Ritalin, Ritalin SR
Generic available

ABOUT THIS DRUG

Methylphenidate is an amphetamine-like drug that works as a mild central nervous system stimulant. It is used primarily for the treatment of attention-deficit hyperactivity disorder (ADHD) in children; for children and adults who have social, psychological, and educational disorders; and for narcolepsy (a condition characterized by sudden collapses into sleep) in adults.

Methylphenidate stimulates the brain stem, which leads to improved alertness, attention span, and concentration. This drug causes an increase in the levels of serotonin and dopamine (nerve transmitters) in the brain, which helps restore the balance between serotonin and other brain chemicals involved in behavior, mood, and thought.

SIDE EFFECTS

Contact your health-care practitioner if you develop side effects while taking this drug. Only he or she can determine if you should continue to take methylphenidate. In some cases, side effects can be controlled by adjusting the dosage or eliminating afternoon or evening doses.

- ➤ *Common in Children:* loss of appetite, weight loss, stomach pain, trouble sleeping, abnormal heart rhythms
- ➤ *Common in Adults:* nervousness and trouble sleeping
- ➤ *Less Common or Rare in Adults:* appetite loss, weight loss, stomach pain, nausea, dizziness, chest pain, abnormal heart rhythms, changes in blood pressure or pulse, fever, arthritis-like symptoms, headache, drowsiness, hair loss, itching, rash, severe jerking or twitching, visual disturbances such as blurred vision, severe psychotic reactions

IMPORTANT PRECAUTIONS

Tell your health-care practitioner if you are sensitive or allergic to methylphenidate or other drugs. Also inform your health-care practitioner about any other medical conditions you suffer from, especially severe anxiety, tension, agitation, glaucoma or other visual problems, high blood pressure, motor tics or spasms, Tourette's syndrome, or a seizure disorder.

Chronic or abusive use of methylphenidate can lead to addiction. This drug should be used with caution in anyone with a history of drug or alcohol abuse or of mental illness.

Before having any type of surgery or dental procedure, inform your surgeon or dentist that you are taking methylphenidate.

This drug may conceal signs of temporary fatigue. Until you know how methylphenidate affects you, do not drive a car, operate machinery, or perform other tasks that require concentration.

Methylphenidate is not an appropriate remedy for children whose symptoms are caused by stress or a psychiatric disorder.

DRUG INTERACTIONS

Inform your health-care practitioner and pharmacist if you are taking any prescription or over-the-counter drugs, as well as any vitamins, herbs, or other supplements. Possible drug interactions include the following:

- Monoamine oxidase inhibitor (MAOI) antidepressants may increase the effects of methylphenidate, leading to adverse reactions.
- Methylphenidate may increase the effects of tricyclic antidepressants.
- Methylphenidate reduces the effectiveness of the antihypertensive drug guanethidine.
- Methylphenidate may also interact with blood thinners such as warfarin, and epilepsy medications including phenobarbital, phenytoin, and primidone.
- Do not combine methylphenidate with alcohol.

FOOD, VITAMIN, AND HERBAL INTERACTIONS

Avoid foods that are rich in the amino acid tyramine while taking methylphenidate. This combination may result in an excessive rise in blood pressure. Tyramine-rich foods include (but are not limited to) aged cheeses, bologna, chicken liver, chocolate, figs, pickled herring, pepperoni, raisins, salami, soy sauce, and yeast extracts. Also avoid beverages that contain meat or meat tenderizers, and alcoholic beverages that may contain tyramine, which include some beers, vermouth, and Chianti wines.

Herbs that affect the central nervous system—including St. John's wort, guarana, ephedra (ma huang), and kola—should be avoided when taking methylphenidate.

Avoid caffeinated beverages, such as coffee, tea, and cola.

RECOMMENDED DOSAGE

Methylphenidate is available in regular and sustained-release tablets. Although the doses given below are typical, only your health-care practitioner can determine the dose and schedule that are most appropriate for you.

- *Children 6 Years and Older:* 5 mg (regular tablets) daily to start, which may be increased as needed to a maximum daily dosage of 60 mg
- *Adults:* 20 to 60 mg daily in divided doses; maximum dosage is 60 mg

Methylphenidate is best taken 30 to 45 minutes before meals. If you miss a dose of the regular tablets, take it as soon as possible and then space out your remaining doses during the rest of the day. Never take two doses at once. Avoid taking methylphenidate within a few hours of bedtime, because it can cause sleeplessness. Do not make dosage changes without your health-care practitioner's knowledge.

The extended-release tablets must be swallowed whole. Do not crush, cut, or chew them.

Methylphenidate must be taken regularly for several weeks before its full effect is felt. Continue to take this drug even if you feel well. Do not discontinue use without consulting your health-care practitioner, especially if you have been taking large doses for a long time. To end treatment, your health-care practitioner will reduce dosage gradually.

SYMPTOMS OF OVERDOSE AND WHAT TO DO

The symptoms of overdose include agitation, confusion, delirium, dry mucous membranes, elevated blood pressure and body temperature, enlarged pupils, euphoria, flushing, hallucinations, headache, muscle twitching, rapid or irregular heartbeat, tremors, vomiting, convulsions, and coma. If overdose occurs, seek immediate medical attention and bring the prescription bottle to the hospital with you.

SPECIAL INFORMATION FOR PREGNANT OR NURSING WOMEN

It is not known whether methylphenidate causes birth defects. If you are or suspect you may be pregnant, consult your health-care practitioner before taking this drug. Methylphenidate should be used only when the benefits of therapy clearly outweigh the potential risks to the fetus.

Small amounts of methylphenidate may pass into breast milk. As a result, your health-care practitioner may advise you to discontinue nursing until you complete treatment with this drug.

SPECIAL INFORMATION FOR SENIORS

Low starting doses are typically used in people age 60 and older. Older individuals may be at greater risk for side effects such as nervousness, agitation, insomnia, high blood pressure, angina, and heart rhythm disturbances.

OPEN QUESTIONS OR CONTROVERSIES

Chronic or abusive use of methylphenidate can potentially lead to tolerance and/or mental or physical dependence. Because some people abuse this drug as a recreational substance, its use should be carefully monitored by parents and health-care prac-

(continued from page 681)

titioners. Methylphenidate must be used with caution in anyone with a history of drug or alcohol abuse or of mental illness.

A number of experts have also questioned the widespread use of methylphenidate in children suspected of having ADHD. Some warn that the drug is overprescribed, while others worry about its side effects. However, the majority of health-care practitioners believe that when a child is carefully and accurately diagnosed, a combination of medication and behavioral therapy can result in dramatic improvement. Moreover, the side effects in children are generally mild, and disappear when methylphenidate is discontinued. If you think your child may have ADHD, consult a developmental pediatrician or child psychiatrist for a thorough evaluation, and discuss whether methylphenidate is an appropriate treatment.

GENERIC NAME

Methylprednisolone *see Corticosteroids, Oral, page 330*

GENERIC NAME

Methyltestosterone *see Testosterone, page 1010*

GENERIC NAME

Methysergide

BRAND NAME

Sansert
No generic available

ABOUT THIS DRUG

Methysergide is used to prevent migraine and cluster headaches. It cannot control attacks once they have begun. Like other ergot alkaloids, methysergide is derived from ergot, a plant fungus. This drug works by blocking the action of the hormone serotonin, which eases the blood vessel constriction that leads to vascular headaches.

SIDE EFFECTS

Side effects are common. If they are severe or persistent, ask your health-care practitioner whether it is possible to adjust your dosage, and whether it is safe for you to continue taking this drug.

- *Common:* impaired circulation to the arms and legs, cold hands and feet, fluid retention, swelling, weight gain
- *Less Common or Rare:* diarrhea, constipation, nausea, vomiting, drowsiness, heartburn, abdominal pain, dizziness, blurred vision, agitation, unsteadiness, rash, flushing, temporary hair loss, sleeplessness, depression

People who take methysergide for long periods of time are more susceptible to fibrosis, or scar tissue formation that may affect the chest, heart, lungs, kidneys, and other vital parts of the body. Tell your health-care practitioner at once if you experience symptoms such as chest pain, fever, fatigue, difficulty breathing, stomach pain, or difficulty urinating.

IMPORTANT PRECAUTIONS

Methysergide should not be taken if you have angina, Buerger's disease, connective tissue disease, heart or blood vessel disease, kidney disease, liver disease, lung disease, a peptic ulcer, peripheral vascular disease, phlebitis, or Raynaud's disease. Do not use this drug if you are pregnant, and tell your health-care practitioner if you have an infection of any kind.

If you have ever experienced an allergic reaction to this or another ergot alkaloid, you should not take methysergide. Regular tablets contain tartrazine dye. If you have asthma or are allergic to aspirin or tartrazine, ask for tartrazine-free tablets.

If you take methysergide and continue to have headaches, this drug probably does not work for you. Ask your health-care practitioner about discontinuing use. If methysergide does effectively prevent migraine and cluster headaches, every 6 months you must discontinue treatment for 3 to 4 weeks. This helps prevent fibrosis (scar tissue formation).

Methysergide may make you drowsy or dizzy. Until you know how this drug affects you, do not drive a car, operate machinery, or perform other tasks that require concentration.

This drug is not for the mild headaches that nearly everyone has from time to time. Methysergide may have serious side effects, and its use is reserved for those with persistent, severe, and otherwise uncontrollable vascular headaches.

DRUG INTERACTIONS

Tell your health-care practitioner and pharmacist if you are taking any other prescription or over-the-counter drugs, as well as any vitamins, herbs, or other supplements. Possible drug interactions include the following:

- Central nervous system depressants such as antihistamines, tranquilizers, sedatives, and sleep aids may increase the depressant effect of methysergide.
- Beta-blockers may further reduce blood flow to the extremities, resulting in cold hands and feet and possibly much more serious circulation problems.
- Do not combine methysergide with triptans such as sumatriptan.
- Do not use alcohol when you are taking methysergide. In some people, alcohol worsens headaches.
- Smoking may increase the harmful effects of this medication.

FOOD, VITAMIN, AND HERBAL INTERACTIONS

Do not combine methysergide with the herb St. John's wort, since both affect serotonin levels.

RECOMMENDED DOSAGE

Methysergide comes in tablet form. The doses given below are typical. However, only your health-care practitioner can determine the dose and schedule that best fit your individual needs.

- *Children:* This drug is not recommended for children under the age of 12.
- *Adults:* 2 to 6 mg daily in divided doses

Methysergide should be taken with meals to reduce stomach irritation. If you forget to take a dose, take it as soon as you remember. If it is almost time for the next dose, skip the one you missed and resume your normal schedule. Never take a double dose. Withdrawal headaches may occur if methysergide is stopped suddenly. Dosage should be gradually tapered off over 2 to 3 weeks.

SYMPTOMS OF OVERDOSE AND WHAT TO DO

Symptoms of methysergide overdose include nausea, vomiting, diarrhea, abdominal pain, dizziness, excitement, and cold hands and feet. If an overdose occurs, seek immediate medical attention and take the prescription bottle to the hospital with you so the health-care practitioner will know exactly what medication was taken.

SPECIAL INFORMATION FOR PREGNANT OR NURSING WOMEN

Do not take methysergide if you are pregnant or planning to become pregnant, or if you are breastfeeding. This medication may cause miscarriage and symptoms such as nausea and vomiting in nursing babies.

SPECIAL INFORMATION FOR SENIORS

Smaller doses are recommended for seniors, who are more susceptible to side effects such as sedation and dizziness.

GENERIC NAME

Metoclopramide

BRAND NAMES

Clopra, Maxolon, Octamide, Reclomide, Reglan
Generic available

ABOUT THIS DRUG

Metoclopramide is used to relieve nausea and vomiting. It is often prescribed to control these and other symptoms of diabetic gastroparesis, including heartburn, indigestion, appetite loss, and a sense of persistent fullness after meals.

This drug works by increasing the movements or contractions of the stomach and intestines. This speeds up the movement of stomach contents into the small intestine.

SIDE EFFECTS

If you develop side effects while taking metoclopramide, ask your health-care practitioner whether it is possible to adjust your dosage, and whether it is safe for you to continue taking this drug.

- *Common:* drowsiness, fatigue, restlessness, diarrhea (with high doses)
- *Less Common or Rare:* nausea, constipation, depression, irritability, blood pressure changes, abnormal heart rhythms, trouble sleeping, visual disturbances, dizziness, dry mouth, breast tenderness and swelling, increased flow of breast milk, tender or oozing nipples, menstrual changes, decreased sex drive and ability, impotence, decreased sperm count, frequent urination, rash, Parkinson-like reactions (such as rigidity, slow movements, tremors, shuffling gait, and mask-like appearance)

IMPORTANT PRECAUTIONS

Always tell your health-care practitioner about all other medical conditions you have. Metoclopramide should not be taken if you have gastrointestinal bleeding, an ulcer, intestinal blockage, a seizure disorder such as epilepsy, or an adrenaline-producing tumor. This drug should be used with caution if you have high blood pressure, liver or kidney problems, or Parkinson's disease.

Metoclopramide may cause mild to severe depression. If you have a history of depression, be sure your health-care practitioner knows about it before you take this drug.

Metoclopramide may make you drowsy or dizzy. Until you know how this drug affects you, do not drive a car, operate machinery, or perform other tasks that require concentration.

DRUG INTERACTIONS

Inform your health-care practitioner and pharmacist if you are taking any other prescription or over-the-counter drugs, as well as any vitamins, herbs, or other supplements. Possible drug interactions include the following:

- Do not take metoclopramide at the same time as or within 14 days of monoamine oxidase inhibitor (MAOI) antidepressants. This combination can cause very high blood pressure.
- Do not combine metoclopramide with antipsychotic drugs such as phenothiazines. This increases the risk of Parkinson-like reactions such as involuntary movements.
- Metoclopramide may increase the sedative effects of central nervous system depressants such as antihistamines, tranquilizers, sedatives, and sleep aids.
- Metoclopramide may also increase the effects of cyclosporine and lithium.
- Metoclopramide may reduce the effects of cimetidine, digoxin, and certain antibiotics.
- Metoclopramide and levodopa interfere with one another.
- Atropinelike drugs may decrease the effects of metoclopramide.
- Combining alcohol with metoclopramide can result in increased side effects such as sedation and intoxication.

FOOD, VITAMIN, AND HERBAL INTERACTIONS

Do not combine metoclopramide with herbs such as hops, kava, passionflower, and valerian. These can increase its sedative effects.

Herbs such as aloe, cascara, and senna may increase the risk of diarrhea.

RECOMMENDED DOSAGE

Metoclopramide comes in tablet form. The doses given below are typical. However, only your health-care practitioner can determine the dose and schedule that best fit your individual needs.

- *Children:* This drug is not recommended for children.
- *Adults:* 20 to 60 mg daily for 2 to 8 weeks

This medication should be taken 30 minutes before meals and at bedtime. If you forget to take a dose, take it as soon as you remember. If it is almost time for the next dose, skip the one you missed and resume your normal schedule. Never take a double dose.

SYMPTOMS OF OVERDOSE AND WHAT TO DO

Symptoms of metoclopramide overdose include drowsiness, confusion, and seizures. If an overdose occurs, seek immediate medical attention and take the prescription bottle to the hospital with you so the health-care practitioner will know exactly what medication was taken.

SPECIAL INFORMATION FOR PREGNANT OR NURSING WOMEN

No studies have adequately investigated the effects of metoclopramide during pregnancy or breastfeeding. If you are pregnant or plan to become pregnant, or if you are breastfeeding or plan to do so, talk with your health-care practitioner before starting this drug. Only a health-care practitioner can determine whether the potential benefits outweigh the potential dangers.

SPECIAL INFORMATION FOR SENIORS

Smaller doses are recommended for seniors, who are more susceptible to Parkinson-like side effects such as trembling and shaky hands.

GENERIC NAME

Metolazone

see Thiazide Diuretics, page 1020

GENERIC NAME
Metoprolol

BRAND NAMES
Lopressor, Toprol XL
Generic available

ABOUT THIS DRUG
Metoprolol is a beta-adrenergic blocking agent (beta-blocker) prescribed to treat mild-to-moderate high blood pressure (hypertension). It is also used to limit the damage caused by heart attacks, and to reduce the risk of repeat heart attacks. Metoprolol is sometimes combined with other high blood pressure medications, such as thiazide diuretics.

Beta-blockers such as metoprolol work by decreasing the force and rate of heart contractions. This in turn reduces the demand for oxygen and lowers blood pressure.

SIDE EFFECTS
Speak to your health-care practitioner if you develop side effects while taking this drug. Only he or she can determine whether it is safe for you to continue taking metoprolol.

- *Common:* depression, dizziness, shortness of breath, fatigue, lethargy, slow heartbeat, cold hands and feet, rash, itching
- *Less Common or Rare:* confusion, short-term memory loss, insomnia, vivid dreams, hallucinations, rapid heartbeat, ringing in the ears, headache, stomach pain, nausea, indigestion, hair loss, excessive tiredness or weakness, heart failure, constipation, swelling, breathing difficulties, chest pain, decreased sex drive and ability, liver damage, worsening of heart difficulties

IMPORTANT PRECAUTIONS
Inform your health-care practitioner about any other medical conditions you suffer from, especially a slow heart rate or serious heart block, congestive heart failure, poor circulation, angina, asthma or other lung ailments, liver or kidney problems, diabetes or hypoglycemia, or a thyroid condition.

Before having any type of surgery or dental procedure, inform your surgeon or dentist that you are taking metoprolol.

This drug may make you more sensitive to the cold. Beta-blockers can decrease blood circulation in the fingers, toes, and skin. Be sure to dress warmly in low temperatures, especially if you already have blood circulation problems.

This drug may make you drowsy. Until you know how metoprolol affects you, do not drive a car, operate machinery, or perform other tasks that demand concentration.

Treatment of high blood pressure also entails certain lifestyle changes, such as weight control, smoking cessation, and a low-sodium diet.

Be extremely careful when you exercise in hot weather. Heavy sweating can lead to dizziness, lightheadedness, vomiting, fainting, dehydration, and a drop in blood pressure.

When you first start taking this drug or when the dosage is increased, you may experience dizziness or faintness when you rise quickly from a sitting or reclining position (postural hypotension). Try to get up slowly, and consult your health-care practitioner if the problem continues.

DRUG INTERACTIONS

Tell your health-care practitioner and pharmacist if you are taking any other prescription or over-the-counter drugs, as well as any vitamins, herbs, or other supplements. Possible drug interactions include the following:

- Drugs that contain aspirin can lessen the blood pressure lowering effects of metoprolol.
- Taking other blood pressure medications (including clonidine, reserpine, and calcium channel blockers) can increase the effects of metoprolol.
- Medications such as cimetidine may increase the effects of metoprolol.
- Metoprolol can interfere with the action of oral antidiabetes medications. It may also change blood glucose levels.
- Metoprolol may interfere with the effectiveness of certain asthma medications, including aminophylline, epinephrine, isoproterenol, and theophylline.
- Metoprolol can increase the effect of antianxiety benzodiazepine drugs.
- If you are also taking ergot alkaloids for migraines, metoprolol may worsen side effects such as cold hands and feet. In rare cases, this drug combination can lead to gangrene.
- Monoamine oxidase inhibitor (MAOI) antidepressants should not be taken at the same time as or within 14 days of metoprolol.

- Metoprolol may interact with anesthetics during surgery, increasing the risk of heart problems. As a result, your health-care practitioner will instruct you to stop taking this drug two days before surgery.
- Alcohol intensifies the drowsiness caused by this drug.
- Cocaine and cigarette smoking may reduce the effectiveness of metoprolol.
- Ask your health-care practitioner about taking over-the-counter cough, cold, sinus, allergy, and weight loss remedies. Many of these can raise blood pressure.

FOOD, VITAMIN, AND HERBAL INTERACTIONS

Do not take herbs that increase blood pressure, including ephedra (ma huang), ginseng, goldenseal, licorice, and saw palmetto. Consult your health-care practitioner before taking substances that may lower blood pressure, such as calcium, soy, or garlic. Your health-care practitioner will probably recommend a low-sodium diet.

RECOMMENDED DOSAGE

Metoprolol is available in regular or extended-release tablets. Although the doses given below are typical, only your health-care practitioner can determine the dose and schedule that are most appropriate for you.

- *Children:* This drug is not recommended for children under the age of 12.
- *Adults:* 25 to 400 mg daily

The regular, short-acting form is best taken on an empty stomach. Extended-release tablets can be taken with food. If you forget to take a dose, take it as soon as you remember. If it is almost time for the next dose, skip the forgotten one, and resume your normal schedule. Never take double doses.

Continue to take this drug even if you feel well. Do not discontinue use without consulting your health-care practitioner. Abrupt withdrawal can cause chest pain, breathing difficulties, increased sweating, irregular heartbeat, and even heart attack in some people. To end treatment, in most cases your health-care practitioner will reduce dosage gradually over a 2-week period.

SYMPTOMS OF OVERDOSE AND WHAT TO DO

The symptoms of metoprolol overdose include slow heart rate, low blood pressure, dizziness, fainting, difficulty breathing, bluish fingernails and palms, and seizures. If overdose occurs, seek immediate medical attention and take the bottle of metoprolol to the hospital with you.

SPECIAL INFORMATION FOR PREGNANT OR NURSING WOMEN

Some studies have shown that women who take beta-blockers during pregnancy give birth to babies with lower birth weight, heart rate, and blood pressure. As a result, metoprolol should be avoided if you are pregnant.

Small amounts of metoprolol can pass into breast milk and cause problems such as slow heart rate, low blood pressure, and trouble breathing. If you must take this drug, your health-care practitioner may recommend bottle-feeding.

SPECIAL INFORMATION FOR SENIORS

Seniors usually require lower doses of metoprolol. Older people are more apt to experience side effects such as heightened sensitivity to the cold, a general feeling of unwellness, chest pain, breathing difficulties, sweating, and variations in heartbeat.

GENERIC NAME

Metronidazole

BRAND NAMES

Flagyl, Protostat
Generic available

ABOUT THIS DRUG

Metronidazole is used to treat infections such as *Trichomonas* (a sexually transmitted disease), amebic dysentery, and giardiasis. When prescribed for *Trichomonas*, both sexual partners should be treated, even if one is asymptomatic.

Metronidazole works by interacting with DNA. It destroys the nucleus of invading cells.

SIDE EFFECTS

Consult your health-care practitioner if you develop side effects while taking metronidazole. Only he or she can determine whether it is safe for you to continue taking this drug.

- *Common:* unpleasant, metallic taste in the mouth, dark urine, vaginal or oral yeast infections, upset stomach, nausea, vomiting, diarrhea, constipation, cramping, appetite loss, dizziness

- *Less Common or Rare:* dry mouth, depression, weakness, irritability, confusion, insomnia, joint pain, numbness and tingling in the extremities, headache, loss of coordination, unsteadiness, incontinence, fever, sore throat, infection, seizures

IMPORTANT PRECAUTIONS

Always tell your health-care practitioner about all other medical conditions you have. Metronidazole should not be taken if you have a history of blood disease or if you have experienced an allergic reaction to this or similar drugs in the past. This medication should be used with caution if you have epilepsy, heart disease, liver problems, a vaginal yeast infection, oral thrush, high blood pressure, liver or kidney problems, or Parkinson's disease.

Metronidazole may cause dizziness and confusion. Until you know how this drug affects you, do not drive a car, operate machinery, or perform other tasks that require concentration.

If metronidazole causes mouth dryness, use sugarless gum or hard candy, ice chips, or a saliva substitute. Consult your health-care practitioner or dentist if the problem continues.

DRUG INTERACTIONS

Inform your health-care practitioner and pharmacist if you are taking any other prescription or over-the-counter drugs, as well as any vitamins, herbs, or other supplements. Possible drug interactions include the following:

- Do not combine metronidazole with alcohol. This can cause nausea, vomiting, cramps, headaches, and flushing.
- Do not take disulfiram while you are taking metronidazole. This combination may lead to increased nervous system effects ranging from confusion to psychotic reactions.
- Cimetidine may increase metronidazole's effects.
- Barbiturates such as phenobarbital may reduce metronidazole's effects.
- Taking blood thinners such as warfarin with metronidazole increases the risk of bleeding.
- Metronidazole may increase the blood levels and effects of lithium and phenytoin.

FOOD, VITAMIN, AND HERBAL INTERACTIONS

Do not combine metronidazole with vitamin B_6 (pyridoxine). This may increase nervous system side effects.

Metronidazole may disturb the balance of friendly bacteria in your body, leading to yeast infections. To counteract this effect, eat yogurt with live cultures or take a *Lactobacillus acidophilus* supplement.

RECOMMENDED DOSAGE

Metronidazole comes as capsules and tablets. The length of treatment varies from one to ten days (and sometimes longer). The doses given below are typical. However, consult your health-care practitioner for the exact dose and schedule that are most appropriate for you.

- *Children:* 35 to 50 mg per 2.2 pounds daily, in divided doses
- *Adults:* Starting dose is 500 mg; your health-care practitioner may increase your dose to 750 mg to 2 g daily in divided doses

To prevent stomach upset, take metronidazole with food or milk. If you forget to take a dose, take it as soon as you remember. If it is almost time for the next dose, skip the forgotten one, and resume your normal schedule. Never take double doses. To cure your infection, continue to take this drug even if you feel well. Do not discontinue use without consulting your health-care practitioner.

SYMPTOMS OF OVERDOSE AND WHAT TO DO

The symptoms of metronidazole overdose include nausea, vomiting, and loss of muscle coordination. If overdose occurs, seek immediate medical attention and take the prescription bottle to the hospital with you.

SPECIAL INFORMATION FOR PREGNANT OR NURSING WOMEN

No studies have adequately investigated the effects of metronidazole during pregnancy or breastfeeding. If you are pregnant or plan to become pregnant, or if you are breastfeeding or plan to do so, talk with your health-care practitioner before starting this drug. Only a health-care practitioner can determine whether the potential benefits outweigh the potential dangers.

SPECIAL INFORMATION FOR SENIORS

Seniors are more apt to experience side effects, and usually require lower doses of this drug.

GENERIC NAME
Miconazole

BRAND NAMES
Micatin, Monistat-3, Monistat-7, Monistat-Derm, Monistat Dual-Pak
Generic available

ABOUT THIS DRUG
Miconazole is an antifungal agent used for skin infections such as athlete's foot and jock itch and for vaginal yeast infections. It is for topical application only. Miconazole products are available both over-the-counter and by prescription.

SIDE EFFECTS
Consult your health-care practitioner if you develop side effects while using miconazole. Only he or she can determine whether it is safe for you to continue using this drug.

- *Common:* rash, irritation, burning sensation, cramping, headache, hives, vaginal itching
- *Less Common or Rare:* If you are taking miconazole for a vaginal infection, stop treatment and consult your health-care practitioner if you experience symptoms such as a foul-smelling discharge, fever, and pain in the lower abdomen, back, or shoulders.

IMPORTANT PRECAUTIONS
Chemicals in Monistat-3 and Monistat-7 can weaken the latex in diaphragms. Use an alternate source of birth control.

Use napkins instead of tampons while using vaginal miconazole.

If a vaginal infection does not respond to treatment, see your health-care practitioner. The problem may be a different type of infection that does not respond to miconazole.

Always tell your health-care practitioner about all other medical conditions you have.

DRUG INTERACTIONS
Although no specific interactions are known, always inform your health-care practitioner and pharmacist if you are taking any other prescription or over-the-counter drugs, as well as any vitamins, herbs, or other supplements.

FOOD, VITAMIN, AND HERBAL INTERACTIONS
No food, vitamin, or herbal interactions have been noted.

RECOMMENDED DOSAGE

Miconazole comes in cream, lotion, powder, spray liquid, and spray powder for application to the skin. It also comes in cream and suppositories for vaginal insertion. The doses given below are typical. However, consult your health-care practitioner for the exact dose and schedule that are most appropriate for you.

Vaginal Cream and Suppositories

- *Children:* Vaginal miconazole is not recommended for girls under the age of 12.
- *Adults:* Insert 1 applicatorful or suppository into the vagina at bedtime for 3 to 7 days.

Skin Products

- *Children and Adults:* Apply to affected skin areas twice daily for up to 1 month.

If you forget a dose, use it as soon as you remember. If it is almost time for the next dose, skip the forgotten one, and resume your normal schedule. Never take double doses. To cure your infection, continue to take this drug even if you feel well. Do not discontinue use without consulting your health-care practitioner.

SYMPTOMS OF OVERDOSE AND WHAT TO DO

Miconazole is for external use only. Accidental ingestion may cause stomach upset. If overdose occurs, seek immediate medical attention and take the miconazole container to the hospital with you.

SPECIAL INFORMATION FOR PREGNANT OR NURSING WOMEN

Pregnant women should not use miconazole in the first trimester. If you are pregnant or plan to become pregnant, or if you are breastfeeding or plan to do so, talk with your health-care practitioner before starting this drug. Only a health-care practitioner can determine whether the potential benefits outweigh the potential dangers.

SPECIAL INFORMATION FOR SENIORS

There are no special instructions for seniors.

GENERIC NAME
Midodrine

BRAND NAME

ProAmatine
No generic available

ABOUT THIS DRUG

Midodrine is used to treat low blood pressure (hypotension). When other measures fail, it may help prevent the dizziness and faintness that overtake some people when rising from a sitting or reclining position.

This drug works by stimulating nerve endings in blood vessels. This causes blood vessels to tighten and blood pressure to rise.

SIDE EFFECTS

Speak to your health-care practitioner if you develop side effects while taking midodrine. Only he or she can determine whether you should continue taking this drug.

- *Common:* blurred vision, headache, pounding in the ears, chills, goose bumps, painful or urgent urination, urinary retention, burning, itching, or prickling of the scalp
- *Less Common or Rare:* high blood pressure when lying down (supine hypertension), anxiety, nervousness, confusion, dry mouth, feeling of pressure in the head, flushing, rash, visual problems, dizziness, upset stomach, nausea, heartburn, gas, tiredness, sleeplessness, dry skin, canker sores, leg cramps

IMPORTANT PRECAUTIONS

Always inform your health-care practitioner about any other medical conditions you suffer from, especially high blood pressure, heart disease, an overactive thyroid, diabetes, urinary retention, or visual problems. Midodrine may aggravate these conditions. If you suffer from liver or kidney problems, your health-care practitioner will probably prescribe a lower dosage.

Do not take this drug after 6 p.m. or if you plan to lie down for a period of time. High blood pressure while lying down (supine hypertension) is one of the most serious side effects of midodrine. Its signs include blurred vision, headache, and pounding in the ears.

This drug may cause blurred vision and dizziness. Until you know how midodrine affects you, do not drive a car, operate machinery, or perform other tasks that demand concentration.

To control low blood pressure, dizziness, and fainting, try to get up slowly when you rise from a sitting or reclining position.

Be extremely careful when you exercise in hot weather. Heavy sweating can lead to dizziness, lightheadedness, fainting, vomiting, dehydration, and low blood pressure.

Midodrine may cause mouth dryness. To counteract this effect, use sugarless gum or candy, ice chips, or a saliva substitute. If the problem continues, consult your health-care practitioner or dentist.

If you have ever experienced an allergic reaction to midodrine or similar drugs, do not take this medication.

DRUG INTERACTIONS

Tell your health-care practitioner and pharmacist if you are taking any other prescription or over-the-counter drugs, as well as any vitamins, herbs, or other supplements. Possible drug interactions include the following:

- Taking midodrine with digitalis, beta-blockers, or similar drugs may increase effects on the heart. Use with caution.
- Steroids such as fludrocortisone and vasoconstrictors such as ephedrine can increase effects on blood pressure.
- Alpha blockers such as prazosin can reduce midodrine's effects.
- Do not drink alcohol, which may further lower blood pressure.
- Consult your health-care practitioner before taking over-the-counter cough, cold, sinus, allergy, or weight loss medications. Many of these can raise blood pressure.

FOOD, VITAMIN, AND HERBAL INTERACTIONS

Do not take herbs that also increase blood pressure, such as ephedra (ma huang), ginseng, goldenseal, licorice, and saw palmetto. Consult your health-care practitioner before taking substances that may lower blood pressure, such as calcium, soy, or garlic. Talk to your health-care practitioner about diet and salt intake.

RECOMMENDED DOSAGE

Midodrine comes in tablet form. Although the doses given below are typical, only your health-care practitioner can determine the dose and schedule that best fit your needs.

- *Children:* This drug is not recommended for children.
- *Adults:* 10 mg 3 times a day

Do not take medication after the evening meal or less than 3 to 4 hours before bedtime. If you miss a dose, take it as soon as you remember. If it is almost time for the next dose, skip the forgotten one, and resume your normal schedule. Never take a double dose.

SYMPTOMS OF OVERDOSE AND WHAT TO DO

The symptoms of midodrine overdose include high blood pressure, goose bumps, difficulty urinating, and feeling cold. If overdose occurs, seek immediate medical attention and take the prescription bottle to the hospital with you.

SPECIAL INFORMATION FOR PREGNANT OR NURSING WOMEN

No studies have adequately investigated the effects of midodrine during pregnancy or breastfeeding. If you are pregnant or plan to become pregnant, or if you are breastfeeding or plan to do so, talk with your health-care practitioner before starting this drug. Only a health-care practitioner can determine whether the potential benefits outweigh the potential dangers.

SPECIAL INFORMATION FOR SENIORS

There are no special instructions for seniors.

GENERIC NAME

Mifepristone

BRAND NAME

Mifeprex

No generic available

ABOUT THIS DRUG

Mifepristone is used to terminate pregnancies of fewer than 49 days in duration. It works by blocking the supply of hormones that sustain the uterus. In the absence of these hormones, pregnancy cannot be supported and uterine contents are expelled.

SIDE EFFECTS

Consult your health-care practitioner if you develop side effects while taking mifepristone. Only he or she can determine whether it is safe for you to continue taking this drug.

- *Common:* uterine cramping, abdominal pain, back pain, nausea, vomiting, diarrhea, headache
- *Less Common or Rare:* fever, chills, pale skin, tiredness, weakness, stomach upset or pain, anxiety, fainting and dizziness upon rising, vaginal itch, excessive vaginal bleeding, increased vaginal discharge, pain during sexual intercourse, flu-like symptoms, runny nose, cough, heartburn, pain around eyes and cheekbones, difficulty breathing, tight chest

IMPORTANT PRECAUTIONS

Before starting this drug, always tell your health-care practitioner about all other medical conditions you have. If you have a bleeding disorder (such as anemia) or a blood clotting disorder (such as hemophilia), mifepristone may cause excessive vaginal bleeding.

Mifepristone does not terminate ectopic pregnancies.

IUDs (intrauterine devices) must be removed before taking this drug.

Call your health-care practitioner if you experience excessive vaginal bleeding. In some cases, you may need surgery to control bleeding or to terminate a pregnancy that this drug did not end.

DRUG INTERACTIONS

Always inform your health-care practitioner and pharmacist if you are taking any other prescription or over-the-counter drugs, as well as any vitamins, herbs, or other supplements. Possible interactions include the following:

- Carbamazepine, dexamethasone, phenobarbital, phenytoin, and rifampin may decrease the effects of mifepristone.
- Erythromycin, itraconazole, and ketoconazole may increase the effects of mifepristone.
- Taking mifepristone with blood thinners such as warfarin can increase the risk of bleeding.
- Corticosteroids may interfere with mifepristone.

FOOD, VITAMIN, AND HERBAL INTERACTIONS

St. John's wort may decrease the effects of mifepristone. Grapefruit juice may increase its effects. Do not combine these substances with mifepristone.

RECOMMENDED DOSAGE

Mifepristone comes in tablet form. The recommended dosage is 600 mg as a single oral dose, followed 2 days later by 400 mg as a single oral dose.

SYMPTOMS OF OVERDOSE AND WHAT TO DO

No specific information on overdose is available. However, if you suspect that an overdose has occurred, seek immediate medical attention and take the mifepristone bottle to the hospital with you.

SPECIAL INFORMATION FOR PREGNANT OR NURSING WOMEN

Mifepristone is used to end an early pregnancy. If pregnancy continues after treatment fails, birth defects may result. It is not known whether this drug passes into breast milk. If you are breastfeeding, your health-care practitioner may advise you to stop while taking mifepristone.

SPECIAL INFORMATION FOR SENIORS

This drug has no application for seniors.

GENERIC NAME

Miglitol

BRAND NAME

Glyset

No generic available

ABOUT THIS DRUG

Miglitol is used to treat the form of diabetes mellitus known as type 2. Type 2 diabetes was formerly known as adult-onset, and is also referred to as noninsulin-dependent. Diet and exercise play a key role in the management of this disease, and often miglitol is used along with other antidiabetes drugs called sulfonylureas.

This drug helps your body regulate the amount of glucose (sugar) in blood. It works by slowing the breakdown and absorption of table sugar and other complex sugars in the small intestine. Miglitol *must* be taken at the beginning of each meal (preferably with the first bite) to be effective.

SIDE EFFECTS

Side effects are most common at the start of treatment. As your body gets used to miglitol, in several weeks there should be few problems. However, all diabetics should learn to recognize the symptoms of low blood sugar and high blood sugar and know what to do if they occur. It is essential to control these symptoms before they progress to more serious conditions.

- *Common:* diarrhea, abdominal pain, gas, low blood iron, rash
- *Hypoglycemia (Low Blood Sugar):* "drunken" behavior, drowsiness, unusual tiredness or weakness, slurred speech, shakiness, dizziness, difficulty concentrating, headache, confusion, anxiety, nervousness, blurred vision, cold sweats, cool pale skin, excessive hunger, restless sleep, nightmares, nausea, fast heartbeat
- *Hyperglycemia (High Blood Sugar):* dry mouth, thirst, frequent urination, dry skin, flushing, appetite loss, difficulty breathing, tiredness

IMPORTANT PRECAUTIONS

Miglitol should not be used if you have intestinal problems such as ulcers or inflammatory bowel disease, intestinal blockage, malabsorption, severe kidney disease, or diabetic ketoacidosis (a life-threatening condition caused by insufficient insulin, with symptoms such as nausea, fatigue, excessive thirst, lower chest pain, and fruity breath). Use this drug with caution if you have an active infection or a history of kidney or liver disease.

Your health-care practitioner will most likely advise you to stop taking this drug for a short time before and after having any type of surgery or dental procedure.

Unlike other oral antidiabetes medications, miglitol does not usually cause low blood sugar (hypoglycemia). However, this condition can occur. The people most susceptible to hypoglycemia are older, weak, or malnourished, or have kidney, liver, adrenal, or hormone problems. Symptoms vary from person to person, so it is essential to learn which symptoms you usually have. As soon as you experience the characteristic signs, address and control them quickly by taking a fast-acting sugar, such as a glucose tablet, glass of fruit juice or nondiet soft drink, tablespoon of corn syrup or honey, or tablespoon of table sugar dissolved in water.

People with uncontrolled diabetes may also experience high blood sugar, or hyperglycemia. (See symptoms above.) If this condition is not treated, it can lead to diabetic coma and death.

In order to prevent these types of complications, carefully follow all diet and exercise recommendations made by your health-care practitioner and nutritionist. In fact, many people with type 2 diabetes are able to successfully control this disease by making healthy lifestyle changes, cutting back on the need for medication.

To monitor the effectiveness of miglitol, measure the amount of glucose in your urine or blood on a regular basis. Your health-care practitioner may also tell you to test your urine for ketones (substances that appear in urine when diabetes is not properly controlled). Carefully follow the instructions of your health-care practitioner and pharmacist when conducting these tests at home. If blood sugar is high or sugar or ketones are present in urine, call your health-care practitioner.

DRUG INTERACTIONS

Inform your health-care practitioner and pharmacist if you are taking any other prescription or over-the-counter drugs, as well as any vitamins, herbs, or other supplements. Possible drug interactions include the following:

- Taking miglitol with a sulfonylurea antidiabetes drug or insulin may increase the risk of hypoglycemia.
- Other drugs—such as clofibrate and large doses of aspirin—may also lead to hypoglycemia.
- Digestive enzymes and activated charcoal may decrease the effectiveness of miglitol.
- Miglitol may decrease the effects of certain drugs, including digoxin, propranolol, and ranitidine.
- Do not drink alcohol while taking miglitol. Alcohol alters blood sugar.

FOOD, VITAMIN, AND HERBAL INTERACTIONS

Supplements such as chromium, garlic, ginger, ginseng, hawthorn, and nettle may affect blood sugar levels. Check with your health-care practitioner before using any dietary supplement.

RECOMMENDED DOSAGE

Miglitol comes in tablet form. Although the doses given below are typical, only your health-care practitioner can determine the dose and schedule that best fit your needs.

- *Children:* This drug is not recommended for children.
- *Adults:* 25 to 100 mg 3 times a day with meals

Take miglitol with the first bite of each main meal. If you forget a dose with your meal, skip it and resume your normal schedule. Never take a double dose.

SYMPTOMS OF OVERDOSE AND WHAT TO DO

Symptoms of miglitol overdose may include gas, diarrhea, and pain. If you suspect that an overdose has occurred, seek immediate medical attention and take the prescription bottle to the hospital with you.

SPECIAL INFORMATION FOR PREGNANT OR NURSING WOMEN

No studies have adequately investigated the effects of miglitol during pregnancy or breastfeeding. If you are pregnant or plan to become pregnant, or if you are breastfeeding or plan to do so, talk with your health-care practitioner before starting this drug. Only a health-care practitioner can determine whether the potential benefits outweigh the potential dangers.

SPECIAL INFORMATION FOR SENIORS

There are no special instructions for seniors.

GENERIC NAME

Minocycline hydrochloride

see Tetracycline Antibiotics, page 1013

GENERIC NAME

Minoxidil

BRAND NAME

Rogaine
Generic available

ABOUT THIS DRUG

Minoxidil is used to stimulate hair growth and to slow balding. It is most effective in people under the age of 40 with recent hair loss. Minoxidil products are available both over-the-counter and by prescription. They are for topical application only. This drug works by stimulating hair follicles.

SIDE EFFECTS

Side effects are generally mild. However, consult your health-care practitioner if they become persistent or severe.

- *Common:* irritation, itching
- *Less Common or Rare:* In the vast majority of cases, not enough minoxidil is absorbed into the bloodstream to cause serious side effects.

IMPORTANT PRECAUTIONS

This treatment can be used on both men and women with hereditary hair loss. However, minoxidil does not cure baldness, and has no effect on receding hairlines. To be effective, hair in the balding area must be at least half an inch long. Most new hair is lost within a few months after the drug is stopped. In some people using this drug, hair loss is only slowed.

Do not apply minoxidil to a sunburned or irritated scalp. Keep it away from your eyes and other body areas. If this drug accidentally comes in contact with your eyes, wash them thoroughly with cool water. If they remain irritated, call your health-care practitioner.

Before taking minoxidil, tell your health-care practitioner about all other medical conditions you have.

DRUG INTERACTIONS

Although no specific interactions are associated with topical minoxidil, always inform your health-care practitioner and pharmacist if you are taking any other prescription or over-the-counter drugs, as well as any vitamins, herbs, or other supplements.

FOOD, VITAMIN, AND HERBAL INTERACTIONS

Vitamin E may reverse hair growth.

RECOMMENDED DOSAGE

Minoxidil comes as a liquid to be applied to the scalp. Apply 1 milliliter to dry scalp and hair twice a day. If you forget to apply a dose, do so as soon as you remember. If it is almost time for the next dose, skip the forgotten one, and resume your normal schedule. Never apply double doses.

SYMPTOMS OF OVERDOSE AND WHAT TO DO

Overdose is unlikely. However, if you suspect that an overdose has occurred, seek immediate medical attention and take the minoxidil container to the hospital with you.

SPECIAL INFORMATION FOR PREGNANT OR NURSING WOMEN

No studies have adequately investigated the effects of topical minoxidil during pregnancy or breastfeeding. If you are pregnant or plan to become pregnant, or if you are breastfeeding or plan to do so, talk with your health-care practitioner before starting this drug. Only a health-care practitioner can determine whether the potential benefits outweigh the potential dangers.

SPECIAL INFORMATION FOR SENIORS

There are no special instructions for seniors.

GENERIC NAME

Mirtazapine

BRAND NAME

Remeron
No generic available

ABOUT THIS DRUG

Mirtazapine is used to treat mental depression. This is more than a simple case of the blues. The symptoms of depression include sleep and appetite changes, sadness, guilt, shame, low self-esteem, anxiety, and extreme fatigue that last for over two weeks.

This drug works by adjusting the levels of two neurotransmitters (chemical messengers in the brain): norepinephrine and serotonin. These chemicals are believed to be low during depression.

SIDE EFFECTS

Inform your health-care practitioner if you develop side effects while taking mirtazapine. If symptoms are severe or prolonged, ask your health-care practitioner whether your dosage requires adjustment, and whether it is safe for you to continue taking this drug.

- *Common:* drowsiness, dizziness, weakness, increased appetite, weight gain, dry mouth, constipation
- *Less Common or Rare:* abnormal dreams, mood or mental changes, agitation, anxiety, confusion, abdominal pain, back pain, nausea, vomiting, trembling, shaking, fluid retention, swelling of hands and ankles, increased thirst, increased urination, difficulty breathing, rash

IMPORTANT PRECAUTIONS

Always inform your health-care practitioner about any other medical conditions you may have, especially dehydration, a history of convulsions or seizures, kidney or liver impairment, heart disease, a history of stroke, or mania (a type of mental illness).

If you plan to undergo surgery or a dental procedure, tell your health-care practitioner or dentist that you are taking mirtazapine.

This drug can make you drowsy and less alert than usual. Until you know how mirtazapine affects you, do not drive a car, operate machinery, or perform other tasks that require concentration.

If this drug causes mouth dryness, use sugarless gum or candy, ice chips, or artificial saliva. If the problem continues, consult your health-care practitioner or dentist.

DRUG INTERACTIONS

Tell your health-care practitioner and pharmacist if you are taking any other prescription or over-the-counter drugs, as well as any vitamins, herbs, or other supplements. Possible drug interactions include the following:

- Do not take monoamine oxidase inhibitor (MAOI) antidepressants at the same time as or within 14 days of mirtazapine. This combination can cause reactions ranging from confusion to seizures, and is potentially fatal.
- Taking other central nervous system depressants along with mirtazapine can result in more drowsiness.
- The combination of mirtazapine and diazepam may cause impaired movement.
- Taking mirtazapine with drugs such as fluoxetine and ritonavir can result in mirtazapine toxicity.
- Do not drink alcohol while taking mirtazapine.

FOOD, VITAMIN, AND HERBAL INTERACTIONS

Do not take mirtazapine with herbs such as hops, kava, passionflower, and valerian. These can increase effects such as drowsiness. Do not take St. John's wort with mirtazapine, since both affect serotonin. Other inappropriate herbs include ginseng, ephedra (ma huang), and yohimbe.

RECOMMENDED DOSAGE

Mirtazapine comes as a tablet. Although the doses given below are typical, only your health-care practitioner can determine the dose and schedule that best fit your needs.

- *Children:* This drug is not recommended for children.
- *Adults:* 15 to 45 mg daily at bedtime

Mirtazapine can be taken with or without food. It must be taken regularly for several weeks before its full effect is felt. If you forget a dose, take it as soon as you remember. If it is almost time for the next dose, skip the missed one and resume your normal schedule. Never take a double dose. Do not stop taking this drug suddenly, especially if you have been taking it a long time. Your health-care practitioner will gradually reduce dosage.

SYMPTOMS OF OVERDOSE AND WHAT TO DO

The symptoms of mirtazapine overdose include drowsiness, confusion, mental impairment, and rapid heartbeat. If overdose occurs, seek immediate medical attention and take the prescription bottle to the hospital with you.

SPECIAL INFORMATION FOR PREGNANT OR NURSING WOMEN

No studies have adequately investigated the effects of mirtazapine during pregnancy or breastfeeding. If you are pregnant or plan to become pregnant, or if you are breastfeeding or plan to do so, talk with your health-care practitioner before starting this drug. Only a health-care practitioner can determine whether the potential benefits outweigh the potential dangers.

SPECIAL INFORMATION FOR SENIORS

Seniors are at higher risk of side effects, and usually require smaller doses.

OPEN QUESTIONS OR CONTROVERSIES

In June 2004, the Food and Drug Administration asked manufacturers of mirtazapine to include in their labeling a warning statement that recommends close observation of adult and pediatric patients for clinical worsening of depression or the emergence of suicidality when being treated with this drug, especially when beginning the drug, or at the time of dose changes, either increases or decreases.

GENERIC NAME
Misoprostol

BRAND NAME
Cytotec
Generic available

ABOUT THIS DRUG
Misoprostol is used to prevent stomach ulcers when you are taking nonsteroidal anti-inflammatory drugs (NSAIDs) such as aspirin. If you must take NSAIDs for a prolonged period of time for a problem such as arthritis, you face an increasing risk of stomach bleeding and ulcers.

Misoprostol helps the stomach defend itself from damage caused by NSAIDs. It protects the lining of the stomach and small intestine by replacing prostaglandins and decreasing the secretion of stomach acid.

SIDE EFFECTS
Side effects are most common at the start of treatment. They usually disappear within several weeks, as your body gets used to misoprostol. However, if symptoms are prolonged or severe, contact your physician. Only he or she can determine whether or not you should continue to take this drug.

- *Common:* nausea, diarrhea, abdominal cramps
- *Less Common or Rare:* headache, constipation, indigestion, gas, vomiting, paleness, stomach or intestinal bleeding, vaginal bleeding

IMPORTANT PRECAUTIONS
Misoprostol should not be taken by pregnant women, since it may cause miscarriage. Women of childbearing age should receive a pregnancy test before taking this drug, and use effective contraception for the duration of treatment.

Always tell your health-care practitioner about any other medical conditions that you may have, especially blood vessel disease, epilepsy, and inflammatory bowel disease.

Misoprostol may cause drowsiness, so limit activities such as driving as necessary.

DRUG INTERACTIONS
Inform your health-care practitioner and pharmacist if you are taking any other prescription or over-the-counter drugs, as well as any vita-

mins, herbs, or other supplements. Possible drug interactions with misoprostol may include the following:

- Antacids may inhibit the absorption and benefits of misoprostol.
- Antacids with magnesium may worsen diarrhea associated with misoprostol.
- Misoprostol may alter the absorption of theophylline and diazepam.

FOOD, VITAMIN, AND HERBAL INTERACTIONS

High-fat meals may reduce the absorption and effects of misoprostol.

RECOMMENDED DOSAGE

Misoprostol is available in tablet form. Although the doses given below are typical, only your health-care practitioner can determine the dose and schedule that are most appropriate for you.

- *Children:* This drug is not recommended for children.
- *Adults:* 100 to 200 micrograms 4 times daily

Misoprostol must be taken with food. If you miss a dose, take it as soon as you remember. However, if it is nearly time for your next scheduled dose, do not take the missed dose. Follow your regular dosing schedule. Never take a double dose.

SYMPTOMS OF OVERDOSE AND WHAT TO DO

Possible symptoms of overdose include drowsiness, diarrhea, changes in heartbeat, low blood pressure, fever, tremor, difficulty breathing, and convulsions. If you suspect an overdose, seek immediate medical attention, and bring the prescription bottle to the hospital with you.

SPECIAL INFORMATION FOR PREGNANT OR NURSING WOMEN

Do not take misoprostol if you are pregnant. This drug causes miscarriage. It is not known whether misoprostol passes into breast milk. However, to be on the safe side, your health-care practitioner will probably advise you to stop breastfeeding while you take this drug.

SPECIAL INFORMATION FOR SENIORS

If side effects are troublesome, lower dosages are recommended for seniors.

GENERIC NAME
Mitoxantrone

BRAND NAME
Novantrone
No generic available

ABOUT THIS DRUG
Mitoxantrone is a neoplastic drug used in the treatment of some types of cancer. It is also prescribed to extend the time between relapses of multiple sclerosis (MS). Even low doses of this drug can prove toxic, so it is prescribed with extreme care.

Mitoxantrone works by suppressing the immune system and destroying cancer cells. Unfortunately, at the same time this medication also affects normal cells, accounting for the great number of side effects.

SIDE EFFECTS
Side effects of mitoxantrone can be extremely serious, and must be promptly reported to your health-care practitioner. Some effects—such as the urine turning blue-green or the whites of the eyes turning blue—are distressing but pose no physical danger. On the other hand, dangerous effects—such as leukemia and other forms of cancer—may develop months or even years after treatment.

- *Common:* nausea, vomiting, diarrhea, constipation, stomach pain, headache, hair loss, mouth and lip sores, mouth bleeding, body aches and pains, cough, sore throat, sneezing, runny nose, swollen glands, congestion, shortness of breath, increased risk of infection, fatigue, irregular menstrual periods
- *Less Common or Rare:* fast or irregular heartbeat, fever, chills, lower back pain, side pain, unusual bleeding or bruising, swelling of lower legs and feet, blood in urine or stools, pinpoint red spots on skin, painful or difficult urination, decreased urination, yellow eyes or skin, sore, reddened eyes, seizures

IMPORTANT PRECAUTIONS
Always tell your health-care practitioner about any other medical conditions you may have, especially active infection, chicken pox, gout, heart disease, kidney stones, liver problems, mouth sores, shingles, or immune system diseases. Mitoxantrone is prescribed with extreme caution in such cases.

Mitoxantrone can cause birth defects if either a man or woman is taking it at the time of conception. It is also associated with miscarriage, impaired fertility, and menstrual irregularities.

Mitoxantrone suppresses the immune system, and may decrease the body's ability to combat infection. Avoid people with infections. If you must go near someone who has received oral polio vaccine, wear a protective face mask.

This drug may cause a number of distressing side effects. Until you know how mitoxantrone affects you, do not drive a car, operate machinery, or perform other tasks that require concentration. Avoid contact sports where bruising and injury might occur.

People taking any dose of mitoxantrone must be closely monitored with regular complete blood counts and other tests.

DRUG INTERACTIONS

Inform your health-care practitioner and pharmacist if you are taking any other prescription or over-the-counter drugs, as well as any vitamins, herbs, or other supplements. Possible drug interactions include the following:

- Do not have live-virus immunizations while taking mitoxantrone without your health-care practitioner's approval. You are at risk of infection from the virus.
- Mitoxantrone may increase the effects of amphotericin B by injection, antithyroid agents, azathioprine, chloramphenicol, colchicines, flucytosine, ganciclovir, interferon, plicamycin, and zidovudine.
- Mitoxantrone may alter the absorption of probenecid and sulfinpyrazone.
- Do not drink alcohol while taking mitoxantrone. This increases the possibility of undesirable liver effects.

FOOD, VITAMIN, AND HERBAL INTERACTIONS

Do not take mitoxantrone with supplements such as echinacea. Drink extra fluids while taking this drug, so it will pass through your body more quickly and prevent kidney problems.

RECOMMENDED DOSAGE

Mitoxantrone is available by injection and is administered in a hospital setting. Dosage is highly individualized and must be determined by your health-care practitioner.

SYMPTOMS OF OVERDOSE AND WHAT TO DO

Mitoxantrone is administered in a hospital setting, and an overdose is unlikely. Severe infection, which results from a dramatic suppression of white blood cells, is a symptom of an overdose. If you suspect that an overdose has occurred, seek immediate medical attention.

SPECIAL INFORMATION FOR PREGNANT OR NURSING WOMEN

Do not take this drug if you are pregnant or think you may be pregnant. Mitoxantrone may cause birth defects or miscarriage. Because of the possibility of serious side effects, breastfeeding is not recommended while you take this drug.

SPECIAL INFORMATION FOR SENIORS

There are no special instructions for seniors.

GENERIC NAME

Modafinil

BRAND NAME

Provigil

No generic available

ABOUT THIS DRUG

Modafinil is a central nervous system stimulant used for the treatment of narcolepsy (a condition characterized by sudden collapses into sleep). To prevent sleep disturbances, this drug should not be taken later than noon. Modafinil does not cure narcolepsy, and must be taken consistently in order to be effective. This drug appears to work by stimulating certain chemicals in the brain.

SIDE EFFECTS

Contact your health-care practitioner if you develop side effects while taking this drug. Only he or she can determine if you should continue to take modafinil.

- *Common:* headache, nausea, runny nose, loss of appetite, anxiety, nervousness, trouble sleeping, dizziness, diarrhea, sore throat, dry mouth
- *Less Common or Rare:* weight loss, stomach pain, nausea, chest pain, abnormal heart rhythms, changes in blood pressure or pulse, fever, arthritis-like symptoms, drowsiness, hair loss, itching, rash, severe jerking or twitching, visual disturbances such as blurred vision, severe psychotic reactions

IMPORTANT PRECAUTIONS

Tell your health-care practitioner if you are sensitive or allergic to modafinil or similar drugs such as methylphenidate. Also inform your health-care practitioner about any other medical conditions you suffer from, especially high blood pressure, a recent heart attack, heart disease, or liver or kidney problems.

Chronic or abusive use of modafinil can lead to addiction. This drug should be used with caution in anyone with a history of drug or alcohol abuse or of psychosis.

Before having any type of surgery or dental procedure, inform your surgeon or dentist that you are taking modafinil.

This drug may impair your judgment. Until you know how modafinil affects you, do not drive a car, operate machinery, or perform other tasks that require concentration.

DRUG INTERACTIONS

Inform your health-care practitioner and pharmacist if you are taking any prescription or over-the-counter drugs, as well as any vitamins, herbs, or other supplements. Possible drug interactions include the following:

- Birth control pills and implants are less effective while you are taking modafinil and for one month afterwards. Use an alternate form of contraception.
- Monoamine oxidase inhibitor (MAOI) antidepressants may increase the effects of modafinil, leading to adverse reactions.
- Modafinil may increase the effects of tricyclic antidepressants.
- Some drugs increase modafinil's central nervous system effects, such as nervousness, irritability, and difficulty sleeping. These include amantadine, amphetamines, diet pills, asthma and sinus medications, cold and allergy remedies, bupropion, caffeine, chlophedianol, methylphenidate, nabilone, and pemoline.
- Modafinil may also interact with cyclosporine, diazepam, propranolol, theophylline, blood thinners such as warfarin, and epilepsy medications such as phenytoin.
- Do not combine modafinil with alcohol.

FOOD, VITAMIN, AND HERBAL INTERACTIONS

Herbs that affect the central nervous system—including St. John's wort, guarana, ephedra (ma huang), and kola—should be avoided when taking modafinil.

Avoid caffeinated beverages, such as coffee, tea, and cola.

RECOMMENDED DOSAGE

Modafinil is available in tablet form. Although the doses given below are typical, only your health-care practitioner can determine the dose and schedule that are most appropriate for you.

- *Children:* This drug is not recommended for children under the age of 17.
- *Adults:* 100 to 200 mg daily in the morning

Modafinil should be taken as a single dose in the morning. If you miss a dose and remember it by noon of that day, take it. Do not take it later, or you may have trouble sleeping that night. If it is later than noon, skip that dose and resume your regular schedule. Never take two doses at once.

SYMPTOMS OF OVERDOSE AND WHAT TO DO

The symptoms of modafinil overdose include nausea, diarrhea, agitation, anxiety, confusion, irritability, aggressiveness, nervousness, insomnia, and tremor. If overdose occurs, seek immediate medical attention and bring the prescription bottle to the hospital with you.

SPECIAL INFORMATION FOR PREGNANT OR NURSING WOMEN

No studies have adequately investigated the effects of modafinil during pregnancy or breastfeeding. If you are pregnant or plan to become pregnant, or if you are breastfeeding or plan to do so, talk with your health-care practitioner before starting this drug. Only a health-care practitioner can determine whether the potential benefits outweigh the potential dangers.

SPECIAL INFORMATION FOR SENIORS

Seniors—especially those with kidney or liver problems—may require lower dosages.

OPEN QUESTIONS OR CONTROVERSIES

Chronic or abusive use of modafinil can potentially lead to tolerance and/or mental or physical dependence. If you have a history of drug or alcohol abuse, use this drug with caution. People with current or past mental illness may also be at increased risk of dependence. To prevent this problem, be very careful to take only the prescribed doses.

GENERIC NAME
Moexipril

BRAND NAME
Univasc
No generic available

ABOUT THIS DRUG
Moexipril is an angiotensin-converting enzyme (ACE) inhibitor used to treat high blood pressure (hypertension). This drug may be prescribed alone or with other high blood pressure medications, such as thiazide diuretics. It works by blocking an enzyme in the body, which relaxes blood vessels and lowers blood pressure.

SIDE EFFECTS
Speak to your health-care practitioner if you develop side effects while taking moexipril. Only he or she can determine whether you should continue taking this drug.

- *Common:* dizziness, flu-like symptoms, dry cough, diarrhea, headache
- *Less Common or Rare:* angina (chest pain), faintness, upset stomach, vomiting, ringing in the ears, tiredness, nausea, constipation, dry mouth, difficulty sleeping, mood changes, anxiety, low blood pressure, rash, breathing difficulties, muscle weakness, joint pain, fluid retention, sensitivity to light, respiratory difficulties, kidney or liver problems, heart rhythm disturbances

IMPORTANT PRECAUTIONS
Always inform your health-care practitioner about any other medical conditions you suffer from, especially congestive heart failure, angina, abnormal heart rhythms, or other heart problems. Also tell your health-care practitioner if you have kidney or liver disease.

Moexipril can affect your kidneys, especially if you have congestive heart failure. If you already have kidney disease, your dosage should be lower than usual.

Before having any type of surgery or dental procedure, tell your surgeon or dentist that you are taking moexipril.

This drug may make you dizzy. Until you know how moexipril affects you, do not drive a car, operate machinery, or perform other tasks that demand concentration.

Treatment of high blood pressure also entails certain lifestyle changes, such as weight control, smoking cessation, and close attention to diet.

When you first start taking this drug or when the dosage is increased, you may experience dizziness or faintness when you rise quickly from a sitting or reclining position (postural hypotension). Try to get up slowly, and consult your health-care practitioner if the problem continues.

Be extremely careful when you exercise in hot weather. Heavy sweating can lead to dizziness, lightheadedness, fainting, vomiting, dehydration, and low blood pressure.

Do not take this drug if you have ever experienced an allergic reaction to it or to other ACE inhibitors. If you have an allergic reaction such as swelling of the face and mouth and a sudden problem with breathing, seek immediate medical attention.

DRUG INTERACTIONS

Tell your health-care practitioner and pharmacist if you are taking any other prescription or over-the-counter drugs, as well as any vitamins, herbs, or other supplements. Possible drug interactions include the following:

- Taking other blood pressure medications can increase the blood pressure lowering effects of moexipril.
- If you are already taking a diuretic, when possible your health-care practitioner will have you stop taking it 2 to 3 days before starting moexipril.
- Moexipril may increase blood levels of potassium, particularly when taken with potassium-sparing diuretics. Too much potassium can cause heart rhythm disturbances.
- Combining moexipril with allopurinol increases the risk of side effects.
- Taking moexipril with lithium can result in toxic levels of lithium in the blood.
- Phenothiazine tranquilizers and antiemetics may increase the effects of moexipril.
- Aspirin and other NSAIDs (such as ibuprofen and indomethacin) can reduce the blood pressure lowering effects of moexipril.
- Separate doses of antacids and moexipril by 2 hours.
- Moexipril increases blood levels of digoxin.
- Alcohol may further lower blood pressure. Use with caution.
- Consult your health-care practitioner before taking over-the-counter cough, cold, sinus, allergy, or weight loss medications. Many of these can raise blood pressure.

FOOD, VITAMIN, AND HERBAL INTERACTIONS

Do not take herbs that increase blood pressure, such as ephedra (ma huang), ginseng, goldenseal, licorice, and saw palmetto. Consult your health-care practitioner before taking substances that may lower blood pressure, such as calcium, soy, or garlic. To minimize possible interactions, take moexipril and iron supplements 2 or 3 hours apart. Because ACE inhibitors raise potassium levels in the body, *do not* take potassium supplements or use salt substitutes containing potassium, and ask your health-care practitioner how many potassium-rich foods (such as bananas, prunes, raisins, melons, tomatoes, citrus fruit, and orange juice) you can safely include in your diet. Also talk to your health-care practitioner about salt intake.

RECOMMENDED DOSAGE

Moexipril is available in oral form as tablets. Although the doses given below are typical, only your health-care practitioner can determine the dose and schedule that best fit your needs.

- *Children:* This drug is not recommended for children.
- *Adults:* 7.5 to 30 mg once daily

Take moexipril one hour before or two hours after meals. Continue to take this drug even if you feel well. Do not discontinue use without consulting your health-care practitioner. If you miss a dose, take it as soon as you remember. If it is almost time for the next dose, skip the forgotten one, and resume your normal schedule. Never take a double dose.

SYMPTOMS OF OVERDOSE AND WHAT TO DO

The symptoms of moexipril overdose may include dizziness and fainting caused by a severe drop in blood pressure. If overdose occurs, seek immediate medical attention and take the prescription bottle to the hospital with you.

SPECIAL INFORMATION FOR PREGNANT OR NURSING WOMEN

Do not take moexipril if you are pregnant (especially during the final six months). This drug can cause fetal injury and death. If you become pregnant while taking moexipril, call your health-care practitioner immediately.

Small amounts of moexipril may pass into breast milk. If you are breastfeeding, your health-care practitioner will likely advise you to stop until your treatment is done.

SPECIAL INFORMATION FOR SENIORS
Seniors usually require lower doses of moexipril.

GENERIC NAME
Mometasone furoate
see Corticosteroids, Nasal Inhalation, page 327; Corticosteroids, Topical, page 337

GENERIC NAME
Montelukast
see Leukotriene Antagonist/Inhibitors, page 600

GENERIC NAME
Morphine
see Codeine, Morphine, Oxycodone, page 313

GENERIC NAME
Moxifloxacin
see Fluoroquinolone Antibiotics, page 468

GENERIC NAME
Mupirocin

BRAND NAME
Bactroban
No generic available

ABOUT THIS DRUG
Mupirocin is a topical antibiotic used to treat *Staphylococcus* and *Streptococcus* skin infections such as impetigo. It is for external application only. Mupirocin works by binding to an enzyme and preventing bacteria from making the proteins they need to survive.

SIDE EFFECTS
Consult your health-care practitioner if you develop side effects while using mupirocin. Only he or she can determine whether it is safe for you to continue applying this drug.

➤ *Common:* skin irritation, burning sensation, stinging, pain

- *Less Common or Rare:* itching, dry skin, inflammation, redness, rash, swelling, tenderness, oozing, nausea

IMPORTANT PRECAUTIONS

If the infection does not begin to heal in 3 to 5 days, or if it gets worse, call your health-care practitioner. Do not use mupirocin if you have ever had an allergic reaction to it or similar drugs. Using this medication for a prolonged period can lead to the growth of resistant bacteria that do not respond to mupirocin. Always tell your health-care practitioner about all other medical conditions you have.

DRUG INTERACTIONS

Although no specific interactions are known, always inform your health-care practitioner and pharmacist if you are taking any other prescription or over-the-counter drugs, as well as any vitamins, herbs, or other supplements.

FOOD, VITAMIN, AND HERBAL INTERACTIONS

No food, vitamin, or herbal interactions have been noted.

RECOMMENDED DOSAGE

Mupirocin comes in cream or ointment form. Apply a small amount to affected skin 3 times daily. If you forget a dose, apply it as soon as you remember. If it is almost time for the next dose, skip the forgotten one, and resume your normal schedule. Never apply double doses.

SYMPTOMS OF OVERDOSE AND WHAT TO DO

Overdosage is unlikely. However, if you suspect overdose, seek immediate medical attention.

SPECIAL INFORMATION FOR PREGNANT OR NURSING WOMEN

No studies have adequately investigated the effects of mupirocin during pregnancy. If you are pregnant or plan to become pregnant, or if you are breastfeeding or plan to do so, talk with your health-care practitioner before starting this drug. Only a health-care practitioner can determine whether the potential benefits outweigh the potential dangers.

SPECIAL INFORMATION FOR SENIORS

There are no special instructions for seniors.

GENERIC NAME
Nabumetone

BRAND NAME
Relafen
No generic available

ABOUT THIS DRUG
Nabumetone is a nonsteroidal anti-inflammatory drug (NSAID) used to relieve the pain and inflammation of rheumatoid arthritis and osteoarthritis. Nabumetone works by reducing the level of prostaglandins, chemicals in the body that produce inflammation and pain.

SIDE EFFECTS
If you develop side effects while taking nabumetone, ask your health-care practitioner whether it is safe for you to continue taking this drug.

- *Common:* diarrhea, constipation, stomach upset or pain, gas, nausea, vomiting, fluid retention, ringing in the ears, appetite loss
- *Less Common or Rare:* headache, dizziness, blurred vision, sensitivity to light, confusion, fainting, tingling in the hands or feet, mouth sores, fatigue, weakness, abnormal bleeding or bruising, rash, hives, itching, heart palpitations, difficulty breathing, gastrointestinal bleeding, ulcers, painful urination, kidney damage

IMPORTANT PRECAUTIONS
Like all NSAIDs, nabumetone can cause gastrointestinal bleeding, ulcers, and stomach perforation. If you take this drug on a regular basis, these types of side effects can occur at any time, with or without warning. People with a history of ulcers, colitis, or any type of gastrointestinal bleeding should be extremely careful when taking nabumetone.

Do not take nabumetone if you have a bleeding disorder or asthma or nasal polyps associated with aspirin use. Use this drug with caution if you have high blood pressure or other heart problems or impaired liver or kidney function. Tell your health-care practitioner if you have ever experienced an allergic reaction to aspirin or related drugs.

Possible side effects of nabumetone include blurred vision and dizziness. Until you know how this drug affects you, do not drive a car, operate machinery, or perform other tasks that require concentration.

Nabumetone may cause increased sun sensitivity. Wear protective clothing and apply sunscreen when using this drug.

DRUG INTERACTIONS

Tell your health-care practitioner and pharmacist if you are taking any other prescription or over-the-counter drugs, as well as any vitamins, herbs, or other supplements. Possible drug interactions include the following:

- Do not combine aspirin, ibuprofen, or other prescription or over-the-counter NSAIDs with nabumetone. This increases the risk of bleeding.
- Other drugs that may increase the risk of bleeding include dipyridamole, sulfinpyrazone, valproic acid, and blood thinners such as warfarin.
- Taking nabumetone with antihypertensive medications such as ACE inhibitors, beta-blockers, and diuretics decreases their blood pressure lowering effects.
- Taking nabumetone with lithium or methotrexate can lead to toxic levels of lithium or methotrexate in the body.
- Do not use alcohol when you are taking nabumetone. Both are stomach irritants, and using them together can increase the risk of stomach bleeding and ulcers.

FOOD, VITAMIN, AND HERBAL INTERACTIONS

Do not combine nabumetone with the herbal remedies clove oil, feverfew, garlic, ginkgo, and ginseng. These herbs may affect clotting.

RECOMMENDED DOSAGE

Nabumetone comes in tablet form. Low starting doses and smallest effective doses are recommended. The doses given below are typical. However, only your health-care practitioner can determine the dose and schedule that best fit your individual needs.

- *Children:* This drug is not recommended for children.
- *Adults:* 1,000 to 2,000 mg daily, in 1 or 2 doses

Nabumetone can be taken with food or milk to prevent stomach upset. Take medication with an 8-ounce glass of water and remain sitting upright or standing (do not lie down) for 30 minutes. If you forget to take a dose, take it as soon as you remember. But if it is almost time for the next dose, skip the one you missed and resume your normal schedule. Never take a double dose.

SYMPTOMS OF OVERDOSE AND WHAT TO DO

Symptoms of nabumetone overdose include nausea, vomiting, diarrhea, abdominal pain, drowsiness, rapid breathing, rapid heartbeat, agitation, confusion, disorientation, sweating, ringing in the ears, stupor, and seizures. If an overdose occurs, seek immediate medical attention and take the prescription bottle to the hospital with you so the health-care practitioner will know exactly what medication was taken.

SPECIAL INFORMATION FOR PREGNANT OR NURSING WOMEN

Use of nabumetone should be avoided in late pregnancy. If you want to take this drug in early pregnancy, ask your health-care practitioner whether the potential benefits outweigh the risks. Because nabumetone may pass into breast milk, it is best to stop breastfeeding while you take this drug.

SPECIAL INFORMATION FOR SENIORS

Smaller doses are recommended for seniors, who are more susceptible to side effects such as diarrhea, dizziness, confusion, fluid retention, stomach ulcers, and kidney or liver effects.

GENERIC NAME

Nadolol

BRAND NAME

Corgard
Generic available

ABOUT THIS DRUG

Nadolol is a beta-adrenergic blocking agent (beta-blocker) prescribed for mild-to-moderate high blood pressure (hypertension). It is also used to treat angina (chest pain). This drug is available in combination with a diuretic (another type of high blood pressure medication).

Nadolol works by decreasing the force and rate of heart contractions. This reduces angina and lowers blood pressure.

SIDE EFFECTS

Speak to your health-care practitioner if you develop side effects while taking this drug. Only he or she can determine whether it is safe for you to continue taking nadolol.

- *Common:* dizziness, drowsiness, tiredness, weakness, changes in heartbeat
- *Less Common or Rare:* lightheadedness, cold hands and feet, fainting, nausea, upset stomach, indigestion, vomiting, diarrhea, cramps, sweating, fatigue, urinary difficulties, impotence, muscle weakness, vivid dreams, excessive tiredness or weakness, constipation, breathing difficulties, cough, fever, blurred vision, dry eyes, rash, stuffy nose, chest pain, slow heartbeat, heart failure

IMPORTANT PRECAUTIONS

Inform your health-care practitioner about any other medical conditions you suffer from, especially a slow heart rate or serious heart block, congestive heart failure, angina, asthma or other lung ailments, liver or kidney problems, diabetes or hypoglycemia, or a thyroid condition.

Before having any type of surgery or dental procedure, inform your surgeon or dentist that you are taking nadolol.

This drug may make you more sensitive to the cold. Beta-blockers can decrease blood circulation in the fingers, toes, and skin. Be sure to dress warmly in low temperatures, especially if you already have blood circulation problems.

This drug may make you drowsy. Until you know how nadolol affects you, do not drive a car, operate machinery, or perform other tasks that demand concentration.

Treatment of high blood pressure also entails certain lifestyle changes, such as weight control, smoking cessation, and a low-sodium diet.

Be extremely careful when you exercise in hot weather. Heavy sweating can lead to dizziness, lightheadedness, vomiting, fainting, dehydration, and a drop in blood pressure.

When you first start taking this drug or when the dosage is increased, you may experience dizziness or faintness when you rise quickly from a sitting or reclining position (postural hypotension). Try to get up slowly, and consult your health-care practitioner if the problem continues.

DRUG INTERACTIONS

Tell your health-care practitioner and pharmacist if you are taking any other prescription or over-the-counter drugs, as well as any vitamins, herbs, or other supplements. Possible drug interactions include the following:

- Drugs that contain aspirin can lessen the blood pressure lowering effects of nadolol.

- Taking other blood pressure medications (including clonidine, reserpine, and calcium channel blockers) can increase the effects of nadolol.
- Nadolol can interfere with the action of oral antidiabetes medications. It may also change blood glucose levels.
- Nadolol may interfere with the effectiveness of certain asthma medications, including aminophylline, epinephrine, isoproterenol, and theophylline.
- Nadolol may increase the effect of antianxiety benzodiazepine drugs.
- If you are also taking ergot alkaloids for migraines, nadolol may worsen side effects such as cold hands and feet. In rare cases, this drug combination may lead to gangrene.
- Nadolol may interact with anesthetics during surgery, increasing the risk of heart problems. As a result, your health-care practitioner will instruct you to stop taking this drug at least two days before surgery.
- Alcohol intensifies the drowsiness caused by this drug.
- Cocaine and cigarette smoking may reduce the effectiveness of nadolol.
- Ask your health-care practitioner about taking over-the-counter cough, cold, sinus, allergy, and weight loss remedies. Many of these can raise blood pressure.

FOOD, VITAMIN, AND HERBAL INTERACTIONS

Do not take herbs that increase blood pressure, including ephedra (ma huang), ginseng, goldenseal, licorice, and saw palmetto. Consult your health-care practitioner before taking substances that may lower blood pressure, such as calcium, soy, or garlic. Your health-care practitioner will probably recommend a low-sodium diet.

RECOMMENDED DOSAGE

Nadolol is available in oral form as tablets. Although the doses given below are typical, only your health-care practitioner can determine the dose and schedule that are most appropriate for you.

- *Children:* This drug is not recommended for children.
- *Adults:* 40 to 320 mg once daily

If nadolol upsets your stomach, take it with food. If you forget to take a dose, take it as soon as you remember. If it is almost time for the next dose, skip the forgotten one, and resume your normal schedule. Never take double doses.

Continue to take this drug even if you feel well. Do not discontinue use without consulting your health-care practitioner. Abrupt withdrawal can cause chest pain, breathing difficulties, increased sweating, irregular heartbeat, and even heart attack in some people. To end treatment, in most cases your health-care practitioner will reduce dosage gradually over a 2-week period.

SYMPTOMS OF OVERDOSE AND WHAT TO DO

The symptoms of nadolol overdose include slow heart rate, low blood pressure, dizziness, fainting, difficulty breathing, bluish fingernails and palms, and seizures. If overdose occurs, seek immediate medical attention and take the prescription bottle to the hospital with you.

SPECIAL INFORMATION FOR PREGNANT OR NURSING WOMEN

Some studies have shown that women who take beta-blockers during pregnancy give birth to babies with lower birth weight, heart rate, and blood pressure. As a result, nadolol should be avoided if you are pregnant.

Small amounts of nadolol can pass into breast milk and cause problems such as slow heart rate, low blood pressure, and trouble breathing. If you must take nadolol, your health-care practitioner may recommend bottle-feeding.

SPECIAL INFORMATION FOR SENIORS

Seniors usually require lower doses of nadolol. Older people are more apt to experience side effects such as heightened sensitivity to the cold, a general feeling of unwellness, chest pain, breathing difficulties, sweating, and variations in heartbeat.

GENERIC NAME

Nafcillin *see Penicillin Antibiotics, page 812*

GENERIC NAME

Naproxen *see Propionic Acid (NSAID) Family, page 880*

GENERIC NAME
Naratriptan
see Triptan-Type Antimigraine Drugs, page 1083

GENERIC NAME
Nedocromil

BRAND NAME
Tilade
No generic available

ABOUT THIS DRUG
Nedocromil is prescribed to treat mild-to-moderate asthma. Taking it may allow you to cut back on or eliminate oral steroids, which have serious side effects. This drug works by inhibiting the release of chemicals in your body that cause the inflammatory symptoms of asthma.

SIDE EFFECTS
Speak to your health-care practitioner if you develop side effects while taking this drug. Only he or she can determine whether you should continue taking nedocromil.

- *Common:* bad taste in mouth, cough, sore throat, hoarseness, headache, nausea, chest pain
- *Less Common or Rare:* dry mouth, dizziness, stomach upset or pain, vomiting, diarrhea, fatigue, itching or burning nasal passages, stuffy nose, sneezing, conjunctivitis, bronchitis, viral infection, wheezing, increased difficulty breathing

IMPORTANT PRECAUTIONS
Tell your health-care practitioner about any other medical conditions you may have, especially impaired kidney function or a heart rhythm disorder.

This drug is not a bronchodilator and should not be used for the immediate relief of an acute asthma attack.

Inform your health-care practitioner if you have experienced allergies to this or similar medications in the past.

Because nedocromil may cause side effects such as dizziness, do not drive a car, operate machinery, or perform other tasks that require concentration until you know how this drug affects you.

To relieve dry mouth or throat irritation, use sugarless gum or hard candy, or rinse your mouth with water. If the problem persists, consult your health-care practitioner or dentist.

DRUG INTERACTIONS

Tell your health-care practitioner if you are taking any other prescription or over-the-counter drugs, as well as any vitamins, herbs, or supplements. Possible drug interactions include the following:

- Nedocromil may allow you to cut back on oral steroid medication.

FOOD, VITAMIN, AND HERBAL INTERACTIONS

No food, vitamin, or herbal interactions have been noted.

RECOMMENDED DOSAGE

Nedocromil comes as an aerosol to inhale by mouth. Although the doses given below are typical, only your health-care practitioner can determine the dose and schedule that best fit your individual needs.

- *Children 6 Years and Older and Adults:* 2 inhalations 4 times daily, for a total daily dosage of 14 mg

If you forget a dose, take it as soon as you remember. Take the rest of the day's doses at evenly spaced intervals, and resume your normal schedule the next day. Never take a double dose.

SYMPTOMS OF OVERDOSE AND WHAT TO DO

Overdosage is unlikely. However, if you suspect overdose, seek immediate medical attention.

SPECIAL INFORMATION FOR PREGNANT OR NURSING WOMEN

No studies have adequately investigated the effects of nedocromil during pregnancy or breastfeeding. If you are pregnant or plan to become pregnant, or if you are breastfeeding or plan to do so, talk with your health-care practitioner before starting this drug. Only a health-care practitioner can determine whether the potential benefits outweigh the potential dangers.

SPECIAL INFORMATION FOR SENIORS

There are no special recommendations for seniors.

GENERIC NAME
Nefazodone

BRAND NAME
Serzone
No generic available

ABOUT THIS DRUG
Nefazodone is used to treat mental depression. This is more than a simple case of the blues. The symptoms of depression include sleep and appetite changes, sadness, guilt, shame, low self-esteem, anxiety, and extreme fatigue that last for over two weeks. Nefazodone works by blocking a chemical messenger in the brain called 5-HT.

SIDE EFFECTS
Inform your health-care practitioner if you develop side effects while taking nefazodone. If symptoms are severe or prolonged, ask your health-care practitioner whether your dosage requires adjustment, and whether it is safe for you to continue taking this drug.

- *Common:* drowsiness, dizziness, lightheadedness, weakness, confusion, dry mouth, constipation, nausea, blurred vision
- *Less Common or Rare:* abnormal dreams, dizziness upon getting up, poor concentration, diarrhea, flu-like symptoms, cough, headache, water retention, increased appetite, lack of coordination, decreased sex drive, difficulty urinating, fever, stiff neck, ringing in ears, thirst, changes in taste

IMPORTANT PRECAUTIONS
Always inform your health-care practitioner about any other medical conditions you may have, especially dehydration, a history of convulsions or seizures, kidney or liver impairment, heart disease, a history of stroke, or mania (a type of mental illness).

If you plan to undergo surgery or a dental procedure, tell your health-care practitioner or dentist that you are taking nefazodone.

This drug can make you drowsy and less alert than usual. Until you know how nefazodone affects you, do not drive a car, operate machinery, or perform other tasks that require concentration.

If this drug causes mouth dryness, use sugarless gum or candy, ice chips, or artificial saliva. If the problem continues, consult your health-care practitioner or dentist.

DRUG INTERACTIONS

Tell your health-care practitioner and pharmacist if you are taking any other prescription or over-the-counter drugs, as well as any vitamins, herbs, or other supplements. Possible drug interactions include the following:

- Do not take monoamine oxidase inhibitor (MAOI) antidepressants at the same time as or within 14 days of nefazodone. This combination can cause reactions ranging from confusion to seizures, and is potentially fatal.
- Taking other central nervous system depressants along with nefazodone can result in increased drowsiness and other effects.
- Nefazodone can increase blood levels and effects of digoxin, haloperidol, propranolol, alprazolam, and triazolam.
- Do not drink alcohol while taking nefazodone.

FOOD, VITAMIN, AND HERBAL INTERACTIONS

Do not take nefazodone with grapefruit juice. Do not combine with herbs such as hops, kava, passionflower, and valerian. These can increase effects such as drowsiness. Do not take St. John's wort with nefazodone, since both affect serotonin. Other inappropriate herbs include ginseng, ephedra (ma huang), and yohimbe.

RECOMMENDED DOSAGE

Nefazodone comes as a tablet. Although the doses given below are typical, only your health-care practitioner can determine the dose and schedule that best fit your needs.

- *Children:* This drug is not recommended for children.
- *Adults:* 200 to 600 mg daily in divided doses

Nefazodone should be taken 1 hour before or 2 hours after meals. It must be taken regularly for several weeks before its full effect is felt. If you forget a dose, take it as soon as you remember. If it is almost time for the next dose, skip the missed one and resume your normal schedule. Never take a double dose. Do not stop taking this drug suddenly, especially if you have been taking it a long time. Your health-care practitioner will gradually reduce your dosage.

SYMPTOMS OF OVERDOSE AND WHAT TO DO

The symptoms of nefazodone overdose include nausea, vomiting, and sleepiness. If overdose occurs, seek immediate medical attention and take the prescription bottle to the hospital with you.

SPECIAL INFORMATION FOR PREGNANT OR NURSING WOMEN

No studies have adequately investigated the effects of nefazodone during pregnancy or breastfeeding. However, decreased fertility and fetal damage occurred in animal studies. If you are pregnant or plan to become pregnant, or if you are breastfeeding or plan to do so, talk with your health-care practitioner before starting this drug. Only a health-care practitioner can determine whether the potential benefits outweigh the potential dangers.

SPECIAL INFORMATION FOR SENIORS

Seniors are at higher risk of side effects, and usually require smaller doses.

OPEN QUESTIONS OR CONTROVERSIES

In June 2004, the Food and Drug Administration asked manufacturers of nefazodone to include in their labeling a warning statement that recommends close observation of adult and pediatric patients for clinical worsening of depression or the emergence of suicidality when being treated with this drug, especially when beginning the drug, or at the time of dose changes, either increases or decreases.

GENERIC NAME

Nelfinavir

BRAND NAME

Viracept
No generic available

ABOUT THIS DRUG

Nelfinavir is a protease inhibitor used to treat HIV, the human immunodeficiency virus that causes acquired immune deficiency syndrome (AIDS). It is commonly prescribed in a triple-drug cocktail in combination with antiretroviral drugs such as zidovudine (AZT). Triple-drug cocktails are credited with reducing the death rate from AIDS in the mid-1990s.

Nelfinavir works by interfering with the reproduction of HIV. It disrupts the process through which proteins are formed and become mature HIV. This in turn slows the progression of the virus and the destruction of the immune system.

SIDE EFFECTS

Side effects are common. Contact your health-care practitioner if they become persistent or severe. Only he or she can determine if you should continue to take nelfinavir.

- *Common:* diarrhea
- *Less Common or Rare:* nausea, intestinal gas, weakness, abdominal pain, rash, liver inflammation, high blood sugar

Serious side effects can occur virtually anywhere in the body when you take nelfinavir. This drug may affect your gastrointestinal tract, sexual function, mental state, kidneys, liver, muscles, and joints. Consult your health-care practitioner if you experience symptoms such as nausea, vomiting, increased hunger, increased thirst, increased urination, dry or itchy skin, confusion, dehydration, fatigue, and fruity mouth odor.

IMPORTANT PRECAUTIONS

Tell your health-care practitioner about any other medical conditions you suffer from, especially liver disease, diabetes, or phenylketonuria (a metabolic problem).

If you are using oral contraceptives, practice other means of contraception while taking nelfinavir.

Nelfinavir does not cure HIV or AIDS, nor does it prevent you from passing the virus on to others. Because your immune system is weakened, opportunistic infections can develop at any time. It is also important to always practice safe sex while taking this drug.

Visit your health-care practitioner on a regular basis to monitor your progress. Periodic blood tests are necessary to investigate unwanted effects, such as high blood sugar.

DRUG INTERACTIONS

Check first with your health-care practitioner before taking any other medication with nelfinavir. To avoid unwanted side effects, tell your health-care practitioner and pharmacist about all other prescription or over-the-counter drugs, vitamins, herbs, or other supplements that you are taking. Possible drug interactions include the following:

- Nelfinavir makes AZT and other anti-HIV drugs more effective.
- Take nelfinavir at least 2 hours before and 1 hour after taking didanosine.

- Nelfinavir may cause birth control pills to be less effective.
- Nelfinavir may interfere with the body's removal of many drugs, including amiodarone, cisapride, ergot medicines, midazolam, quinidine, rifabutin, rifampin, and triazolam. This can lead to serious side effects.

FOOD, VITAMIN, AND HERBAL INTERACTIONS

When taking the triple-drug cocktail, it is particularly important to follow your health-care practitioner's dietary recommendations.

RECOMMENDED DOSAGE

Nelfinavir is available as powder and tablets. The doses given below are typical. However, doses are different for different patients, and only your health-care practitioner can determine the dose and schedule that are most appropriate for you.

- *Children 2 to 13 Years:* 20 to 30 mg per 2.2 pounds of body weight, 3 times a day
- *Children Older than 13 Years and Adults:* 750 mg 3 times a day

Nelfinavir must be taken with food. It is essential to take this drug exactly as prescribed. If you miss a dose, take it as soon as you remember. However, if it is nearly time for your next scheduled dose, do not take the missed dose. Follow your regular dosing schedule. Never take a double dose.

SYMPTOMS OF OVERDOSE AND WHAT TO DO

No specific information on overdosing with nelfinavir is available. However, if you suspect overdose, seek medical attention immediately, and bring the prescription bottle with you to the hospital so that health-care practitioners will know exactly what drug was taken.

SPECIAL INFORMATION FOR PREGNANT OR NURSING WOMEN

No studies have adequately investigated the effects of nelfinavir during pregnancy or breastfeeding. If you are pregnant or plan to become pregnant, consult with your health-care practitioner before taking this medication. It is not known whether nelfinavir passes into breast milk. However, HIV can be transferred by breast milk, so bottle-feeding is recommended.

SPECIAL INFORMATION FOR SENIORS

There are no special instructions for seniors.

GENERIC NAME
Neomycin sulfate

BRAND NAMES
AK-Spore, Neosporin Ophthalmic
Generic available

ABOUT THIS DRUG
Neomycin sulfate is an antibiotic used in combination with two other antibiotics—gramicidin and polymyxin B sulfate—in the eye medication Neosporin Ophthalmic. This remedy is prescribed to treat superficial eye infections. Neomycin sulfate works by destroying many common bacteria responsible for eye infections.

SIDE EFFECTS
Consult your health-care practitioner if you develop side effects while using this product. Only he or she can determine whether it is safe for you to continue using neomycin sulfate.

- *Common:* eye irritation, itching, redness, swelling
- *Less Common or Rare:* burning, stinging, allergic reaction, development of secondary eye infection

IMPORTANT PRECAUTIONS
Do not use this product if you have ever experienced an allergic reaction to neomycin sulfate, gramicidin, polymyxin B sulfate, or similar antibiotics. Antibiotics should not be used for prolonged periods of time, or there is a greater risk of the growth of other resistant bacteria. If the infection does not clear up within a few days, or if symptoms worsen, call your health-care practitioner. Also ask your health-care practitioner whether you should stop wearing contact lenses for the duration of the infection.

DRUG INTERACTIONS
Although no specific drug interactions are associated with this neomycin sulfate eyedrops, always tell your health-care practitioner and pharmacist if you are taking other prescription or over-the-counter drugs, as well as any vitamins, herbs, or other supplements.

FOOD, VITAMIN, AND HERBAL INTERACTIONS
No food, vitamin, or herbal interactions have been noted.

RECOMMENDED DOSAGE

This product comes as an eyedrop solution. The dosage below is typical.

- *Children and Adults:* Apply 1 to 2 drops to the affected eye 2 to 4 times daily.

Remove contact lenses before using eyedrops, and do not reinsert them for at least 15 minutes. To avoid infection, do not touch the dropper to the eye.

If you miss a dose, administer it as soon as you remember. However, if it is nearly time for your next scheduled dose, do not administer the missed dose. Follow your regular dosing schedule. Never administer a double dose.

SYMPTOMS OF OVERDOSE AND WHAT TO DO

Overdose is unlikely. However, if you suspect an overdose, seek immediate medical attention.

SPECIAL INFORMATION FOR PREGNANT OR NURSING WOMEN

This drug is considered safe for pregnant and nursing women.

SPECIAL INFORMATION FOR SENIORS

There are no special instructions for seniors.

GENERIC NAME

Nesiritide

BRAND NAME

Natrecor

No generic available

ABOUT THIS DRUG

Nesiritide is a cardiotonic drug prescribed for the treatment of severe congestive heart failure that has recently worsened. Its use is reserved for those who are short of breath even while engaging in only minimal activity or while at rest. This drug works by stimulating the heart.

SIDE EFFECTS

Consult your health-care practitioner if you develop side effects while taking this drug. Only he or she can determine whether it is safe for you to continue taking nesiritide.

- *Common:* headache, low blood pressure
- *Less Common or Rare:* chest pain or tightness, bluish lips or skin, shortness of breath, difficulty breathing, changes in heartbeat, unusual tiredness, weakness, cool, clammy skin, stomach or back pain, leg cramps, pins and needles, numbness, anxiety, confusion, cough, fever, nausea, vomiting, pale skin, vision changes, unusual bleeding or bruising, coughing up blood

IMPORTANT PRECAUTIONS

Always tell your health-care practitioner about any other medical conditions you may have, especially heart disease and low blood pressure. Nesiritide may make these problems worse.

This drug may cause side effects such as unusual tiredness. Until you know how nesiritide affects you, do not drive a car, operate machinery, or perform other tasks that require concentration.

People taking nesiritide must be closely monitored with regular complete blood counts and other tests.

DRUG INTERACTIONS

Inform your health-care practitioner and pharmacist if you are taking any other prescription or over-the-counter drugs, as well as any vitamins, herbs, or other supplements. Possible drug interactions include the following:

- Heart medicine such as ACE inhibitors may increase the risk of low blood pressure.

FOOD, VITAMIN, AND HERBAL INTERACTIONS

Consult your health-care practitioner regarding any special dietary recommendations.

RECOMMENDED DOSAGE

Nesiritide is available by injection and is administered in a health facility setting. Dosage is highly individualized and must be determined by your health-care practitioner.

SYMPTOMS OF OVERDOSE AND WHAT TO DO

No specific information is available regarding nesiritide overdose. If you suspect that an overdose has occurred, seek immediate medical attention.

SPECIAL INFORMATION FOR PREGNANT OR NURSING WOMEN

No studies have adequately investigated the effects of nesiritide during pregnancy or breastfeeding. If you are pregnant or plan to become pregnant, or if you are breastfeeding or plan to do so, consult your health-care practitioner before taking this medication. Only a health-care practitioner can determine whether the potential benefits outweigh the risks.

SPECIAL INFORMATION FOR SENIORS

There are no special instructions for seniors.

GENERIC NAME

Nevirapine

BRAND NAME

Viramune

No generic available

ABOUT THIS DRUG

Nevirapine is prescribed for the treatment of advanced cases of HIV, the human immunodeficiency virus that causes acquired immune deficiency syndrome (AIDS). This drug is also used to prevent mother-to-child transmission of HIV during labor and childbirth. It is commonly taken with other anti-HIV medication.

Nevirapine works by interfering with the reproduction of HIV. This slows the progression of the virus and the destruction of the immune system.

SIDE EFFECTS

Contact your health-care practitioner if you develop side effects while taking this drug. Only he or she can determine if you should continue to take nevirapine.

- *Common:* diarrhea, nausea, vomiting, fatigue, headache, fever, rash
- *Less Common or Rare:* abdominal pain, joint or muscle pain, tingling sensation, mouth sores, liver inflammation

The most serious side effect of nevirapine is a severe and potentially life-threatening rash that strikes as many as one in three people taking this drug. This rash usually appears in the first six weeks of treatment, and may be accompanied by fever, mouth sores, blisters, muscle and joint pain, swelling, reddened eyes, and fatigue. If you experience these symptoms, stop taking medication at once and call your health-care practitioner.

IMPORTANT PRECAUTIONS

Nevirapine should not be taken if you have liver or kidney problems.

If you are using oral contraceptives, practice other means of contraception while taking nevirapine.

Nevirapine does not cure HIV or AIDS, nor does it prevent you from passing on the virus on to others. Opportunistic infections may still occur, and it is important to always practice safe sex while taking this drug.

Visit your health-care practitioner on a regular basis to monitor your progress. Periodic blood tests are necessary to investigate unwanted effects, such as liver problems.

DRUG INTERACTIONS

To avoid unwanted side effects, tell your health-care practitioner and pharmacist about all other prescription or over-the-counter drugs, vitamins, herbs, or other supplements that you are taking. Possible drug interactions include the following:

- Ask your health-care practitioner before taking nevirapine with protease-inhibitor drugs, because it can limit their effectiveness.
- Nevirapine may cause birth control pills to be less effective.
- Nevirapine may interfere with many other drugs, including macrolide antibiotics, cimetidine, ketoconazole, rifabutin, and rifampin. Check first with your health-care practitioner before taking any other medication with nevirapine.

FOOD, VITAMIN, AND HERBAL INTERACTIONS

When taking drugs for HIV infection, it is particularly important to follow your health-care practitioner's dietary recommendations.

RECOMMENDED DOSAGE

Nevirapine is available as oral suspension and tablets. The doses given below are typical. However, doses are different for different patients, and only your health-care practitioner can determine the dose and schedule that are most appropriate for you.

- *Children 2 Months to 8 Years:* Consult your health-care practitioner.
- *Children Older than 8 Years:* 4 mg per 2.2 pounds of body weight once daily for 14 days, followed by 4 mg per 2.2 pounds of body weight twice a day

- *Adults:* 200 mg once daily for 14 days, followed by 200 mg twice a day

Nevirapine may be taken with or without food. In order to prevent the development of drug-resistant HIV, it is essential to take this drug exactly as prescribed by your health-care practitioner. If you develop a rash early in treatment, stop taking nevirapine and call your health-care practitioner.

If you miss a dose of nevirapine, take it as soon as you remember. However, if it nearly time for your next scheduled dose, do not take the missed dose. Follow your regular dosing schedule. Never take a double dose.

SYMPTOMS OF OVERDOSE AND WHAT TO DO

Symptoms of nevirapine overdose may include nausea, vomiting, fever, headache, fatigue, sleeplessness, and breathing difficulties. If you suspect overdose, seek medical attention immediately, and bring the prescription bottle with you to the hospital so that health-care practitioners will know exactly what drug was taken.

SPECIAL INFORMATION FOR PREGNANT OR NURSING WOMEN

No studies have adequately investigated the effects of nevirapine during pregnancy or breastfeeding. If you are pregnant or plan to become pregnant, consult with your health-care practitioner before taking this medication. Nevirapine passes into breast milk and HIV can be transferred by breast milk, so bottle-feeding is recommended.

SPECIAL INFORMATION FOR SENIORS

There are no special instructions for seniors.

GENERIC NAME

Niacin

BRAND NAMES

Endur-Acin, Nia-Bid, Niac, Niacels, Niacor, Niaspan, Nico-400, Nicobid Tempules, Nicolar, Nicotinex Elixir, Slo-Niacin
Generic available

ABOUT THIS DRUG

Also known as nicotinic acid and vitamin B_3, niacin is used to lower abnormally high levels of blood cholesterol and triglycerides. This helps to prevent medical problems brought on by plaque and fat clogging arteries. Niacin works by inhibiting the production of triglycerides and preventing fatty tissue from converting to cholesterol and triglycerides.

SIDE EFFECTS

Speak to your health-care practitioner if you develop side effects while taking this drug. Only he or she can determine if you should continue to take niacin.

- *Common:* flushing, itching, tingling, feeling of warmth in face and neck, dizziness and faintness upon rising
- *Less Common or Rare:* headache, dizziness, faintness, fever, nausea, vomiting, diarrhea, stomach or lower back pain, joint pain, muscle cramps, muscle damage, dry skin, frequent urination, unusual thirst, swelling of feet and lower legs, darkening of urine, yellow eyes or skin

IMPORTANT PRECAUTIONS

Always tell your health-care practitioner about any other medical conditions you may have, especially bleeding problems, diabetes, glaucoma, gout, liver problems, low blood pressure, or stomach ulcer. Niacin may make these problems worse.

This drug may cause side effects such as dizziness. Until you know how niacin affects you, do not drive a car, operate machinery, or perform other tasks that require concentration.

Treatment for high cholesterol also entails careful attention to diet and exercise. Your health-care practitioner will most likely recommend a diet that is low in saturated fat, cholesterol, and sugar. It is also important to maintain a healthy weight.

People taking niacin must be closely monitored with regular blood tests.

Large doses of niacin may raise blood levels of glucose and uric acid. People with diabetes or gout should regularly monitor these levels as well.

DRUG INTERACTIONS

Inform your health-care practitioner and pharmacist if you are taking any other prescription or over-the-counter drugs, as well as any vitamins, herbs, or other supplements. Possible drug interactions include the following:

- Taking a children's aspirin tablet with each dose of niacin may prevent facial flushing. However, aspirin may increase absorption of niacin. Consult your health-care practitioner for advice.

- Niacin may increase the effect of antihypertensive drugs, resulting in very low blood pressure.
- Niacin may decrease the effects of aspirin, antidiabetic drugs, probenecid, and sulfinpyrazone.
- Taking niacin with isoniazid may result in decreased absorption and effects of niacin.
- Combining niacin with other cholesterol-lowering drugs such as lovastatin increases the risk of muscle problems.
- Alcohol may cause excessive lowering of blood pressure.
- Smoking may increase dizziness and flushing.

FOOD, VITAMIN, AND HERBAL INTERACTIONS

Following a special diet low in saturated fat and cholesterol can make medication more effective and also reduce your need for medication. Do not combine the over-the-counter dietary supplement Cholestin with niacin. This may worsen the risk of muscle damage.

RECOMMENDED DOSAGE

Niacin is available as tablets, extended-release tablets, extended-release capsules, and solution. The doses given below are typical. However, doses are different for different patients, and only your health-care practitioner can determine the dose and schedule that are most appropriate for you.

- *Children:* Consult your health-care practitioner.
- *Teenagers and Adults:* 100 mg 3 times a day to start, which may be increased to the usual ongoing dose of 1 to 2 g daily in divided doses.

If niacin upsets your stomach, take it with food or milk. Swallow extended-release tablets and capsules whole. If you miss a dose, take it as soon as you remember. However, if it is nearly time for your next scheduled dose, do not take the missed dose. Follow your regular dosing schedule. Never take a double dose. Do not stop taking niacin without consulting your health-care practitioner. This may cause cholesterol levels to rise again.

SYMPTOMS OF OVERDOSE AND WHAT TO DO

Symptoms of niacin overdose may include nausea, vomiting, diarrhea, cramps, weakness, and flushing. If you suspect that an overdose has occurred, seek immediate medical attention and take the prescription bottle to the hospital with you.

SPECIAL INFORMATION FOR PREGNANT OR NURSING WOMEN

No studies have adequately investigated the effects of niacin during pregnancy or breastfeeding. However, birth defects have occurred in animal studies. Avoid taking niacin in the first three months of pregnancy, and consult your health-care practitioner before taking this medication in your second or third trimester. Only a health-care practitioner can determine whether the potential benefits outweigh the risks. Since niacin passes into breast milk, your health-care practitioner will probably advise you to stop breastfeeding while taking this drug.

SPECIAL INFORMATION FOR SENIORS

Seniors may be more prone to side effects such as low blood pressure and dizziness.

OPEN QUESTIONS OR CONTROVERSIES

Recent studies have suggested that the extended-release forms of niacin may be more likely to cause liver damage than the short-acting forms. Ask your health-care practitioner which is the best choice for you.

GENERIC NAME

Nicardipine

BRAND NAMES

Cardene, Cardene SR

No generic available

ABOUT THIS DRUG

Nicardipine is a calcium channel blocker used to treat angina (chest pain) and mild-to-moderate high blood pressure (hypertension). If you have clogged arteries, you may experience chest pain when you exert yourself, because of a lack of oxygen supply to the heart. Left untreated, over time high blood pressure can damage blood vessels and lead to problems such as stroke and heart failure.

This drug may be used alone or in combination with other blood pressure medications (especially beta-blockers such as atenolol). Cardene SR (the extended-release form) is prescribed only for high blood pressure.

Calcium channel blockers such as nicardipine work by blocking the passage of calcium into the cells of the heart and blood vessels. This reduces the heart's workload, relaxes blood vessels, and increases the supply of oxygen and blood to the heart.

SIDE EFFECTS

Consult your health-care practitioner if you develop side effects while taking this drug. Only he or she can determine whether it is safe for you to continue taking nicardipine.

- *Common:* headache, low blood pressure, dizziness, nausea, indigestion, weakness, pounding heart, swelling of feet, sleepiness, increased angina (chest pain) at the start of treatment, swelling, tenderness, or bleeding of the gums
- *Less Common or Rare:* flushing and feeling of warmth, faintness, vomiting, constipation, drowsiness, difficulty sleeping

IMPORTANT PRECAUTIONS

This drug should not be taken if you have advanced aortic stenosis (a narrowing of the aorta), or if you have ever experienced an allergic reaction to this or other calcium channel blockers in the past. Use nicardipine with caution if you have liver or kidney problems, muscular dystrophy, impaired circulation to the fingers, heart rhythm disturbances, or a history of heart attack, stroke, or congestive heart failure.

You may experience a brief headache shortly after you take a dose of nicardipine. This side effect is less troublesome after you have been taking the drug for a while. But if headaches are severe, consult your health-care practitioner.

This drug may cause side effects such as drowsiness and dizziness. Until you know how nicardipine affects you, do not drive a car, operate machinery, or perform other tasks that require concentration.

When you first start taking this drug or when the dosage is increased, you may experience dizziness or faintness when you rise quickly from a sitting or reclining position (postural hypotension). Try to get up slowly, and consult your health-care practitioner if the problem continues.

Chest pain resulting from exercise is usually prevented by this drug. This may tempt you to be more active than you should. Ask your health-care practitioner what amount of exercise is appropriate. When you exercise in hot weather, do so with much caution. Heavy sweating can lead to dizziness, lightheadedness, fainting, vomiting, dehydration, and low blood pressure.

Treatment for high blood pressure also entails careful attention to other aspects of your lifestyle. Your health-care practitioner will most likely recommend a diet that is low in salt and saturated fat. It is also important to maintain a healthy weight and to refrain from smoking. People taking nicardipine must be closely monitored with regular blood tests, and should learn to check their pulses to monitor heart rate.

Before having any type of surgery or dental procedure, tell your surgeon or dentist that you are taking nicardipine.

DRUG INTERACTIONS

Inform your health-care practitioner and pharmacist if you are taking any other prescription or over-the-counter drugs, as well as any vitamins, herbs, or other supplements. Possible drug interactions include the following:

- Taking other blood pressure medications such as beta-blockers and digitalis can increase the blood pressure lowering effects of nicardipine. This type of combination must be carefully monitored by your health-care practitioner.
- Taking amiodarone with this drug may cause the heart to stop.
- Cimetidine, ranitidine, ritonavir, delavirdine, and antifungal drugs such as ketoconazole may increase the effects of nicardipine.
- Rifampin and NSAIDs (such as aspirin, ibuprofen, and indomethacin) can reduce the blood pressure lowering effects of nicardipine.
- Nicardipine can increase blood levels of cyclosporine to toxic levels, resulting in kidney damage.
- Other drugs that may interact with nicardipine include blood thinners such as warfarin and phenytoin.
- Phenytoin may result in phenytoin toxicity or decreased efficacy of nicardipine.
- Alcohol may further lower blood pressure. Use with caution.
- Consult your health-care practitioner before taking over-the-counter cough, cold, sinus, allergy, or weight loss medications. Many of these can raise blood pressure.

FOOD, VITAMIN, AND HERBAL INTERACTIONS

Do not take nicardipine with grapefruit juice or with high-fat meals. Do not take herbs that increase blood pressure, such as ephedra (ma huang), ginseng, goldenseal, licorice, and saw palmetto. Consult your health-care practitioner before taking substances that may lower blood pressure, such as magnesium, calcium, soy, or garlic.

RECOMMENDED DOSAGE

Nicardipine is available as regular and extended-release tablets, extended-release capsules, and solution. The doses given below are typical. However, doses are different for different patients, and only your health-care practitioner can determine the dose and schedule that are most appropriate for you.

- *Children:* This drug is not recommended for children.
- *Adults:* 60 to 120 mg daily in divided doses

If nicardipine upsets your stomach, take it with food or milk. Swallow the capsules whole. If you miss a dose, take it as soon as you remember. However, if it is nearly time for your next scheduled dose, do not take the missed dose. Follow your regular dosing schedule. Never take a double dose. Do not suddenly stop taking nicardipine without consulting your health-care practitioner. This may cause angina. A gradual reduction in dosage is safest.

SYMPTOMS OF OVERDOSE AND WHAT TO DO

Symptoms of nicardipine overdose may include low blood pressure, reduced heart rate, weakness, lightheadedness, slurred speech, confusion, drowsiness, shortness of breath, flushed skin, tremors, and fainting. If you suspect that an overdose has occurred, seek immediate medical attention and take the prescription bottle to the hospital with you.

SPECIAL INFORMATION FOR PREGNANT OR NURSING WOMEN

No studies have adequately investigated the effects of nicardipine during pregnancy or breastfeeding. However, birth defects have occurred in animal studies. Avoid taking nicardipine during the first three months of pregnancy, and consult your health-care practitioner before taking this medication during your second or third trimester. Only a health-care practitioner can determine whether the potential benefits outweigh the risks. Since nicardipine may pass into breast milk, your health-care practitioner may advise you to stop breastfeeding while taking this drug.

SPECIAL INFORMATION FOR SENIORS

Seniors may be more prone to side effects such as weakness, dizziness, and fainting, and may benefit from a lower dosage.

> **OPEN QUESTIONS OR CONTROVERSIES**
> Some studies have suggested that people taking calcium channel blockers several times a day (rather than once a day) are more likely to have a heart attack than those who take beta-blockers or similar medications. Ask your health-care practitioner which drug is the best choice for you.

GENERIC NAME

Nicotine

BRAND NAMES

Habitrol, Nicoderm, Nicotrol, Nicotrol Inhaler, ProStep
No generic available

ABOUT THIS DRUG

Nicotine patches and nasal sprays are used to treat addiction to cigarettes and other tobacco products. Because nicotine is a stimulant and a habit-forming substance, these products should be utilized only on a short-term basis. Since the addiction to cigarettes is psychological as well as physical, health-care practitioners recommend combining medication with counseling, education, and psychological support.

Nicotine products work by furnishing an alternate source of nicotine for people who are nicotine-dependent. They lessen withdrawal symptoms (such as headache, anxiety, irritability, anger, frustration, concentration difficulties, restlessness, and insomnia) and reduce your craving for cigarettes.

SIDE EFFECTS

If you experience side effects while using a nicotine patch or spray, consult your health-care practitioner. Only he or she can determine whether it is safe for you to continue taking this drug. Nicotine use should be completely avoided in children under 12.

Skin Patches

- *Common:* fatigue, local irritation and rashes
- *Less Common or Rare:* back pain, body aches, muscle and joint pain, headache, weakness, upset stomach, diarrhea, dizziness, nervousness, insomnia, cough, sore throat, changes in taste, painful menstruation, abdominal pain, vomiting, chest pain, hypertension, dry mouth, si-

nus irritation, sweating, tingling sensations, lapses in concentration, allergic reactions, heart palpitations, irregular heartbeat

Nasal Sprays

- *Common:* nose, throat, and eye irritation
- *Less Common or Rare:* back pain, flu-like symptoms, coughing, fever, headache, upset stomach, nausea, gas, hiccups, diarrhea, changes in taste, jaw and neck pain, nasal and sinus inflammation, allergies, toothache

If you develop palpitations or an irregular heartbeat, stop taking nicotine immediately and call your health-care practitioner.

IMPORTANT PRECAUTIONS

Do not smoke cigarettes or use other tobacco products while using this drug; this can result in an overdose of nicotine. Tell your health-care practitioner if you are sensitive or allergic to nicotine or other drugs. If you are allergic to nicotine or menthol, do not use the inhaler. If you are interested in using the patches, also inform your health-care practitioner of any sensitivity or allergy to adhesive tape or bandages.

Inform your health-care practitioner about any other medical conditions you suffer from, especially angina (chest pain), arrhythmia (irregular heartbeat), insulin-dependent diabetes, heart disease, a history of heart attack, severe hypertension, kidney or liver disease, stomach ulcers, or an overactive thyroid. If you are using nicotine patches, also inform your health-care practitioner of any skin problems such as eczema. The inhaler should be used with caution if you have respiratory disease, adrenal tumors, Buerger's disease (circulatory problems in the legs), or Raynaud's disease (circulatory problems in the fingers and toes).

Before having any type of surgery or dental procedure, inform your surgeon or dentist that you are taking nicotine.

Nicotine can be toxic to children and pets. To avoid accidental poisoning, always store and dispose of all nicotine products in a safe place, out of the reach of children and animals. Even used patches still contain enough nicotine to be poisonous. Wrap them in their original wrapper or in aluminum foil before placing in an out-of-reach trash receptacle.

DRUG INTERACTIONS

When you stop smoking, the effects of medications on your body may be altered. Be sure to tell your health-care practitioner that you have quit so that he or she can make the necessary dosage adjustments. Also inform your health-care practitioner and pharmacist about all other medications you take, including prescription and over-the-counter drugs, vitamins, and alternative treatments such as herbal supplements. Possible drug interactions include the following:

- If you stop smoking, the effects of acetaminophen, glutethimide, imipramine, oxazepam, pentazocine, propoxyphene, propranolol, and theophylline may be increased.
- Cessation of smoking may cause more insulin to be absorbed from injections.
- When you stop smoking, you may become more sensitive to the caffeine in many over-the-counter remedies, such as cough and cold remedies and diet aids.
- Nicotine can also affect the absorption of nervous system drugs and diuretics.

FOOD, VITAMIN, AND HERBAL INTERACTIONS

When you stop smoking, you may become more sensitive to the caffeine in coffee and tea.

RECOMMENDED DOSAGE

Nicotine is available by prescription as skin patches and nasal sprays. (Another option is nonprescription nicotine gum.)

Skin Patches

- Nicotine skin patches come in various strengths and with different applications. Some are worn 24 hours a day; others are not worn while you sleep. Nicotine patches are applied once a day, usually at the same time, to hairless skin.

Nasal Spray

- Tilt your head back, do not sniff or inhale, and administer 1 to 2 sprays in each nostril. This can be done up to 5 times hourly. To ease the symptoms of nicotine withdrawal, use the spray at least 8 times daily. Do not use more than 40 times a day. Gradually cut back on inhaler use after 3 months. Do not use for longer than 6 months because of the risk of addiction. Clean the mouthpiece regularly with soap and water.

SYMPTOMS OF OVERDOSE AND WHAT TO DO

If you suspect a nicotine overdose, seek immediate medical attention. The symptoms include nausea, vomiting, trouble breathing, excessive salivation, stomach pain, diarrhea, headache, blurred vision, dizziness, cold sweat, pallor, weakness, confusion, hearing difficulties, low blood pressure, and weak pulse. These symptoms may progress to fainting, convulsions, and death. Take the nicotine container to the hospital so that health-care practitioners will know exactly what drug was used.

SPECIAL INFORMATION FOR PREGNANT OR NURSING WOMEN

Nicotine is associated with miscarriage, fetal harm (when used in the third trimester), and breathing difficulties in newborns. It is not safe for use during pregnancy. However, in pregnant women who cannot quit smoking (even with the help of counseling), health-care practitioners may consider which risk poses more danger to the fetus: continued smoking, or use of nicotine products to help the mother quit. Nicotine passes into breast milk and should not be used when breastfeeding.

SPECIAL INFORMATION FOR SENIORS

Seniors are often more sensitive to side effects of nicotine such as weakness, dizziness, and body aches.

OPEN QUESTIONS OR CONTROVERSIES

Nicotine in any form can be addictive, so long-term use of these products is not recommended. In addition, nicotine is a poison, and high levels can be fatal. Pay close attention to your health-care practitioner's instructions and package directions when using any nicotine product. Never exceed recommended dosages, and use for only limited periods of time.

GENERIC NAME

Nifedipine

BRAND NAMES

Adalat, Adalat CC, Procardia, Procardia XL
Generic available

ABOUT THIS DRUG

Nifedipine is a calcium channel blocker used to treat angina (chest pain). The long-acting forms may also be prescribed for mild-to-moderate high blood pressure (hypertension). However, the regular, immediate-release forms *must not* be used to treat hypertension or heart attacks.

This drug may be used alone or in combination with other blood pressure medications. If you have clogged arteries, you may experience chest pain when you exert yourself, because of a lack of oxygen supply to the heart. Left untreated, high blood pressure can eventually damage blood vessels and lead to problems such as stroke and heart failure.

Calcium channel blockers such as nifedipine work by blocking the passage of calcium into the cells of the heart and blood vessels. This reduces the heart's workload, relaxes blood vessels, and increases the supply of oxygen and blood to the heart.

SIDE EFFECTS

Consult your health-care practitioner if you develop side effects while taking this drug. Only he or she can determine whether it is safe for you to continue taking nifedipine.

- *Common:* low blood pressure, fast heartbeat, swelling of ankles and feet, flushing and feeling warm, sweating
- *Less Common or Rare:* headache, dizziness, nausea, trouble with vision, swollen joints, indigestion, weakness, pounding heart, shakiness, giddiness, sleepiness, increased angina (chest pain) at the start of treatment, mood changes, faintness, vomiting, constipation, drowsiness, taste and smell disturbances, difficulty sleeping, muscle cramps, stuffy nose, breathing difficulties, cough, wheezing, swelling, tenderness, or bleeding of the gums, unusual bruising, heart palpitations, heart failure

IMPORTANT PRECAUTIONS

This drug should not be taken if you have advanced aortic stenosis (a narrowing of the aorta), liver disease, or low blood pressure, or if you have ever experienced an allergic reaction to this or other calcium channel blockers in the past. Immediate-release nifedipine has also been associated with a significantly increased risk in mortality for people over the age of 71. People in this age group *should not* take this drug.

Use nifedipine with caution if you have liver or kidney problems, muscular dystrophy, impaired circulation to the fingers, heart rhythm disturbances, atrial fibrillation, cardiomyopathy, or a history of heart attack, stroke, or congestive heart failure.

This drug may cause side effects such as trouble with vision, drowsiness, and dizziness. Until you know how nifedipine affects you, do not drive a car, operate machinery, or perform other tasks that require concentration.

When you first start taking this drug or when the dosage is increased, you may experience dizziness or faintness when you rise quickly from a sitting or reclining position (postural hypotension). Try to get up slowly, and consult your health-care practitioner if the problem continues.

Chest pain resulting from exercise is usually prevented by this drug. This may tempt you to be more active than you should. Ask your health-care practitioner what amount of exercise is appropriate. When you exercise in hot weather, take even greater care. Heavy sweating can lead to dizziness, lightheadedness, fainting, vomiting, dehydration, and low blood pressure.

Treatment for high blood pressure also entails careful attention to other aspects of your lifestyle. Your health-care practitioner will most likely recommend a diet that is low in salt and saturated fat. It is also important to maintain a healthy weight and to refrain from smoking. People taking nifedipine must be closely monitored with regular blood tests, and should learn to check their pulses to monitor heart rate.

Before having any type of surgery or dental procedure, tell your surgeon or dentist that you are taking nifedipine.

DRUG INTERACTIONS

Inform your health-care practitioner and pharmacist if you are taking any other prescription or over-the-counter drugs, as well as any vitamins, herbs, or other supplements. Possible drug interactions include the following:

- Taking other blood pressure medications such as beta-blockers and digitalis can increase the blood pressure lowering effects of nifedipine. This type of combination must be carefully monitored by your health-care practitioner.
- Taking amiodarone with this drug may cause the heart to stop.
- Cimetidine, ranitidine, ritonavir, and antifungal drugs such as ketoconazole may increase the effects of nifedipine.
- Drugs such as rifampin can reduce the blood pressure lowering effects of nifedipine.
- Nifedipine can increase blood levels and effects of phenytoin to toxic levels.
- Other drugs that may interact with nifedipine include blood thinners such as warfarin, cyclosporine, quinidine, and oral antidiabetic drugs.

- Alcohol may further lower blood pressure. Use with caution.
- Consult your health-care practitioner before taking over-the-counter cough, cold, sinus, allergy, or weight loss medications. Many of these can raise blood pressure.

FOOD, VITAMIN, AND HERBAL INTERACTIONS

Do not take nifedipine with grapefruit juice, which greatly increases the absorption and effects of this drug. Do not take herbs that increase blood pressure, such as ephedra (ma huang), ginseng, goldenseal, licorice, and saw palmetto. Consult your health-care practitioner before taking substances that may lower blood pressure, such as magnesium, calcium, soy, or garlic.

RECOMMENDED DOSAGE

Nifedipine is available as regular and extended-release or sustained-release tablets, and capsules. The doses given below are typical. However, doses are different for different patients, and only your health-care practitioner can determine the dose and schedule that are most appropriate for you.

- *Children:* This drug is not recommended for children.
- *Adults:* 30 to 120 mg daily, which may be taken in 1 dose or in divided doses, depending on which brand your health-care practitioner prescribes

Take nifedipine exactly as prescribed by your health-care practitioner. Procardia can be taken with or without food, while Adalat CC is best taken on an empty stomach. Swallow the tablets whole. If you miss a dose, take it as soon as you remember. However, if it is nearly time for your next scheduled dose, do not take the missed dose. Follow your regular dosing schedule. Never take a double dose. Do not suddenly stop taking nifedipine without consulting your health-care practitioner. This may cause angina. A gradual reduction in dosage is safest.

SYMPTOMS OF OVERDOSE AND WHAT TO DO

Symptoms of nifedipine overdose may include low blood pressure, reduced heart rate, weakness, lightheadedness, slurred speech, confusion, drowsiness, shortness of breath, flushed skin, tremors, and fainting. If you suspect that an overdose has occurred, seek immediate medical attention and take the prescription bottle to the hospital with you.

SPECIAL INFORMATION FOR PREGNANT OR NURSING WOMEN

No studies have adequately investigated the effects of nifedipine during pregnancy or breastfeeding. However, birth defects have occurred in animal studies. Avoid taking nifedipine during the first three months of pregnancy, and consult your health-care practitioner before taking this medication in your second or third trimester. Only a health-care practitioner can determine whether the potential benefits outweigh the risks. Since nifedipine may pass into breast milk, your health-care practitioner may advise you to stop breastfeeding while taking this drug.

SPECIAL INFORMATION FOR SENIORS

Immediate-release nifedipine has been linked with a significantly increased risk in mortality for people over the age of 71. People in this age group *should not* take this form of drug. Seniors may also be more prone to side effects such as weakness, dizziness, and fainting, and may benefit from a lower dosage of extended-release forms.

OPEN QUESTIONS OR CONTROVERSIES

Some studies have suggested that people taking calcium channel blockers several times a day (rather than once a day) are more likely to have a heart attack than those who take beta-blockers or similar medications. Ask your health-care practitioner which drug is the best choice for you.

GENERIC NAME

Nilutamide

BRAND NAME

Nilandron
No generic available

ABOUT THIS DRUG

Nilutamide is a neoplastic drug used in the treatment of advanced prostate cancer. It is usually prescribed when cancer has begun to spread beyond the prostate. Treatment begins immediately following removal of the testes.

This drug, an antiandrogen, works by blocking the effect of the male hormone testosterone, which encourages prostate cancer. It is usually taken with other treatment that decreases the production of testosterone.

SIDE EFFECTS

Side effects of nilutamide can be extremely serious, and must be promptly reported to your health-care practitioner. Be on the lookout for any signs of lung damage (such as chest pain, shortness of breath, and cough) or liver damage (such as jaundice, tenderness in the upper right side of the abdomen, and fatigue). Only your health-care practitioner can determine whether or not it is safe for you to continue taking this drug.

- *Common:* abnormal vision, poor adaptation to the dark, headache, nausea, constipation, appetite loss, diarrhea, dizziness, trouble sleeping, low sperm count, impotence, hot flashes, swollen breasts, inability to tolerate alcohol, cough, hoarseness, fever, runny nose, sneezing, sore throat, tightness in chest, wheezing
- *Less Common or Rare:* chest pain, shortness of breath, lung damage, fainting, inflammation of nasal passages, heightened sensitivity to light, dry mouth, overall feeling of unwellness, itching, nervousness, tingling, urinary tract infection, jaundice, tenderness in the upper right side of the abdomen, fatigue, liver damage, arthritis, cataracts, abdominal bleeding, tarry stools

IMPORTANT PRECAUTIONS

Always tell your health-care practitioner about any other medical conditions you may have, especially blood deficiencies or disorders, lung problems, and liver disease. Nilutamide is prescribed with extreme caution in such cases.

This drug may cause a low sperm count, infertility, and impotence. Before starting treatment, it is best to discuss these issues with your health-care practitioner.

Nilutamide may cause side effects such as abnormal vision. It temporarily changes the way your eyes react to light. Wearing tinted glasses or sunglasses may reduce this effect. However, until you know how nilutamide affects you, do not drive a car, operate machinery, or perform other tasks that require accurate vision.

People taking this drug must be closely monitored with regular complete blood counts and other tests.

DRUG INTERACTIONS

Inform your health-care practitioner and pharmacist if you are taking any other prescription or over-the-counter drugs, as well as any vitamins, herbs, or other supplements. Possible drug interactions include the following:

- Nilutamide may increase the effects of blood thinners such as warfarin, phenytoin, and theophylline.
- Do not drink alcohol while taking nilutamide. This combination can cause facial flushing, flu-like symptoms, and a drop in blood pressure.
- Smoking tobacco may increase your risk of anemia and other blood disorders.

FOOD, VITAMIN, AND HERBAL INTERACTIONS

Do not take nilutamide with supplements such as echinacea.

RECOMMENDED DOSAGE

Nilutamide comes in tablet form. Although the doses given below are typical, doses are different for different patients. Only your health-care practitioner can determine the dose and schedule that best fit your particular needs. This drug is only for use by men.

- *Adults:* 300 mg once a day for 30 days, followed by 150 mg once a day for a time period to be determined by your health-care practitioner

This drug can be taken with food or on an empty stomach. If you miss a dose, take it as soon as you remember. However, if it is nearly time for your next scheduled dose, do not take the missed dose. Follow your regular dosing schedule. Never take a double dose.

Unwanted side effects such as hot flashes and decreased sexual ability are common, and men with prostate cancer are susceptible to problems such as urinary tract infections and painful urination. Nevertheless, it is essential to adhere to your treatment schedule, and to take nilutamide exactly as prescribed by your health-care practitioner.

SYMPTOMS OF OVERDOSE AND WHAT TO DO

Symptoms of nilutamide overdose may include nausea, vomiting, headache, dizziness, and general discomfort. If you suspect that an overdose has occurred, seek immediate medical attention and take the prescription bottle to the hospital with you.

SPECIAL INFORMATION FOR PREGNANT OR NURSING WOMEN

This drug is for men only.

SPECIAL INFORMATION FOR SENIORS

There are no special instructions for seniors.

GENERIC NAME
Nimodipine

BRAND NAME
Nimotop
No generic available

ABOUT THIS DRUG
Nimodipine is a calcium channel blocker used to treat a stroke, or burst blood vessels in the brain. This drug differs from other calcium channel blockers in that it has little effect on the heart. Its major impact is on the blood vessels of the brain, through which it can improve neurological function after a stroke.

SIDE EFFECTS
Speak to your health-care practitioner if you develop side effects while taking this drug. Only he or she can determine whether it is safe for you to continue taking nimodipine.

- *Common:* low blood pressure, diarrhea, headache
- *Less Common or Rare:* swelling of arms or legs, dizziness, depression, memory loss, hallucinations, paranoia, psychosis, nausea, vomiting, stomach bleeding, muscle cramps, breathing difficulties, flushing, sexual difficulties, jaundice, liver inflammation, fast heartbeat, high blood pressure, heart attack, heart failure

IMPORTANT PRECAUTIONS
Use nimodipine with caution if you have liver disease or if you have ever experienced an allergic reaction to this or other calcium channel blockers.

This drug may cause side effects such as dizziness. Until you know how nimodipine affects you, do not drive a car, operate machinery, or perform other tasks that require concentration.

Before having any type of surgery or dental procedure, tell your surgeon or dentist that you are taking nimodipine.

DRUG INTERACTIONS
Inform your health-care practitioner and pharmacist if you are taking any other prescription or over-the-counter drugs, as well as any vitamins, herbs, or other supplements. Possible drug interactions include the following:

- Combining nimodipine with beta-blockers may lead to heart failure in susceptible individuals.

- Nimodipine may lead to increased bleeding, especially when combined with aspirin.
- Nimodipine may add to the effects of digoxin.

FOOD, VITAMIN, AND HERBAL INTERACTIONS

Do not take nimodipine with grapefruit juice, which greatly increases the absorption and effects of this drug.

RECOMMENDED DOSAGE

Nimodipine comes as capsules. Although the doses given below are typical, only your health-care practitioner can determine the dose and schedule that are best for you.

- *Children:* This drug is not recommended for children.
- *Adults:* 60 mg 4 times daily, starting within 96 hours of a stroke and continuing for 21 days

Nimodipine should be taken 1 hour before or 2 hours after meals. However, if this drug upsets your stomach, take it with food or milk. If you miss a dose, take it as soon as you remember. If it is nearly time for your next scheduled dose, do not take the missed dose. Follow your regular dosing schedule. Never take a double dose, and call your health-care practitioner if you miss more than 2 consecutive doses.

SYMPTOMS OF OVERDOSE AND WHAT TO DO

Symptoms of nimodipine overdose may include weakness, slurred speech, confusion, drowsiness, and nausea. If you suspect that an overdose has occurred, seek immediate medical attention and take the prescription bottle to the hospital with you.

SPECIAL INFORMATION FOR PREGNANT OR NURSING WOMEN

No studies have adequately investigated the effects of nimodipine during pregnancy or breastfeeding. However, birth defects have occurred in animal studies. Consult your health-care practitioner before starting this medication. Only a health-care practitioner can determine whether the potential benefits outweigh the risks. Since nimodipine may pass into breast milk, your health-care practitioner will most likely advise you to stop breastfeeding while taking this drug.

SPECIAL INFORMATION FOR SENIORS

Seniors may be more prone to side effects and may benefit from a lower dosage.

GENERIC NAME
Nisoldipine

BRAND NAME
Sular
No generic available

ABOUT THIS DRUG
Nisoldipine is a calcium channel blocker used to high blood pressure (hypertension). Left untreated, over time high blood pressure can damage blood vessels and lead to problems such as stroke and heart failure.

Calcium channel blockers such as nisoldipine work by blocking the passage of calcium into the cells of the heart and blood vessels. This reduces the heart's workload, relaxes blood vessels, and increases the supply of oxygen and blood to the heart.

SIDE EFFECTS
Speak to your health-care practitioner if you develop side effects while taking this drug. Only he or she can determine whether it is safe for you to continue taking nisoldipine.

➤ *Common:* swelling of arms and legs, headache, flushing, sore throat, sinus irritation, heart palpitations

➤ *Less Common or Rare:* increased chest pain (angina) at the start of treatment, dizziness, low blood pressure, nausea, rash, indigestion, weakness, pounding heart, shakiness, giddiness, sleepiness, mood changes, faintness, vomiting, constipation, drowsiness, taste and smell disturbances, difficulty sleeping, muscle cramps, stuffy nose, breathing difficulties, cough, wheezing, heart failure

IMPORTANT PRECAUTIONS
This drug should not be taken if you have severe liver disease or low blood pressure, or if you have ever experienced an allergic reaction to this or other calcium channel blockers in the past. Use nisoldipine with caution if you have liver or kidney problems, or a history of heart attack, stroke, or congestive heart failure.

This drug may cause side effects such as drowsiness and dizziness. Until you know how nisoldipine affects you, do not drive a car, operate machinery, or perform other tasks that require concentration.

Chest pain resulting from exercise is usually prevented by this drug. This may tempt you to be more active than you should. Ask your health-care practitioner what amount of exercise is appropriate. When you exercise in hot weather, take even greater care. Heavy sweating can lead to dizziness, lightheadedness, fainting, vomiting, dehydration, and low blood pressure.

Treatment for high blood pressure also entails careful attention to other aspects of your lifestyle. Your health-care practitioner will most likely recommend a diet that is low in salt and saturated fat. It is also important to maintain a healthy weight and to refrain from smoking. People taking nisoldipine must be closely monitored with regular blood tests, and should learn to check their pulses to monitor heart rate.

Before having any type of surgery or dental procedure, tell your surgeon or dentist that you are taking nisoldipine.

DRUG INTERACTIONS

Inform your health-care practitioner and pharmacist if you are taking any other prescription or over-the-counter drugs, as well as any vitamins, herbs, or other supplements. Possible drug interactions include the following:

- Taking other blood pressure medications such as beta-blockers and digitalis can increase the blood pressure lowering effects of nisoldipine. This type of combination must be carefully monitored by your health-care practitioner.
- Cimetidine, ranitidine, and antifungal drugs such as ketoconazole may increase the effects of nisoldipine.
- Drugs such as rifampin may reduce the blood pressure lowering effects of nisoldipine.
- Nisoldipine may increase blood levels and effects of phenytoin.
- Other drugs that may interact with nisoldipine include blood thinners such as warfarin, amiodarone, cyclosporine, quinidine, and oral antidiabetic drugs.
- Alcohol may further lower blood pressure. Use with caution.
- Consult your health-care practitioner before taking over-the-counter cough, cold, sinus, allergy, or weight loss medications. Many of these can raise blood pressure.

FOOD, VITAMIN, AND HERBAL INTERACTIONS

Do not take nisoldipine with grapefruit juice, which greatly increases the absorption and effects of this drug. Avoid fatty foods. Do not take herbs that increase blood pressure, such as ephedra (ma huang), ginseng, goldenseal, licorice, and saw palmetto. Consult your health-care practitioner before taking substances that may lower blood pressure, such as magnesium, calcium, soy, or garlic.

RECOMMENDED DOSAGE

Nisoldipine is available in tablet form. The doses given below are typical. However, doses are different for different patients, and only your health-care practitioner can determine the dose and schedule that are most appropriate for you.

- *Children:* This drug is not recommended for children.
- *Adults:* 20 to 60 mg daily

Nisoldipine can be taken with or without food. Swallow the tablets whole. If you miss a dose, take it as soon as you remember. However, if it is nearly time for your next scheduled dose, do not take the missed dose. Follow your regular dosing schedule. Never take a double dose. Do not suddenly stop taking nisoldipine without consulting your health-care practitioner. This may cause angina. A gradual reduction in dosage is safest.

SYMPTOMS OF OVERDOSE AND WHAT TO DO

Symptoms of nisoldipine overdose may include low blood pressure, reduced heart rate, weakness, lightheadedness, slurred speech, confusion, drowsiness, shortness of breath, flushed skin, tremors, and fainting. If you suspect that an overdose has occurred, seek immediate medical attention and take the prescription bottle to the hospital with you.

SPECIAL INFORMATION FOR PREGNANT OR NURSING WOMEN

No studies have adequately investigated the effects of nisoldipine during pregnancy or breastfeeding. However, birth defects have occurred in animal studies. Consult your health-care practitioner before starting this medication. Only a health-care practitioner can determine whether the potential benefits outweigh the risks. Since nisoldipine may pass into breast milk, your health-care practitioner will most likely advise you to stop breastfeeding while taking this drug.

SPECIAL INFORMATION FOR SENIORS

Seniors may also be more prone to side effects such as weakness, dizziness, and faintness, and may benefit from a lower dosage.

OPEN QUESTIONS OR CONTROVERSIES
Some studies have suggested that people taking calcium channel blockers several times a day (rather than once a day) are more likely to have a heart attack than those who take betablockers or similar medications. Ask your health-care practitioner which drug is the best choice for you.

GENERIC NAME
Nitrofurantoin

BRAND NAMES
Furadantin, Macrobid, Macrodantin
Generic available

ABOUT THIS DRUG
Nitrofurantoin is used to treat or prevent urinary tract infections. Because this drug may cause a variety of severe side effects, your health-care practitioner will closely monitor your health while you are taking it.

Nitrofurantoin works by interfering with the bacteria that cause infection.

SIDE EFFECTS
Consult your health-care practitioner if you develop side effects while taking nitrofurantoin. Only he or she can determine whether it is safe for you to continue taking this drug.

- *Common:* nausea, vomiting, diarrhea, gas, stomach pain, appetite loss, brown urine
- *Less Common or Rare:* fever, chills, blue skin, dizziness, drowsiness, difficulty breathing, cough, chest pain, hoarseness, depression, confusion, numbness, tingling, muscle weakness, joint or muscle pain, eye problems, temporary hair loss, jaundice, allergic reactions, rash, itching, hives, changes in white and red blood cells

Nitrofurantoin may cause serious lung problems in the first week of treatment. Contact your health-care practitioner immediately if you experience symptoms such as breathing difficulties, cough, fever, chills, and chest pain.

In rare cases, long-term treatment with this drug may lead to a variety of severe lung problems, including inflammation of the lungs and pulmonary fibrosis. Consult your health-care practitioner at once if you experience difficulty breathing, coughing, and wheezing.

IMPORTANT PRECAUTIONS

Always tell your health-care practitioner about all other medical conditions you have, especially anemia, diabetes mellitus, kidney or lung disease, or vitamin B_6 deficiency. These conditions may increase the risk of side effects. Nitrofurantoin may also cause false test results in diabetics' urine sugar tests. It may lead to anemia in people who have G6PD deficiency.

Do not take nitrofurantoin if you have ever experienced an allergic reaction to it or similar drugs.

Tell your health-care practitioner if you have diarrhea, which may be a sign of potentially serious intestinal inflammation.

Nitrofurantoin may cause side effects such as dizziness and confusion. Until you know how this drug affects you, do not drive a car, operate machinery, or perform other tasks that require concentration.

Long-term treatment with nitrofurantoin is associated with a variety of rare but potentially very serious health conditions, including lung problems, hepatitis, peripheral neuropathy (a nerve disease), hemolytic anemia (the destruction of red blood cells), and the growth of drug-resistant bacteria. As a result, your health-care practitioner will carefully monitor your condition while you take this drug. If you experience any unusual or troublesome side effects, consult your health-care practitioner.

DRUG INTERACTIONS

Inform your health-care practitioner and pharmacist if you are taking any other prescription or over-the-counter drugs, as well as any vitamins, herbs, or other supplements. Possible drug interactions include the following:

- A number of drugs may increase the side effects of nitrofurantoin, including those that affect the blood. These include acetohydroxamic acid, dapsone, furazolidone, methyldopa, primaquine, procainamide, quinidine, sulfa drugs, and oral antidiabetes medications.
- Numerous drugs increase the risk of nervous system side effects. Among these are carbamazepine, chloroquine, cisplatin, cytarabine, DTP vaccine, disulfiram, ethotoin, hydroxychloroquine, lindane, lithium, mephenytoin, mexiletine, pemoline, phenytoin, pyroxidine, and vincristine.

- Probenecid and sulfinpyrazone may increase side effects and reduce nitrofurantoin's effectiveness.

FOOD, VITAMIN, AND HERBAL INTERACTIONS

Consult your health-care practitioner before combining nitrofurantoin with any supplements, especially magnesium and vitamins B_6 (pyridoxine) and K.

This drug may disturb the balance of friendly bacteria in your body, leading to yeast infections. To counteract this effect, eat yogurt with live cultures or take a *Lactobacillus acidophilus* supplement.

RECOMMENDED DOSAGE

Nitrofurantoin comes as capsules, extended-release capsules, tablets, and oral suspension. Therapy can be for short-term treatment (7 days) or long-term prevention (for a period of months). The doses given below are typical. However, consult your health-care practitioner for the exact dose and schedule that are most appropriate for you.

- *Children 1 Month to 12 Years:* 5 to 7 mg per 2.2 pounds of body weight daily, in divided doses; long-term dosage is lower
- *Children Older than 12 Years and Adults:* 200 mg to 400 mg daily, in single or divided doses depending on the brand your health-care practitioner prescribes; long-term dosage is lower

To prevent stomach upset and improve your body's absorption of this drug, take nitrofurantoin with food or milk. Swallow the capsules whole. Do not open, crush, or chew them. If you forget to take a dose, take it as soon as you remember. If it is almost time for the next dose, skip the forgotten one, and resume your normal schedule. Never take double doses. To cure your infection, continue to take this drug even if you feel well. Do not discontinue use without consulting your health-care practitioner.

SYMPTOMS OF OVERDOSE AND WHAT TO DO

Vomiting is the most common symptom of overdose. If you suspect that an overdose has occurred, seek immediate medical attention and take the prescription bottle to the hospital with you.

SPECIAL INFORMATION FOR PREGNANT OR NURSING WOMEN

No studies have adequately investigated the effects of this drug during pregnancy or breastfeeding. However, nitrofurantoin does appear in breast milk. If you are pregnant or plan to become pregnant, or if you are breastfeeding or plan to do so, talk with your health-care practitioner before starting this drug. Only a health-care practitioner can determine whether the potential benefits outweigh the potential dangers.

SPECIAL INFORMATION FOR SENIORS

Seniors are more apt to experience side effects, and usually require lower doses of nitrofurantoin.

GENERIC NAME

Nitroglycerin

BRAND NAMES

Deponit, Minitran, Nitrek, Nitro-Bid, Nitro-Derm, Nitrodisc, Nitro-Dur, Nitrogard, Nitroglyn, Nitrol, Nitrolingual, Nitrong, NitroQuick, Nitrostat, Nitro-Time, Transderm-Nitro
Generic available

ABOUT THIS DRUG

Nitroglycerin is prescribed for chest pain (angina). Depending on the type that is used, this drug can relieve an attack of angina; prevent an attack that is likely to occur (for example, due to exertion); or reduce the overall number of angina attacks, when it is taken on a regular, long-term basis. The type of nitroglycerin your health-care practitioner prescribes will depend on your condition. Do not change types or brands without consulting your health-care practitioner.

Nitroglycerin works by relaxing blood vessels and increasing the blood and oxygen supply to the heart. This reduces the heart's workload.

SIDE EFFECTS

Speak to your health-care practitioner if you develop side effects while taking this drug. If you experience blurred vision or dry mouth, stop taking the medication and contact your health-care practitioner. Only he or she can determine whether it is safe for you to continue taking nitroglycerin.

- *Common:* flushing, headache, dizziness, lightheadedness, worsened chest pain
- *Less Common or Rare:* faintness, pounding heart, nausea, vomiting, diarrhea, weakness, sweating, pallor, restlessness, numbness, vertigo, discoloration of urine, allergic reactions, rash

IMPORTANT PRECAUTIONS

Always tell your health-care practitioner about any other medical conditions you may have, especially a recent heart attack, stroke, or head injury, kidney or liver disease, anemia, increased intraocular pressure, hyperthyroidism, or a previous allergic reaction to this drug. Your health-care practitioner will most likely advise you not to use nitroglycerin in these cases.

This medication should be used with caution if you have low blood pressure, glaucoma, an overactive thyroid, or malabsorption, or if you have had a previous allergic reaction to nitrates or nitrites (or to adhesives, if you are using the patch).

Since nitroglycerin may increase your tolerance for exercise, ask your health-care practitioner what level and type of exertion are safe for you. It is also important to avoid extreme temperatures while you are taking this drug. Be careful when you exercise in hot weather. Heavy sweating can lead to dizziness, lightheadedness, fainting, vomiting, dehydration, and low blood pressure.

This drug may cause side effects such as dizziness and fainting. Until you know how nitroglycerin affects you, do not drive a car, operate machinery, or perform other tasks that require concentration.

When you first start taking this drug or when the dosage is increased, you may experience dizziness or faintness when you rise quickly from a sitting or reclining position (postural hypotension). Try to get up slowly, and consult your health-care practitioner if the problem continues.

If you have high blood pressure, your health-care practitioner will also advise you to make certain lifestyle changes, such as weight control, smoking cessation, and close attention to diet.

People taking nitroglycerin require regular monitoring by their health-care practitioners.

DRUG INTERACTIONS

Inform your health-care practitioner and pharmacist if you are taking any other prescription or over-the-counter drugs, as well as any vitamins, herbs, or other supplements. Possible drug interactions include the following:

- Do not combine nitroglycerin with sildenafil. This may cause very low blood pressure.
- Exercise extreme caution when taking nitroglycerin with antihypertensive drugs such as diuretics. This can result in excessive lowering of blood pressure.
- Aspirin and other NSAIDs may increase the effects of nitroglycerin.

- A number of drugs increase the effects of nitroglycerin. These include mononitrate and isosorbide dinitrate.
- Taking nitroglycerin with ergot medications, alteplase, and heparin may result in reduced therapeutic benefits of ergot medications, alteplase, and heparin.

FOOD, VITAMIN, AND HERBAL INTERACTIONS

Consult your health-care practitioner before taking dietary supplements such as hawthorn and co-enzyme Q-10.

RECOMMENDED DOSAGE

Nitroglycerin comes as sublingual or transmucosal tablets, spray, sustained-release capsules or tablets, patches, and ointment. Although the doses given below are typical, only your health-care practitioner can determine the type of nitroglycerin and the dosage that best fit your individual needs. This drug is not recommended for children.

Sublingual or Transmucosal Tablets

- At the first sign of chest pain, dissolve 1 tablet under the tongue or inside the cheek. Repeat this dose every 5 minutes until pain is relieved. If pain continues longer than 15 minutes, and you have taken 3 tablets, seek immediate medical attention. For prevention, you can also take 1 tablet 5 to 10 minutes before activity that is likely to cause chest pain.

Spray

- At the first sign of chest pain, spray 1 to 2 pre-measured doses under the tongue. Repeat this dose every 5 minutes until pain is relieved. If pain continues longer than 15 minutes, and you have taken 3 doses, seek immediate medical attention. For prevention, you can also take 1 dose 5 to 10 minutes before activity that is likely to cause chest pain.

Sustained-Release Capsules or Tablets

- The typical dosage is 1 capsule or tablet every 8 to 12 hours. This form of medication may reduce the number of angina attacks, but it does not relieve an attack that has already begun because it works more slowly.

Skin Patches

- To prevent angina, apply 1 patch to hairless skin every 24 hours.

Ointment

- To prevent angina, apply 0.5 to 2 inches of ointment to hairless skin at 3- to 4-hour intervals. Rotate application sites to prevent rash.

If you are using nitroglycerin to relieve chest pain, take only the smallest amount necessary. People who take excessive amounts are more likely to experience headaches and may become more tolerant to this drug, rendering it less effective. To avoid tolerance from developing, your health-care practitioner will also advise you to have regular nitroglycerin-free intervals of 6 to 12 hours.

Sublingual tablets lose their effectiveness when exposed to air. Open the container only when you need a dose, and close it immediately afterward. These tablets frequently cause a burning sensation under the tongue, but this is not necessarily an indication of their effectiveness.

Carefully dispose of patches. Enough medication is left on them to be harmful to children and pets.

Oral forms of nitroglycerin should be taken 1 hour before or 2 hours after meals with a full (8-ounce) glass of water. However, if they upset your stomach, take them with milk. To avoid dizziness and falls, take nitroglycerin sitting down.

Do not suddenly stop taking nitroglycerin. This can cause angina. If necessary, your health-care practitioner will gradually reduce dosage over 4 to 6 weeks.

SYMPTOMS OF OVERDOSE AND WHAT TO DO

Symptoms of nitroglycerin overdose may include low blood pressure, blurred vision, heart palpitations, rapid heartbeat, slow pulse, difficulty breathing, dizziness, headache, confusion, cold and clammy skin, bluish skin, nausea, vomiting, fever, and paralysis. If you suspect that an overdose has occurred, seek immediate medical attention and take the prescription bottle to the hospital with you.

SPECIAL INFORMATION FOR PREGNANT OR NURSING WOMEN

No studies have adequately investigated the effects of nitroglycerin during pregnancy or breastfeeding. If you are pregnant or planning to become pregnant, or if you are breastfeeding or plan to do so, talk with your health-care practitioner before starting this drug. Only a health-care practitioner can determine whether the potential benefits outweigh the potential dangers.

SPECIAL INFORMATION FOR SENIORS

Seniors may be more prone to side effects such as headache, dizziness, flushing, fainting, and falling. Treatment should begin with small doses.

GENERIC NAME

Nizatidine

BRAND NAMES

Axid, Axid-AR
Generic available

ABOUT THIS DRUG

Nizatidine is used to prevent or treat gastric (stomach) and duodenal (upper intestinal) ulcers. This drug may also be prescribed for other conditions in which the stomach makes too much acid, such as heartburn or acid indigestion. It is available both with and without a prescription.

Nizatidine is a type of drug known as a histamine H_2 antagonist or blocker. It works by decreasing the amount of acid produced by the stomach.

SIDE EFFECTS

Inform your health-care practitioner if you experience any severe or persistent side effects. If symptoms such as heartburn and acid indigestion last for 2 weeks while you are taking nizatidine, consult your health-care practitioner. Only he or she can determine whether or not you should continue to take this drug.

- *Common:* nausea, vomiting, abdominal pain, gas, indigestion, headache, fatigue, nasal inflammation, sore throat, dizziness, increased sweating, weakness
- *Less Common or Rare:* chest pain, back pain, muscle pain, stomach or intestinal problems, constipation, appetite loss, visual disturbances, teeth problems, anxiety, nervousness, trouble sleeping, sleepiness, cough, fever, dry mouth, infection, rash

IMPORTANT PRECAUTIONS

Always tell your health-care practitioner about any other medical conditions that you may have, especially kidney or liver disease. Also inform your health-care practitioner if you have ever experienced an allergic reaction to this or similar drugs, such as cimetidine.

Nizatidine is intended for the treatment of noncancerous stomach ulcers, and may conceal warning signs of a malignancy. Contact your health-care practitioner if you experience any problems while taking this drug.

DRUG INTERACTIONS

Inform your health-care practitioner and pharmacist if you are taking any other prescription or over-the-counter drugs, as well as any vitamins, herbs, or other supplements. Possible drug interactions with nizatidine may include the following:

- Consult your health-care practitioner about combining antacids with nizatidine. You will probably be advised to separate the times you take them by half an hour to an hour.
- Nizatidine may increase the effects of high-dose aspirin, amoxicillin, and theophylline.
- Alcohol use and cigarette smoking decrease the effect of nizatidine, by increasing the amount of acid produced by the stomach.

FOOD, VITAMIN, AND HERBAL INTERACTIONS

Certain foods—such as garlic, onions, and tomatoes—may increase stomach acid production, and spicy or deep-fried foods are likely to cause heartburn. Ask your health-care practitioner about any special dietary recommendations.

Do not use herbs such as kola and ephedra (ma huang), which may increase stomach acid.

RECOMMENDED DOSAGE

Nizatidine is available in capsule or tablet form. Most ulcers respond well to 4 to 6 weeks of treatment. If this drug is prescribed for longer periods (for example, to prevent duodenal ulcers), it is usually at a lower dosage. Although the doses given below are typical, only your health-care practitioner can determine the dose and schedule that are most appropriate for you.

- *Children:* This drug is not recommended for children.
- *Adults:* 300 mg once a day at bedtime, or 150 mg twice a day; lower preventive doses of 75 to 150 mg daily are prescribed for long-term use

Nizatidine may be taken with or without food. If you miss a dose, take it as soon as you remember. However, if it is nearly time for your next scheduled dose, do not take the missed dose. Follow your regular dosing schedule. Never take a double dose. Do not stop taking medication suddenly.

SYMPTOMS OF OVERDOSE AND WHAT TO DO

No specific information on nizatidine overdose is available. If you suspect an overdose, seek immediate medical attention, and bring the prescription bottle to the hospital with you.

SPECIAL INFORMATION FOR PREGNANT OR NURSING WOMEN

No studies have adequately investigated the effects of nizatidine during pregnancy or breastfeeding. If you are pregnant or planning to become pregnant, or if you are breastfeeding or plan to do so, talk with your health-care practitioner before starting this drug. Only a health-care practitioner can determine whether the potential benefits outweigh the potential dangers.

SPECIAL INFORMATION FOR SENIORS

Side effects are more common in seniors, and lower dosages are usually recommended.

GENERIC NAME

Norethindrone acetate *see Progestins, page 876*

GENERIC NAME

Norfloxacin *see Fluoroquinolone Antibiotics, page 468*

GENERIC NAME

Norgestimate *see Estrogens, page 436*

GENERIC NAME

Nortriptyline *see Tricyclic Antidepressants, page 1076*

GENERIC NAME
Nystatin

BRAND NAMES

Mycostatin, Nilstat, Nystex
Generic available

ABOUT THIS DRUG

Nystatin is used to treat fungal infections of the skin, mouth, vagina, and intestinal tract. It works by eradicating the underlying cause of infection.

SIDE EFFECTS

Consult your health-care practitioner if you develop side effects while taking nystatin. Only he or she can determine whether it is safe for you to continue taking this drug.

➤ *Common:* rash, irritation, burning sensation, cramping, headache, hives, vaginal itching

➤ *Less Common or Rare:* nausea, vomiting, diarrhea, stomach pain

IMPORTANT PRECAUTIONS

Always tell your health-care practitioner about all other medical conditions you have, and if you have ever experienced an allergic reaction to this or similar medications.

Use napkins instead of tampons while using vaginal nystatin. If a vaginal infection does not respond to treatment, see your health-care practitioner. The problem may be a different type of infection that does not respond to this treatment.

DRUG INTERACTIONS

Although no specific interactions are known, always inform your health-care practitioner and pharmacist if you are taking any other prescription or over-the-counter drugs, as well as any vitamins, herbs, or other supplements.

FOOD, VITAMIN, AND HERBAL INTERACTIONS

No food, vitamin, or herbal interactions have been noted.

RECOMMENDED DOSAGE

Nystatin comes as ointment, cream, lozenges (pastilles), oral tablets, oral suspension, and vaginal tablets. Treatment ranges in length from one to 14 days. The doses given below are typical. However, consult your health-care practitioner for the exact dose and schedule that are most appropriate for you.

Ointment and Cream

- *Children and Adults:* Apply a small amount to the skin several times daily, as directed by your health-care practitioner.

Lozenges and Oral Tablets

- *Children 5 Years and Older and Adults:* 1 to 2 lozenges or tablets 3 to 5 times a day

Oral Suspension

- *Older Infants to Children 5 Years:* 2 milliliters 4 times a day
- *Children 5 Years and Older and Adults:* 4 to 6 milliliters 4 times a day

Vaginal Tablets

- *Adult Women:* Insert 1 tablet high in the vagina once daily.

If you forget to take a dose, take it as soon as you remember. If it is almost time for the next dose, skip the forgotten one, and resume your normal schedule. Never take double doses. To cure your infection, continue to take this drug even if you feel well. Do not discontinue use without consulting your health-care practitioner.

SYMPTOMS OF OVERDOSE AND WHAT TO DO

Stomach upset is the most common symptom of overdose. If you suspect that an overdose has occurred, seek immediate medical attention and take the prescription bottle to the hospital with you.

SPECIAL INFORMATION FOR PREGNANT OR NURSING WOMEN

Nystatin is considered safe for use in pregnant and nursing women.

SPECIAL INFORMATION FOR SENIORS

There are no special instructions for seniors.

GENERIC NAME

Ofloxacin

see Fluoroquinolone Antibiotics, page 468

GENERIC NAME
Olanzapine

BRAND NAMES

Zyprexa, Zydis
No generic available

ABOUT THIS DRUG

Olanzapine is an antipsychotic drug used on a short-term basis to control acute mental disorders. It has positive effects on mood, behavior, and thinking. This drug may also be prescribed to ease mania in bipolar disorder.

Olanzapine works by blocking the action of two important nerve transmitters in the brain, dopamine and serotonin. This corrects an underlying imbalance believed to be responsible for a number of mental disorders.

SIDE EFFECTS

Talk to your health-care practitioner if you develop side effects while taking olanzapine. Only he or she can determine whether it is safe for you to continue taking this drug and whether it is necessary to readjust your dosage.

- *Common:* headache, fatigue, sleeplessness, dizziness, agitation, hostility, runny nose
- *Less Common or Rare:* low blood pressure, rapid heart rate, trouble swallowing, fever, dizziness or fainting upon rising, dry mouth, increased appetite, weight gain, personality changes, memory loss, difficulty speaking, stuttering, anxiety, euphoria, constipation, cough, joint pain, muscle stiffness, rigid neck, restlessness, tremor, twitching, swelling in the arms and legs, arm or leg pain, visual disturbances, abdominal, back, or chest pain, vaginal infection, vomiting, Parkinson-like reactions (such as uncontrollable jerking movements), symptoms of tardive dyskinesia (such as lip smacking, wormlike movements of the tongue, and slow, rhythmical, involuntary movements), seizures

When you first start taking olanzapine, consult your health-care practitioner if you experience side effects such as low blood pressure, faintness upon rising, dizziness, and a rapid heart rate. If you have heart disease, are dehydrated, or take blood pressure medication, you are more likely to have these problems. Your health-care practitioner will probably lower your dosage.

People taking antipsychotic drugs may experience a rare but life-threatening set of side effects known as neuroleptic malignant syndrome (NMS). Symptoms include fever, difficulty breathing, rapid heartbeat, rigid muscles, mental changes, increased sweating, irregular blood pressure, and convulsions. Immediate medical attention is required.

Side effects such as lip smacking, wormlike movements of the tongue, and slow, rhythmical, involuntary movements are characteristic of a disorder known as tardive dyskinesia. Older adults (especially women) are more susceptible to this condition, which may become permanent. If you experience tardive dyskinesia, your health-care practitioner will probably advise you to stop taking this drug.

IMPORTANT PRECAUTIONS

You should not take olanzapine if you have neuroleptic malignant syndrome or if you have experienced a previous allergic reaction to this drug.

Use olanzapine with caution if you have liver disease, a seizure disorder, low blood pressure, heart disease, a history of heart attack, dehydration, narrow-angle glaucoma, an enlarged prostate, Alzheimer's disease, phenylketonuria, constipation, trouble swallowing, or a history of breast cancer.

Before having any type of surgery or dental procedure, tell your surgeon or dentist that you are taking olanzapine.

This drug may impair your physical coordination and mental alertness. Until you know how olanzapine affects you, do not drive a car, operate machinery, or perform other tasks that demand concentration.

Drink plenty of fluids and avoid extreme heat while you take this drug. Be especially careful when you exercise in hot weather, take a hot bath, or enter a sauna. Heavy sweating can lead to dizziness, lightheadedness, fainting, vomiting, and dehydration.

When you first start taking this drug or when the dosage is increased, you may experience dizziness or faintness when you rise quickly from a sitting or reclining position (postural hypotension). Try to get up slowly, and consult your health-care practitioner if the problem continues.

Women metabolize olanzapine 30% more slowly than men, so they experience its effects for a longer period of time.

DRUG INTERACTIONS

Inform your health-care practitioner and pharmacist if you are taking any other prescription or over-the-counter drugs, as well as any vita-

mins, herbs, or other supplements. Possible drug interactions include the following:

- Since olanzapine may cause low blood pressure, be cautious about combining this medication with high blood pressure drugs.
- Antianxiety benzodiazepines such as diazepam may also increase the risk of low blood pressure.
- Do not combine olanzapine with lithium. This increases the risk of serious nerve side effects.
- Sedative drugs (either prescription or over-the-counter) may cause increased drowsiness.
- Taking olanzapine with fluoroquinolone antibiotics or fluvoxamine may lead to olanzapine toxicity.
- Carbamazepine reduces the amount of olanzapine absorbed by the body.
- Other drugs that may reduce the effects of olanzapine include omeprazole and rifampin.
- Smoking cigarettes may accelerate the removal of olanzapine from your body.
- Avoid alcohol while taking olanzapine.

FOOD, VITAMIN, AND HERBAL INTERACTIONS

Do not take olanzapine with grapefruit juice. This can lead to toxic amounts of medication in the blood.

Do not combine olanzapine with herbs that produce sedative effects, such as catnip, elecampane, goldenseal, gotu kola, hops, kava, lemon balm, skullcap, St. John's wort, and valerian. Also do not use ginseng, kola, or ephedra (ma huang) while taking this drug.

RECOMMENDED DOSAGE

Olanzapine comes as a tablet and can also be administered as an intramuscular (IM) injection (dosage for IM form not given here). The doses given below are typical, but dosage is always carefully individualized according to a person's particular needs and reactions to therapy.

- *Children:* This drug is not recommended for children.
- *Adults:* 5 to 10 mg daily to start, to a maximum of 20 mg daily

Olanzapine tablets can be crushed and taken with food. If you forget a dose, take it as soon as you remember. If it is almost time for the next dose, skip it and resume your normal schedule. Never take a double dose. You must use this drug for at least a week for it to be effective.

SYMPTOMS OF OVERDOSE AND WHAT TO DO

The symptoms of olanzapine overdose include drowsiness and slurred speech. If overdose occurs, seek immediate medical attention and take the prescription bottle to the hospital with you.

SPECIAL INFORMATION FOR PREGNANT OR NURSING WOMEN

No studies have adequately investigated the effects of olanzapine during pregnancy or breastfeeding. If you are pregnant or planning to become pregnant, or if you are breastfeeding or plan to do so, talk with your health-care practitioner before starting this drug. Only a health-care practitioner can determine whether the potential benefits outweigh the potential dangers.

SPECIAL INFORMATION FOR SENIORS

Seniors require lower doses of olanzapine. This age group is more likely to experience effects such as drowsiness, dizziness, low blood pressure, Parkinson-like reactions (such as uncontrollable jerking movements), and tardive dyskinesia (with symptoms such as lip smacking, wormlike movements of the tongue, and slow, rhythmical, involuntary movements).

GENERIC NAME

Olanzapine and Fluoxetine

BRAND NAME

Symbyax
No generic available

ABOUT THIS DRUG

Olanzapine/fluoxetine is the first medication approved by the Food and Drug Administration (FDA) for treatment of bipolar depression. The olanzapine component is an antipsychotic drug used to control acute mental disorders, including mania in bipolar disorder, while the fluoxetine component is a selective serotonin reuptake inhibitor (SSRI) antidepressant that is prescribed for individuals who have major depression.

The properties of olanzapine and fluoxetine work together to treat bipolar depression. That is, they activate three chemical systems in the brain—serotonin, norepinephrine, and dopamine—which enhance the antidepressant effect.

SIDE EFFECTS

Be sure to tell your health-care practitioner if you experience any side effects while taking olanzapine/fluoxetine. Only your health-care practitioner can determine whether it is safe for you to continue taking this drug. The following side effects are those associated with the use of olanzapine and/or fluoxetine.

- ➤ *Most Common:* abnormal dreams, amnesia, anxiety, bronchitis, chills, confusion, conjunctivitis, cough, diarrhea, dilated pupils, dizziness, drowsiness, dry eyes, dry mouth, ear pain, excessive sweating, fatigue, headache, high blood pressure, impotence, light intolerance, insomnia, mood swings, nervousness, nausea, rash, ringing in the ears, runny nose, sore throat, tremors, vomiting, weakness, weight gain, yawning, swelling in hands or feet
- ➤ *Less Common:* abnormal gait, abnormal cessation of menstrual flow, acne, apathy, arthritis, asthma, bone pain, breast pain, bursitis, convulsions, dark stool, euphoria, facial swelling, fever, hair loss, hallucinations, hiccups, hives, hostility, infection, inflamed esophagus, inflamed stomach lining, involuntary movements, irregular heartbeat, lack of muscle coordination, low blood pressure when standing from a seated or lying position, migraine, inflamed mouth, muscle spasm, nosebleed, swallowing difficulties, pelvic pain, rapid breathing, inflamed skin, thirst, twitching, urinary problems, vertigo, vision problems
- ➤ *Rare:* belching, bleeding gums, bloody urine, bloody diarrhea, breast enlargement, breathing difficulties, coma, dehydration, deafness, delusions, diabetes, double vision, duodenal ulcer, enlarged liver, enlarged thyroid gland, eye bleeding, female milk production, gallstones, gastrointestinal bleeding, glaucoma, gout, heart attack, heart failure, hepatitis, high blood sugar, increased salivation, inflamed eyes, inflamed intestinal tract, loss of taste, muscle spasms, psoriasis, rash, rheumatoid arthritis, skin discoloration, slurred speech, tongue swelling, vomiting blood, weakness

People taking antipsychotic drugs may experience a rare but life-threatening set of side effects known as neuroleptic malignant syndrome (NMS). Symptoms include fever, difficulty breathing, rapid heartbeat, rigid muscles, mental changes, increased sweating, irregular blood pressure, and convulsions. Immediate medical attention is required.

Side effects such as lip smacking, wormlike movements of the tongue, and slow, rhythmical, involuntary movements are characteristic of a disorder known as tardive dyskinesia. Older adults (especially women) are more susceptible to this condition, which may become permanent. If you experience tardive dyskinesia, your health-care practitioner may advise you to stop taking this drug.

IMPORTANT PRECAUTIONS

Tell your health-care practitioner if you are sensitive or allergic to olanzapine and/or fluoxetine or to any other drugs.

Olanzapine/fluoxetine should not be taken along with MAO inhibitors (e.g., phenelzine, furazolidone, linezolid), and do not take this combination within at least 14 days of stopping treatment with an MAOI. If you want to start taking an MAOI after stopping olanzapine/fluoxetine, wait at least five weeks to start the MAOI. Serious and even fatal reactions can occur if MAOIs are mixed with olanzapine/fluoxetine.

Before taking olanzapine/fluoxetine, tell your health-care practitioner if you have a history of high blood sugar or diabetes, liver problems, seizures, low or high blood pressure, heart problems or heart attack, stroke or transient ischemic attack (TIA), an enlarged prostate, narrow angle glaucoma, or paralytic ileus, or if you smoke cigarettes, drink alcohol, exercise often, or are often in hot places.

The safety and effectiveness of this drug has not been determined for children.

Because olanzapine/fluoxetine can cause drowsiness and dizziness, you should make sure you know how you react to the drug before you drive or operate hazardous equipment. Olanzapine/fluoxetine may cause dizziness, or increased or abnormal heart rate upon standing, particularly during the initial dosing phase.

Weight gain may be a problem for some individuals. Fourteen percent of patients who use olanzapine/fluoxetine typically gain more than 10 percent of their baseline weight (weight before starting treatment).

DRUG INTERACTIONS

Tell your health-care practitioner and pharmacist if you are taking any prescription or nonprescription drugs, as well as any vitamins, herbs, or other supplements. Possible drug interactions include the following:

- Since olanzapine may cause low blood pressure, be cautious about combining olanzapine/fluoxetine with antihypertensive drugs.
- The effects of levodopa and dopamine agonists may be inhibited by olanzapine/fluoxetine.

- Use of diazepam may increase the risk of orthostatic hypotension.
- Carbamazepine reduces the amount of olanzapine absorbed by the body.
- Blood levels of clozapine may increase when taken with this combination drug.
- Fluvoxamine increases the amount of olanzapine absorbed by the body.
- Fluoxetine may increase the amount of haloperidol and phenytoin the body absorbs.
- MAOIs should not be used with olanzapine/fluoxetine, and this combination medication should not be used within at least 14 days of discontinuing an MAOI.
- Thioridazine should not be used with olanzapine/fluoxetine or within at least five weeks after stopping the combination medication.
- Sumatriptan taken with an SSRI (e.g., fluoxetine) has been known to cause weakness and incoordination.
- Tryptophan taken with fluoxetine can cause agitation, restlessness, and gastrointestinal distress.
- Use of aspirin and/or NSAIDs can increase the risk of gastrointestinal bleeding.

FOOD, VITAMIN, AND HERBAL INTERACTIONS

Do not take olanzapine/fluoxetine with grapefruit or grapefruit juice. This can lead to toxic amounts of medication in the blood.

Do not combine olanzapine/fluoxetine with herbs that produce sedative effects, such as catnip, elecampane, goldenseal, gotu kola, hops, kava, lemon balm, skullcap, St. John's wort, and valerian. Also do not use ginseng, kola, or ephedra (ma huang) while taking this combination drug.

RECOMMENDED DOSAGE

The olanzapine/fluoxetine combination is available in capsules in several formulations: 6 mg/25 mg, 6 mg/50 mg, 12 mg/25 mg, and 12 mg/50 mg. The dosages given here are typical. However, your health-care practitioner will determine the most appropriate dose and schedule for your needs.

- *Children*: Not indicated for use in children
- *Adults*: 6 mg/25 mg once daily in the evening as a starting dose. Your health-care practitioner may increase your dose as needed.

Olanzapine/fluoxetine can be taken with or without food. If you miss a dose, take it as soon as you remember. If it is nearly time for your next dose, skip the missed dose and return to your normal dosing schedule. Never take a double dose.

SYMPTOMS OF OVERDOSE AND WHAT TO DO

Symptoms of overdose may include arrhythmia, coma, confusion, convulsions, drowsiness, and lethargy. If overdose occurs, seek immediate medical attention and bring the prescription container with you to the hospital.

SPECIAL INFORMATION FOR PREGNANT OR NURSING WOMEN

No adequate studies of the effects of olanzapine or fluoxetine on pregnant or breastfeeding women have been done. One study found that some children born to mothers who took fluoxetine were born prematurely, had breathing problems or nursing difficulties, or experienced jitteriness. Four other studies, however, did not have these findings. If you are pregnant or plan to become pregnant and this drug combination is crucial for your health, you and your health-care practitioner must weigh the potential benefits against the potential risks to the fetus.

Fluoxetine appears in breast milk. If you are breastfeeding, your health-care practitioner will likely advise you to switch to bottle feeding until your treatment is complete.

SPECIAL INFORMATION FOR SENIORS

Older adults may experience more side effects and more serious ones. Dosages also may need to be reduced. In particular, olanzapine/fluoxetine should be used cautiously in elderly patients with dementia.

GENERIC NAME

Olopatadine

BRAND NAME

Patanol

No generic available

ABOUT THIS DRUG

Olopatadine ophthalmic eye solution is an antihistamine used to prevent eye itching, swelling, and tearing due to allergies and conjunctivitis (pinkeye). This drug works by preventing mast cells in the body from releasing substances that cause inflammation and other allergic reactions.

SIDE EFFECTS

Consult your health-care practitioner if you experience side effects while using olopatadine. Only he or she can determine whether or not you should continue to use this drug.

- *Common:* headache
- *Less Common or Rare:* eye irritation, burning, stinging, dryness, itching, redness, swelling, feeling of something in the eye, sore throat, runny nose, cold symptoms, sinus inflammation, changes in taste

IMPORTANT PRECAUTIONS

Before using this drug, tell your health-care practitioner if you have ever experienced an allergic reaction to olopatadine or similar drugs.

DRUG INTERACTIONS

Although no specific interactions are known, always tell your health-care practitioner and pharmacist if you are taking any other prescription or over-the-counter drugs, as well as any vitamins, herbs, or other supplements.

FOOD, VITAMIN, AND HERBAL INTERACTIONS

No food, vitamin, or herbal interactions have been noted.

RECOMMENDED DOSAGE

Olopatadine comes as an eyedrop solution. Although the dosage below is typical, consult your health-care practitioner for exact instructions. This drug is not recommended for children under age three.

- *Children 3 Years and Older and Adults:* Apply 1 to 2 drops in each eye 2 times daily, 6 to 8 hours apart.

Remove contact lenses before using olopatadine, and do not reinsert them for at least 15 minutes. Be careful not to touch the dropper to the eye. If you miss a dose of medication, administer it as soon as you remember. However, if it is nearly time for your next scheduled dose, do not administer the missed dose. Follow your regular dosing schedule. Never use a double dose.

SYMPTOMS OF OVERDOSE AND WHAT TO DO
Overdose is unlikely. However, if you suspect an overdose, seek immediate medical attention, and bring the prescription bottle to the hospital with you.

SPECIAL INFORMATION FOR PREGNANT OR NURSING WOMEN
Little olopatadine is absorbed into the body. However, if you are pregnant or plan to become pregnant, or if you are breastfeeding or plan to do so, talk with your health-care practitioner before starting this drug. Only a health-care practitioner can determine whether the potential benefits outweigh the potential dangers.

SPECIAL INFORMATION FOR SENIORS
No special instructions are provided for seniors.

GENERIC NAME

Olsalazine

BRAND NAME
Dipentum
No generic available

ABOUT THIS DRUG
Olsalazine is an anti-inflammatory medicine used to treat inflammatory bowel disease such as ulcerative colitis. This drug reduces symptoms including diarrhea, rectal bleeding, and stomach pain. It is generally prescribed for people who cannot take sulfasalazine.

Olsalazine works by controlling inflammation in the bowel. It reduces the formation of prostaglandins, substances that play a major role in inflammation.

SIDE EFFECTS
Speak to your health-care practitioner if you experience side effects while taking this drug. Only he or she can determine whether it is safe for you to continue taking olsalazine.

- *Common:* diarrhea, loose stools
- *Less Common or Rare:* nausea, vomiting, abdominal pain, bloating, cramps, indigestion, loss of appetite, headache, sluggishness, drowsiness, dizziness, vertigo, lightheadedness, insomnia, rectal bleeding, rash, itching, upper respiratory infection, joint pain, photosensitivity

IMPORTANT PRECAUTIONS

Inform your health-care practitioner if you have experienced any previous allergic reactions to this drug or to aspirin (or other salicylates), mesalamine, or sulfasalazine. Also tell your health-care practitioner about any other medical conditions you may have, especially allergies or liver or kidney impairment. If you have kidney disease, taking olsalazine may cause further kidney damage. In rare cases, people taking this drug have developed hepatitis. Some people using olsalazine have also had flare-ups of colitis. Consult your health-care practitioner if you experience diarrhea.

This drug may cause drowsiness or dizziness. Until you know how olsalazine affects you, do not drive a car, operate machinery, or perform other tasks that demand concentration.

Olsalazine may cause increased sensitivity to the sun. To counteract this effect, wear protective clothing and apply sunscreen.

DRUG INTERACTIONS

Inform your health-care practitioner if you are taking any other prescription or over-the-counter drugs, as well as any vitamins, herbs, or supplements. Possible drug interactions include the following:

- Combining olsalazine with alendronate may increase the risk of stomach upset.
- Taking enoxaprin with olsalazine may increase the risk of bleeding.
- Consult your health-care practitioner before combining olsalazine with warfarin.
- Tell your health-care practitioner if you are taking sulfasalazine.
- Do not take this drug for 6 weeks after having varicella vaccine.

FOOD, VITAMIN, AND HERBAL INTERACTIONS

Do not take olsalazine with dietary supplements that may cause photosensitivity, such as St. John's wort.

RECOMMENDED DOSAGE

Olsalazine comes in capsule form. The doses given below are typical, but only your health-care practitioner can determine the best dose and schedule for you.

- *Children:* This drug is not recommended for children under the age of 12.
- *Adults:* 1,000 mg daily, divided into 2 equal doses

Take olsalazine with food to prevent stomach upset. If you forget a dose, take it as soon as you remember. If it is almost time for the next dose, skip the missed one and resume your normal schedule. Never take a double dose.

SYMPTOMS OF OVERDOSE AND WHAT TO DO

Symptoms of overdose may include diarrhea, nausea, vomiting, and cramping. If you suspect an overdose, seek immediate medical attention and take the prescription bottle to the hospital with you.

SPECIAL INFORMATION FOR PREGNANT OR NURSING WOMEN

No studies have adequately investigated the effects of olsalazine during pregnancy or breastfeeding. However, this drug has caused birth defects in animal studies. If you are pregnant or plan to become pregnant, or if you are breastfeeding or plan to do so, talk with your health-care practitioner before starting this drug. Only a health-care practitioner can determine whether the potential benefits outweigh the potential dangers.

SPECIAL INFORMATION FOR SENIORS

There are no special instructions for seniors.

GENERIC NAME

Omeprazole

BRAND NAME

Prilosec

No generic available

ABOUT THIS DRUG

Omeprazole is used to treat conditions in which there is too much acid in the stomach. It is prescribed for duodenal and gastric ulcers, gastritis, erosive esophagitis, gastroesophageal reflux disease (GERD), Zollinger-Ellison syndrome, mastocytosis, and endocrine adenoma. In some cases, omeprazole is used in combination with antibiotics to treat ulcers associated with *H. pylori* bacteria.

This drug works by blocking an enzyme system that enables the stomach to produce acid. This eliminates an important cause of acid-related conditions, and creates a better environment for healing.

SIDE EFFECTS

Contact your health-care practitioner if you experience side effects while taking omeprazole. Only he or she can determine whether or not you should continue to take this drug.

- *Common:* nausea, vomiting, diarrhea, abdominal pain, headache
- *Less Common or Rare:* changes in appetite, joint or muscle pain, bruising, drowsiness, dizziness, fatigue, anxiety, depression, constipation, cough, fever, dry mouth, ringing in the ears, nosebleeds, fluid retention, itching, back pain, chest pain, changes in liver function, high blood pressure

The reduction of stomach acid may make you more susceptible to bacterial infections such as *Campylobacter*. Promptly report symptoms such as fever and loose, mucousy stools to your health-care practitioner.

IMPORTANT PRECAUTIONS

Always inform your health-care practitioner about all other medical conditions you suffer from, especially liver problems or blood cell or bone marrow disorders. Tell your health-care practitioner if you have ever experienced an allergic reaction to this or similar medications.

Omeprazole may cause drowsiness, so limit activities such as driving as necessary.

DRUG INTERACTIONS

Inform your health-care practitioner and pharmacist if you are taking any other prescription or over-the-counter drugs, as well as any vitamins, herbs, or other supplements. Possible drug interactions with omeprazole may include the following:

- Omeprazole may increase the effects of carbamazepine, cyclosporine, diazepam, digoxin, disulfiram, fluvastatin, methotrexate, phenytoin, and warfarin.
- Omeprazole may decrease the effects of amoxicillin, ampicillin, itraconazole, ketoconazole, olanzapine, ritonavir, and trovafloxacin.
- If omeprazole is taken with an antibiotic, also be certain to refer to the drugs that interact with that particular antibiotic.
- Do not smoke cigarettes. This can worsen acid secretion.

FOOD, VITAMIN, AND HERBAL INTERACTIONS

Omeprazole may interfere with the absorption of iron, zinc, and B vitamins such as folate. Taking a daily multivitamin-multimineral supplement is recommended. Do not use the herbs St. John's wort, kola, or ephedra (ma huang) while taking omeprazole.

RECOMMENDED DOSAGE

Omeprazole is available in capsule form. Although the doses given below are typical, only your health-care practitioner can determine the dose and schedule that are most appropriate for you.

Gastroesophageal Reflux Disease (GERD)

- *Children:* This drug is not recommended for children.
- *Adults:* 20 mg once a day for 4 weeks

Duodenal Ulcers

- *Children:* This drug is not recommended for children.
- *Adults:* 20 mg once a day for 4 to 8 weeks

Duodenal Ulcers Associated with *H. pylori* Bacteria

- *Children:* This drug is not recommended for children.
- *Adults:* 40 mg omeprazole once daily and 500 mg clarithromycin 3 times a day for 14 days, followed by 20 mg omeprazole once daily for an additional 18 days

Gastric Ulcers

- *Children:* This drug is not recommended for children.
- *Adults:* 40 mg once a day for 4 to 8 weeks

Erosive Esophagitis

- *Children:* This drug is not recommended for children.
- *Adults:* 20 mg once a day for up to 8 weeks

Other Excess Acid Conditions

- *Children:* This drug is not recommended for children.
- *Adults:* 60 to 80 mg once a day

Omeprazole should be taken on an empty stomach, preferably in the morning. The capsules should be swallowed whole. If you miss a dose, take it as soon as you remember. However, if it is nearly time for your next scheduled dose, do not take the missed dose. Follow your regular dosing schedule dose. Never take a double dose.

SYMPTOMS OF OVERDOSE AND WHAT TO DO

Possible symptoms of overdose include nausea, abdominal pain, drowsiness, dizziness, and lethargy. If you suspect an overdose, seek immediate medical attention, and bring the prescription bottle with you.

SPECIAL INFORMATION FOR PREGNANT OR NURSING WOMEN

No studies have adequately investigated the effects of omeprazole during pregnancy or breastfeeding. If you are pregnant or plan to become pregnant, or if you are breastfeeding or plan to do so, talk with your health-care practitioner before starting this drug. Only a health-care practitioner can determine whether the potential benefits outweigh the potential dangers.

SPECIAL INFORMATION FOR SENIORS

Smaller doses are appropriate for seniors.

GENERIC NAME

Ondansetron *see Antiemetics, page 128*

GENERIC NAME

Orlistat

BRAND NAME

Xenical
No generic available

ABOUT THIS DRUG

Orlistat is used in the treatment of obesity. This drug should be used on a short-term basis only and under a health-care practitioner's close supervision. Weight-loss medications are not a substitute for a sensible, healthy, overall weight loss program.

Orlistat works by blocking the absorption of dietary fat into the bloodstream. It cuts fat absorption by approximately 33 percent.

SIDE EFFECTS

If you develop side effects while taking orlistat, ask your health-care practitioner whether it is safe for you to continue taking this drug.

- *Common:* nausea, vomiting, diarrhea, fatty or oily stools, fecal urgency, increased defecation, incontinence, rectal discomfort or pain, gas, oily discharge, abdominal discomfort or pain, sleep problems, fatigue, anxiety, dizziness, back pain, muscle pain, urinary or respiratory tract infections, gum problems, earache, menstrual problems, vaginal inflammation, rash
- *Less Common or Rare:* depression, dry skin, joint disorders, ear, nose, or throat problems

IMPORTANT PRECAUTIONS

This drug is not an appropriate remedy for people who have malabsorption or cholestasis (a blockage in the supply of bile required for digestion). Do not use orlistat if you have experienced an allergic reaction to this or similar medications. People who are prone to kidney stones should use this drug with caution.

In order to lose weight, exercise regularly and follow a reduced-calorie diet while taking orlistat. To keep weight off, continue to follow a sensible program of diet and exercise under the supervision of your health-care practitioner.

Orlistat has been associated with a loss of vitamins A, D, E, and K. Without supplementation, this may lead to an increased risk of bleeding.

Orlistat may cause side effects such as dizziness. Until you know how this drug affects you, do not drive a car, operate machinery, or engage in other actions that require concentration.

Before having surgery or a dental procedure, tell your health-care practitioner or dentist that you take orlistat.

DRUG INTERACTIONS

Tell your health-care practitioner and pharmacist if you are taking any other prescription or over-the-counter drugs, as well as any vitamins, herbs, or other supplements. Drug interactions may include the following:

- Taking orlistat with pravastatin may result in an increased effect in lowering cholesterol.
- Combining orlistat with warfarin may cause increased warfarin effects.

FOOD, VITAMIN, AND HERBAL INTERACTIONS

Vitamin and mineral deficiencies have been associated with orlistat. This drug may reduce the effects of fat-soluble vitamins and beta-carotene. Ask your health-care practitioner to recommend a daily vitamin and mineral supplement.

Do not take any herbal weight loss products while you are taking orlistat. Avoid foods that cause gas.

RECOMMENDED DOSAGE

Orlistat comes in capsule form. The doses given below are typical, but only your health-care practitioner can determine the dose and schedule that best fit your particular needs.

- *Children:* This drug is not recommended for children.

➤ *Adults:* one 120-mg capsule 3 times a day before or with each meal that contains fat

Take orlistat with or up to an hour before each meal that contains fat. If you eat a meal that doesn't contain fat or if you skip a meal, do not take orlistat. Never take double doses.

SYMPTOMS OF OVERDOSE AND WHAT TO DO
No specific information on orlistat overdose is available. If you suspect an overdose, seek immediate medical attention, and bring the prescription bottle to the hospital with you.

SPECIAL INFORMATION FOR PREGNANT OR NURSING WOMEN
No studies have adequately investigated the effects of orlistat during pregnancy or breastfeeding. If you are pregnant or plan to become pregnant, or if you are breastfeeding or plan to do so, talk with your health-care practitioner before starting this drug. Only a health-care practitioner can determine whether the potential benefits outweigh the potential dangers.

SPECIAL INFORMATION FOR SENIORS
There are no special guidelines for seniors.

GENERIC NAME

Oseltamivir

BRAND NAME
Tamiflu
No generic available

ABOUT THIS DRUG
Oseltamivir is an antiviral drug used to shorten the duration of the flu. This drug is prescribed for influenza types A and B. In order to be effective, it must be taken within the first 2 days of the appearance of flu symptoms. Although oseltamivir cannot cure the flu, it may shorten its duration by at least a day. In some cases, this medication is taken to prevent infection after coming into contact with someone who has the flu.

Oseltamivir is a new type of antiviral drug. It works by blocking the flu virus from making copies of itself and infecting new cells.

SIDE EFFECTS

If you develop side effects while taking oseltamivir, ask your health-care practitioner whether it is safe for you to continue taking this drug.

- *Common:* nausea, vomiting
- *Less Common or Rare:* insomnia, dizziness, vertigo, headache, cough, bronchitis, fatigue, fainting

IMPORTANT PRECAUTIONS

Oseltamivir is not a cure for the flu. Older people and others at risk should continue to receive yearly flu shots to prevent this virus.

Always tell your health-care practitioner about all other medical conditions from which you suffer, including kidney, heart, lung, and liver problems. Do not use oseltamivir if you have experienced an allergic reaction to this or any similar medication. People with kidney disease should receive lower doses.

Oseltamivir may cause side effects such as dizziness and vertigo. Until you know how this drug affects you, do not drive a car, operate machinery, or engage in other actions that require concentration.

DRUG INTERACTIONS

Tell your health-care practitioner and pharmacist if you are taking any other prescription or over-the-counter drugs, as well as any vitamins, herbs, or other supplements. At present, the only drug-drug interaction concerns probenecide, which may result in an increased effect of oseltamivir.

FOOD, VITAMIN, AND HERBAL INTERACTIONS

No food, vitamin, or herbal interactions have been noted.

RECOMMENDED DOSAGE

Oseltamivir comes in capsule form. The doses given below are typical, but only your health-care practitioner can determine the dose and schedule that best fit your particular needs.

- *Children:* This drug is not recommended for children.
- *Adults:* 75 mg twice a day for 5 days

If it upsets your stomach, take oseltamivir with food. If you miss a dose, take it as soon as you remember. However, if it is nearly time for your next scheduled dose, do not take the missed dose. Follow your regular dosing schedule. Never take a double dose.

SYMPTOMS OF OVERDOSE AND WHAT TO DO

Symptoms of oseltamivir overdose may include nausea and vomiting. If you suspect an overdose, seek immediate medical attention, and bring the prescription bottle to the hospital with you.

SPECIAL INFORMATION FOR PREGNANT OR NURSING WOMEN

No studies have adequately investigated the effects of oseltamivir during pregnancy or breastfeeding. If you are pregnant or plan to become pregnant, or if you are breastfeeding or plan to do so, talk with your health-care practitioner before starting this drug. Only a health-care practitioner can determine whether the potential benefits outweigh the potential dangers.

SPECIAL INFORMATION FOR SENIORS

Oseltamivir may be less effective in seniors. All older people should get annual flu shots.

GENERIC NAME

Oxacillin *see Penicillin Antibiotics, page 812*

GENERIC NAME

Oxaliplatin

BRAND NAME

Eloxatin
No generic available

ABOUT THIS DRUG

Oxaliplatin is an anticancer drug that is prescribed along with 5-fluorouracil and leucovorin for the treatment of advanced colorectal cancer in adults.

This drug can help shrink tumors, slow the progression of cancer, and help prolong survival in people who have advanced colorectal cancer.

SIDE EFFECTS

Side effects are common. Consult your health-care practitioner if they are persistent or severe. Only he or she can determine whether it is safe for you to continue receiving oxaliplatin treatments.

- *Most Common:* diarrhea, fatigue, nausea, sores in the mouth, pain, tingling or numbness in the fingers or toes, vomiting
- *Less Common:* back pain, cough, dehydration, edema, tightness in base of throat (occurs and passes quickly during infusion or shortly after)
- *Rare:* allergic reaction (closed throat, difficulty breathing, hives, swollen lips, tongue, or face)

IMPORTANT PRECAUTIONS

Tell your health-care practitioner if you are sensitive or allergic to oxaliplatin, platinum (oxaliplatin is a platinum-containing drug), or to any other drugs.

Extreme allergic reactions have been reported and may occur within minutes of receiving oxaliplatin. Your health-care practitioner will need to administer epinephrine, corticosteroids, or antihistamines to alleviate symptoms.

Your health-care practitioner will likely conduct blood tests before each administration of oxaliplatin to monitor blood cell count, as this form of anticancer therapy can cause a decline in red and white blood cell levels, as well as platelets.

As much as possible, avoid contact with people who have an infection. If you think you are getting an infection or if you experience fever, chills, cough, hoarseness, lower back or side pain, persistent diarrhea, persistent vomiting, difficulty breathing, or painful or difficult urination, or if you notice any unusual bleeding or bruising, blood in stools or urine, or pinpoint red spots on your skin, contact your health-care practitioner immediately.

Avoid cold drinks, cold temperatures, and cold objects, such as ice packs. Wear gloves when taking things out of the freezer or refrigerator.

Talk to your health-care practitioner before you have any dental work done while taking oxaliplatin. Be cautious when using a toothbrush, toothpick, or dental floss.

Premedication with antiemetics (antivomiting) drugs is recommended when using oxaliplatin.

DRUG INTERACTIONS

No drug-drug interactions have been documented. However, you should still tell your health-care practitioner and pharmacist if you are taking any prescription or nonprescription drugs, as well as any vitamins, herbs, or other supplements.

FOOD, VITAMIN, AND HERBAL INTERACTIONS
No food, vitamin, or herbal interactions have been noted.

RECOMMENDED DOSE
Oxaliplatin is administered by intravenous (IV) infusion under the supervision of a qualified health-care practitioner experienced in the use of cancer chemotherapy. It is typically given on the first day only of a two-day treatment cycle along with leucovorin, and the cycle is usually repeated every 14 days. Your health-care practitioner will determine the most appropriate dose and schedule for your needs.

SYMPTOMS OF OVERDOSE AND WHAT TO DO
Symptoms of overdose can include any of the following: agitation, black tarry stools, bleeding gums, blood in urine or stool, burning or itching skin, chest pain, confusion, cough or hoarseness, diarrhea, difficult urination, dizziness, fever or chills, incoordination, lack of sensation, lower back or side pain, muscle twitching, paralysis, respiratory failure, seizures, severe weakness, shortness of breath, slow or irregular heartbeat, slurred speech, tremors, and profuse vomiting. If overdose occurs, seek immediate medical attention.

SPECIAL INFORMATION FOR PREGNANT OR NURSING WOMEN
Oxaliplatin can harm the fetus. Use effective contraception to make sure that you do not become pregnant while taking this drug. If you are already pregnant, talk with your health-care practitioner before treatment with oxaliplatin. Only a health-care practitioner can determine whether the potential benefits of treatment outweigh its dangers.

It is not known whether oxaliplatin passes into breast milk. However, your health-care practitioner will likely recommend you switch to bottle feeding if you are treated with this drug.

SPECIAL INFORMATION FOR SENIORS
No special instructions are provided for seniors.

GENERIC NAME

Oxaprozin *see Propionic Acid (NSAID) Family, page 880*

GENERIC NAME
Oxiconazole

BRAND NAME
Oxistat
No generic available

ABOUT THIS DRUG
Oxiconazole is an antifungal agent used for fungal skin infections such as athlete's foot, jock itch, and ringworm of the body (tinea corporis). It is for topical application only. This drug works by killing the fungus or preventing its growth.

SIDE EFFECTS
Consult your health-care practitioner if you develop side effects while using oxiconazole. Only he or she can determine whether it is safe for you to continue using this drug.

- *Common:* itching, burning
- *Less Common or Rare:* rash, inflammation, swelling, irritation, tingling, pain, redness, scaling, eczema, skin eruptions

IMPORTANT PRECAUTIONS
Keep oxiconazole away from your eyes, mouth, and nose. This drug is not for vaginal inflammation. Always tell your health-care practitioner about all other medical conditions you have, and if you have ever experienced an allergic reaction to this or similar medications.

DRUG INTERACTIONS
Although no specific interactions are known, always inform your health-care practitioner and pharmacist if you are taking any other prescription or over-the-counter drugs, as well as any vitamins, herbs, or other supplements.

FOOD, VITAMIN, AND HERBAL INTERACTIONS
No food, vitamin, or herbal interactions have been noted.

RECOMMENDED DOSAGE
Oxiconazole comes in cream and lotion form. The doses given below are typical. However, consult your health-care practitioner for the exact dose and schedule that are most appropriate for you.

- ➤ *Children and Adults:* Apply to affected skin areas once or twice daily for 2 to 4 weeks

If you forget a dose, use it as soon as you remember. If it is almost time for the next dose, skip the forgotten one, and resume your normal schedule. Never take double doses. To cure your infection, continue to take this drug even if you feel well. Do not discontinue use without consulting your health-care practitioner.

SYMPTOMS OF OVERDOSE AND WHAT TO DO
Oxiconazole is for external use only. Accidental ingestion may cause stomach upset. If overdose occurs, seek immediate medical attention and take the prescription container to the hospital with you.

SPECIAL INFORMATION FOR PREGNANT OR NURSING WOMEN
Little oxiconazole is absorbed into the bloodstream. However, if you are pregnant or plan to become pregnant, or if you are breastfeeding or plan to do so, talk with your health-care practitioner before starting this drug. Only a health-care practitioner can determine whether the potential benefits outweigh the potential dangers.

SPECIAL INFORMATION FOR SENIORS
There are no special instructions for seniors.

GENERIC NAME

Oxtriphylline

see Xanthine Bronchodilators, page 1116

GENERIC NAME

Oxybutynin

BRAND NAMES
Ditropan, Oxytrol
Generic available

ABOUT THIS DRUG
Oxybutynin is an antispasmodic drug used to decrease muscle spasms in the bladder and the consequent frequent urge to urinate. It is also prescribed to manage the urgent need to urinate, painful

urination, and urinary leakage. This drug works by controlling the smooth muscle that opens and closes the bladder.

SIDE EFFECTS

Speak to your health-care practitioner if you develop side effects while using oxybutynin. Only he or she can determine whether or not you should continue taking this drug.

- *Common:* decreased sweating, constipation, drowsiness, dry mouth, throat, and nose
- *Less Common or Rare:* difficulty urinating, sleep disturbances, restlessness, dizziness, weakness, impotence, visual disturbances, nausea, palpitations, rapid heart rate, photosensitivity, rash

IMPORTANT PRECAUTIONS

Always tell your health-care practitioner about all other medical conditions you have, especially bleeding, colitis, an ileostomy or colostomy, dry mouth, an enlarged prostate, glaucoma, heart disease, hiatal hernia, high blood pressure, intestinal blockage, myasthenia gravis, an overactive thyroid, pregnancy-related toxemia, and urinary tract problems or blockage. Oxybutynin may make these problems worse. If you have liver or kidney disease, your health-care practitioner will probably prescribe a lower dosage. Also inform your health-care practitioner if you have ever experienced an allergic reaction to this or similar medications.

Oxybutynin may make you sweat less, which can cause your temperature to rise. Be extremely careful when you exercise in hot weather or enter a sauna. Heavy sweating can lead to fever, dizziness, lightheadedness, vomiting, fainting, dehydration, and heat stroke.

This drug may cause side effects such as blurred vision, drowsiness, and dizziness. Until you know how oxybutynin affects you, do not drive a car, operate machinery, or perform other tasks that demand concentration.

Oxybutynin may lead to mouth dryness. To counteract this effect, use sugarless gum or candy, ice chips, or a saliva substitute. If the problem continues, consult your health-care practitioner or dentist.

Oxybutynin may cause increased sensitivity to the sun. Wear protective clothing and apply sunscreen while you take this drug.

DRUG INTERACTIONS

Inform your health-care practitioner and pharmacist if you are taking any other prescription or over-the-counter drugs, as well as any vitamins, herbs, or other supplements. Possible drug interactions include the following:

- Oxybutynin may add to the effects of central nervous system depressants, such as antihistamines, barbiturates, muscle relaxants, narcotics, sedatives, tranquilizers, and sleeping pills. Consult your health-care practitioner before combining these drugs.
- Amantadine and atenolol may increase the effects of oxybutynin.
- Oxybutynin may interfere with digoxin, haloperidol, levodopa, phenothiazine drugs, and nitrofurantoin.
- Avoid alcohol while taking this drug.

FOOD, VITAMIN, AND HERBAL INTERACTIONS

Consult your health-care practitioner before combining oxybutynin with any herbs with sedative effects, such as catnip, elecampane, goldenseal, gotu kola, hops, kava, lemon balm, skullcap, St. John's wort, and valerian.

RECOMMENDED DOSAGE

Oxybutynin comes as a tablet, syrup, and patch. The doses given below are typical. However, consult your health-care practitioner for the exact dose and schedule that are most appropriate for you. A longer-acting form of this drug can also be taken once daily.

- *Children Older than 5 Years:* 5 mg 2 to 3 times a day
- *Adults:* 5 mg 2 to 4 times a day. To use the patch, apply one twice weekly.

Oxybutynin may be taken with or without food. If you forget a dose, take it as soon as you remember. If it is almost time for the next dose, skip the forgotten one, and resume your normal schedule. Never take double doses. When using the patch, always change it on the same two days each week.

SYMPTOMS OF OVERDOSE AND WHAT TO DO

Symptoms of oxybutynin overdose may include dehydration, nausea, vomiting, difficulty breathing, rapid heartbeat, fever, flushing, tremor, hallucinations, delirium, coma, and convulsions. If overdose occurs, seek immediate medical attention and take the prescription container to the hospital with you.

SPECIAL INFORMATION FOR PREGNANT OR NURSING WOMEN

No studies have adequately investigated the effects of oxybutynin during pregnancy or breastfeeding. If you are pregnant or plan to become pregnant, or if you are breastfeeding or plan to do so, talk with your health-care practitioner before starting this drug. Only a health-care practitioner can determine whether the potential benefits outweigh the potential dangers.

SPECIAL INFORMATION FOR SENIORS

Seniors are more susceptible to side effects, and may require lower doses.

GENERIC NAME

Oxycodone hydrochloride

see Acetaminophen plus Narcotic, page 56; Aspirin Combinations, page 149

GENERIC NAME

Oxytetracycline

see Tetracycline Antibiotics, page 1013

GENERIC NAME

Paclitaxel

BRAND NAME

Taxol
No generic available

ABOUT THIS DRUG

Paclitaxel is a neoplastic (anticancer) drug used to treat many forms of cancer, including ovarian, breast, and lung cancer. It may also be prescribed for other types of cancer and for Kaposi's sarcoma associated with acquired immunodeficiency syndrome (AIDS).

This drug works by destroying cancer cells. Unfortunately, at the same time paclitaxel also affects normal cells, accounting for the great number of side effects.

SIDE EFFECTS

Side effects of paclitaxel can be extremely serious, and must be promptly reported to your health-care practitioner. Some effects—such as hair loss (including eyebrows, eyelashes, and pubic hair)—are distressing but pose no physical danger. The most serious effects are due to lowered white blood cell and platelet counts which can result in infection or bleeding. Immediately report signs of infection (fever, chills) or bleeding, such as tarry stools and pinpoint red spots on your skin. Prolonged treatment with paclitaxel can cause nerve damage, resulting in numbness, pain, or decreased sensation in the extremities. These symptoms may improve after the drug is discontinued.

- *Common:* nausea, vomiting, diarrhea, headache, hair loss, lower back or side pain, muscle and joint pain, cough, hoarseness, fever, chills, flushing of face, dizziness, fainting, shortness of breath, increased risk of infection, difficult or painful urination, swelling, fluid retention, rash, itching, numbness and tingling in the hands and feet, liver or kidney damage, changed platelet and white blood cell counts, anemia, fatigue
- *Less Common or Rare:* slow heartbeat, low blood pressure, black, tarry stools, unusual bleeding or bruising, mouth and lip sores, blood in urine or stools, pinpoint red spots on skin, severe shortness of breath, severe skin reactions, severe heart problems

IMPORTANT PRECAUTIONS

Always tell your health-care practitioner about any other medical conditions you may have, especially active infection, chicken pox, heart disease, liver problems, shingles, or immune system diseases. Paclitaxel is prescribed with extreme caution in such cases.

Paclitaxel suppresses the immune system, and may decrease the body's ability to combat infection. Avoid people with infections. If you must go near someone who has received oral polio vaccine, wear a protective face mask.

This drug may cause a number of distressing side effects. Until you know how paclitaxel affects you, do not drive a car, operate machinery, or perform other tasks that require concentration.

Avoid contact sports where bruising and injury might occur. Ask your health-care practitioner how to safely brush your teeth and floss. Before having dental work, tell your dentist that you are having chemotherapy.

People taking any dose of paclitaxel must be closely monitored with regular complete blood counts and other tests.

DRUG INTERACTIONS

Inform your health-care practitioner and pharmacist if you are taking any other prescription or over-the-counter drugs, as well as any vitamins, herbs, or other supplements. Possible drug interactions include the following:

- Do not have live-virus immunizations while taking paclitaxel without your health-care practitioner's approval. You are at risk of infection from the virus.
- Paclitaxel may increase the effects of amphotericin B by injection, antithyroid agents, azathioprine, chloramphenicol, colchicine, flucytosine, ganciclovir, interferon, plicamycin, and zidovudine.
- Many drugs increase the risk of side effects from paclitaxel. These include cyclosporine, dexamethasone, diazepam, estradiol, ketoconazole, quinidine, testosterone, and verapamil.
- Do not drink alcohol while taking paclitaxel. This increases the possibility of undesirable effects on the bone marrow and liver.

FOOD, VITAMIN, AND HERBAL INTERACTIONS

Do not take paclitaxel with supplements such as echinacea.

RECOMMENDED DOSAGE

Paclitaxel is available by injection and is administered in a health-care facility. Dosage is highly individualized and must be determined by your health-care practitioner.

SYMPTOMS OF OVERDOSE AND WHAT TO DO

High doses of paclitaxel over a prolonged period of time may cause fatigue, numbness or tingling in the extremities, weakness, and increased inflammation of the mucous membranes. If you suspect that an overdose has occurred, seek immediate medical attention.

SPECIAL INFORMATION FOR PREGNANT OR NURSING WOMEN

Do not take this drug if you are pregnant or think you may be pregnant. Paclitaxel may cause birth defects or miscarriage. Because of the possibility of serious side effects, breastfeeding is not recommended while you take this drug.

SPECIAL INFORMATION FOR SENIORS

There are no special instructions for seniors.

GENERIC NAME

Pantoprazole

BRAND NAME

Protonix
No generic available

ABOUT THIS DRUG

Pantoprazole is prescribed for the short-term treatment (eight weeks) of erosion or sores in the esophagus, which may be caused by gastroesophageal reflux disease (GERD) and Zollinger-Ellison syndrome.

This medication inhibits the secretion of gastric acid.

SIDE EFFECTS

Be sure to tell your health-care practitioner if you experience any side effects while taking pantoprazole. Only your health-care practitioner can determine whether it is safe for you to continue taking this drug.

- *Most Common:* constipation, diarrhea, headache, insomnia, nausea, rash, vomiting
- *Rare:* abnormal heartbeat, allergic reaction (closing of throat, difficulty breathing, hives, swelling of lips, mouth, or face), dizziness, leg cramps, muscle pain, nervousness, water retention

IMPORTANT PRECAUTIONS

Tell your health-care practitioner if you are sensitive or allergic to pantoprazole or to any other drugs.

Tell your health-care practitioner if you have liver disease, as you may need an adjustment to your dosage of pantoprazole.

An improvement in symptoms in response to pantoprazole does not mean you do not have other gastric conditions. Because erosive esophagitis is a chronic condition, you may need prolonged treatment. In long-term studies of rats given pantoprazole, the drug caused rare types of gastrointestinal tumors, but the relevance of these findings to humans is not known.

Long-term treatment with pantoprazole may result in decreased absorption of cyanocobalamin (vitamin B_{12}).

Do not crush, chew, or split the tablets; they are slow-release formulations and designed to be taken whole.

DRUG INTERACTIONS

Tell your health-care practitioner and pharmacist if you are taking any prescription or nonprescription drugs, as well as any vitamins, herbs, or other supplements. Possible drug interactions include the following:

- Taking digoxin with pantoprazole may increase digoxin toxicity.
- Effectiveness of ketoconazole and other drugs where acid in the stomach is important for absorption may be reduced when taken with pantoprazole.

FOOD, VITAMIN, AND HERBAL INTERACTIONS

Do not use ginger or yarrow when taking pantoprazole, as they interfere with the drug's effectiveness.

RECOMMENDED DOSAGE

Pantoprazole is available in 20- and 40-mg tablets. The dosages given here are typical. However, your health-care practitioner will determine the most appropriate dose and schedule for your needs.

- *Children:* This drug is not recommended for children.
- *Adults:* 40 mg once a day for 4 to 8 weeks

Pantoprazole tablets are slow-release and so should not be chewed, crushed, or split. Take this drug with 8 ounces of water.

If you miss a dose, take it as soon as you remember. If it is nearly time for your next dose, do not take the missed dose. Continue with your regular dosing schedule. Never take a double dose.

SYMPTOMS OF OVERDOSE AND WHAT TO DO

Symptoms of overdose are not known. If overdose occurs, seek immediate medical attention and bring the prescription container with you to the hospital.

SPECIAL INFORMATION FOR PREGNANT OR NURSING WOMEN

No adequate studies of the effects of pantoprazole on pregnant or nursing women have been done. If you are pregnant or plan to become pregnant, talk to your health-care practitioner.

Pantoprazole has been detected in breast milk in a single nursing mother. If you are breastfeeding, your health-care practitioner may advise you to stop until treatment is complete.

SPECIAL INFORMATION FOR SENIORS

No special precautions have been noted for older adults.

GENERIC NAME

Paroxetine

BRAND NAMES

Paxil, Paxil CR

No generic available

ABOUT THIS DRUG

Paroxetine is used to treat mental depression. This is more than a simple case of the blues. The symptoms of depression include sleep and appetite changes, sadness, guilt, shame, low self-esteem, anxiety, and extreme fatigue that last for over two weeks. Paroxetine is also used to treat social anxiety, panic, generalized anxiety, and panic disorder.

Paroxetine is a type of drug known as a selective serotonin reuptake inhibitor (SSRI). It works by making more serotonin available in the brain.

SIDE EFFECTS

Inform your health-care practitioner if you develop side effects while taking paroxetine. If symptoms are severe or prolonged, ask your health-care practitioner whether your dosage requires adjustment, and whether it is safe for you to continue taking this drug. Side effects generally become less troublesome after 4 to 6 weeks of treatment.

- *Common:* drowsiness, dizziness, weakness, decreased appetite, dry mouth, nausea, diarrhea, constipation, gas, nervousness, male genital disorders
- *Less Common or Rare:* agitation, blurred vision, drugged feeling, pounding heartbeat, decreased sex drive, increased appetite, muscle tenderness or weakness, upset stomach, vomiting, yawning, twitching, tightness in throat, altered sense of taste, burning or tingling sensation, urinary disorders, rash

IMPORTANT PRECAUTIONS

Always inform your health-care practitioner about any other medical conditions you may have, especially a history of convulsions or seizures, kidney or liver impairment, dehydration, a problem with metabolism or blood circulation, or mania (a type of mental illness). Tell your health-care practitioner if you have ever experienced an allergic reaction to this or similar drugs.

If you plan to undergo surgery or a dental procedure, tell your health-care practitioner or dentist that you are taking paroxetine.

This drug can make you dizzy and less alert than usual. Until you know how paroxetine affects you, do not drive a car, operate machinery, or perform other tasks that require concentration.

If this drug causes mouth dryness, use sugarless gum or candy, ice chips, or artificial saliva. If the problem continues, consult your health-care practitioner or dentist.

Paroxetine may cause excessive sweating. If you work or exercise in hot weather, drink plenty of fluids to prevent dehydration.

DRUG INTERACTIONS

Tell your health-care practitioner and pharmacist if you are taking any other prescription or over-the-counter drugs, as well as any vitamins, herbs, or other supplements. Possible drug interactions include the following:

- Do not take monoamine oxidase inhibitor (MAOI) antidepressants at the same time as or within 14 days of paroxetine. This combination can cause potentially fatal serotonin syndrome.
- Other drugs that may lead to serotonin syndrome include dextromethorphan (an ingredient in many over-the-counter cough suppressants), fenfluramine, sibutramine, and venlafaxine.
- Taking other central nervous system depressants along with paroxetine can result in more drowsiness.
- Combining paroxetine with drugs such as ritonavir can result in paroxetine toxicity.
- Taking paroxetine with warfarin may result in increased bleeding.
- Cimetidine may increase the effects of paroxetine.
- The combination of lithium and paroxetine may cause increased adverse effects.
- Quinidine may increase the effects of paroxetine.
- Phenobarbital decreases the effects of paroxetine.
- Do not drink alcohol while taking paroxetine.

FOOD, VITAMIN, AND HERBAL INTERACTIONS

Do not combine paroxetine with herbs such as hops, kava, passionflower, and valerian. These can increase effects such as drowsiness. Do not take St. John's wort with paroxetine, since both affect serotonin. Other inappropriate herbs include ginseng, ephedra (ma huang), and yohimbe.

RECOMMENDED DOSAGE

Paroxetine comes as a capsule or an oral suspension. Although the doses given below are typical, only your health-care practitioner can determine the dose and schedule that best fit your needs.

- *Children:* This drug is not recommended for children.
- *Adults:* 20 mg daily to start, which may be gradually increased as needed to a maximum daily dose of 50 mg; the controlled-release

form dosage of Paxil CR is 25 mg to start, which may be gradually increased to a maximum daily dose of 62.5 mg

Paroxetine can be taken with or without food. It must be taken regularly for several weeks before its full effect is felt. If you forget a dose, take it as soon as you remember. If it is almost time for the next dose, skip the missed one and resume your normal schedule. Never take a double dose. Do not stop taking this drug suddenly, especially if you have been taking it a long time. Your health-care practitioner will gradually reduce your dosage.

SYMPTOMS OF OVERDOSE AND WHAT TO DO

The symptoms of paroxetine overdose include dizziness, confusion, sweating, drowsiness, nausea, vomiting, facial flushing, and tremor. If overdose occurs, seek immediate medical attention and take the prescription bottle to the hospital with you.

SPECIAL INFORMATION FOR PREGNANT OR NURSING WOMEN

No studies have adequately investigated the effects of paroxetine during pregnancy or breastfeeding. If you are pregnant or plan to become pregnant, or if you are breastfeeding or plan to do so, talk with your health-care practitioner before starting this drug. Only a health-care practitioner can determine whether the potential benefits outweigh the potential dangers.

SPECIAL INFORMATION FOR SENIORS

Seniors are at higher risk of side effects, and usually require smaller doses.

OPEN QUESTIONS OR CONTROVERSIES

In June 2004, the Food and Drug Administration asked manufacturers of paroxetine to include in their labeling a warning statement that recommends close observation of adult and pediatric patients for clinical worsening of depression or the emergence of suicidality when being treated with this drug, especially when beginning the drug, or at the time of dose changes, either increases or decreases.

GENERIC NAME
Pemoline

BRAND NAME
Cylert
Generic available

ABOUT THIS DRUG
Pemoline is used for the treatment of attention-deficit hyperactivity disorder (ADHD) in children.

Pemoline stimulates the brain stem, which leads to improved alertness, attention span, and concentration. This drug causes an increase in the levels of serotonin and dopamine (nerve transmitters) in the brain, which helps restore the balance between serotonin and other brain chemicals involved in behavior, mood, and thought.

SIDE EFFECTS
Contact your health-care practitioner if you develop side effects while taking this drug. Only he or she can determine if you should continue to take pemoline.

- *Common:* insomnia
- *Less Common or Rare:* appetite loss, stomach pain, nausea, dizziness, chest pain, abnormal heart rhythms, changes in blood pressure or pulse, fever, arthritis-like symptoms, headache, drowsiness, hair loss, itching, rash, severe jerking or twitching, visual disturbances such as blurred vision, severe psychotic reactions

IMPORTANT PRECAUTIONS
Tell your health-care practitioner if you are allergic to pemoline or similar drugs. Also inform your health-care practitioner about any other medical conditions you suffer from, especially liver or kidney disease, severe anxiety, tension, agitation, glaucoma or other visual problems, high blood pressure, motor tics or spasms, Tourette's syndrome, or a seizure disorder.

Chronic or abusive use of pemoline can lead to addiction. This drug should be used with caution in anyone with a history of drug or alcohol abuse or of mental illness.

Before having any type of surgery or dental procedure, inform your surgeon or dentist that you are taking pemoline.

This drug may conceal signs of temporary fatigue. Until you know how pemoline affects you, do not operate machinery or perform other tasks that require concentration.

Pemoline is not an appropriate remedy for children whose symptoms are caused by stress or a psychiatric disorder.

DRUG INTERACTIONS

Inform your health-care practitioner and pharmacist if you are taking any prescription or over-the-counter drugs, as well as any vitamins, herbs, or other supplements. Possible drug interactions include the following:

- Pemoline may increase the effects of other nervous system stimulants, leading to nervousness, insomnia, and irritability.
- When taking pemoline, the dosage of anticonvulsants may need to be increased.

FOOD, VITAMIN, AND HERBAL INTERACTIONS

Avoid foods that are rich in the amino acid tyramine while taking pemoline. This combination may result in an excessive rise in blood pressure. Tyramine-rich foods include (but are not limited to) aged cheeses, bologna, chicken liver, chocolate, figs, pickled herring, pepperoni, raisins, salami, soy sauce, and yeast extracts. Also avoid beverages that contain meat or meat tenderizers, and alcoholic beverages that may contain tyramine, which include some beers, vermouth, and Chianti wines.

Herbs that affect the central nervous system—including St. John's wort, guarana, ephedra (ma huang), and kola—should be avoided when taking pemoline.

Avoid caffeinated beverages, such as tea or cola.

RECOMMENDED DOSAGE

Pemoline is available in tablet form. Although the doses given below are typical, only your health-care practitioner can determine the dose and schedule that are most appropriate for you.

- *Children 6 Years and Older:* 37.5 mg daily to start, which may be gradually increased as needed to a maximum daily dosage of 112.5 mg
- *Adults:* This drug is not generally recommended for adults.

Pemoline is taken once daily, in the morning. If it causes stomach upset, it can be taken with food. Do not take pemoline late in the day, as it may cause sleeplessness. Never take two doses at once.

Pemoline must be taken regularly for several weeks before its full effect is felt. Continue to take this drug even if you feel well. Do not discontinue use without consulting your health-care practitioner, especially if you have been taking large doses for a long time. To end treatment, your health-care practitioner will reduce dosage gradually.

SYMPTOMS OF OVERDOSE AND WHAT TO DO

The symptoms of pemoline overdose include agitation, confusion, delirium, elevated blood pressure and body temperature, enlarged pupils, euphoria, flushing, hallucinations, headache, muscle twitching, rapid or irregular heartbeat, tremors, vomiting, convulsions, and coma. If overdose occurs, seek immediate medical attention and bring the prescription bottle to the hospital with you.

SPECIAL INFORMATION FOR PREGNANT OR NURSING WOMEN

This drug is recommended primarily for children. No studies have adequately investigated the effects of pemoline during pregnancy or breastfeeding.

SPECIAL INFORMATION FOR SENIORS

This drug is recommended primarily for children.

GENERIC NAME

Penbutolol

BRAND NAME

Levatol
No generic available

ABOUT THIS DRUG

Penbutolol is a beta-adrenergic blocking agent (beta-blocker) prescribed to treat mild-to-moderate high blood pressure (hypertension). It is also used to limit the damage caused by heart attacks, and to reduce attacks of angina (chest pain).

This drug works by interfering with nerve impulses that increase heart rate and contractions, thus lowering blood pressure. Penbutolol causes less slowing of the heart rate than many other beta-blockers.

SIDE EFFECTS

Speak to your health-care practitioner if you develop side effects while taking this drug. Only he or she can determine whether it is safe for you to continue taking penbutolol.

- *Common:* fatigue, lethargy, lightheadedness, slow heart rate, cold hands and feet
- *Less Common or Rare:* dizziness, headache, nausea, upset stomach, indigestion, vomiting, diarrhea, constipation, muscle and joint pain, rash, hair loss, bronchial spasm, disorientation, confusion, anxiety, depression, short-term memory loss, insomnia, vivid dreams, hallucinations, carpal tunnel syndrome, impotence, chest pain, shortness of breath, heart failure

IMPORTANT PRECAUTIONS

Always inform your health-care practitioner about any other medical conditions you suffer from, especially a slow heart rate or serious heart block, congestive heart failure, angina, abnormal growth of the left side of the heart, asthma or other lung ailments, a history of allergies, liver or kidney problems, diabetes or hypoglycemia, or a thyroid condition. Tell your health-care practitioner if you have ever experienced an allergic reaction to penbutolol or other beta-blocker.

Before having any type of surgery or dental procedure, inform your surgeon or dentist that you are taking penbutolol.

This drug may make you more sensitive to the cold. Beta-blockers including penbutolol can decrease blood circulation in the fingers, toes, and skin. Be sure to dress warmly in low temperatures, especially if you already have blood circulation problems.

This drug may cause side effects such as lightheadedness and dizziness. Until you know how penbutolol affects you, do not drive a car, operate machinery, or perform other tasks that demand concentration.

Some beta-blockers cause dizziness or faintness when you rise quickly from a sitting or reclining position (postural hypotension). When you first start taking this drug or when the dosage is increased, try to get up slowly, and consult your health-care practitioner if the problem continues.

Treatment of high blood pressure also entails certain lifestyle changes, such as weight control, smoking cessation, and close attention to diet.

Be extremely careful when you exercise in hot weather. Heavy sweating can lead to dizziness, lightheadedness, fainting, vomiting, dehydration, and low blood pressure.

DRUG INTERACTIONS

Tell your health-care practitioner and pharmacist if you are taking any other prescription or over-the-counter drugs, as well as any vita-

mins, herbs, or other supplements. Possible drug interactions include the following:

- Drugs that contain aspirin can lessen the blood pressure lowering effects of penbutolol.
- Taking other blood pressure medications (including clonidine, reserpine, and calcium channel blockers) can increase the effects of penbutolol.
- Medications such as birth control pills, methimazole, propylthiouracil, and ritonavir may increase the effects of labetalol.
- Penbutolol can interfere with the action of oral antidiabetes medications. It may also change blood glucose levels.
- Penbutolol may interfere with the effectiveness of epinephrine.
- Taking penbutolol with fluvoxamine or fluoxetine may cause a slow heartbeat and excessive lowering of blood pressure.
- Do not combine penbutolol with amiodarone.
- Taking penbutolol with digoxin increases the risk of heart problems.
- Alcohol intensifies the drowsiness caused by this drug.
- Consult your health-care practitioner before taking over-the-counter nasal decongestant, cough, cold, allergy, and weight loss remedies. Many of these can raise blood pressure.

FOOD, VITAMIN, AND HERBAL INTERACTIONS

Do not take herbs that increase blood pressure, including ephedra (ma huang), ginseng, goldenseal, licorice, and saw palmetto. Consult your health-care practitioner before taking substances that may lower blood pressure, such as calcium, soy, or garlic. Your health-care practitioner will probably recommend a low-sodium diet.

RECOMMENDED DOSAGE

Penbutolol comes in tablet form. Although the doses given below are typical, only your health-care practitioner can determine the dose and schedule that are most appropriate for you.

- *Children:* This drug is not recommended for children.
- *Adults:* 20 mg to start, which may be gradually increased as needed to a maximum of 80 mg daily

Penbutolol may be taken with or without food. If you forget to take a dose, take it as soon as you remember. If it is almost time for the next dose, skip the forgotten one, and resume your normal schedule. Never take double doses.

Continue to take this drug even if you feel well. Do not abruptly discontinue use without consulting your health-care practitioner. To end treatment, your health-care practitioner will reduce your dosage gradually.

SYMPTOMS OF OVERDOSE AND WHAT TO DO

The symptoms of penbutolol overdose include slow pulse, low blood pressure, weakness, fainting, congestive heart failure, coma, and seizures. If overdose occurs, seek immediate medical attention and take the prescription bottle to the hospital with you so the health-care practitioner will know what medication was taken.

SPECIAL INFORMATION FOR PREGNANT OR NURSING WOMEN

Some studies have shown that women who take beta-blockers during pregnancy give birth to babies with lower birth weight, heart rate, and blood pressure. As a result, penbutolol should be avoided if you are pregnant.

Small amounts of beta-blockers may pass into breast milk and cause problems such as slow heart rate, low blood pressure, and trouble breathing. If you must take this drug, your health-care practitioner may recommend bottle-feeding.

SPECIAL INFORMATION FOR SENIORS

Seniors require lower doses of penbutolol, and frequent blood pressure checks are needed to prevent excessive lowering of blood pressure. Be on the alert for problems such as unsteadiness, falls, dizziness, confusion, depression, and hallucinations.

GENERIC NAME

Penciclovir

BRAND NAME

Denavir

No generic available

ABOUT THIS DRUG

Penciclovir is an antiviral drug prescribed for cold sores. In order to be effective, this drug must be applied at the very first sign of a cold sore. Although it does not cure these lesions, it may lessen their pain and duration. Penciclovir works by blocking the formation, multiplication, and spread of the herpes simplex virus that causes cold sores.

SIDE EFFECTS

Side effects are generally mild. However, consult your health-care practitioner if they become persistent or severe.

- *Common:* swelling, redness
- *Less Common or Rare:* headache, numbness, skin reaction, change in sense of taste

IMPORTANT PRECAUTIONS

Keep penciclovir away from your eyes and other body areas. Before using this drug, tell your health-care practitioner about any other medical conditions you have, and whether you have ever experienced an allergic reaction to this or similar drugs.

DRUG INTERACTIONS

Although no specific interactions are associated with penciclovir, always inform your health-care practitioner and pharmacist if you are taking any other prescription or over-the-counter drugs, as well as any vitamins, herbs, or other supplements.

FOOD, VITAMIN, AND HERBAL INTERACTIONS

Do not take echinacea while using this drug.

RECOMMENDED DOSAGE

Penciclovir comes as an ointment or cream. Although the doses given below are typical, only your health-care practitioner can determine the dose and schedule that are most appropriate for you.

- *Children:* This drug is not recommended for children.
- *Adults:* Apply to all infected areas every 2 hours while awake for 4 consecutive days.

Treatment must begin at the first sign of infection. If you forget to apply a dose, do so as soon as you remember. If it is almost time for the next dose, skip the forgotten one, and resume your normal schedule. Never apply double doses.

SYMPTOMS OF OVERDOSE AND WHAT TO DO

Overdose is unlikely. However, if you suspect that an overdose has occurred, seek immediate medical attention and take the penciclovir container to the hospital with you.

SPECIAL INFORMATION FOR PREGNANT OR NURSING WOMEN

No studies have adequately investigated the effects of penciclovir during pregnancy or breastfeeding. If you are pregnant or plan to become pregnant, or if you are breastfeeding or plan to do so, talk with your health-care practitioner before starting this drug. Only a health-care practitioner can determine whether the potential benefits outweigh the potential dangers.

SPECIAL INFORMATION FOR SENIORS

Dosage must be adjusted for seniors with kidney damage.

GENERIC NAME

Class: Penicillin antibiotics

Generics: (1) amoxicillin; (2) ampicillin; (3) bacampicillin; (4) carbenicillin indanyl sodium; (5) cloxacillin; (6) dicloxacillin sodium; (7) nafcillin; (8) oxacillin; (9) penicillin V

BRAND NAMES

(1) Amoxil, Trimox, Wymox; also available in combination with potassium clavulanate as Augmentin; (2) Marcillin, Omnipen, Principen, Totacillin; (3) Spectrobid; (4) Geocillin; (5) Cloxapen; (6) Dycill, Dynapen, Pathocil; (7) Unipen; (8) Bactocill; (9) Beepen-VK, Betapen-VK, Ledercillin VK, Penicillin VK, Pen-Vee K, V-Cillin K, Veetids

All available as generic except carbenicillin and nafcillin

ABOUT THIS DRUG

Penicillin antibiotics are used to treat a wide variety of infections, including those that affect the ears, sinuses, throat, respiratory tract, heart, and genitourinary tract. These drugs are prescribed for problems such as middle ear infections, sinusitis, strep throat, pneumonia, ulcers, Lyme disease, dental abscesses, scarlet fever, gonorrhea, and syphilis.

Penicillin antibiotics kill invading bacteria by destroying their cell walls. These drugs are not effective against other types of microorganisms, such as viruses, fungi, and parasites. Antibiotics should not be prescribed for colds or flu. Numerous bacteria are also resistant to penicillin antibiotics.

SIDE EFFECTS

Consult your health-care practitioner if you develop side effects while taking one of these drugs. Only he or she can determine whether it is safe for you to continue taking a penicillin antibiotic.

- *Common:* diarrhea, upset stomach, nausea, vomiting, abdominal pain, colitis, sore mouth, coated tongue, vaginal irritation, oral or rectal fungal infection
- *Less Common or Rare:* superinfection, itchy eyes, appetite loss, yellow eyes and skin, bleeding abnormalities, anemia, black tongue, severe skin reactions, abnormal lowering of white blood cells

Serious and potentially fatal allergic reactions may occur in one in ten people who take a penicillin antibiotic. Stop taking medication and contact your health-care practitioner immediately if you develop symptoms such as difficulty breathing, rash, itching, swelling, low blood pressure, chills, fever, abnormal bleeding or bruising, and a general feeling of unwellness.

IMPORTANT PRECAUTIONS

Tell your health-care practitioner if you have ever experienced an allergic reaction to a penicillin or cephalosporin antibiotic. If so, he or she will most likely prescribe a different antibiotic for you. If you are allergic to penicillin antibiotics, you may also be allergic to cephalosporins.

Always inform your health-care practitioner about any other medical conditions you suffer from, especially kidney or liver disease, allergies, asthma, colitis, stomach problems, cystic fibrosis, or blood disease.

If you are using oral contraceptives, practice other means of contraception while taking penicillin antibiotics.

Ampicillin may cause increased sensitivity to the sun. Wear protective clothing and apply sunscreen while taking this drug.

DRUG INTERACTIONS

Check first with your health-care practitioner before taking any other medication with a penicillin antibiotic. To avoid unwanted side effects, tell your health-care practitioner and pharmacist about all other prescription or over-the-counter drugs, vitamins, herbs, or other supplements that you are taking. Possible drug interactions include the following:

- Penicillin antibiotics may decrease the effects of oral contraceptives.

- A number of drugs may decrease the effects of penicillin antibiotics. These include antacids, chloramphenicol, erythromycin, neomycin, and tetracyclines.
- Beta-blockers may increase the risk of penicillin reactions.
- Taking ampicillin with atenolol may decrease the effects of atenolol.
- Combining ampicillin with allopurinol may increase the risk of rashes.
- Do not combine bacampicillin with disulfiram.
- Other drugs that may interact with penicillins include cyclosporine, methotrexate, NSAIDs, probenecid, sulfa drugs, and warfarin.

FOOD, VITAMIN, AND HERBAL INTERACTIONS

When taking penicillin antibiotics, you also destroy friendly bacteria such as *Lactobacillus acidophilus* that normally reside in the intestine. This can result in yeast infections. To prevent this problem, eat yogurt with live cultures or take *Lactobacillus acidophilus* supplements.

Do not take penicillin antibiotics with carbonated beverages or fruit juice. In order to prevent any vitamin deficiencies, it may also be beneficial to take a daily multivitamin.

RECOMMENDED DOSAGE

Penicillin antibiotics are available in a wide variety of forms, including tablets, capsules, and oral suspension. Take only the exact type, brand, and strength of medication prescribed by your health-care practitioner. Different forms are not interchangeable. The doses given below are average. However, doses vary from person to person, and according to the condition being treated. Only your health-care practitioner can determine the dose and schedule that are most appropriate for you.

Amoxicillin

- *Children:* 10 to 20 mg per pound daily, in 3 divided doses
- *Adults:* 250 to 500 mg every 8 hours

Amoxicillin/Clavulanate

- *Children:* 10 to 20 mg per pound daily, in 3 divided doses
- *Adults:* 250 mg every 8 hours; or 500 to 875 mg every 12 hours

Ampicillin

- *Children:* 25 to 100 mg per pound daily, in 4 to 6 doses
- *Adults:* 250 to 1,000 mg every 6 hours

Bacampicillin

- *Children:* 12 to 25 mg per pound daily, divided into 2 doses
- *Adults:* 400 to 800 mg every 12 hours

Carbenicillin Indanyl Sodium

- *Children:* This drug is not recommended for children.
- *Adults:* 380 to 760 mg every 6 hours

Cloxacillin Sodium

- *Children:* 25 mg per pound daily, divided into 4 doses
- *Adults:* 250 to 500 mg every 6 hours

Dicloxacillin

- *Children:* 6 to 12 mg per pound daily, divided into 4 doses
- *Adults:* 125 to 250 mg every 6 hours

Nafcillin

- *Children:* 5 to 25 mg per pound daily, every 6 to 8 hours
- *Adults:* 250 to 1,000 mg every 4 to 6 hours

Oxacillin

- *Children:* 25 to 50 mg per pound daily, in 4 to 6 doses
- *Adults:* 500 to 1,000 mg every 4 to 6 hours

Penicillin V

- *Children:* 12 to 25 mg per pound daily, in 3 or 4 doses
- *Adults:* 125 to 500 mg every 6 to 8 hours

Most penicillin antibiotics are best absorbed on an empty stomach. However, if an antibiotic upsets your stomach, ask your health-care practitioner about taking it with food. If you miss a dose, take it as soon as you remember. If it is nearly time for your next scheduled dose, do not take the missed dose. Follow your regular dosing schedule. Never take a double dose.

It is essential to take penicillin antibiotics exactly as prescribed. In order to receive their full benefits, continue to take antibiotics for the full number of days prescribed. Failing to do so can result in even more serious and drug-resistant infection.

SYMPTOMS OF OVERDOSE AND WHAT TO DO

Symptoms of overdose may include diarrhea and stomach upset. If you suspect overdose, seek medical attention immediately, and bring the prescription bottle with you to the hospital so that health-care practitioners will know exactly what drug was taken.

SPECIAL INFORMATION FOR PREGNANT OR NURSING WOMEN

Penicillin antibiotics are generally considered safe to use during pregnancy. However, if you are pregnant or plan to become pregnant, consult with your health-care practitioner before taking these medications. Only a health-care practitioner can determine whether the potential benefits outweigh the potential dangers. Because penicillin antibiotics may pass into breast milk, your health-care practitioner may advise you to stop breastfeeding while you take these drugs.

SPECIAL INFORMATION FOR SENIORS

There are no special instructions for seniors.

GENERIC NAME

Pentazocine

see Aspirin Combinations, page 149

GENERIC NAME

Pentosan polysulfate sodium

BRAND NAME

Elmiron

No generic available

ABOUT THIS DRUG

Pentosan polysulfate sodium is prescribed to relieve bladder pain or discomfort due to interstitial cystitis. This is a long-term, painful bladder infection. It may be necessary to take pentosan for 3 to 6 months before you feel better.

This drug works by preventing irritating substances from reaching bladder cells. Pentosan may relieve symptoms, but it does not cure interstitial cystitis.

SIDE EFFECTS

Inform your health-care practitioner if you develop side effects while taking pentosan. If symptoms are severe or prolonged, ask your health-care practitioner whether your dosage requires adjustment, and whether it is safe for you to continue taking this drug.

- *Common:* patchy hair loss, nausea, diarrhea, stomach upset, abdominal pain, headache, dizziness, depression, emotional upset
- *Less Common or Rare:* bleeding gums, black and blue marks, nosebleeds, constipation, difficulty swallowing, dry throat, heartburn, increased sensitivity to sunlight, red eyes, itching, appetite loss, ringing in the ears, runny nose, mouth sores, gas

IMPORTANT PRECAUTIONS

Always inform your health-care practitioner about any other medical conditions you may have, especially blood or blood vessel disease, intestinal blockage, polyps, or ulcers. Pentosan may increase the risk of bleeding.

If you have liver or spleen problems, you may be at a higher risk of side effects.

Because pentosan has anticoagulant effects, you may experience side effects such as nosebleeds and black and blue marks while taking this drug.

If you plan to undergo surgery or a dental procedure, tell your health-care practitioner or dentist that you are taking pentosan.

DRUG INTERACTIONS

Tell your health-care practitioner and pharmacist if you are taking any other prescription or over-the-counter drugs, as well as any vitamins, herbs, or other supplements. Pentosan may interact with the folllowing drugs:

- Exercise caution when combining pentosan with drugs such as aspirin, heparin, alteplase, streptokinase, and warfarin. This may increase the risk of bleeding.

FOOD, VITAMIN, AND HERBAL INTERACTIONS

Follow any special dietary instructions recommended by your health-care practitioner or nutritionist. Certain foods and beverages may aggravate your condition.

RECOMMENDED DOSAGE

Pentosan comes as a capsule. Although the doses given below are typical, only your health-care practitioner can determine the dose and schedule that best fit your needs.

- ➤ *Children:* This drug is not recommended for children.
- ➤ *Adults:* 100 mg 3 times a day

Pentosan should be taken 1 hour before or 2 hours after meals. Take this medication with a full glass (8 ounces) of water. If you forget a dose, take it as soon as you remember. If it is almost time for the next dose, skip the missed one and resume your normal schedule. Never take a double dose.

SYMPTOMS OF OVERDOSE AND WHAT TO DO

The symptoms of pentosan overdose may include bleeding, upset stomach, and liver problems. If overdose occurs, seek immediate medical attention and take the prescription bottle to the hospital with you.

SPECIAL INFORMATION FOR PREGNANT OR NURSING WOMEN

No studies have adequately investigated the effects of pentosan during pregnancy or breastfeeding. If you are pregnant or plan to become pregnant, or if you are breastfeeding or plan to do so, talk with your health-care practitioner before starting this drug. Only a health-care practitioner can determine whether the potential benefits outweigh the potential dangers.

SPECIAL INFORMATION FOR SENIORS

There are no special instructions for seniors.

GENERIC NAME

Pergolide

BRAND NAME

Permax

No generic available

ABOUT THIS DRUG

Pergolide is used to treat Parkinson's disease. It is often combined with levodopa or carbidopa. Like these drugs, pergolide works by correcting the dopamine deficiency that is believed to be the cause of Parkinson's disease. It stimulates a nerve ending in the central nervous system that is normally stimulated by dopamine.

SIDE EFFECTS

Side effects from pergolide are common. Call your health-care practitioner if symptoms become severe or do not go away. Contact your health-care practitioner immediately if you experience alarming side effects such as hallucinations, chest pain, low blood pressure, dizziness, fainting, uncontrolled body movements, difficulty breathing, or severe headache. Only your health-care practitioner can determine if you should continue to take this drug.

- *Common:* hallucinations, nausea, upset stomach, diarrhea, constipation, confusion, fatigue, difficulty sleeping, twisting body movements
- *Less Common or Rare:* loss of appetite, heartburn, rash, dry mouth, hiccups, dizziness, restlessness, muscle twitching, tremor, weakness, numbness, blurred or double vision, difficulty urinating, changes in mental state, sleepiness, decreased alertness, anxiety, depression, psychosis, body aches and pains, infection, swelling of the hands and feet, painful menstruation, buzzing or ringing in the ears, deafness, dizziness upon rising, changes in blood pressure and heart rhythm, heart failure, thyroid tumor, diabetes, loss of bowel control, colitis, muscular rigidity or stiffness

IMPORTANT PRECAUTIONS

Always inform your health-care practitioner of any other medical conditions you have, especially abnormal heart rhythms, a history of confusion, or difficulty with movement (dyskinesia).

Because pergolide may cause side effects such as dizziness and fatigue, do not drive a car, operate machinery, or perform other tasks that require concentration until you know how this drug affects you.

Pergolide may cause dizziness or faintness when you rise quickly from a sitting or reclining position (postural hypotension). When you first start taking this drug or when the dosage is increased, try to get up slowly, and consult your health-care practitioner if the problem continues.

Pergolide may cause mouth dryness. To counteract this effect, use sugarless gum or candy, ice chips, or a saliva substitute. If the problem continues, consult your health-care practitioner or dentist.

DRUG INTERACTIONS

Tell your health-care practitioner and pharmacist if you are taking any other prescription or over-the-counter drugs, as well as any vitamins, herbs, or other supplements. Possible drug interactions include the following:

- Pergolide may interact with high blood pressure medications by further reducing pressure.
- Alcohol, tranquilizers, antidepressants, and other central nervous system depressants may increase the effects of pergolide.
- Many drugs decrease the effects of pergolide. These include droperidol, haloperidol, phenothiazines, thioxanthenes, loxapine, metoclopramide, methyldopa, molindone, papaverine, and reserpine.

FOOD, VITAMIN, AND HERBAL INTERACTIONS

Consult your health-care practitioner before combining pergolide with any herbs with sedative effects, such as catnip, elecampane, goldenseal, gotu kola, hops, kava, lemon balm, skullcap, St. John's wort, and valerian.

RECOMMENDED DOSAGE

Pergolide is available in tablet form. Although the doses given below are typical, only your health-care practitioner can determine the dose and schedule that are most appropriate for you.

- *Children:* This drug is not recommended for children.
- *Adults:* 0.5 to 5 mg daily

To prevent stomach upset, take pergolide with food. If you miss a dose, take it as soon as you remember. However, if it is almost time for the next dose, skip the one you missed and go back to your regular dosing schedule. Never take a double dose. Do not stop taking pergolide suddenly. This may cause severe Parkinson's symptoms to return.

SYMPTOMS OF OVERDOSE AND WHAT TO DO

Symptoms of pergolide overdose may include nausea, vomiting, muscle twitching, involuntary movements, agitation, hallucinations, heart palpitations, and low blood pressure. If overdose does occur, seek medical attention immediately, and bring the prescription bottle with you to the hospital so that health-care practitioners will know exactly what drug was used.

SPECIAL INFORMATION FOR PREGNANT OR NURSING WOMEN

No studies have adequately investigated the effects of pergolide during pregnancy or breastfeeding. If you are pregnant or plan to become pregnant, or if you are breastfeeding or plan to do so, talk with your health-care practitioner before starting this drug. Only a health-care practitioner can determine whether the potential benefits outweigh the potential dangers.

SPECIAL INFORMATION FOR SENIORS

There are no special instructions for seniors.

GENERIC NAME

Perindopril *see Quinapril, page 894*

GENERIC NAME

Permethrin

BRAND NAMES

Acticin, Elimite, Nix, Rid
Generic available

ABOUT THIS DRUG

Permethrin is used to treat head lice and scabies. The lotion destroys both the lice and their eggs, while the cream kills the mites that cause scabies. This drug works by interfering with the parasites' nervous systems.

SIDE EFFECTS

Consult your health-care practitioner if you experience side effects when using permethrin. If stinging or skin irritation are severe, you will probably be advised to discontinue use.

- *Common:* burning, stinging, itching
- *Less Common or Rare:* numbness, tingling, swelling, redness, rash

IMPORTANT PRECAUTIONS

Do not apply lotion or cream around the eyes, nose, or mouth. If permethrin accidentally gets in the eyes, flush them immediately with plenty of water. Call your health-care practitioner if any irritation persists.

Do not apply permethrin to broken skin or open sores. Use only on hairy areas of the body with intact skin.

Always inform your health-care practitioner about any other medical conditions you suffer from, especially severe inflammation of the scalp.

Parasites are easily transferred from one person to another via direct contact or by touching the clothing, hats, hairbrushes, or other items of infected people. To prevent infection or reinfection, wash clothing, bedding, and towels in very hot water; soak hairbrushes and combs in hot water and do not share them with others; and thoroughly vacuum your home (including upholstered furniture).

DRUG INTERACTIONS

Inform your health-care practitioner and pharmacist if you are taking any other prescription or over-the-counter drugs, as well as any vitamins, herbs, or other supplements. Do not apply permethrin with other topical medications.

FOOD, VITAMIN, AND HERBAL INTERACTIONS

No food, vitamin, or herbal interactions have been noted.

RECOMMENDED DOSAGE

Permethrin comes as a 1% lotion to treat head lice and a 5% cream for scabies. Follow dosage instructions exactly. The lotion can be used on children age 2 and over; the cream is appropriate for infants age 2 months and over.

Head Lice

- Shampoo your hair and scalp with regular shampoo.
- Rinse and towel dry your hair and scalp.
- Allow hair to air dry for several minutes.
- Lean over a sink to apply permethrin. Do not stand in a shower or sit in a bathtub.
- After shaking the bottle, thoroughly wet hair and scalp with the lotion. Cover the areas behind your ears and the back of your neck.
- Leave permethrin on the hair 10 minutes.
- Rinse hair thoroughly, and towel dry.
- Use a fine-toothed comb to remove any nits (lice eggs).
- Wash your hands to remove all traces of medication.

Scabies

- Take a shower or bath.
- Massage cream over your entire body, from head to toe. Be sure to reach creases in the skin.
- Infants (age 2 months and over) should be treated on the scalp, side of the head, and forehead.
- Leave cream on 8 to 14 hours.
- Wash cream off in a shower or bath.

SYMPTOMS OF OVERDOSE AND WHAT TO DO

Permethrin is for external use only. If it is accidentally swallowed, proceed to the nearest hospital and bring the prescription container with you.

SPECIAL INFORMATION FOR PREGNANT OR NURSING WOMEN

No studies have adequately investigated the effects of permethrin during pregnancy or breastfeeding. However, if you are or think you may be pregnant, or if you are breastfeeding, consult your health-care practitioner before applying this medication on yourself or others. Only your health-care practitioner can determine if the benefits outweigh the potential dangers.

SPECIAL INFORMATION FOR SENIORS

There are no special guidelines for seniors.

GENERIC NAME

Perphenazine

see Tricyclic Antidepressants, page 1076

BRAND NAMES

Trilafon, Trilafon Concentrate
Generic available

ABOUT THIS DRUG

Perphenazine is a phenothiazine antipsychotic drug used to treat psychotic disorders, such as schizophrenia, and other severe mental conditions characterized by distorted thoughts, emotions, and perceptions.

This drug and other phenothiazines affect the hypothalamus, a portion of the brain that controls body temperature, alertness, muscle tone, hormone balance, vomiting, and metabolism.

SIDE EFFECTS

Contact your health-care practitioner if you experience any side effects while taking perphenazine. Only he or she can determine whether you should continue to take this drug.

- *More Common:* dry mouth, blurred vision, drowsiness, nausea, reduced sweating, hand tremor, stiffness, stooped posture
- *Less Common:* difficulty urinating, menstrual irregularities, breast swelling or pain, unusual bruising or bleeding, heart palpitations, rash, itching, uncontrolled movements of the tongue, fever, chills, sore throat, photosensitivity

People taking antipsychotic drugs may experience a rare but life-threatening set of side effects known as neuroleptic malignant syndrome (NMS). Symptoms include fever, difficulty breathing, rapid heartbeat, rigid muscles, mental changes, increased sweating, irregular blood pressure, and convulsions. Immediate medical attention is required.

Side effects such as lip smacking, wormlike movements of the tongue, and slow, rhythmical, involuntary movements are characteristic of a disorder known as tardive dyskinesia. Older adults (especially women) are more susceptible to this condition, which may become permanent. If you experience tardive dyskinesia, your health-care practitioner will probably advise you to stop taking this drug.

IMPORTANT PRECAUTIONS

Do not take perphenazine if you have had an allergic reaction to this drug or to any other drugs in the past.

Do not take perphenazine if you have very low blood pressure; heart, liver, kidney, or blood disease; or Parkinson's disease.

Perphenazine should be used under strict medical supervision if you have glaucoma, epilepsy, urinary problems, breast cancer, benign prostatic hyperplasia, or stomach ulcers.

This drug affects the temperature control center of your brain. Therefore, do not become overheated during exercise or hot weather or in other hot environments (e.g., saunas, hot baths).

Because perphenazine can cause blurred vision and drowsiness, make sure you know how you react to the drug before you drive or operate any type of hazardous equipment.

Perphenazine can increase your skin's sensitivity to the sun. Take precautions to avoid overexposure, such as wearing sunscreen, long-sleeved shirts, long pants, and a hat.

DRUG INTERACTIONS

Tell your health-care practitioner and pharmacist about any prescription and over-the-counter drugs you are taking, as well as any vitamins, herbs, or other supplements. Perphenazine can interact with other medications.

- Alcohol and other drugs that depress the central nervous system (e.g., barbiturates, sleeping pills, narcotics, tranquilizers) may produce additional sedative effects.
- Antithyroid medications increase the risk of developing serious blood conditions.
- Antacids that contain aluminum may reduce the effectiveness of perphenazine. They should be taken at least 2 hours before or after taking a dose of perphenazine.
- Bromocriptine and appetite suppressants may be less effective.
- Guanethidine's ability to lower blood pressure may be reduced.
- Lithium, metoclopramide, pemoline, and rauwolfia alkaloids may cause uncontrolled muscle movements.
- Amantadine, bromocriptine, diuretics, levobunolol, narcotics, and propranolol may result in very low blood pressure.
- Disopyramide, erythromycin, procainamide, and quinidine may cause serious changes in heart rhythm.
- Tricyclic antidepressants (e.g., amitriptyline, imipramine) may cause antidepressant side effects.

FOOD, VITAMIN, AND HERBAL INTERACTIONS

Herbs that produce a sedative effect may cause potentially serious depressant interactions when used with perphenazine. Some of those herbs include calendula, capsicum, catnip, goldenseal, gotu kola, hops, kava, lady's slipper, passionflower, sage, Siberian ginseng, skullcap, St. John's wort, and valerian, among others.

RECOMMENDED DOSAGE

Perphenazine is available in tablets and oral solution. The dosage recommendations given here are typical. However, your health-care practitioner will determine the most appropriate dose and schedule for your particular needs.

Tablets

- *Children up to 12 Years:* Your health-care practitioner will determine whether it is appropriate for your child.
- *Children 12 Years and Older and Adults:* 4 to 16 mg, 2 to 4 times daily

Oral Solution

- *Children up to 12 Years:* Your health-care practitioner will determine whether it is appropriate for your child.
- *Children 12 Years and Older and Adults:* 8 to 16 mg, 2 to 4 times daily

Perphenazine can be taken with food or with a full glass of water or milk to reduce stomach irritation. If you miss a dose, take it as soon as you remember. If it is nearly time for your next dose, do not take the missed dose. Continue with your regular dosing schedule. Never take a double dose.

SYMPTOMS OF OVERDOSE AND WHAT TO DO

Symptoms of overdose include agitation, coma, convulsions, breathing difficulties, dry mouth, extreme sleepiness, fever, intestinal blockage, irregular heart rate, low blood pressure, restlessness, and swallowing difficulties. If an overdose occurs, seek immediate medical attention and bring the prescription container with you to the hospital.

SPECIAL INFORMATION FOR PREGNANT OR NURSING WOMEN

Adequate studies of the effects of perphenazine on pregnant or nursing women have not been done. If you are pregnant or plan to become pregnant, talk to your health-care practitioner. This drug should not be used during pregnancy unless your health-care practitioner determines it is essential for your health.

Perphenazine passes into breast milk. Your health-care practitioner will advise you to stop breastfeeding until you have completed treatment.

SPECIAL INFORMATION FOR SENIORS

Seniors are more likely to experience constipation, trouble urinating, dry mouth, confusion, memory difficulties, dizziness, drowsiness, trembling of the hands, and problems with muscle movement.

GENERIC NAME
Phendimetrazine

BRAND NAMES
Adipost, Bontril, Melfiat, Obezine, Phendiet, Plegine, Prelu-2, PT 105

Generic available

ABOUT THIS DRUG
Phendimetrazine is an appetite suppressant used in the treatment of obesity. This drug should be used on a short-term basis only and under a health-care practitioner's close supervision. Appetite suppressants are not a substitute for a sensible, healthy, overall weight loss program. Phendimetrazine works by stimulating the central nervous system.

SIDE EFFECTS
If you develop side effects while taking phendimetrazine, ask your health-care practitioner whether it is safe for you to continue taking this drug.

- *Common:* overstimulation, nervousness, restlessness, difficulty sleeping, a sense of euphoria, false sense of well-being, "feeling high"
- *Less Common or Rare:* high blood pressure, palpitations, dizziness, blurred vision, tremors, headache, sweating, chills, fever, weakness, changes in sex drive, nausea, vomiting, diarrhea, dry mouth, difficulty urinating, rash, itching, hair loss, muscle pain

IMPORTANT PRECAUTIONS
This drug is not an appropriate remedy for people who have heart disease, high blood pressure, glaucoma, or thyroid disease. Do not use phendimetrazine if you have experienced an allergic reaction to this or other appetite suppressants. Because appetite suppressants have habit-forming potential, inform your health-care practitioner if you have a history of mental illness or substance abuse. If you have diabetes, phendimetrazine may alter the amount of medication you require.

In order to lose weight, follow a reduced-calorie diet and an exercise program while taking phendimetrazine. To keep weight off, continue to follow a sensible program of diet and exercise under the supervision of your health-care practitioner.

Phendimetrazine makes some people dizzy, lightheaded, and

less alert than usual. Until you know how this drug affects you, do not drive a car, operate machinery, or engage in other actions that require concentration.

Because phendimetrazine may cause dry mouth, use sugarless candy or gum, ice chips, or a saliva substitute. If the problem continues, consult your health-care practitioner or dentist.

Before having surgery or a dental procedure, tell your health-care practitioner or dentist that you take phendimetrazine.

If you have a urine test while taking phendimetrazine, you may test positive for amphetamines.

DRUG INTERACTIONS

Tell your health-care practitioner and pharmacist if you are taking any other prescription or over-the-counter drugs, as well as any vitamins, herbs, or other supplements. Possible drug interactions include the following:

- Do not take phendimetrazine with or within 14 days of taking a monoamine oxidase (MAO) inhibitor. This combination can cause very high blood pressure.
- Diabetes, asthma, and antidepressant medication doses may require adjustment when you take phendimetrazine.
- Phendimetrazine may reduce the effects of high blood pressure medications.
- Combining phendimetrazine with other stimulants (such as other appetite suppressants, amphetamines, methylphenidate, caffeine, or cocaine) can result in unwanted effects ranging from overstimulation to heart problems.
- Taking tricyclic antidepressants with phendimetrazine may cause high blood pressure or an irregular heartbeat.
- Be careful when you use over-the-counter remedies while taking phendimetrazine. Many cough, cold, sinus, and allergy remedies raise blood pressure.

FOOD, VITAMIN, AND HERBAL INTERACTIONS

Do not take phendimetrazine with herbs that raise blood pressure, such as ephedra (ma huang), ginseng, goldenseal, licorice, or saw palmetto.

Moderate your consumption of caffeinated beverages such as coffee, tea, and cola.

RECOMMENDED DOSAGE

Phendimetrazine comes in regular or extended-release tablets. The doses given below are typical, but only your health-care practitioner can determine the dose and schedule that best fit your particular needs.

- ➤ *Children:* This drug is not recommended for children under the age of 16.
- ➤ *Adults:* 17.5 to 35 mg 2 to 3 times daily, 1 hour before meals; extended-release tablets (105 mg) are taken once daily before breakfast

To prevent trouble sleeping, take single-dose medication 10 to 14 hours before bedtime, or the last dose of the day 4 to 6 hours before bedtime. Swallow extended-release tablets whole; do not break, crush, or chew them. If you find that several weeks of therapy do not affect your appetite, do not increase the dose. Consult your health-care practitioner. If you miss a dose, skip it. Never take double doses.

SYMPTOMS OF OVERDOSE AND WHAT TO DO

The symptoms of phendimetrazine overdose include nausea, vomiting, diarrhea, blood pressure changes, confusion, restlessness, panic, clammy skin, tremors, hallucinations, and fever. If overdose occurs, seek immediate medical attention and take the bottle of phendimetrazine to the hospital with you.

SPECIAL INFORMATION FOR PREGNANT OR NURSING WOMEN

Large doses of phendimetrazine may cause birth defects. If you are or think you may be pregnant, consult your health-care practitioner before using this drug. Only your health-care practitioner can determine if the benefits outweigh the potential dangers. It is not known whether phendimetrazine passes into breast milk. However, if you are breastfeeding, your health-care practitioner will likely advise you to stop until your treatment is done.

SPECIAL INFORMATION FOR SENIORS

Phendimetrazine may aggravate many diseases associated with advanced age, including heart disease, high blood pressure, and diabetes.

OPEN QUESTIONS OR CONTROVERSIES

Appetite suppressants can cause dependence. They should be used on a short-term basis only, and should be avoided by those with a history of mental illness or drug or alcohol abuse. Signs of dependence include a strong need for medication, a desire to increase the dosage, and withdrawal symptoms (such as depression, cramps, nausea, and fatigue) when you stop taking phendimetrazineg.

GENERIC NAME

Phenelzine

BRAND NAME

Nardil
No generic available

ABOUT THIS DRUG

Phenelzine is a monoamine oxidase inhibitor (MAOI) used to treat mental depression, and associated anxiety and phobias. MAOIs were the first antidepressants developed. These drugs increase levels of neurotransmitters (chemical messengers in the brain) by interfering with their normal breakdown in the body. Phenelzine and other MAOI antidepressants are less frequently prescribed today, as newer medications with fewer side effects and interactions have become widely available.

SIDE EFFECTS

Because phenelzine has been associated with potentially fatal high blood pressure, stop taking medication and contact your health-care practitioner immediately if you experience symptoms such as a severe headache or heart palpitations. Also inform your health-care practitioner of other side effects, particularly if they are severe or prolonged. Only your health-care practitioner can determine whether it is safe for you to continue taking this drug.

- *Common:* drowsiness, dizziness, weakness, dry mouth, itching, constipation, stomach disorders, fatigue, headache, sleep disturbances, twitching, tremor, muscle spasms, low blood pressure when rising, fluid retention, weight gain, sexual difficulties
- *Less Common or Rare:* anxiety, sweating, fever, jitteriness, tingling, rapid breathing and heart rate, false sense of well-being, blurred vi-

sion, glaucoma, involuntary eye movements, lack of coordination, rash, yellow skin and eyes, liver damage, inability to urinate, mania, onset of schizophrenia, delirium, swelling in throat, heart palpitations, high blood pressure, convulsions, coma

IMPORTANT PRECAUTIONS

Always inform your health-care practitioner about any other medical conditions you may have, especially congestive heart failure, high blood pressure, a history of heart attack or stroke, diabetes, kidney or liver impairment, or an adrenal gland tumor. Tell your health-care practitioner if you have ever had an allergic reaction to this or another MAOI antidepressant.

Many drugs and foods interact with phenelzine, and can result in potentially fatal reactions. Pay careful attention to the interactions listed below.

If you plan to undergo surgery or a dental procedure, tell your health-care practitioner or dentist that you are taking phenelzine.

This drug can make you drowsy and less alert than usual. Until you know how phenelzine affects you, do not drive a car, operate machinery, or perform other tasks that require concentration.

When you first start taking this drug or when the dosage is increased, you may experience dizziness or faintness when you rise quickly from a sitting or reclining position (postural hypotension). Try to get up slowly, and consult your health-care practitioner if the problem continues.

If this drug causes mouth dryness, use sugarless gum or candy, ice chips, or artificial saliva. If the problem continues, consult your health-care practitioner or dentist.

DRUG INTERACTIONS

Phenelzine may have dangerous interactions with many drugs. Always tell your health-care practitioner and pharmacist if you are taking any other prescription or over-the-counter drugs, as well as any vitamins, herbs, or other supplements. Possible drug interactions include the following:

- Do not take phenelzine at the same time as or within 14 days of amphetamines, appetite suppressants, methylphenidate, other stimulants, or other MAOI antidepressants. These combinations can cause potentially fatal high blood pressure.
- Do not combine phenelzine with over-the-counter decongestants such as cold, sinus, asthma, hay fever, or allergy remedies. Many of these medications raise blood pressure.

- Do not take phenelzine at the same time as or within 14 days of SSRI or tricyclic antidepressants. These combinations can result in severe and potentially fatal reactions.
- Taking phenelzine with disulfiram or tranylcypromine sulfate may lead to reactions such as agitation, delirium, and hallucinations.
- Phenelzine increases the effects of beta-blockers, barbiturates, sulfa drugs, levodopa, methyldopa, meperidine, sumatriptan, L-tryptophan, thiazide-type diuretics, sulfonylurea-type antidiabetic drugs, and stimulants.
- Phenelzine interferes with the effects of guanethidine.
- Do not drink alcohol while taking phenelzine.
- Cigarette smoking may decrease the effectiveness of this drug.

FOOD, VITAMIN, AND HERBAL INTERACTIONS

It is essential to avoid foods that are rich in the amino acid tyramine while taking and for 2 weeks after taking phenelzine. This combination may result in an excessive and potentially fatal rise in blood pressure. Tyramine-rich foods include (but are not limited to) aged cheeses, bologna, chicken liver, chocolate, figs, pickled herring, pepperoni, raisins, salami, soy sauce, and yeast extracts. Also avoid beverages that contain meat or meat tenderizers, and alcoholic beverages that may contain tyramine, which include some beers, vermouth, and Chianti wines.

Herbs that affect the central nervous system—including St. John's wort, guarana, ephedra (ma huang), ginseng, scotch broom, and kola—must also be avoided when taking phenelzine. In addition, avoid caffeinated beverages, such as coffee, tea, and cola.

RECOMMENDED DOSAGE

Phenelzine comes as a tablet. Although the doses given below are typical, only your health-care practitioner can determine the dose and schedule that best fit your needs.

- *Children:* This drug is not recommended for children under the age of 16.
- *Adults:* 15 mg 3 times a day to start, which may be gradually increased as needed to a maximum daily dose of 90 mg

Phenelzine can be taken with or without food. This drug must be taken regularly for approximately 4 weeks before its full effect is felt. If you forget a dose, take it as soon as you remember. If it is almost time for the next dose, skip the missed one and resume your normal schedule. Never take a double dose. In order to avoid withdrawal symptoms such as agitation and nightmares, you must stop taking phenelzine gradually.

SYMPTOMS OF OVERDOSE AND WHAT TO DO

An overdose of phenelzine can be fatal. Its symptoms may include changes in blood pressure, severe headache, sweating, fever, faintness, agitation, difficulty breathing, drowsiness, dizziness, rapid pulse, hallucinations, hyperactivity, irritability, jaw muscle spasms, backward arching, rigidity, convulsions, and coma. If overdose occurs, seek immediate medical attention and take the prescription bottle to the hospital with you.

SPECIAL INFORMATION FOR PREGNANT OR NURSING WOMEN

No studies have adequately investigated the effects of phenelzine during pregnancy or breastfeeding. If you are pregnant or plan to become pregnant, or if you are breastfeeding or plan to do so, talk with your health-care practitioner before starting this drug. Only a health-care practitioner can determine whether the potential benefits outweigh the potential dangers.

SPECIAL INFORMATION FOR SENIORS

Seniors are at higher risk of side effects, and usually require smaller doses.

GENERIC NAME

Phenindamine

see Antihistamine-Decongestant Combination, page 132

GENERIC NAME

Pheniramine

see Antihistamine-Decongestant Combination, page 132

GENERIC NAME

Phenobarbital

BRAND NAMES

Bellatal, Solfoton

Generic available

ABOUT THIS DRUG

Phenobarbital, a barbiturate, is used as a sedative to relieve anxiety and nervous tension, and to control tonic-clonic, partial, and childhood febrile seizures. When prescribed for epileptic seizures, phenobarbital is far more effective when combined with anticonvulsants such as phenytoin.

Phenobarbital acts on the central nervous system, blocking select nerve impulses in the brain. If this drug is taken in excessive doses or for long periods of time, physical and/or psychological dependence may develop.

SIDE EFFECTS

Inform your health-care practitioner if you develop side effects while taking phenobarbital. If symptoms are severe or prolonged, ask your health-care practitioner whether your dosage requires adjustment, and whether it is safe for you to continue taking this drug.

- *Common:* drowsiness, lethargy, impaired concentration, mental and physical sluggishness
- *Less Common or Rare:* dizziness, unsteadiness, an intoxicated appearance, visual disturbances, nausea, vomiting, constipation, diarrhea, photosensitivity, difficulty breathing, runny nose, watery eyes, sneezing, rash, sexual difficulties, yellow eyes and skin, anemia, osteoporosis, seizures, irritability and hyperactivity in children

IMPORTANT PRECAUTIONS

Always inform your health-care practitioner about any other medical conditions you may have. Phenobarbital should not be taken if you have severe liver disease, a respiratory condition, or porphyria. Use this drug with caution if you have mild-to-moderate kidney or liver impairment, a history of depression, myasthenia gravis, or a seizure disorder. Tell your health-care practitioner if you have ever experienced an allergic reaction to this or other barbiturates.

Phenobarbital can lead to physical and/or psychological addiction. This drug should be used with caution in anyone with a history of drug or alcohol abuse.

If you plan to undergo surgery or a dental procedure, tell your health-care practitioner or dentist that you are taking phenobarbital.

This drug can make you drowsy and less alert than usual. Until you know how phenobarbital affects you, do not drive a car, operate machinery, or perform other tasks that require concentration.

Phenobarbital may reduce the effectiveness of oral contraceptives. Use other forms of contraception while you take this drug.

Irritability and hyperactivity may occur in children who take phenobarbital to control seizures. During puberty, as metabolism slows, more medication may be absorbed. Regular blood tests are necessary to monitor the absorption of phenobarbital.

This drug may cause increased sensitivity to the sun. Wear protective clothing and apply sunscreen.

DRUG INTERACTIONS

Tell your health-care practitioner and pharmacist if you are taking any other prescription or over-the-counter drugs, as well as any vitamins, herbs, or other supplements. Possible drug interactions include the following:

- When phenobarbital is prescribed for seizures, it is more effective when combined with anticonvulsants such as phenytoin.
- Taking other central nervous system depressants (such as sedatives, antidepressants, narcotics, or tranquilizers) with phenobarbital can result in increased drowsiness and excessive sedation.
- The flu vaccine may lead to toxic levels of phenobarbital.
- Phenobarbital reduces the effectiveness of many other drugs. These include oral contraceptives, blood thinners such as warfarin, beta-blockers, protease inhibitors, bupropion, carbamazepine, cortisone-like drugs, delavirdine, dexamethasone, diltiazem, disopyramide, donepezil, doxycycline, felodipine, griseofulvin, lamotrigine, levonorgestrel, metoprolol, montelukast, nimodipine, quinidine, paroxetine, propafenone, propranolol, ritonavir, theophylline, tretinoin, tricyclic antidepressants, verapamil, and venlafaxine.
- Do not combine phenobarbital and chloramphenicol.
- Do not drink alcohol or smoke cigarettes while taking phenobarbital.
- Marijuana causes increased drowsiness and unsteadiness, significantly impairing mental and physical function.

FOOD, VITAMIN, AND HERBAL INTERACTIONS

Do not take phenobarbital with herbs such as hops, kava, passionflower, and valerian. These can increase its sedative effects. Phenobarbital should not be combined with dong quai, ephedra (ma huang), ginkgo, ginseng, kola, St. John's wort, glutamine, and nicotinamide.

Phenobarbital may increase your need for folic acid, vitamin D, and calcium. To counteract this effect, follow a well-balanced diet and consider a daily vitamin and mineral supplement.

RECOMMENDED DOSAGE

Phenobarbital comes as a capsule, tablet, or elixir. Although the doses given below are typical, only your health-care practitioner can determine the dose and schedule that best fit your needs.

Sedation

- *Children:* Phenobarbital is not recommended for sedation in children.
- *Adults:* 30 to 120 mg daily, divided into 2 or 3 doses

Anticonvulsant Use

- *Children:* 3 to 6 mg per 2.2 pounds of body weight daily
- *Adults:* 60 to 200 mg daily

To prevent stomach upset, phenobarbital may be taken with milk or fruit juice. If you forget a dose, take it as soon as you remember. If it is almost time for the next dose, skip the missed one and resume your normal schedule. Never take a double dose. If you have been taking phenobarbital for a long period of time, to prevent seizures you must stop taking it gradually.

SYMPTOMS OF OVERDOSE AND WHAT TO DO

Barbiturate overdose can be fatal. The symptoms of phenobarbital overdose may resemble intoxication. They include confusion, slurred speech, dizziness, loss of coordination, depression, and impaired vision. If overdose occurs, seek immediate medical attention and take the prescription bottle to the hospital with you.

SPECIAL INFORMATION FOR PREGNANT OR NURSING WOMEN

Barbiturates should not be used during pregnancy. If phenobarbital must be taken while pregnant, the mother should receive vitamin K shortly before childbirth, and the infant should receive it immediately afterward. Because phenobarbital may pass into breast milk, breastfeeding is not advisable while taking this drug.

SPECIAL INFORMATION FOR SENIORS

Barbiturates are not recommended for seniors. If phenobarbital is prescribed, low starting doses are necessary. Beware of side effects such as agitation, confusion, and hypothermia.

GENERIC NAME

Phentermine hydrochloride

BRAND NAMES

Adipex-P, Fastin, Ionamin, Obenix, Phentercot, Pheneturide, Pro-Fast, Teramine, Zantryl
Generic available

ABOUT THIS DRUG

Phentermine is an appetite suppressant used in the treatment of obesity. This drug should be used on a short-term basis only and under a health-care practitioner's close supervision. Appetite suppressants are not a substitute for a sensible, healthy, overall weight loss program. Phentermine works by stimulating the central nervous system.

SIDE EFFECTS

If you develop side effects while taking phentermine, ask your health-care practitioner whether it is safe for you to continue taking this drug.

- *Common:* overstimulation, nervousness, restlessness, difficulty sleeping, a sense of euphoria, false sense of well-being, "feeling high"
- *Less Common or Rare:* high blood pressure, palpitations, dizziness, blurred vision, tremors, headache, sweating, chills, fever, weakness, changes in sex drive, nausea, vomiting, diarrhea, dry mouth, difficulty urinating, rash, itching, hair loss, muscle pain

IMPORTANT PRECAUTIONS

This drug is not an appropriate remedy for people who have heart disease, high blood pressure, glaucoma, or thyroid disease. Do not use phentermine if you have experienced an allergic reaction to this or other appetite suppressants. Because appetite suppressants have habit-forming potential, inform your health-care practitioner if you have a history of mental illness or substance abuse. If you have diabetes, phentermine may alter the amount of medication you require.

In order to lose weight, follow a reduced-calorie diet and an exercise program while taking phentermine. To keep weight off, continue to follow a sensible program of diet and exercise under the supervision of your health-care practitioner.

Phentermine makes some people dizzy, lightheaded, and less alert than usual. Until you know how this drug affects you, do not drive a car, operate machinery, or engage in other actions that require concentration.

Because phentermine may cause dry mouth, use sugarless candy or gum, ice chips, or a saliva substitute. If the problem continues, consult your health-care practitioner or dentist.

Before having surgery or a dental procedure, tell your health-care practitioner or dentist that you take phentermine.

If you have a urine test while taking phentermine, you may test positive for amphetamines.

DRUG INTERACTIONS

Tell your health-care practitioner and pharmacist if you are taking any other prescription or over-the-counter drugs, as well as any vitamins, herbs, or other supplements. Possible drug interactions include the following:

- Do not take phentermine with or within 14 days of taking a monoamine oxidase (MAO) inhibitor. This combination can cause very high blood pressure.
- Diabetes, asthma, and antidepressant medications may require adjustment when you take phentermine.
- Phentermine may reduce the effects of high blood pressure medications.
- Combining phentermine with other stimulants (such as other appetite suppressants, amphetamines, methylphenidate, caffeine, or cocaine) can result in unwanted effects ranging from overstimulation to heart problems.
- Taking tricyclic antidepressants with phentermine may cause high blood pressure or an irregular heartbeat.
- Be careful when you use over-the-counter remedies while taking phentermine. Many cough, cold, sinus, and allergy remedies raise blood pressure.

FOOD, VITAMIN, AND HERBAL INTERACTIONS

Do not take phentermine with herbs that raise blood pressure, such as ephedra (ma huang), ginseng, goldenseal, licorice, or saw palmetto.

Moderate your consumption of caffeinated beverages such as coffee, tea, and cola.

RECOMMENDED DOSAGE

Phentermine comes in capsules, resin capsules, and tablets. The doses given below are typical, but only your health-care practitioner can determine the dose and schedule that best fit your particular needs.

- *Children:* This drug is not recommended for children under the age of 16.
- *Adults:* 15 to 37.5 mg once a day, before breakfast or 1 to 2 hours after breakfast; in some cases, your health-care practitioner may recommend taking smaller doses 30 minutes before meals

To prevent trouble sleeping, take single-dose medication 10 to 14 hours before bedtime, or the last dose of the day 4 to 6 hours before bedtime. Swallow extended-release capsules or tablets whole; do not break, crush, or chew them. If you find that several weeks of therapy do not affect your appetite, do not increase the dose. Consult your health-care practitioner. If you miss a dose, skip it. Never take double doses.

SYMPTOMS OF OVERDOSE AND WHAT TO DO

The symptoms of phentermine overdose include nausea, vomiting, diarrhea, blood pressure changes, confusion, restlessness, panic, clammy skin, tremors, hallucinations, and fever. If overdose occurs, seek immediate medical attention and take the bottle of phentermine to the hospital with you.

SPECIAL INFORMATION FOR PREGNANT OR NURSING WOMEN

Large doses of phentermine may cause birth defects. If you are or think you may be pregnant, consult your health-care practitioner before using this drug. Only your health-care practitioner can determine if the benefits outweigh the potential dangers. It is not known whether phentermine passes into breast milk. However, if you are breastfeeding, your health-care practitioner will likely advise you to stop until your treatment is done.

SPECIAL INFORMATION FOR SENIORS

Phentermine may aggravate many diseases associated with advanced age, including heart disease, high blood pressure, and diabetes.

OPEN QUESTIONS OR CONTROVERSIES

In 1997, the FDA alerted health-care practitioners to reports of valvular heart disease in women treated for obesity with "fen-phen"—the combination of fenfluramine and phentermine. Although each of these two drugs was approved individually for the short-term treatment of obesity, "off-label" use of the

(continued from page 839)
combination (often for longer than recommended periods of time) had become widespread, with disastrous results. Always take drugs only in the recommended dosages and for the periods of time approved by the FDA, and pay close attention to possible drug interactions.

Another concern is that appetite suppressants can cause dependence. Again, they should be used on a short-term basis only—and should be avoided by those with a history of mental illness or drug or alcohol abuse. Signs of dependence include a strong need for medication, a desire to increase the dosage, and withdrawal symptoms (such as depression, cramps, nausea, and fatigue) when you stop taking phentermine.

GENERIC NAME

Phenylephrine

see Antihistamine-Decongestant Combination, page 132

GENERIC NAME

Phenylpropanolamine

see Antihistamine-Decongestant Combination, page 132

GENERIC NAME

Phenyltoloxamine

see Antihistamine-Decongestant Combination, page 132

GENERIC NAME

Phenytoin

BRAND NAME

Dilantin

Generic available

Note: The information in this profile also applies to ethotoin, fosphenytoin, and mephenytoin.

ABOUT THIS DRUG

Phenytoin is a hydantoin anticonvulsant used to relieve epileptic seizures. It is also prescribed for the prevention of seizures following surgery in people who do not have epilepsy.

Phenytoin works by inhibiting activity in the part of the brain associated with grand mal seizures. This drug is often taken in combination with phenobarbital or other anticonvulsants.

SIDE EFFECTS

Side effects are usually most common at the beginning of therapy, and tend to disappear as time goes on. However, if symptoms are severe or prolonged, ask your health-care practitioner whether your dosage can be reduced, and whether it is safe for you to continue taking this drug.

- *Common:* constipation, dizziness, drowsiness, impaired coordination, mental confusion, nervousness, irritability, involuntary eye movements
- *Less Common or Rare:* enlarged or bleeding gums, swollen glands, breast development in males, balding, muscle twitching, learning difficulties, confusion, clumsiness, unsteadiness, headache, fever, nausea, vomiting, diarrhea, sexual difficulties, weight gain, joint or muscle pain, enlargement of the jaw, shallow breathing, sensitivity to light, rash, itching, slurred speech, stuttering, yellow eyes or skin, liver damage

Contact your health-care practitioner at once if you develop symptoms such as a rash, severe nausea or vomiting, unusual bleeding or bruising, yellow eyes or skin, slurred speech, or loss of coordination.

IMPORTANT PRECAUTIONS

Always inform your health-care practitioner about any other medical conditions you may have, especially blood disease, diabetes, liver or kidney disease, porphyria, lupus, thyroid disease, low blood pressure, a slow heart rate, heart disease, or a history of alcohol abuse. If you have a fever for more than 24 hours, consult your health-care practitioner. This may decrease the effects of phenytoin. Tell your health-care practitioner if you have ever experienced an allergic reaction to this or similar drugs.

If you undergo surgery, a medical test, emergency medical treatment, or a dental procedure, tell the health-care practitioner or dentist that you are taking phenytoin.

This drug can make you drowsy and less alert than usual. Until you know how phenytoin affects you, do not drive a car, operate machinery, or perform other tasks that require concentration.

Because phenytoin may reduce the effectiveness of oral contraceptives, use alternate means of contraception.

Phenytoin may cause hyperglycemia (high blood sugar), which blocks the effects of insulin. Diabetics must carefully monitor their blood sugar levels, and may require adjustments in medication dosage.

This drug may cause increased sensitivity to the sun. Wear protective clothing and apply sunscreen.

Because phenytoin may affect the gums, good oral hygiene and regular visits to the dentist are essential.

Regular blood tests are necessary to monitor the absorption of phenytoin, especially during the first months of treatment. Older people and those with liver damage are more prone to dangerous side effects and usually require lower doses.

DRUG INTERACTIONS

Tell your health-care practitioner and pharmacist if you are taking any other prescription or over-the-counter drugs, as well as any vitamins, herbs, or other supplements. Possible drug interactions include the following:

- Phenytoin may increase the effectiveness of other anticonvulsants, such as phenobarbital.
- Taking other central nervous system depressants (such as sedatives, antidepressants, narcotics, or tranquilizers) with phenytoin can result in increased drowsiness and excessive sedation.
- Do not take phenytoin within 2 to 3 hours of antacids or antidiarrhea medication.
- Phenytoin reduces the effectiveness of many other drugs. These include oral contraceptives, digitalis drugs, corticosteroids, amiodarone, carbamazepine, disopyramide, doxycycline, estrogens, haloperidol, methadone, quinine, theophylline, and valproic acid.
- Phenytoin also interacts with many other prescription and nonprescription drugs, including acetaminophen, aspirin, cyclosporine, insulin, lidocaine, lithium, mebendazole, meperidine, tricyclic antidepressants, and warfarin. Do not start or stop taking any other medicines with phenytoin without consulting your health-care practitioner.
- Do not drink alcohol while taking phenytoin.
- Marijuana causes increased drowsiness and unsteadiness, significantly impairing mental and physical function.

FOOD, VITAMIN, AND HERBAL INTERACTIONS

Do not take phenytoin within 2 to 3 hours of calcium supplements, or 1 to 2 hours of high-calcium foods (such as milk, cheese, and other dairy products). Do not combine with herbs such as hops, kava, passionflower, and valerian. These can increase phenytoin's sedative effects. Folic acid and vitamin D supplements are recommended.

RECOMMENDED DOSAGE

Phenytoin comes in oral form as chewable tablets, immediate-release and extended-release capsules, and an oral suspension. Dosage is very carefully tailored to fit individual needs.

- *Children:* 2.5 mg per pound of body weight to start, which may be gradually increased as needed to a maximum daily dosage of 300 mg
- *Adults:* 300 mg daily to start, divided into 3 doses; maximum daily dosage is 600 mg

If your seizures are successfully controlled with 3 doses of medication a day, your health-care practitioner may allow you to try a once-daily dosage. To prevent stomach upset, phenytoin may be taken with food. If you forget a dose, take it as soon as you remember. If it is within 4 hours of the next dose, skip the missed one and resume your normal schedule. Never take a double dose. If you have been taking phenytoin for a long period of time, to prevent seizures you must stop taking it gradually. Do not switch phenytoin brands without consulting your health-care practitioner.

SYMPTOMS OF OVERDOSE AND WHAT TO DO

Overdose can be fatal. The symptoms of phenytoin overdose may resemble intoxication. They include confusion, slurred speech, dizziness, unsteadiness, clumsiness, loss of coordination, staggering, and blurred or double vision. If overdose occurs, seek immediate medical attention and take the prescription bottle to the hospital with you.

SPECIAL INFORMATION FOR PREGNANT OR NURSING WOMEN

Antiepileptic drugs are associated with an increased risk of birth defects, and whenever possible should not be used during pregnancy. Because phenytoin may pass into breast milk, breastfeeding is not advisable while taking this drug.

SPECIAL INFORMATION FOR SENIORS

Seniors are more sensitive to side effects, and usually require lower doses.

GENERIC
Pimozide

BRAND NAME
Orap
No generic available

ABOUT THIS DRUG
Pimozide is used to treat individuals who have severe symptoms of Tourette's syndrome who cannot take or have not been helped by other medications.

Pimozide works in the central nervous system to help control the uncontrollable, repeated tics (body movements) and vocal outbursts associated with this disease. Although it cannot cure the tics, it can reduce their severity and number.

SIDE EFFECTS
Contact your health-care practitioner if you experience any side effects while taking pimozide. Only a doctor can determine whether you should continue to take this drug.

- *More Common:* blurred vision or other vision problems, constipation, dizziness, lightheadedness or fainting when rising from a seated or lying position, drowsiness, dry mouth, discolored skin, difficulty speaking, irregular heartbeat, behavior or mood changes, restlessness, shuffling walk, slowed movements, stiff legs or arms, swollen or sore breasts, trembling of hands and fingers, lack of facial expression
- *Less Common or Rare:* diarrhea, decreased sexual performance, headache, loss of appetite, weight loss, depression, nausea and vomiting, weakness or tiredness, difficulty swallowing, increased blinking or eyelid spasm, sore throat, swelling of the face, jaundice, unusual bruising or bleeding

A rare but life-threatening set of side effects known as neuroleptic malignant syndrome (NMS) may occur when you are taking pimozide. Symptoms include fever, difficulty breathing, rapid heartbeat, rigid muscles, mental changes, increased sweating, irregular blood pressure, and convulsions. Immediate medical attention is required.

In rare cases, pimozide has been associated with side effects such as lip smacking, wormlike movements of the tongue, and slow, rhythmical, involuntary movements. These are characteristic of a disorder known as tardive dyskinesia. If you experience tardive dyskinesia, your doctor will probably advise you to stop taking this drug.

IMPORTANT PRECAUTIONS

Tell your health-care practitioner if you have ever had any unusual or allergic reaction to pimozide, haloperidol, or other medicines used to treat mental illness.

Children are especially sensitive to the effects of pimozide and as a result may experience more or more severe side effects.

Sudden deaths have been associated with use of this drug when patients have taken more than 10 mg daily.

Because pimozide can cause dizziness and drowsiness, do not drive a car, operate machinery, or perform other tasks that require concentration until you know how the drug affects you.

Before undergoing any type of dental or medical surgery or emergency treatment, tell the health-care practitioner that you are taking pimozide. Use of pimozide along with drugs used during such procedures may increase depressant effects on the central nervous system.

Pimozide can cause dry mouth, which can be alleviated by chewing sugarless gum, melting ice in your mouth, or using a saliva substitute. If dry mouth continues for more than 2 weeks despite attempts to eliminate it, consult with your health-care practitioner.

Tell your health-care practitioner if you have any of the following medical conditions, as taking pimozide may make them worse or increase the chance of side effects: history of breast cancer, narrow-angle glaucoma, heart disease, intestinal blockage, liver or kidney disease, difficult urination, or urinary tract blockage.

If you have low blood potassium levels, use of pimozide may increase your chance of developing serious arrhythmias.

If you have a history of seizures, use of pimozide may increase the chance of having seizures.

DRUG INTERACTIONS

Inform your health-care practitioner if you are taking any other prescription or over-the-counter drugs, as well as any vitamins, herbs, or other supplements. Possible drug interactions include the following:

- Amoxapine, antipsychotics, metoclopramide, paroxetine, promethazine, rauwolfia, reserpine, and tacrine may increase the chance of developing unusual movements.
- Amphetamines, methylphenidate, and pemoline may cause tics to develop.
- Anticholinergics (medicine for abdominal or stomach spasms or cramps) may increase the chance of dry mouth, constipation, and unusual excitement.

- Azithromycin, clarithromycin, dirithromycin, disopyramide, erythromycin, indinavir, itraconazole, ketoconazole, maprotiline, nefazodone, nelfinavir, phenothiazines (e.g., chlorpromazine, perphenazine), probucol, procainamide, quinidine, ritonavir, saquinavir, tricyclic antidepressants (e.g., amitriptyline, desipramine), or zileuton may increase the chance of developing serious and potentially deadly changes in heart rhythm.
- Central nervous system depressants, such as antihistamines or sedatives, may increase CNS effects.

FOOD, VITAMIN, AND HERBAL INTERACTIONS

Do not combine pimozide with herbs that produce sedative effects, such as catnip, elecampane, goldenseal, gotu kola, hops, kava, lemon balm, skullcap, St. John's wort, and valerian.

Do not take pimozide with grapefruit juice.

RECOMMENDED DOSAGE

Pimozide comes as a tablet. The doses given below are typical, but dosage is always carefully individualized according to a person's particular needs and reactions to therapy.

- *Children Up to 12 Years:* Dose to be determined by the health-care practitioner
- *Children 12 Years and Older:* 0.023 mg per pound of body weight to start. Your health-care practitioner may increase the dose as needed.
- *Adults:* 1 to 2 mg daily to start. Your health-care practitioner may increase the dose if needed. The maximum dose is 10 mg daily.

Pimozide can be taken with food. If you miss a dose, take it as soon as you remember. However, if it is nearly time for your next scheduled dose, do not take the missed dose. Follow your regular dosing schedule. Never take a double dose.

SYMPTOMS OF OVERDOSE AND WHAT TO DO

Symptoms of overdose may include convulsions, severe dizziness, muscle trembling, jerking, or stiffness, severe difficulty breathing, severe uncontrollable movements, and coma. If an overdose occurs, seek medical attention immediately, and bring the prescription bottle with you to the hospital so the doctors will know exactly what drug was taken.

SPECIAL INFORMATION FOR PREGNANT OR NURSING WOMEN

In animal studies, rats and rabbits given more than the highest recommended human dose of pimozide have shown fewer pregnancies, retarded development of the fetus, and toxic effects in the mother and fetus. If you are pregnant or plan to become pregnant, talk with your doctor before starting this drug. Only a physician can determine whether the potential benefits outweigh the potential dangers.

It is not known whether pimozide passes into breast milk. If you are breastfeeding, your doctor will likely advise you to stop until your treatment is done.

SPECIAL INFORMATION FOR SENIORS

Because they are more sensitive to the effects of pimozide, seniors are more likely to experience constipation, dizziness or fainting, drowsiness, dry mouth, trembling of the hands and fingers, and symptoms of tardive dyskinesia (e.g., rapid, worm-like movements of the tongue or any other uncontrolled movements of the mouth, tongue, jaw, and/or arms and legs).

GENERIC NAME

Pindolol

BRAND NAME

Visken

Generic available

ABOUT THIS DRUG

Pindolol is a beta-adrenergic blocking agent (beta-blocker) prescribed to treat mild-to-moderate high blood pressure (hypertension). It may also relieve chest pain (angina).

Pindolol works by decreasing the force and rate of heart contractions. This in turn reduces the demand for oxygen and lowers blood pressure.

SIDE EFFECTS

Speak to your health-care practitioner if you develop side effects while taking this drug. Only he or she can determine whether it is safe for you to continue taking pindolol.

- *Common:* scalp tingling, dizziness, lightheadedness, fainting, nausea, upset stomach, indigestion, vomiting, diarrhea, cramps, sweating, fatigue, urinary difficulties, impotence, muscle weakness, blurred vision, dry eyes, rash, hair loss, bronchial spasm, stuffy nose
- *Less Common or Rare:* disorientation, confusion, anxiety, depression, short-term memory loss, insomnia, vivid dreams, hallucina-

tions, excessive tiredness or weakness, slow heartbeat, constipation, cold hands and feet, breathing difficulties, fever with sore throat, heart failure

IMPORTANT PRECAUTIONS

Always inform your health-care practitioner about any other medical conditions you suffer from, especially a slow heart rate or serious heart block, congestive heart failure, angina, asthma or other lung ailments, liver or kidney problems, diabetes or hypoglycemia, or a thyroid condition. Tell your health-care practitioner if you have ever experienced an allergic reaction to pindolol or another beta-blocker.

Before having any type of surgery or dental procedure, inform your surgeon or dentist that you are taking pindolol.

This drug may make you more sensitive to the cold. Beta-blockers including pindolol can decrease blood circulation in the fingers, toes, and skin. Be sure to dress warmly in low temperatures, especially if you already have blood circulation problems.

This drug may make you drowsy. Until you know how pindolol affects you, do not drive a car, operate machinery, or perform other tasks that demand concentration.

When you first start taking this drug or when the dosage is increased, you may experience dizziness or faintness when you rise quickly from a sitting or reclining position (postural hypotension). Try to get up slowly, and consult your health-care practitioner if the problem continues.

Treatment of high blood pressure also entails certain lifestyle changes, such as weight control, smoking cessation, and close attention to diet.

Be extremely careful when you exercise in hot weather. Heavy sweating can lead to dizziness, lightheadedness, fainting, vomiting, dehydration, and low blood pressure.

DRUG INTERACTIONS

Tell your health-care practitioner and pharmacist if you are taking any other prescription or over-the-counter drugs, as well as any vitamins, herbs, or other supplements. Possible drug interactions include the following:

- Drugs that contain aspirin can lessen the blood pressure lowering effects of pindolol.
- Taking other blood pressure medications (including clonidine, reserpine, and calcium channel blockers) can increase the effects of pindolol.

- Medications such as cimetidine may increase the effects of pindolol.
- Pindolol can interfere with the action of oral antidiabetes medications. It may also change blood glucose levels.
- Pindolol may interfere with the effectiveness of certain asthma medications, including aminophylline, epinephrine, isoproterenol, and theophylline.
- Pindolol can increase the effect of antianxiety benzodiazepine drugs.
- If you are also taking ergot alkaloids for migraines, pindolol may worsen side effects such as cold hands and feet. In rare cases, this drug combination can lead to gangrene.
- Monoamine oxidase inhibitor (MAOI) antidepressants should not be taken at the same time as or within 14 days of pindolol.
- Pindolol may interact with anesthetics during surgery, increasing the risk of heart problems. As a result, your health-care practitioner will instruct you how to stop taking this drug two days before surgery.
- Alcohol intensifies the drowsiness caused by this drug.
- Cocaine and cigarette smoking may reduce the effectiveness of pindolol.
- Ask your health-care practitioner about taking over-the-counter cough, cold, allergy, and weight loss remedies. Many of these can raise blood pressure.

FOOD, VITAMIN, AND HERBAL INTERACTIONS

Do not take herbs that increase blood pressure, including ephedra (ma huang), ginseng, goldenseal, licorice, and saw palmetto. Consult your health-care practitioner before taking substances that may lower blood pressure, such as calcium, soy, or garlic. Your health-care practitioner will probably recommend a low-sodium diet.

RECOMMENDED DOSAGE

Pindolol comes as a tablet. Although the doses given below are typical, only your health-care practitioner can determine the dose and schedule that are most appropriate for you.

- *Children:* This drug is not recommended for children under the age of 12.
- *Adults:* 10 mg daily to start, which may be gradually increased as needed to a maximum daily dose of 60 mg

If pindolol upsets your stomach, take it with food. If you forget to take a dose, take it as soon as you remember. If it is almost time for the next dose, skip the forgotten one, and resume your normal schedule. Never take double doses.

Continue to take this drug even if you feel well. Do not discontinue use without consulting your health-care practitioner. Abrupt withdrawal can cause chest pain, breathing difficulties, increased sweating, and an irregular heartbeat. To end treatment, in most cases your health-care practitioner will reduce dosage gradually over 2 to 3 weeks.

SYMPTOMS OF OVERDOSE AND WHAT TO DO

The symptoms of pindolol overdose include slow heart rate, low blood pressure, dizziness, fainting, difficulty breathing, bluish fingernails and palms, and seizures. If overdose occurs, seek immediate medical attention and take the bottle of pindolol to the hospital with you.

SPECIAL INFORMATION FOR PREGNANT OR NURSING WOMEN

Some studies have shown that women who take beta-blockers during pregnancy give birth to babies with lower birth weight, heart rate, and blood pressure. As a result, pindolol should be avoided if you are pregnant.

Small amounts of pindolol can pass into breast milk and cause problems such as slow heart rate, low blood pressure, and trouble breathing. If you must take pindolol, your health-care practitioner may recommend bottle-feeding.

SPECIAL INFORMATION FOR SENIORS

Seniors usually require lower doses of pindolol. Older people are more apt to experience side effects such as heightened sensitivity to the cold, a general feeling of unwellness, chest pain, breathing difficulties, sweating, and variations in heartbeat.

GENERIC NAME

Pioglitazone

BRAND NAME

Actos

No generic available

ABOUT THIS DRUG

Pioglitazone is used to treat the form of diabetes mellitus known as type 2. Type 2 diabetes was formerly known as adult-onset, and is also referred to as noninsulin-dependent. Pioglitazone may be prescribed alone, or with metformin, insulin, or antidiabetes drugs called sulfonylureas. Diet and exercise also play a key role in the management of diabetes.

Pioglitazone helps your body regulate the amount of glucose (sugar) in blood. It works by making cells more sensitive to insulin.

SIDE EFFECTS

Consult your health-care practitioner if you develop side effects while taking this drug. Only he or she can determine whether it is safe for you to continue taking pioglitazone.

- *Common:* teeth problems, sinus irritation, headache, respiratory infection, sore throat, muscle aches
- *Less Common or Rare:* swollen arms and legs, weight gain, anemia, yellow eyes and skin, liver problems

IMPORTANT PRECAUTIONS

Pioglitazone should not be taken if you have liver impairment, hepatitis, anemia, swollen arms and legs, heart failure, type 1 diabetes, or diabetic ketoacidosis (a life-threatening condition caused by insufficient insulin, with symptoms such as nausea, fatigue, excessive thirst, lower chest pain, and fruity breath). Also inform your health-care practitioner if you have ever experienced an allergic reaction to this or similar drugs.

Pioglitazone does not cause low blood sugar (hypoglycemia). However, this condition can occur, especially if you take pioglitazone with other antidiabetes medications. The people most susceptible to hypoglycemia are older, weak, or malnourished, or have kidney, liver, adrenal, or hormone problems. Symptoms vary from person to person, so it is essential to learn which symptoms you usually have. As soon as you experience the characteristic signs, address and control them quickly by taking a fast-acting sugar, such as a glucose tablet, glass of fruit juice or nondiet soft drink, tablespoon of corn syrup or honey, or tablespoon of table sugar dissolved in water.

People with uncontrolled diabetes may also experience high blood sugar, or hyperglycemia. Symptoms include drowsiness, blurred vision, loss of appetite, nausea, unusual thirst, dry mouth, and flushed skin. Check your blood sugar level and call your health-care practitioner. If this condition is not treated, it can lead to diabetic coma and death.

Carefully follow all diet and exercise recommendations made by your health-care practitioner and nutritionist. In fact, many people with type 2 diabetes are able to successfully control their disease by making healthy lifestyle changes, cutting back on the need for medication.

To monitor the effectiveness of pioglitazone, visit your health-care practitioner on a regular basis. Promptly report symptoms such as yellow skin and eyes, fatigue, appetite loss, dark-colored urine, and abdominal pain; these may be signs of liver damage. Consult your health-care practitioner during illness or stressful periods, or if you must have surgery. Your dosage may require adjustment.

Pioglitazone may reduce the effectiveness of oral contraceptives. Use alternate methods of contraception.

DRUG INTERACTIONS

Inform your health-care practitioner and pharmacist if you are taking any other prescription or over-the-counter drugs, as well as any vitamins, herbs, or other supplements. Possible drug interactions include the following:

- Pioglitazone increases the blood-sugar-lowering effects of insulin and other antidiabetes medications. Careful adjustment of dosage is necessary.
- This drug may reduce the effectiveness of oral contraceptives.
- Ketoconazole decreases the effects of pioglitazone.
- Pioglitazone may interfere with the effects of many other drugs. These include calcium channel blockers, erythromycin, astemizole, cisapride, corticosteroids, cyclosporine, statin cholesterol-lowering drugs, tacrolimus, triazolam, and trimetrexate.
- Do not drink alcohol while taking pioglitazone. Alcohol affects blood sugar levels.

FOOD, VITAMIN, AND HERBAL INTERACTIONS

Herbs such as garlic, ginger, ginseng, hawthorn, and nettle may affect blood sugar levels, and some experts recommend chromium for diabetics. However, always check with your health-care practitioner before using any dietary supplement.

RECOMMENDED DOSAGE

Pioglitazone comes in tablet form. Although the doses given below are typical, only your health-care practitioner can determine the dose and schedule that best fit your needs.

- *Children:* This drug is not recommended for children.
- *Adults:* 15 to 45 mg once daily.

Pioglitazone may be taken with or without food. If you forget a dose, take it as soon as you remember. If it is almost time for the next dose, skip the missed one and resume your normal schedule. Never take a double dose.

SYMPTOMS OF OVERDOSE AND WHAT TO DO

Little is known about pioglitazone overdose. If you suspect that an overdose has occurred, seek immediate medical attention and take the prescription bottle to the hospital with you.

SPECIAL INFORMATION FOR PREGNANT OR NURSING WOMEN

Pioglitazone should not be used during pregnancy. It is critically important to monitor and control blood sugar when you are pregnant. However, it is safer to accomplish this through diet or a combination of diet and insulin. Consult your health-care practitioner as soon as you think you may be pregnant or if you are planning to become pregnant.

If you are breastfeeding or plan to do so, talk with your health-care practitioner before starting this drug. Only a health-care practitioner can determine whether the potential benefits outweigh the potential dangers.

SPECIAL INFORMATION FOR SENIORS

There are no special instructions for seniors.

GENERIC NAME

Pirbuterol

BRAND NAME

Maxair

No generic available

ABOUT THIS DRUG

Pirbuterol is a bronchodilator medication used to prevent and treat wheezing, shortness of breath, and troubled breathing caused by asthma, chronic bronchitis, emphysema, and other lung diseases. An advantage of this drug is that it works more quickly and has more lasting effects than similar drugs.

Pirbuterol works by dilating bronchial tubes that are in constriction. It relaxes and opens air passages in the lungs, making it easier to breathe.

SIDE EFFECTS

Speak to your health-care practitioner if you develop side effects while taking this drug. Only he or she can determine whether you should continue taking pirbuterol.

- *Common:* dry mouth, throat irritation, changes in taste, nervousness, fast or irregular heartbeat, heart palpitations, nervousness, trembling
- *Less Common or Rare:* bad taste in mouth, cough, dizziness, tiredness, headache, stomach upset, nausea, vomiting, diarrhea, tremors, insomnia, heart rhythm disturbances, high blood pressure, worsening of asthma

IMPORTANT PRECAUTIONS

Tell your health-care practitioner about any other medical conditions you may have, especially heart disease, an irregular heartbeat, increased heart rate, high blood pressure, an overactive thyroid, glaucoma, diabetes, or seizures.

Inform your health-care practitioner if you have experienced allergies to this or similar medications in the past.

Because pirbuterol may cause side effects such as nervousness and dizziness, do not drive a car, operate machinery, or perform other tasks that require concentration until you know how this drug affects you.

To relieve dry mouth or throat irritation, use sugarless gum or hard candy, or rinse your mouth with water. If the problem continues, consult your health-care practitioner or dentist.

DRUG INTERACTIONS

Tell your health-care practitioner if you are taking any other prescription or over-the-counter drugs, as well as any vitamins, herbs, or supplements. Possible drug interactions include the following:

- Taking pirbuterol at the same time as or within 14 days of monoamine oxidase inhibitor (MAOI) antidepressants can cause a dangerous increase in blood pressure.
- Do not use other inhaled medications without consulting your health-care practitioner. This can result in increased cardiovascular side effects.
- Medications such as beta-blockers may decrease the effects of pirbuterol.

- Phenothiazines, disopyramide, procainamide, and quinidine may increase the risk of heart problems.
- Inform your health-care practitioner if you are taking digitalis or any form of stimulant drug.
- Check with your health-care practitioner before using over-the-counter drugs. Many cold, cough, allergy, sinus, and weight loss remedies can raise blood pressure.

FOOD, VITAMIN, AND HERBAL INTERACTIONS

Do not take herbs that increase blood pressure, such as ephedra (ma huang), ginseng, goldenseal, licorice, and saw palmetto. Combining pirbuterol with herbs including St. John's wort and kola can cause nervousness. Avoid caffeinated beverages such as coffee, tea, and cola while you are taking this drug.

RECOMMENDED DOSAGE

Pirbuterol comes as an aerosol. Although the doses given below are typical, only your health-care practitioner can determine the dose and schedule that best fit your individual needs.

Prevention and Treatment of Bronchospasm

- *Children:* This drug is not recommended for children under the age of 12.
- *Adults:* 1 to 2 inhalations every 4 to 6 hours, for a maximum daily dosage of 12 inhalations

Prevention of Exercise-Related Bronchospasm

- *Children:* This drug is not recommended for children under the age of 12.
- *Adults:* 2 inhalations taken 5 minutes before exercise

It is important to take pirbuterol exactly as prescribed. Taking it more often than recommended can result in a loss in effectiveness and heart rhythm disturbances. If you forget a dose, take it as soon as you remember. Take the rest of the day's doses at evenly spaced intervals, and resume your normal schedule the next day. Never take a double dose.

SYMPTOMS OF OVERDOSE AND WHAT TO DO

Symptoms of pirbuterol overdose may include chest pain, rapid heart rate, heart palpitations, nervousness, tremor, sweating, vomiting, and headache. If overdose occurs, seek immediate medical attention and take the prescription bottle to the hospital with you.

SPECIAL INFORMATION FOR PREGNANT OR NURSING WOMEN

No studies have adequately investigated the effects of pirbuterol during pregnancy or breastfeeding. If you are pregnant or plan to become pregnant, or if you are breastfeeding or plan to do so, talk with your health-care practitioner before starting this drug. Only a health-care practitioner can determine whether the potential benefits outweigh the potential dangers.

SPECIAL INFORMATION FOR SENIORS

Seniors may be more susceptible to side effects such as nervousness, heart rhythm disturbances, heart palpitations, and muscle tremors. Pirbuterol should be used with extreme caution in older people who have heart problems or high blood pressure.

GENERIC NAME

Piroxicam

BRAND NAME

Feldene
Generic available

ABOUT THIS DRUG

Piroxicam is a nonsteroidal anti-inflammatory drug (NSAID) used to relieve the pain and inflammation of rheumatoid arthritis, juvenile rheumatoid arthritis, osteoarthritis, and menstrual pain. Like all NSAIDs, piroxicam can cause gastrointestinal bleeding and ulcers.

This drug works by reducing the level of prostaglandins, chemicals in the body that produce inflammation and pain.

SIDE EFFECTS

Tell your health-care practitioner if you develop side effects while taking piroxicam. Only he or she can determine whether it is safe for you to continue taking this drug.

- *Common:* diarrhea, constipation, stomach upset, abdominal pain, indigestion, heartburn, gas, nausea, vomiting
- *Less Common or Rare:* gastrointestinal bleeding, ulcers, confusion, nervousness, sleep disturbances, dry mouth, sun sensitivity, head-

ache, dizziness, blurred vision, fainting, tingling in the hands or feet, fatigue, weakness, skin eruptions, hives, heart problems, difficulty breathing, painful urination, kidney damage, bloody or black, tarry stools

In rare instances, long-term treatment with piroxicam may cause stomach ulcers and bleeding. Seek immediate medical attention if you experience symptoms such as severe stomach pain, black, tarry stools, or vomiting material that looks like coffee grounds.

IMPORTANT PRECAUTIONS

Like all NSAIDs, piroxicam can cause gastrointestinal bleeding, ulcers, and stomach perforation. If you take this drug on a regular basis, these types of side effects can occur at any time, with or without warning. People with a history of gastrointestinal disorders such as ulcers, colitis, or bleeding should be extremely careful when taking piroxicam.

Do not take piroxicam if you have asthma or nasal polyps associated with aspirin use, ulcers, colitis, gastrointestinal bleeding, or a bleeding or blood cell disorder. Use this drug with caution if you have congestive heart failure, high blood pressure or other heart problems, dehydration or fluid retention, impaired liver or kidney function, or a bleeding disorder. Tell your health-care practitioner if you have ever experienced an allergic reaction to aspirin or related drugs.

Piroxicam may cause side effects such as blurred vision. Until you know how this drug affects you, do not drive a car, operate machinery, or perform other tasks that require concentration. Report visual problems to your health-care practitioner.

This drug may cause fluid retention and kidney or liver damage. Contact your health-care practitioner at once if you experience symptoms such as yellow skin and eyes, fatigue, appetite loss, dark-colored urine, abdominal pain, and swelling in the arms and legs.

Piroxicam may cause increased sun sensitivity. Wear protective clothing and apply sunscreen when using this drug.

DRUG INTERACTIONS

Tell your health-care practitioner and pharmacist if you are taking any other prescription or over-the-counter drugs, as well as any vitamins, herbs, or other supplements. Possible drug interactions include the following:

- Do not combine aspirin, ibuprofen, or other prescription or over-the-counter NSAIDs with piroxicam. These combinations increase the risk of bleeding.

- Other drugs that may increase the risk of bleeding include blood thinners such as warfarin.
- Taking piroxicam with antihypertensive medications such as beta-blockers and ACE inhibitors may decrease their blood pressure lowering effects.
- Taking piroxicam with lithium can lead to toxic levels of lithium in the body.
- Piroxicam may increase methotrexate and phenytoin side effects.
- Combining piroxicam with alcohol increases the risk of stomach bleeding and ulcers.

FOOD, VITAMIN, AND HERBAL INTERACTIONS

Do not combine piroxicam with the herbal remedies clove oil, feverfew, garlic, ginkgo, and ginseng. Like piroxicam, these herbs may affect clotting.

RECOMMENDED DOSAGE

Piroxicam comes in capsule form. Low starting doses and smallest effective doses are recommended. Although the dose given below is typical, only your health-care practitioner can determine the dose and schedule that best fit your individual needs.

- *Children:* This drug is not recommended for children.
- *Adults:* 20 mg once daily

Take piroxicam with food or an antacid to prevent stomach upset. If you forget to take a dose, take it as soon as you remember. But if it is almost time for the next dose, skip the one you missed and resume your normal schedule. Never take double doses.

SYMPTOMS OF OVERDOSE AND WHAT TO DO

Symptoms of piroxicam overdose include drowsiness, nausea, vomiting, and stomach pain. If an overdose occurs, seek immediate medical attention and take the bottle of piroxicam to the hospital with you so the health-care practitioner will know exactly what medication was taken.

SPECIAL INFORMATION FOR PREGNANT OR NURSING WOMEN

No studies have adequately investigated the effects of piroxicam during pregnancy. If you are pregnant or plan to become pregnant, talk with your health-care practitioner before starting this drug. Only a health-care practitioner can determine whether the potential benefits outweigh the risks. In animal studies, piroxicam has decreased the amount of milk. Your health-care practitioner will most likely recommend that you forego breastfeeding while taking this drug.

SPECIAL INFORMATION FOR SENIORS

Seniors may be more susceptible to side effects.

GENERIC NAME
Podofilox

BRAND NAME

Condylox
No generic available

ABOUT THIS DRUG

Podofilox is used to treat external genital warts. These warts can appear in the genital and anal areas and on the abdomen. They are caused by the human papillomavirus.

Podofilox is for topical application only, and is not used for internal warts. This drug works by destroying the skin of the wart.

SIDE EFFECTS

Consult your health-care practitioner if you develop side effects while using podofilox. Only he or she can determine whether it is safe for you to continue using this drug.

- *Common:* blistering, crusting, scabbing, burning, itching, dryness, peeling, soreness, tenderness, stinging, tingling, bleeding, skin erosion
- *Less Common or Rare:* sleeplessness, dizziness, bad odor, pain during intercourse, scarring, blood in the urine, headache, vomiting

IMPORTANT PRECAUTIONS

Proper diagnosis is necessary before using this treatment. Do not get medication in your eyes, and wash your hands thoroughly after application. Do not use this medication if you have ever experienced an allergic reaction to it or similar medications. Always tell your health-care practitioner about all other medical conditions you have.

DRUG INTERACTIONS

Although no specific interactions are known, always inform your health-care practitioner and pharmacist if you are taking any other prescription or over-the-counter drugs, as well as any vitamins, herbs, or other supplements.

FOOD, VITAMIN, AND HERBAL INTERACTIONS

No food, vitamin, or herbal interactions have been noted.

RECOMMENDED DOSAGE

Podofilox comes as a gel and solution. The doses given below are typical. However, consult your health-care practitioner for the exact dose and schedule that are most appropriate for you.

- *Children:* This drug is not recommended for children.
- *Adults:* Apply a small amount to warts twice daily for 3 days. Skip 4 days. If warts are still apparent, this cycle can be repeated for up to 4 weeks.

If you forget a dose, use it as soon as you remember. If it is within 4 hours of the next dose, skip the forgotten one, and resume your normal schedule. Never apply double doses.

SYMPTOMS OF OVERDOSE AND WHAT TO DO

Symptoms of overdose may include nausea, vomiting, diarrhea, chills, fever, sore throat, unusual bleeding, and oral ulcers. If overdose occurs, seek immediate medical attention and take the prescription container to the hospital with you.

SPECIAL INFORMATION FOR PREGNANT OR NURSING WOMEN

High doses of podofilox have caused birth defects in animal studies. If you are pregnant or plan to become pregnant, or if you are breastfeeding or plan to do so, talk with your health-care practitioner before starting this drug. Only a health-care practitioner can determine whether the potential benefits outweigh the potential dangers.

SPECIAL INFORMATION FOR SENIORS

There are no special instructions for seniors.

GENERIC NAME

Polythiazide

see Thiazide Diuretics, page 1020

GENERIC NAME

Potassium

BRAND NAMES

Cena-K, Effer-K, Gen-K, Kaochlor 10%, Kaochlor S-F, Kaon, Kaon-Cl 20%, K+Care, Kay Ciel, Kaylixir, K-Dur 10, K-Dur 20, K-G Elixir, K-Lease, K-Lor, Klor-Con, Klorvess, Klotrix, K-Lyte, K-Norm, Kolyum, K-Tab, Micro K Extencaps, Potosalan, Rum-K, Slow-K, Ten-K, Tri-K, Twin-K

Generic available

ABOUT THIS DRUG

Potassium is used to treat low levels of potassium in the body (hypokalemia) and mild high blood pressure (hypertension). Normally a well-balanced diet provides all the potassium you need for good health. However, certain diseases (such as kidney disease or gastrointestinal problems accompanied by vomiting and diarrhea) and medications (such as diuretics or "water pills") deplete your body's supply of this vital mineral.

Potassium is essential for the proper functioning of the kidneys, heart, and other organs. A shortage can lead to problems such as nausea, vomiting, muscle weakness, mood changes, and irregular heartbeat. Supplements make up for any depletion of potassium. They are available in a wide variety of brands, types, and forms. Depending on your particular needs, your health-care practitioner may prescribe potassium chloride, potassium gluconate, or potassium-containing salt substitutes.

SIDE EFFECTS

Speak to your health-care practitioner if you develop side effects while taking this drug. Only he or she can determine if you should continue to take potassium.

- ➤ *Common:* diarrhea, nausea, gas, stomach discomfort or pain, vomiting
- ➤ *Less Common or Rare:* low blood pressure, muscle weakness, heaviness in the legs, tingling in the hands and feet, confusion, rash, abnormal heart rhythms

In rare cases, people taking potassium develop hyperkalemia (high blood potassium levels). Those with kidney disease are especially susceptible to this problem. Stop taking potassium and contact your health-care practitioner at once if you develop symptoms such as low blood pressure, muscle weakness, tingling, heaviness in the legs, breathing difficulties, confusion, listlessness, abnormal heart rhythms, restlessness, and pallor.

IMPORTANT PRECAUTIONS

Always tell your health-care practitioner about any other medical conditions you may have, especially Addison's disease, dehydration, heat cramps, diabetes, esophageal blockage, kidney or liver disease, diarrhea, heart disease, intestinal blockage, stomach ulcers, or severe burns. People with heart problems will most likely be advised to avoid slow-release forms of potassium.

Check with your health-care practitioner before starting any new exercise program. Exercise can increase the amount of potassium in the body. If you become dehydrated or your muscles cramp up, do not take potassium.

DRUG INTERACTIONS

Inform your health-care practitioner and pharmacist if you are taking any other prescription or over-the-counter drugs, as well as any vitamins, herbs, or other supplements. Possible drug interactions include the following:

- Taking potassium with ACE inhibitors may result in hyperkalemia (high blood potassium levels).
- Do not take potassium with potassium-sparing diuretics.
- When combined with potassium, certain drugs may cause or worsen stomach or intestinal problems. These include amantadine, anticholinergics, antidepressants, antihistamines, antipsychotics, buclizine, carbamazepine, disopyramide, flavoxate, meclizine, methylphenidate, oxybutynin, procainamide, promethazine, quinidine, and trimeprazine.
- Taking digitalis with potassium may worsen heart problems.

FOOD, VITAMIN, AND HERBAL INTERACTIONS

For good health, follow a balanced diet. Do not use excess salt, which can cause potassium depletion. Do not use low-salt products (which often contain potassium) without consulting your health-care practitioner.

RECOMMENDED DOSAGE

Potassium is available in a wide variety of forms, including oral liquid, powder, granules, effervescent tablets, regular tablets, and sustained-release tablets or capsules. Do not change from one potassium product to another without consulting your health-care practitioner. The doses given below are typical. However, doses are different for different patients, and only your health-care practitioner can determine the dose and schedule that are most appropriate for you.

- *Children:* Consult your health-care practitioner.
- *Adults:* 1,600 to 2,000 mg daily

Closely follow the directions for taking any potassium supplement. All forms of potassium should be taken with a full glass of water or fruit juice, with or immediately after meals. Swallow sustained-release tablets and capsules whole. If you miss a dose, take it as soon as you remember. However, if it is nearly time for your next scheduled dose, do not take the missed dose. Follow your regular dosing schedule. Never take a double dose.

SYMPTOMS OF OVERDOSE AND WHAT TO DO

Symptoms of potassium overdose may include low blood pressure, muscle weakness, heaviness in the legs, breathing difficulties, confusion, listlessness, abnormal heart rhythms, and heart attack. If you suspect that an overdose has occurred, seek immediate medical attention and take the prescription bottle to the hospital with you.

SPECIAL INFORMATION FOR PREGNANT OR NURSING WOMEN

Potassium supplements are considered safe to use during pregnancy and breastfeeding. However, always consult your health-care practitioner before taking any drug while pregnant or breastfeeding.

SPECIAL INFORMATION FOR SENIORS

There are no special instructions for seniors.

GENERIC NAME

Pramipexole

BRAND NAME

Mirapex

No generic available

ABOUT THIS DRUG

Pramipexole is used to treat Parkinson's disease. It is often combined with levodopa or carbidopa. An advantage of pramipexole is that if you experience the "on-off" phenomenon—in which symptom-free periods alternate with periods in which medication loses its effect—pramipexole extends the positive "on" periods and shortens the negative "off" ones.

Like other antiparkinsonian drugs, pramipexole works by correcting the dopamine deficiency that is believed to be the cause of Parkinson's disease. It works by enhancing the activity of the dopamine that is available.

SIDE EFFECTS

Side effects from pramipexole are common. Call your health-care practitioner if they become severe or do not go away. Contact your health-care practitioner immediately if you experience alarming side effects such as hallucinations, eye problems, or muscle wasting. Only your health-care practitioner can determine if you should continue to take this drug.

- *Common:* hallucinations, abnormal dreams, memory loss, nausea, lack of appetite, dry mouth, constipation, confusion, fatigue, dizziness, dizziness upon standing, weakness, difficulty sleeping, involuntary or jerky body movements, difficulty walking, increased urination, urinary tract infections, chest pain, difficulty breathing, arthritis, vision abnormalities
- *Less Common or Rare:* overall feeling of unwellness, impotence, reduced sex drive, restlessness, muscle spasms or twitching, delusions, thinking abnormalities, difficulty swallowing, urinary incontinence, circulation problems, skin disorders, eye disorders, pneumonia, blood clots, heart or lung problems, mental illness, convulsions

IMPORTANT PRECAUTIONS

Always inform your health-care practitioner of any other medical conditions you have, especially kidney problems, eye problems, low blood pressure, or hallucinations.

Older people and those with advanced Parkinson's disease are more susceptible to side effects such as hallucinations and drowsiness. Contact your health-care practitioner if you experience problems such as falling asleep while going about your daily activities.

Because pramipexole may cause side effects such as dizziness and fatigue, do not drive a car, operate machinery, or perform other tasks that require concentration until you know how this drug affects you.

When you first start taking this drug or when the dosage is increased, you may experience dizziness or faintness when you rise quickly from a sitting or reclining position (postural hypotension). Try to get up slowly, and consult your health-care practitioner if the problem continues.

Pramipexole may cause dry mouth. To counteract this effect, use sugarless gum or candy, ice chips, or a saliva substitute. If the problem continues, consult your health-care practitioner or dentist.

To monitor treatment, visit your health-care practitioner on a regular basis.

DRUG INTERACTIONS

Tell your health-care practitioner and pharmacist if you are taking any other prescription or over-the-counter drugs, as well as any vitamins, herbs, or other supplements. Possible drug interactions include the following:

- Combining pramipexole with levodopa or carbidopa may cause twitching or jerky movements. To prevent these effects, your health-care practitioner will adjust the dosage of medications.
- Cimetidine increases the effects of pramipexole.
- Drugs that are eliminated through the kidneys—such as ranitidine and verapamil—reduce the body's ability to clear pramipexole.
- Many drugs decrease the effects of pramipexole. These include haloperidol, phenothiazines, thioxanthenes, and metoclopramide.
- Pramipexole may increase the effects of central nervous system depressants such as tranquilizers.

FOOD, VITAMIN, AND HERBAL INTERACTIONS

Consult your health-care practitioner before combining pramipexole with any herbs with sedative effects, such as catnip, elecampane, goldenseal, gotu kola, hops, kava, lemon balm, skullcap, St. John's wort, and valerian.

RECOMMENDED DOSAGE

Pramipexole is available in tablet form. Although the doses given below are typical, only your health-care practitioner can determine the dose and schedule that are most appropriate for you.

- *Children:* This drug is not recommended for children.
- *Adults:* 0.125 mg 3 times daily to start, which can be gradually increased as needed to a maximum daily dose of 4.5 mg

To prevent stomach upset, take pramipexole with food. If you miss a dose, take it as soon as you remember. However, if it is almost time for the next dose, skip the one you missed and go back to your regular dosing schedule. Never take a double dose. Do not stop taking pramipexole suddenly. This may cause severe Parkinson's symptoms to return.

SYMPTOMS OF OVERDOSE AND WHAT TO DO

Little is known about pramipexole overdose. However, if you suspect an overdose, seek medical attention immediately, and bring the prescription bottle with you to the hospital so that health-care practitioners will know exactly what drug was used.

SPECIAL INFORMATION FOR PREGNANT OR NURSING WOMEN

No studies have adequately investigated the effects of pramipexole during pregnancy or breastfeeding. If you are pregnant or plan to become pregnant, or if you are breastfeeding or plan to do so, talk with your health-care practitioner before starting this drug. Only a health-care practitioner can determine whether the potential benefits outweigh the potential dangers.

SPECIAL INFORMATION FOR SENIORS

Seniors may be more susceptible to side effects such as hallucinations and drowsiness.

GENERIC NAME

Pravastatin

see Statin Cholesterol-Lowering Drugs, page 959

GENERIC NAME

Prazosin

BRAND NAME

Minipress
Generic available

ABOUT THIS DRUG

Prazosin is used to treat high blood pressure (hypertension). It may be prescribed alone or with other antihypertensive medications, such as thiazide diuretics or beta-blockers. This drug must be taken regularly in order to be effective.

Prazosin works by controlling impulses along select nerve pathways in the body. This action relaxes and expands blood vessels, thus lowering blood pressure.

SIDE EFFECTS

Side effects such as dizziness are most common when you first start taking prazosin. However, if any side effects become persistent or severe, speak to your health-care practitioner. Only he or she can determine whether it is safe for you to continue taking this drug.

- *Common:* drowsiness, dizziness, headache, weakness, lack of energy, nausea, heart palpitations
- *Less Common or Rare:* dizziness upon standing, fainting, vertigo, shortness of breath, confusion, nervousness, depression, blurred vision, red eyes, constipation, diarrhea, dry mouth, nasal congestion, fluid retention, frequent urination, nosebleeds, rash, ringing in ears, pins and needles, painful erection, impotence, urinary problems, joint pain, rapid heartbeat

IMPORTANT PRECAUTIONS

Always inform your health-care practitioner about any other medical conditions you suffer from, especially angina (chest pain), kidney disease, or severe heart disease. Tell your health-care practitioner if you have ever experienced an allergic reaction to this or similar medications.

This drug may make you dizzy or drowsy. Until you know how prazosin affects you, do not drive a car, operate machinery, or perform other tasks that demand concentration.

When you first start taking this drug, you may experience dizziness or faintness when you rise quickly from a sitting or reclining position (postural hypotension). Try to get up slowly, and consult your health-care practitioner if the problem continues.

Be extremely careful when you exercise in hot weather. Heavy sweating can lead to dizziness, lightheadedness, fainting, vomiting, dehydration, and low blood pressure.

Prazosin may cause dry mouth. To counteract this effect, use sugarless gum or candy, ice chips, or a saliva substitute. If the problem continues, consult your health-care practitioner or dentist.

Treatment of high blood pressure also entails certain lifestyle changes, such as weight control, smoking cessation, and close attention to diet. Before having any type of surgery or dental procedure, tell your surgeon or dentist that you are taking prazosin.

DRUG INTERACTIONS

Tell your health-care practitioner and pharmacist if you are taking any other prescription or over-the-counter drugs, as well as any vitamins, herbs, or other supplements. Possible drug interactions include the following:

- Prazosin adds to the effects of other blood-pressure-lowering medications.
- Indomethacin may decrease the effects of prazosin.
- Alcohol may further lower blood pressure and increase the risk of side effects such as dizziness and lightheadedness.
- Consult your health-care practitioner before taking over-the-counter cough, cold, sinus, allergy, or weight loss medications. Many of these can raise blood pressure.

FOOD, VITAMIN, AND HERBAL INTERACTIONS

Do not take herbs that increase blood pressure, such as ephedra (ma huang), ginseng, goldenseal, licorice, and saw palmetto. Consult your health-care practitioner before taking substances that may lower blood pressure, such as calcium, soy, or garlic. Talk to your health-care practitioner about diet and salt intake.

RECOMMENDED DOSAGE

Prazosin is available in capsule form. Although the doses given below are typical, only your health-care practitioner can determine the dose and schedule that best fit your needs.

- *Children:* This drug is not recommended for children.
- *Adults:* 0.5 to 1 mg 2 to 3 times daily to start, which may be gradually increased as needed to a total daily dosage of 6 to 15 mg. The maximum daily dosage is 40 mg.

Prazosin can be taken with or without food. Continue to take this drug even if you feel well. Do not discontinue use without consulting your health-care practitioner. If you miss a dose, take it as soon as you remember. If it is almost time for the next dose, skip the forgotten one, and resume your normal schedule. Never take a double dose.

SYMPTOMS OF OVERDOSE AND WHAT TO DO

The symptoms of prazosin overdose include drowsiness and low blood pressure. If overdose occurs, seek immediate medical attention and take the prescription bottle to the hospital with you.

SPECIAL INFORMATION FOR PREGNANT OR NURSING WOMEN

No studies have adequately investigated the effects of prazosin during pregnancy or breastfeeding. If you are pregnant or plan to become pregnant, or if you are breastfeeding or plan to do so, talk with your health-care practitioner before starting this drug. Only a

health-care practitioner can determine whether the potential benefits outweigh the potential dangers.

SPECIAL INFORMATION FOR SENIORS
Seniors are more susceptible to side effects such as drowsiness, lightheadedness, and dizziness upon rising. Lower doses are recommended.

GENERIC NAME
Prednicarbate
see Corticosteroids, Topical, page 337

GENERIC NAME
Prednisolone
see Corticosteroids, Oral, page 330

GENERIC NAME
Prednisone
see Corticosteroids, Oral, page 330

GENERIC NAME
Procainamide

BRAND NAMES
Procan, Procan SR, Procanbid, Promine, Pronestyl, Pronestyl-SR
Generic available

ABOUT THIS DRUG
Procainamide is used to treat abnormal heart rhythms (arrhythmias). There are two types of arrhythmias. In tachycardia, heartbeats are faster than normal. In bradycardia, they are slower than normal.

This drug works by slowing the transmission of nerve impulses through the heart.

When irregular heartbeats are restored to a normal rhythm, the heart is able to function more efficiently.

SIDE EFFECTS
Because this drug may cause a number of serious side effects, you should be closely monitored by your health-care practitioner while

taking it. Immediately report any signs of infection or other unusual side effects to your health-care practitioner. Only he or she can determine whether it is safe for you to continue taking procainamide.

- *Common:* nausea, vomiting, abdominal pain, diarrhea, loss of appetite, bitter taste, lupus-like symptoms (abdominal and chest pain, joint pain and inflammation, muscle pain, fever, chills, skin lesions)
- *Less Common or Rare:* dizziness, weakness, giddiness, hallucinations, depression, flushing, rash, hives, itching, low blood pressure, changes in blood counts, anemia

Lupus-like reactions may occur in as many as 30% of the people who take procainamide. It is also possible to develop bone marrow suppression (a dangerous condition that prevents your body from making blood cells), especially in the first 3 months of taking this drug. Notify your health-care practitioner immediately if you experience symptoms such as appetite loss, dizziness, fever, chills, nausea, vomiting, sore throat, diarrhea, easy bleeding or bruising, cough, wheezing, joint or muscle pain, yellow skin or eyes, chest or abdominal pain, tremor, hallucinations, palpitations, or mouth ulcers.

IMPORTANT PRECAUTIONS

Always inform your health-care practitioner about any other medical conditions you suffer from, especially a heart block, heart failure, asthma or other lung ailments, liver or kidney problems, lupus erythematosus, or myasthenia gravis. Tell your health-care practitioner if you have ever experienced an allergic reaction to procainamide, procaine or other local anesthetics, or aspirin.

This drug may make you dizzy and weak. Until you know how procainamide affects you, do not drive a car, operate machinery, or perform other tasks that demand concentration.

Before having any type of surgery or dental procedure, inform your surgeon or dentist that you are taking procainamide. See your health-care practitioner on a regular basis while taking this medication.

DRUG INTERACTIONS

Tell your health-care practitioner and pharmacist if you are taking any other prescription or over-the-counter drugs, as well as any vitamins, herbs, or other supplements. Possible drug interactions include the following:

- Taking other antiarrhythmic drugs with procainamide may depress heart function.

- Combining procainamide with blood pressure medications (such as beta-blockers) increases the risk of side effects of procainamide.
- The effects of medications such as ambenonium, neostigmine, and pyridostigmine may be blocked by procainamide.
- Pimozide may increase the risk of heart rhythm disturbances.
- Do not use alcohol while taking procainamide.
- Consult your health-care practitioner before taking over-the-counter cough, cold, sinus, allergy, or weight loss medications. Many of these are stimulants.

FOOD, VITAMIN, AND HERBAL INTERACTIONS

Consult your health-care practitioner before taking herbal remedies that may affect the cardiovascular system, such as ephedra (ma huang), ginseng, goldenseal, hawthorn, licorice, and saw palmetto. Your health-care practitioner will probably recommend a low-fat, low-sodium, high-fiber, heart-healthy diet.

RECOMMENDED DOSAGE

Procainamide comes as a capsule, tablet, and extended-release tablet. Although the doses given below are typical, real doses are highly individualized according to the nature of your particular heart problem, age, and level of kidney function.

- *Children:* This drug is not recommended for children.
- *Adults:* 23 mg per pound of body weight daily, in divided doses

Procainamide should be taken on an empty stomach, 1 hour before or 2 hours after eating. However, if it upsets your stomach, ask your health-care practitioner about taking this drug with food.

It is particularly important to take procainamide on a regular basis at evenly spaced times. Try not to forget any doses. Procainamide works best when there is a constant amount in the blood. However, if you forget to take a dose and remember it within 2 hours (or 4 hours of the extended-release tablets), take it as soon as you remember. Otherwise skip the forgotten one, and resume your normal schedule. Never take double doses.

Continue to take procainamide even if you feel well. Do not discontinue use without consulting your health-care practitioner. Abrupt withdrawal can cause potentially serious changes in heart activity. To end treatment, in most cases your health-care practitioner will reduce dosage gradually.

SYMPTOMS OF OVERDOSE AND WHAT TO DO

The symptoms of procainamide overdose include changes in heart function and heartbeat. If overdose occurs, seek immediate medical attention and take the bottle of procainamide to the hospital with you.

SPECIAL INFORMATION FOR PREGNANT OR NURSING WOMEN

No studies have adequately investigated the effects of procainamide during pregnancy or breastfeeding. If you are pregnant or planning to become pregnant, or if you are breastfeeding or plan to do so, talk with your health-care practitioner before starting this drug. Only a health-care practitioner can determine whether the potential benefits outweigh the potential dangers.

SPECIAL INFORMATION FOR SENIORS

Seniors are more apt to experience side effects such as dizziness or lightheadedness, and usually require lower doses.

GENERIC NAME

Prochlorperazine

BRAND NAME

Compazine
Generic available

ABOUT THIS DRUG

Prochlorperazine is used to treat severe nausea and vomiting caused by radiation therapy, cancer chemotherapy, surgery, and other conditions. It is also prescribed for psychotic symptoms such as hostility and hallucinations, and for mental disorders including schizophrenia.

This drug is known as a phenothiazine. It works by affecting a part of the brain called the hypothalamus, which controls vital functions such as alertness, hormone balance, body temperature, metabolism, muscle tone, and vomiting.

SIDE EFFECTS

Drowsiness and yellow eyes and skin are common at the outset of therapy. Although they usually disappear within the first 4 weeks of treatment, consult your health-care practitioner if any side effects become persistent or severe while taking prochlorperazine. Only he or she can determine whether it is safe for you to continue taking this drug and whether it is necessary to readjust your dosage.

- *Common:* drowsiness, yellow eyes and skin (especially in the first weeks of treatment)
- *Less Common or Rare:* increase in psychotic symptoms, low blood pressure, rapid heart rate, heart attack, trouble swallowing, fever, headache, nausea, dizziness, dizziness or fainting upon rising, drowsiness, dry mouth, increased appetite, weight gain, agitation, insomnia, shoulder and neck pain, painful muscle spasms, jitteriness, swelling and itching skin, blurred vision, dilated pupils, menstrual irregularities, painful and persistent erections, impotence, infection, urinary problems, dark urine, slow or difficult speech, Parkinson-like reactions (such as rigidity, tremors, a shuffling gait, a mask-like appearance, and uncontrollable jerking movements), symptoms of tardive dyskinesia (such as lip smacking, wormlike movements of the tongue, and slow, rhythmical, involuntary movements), seizures

Contact your health-care practitioner immediately if you have an increase in psychotic symptoms or paranoid reactions. People taking antipsychotic drugs may also experience a rare but life-threatening set of side effects known as neuroleptic malignant syndrome (NMS). Symptoms include fever, difficulty breathing, rapid heartbeat, rigid muscles, mental changes, increased sweating, irregular blood pressure, and convulsions. Seek immediate medical attention.

Side effects such as lip smacking, wormlike movements of the tongue, and slow, rhythmical, involuntary movements are characteristic of a disorder known as tardive dyskinesia. Older adults (especially women) are more susceptible to this condition. If you experience tardive dyskinesia, your health-care practitioner will probably advise you to stop taking this drug.

IMPORTANT PRECAUTIONS

Prochlorperazine suppresses the natural gag reflex. As a result, some people taking this drug have accidentally choked to death.

You should not take prochlorperazine if you have neuroleptic malignant syndrome or if you have experienced a previous allergic reaction to this drug or other phenothiazines.

Tell your health-care practitioner if you have other medical conditions, especially kidney or liver disease, a seizure disorder, brain tumor, low blood pressure, heart disease, a history of heart attack, a blood disorder, dehydration, glaucoma, asthma or other lung disease, Parkinson's disease, an enlarged prostate, difficulty urinating, or intestinal blockage.

Before having any type of surgery or dental procedure, tell your surgeon or dentist that you are taking prochlorperazine.

This drug may impair your physical coordination and mental alertness. Until you know how prochlorperazine affects you, do not drive a car, operate machinery, or perform other tasks that demand concentration.

Drink plenty of fluids and avoid extreme heat. Be especially careful when you exercise in hot weather or enter a hot bath or sauna. Heavy sweating can lead to dizziness, lightheadedness, fainting, vomiting, and dehydration.

When you first start taking this drug or when the dosage is increased, you may experience dizziness or faintness when you rise quickly from a sitting or reclining position (postural hypotension). Try to get up slowly, and consult your health-care practitioner if the problem continues.

This drug may cause heightened sun sensitivity. Wear sunglasses and protective clothing, and apply sunscreen.

If prochlorperazine causes dry mouth, use sugarless gum or hard candy, ice chips, or a saliva substitute. Consult your health-care practitioner or dentist if the problem continues.

DRUG INTERACTIONS

Inform your health-care practitioner and pharmacist if you are taking any other prescription or over-the-counter drugs, as well as any vitamins, herbs, or other supplements. Possible drug interactions include the following:

- Taking central nervous system depressants such as tranquilizers, sleep aids, or antidepressants increases the effects of prochlorperazine.
- This drug may increase the effects of tricyclic antidepressants.
- Since prochlorperazine may cause low blood pressure, be cautious about combining this medication with antihypertensive drugs such as propranolol.
- Antianxiety benzodiazepines such as diazepam may also increase the risk of low blood pressure.
- Aluminum antacids and anticholinergic drugs reduce the effects of prochlorperazine.
- Do not combine prochlorperazine with lithium. This increases the risk of serious nerve side effects.
- Taking metoclopramide with prochlorperazine increases the risk of Parkinson-like reactions.

- Prochlorperazine reduces the blood-pressure-lowering effects of guanethidine.
- Prochlorperazine reduces the effects of appetite suppressants.
- Avoid alcohol while taking prochlorperazine.

FOOD, VITAMIN, AND HERBAL INTERACTIONS

Do not combine prochlorperazine with herbs that produce sedative effects, such as catnip, elecampane, goldenseal, gotu kola, hops, kava, lemon balm, skullcap, St. John's wort, and valerian. Stimulants such as ginseng, ephedra (ma huang), or caffeine may reduce the effectiveness of this drug.

RECOMMENDED DOSAGE

Prochlorperazine comes as a tablet, extended-release capsule, oral liquid, and rectal suppository. The doses given below are typical, but dosage is always carefully individualized according to a person's particular needs and reactions to therapy.

Severe Nausea and Vomiting

- *Children (20 to 29 Pounds):* 2 mg once or twice daily; maximum daily dosage is 7.5 mg
- *Children (30 to 39 Pounds):* 2 mg 2 or 3 times daily; maximum daily dosage is 10 mg
- *Children (40 to 85 Pounds):* 2 mg 3 times daily, or 5 mg 2 times daily; maximum daily dosage is 15 mg
- *Adults:* 15 to 40 mg daily, in single or divided doses; rectal dose is one 25-mg suppository twice daily

Psychosis

- *Children 2 to 5 Years:* 4 to 6 mg daily in divided doses to start; this dosage may be gradually increased as needed to a maximum daily dosage of 20 mg
- *Children 6 to 12 Years:* 4 to 6 mg daily in divided doses to start; this dosage may be gradually increased as needed to a maximum daily dosage of 25 mg
- *Adults:* 15 to 150 mg daily in divided doses

Prochlorperazine capsules must be swallowed whole. Do not allow liquid medication to touch your skin. If you forget a dose, take it as soon as you remember. If it is almost time for the next dose, skip it and resume your normal schedule. Never take a double dose. Although this drug is not habit-forming, dosage must be reduced gradually.

SYMPTOMS OF OVERDOSE AND WHAT TO DO

The symptoms of prochlorperazine overdose include weakness, fatigue, depression, low blood pressure, muscle spasms, fever, agitation, convulsions, and coma. If overdose occurs, seek immediate medical attention and take the prescription bottle to the hospital with you.

SPECIAL INFORMATION FOR PREGNANT OR NURSING WOMEN

Prochlorperazine is not generally recommended during pregnancy. However, if you experience severe nausea and vomiting, your health-care practitioner may prescribe this drug. Prochlorperazine may pass into breast milk, so breastfeeding is not recommended while you take it.

SPECIAL INFORMATION FOR SENIORS

Seniors require lower doses of prochlorperazine. Older people (especially women) are more likely to experience effects such as drowsiness, dizziness, low blood pressure, and tardive dyskinesia (with symptoms such as lip smacking, wormlike movements of the tongue, and slow, rhythmical, involuntary movements).

GENERIC NAME

Progesterone *see Progestins, page 876*

GENERIC NAME

Class: Progestins

Generics: (1) medroxyprogesterone acetate; (2) megestrol; (3) norethindrone acetate; (4) progesterone

BRAND NAMES

(1) Amen, Curretab, Cycrin, Provera; (2) Megace; (3) Aygestin; (4) Crinone, Gesterol, Prometrium
All available as generic except norethindrone acetate

ABOUT THESE DRUGS

Progestins are used to treat a variety of conditions, including irregular menstrual bleeding; breast, uterine, or kidney cancer; menopausal symptoms, in combination with estrogen replacement therapy (ERT); premenstrual tension; endometriosis (heavy uterine bleeding); and appetite and weight loss in people with AIDS (acquired immunodeficiency syndrome). High doses of progestins help some women become pregnant and successfully maintain their pregnancies, while low doses in oral contraceptives can prevent a pregnancy from occurring. These drugs are also used in egg donor and infertility procedures.

Progestins are hormones. Although used by both men and women for different purposes, they are derived from the female hormone progesterone. Progesterone, the primary hormone in pregnancy, prepares the womb for a fertilized egg and supports the continuing development of the fetus. Progestins direct other hormones to correctly start and stop the menstrual cycle. During ERT, progestins prevent estrogen from improperly thickening the lining of the uterus. In the treatment of cancer, progestins change cancer cells' ability to react to other chemicals that promote tumor growth. These drugs trigger the production of proteins that stimulate appetite in people with AIDS. Because of their many different effects, it is essential to take progestins exactly as prescribed by your health-care practitioner.

SIDE EFFECTS

Speak to your health-care practitioner if you develop side effects while taking this drug. Only he or she can determine if you should continue to take progestins.

- *Common:* abdominal pain, cramps, water retention, swollen feet and ankles, increase in blood pressure, dizziness, headache, mood changes, nervousness, weight loss or gain, fatigue, changes in vaginal bleeding (such as spotting or breakthrough bleeding), breast tenderness, dry mouth, frequent urination, loss of appetite, unusual thirst, acne, mental depression, rash
- *Less Common or Rare:* breast pain, backache, hot flashes, loss or gain of body hair, loss of sexual desire, unexpected or increased flow of breast milk, nervousness, trouble sleeping, headache, itching, unusual rashes, urinary infections, swollen or bleeding gums

Consult your health-care practitioner at once if you experience symptoms such as swelling or pain in a leg vein, shortness of breath, coughing, vision problems, migraine, or weakness or numbness in an arm or leg. These may be signs of a life-threatening blood clot.

IMPORTANT PRECAUTIONS

Always tell your health-care practitioner about any other medical conditions you may have, especially asthma, epilepsy, bleeding problems, blood clots, varicose veins, a history of stroke, heart or circulation problems, high cholesterol, kidney or liver disease, mental depression, diabetes, osteoporosis, or breast disease.

If you are sexually active, use another method of birth control while taking progestins for noncontraceptive use. If you suspect that you are pregnant, stop taking medication immediately and consult your health-care practitioner.

Unexpected vaginal bleeding (such as spotting or breakthrough bleeding) may occur while you are taking progestins. If this is persistent or severe, or if it is more than 45 days since your last period, see your health-care practitioner.

By changing your hormone balance, progestins may cause temporary thinning of the bones. These drugs may also mask the symptoms of menopause.

Low-dose progestin-only oral contraceptives are usually prescribed for women who cannot take estrogen. However, they are typically not as effective as estrogen-progestin combinations. Keep in mind too that no method of birth control is 100% effective. (For further information, see CONTRACEPTIVES, ORAL.)

Progestins may cause side effects such as dizziness. Until you know how this medication affects you, do not drive a car, operate machinery, or perform other tasks that demand concentration.

Because progestins may affect the gums, good oral hygiene and regular visits to the dentist are essential.

Progestins may increase your sensitivity to the sun. Wear protective clothing and apply sunscreen.

Before having any type of surgery, medical test, or dental procedure, tell your surgeon or dentist that you are taking progestins. To monitor your progress, your health-care practitioner will want to see you at least once every 6 to 12 months.

DRUG INTERACTIONS

Inform your health-care practitioner and pharmacist if you are taking any other prescription or over-the-counter drugs, as well as any vitamins, herbs, or other supplements. Possible drug interactions include the following:

- A number of medications may decrease the effects of progestins. These include aminoglutethimide, carbamazepine, phenobarbital, phenytoin, rifabutin, and rifampin.

➤ If you have diabetes, a decrease in glucose tolerance may require an alteration in your medication.

FOOD, VITAMIN, AND HERBAL INTERACTIONS

Calcium and vitamin D supplements may counteract effects such as temporary thinning of the bones.

RECOMMENDED DOSAGE

Progestins are available in a wide variety of forms, including tablets, injections, suppositories, and gel. The dose and schedule your health-care practitioner prescribes will depend on the type of medicine prescribed, the brand, and the medical condition being treated. Never change the type or brand you take without consulting your health-care practitioner.

If progestins upset your stomach, take them with food. If you miss a dose, take it as soon as you remember. However, if it nearly time for your next scheduled dose, do not take the missed dose. Follow your regular dosing schedule. Never take a double dose.

SYMPTOMS OF OVERDOSE AND WHAT TO DO

No specific information is available regarding overdose. However, if you suspect that an overdose has occurred, seek immediate medical attention and take the prescription bottle to the hospital with you.

SPECIAL INFORMATION FOR PREGNANT OR NURSING WOMEN

Progestins may cause birth defects, especially in the first 4 months of pregnancy. Notify your health-care practitioner at once if you become pregnant while taking these drugs. Progestins may increase or decrease the amount of breast milk produced. Your health-care practitioner may advise you to refrain from breastfeeding while taking this medication.

SPECIAL INFORMATION FOR SENIORS

There are no special instructions for seniors.

GENERIC NAME

Promethazine

see Antihistamine-Decongestant Combination, page 132

GENERIC NAME

Class: Propionic acid (NSAID) family

Generics: (1) fenoprofen; (2) flurbiprofen; (3) ibuprofen; (4) ketoprofen; (5) naproxen; (6) oxaprozin

BRAND NAMES

(1) Nalfon, Nalfon 200; (2) Ansaid, Ocufen; (3) Advil, Dolgesic, Genpril, Haltran, Ibren, Ibu, Ibuprin, Ibuprohm, Medipren, Motrin, Nuprin, Q-Profen, Rufen, Trendar; (4) Actron, Orudis, Oruvail; (5) Aleve, Anaprox, EC-Naprosyn, Naprelan, Napron X, Naprosyn; (6) Daypro
All available as generic except oxaprozin

ABOUT THESE DRUGS

Nonsteroidal anti-inflammatory drugs (NSAIDs) are used to relieve the pain and inflammation of rheumatoid arthritis and osteoarthritis. They may also be recommended for other conditions, including menstrual cramps, muscle sprains and strains, bursitis, tendonitis, gout attacks, and other types of pain. In addition, ibuprofen and naproxen are used to reduce fever. NSAIDs are available both by prescription and over-the-counter. They work by reducing the level of prostaglandins, chemicals in the body that produce inflammation and pain.

SIDE EFFECTS

NSAIDs may cause potentially serious side effects, especially when used for a long time and in large doses. If you develop side effects while taking one of these drugs, ask your health-care practitioner whether it is safe for you to continue taking it.

- *Common:* diarrhea, constipation, stomach upset or pain, gas, nausea, vomiting, fluid retention, ringing in the ears, appetite loss
- *Less Common or Rare:* headache, dizziness, blurred vision, sensitivity to light, confusion, fainting, tingling in the hands or feet, mouth sores, fatigue, weakness, abnormal bleeding or bruising, rash, hives, itching, heart palpitations, difficulty breathing, gastrointestinal bleeding, ulcers, painful urination, kidney damage

Stop taking NSAIDs and consult your health-care practitioner immediately if you experience symptoms such as abdominal pain, stomach cramps, diarrhea, nausea, heartburn, indigestion, visual disturbances, vomiting of blood or material that looks like coffee grounds, or black, tarry stools. These may be signs of dangerous reactions such as ulcers or internal bleeding.

IMPORTANT PRECAUTIONS

NSAIDs can cause gastrointestinal bleeding, ulcers, and stomach perforation. If you take NSAIDs on a regular basis, these types of side effects can occur at any time, with or without warning. People with a history of ulcers, colitis, or any type of gastrointestinal bleeding should be extremely careful when taking any NSAID.

Do not take an NSAID if you have a bleeding disorder or asthma or nasal polyps associated with aspirin use. Use these drugs with caution if you have high blood pressure or other heart problems, or impaired liver or kidney function. Tell your health-care practitioner if you have ever experienced an allergic reaction to aspirin or related drugs.

Drinking 3 or more alcoholic beverages a day increases the risk of side effects such as bleeding.

Other possible side effects of NSAIDs include blurred vision and dizziness. Until you know how a drug affects you, do not drive a car, operate machinery, or perform other tasks that require concentration.

NSAIDs may cause increased sun sensitivity. Wear protective clothing and apply sunscreen when using these drugs.

Before undergoing any type of surgery or dental procedure, inform your health-care practitioner or dentist that you are taking an NSAID. Visit your health-care practitioner on a regular basis while taking these drugs.

DRUG INTERACTIONS

Tell your health-care practitioner and pharmacist if you are taking any other prescription or over-the-counter drugs, as well as any vitamins, herbs, or other supplements. Possible drug interactions include the following:

- Do not use more than 1 NSAID at a time. Combining NSAIDs increases the risk of bleeding.
- Other drugs that may increase the risk of bleeding include dipyridamole, sulfinpyrazone, valproic acid, and blood thinners such as warfarin.
- Taking NSAIDs with antihypertensive medications such as ACE inhibitors, beta-blockers, and diuretics decreases their blood-pressure-lowering effects.
- Mixing NSAIDs with cyclosporine may increase the negative kidney effects of both drugs.

- Taking NSAIDs with lithium or methotrexate can lead to toxic levels of lithium or methotrexate in the body.
- Do not use alcohol when you are taking an NSAID. Both are stomach irritants, and using them together can increase the risk of stomach bleeding and ulcers.

FOOD, VITAMIN, AND HERBAL INTERACTIONS

Do not combine NSAIDs with herbal remedies such as clove oil, feverfew, garlic, ginkgo, and ginseng. These herbs may affect clotting.

RECOMMENDED DOSAGE

NSAIDs come in a variety of forms, including tablets, extended-release tablets, caplets, capsules, extended-release capsules, gelcaps, and oral suspension. Low starting doses and smallest effective doses are recommended. The doses given below are typical. However, only your health-care practitioner can determine the dose and schedule that best fit your individual needs.

Fenoprofen

- *Children:* This drug is not recommended for children.
- *Adults:* 800 to 3,200 mg daily in divided doses

Flurbiprofen

- *Children:* This drug is not recommended for children.
- *Adults:* 200 to 300 mg daily in divided doses

Ibuprofen

- *Children:* Consult your health-care practitioner.
- *Adults:* 1,200 to 3,200 mg daily in divided doses

Ketoprofen

- *Children:* This drug is not recommended for children.
- *Adults:* 150 to 300 mg daily in divided doses

Naproxen

- *Children:* Consult your health-care practitioner.
- *Adults:* 500 to 1,250 mg daily in divided doses

Oxaprozin

- *Children:* This drug is not recommended for children.
- *Adults:* 1,200 to 1,800 mg daily in divided doses

NSAIDs may be taken with food, milk, or an antacid to prevent stomach upset. Your health-care practitioner may also advise you to take medication with a full (8-ounce) glass of water, and remain upright (do not lie down) for 15 to 30 minutes afterward. If you forget to take a dose, take it as soon as you remember. But if it is almost time for the next dose, skip the one you missed and resume your normal schedule. Never take a double dose.

SYMPTOMS OF OVERDOSE AND WHAT TO DO

Symptoms of NSAID overdose may include nausea, vomiting, diarrhea, abdominal pain, drowsiness, rapid breathing, rapid heartbeat, agitation, confusion, disorientation, sweating, ringing in the ears, stupor, and seizures. If an overdose occurs, seek immediate medical attention and take the prescription bottle to the hospital with you so the health-care practitioner will know exactly what medication was taken.

SPECIAL INFORMATION FOR PREGNANT OR NURSING WOMEN

Use of NSAIDs should be avoided in late pregnancy. If you want to take one of these drugs in early pregnancy, ask your health-care practitioner whether the potential benefits outweigh the risks. Because NSAIDs may pass into breast milk, it is best to stop breastfeeding while you take them.

SPECIAL INFORMATION FOR SENIORS

Smaller doses are recommended for seniors, who are more susceptible to side effects such as confusion, fluid retention, swelling of the feet and lower legs, stomach ulcers, and kidney or liver effects.

GENERIC NAME

Propoxyphene hydrochloride, propoxyphene napsylate

BRAND NAMES

Darvon, Darvon-N
Generic available

ABOUT THIS DRUG

Propoxyphene is an analgesic prescribed to relieve mild-to-moderate pain. It is considered to be as effective as aspirin in this regard, and about half as effective as codeine. There are two forms of propoxyphene: propoxyphene hydrochloride and propoxyphene napsylate.

This drug is a chemical derivative of the narcotic pain reliever methadone. It is more effective when combined with aspirin or acetaminophen.

SIDE EFFECTS

Inform your health-care practitioner if you develop side effects while taking propoxyphene. If symptoms are severe or prolonged, ask your health-care practitioner whether your dosage requires adjustment, and whether it is safe for you to continue taking this drug.

- *Common:* drowsiness, dizziness, nausea, vomiting
- *Less Common or Rare:* stomach pain, constipation, headache, lightheadedness, a false sense of well-being, weakness, visual disturbances

IMPORTANT PRECAUTIONS

Always inform your health-care practitioner about any other medical conditions you may have, especially emotional problems, mental depression, suicidal tendencies, a history of drug or alcohol abuse, a head injury or brain disease, a history of convulsions, kidney or liver impairment, asthma or other lung diseases, thyroid disease, urinary problems, an enlarged prostate, colitis, or heart disease. Do not take propoxyphene if you have ever experienced an allergic reaction to it or similar drugs.

Propoxyphene can lead to physical and/or psychological addiction. This drug should be used with caution in anyone with a history of drug or alcohol abuse, or of mental depression and suicidal tendencies.

If you plan to undergo surgery or a dental procedure, tell your health-care practitioner or dentist that you are taking propoxyphene.

This drug can make you drowsy and less alert than usual. Until you know how propoxyphene affects you, do not drive a car, operate machinery, or perform other tasks that require concentration.

DRUG INTERACTIONS

Tell your health-care practitioner and pharmacist if you are taking any other prescription or over-the-counter drugs, as well as any vita-

mins, herbs, or other supplements. Possible drug interactions include the following:

- Do not take monoamine oxidase inhibitor (MAOI) antidepressants at the same time as or within 14 days of propoxyphene.
- Do not take other central nervous system depressants (such as tranquilizers, barbiturates, sleep aids, antidepressants, or alcohol) with propoxyphene. This combination causes increased drowsiness, and in some cases has resulted in drug-related deaths.
- Drugs such as cimetidine increase blood levels and thus effects of propoxyphene.
- Naltrexone may reduce the effectiveness of propoxyphene.
- Propoxyphene may increase the blood-thinning effects of warfarin.
- Do not smoke cigarettes while taking propoxyphene.

FOOD, VITAMIN, AND HERBAL INTERACTIONS

Do not take propoxyphene with herbs such as hops, kava, passionflower, and valerian. These can increase its sedative effects.

RECOMMENDED DOSAGE

Propoxyphene comes as a capsule, tablet, or oral suspension. One hundred mg of propoxyphene napsylate provides the equivalent pain relief as 65 mg of propoxyphene hydrochloride. Although the doses given below are typical, only your health-care practitioner can determine the dose and schedule that best fit your needs.

Propoxyphene Hydrochloride

- *Children:* This drug is not recommended for children.
- *Adults:* 65 mg every 4 hours as needed, with a maximum daily dose of 390 mg

Propoxyphene Napsylate

- *Children:* This drug is not recommended for children.
- *Adults:* 100 mg every 4 hours as needed, with a maximum daily dose of 600 mg

To prevent stomach upset, propoxyphene may be taken with food. Take it with a full (8-ounce) glass of water. If you forget a dose, take it as soon as you remember. If it is almost time for the next dose, skip the missed one and resume your normal schedule. Never take a double dose. Because of the potential for addiction, never take more of this drug than is prescribed by your health-care practitioner.

SYMPTOMS OF OVERDOSE AND WHAT TO DO

The symptoms of propoxyphene overdose may include drowsiness, sluggishness, pinpoint pupils, breathing problems, convulsions, stupor, and coma. If overdose occurs, seek immediate medical attention and take the prescription bottle to the hospital with you.

SPECIAL INFORMATION FOR PREGNANT OR NURSING WOMEN

If you are pregnant or planning to become pregnant, discuss the potential risks versus the benefits of propoxyphene with your health-care practitioner. In animal studies, high doses of this drug have caused birth defects. Because propoxyphene may pass into breast milk, breastfeeding is not advisable while taking it.

SPECIAL INFORMATION FOR SENIORS

Seniors are at a higher risk of side effects such as drowsiness and dizziness. Smaller doses are preferable.

OPEN QUESTIONS OR CONTROVERSIES

Excessive doses of this drug—alone or with central nervous system depressants such as alcohol or tranquilizers—have resulted in drug-related deaths. In addition, propoxyphene can cause psychological and/or physical dependence. Do not take a larger dose of propoxyphene, take it more often, or use it for a longer period than your health-care practitioner recommends. Do not use it in combination with other drugs that cause drowsiness.

GENERIC NAME

Propranolol

BRAND NAMES

Betachron ER, Inderal, Inderal LA

Generic available

ABOUT THIS DRUG

Propranolol is a beta-adrenergic blocking agent (beta-blocker) prescribed to treat high blood pressure, angina pectoris (chest pain), and abnormal heart rhythms. It is also used to prevent second heart attacks, migraine headaches, and tremors.

Beta-blockers such as propranolol work by interfering with nerve impulses. They reduce the heart's workload and help it to beat more regularly.

SIDE EFFECTS

Contact your health-care practitioner if you develop side effects while taking this drug. Only he or she can determine whether it is safe for you to continue taking propranolol.

- *Common:* impotence
- *Less Common or Rare:* dizziness, lightheadedness, disorientation, confusion, anxiety, depression, short-term memory loss, insomnia, vivid dreams, hallucinations, excessive tiredness or weakness, slow heartbeat, heart failure, upset stomach, nausea and vomiting, constipation or diarrhea, rash, cold hands and feet, tingling, breathing difficulties, bronchospasm (wheezing cough associated with asthma and bronchitis), dry eyes, visual changes, hair loss, fever with sore throat, stuffy nose

IMPORTANT PRECAUTIONS

Always inform your health-care practitioner about any other medical conditions you suffer from, especially a slow heart rate or serious heart block, congestive heart failure, asthma or other lung ailments, liver or kidney problems, depression, diabetes or hypoglycemia, psoriasis, or a thyroid condition. Tell your health-care practitioner if you have ever experienced an allergic reaction to this or other beta-blockers.

Before having any type of surgery or dental procedure, inform your surgeon or dentist that you are taking propranolol.

This drug may make you more sensitive to the cold. Beta-blockers including propranolol can decrease blood circulation in the fingers, toes, and skin. Be sure to dress warmly in low temperatures, especially if you already have circulation problems.

Propranolol may make you drowsy. Until you know how this drug affects you, do not drive a car, operate machinery, or perform other tasks that demand concentration.

Treatment of high blood pressure also entails certain lifestyle changes, such as weight control, smoking cessation, and a low-sodium diet. Because taking propranolol can reduce or prevent chest pain, consult your health-care practitioner about what constitutes the right amount of exercise for you.

DRUG INTERACTIONS

Tell your health-care practitioner and pharmacist if you are taking any prescription or over-the-counter drugs, as well as any vitamins, herbs, or other supplements. Possible drug interactions include the following:

- Drugs that contain aspirin can lessen the blood-pressure-lowering effects of propranolol.
- Taking other blood pressure medications (including clonidine, reserpine, and calcium channel blockers) can increase the effects of propranolol.
- Medications such as quinolone antibiotics, oral contraceptives, tranquilizers, and cimetidine may increase the effects of propranolol.
- Propranolol can interfere with the action of oral antidiabetes medications. It may also change blood glucose levels.
- Propranolol may interfere with the effectiveness of certain asthma medications, including aminophylline, epinephrine, isoproterenol, and theophylline.
- Propranolol can increase the effect of antianxiety benzodiazepine drugs.
- If you are also taking ergot alkaloids for migraines, propranolol may worsen side effects such as cold hands and feet. In rare cases, this drug combination can lead to gangrene.
- Monoamine oxidase inhibitor (MAOI) antidepressants should not be taken within 14 days of propranolol.
- Propranolol may interact with anesthetics during surgery, increasing the risk of heart problems. As a result, your health-care practitioner will instruct you how to stop taking this drug two days before surgery.
- Alcohol intensifies the drowsiness caused by this drug.
- Cocaine and cigarette smoking may reduce the effectiveness of propranolol.

FOOD, VITAMIN, AND HERBAL INTERACTIONS

Do not take herbs that increase blood pressure, including ephedra (ma huang), ginseng, or licorice. Consult your health-care practitioner before taking substances that may lower blood pressure, such as calcium or garlic.

RECOMMENDED DOSAGE

Propranolol comes as a tablet, capsule, solution, or concentrate. Dosage depends on the condition being treated.

Hypertension

- *Children:* This drug is not recommended for children under the age of 12.
- *Adults:* 80 to 240 mg daily, divided into 2 or 3 doses

Angina Pectoris

- *Children:* This drug is not recommended for children under the age of 12.
- *Adults:* 80 to 320 mg daily, divided into 2, 3, or 4 doses

Arrhythmias (Irregular Heartbeats)

- *Children:* This drug is not recommended for children under the age of 12.
- *Adults:* 30 to 120 mg daily, divided into 3 or 4 doses, taken before meals and at bedtime

Heart Attacks

- *Children:* This drug is not recommended for children under the age of 12.
- *Adults:* 180 to 240 mg daily, divided into smaller doses

Migraines

- *Children:* This drug is not recommended for children under the age of 12.
- *Adults:* 80 to 240 mg daily, divided into smaller doses. If propranolol fails to relieve symptoms in 4 to 6 weeks, your health-care practitioner will gradually take you off this drug.

Tremors

- *Children:* This drug is not recommended for children under the age of 12.
- *Adults:* 80 to 320 mg, divided into smaller doses

It is best to take propranolol on an empty stomach. The extended-release tablets must be swallowed whole; do not crush, cut, or chew them. Dilute the concentrate with water, juice, or a soft drink, or mix with applesauce or pudding directly before taking. Continue to take propranolol even if you feel well. Do not discontinue use without consulting your health-care practitioner. Abrupt withdrawal can cause chest pain, breathing difficulties, increased sweating, irregular heartbeat, and even heart attack in some people. To end treatment, in most cases your health-care practitioner will reduce dosage gradually over a 2-week period.

SYMPTOMS OF OVERDOSE AND WHAT TO DO

If you suspect a propranolol overdose, seek immediate medical attention. The symptoms include slow heart rate, low blood pressure, dizziness, fainting, difficulty breathing, bluish fingernails and palms, and seizures. Take the bottle of propranolol with you to the hospital so that health-care practitioners will know exactly what drug was used.

SPECIAL INFORMATION FOR PREGNANT OR NURSING WOMEN

Some studies have shown that women who take beta-blockers during pregnancy give birth to babies with lower birth weight, heart rate, and blood pressure. As a result, propranolol should be avoided if you are pregnant.

Small amounts of propranolol can pass into breast milk and cause problems such as slow heart rate, low blood pressure, and trouble breathing. Your health-care practitioner may advise you to discontinue nursing until you complete treatment with this drug.

SPECIAL INFORMATION FOR SENIORS

Seniors usually require lower doses of propranolol. Older people are more apt to experience side effects such as sensitivity to the cold.

GENERIC NAME

Protriptyline

see Tricyclic Antidepressants, page 1076

GENERIC NAME

Pseudoephedrine

see Antihistamine-Decongestant Combination, page 132

GENERIC NAME

Pyrilamine

see Antihistamine-Decongestant Combination, page 132

GENERIC NAME
Quetiapine

BRAND NAME
Seroquel
No generic available

ABOUT THIS DRUG
Quetiapine is an antipsychotic drug used to treat psychotic disorders such as schizophrenia, as well as bipolar disease. Schizophrenia is characterized by disturbances in thinking, emotional reactions, and behavior.

This drug, the first in a new class of antipsychotics, works by lessening the action of two important nerve transmitters in the brain: dopamine and serotonin. This corrects an underlying imbalance believed to be responsible for a number of mental disorders.

SIDE EFFECTS
Side effects are common. If they become persistent or severe, talk to your health-care practitioner. Only he or she can determine whether it is safe for you to continue taking this drug and whether it is necessary to readjust your dosage.

- *Common:* headache, drowsiness, dizziness, weakness, dry mouth, upset stomach, indigestion, abdominal pain, constipation, weight gain, diminished or uncontrollable movement, low blood pressure, excessive muscle tone, nasal inflammation, neck rigidity, rash
- *Less Common or Rare:* rapid heartbeat, trouble swallowing, fever, cough, ear pain, flu, dehydration, sore throat, sweating, chills, palpitations, dizziness or fainting upon rising, loss of appetite, lack of emotion, hallucinations, delusions, paranoia, abnormal thinking or dreams, amnesia, confusion, stupor, difficulty breathing or speaking, asthma, underactive thyroid, bone pain, joint pain, back pain, arthritis, muscle weakness, trembling, twitching, swelling or stiffness in the feet and legs, heavy menstruation, loss of menstruation, vaginal inflammation or infection, rectal bleeding, hemorrhoids, intestinal inflammation, uncontrollable bowel movements, increased sex drive, abnormal ejaculation, impotence, visual disturbances, eye pain, sensitivity to light, ear ringing, seborrhea, eczema, itching, low blood sugar, diabetes, urinary frequency or incontinence, taste disturbances, teeth grinding, fungal infection, symptoms of tardive dyskinesia (such as lip smacking, wormlike movements of the tongue, and slow, rhythmical, involuntary movements)

People taking antipsychotic drugs may experience a rare but life-threatening set of side effects known as neuroleptic malignant syndrome (NMS). Symptoms include fever, difficulty breathing, rapid heartbeat, rigid muscles, mental changes, increased sweating, irregular blood pressure, and convulsions. Immediate medical attention is required.

Side effects such as lip smacking, wormlike movements of the tongue, and slow, rhythmical, involuntary movements are characteristic of a disorder known as tardive dyskinesia. Older adults (especially women) are more susceptible to this condition, which may become permanent. If you experience tardive dyskinesia, your health-care practitioner will probably advise you to stop taking this drug.

IMPORTANT PRECAUTIONS

You should not take quetiapine if you have neuroleptic malignant syndrome. Inform your health-care practitioner if you have ever experienced a previous allergic reaction to this or other antipsychotic drugs. Use quetiapine with caution if you have kidney or liver disease, a seizure disorder, heart disease, a history of heart attack or stroke, low blood pressure, dehydration, Alzheimer's disease, an underactive thyroid, or a history of breast cancer.

Before having any type of surgery or dental procedure, or undergoing anesthesia, tell your surgeon or dentist that you are taking quetiapine.

This drug may cause drowsiness, especially when you first start using it. Until you know how quetiapine affects you, do not drive a car, operate machinery, or perform other tasks that demand concentration.

Drink plenty of fluids and avoid extreme heat. Some antipsychotic drugs make it more difficult for your body to cool down. Be especially careful when you exercise in hot weather or enter a hot bath or sauna. Heavy sweating can lead to dizziness, lightheadedness, fainting, vomiting, and dehydration.

When you first start taking this drug or when the dosage is increased, you may experience dizziness or faintness when you rise quickly from a sitting or reclining position (postural hypotension). Try to get up slowly, and consult your health-care practitioner if the problem continues.

Your health-care practitioner will monitor your treatment at regular visits, especially during the first months of therapy. Eye exams are necessary, because in rare cases this drug has been associated with cataracts. Quetiapine may increase blood levels of cholesterol and triglycerides.

DRUG INTERACTIONS

Inform your health-care practitioner and pharmacist if you are taking any other prescription or over-the-counter drugs, as well as any vitamins, herbs, or other supplements. Possible drug interactions include the following:

- Quetiapine adds to the effects of central nervous system depressants such as tranquilizers, sleep aids, narcotics, antihistamines, anesthesia, and antidepressants.
- Drugs such as clarithromycin, diltiazem, erythromycin, fluconazole, itraconazole, ketoconazole, nefazodone, and verapamil may increase the effects of quetiapine.
- Drugs including carbamazepine, griseofulvin, phenylbutazone, phenytoin, primidone, rifampin, and saquinavir may reduce the effects of quetiapine.
- Quetiapine may interfere with the effects of antiparkinsonian drugs such as levodopa.
- Avoid alcohol while taking quetiapine.

FOOD, VITAMIN, AND HERBAL INTERACTIONS

Do not combine quetiapine with herbs that produce sedative effects, such as catnip, elecampane, goldenseal, gotu kola, hops, kava, lemon balm, skullcap, St. John's wort, and valerian. Also do not use ginseng, kola, or ephedra (ma huang) while taking this drug.

RECOMMENDED DOSAGE

Quetiapine comes as a tablet. The doses given below are typical, but dosage is always carefully individualized according to a person's particular needs and reactions to therapy.

- *Children:* This drug is not recommended for children.
- *Adults:* 150 to 750 mg daily

Quetiapine may be taken with or without food. If you forget a dose, take it as soon as you remember. If it is almost time for the next dose, skip it and resume your normal schedule. Never take a double dose.

SYMPTOMS OF OVERDOSE AND WHAT TO DO

The symptoms of quetiapine overdose include drowsiness, dizziness, rapid heartbeat, and fainting. If overdose occurs, seek immediate medical attention and take the prescription bottle to the hospital with you.

SPECIAL INFORMATION FOR PREGNANT OR NURSING WOMEN

No studies have adequately investigated the effects of quetiapine during pregnancy or breastfeeding. If you are pregnant or planning to become pregnant, or if you are breastfeeding or plan to do so, talk with your health-care practitioner before starting this drug. Only a health-care practitioner can determine whether the potential benefits outweigh the potential dangers.

SPECIAL INFORMATION FOR SENIORS

Seniors may be more sensitive to side effects such as drowsiness, dizziness, and fainting. Lower doses are recommended.

GENERIC NAME

Quinapril

BRAND NAME

Accupril
No generic available

ABOUT THIS DRUG

Quinapril is an angiotensin-converting enzyme (ACE) inhibitor used to treat high blood pressure (hypertension). This drug may be prescribed alone or with other high blood pressure medications, such as thiazide diuretics. It works by blocking an enzyme in the body, which relaxes blood vessels and lowers blood pressure.

SIDE EFFECTS

Speak to your health-care practitioner if you develop side effects while taking quinapril. Only he or she can determine whether you should continue taking this drug.

- *Common:* dizziness, lightheadedness, headache, cough, tiredness
- *Less Common or Rare:* angina (chest pain), faintness, vertigo, upset stomach, abdominal pain, nausea, vomiting, bleeding in the stomach or intestines, overall feeling of unwellness, dizziness upon standing, sleepiness, insomnia, constipation, dry mouth, sore throat, hair loss, nervousness, numbness, tingling, skin peeling, sensitivity to light, high potassium, kidney or liver problems, yellow eyes or skin, hepatitis, inflammation of the pancreas, increased sweating, heart rhythm disturbances, rapid heartbeat, high blood pressure, heart failure, heart attack, severe allergic reactions

IMPORTANT PRECAUTIONS

Always inform your health-care practitioner about any other medical conditions you suffer from, especially congestive heart failure, angina (chest pain), abnormal heart rhythms, or other heart problems. Also tell your health-care practitioner if you have kidney or liver disease.

Quinapril can affect your kidneys, especially if you have congestive heart failure. If you already have kidney disease, your dosage should be lower than usual. Your kidneys must be monitored while you take this drug.

Before having any type of surgery, anesthesia, or dental procedure, tell your surgeon or dentist that you are taking quinapril.

This drug may make you dizzy or drowsy. Until you know how quinapril affects you, do not drive a car, operate machinery, or perform other tasks that demand concentration.

Treatment of high blood pressure also entails certain lifestyle changes, such as weight control, smoking cessation, and close attention to diet.

When you first start taking this drug, you may feel lightheaded, and experience dizziness or faintness when you rise quickly from a sitting or reclining position (postural hypotension). Try to get up slowly, and consult your health-care practitioner if the problem continues.

Be extremely careful when you exercise in hot weather. Heavy sweating can lead to dizziness, lightheadedness, fainting, vomiting, dehydration, and low blood pressure.

Do not take this drug if you have ever experienced an allergic reaction to it or to other ACE inhibitors. If you have an allergic reaction such as swelling of the face and mouth and a sudden problem with breathing, seek immediate medical attention. Also contact your health-care practitioner immediately if you develop a sore throat and fever, or yellow eyes or skin.

Your health-care practitioner will monitor your response to this drug with regular blood counts and other tests.

DRUG INTERACTIONS

Tell your health-care practitioner and pharmacist if you are taking any other prescription or over-the-counter drugs, as well as any vitamins, herbs, or other supplements. Possible drug interactions include the following:

- ➤ Taking other blood pressure medications can increase the blood-pressure-lowering effects of quinapril.

- If you are already taking a diuretic, when possible your health-care practitioner will have you stop taking it 2 to 3 days before starting quinapril.
- Quinapril may increase blood levels of potassium, particularly when taken with potassium-sparing diuretics. Too much potassium can cause heart rhythm disturbances.
- Combining quinapril with allopurinol increases the risk of side effects.
- Taking quinapril with lithium can result in toxic levels of lithium in the blood.
- Phenothiazine tranquilizers and antiemetics may increase the effects of quinapril.
- Indomethacin may reduce the blood-pressure-lowering effects of quinapril.
- Separate doses of antacids and quinapril by 2 hours.
- Quinapril increases blood levels of digoxin.
- Avoid alcoholic beverages. Alcohol may further lower blood pressure, and increase the risk of dizziness and fainting.
- Consult your health-care practitioner before taking over-the-counter cough, cold, sinus, allergy, or weight loss medications. Many of these can raise blood pressure.

FOOD, VITAMIN, AND HERBAL INTERACTIONS

Do not take herbs that increase blood pressure, such as ephedra (ma huang), ginseng, goldenseal, licorice, and saw palmetto. Consult your health-care practitioner before taking substances that may lower blood pressure, such as calcium, soy, or garlic. To minimize possible interactions, take quinapril and iron supplements 2 to 3 hours apart. Because ACE inhibitors raise potassium levels in the body, *do not* take potassium supplements or use salt substitutes containing potassium, and ask your health-care practitioner how many potassium-rich foods (such as bananas, prunes, raisins, melons, tomatoes, citrus fruit, and orange juice) you can safely include in your diet. Also talk to your health-care practitioner about salt intake.

RECOMMENDED DOSAGE

Quinapril is available in oral form as tablets. Although the doses given below are typical, only your health-care practitioner can determine the dose and schedule that best fit your needs.

- *Children:* This drug is not recommended for children.
- *Adults:* 10 to 80 mg in single or divided doses

Take quinapril one hour before or two hours after meals. Continue to take this drug even if you feel well. Do not discontinue use without consulting your health-care practitioner. If you miss a dose, take it as soon as you remember. If it is almost time for the next dose, skip the forgotten one, and resume your normal schedule. Never take a double dose.

SYMPTOMS OF OVERDOSE AND WHAT TO DO

The symptoms of quinapril overdose may include dizziness and fainting caused by a severe drop in blood pressure. If overdose occurs, seek immediate medical attention and take the prescription bottle to the hospital with you.

SPECIAL INFORMATION FOR PREGNANT OR NURSING WOMEN

Do not take quinapril if you are pregnant (especially during the final six months). This drug can cause fetal injury and death. If you become pregnant while taking quinapril, call your health-care practitioner immediately.

Small amounts of quinapril may pass into breast milk. If you are breastfeeding, your health-care practitioner will likely advise you to stop until your treatment is done.

SPECIAL INFORMATION FOR SENIORS

Seniors usually require lower doses of quinapril.

GENERIC NAME

Quinethazone *see Thiazide Diuretics, page 1020*

GENERIC NAME

Quinidine

BRAND NAMES

Cardioquin, Quinaglute Dura-Tabs, Quinalan, Quinidex Extentabs, Quinora

Generic available

ABOUT THIS DRUG

Quinidine is used to treat arrhythmias (abnormal heart rhythms). Its use is reserved for certain types of dangerous heart irregularities.

This drug works by altering the flow of potassium in the heart. This allows the heart to beat at a normal, even rate.

SIDE EFFECTS

Because this drug may cause a number of serious side effects, you should be closely monitored by your health-care practitioner while taking it. Immediately report any signs of infection or other unusual side effects to your health-care practitioner. Only he or she can determine whether it is safe for you to continue taking quinidine.

- *Common:* nausea, vomiting, abdominal pain, diarrhea, appetite loss
- *Less Common or Rare:* dizziness, hallucinations, delirium, confusion, depression, apprehension, excitement, fainting, vertigo, lack of coordination, flushing, dilated pupils, intolerance to light, blurred or double vision, night blindness, ringing in the ears, joint or muscle pain, difficulty swallowing, rash, hives, eczema, itching, change in skin pigmentation, skin sensitivity to light, low blood pressure, changes in blood counts, anemia, swelling of the face, sore throat, fever, chills, hepatitis, asthma attack, wheezing, lupus, blood clots

High doses of quinidine are associated with a reaction known as cinchonism. Contact your health-care practitioner at once if you experience symptoms such as headache, nausea, ringing in the ears, hearing loss, visual disturbances, dizziness, and rash.

IMPORTANT PRECAUTIONS

Always inform your health-care practitioner about any other medical conditions you suffer from, especially heart block, low blood pressure, low potassium or magnesium levels, or a history of heart attack. In these types of circumstances, quinidine can actually *cause* heart irregularities.

In rare cases, people using this drug for long periods have experienced abnormal heart rhythms and fainting. These episodes are potentially fatal.

Tell your health-care practitioner if you have ever experienced an allergic reaction to quinidine, or to related drugs such as quinine. If you bruise easily when taking quinidine (or quinine), this drug is not for you. There have been rare cases of severe allergic reactions to quinidine, especially at the start of therapy. If you have asthma, myasthenia gravis, or an infection, the allergic reaction may not be readily apparent.

People with kidney or liver disease generally require lower doses of quinidine.

This drug may cause side effects such as blurred or double vision.

Until you know how quinidine affects you, do not drive a car, operate machinery, or perform other tasks that demand concentration.

Before having any type of surgery, dental procedure, or emergency treatment, inform your surgeon or dentist that you are taking quinidine. It is also essential that you visit your health-care practitioner on a regular basis to make certain that this drug is benefiting your condition without causing harmful side effects.

DRUG INTERACTIONS

Tell your health-care practitioner and pharmacist if you are taking any other prescription or over-the-counter drugs, as well as any vitamins, herbs, or other supplements. Possible drug interactions include the following:

- Quinidine may lead to toxic levels of digoxin in the body.
- Taking other antiarrhythmic drugs with quinidine may alter heart function.
- Quinidine may increase the effects of warfarin, beta-blockers such as metoprolol, propafenone, benztropine and other anticholinergic drugs, and tricyclic antidepressants.
- Many drugs decrease the effects of quinidine. These include barbiturates such as phenobarbital, phenytoin, nifedipine, rifampin, sucralfate, and bethanechol.
- Other drugs increase the effects of quinidine. These include some antacids, amiodarone, cimetidine, verapamil, and drugs that decrease urine acid levels.
- Do not use alcohol or tobacco while taking quinidine.
- Consult your health-care practitioner before taking over-the-counter cough, cold, sinus, allergy, or weight loss medications. Many of these are stimulants.

FOOD, VITAMIN, AND HERBAL INTERACTIONS

Caffeinated beverages may increase the irritability of your heart. Consult your health-care practitioner before taking any herbal remedies that may affect the cardiovascular system, such as ephedra (ma huang), ginseng, goldenseal, hawthorn, licorice, and saw palmetto. Your health-care practitioner will probably recommend a low-fat, low-sodium, high-fiber, heart-healthy diet.

RECOMMENDED DOSAGE

Quinidine comes as a regular or extended-release tablet. Although the doses given below are typical, actual doses are highly individualized according to the nature of your particular heart problem, age, and level of kidney function.

- *Children:* Consult your health-care practitioner.
- *Adults:* 600 to 1,800 mg daily, in single or divided doses.

If it upsets your stomach, quinidine can be taken with food. It is particularly important to take this drug on a regular basis at evenly spaced times. Try not to forget any doses. However, if you forget to take a dose and remember it within 2 hours of the regular time, take it. Otherwise skip the forgotten dose, and resume your normal schedule. Never take double doses. Do not change types or brands of quinidine or discontinue use without consulting your health-care practitioner.

SYMPTOMS OF OVERDOSE AND WHAT TO DO

Symptoms of quinidine overdose may include abnormal heart rhythms, blurred vision, confusion, headache, diarrhea, ringing in the ears, lethargy, seizures, and coma. If overdose occurs, seek immediate medical attention and take the prescription bottle to the hospital with you.

SPECIAL INFORMATION FOR PREGNANT OR NURSING WOMEN

No studies have adequately investigated the effects of quinidine during pregnancy or breastfeeding. If you are pregnant or planning to become pregnant, or if you are breastfeeding or plan to do so, talk with your health-care practitioner before starting this drug. Only a health-care practitioner can determine whether the potential benefits outweigh the potential dangers.

SPECIAL INFORMATION FOR SENIORS

Seniors are more apt to experience side effects and usually require lower doses.

OPEN QUESTIONS OR CONTROVERSIES

Quinidine relieves the symptoms of many people with severe heart rhythm disturbances. However, studies have shown that on average antiarrhythmic drugs do not improve the probability of long-term survival, and in some cases may even lower the chances.

GENERIC NAME
Rabeprazole

BRAND NAME
Aciphex
No generic available

ABOUT THIS DRUG
Rabeprazole is used to treat or prevent conditions in which there is too much acid in the stomach. It is prescribed for duodenal ulcers, gastroesophageal reflux disease (GERD), and Zollinger-Ellison syndrome. Rabeprazole works by blocking an enzyme that causes the stomach to produce excess acid. This eliminates an important cause of acid-related conditions, and creates a better environment for healing.

SIDE EFFECTS
Contact your health-care practitioner if you experience side effects while taking rabeprazole. Only he or she can determine whether you should continue to take this drug.

- *Common:* headache
- *Less Common or Rare:* changes in appetite, nausea, vomiting, diarrhea, constipation, gas, heartburn, stomach pain, joint or muscle pain, weakness, numbness, tingling or pain in the extremities, bruising, dizziness, fatigue, sleepiness, anxiety, depression, fever, fainting, dry mouth, ringing in the ears, nosebleeds, fluid retention, itching, chest pain, changes in liver function, high blood pressure

The reduction of stomach acid may make you more susceptible to bacterial infections such as *Campylobacter*. Promptly report symptoms such as fever and loose, mucousy stools to your health-care practitioner.

IMPORTANT PRECAUTIONS
Always inform your health-care practitioner about all other medical conditions you suffer from. Liver disease may increase the risk of side effects of this drug, and rabeprazole may worsen stomach infection. Tell your health-care practitioner if you have ever experienced an allergic reaction to this or similar medications.

Because rabeprazole may mask the symptoms of stomach cancer, cancer should be ruled out before taking it.

Rabeprazole may cause sleepiness, so limit activities such as driving as necessary.

DRUG INTERACTIONS

Inform your health-care practitioner and pharmacist if you are taking any other prescription or over-the-counter drugs, as well as any vitamins, herbs, or other supplements. Possible drug interactions include the following:

- Rabeprazole may increase the effects of digoxin.
- Rabeprazole may decrease the effects of drugs such as ketoconazole.
- Do not smoke cigarettes. This can worsen acid secretion.

FOOD, VITAMIN, AND HERBAL INTERACTIONS

Rabeprazole may interfere with the absorption of iron, zinc, and B vitamins such as folate. Taking a daily multivitamin-multimineral supplement is recommended. Do not use the herbs St. John's wort, kola, or ephedra (ma huang) while taking rabeprazole.

RECOMMENDED DOSAGE

Rabeprazole is available in tablet form. Although the doses given below are typical, only your health-care practitioner can determine the dose and schedule that are most appropriate for you.

Gastroesophageal Reflux Disease (GERD)

- *Children:* This drug is not recommended for children.
- *Adults:* 20 mg once a day for 4 to 8 weeks (or longer to prevent a relapse)

Duodenal Ulcers

- *Children:* This drug is not recommended for children.
- *Adults:* 20 mg once a day after the morning meal for 4 to 8 weeks

Zollinger-Ellison Syndrome

- *Children:* This drug is not recommended for children.
- *Adults:* 60 mg once a day to start, which may be gradually increased as needed

If you have a duodenal ulcer, take rabeprazole after your morning meal. The capsules should be swallowed whole. If you miss a dose, take it as soon as you remember. However, if it is nearly time for your next scheduled dose, do not take the missed dose. Follow your regular dosing schedule. Never take a double dose.

SYMPTOMS OF OVERDOSE AND WHAT TO DO

No specific information is available regarding overdose. However, if you suspect an overdose, seek immediate medical attention, and bring the prescription bottle with you.

SPECIAL INFORMATION FOR PREGNANT OR NURSING WOMEN

No studies have adequately investigated the effects of rabeprazole during pregnancy. If you are pregnant or plan to become pregnant, talk with your health-care practitioner before starting this drug. Only a health-care practitioner can determine whether the potential benefits outweigh the potential dangers. Because rabeprazole may pass into breast milk, your health-care practitioner may advise you to stop breastfeeding while you take this drug.

SPECIAL INFORMATION FOR SENIORS

There are no special guidelines for seniors.

GENERIC NAME

Raloxifene

BRAND NAME

Evista

No generic available

ABOUT THIS DRUG

Raloxifene is used to prevent and treat osteoporosis (thinning of the bones) in postmenopausal women. Risk factors for osteoporosis include family history, an inactive lifestyle, slim build, early menopause, insufficient calcium in the diet, and smoking or alcohol use.

This drug is similar to the hormone estrogen in that it increases bone density and reduces bone loss. An advantage is that raloxifene does not have the estrogen-like effects on the breasts and uterus that appear to increase cancer risk.

SIDE EFFECTS

Speak to your health-care practitioner if you develop side effects while taking raloxifene. Only he or she can determine whether you should continue taking this drug.

- *Common:* hot flashes, bloody or cloudy urine, chest pain, painful urination, frequent urge to urinate, vaginal itching, vaginal discharge, fever, infection, flu-like symptoms, body aches, congestion, sinus irritation, joint or muscle pain, swollen joints, leg cramps, upset stomach, gas, vomiting, mental depression, trouble sleeping, rash, unexplained weight gain, swelling of the hands, ankles, or feet
- *Less Common or Rare:* abdominal pain, body pain, lung congestion, visual disturbances, difficulty breathing, hoarseness, trouble swallowing, nausea, appetite loss, weakness, coughing blood, headache, migraine, numbness, shortness of breath, lost coordination, visual or speech disturbances

IMPORTANT PRECAUTIONS

Only postmenopausal women should use this drug. Do not take raloxifene if you are or are able to become pregnant, have blood-clotting problems, or have experienced a previous allergic reaction to this or similar medications. Women with liver disease should use this drug with caution. Always inform your health-care practitioner about any other medical conditions you suffer from, including cancer or congestive heart failure.

Raloxifene may cause hot flashes to occur. Contact your health-care practitioner if this happens.

Unlike estrogen, raloxifene does not stimulate the breasts or uterus. Call your health-care practitioner immediately if you experience breast pain, vaginal bleeding, or swelling of the hands and feet.

Because raloxifene increases the risk of blood clots, you will probably need to stop taking this drug at least several days before and following surgery (or any period of restricted activity or bed rest). When taking long car or plane trips, get up and walk around on a regular basis.

DRUG INTERACTIONS

Tell your health-care practitioner and pharmacist if you are taking any other prescription or over-the-counter drugs, as well as any vitamins, herbs, or other supplements. Possible drug interactions include the following:

- Raloxifene should not be used with estrogens.
- Cholestyramine reduces the absorption and effects of raloxifene.
- Raloxifene may reduce the effects of warfarin.
- Raloxifene may increase the effects of clofibrate, diazepam, ibuprofen, indomethacin, and naproxen.

FOOD, VITAMIN, AND HERBAL INTERACTIONS

It is essential for postmenopausal women to get adequate amounts of calcium and vitamin D. Calcium is critical for healthy bones, and vitamin D helps your body absorb calcium. Ask your health-care practitioner about a daily vitamin and mineral supplement.

RECOMMENDED DOSAGE

Raloxifene comes as a tablet. The doses given below are typical. However, only your health-care practitioner can determine the dosage and schedule that are best for you.

- *Children:* This drug is not recommended for children.
- *Adults:* 60 mg once daily

Raloxifene can be taken with or without food. If you forget to take a dose, take it as soon as you remember. If it is almost time for the next dose, skip the forgotten one, and resume your normal schedule. Never take double doses.

SYMPTOMS OF OVERDOSE AND WHAT TO DO

Little information is available regarding raloxifene overdose. However, if overdose occurs, seek immediate medical attention and take the prescription bottle to the hospital with you.

SPECIAL INFORMATION FOR PREGNANT OR NURSING WOMEN

Raloxifene is used in postmenopausal women. It is not considered safe to use during pregnancy or breastfeeding.

SPECIAL INFORMATION FOR SENIORS

There are no special instructions for seniors.

GENERIC NAME

Ramipril

BRAND NAME

Altace

No generic available

ABOUT THIS DRUG

Ramipril is an angiotensin-converting enzyme (ACE) inhibitor used to treat high blood pressure (hypertension). This drug may be prescribed alone or with other high blood pressure medications, such as thiazide diuretics. It works by blocking an enzyme in the body, which relaxes blood vessels and lowers blood pressure.

SIDE EFFECTS

Speak to your health-care practitioner if you develop side effects while taking ramipril. Only he or she can determine whether you should continue taking this drug.

- *Common:* dizziness, lightheadedness, headache, cough, tiredness
- *Less Common or Rare:* angina (chest pain), faintness, vertigo, upset stomach, abdominal pain, nausea, vomiting, bleeding in the stomach or intestines, overall feeling of unwellness, dizziness upon standing, sleepiness, insomnia, constipation, dry mouth, sore throat, hair loss, nervousness, numbness, tingling, skin peeling, sensitivity to light, high potassium, kidney or liver problems, yellow eyes or skin, hepatitis, inflammation of the pancreas, increased sweating, heart rhythm disturbances, rapid heartbeat, high blood pressure, heart failure, heart attack, severe allergic reactions

IMPORTANT PRECAUTIONS

Always inform your health-care practitioner about any other medical conditions you suffer from, especially congestive heart failure, angina (chest pain), abnormal heart rhythms, or other heart problems. Also tell your health-care practitioner if you have kidney or liver disease.

Ramipril can affect your kidneys, especially if you have congestive heart failure. If you already have kidney disease, your dosage should be lower than usual. Your kidneys must be monitored while you take this drug.

Before having any type of surgery, anesthesia, or dental procedure, tell your surgeon or dentist that you are taking ramipril.

This drug may make you dizzy or drowsy. Until you know how ramipril affects you, do not drive a car, operate machinery, or perform other tasks that demand concentration.

Treatment of high blood pressure also entails certain lifestyle changes, such as weight control, smoking cessation, and close attention to diet.

When you first start taking this drug, you may feel lightheaded, and experience dizziness or faintness when you rise quickly from a sitting or reclining position (postural hypotension). Try to get up slowly, and consult your health-care practitioner if the problem continues.

Be extremely careful when you exercise in hot weather. Heavy sweating can lead to dizziness, lightheadedness, fainting, vomiting, dehydration, and low blood pressure.

Do not take this drug if you have ever experienced an allergic reaction to it or to other ACE inhibitors. If you have an allergic reaction such as swelling of the face and mouth and a sudden problem with breathing, seek immediate medical attention. Also contact your health-care practitioner immediately if you develop a sore throat and fever, or yellow eyes or skin.

Your health-care practitioner will monitor your response to this drug with regular blood counts and other tests.

DRUG INTERACTIONS

Tell your health-care practitioner and pharmacist if you are taking any other prescription or over-the-counter drugs, as well as any vitamins, herbs, or other supplements. Possible drug interactions include the following:

- Taking other blood pressure medications can increase the blood-pressure-lowering effects of ramipril.
- If you are already taking a diuretic, when possible your health-care practitioner will have you stop taking it 2 to 3 days before starting ramipril.
- Ramipril may increase blood levels of potassium, particularly when taken with potassium-sparing diuretics. Too much potassium can cause heart rhythm disturbances.
- Combining ramipril with allopurinol increases the risk of side effects.
- Taking ramipril with lithium can result in toxic levels of lithium in the blood.
- Phenothiazine tranquilizers and antiemetics may increase the effects of ramipril.
- Indomethacin may reduce the blood pressure lowering effects of ramipril.
- Separate doses of antacids and ramipril by 2 hours.
- Ramipril increases blood levels of digoxin.
- Avoid alcoholic beverages. Alcohol may further lower blood pressure, and increase the risk of dizziness and fainting.
- Consult your health-care practitioner before taking over-the-counter cough, cold, sinus, allergy, or weight loss medications. Many of these can raise blood pressure.

FOOD, VITAMIN, AND HERBAL INTERACTIONS

Do not take herbs that increase blood pressure, such as ephedra (ma huang), ginseng, goldenseal, licorice, and saw palmetto. Consult your health-care practitioner before taking substances that may lower blood pressure, such as calcium, soy, or garlic. To minimize possible interactions, take ramipril and iron supplements 2 to 3 hours apart. Because ACE inhibitors raise potassium levels in the body, *do not* take potassium supplements or use salt substitutes containing potassium, and ask your health-care practitioner how many potassium-rich foods (such as bananas, prunes, raisins, melons, tomatoes, citrus fruit, and orange juice) you can safely include in your diet. Also talk to your health-care practitioner about salt intake.

RECOMMENDED DOSAGE

Ramipril is available in oral form as capsules. Although the doses given below are typical, only your health-care practitioner can determine the dose and schedule that best fit your needs.

- *Children:* This drug is not recommended for children.
- *Adults:* 2.5 to 20 mg in single or divided doses

Take ramipril one hour before or two hours after meals. Continue to take this drug even if you feel well. Do not discontinue use without consulting your health-care practitioner. If you miss a dose, take it as soon as you remember. If it is almost time for the next dose, skip the forgotten one, and resume your normal schedule. Never take a double dose.

SYMPTOMS OF OVERDOSE AND WHAT TO DO

The symptoms of ramipril overdose may include dizziness and fainting caused by a severe drop in blood pressure. If overdose occurs, seek immediate medical attention and take the prescription bottle to the hospital with you.

SPECIAL INFORMATION FOR PREGNANT OR NURSING WOMEN

Do not take ramipril if you are pregnant (especially during the final six months). This drug can cause fetal injury and death. If you become pregnant while taking ramipril, call your health-care practitioner immediately.

Small amounts of ramipril may pass into breast milk. If you are breastfeeding, your health-care practitioner will likely advise you to stop until your treatment is done.

SPECIAL INFORMATION FOR SENIORS

Seniors usually require lower doses of ramipril.

GENERIC NAME
Ranitidine

BRAND NAMES

Zantac, Zantac 75
Generic available

ABOUT THIS DRUG

Ranitidine is used to prevent or treat gastric (stomach) and duodenal (upper intestinal) ulcers. This drug may also be prescribed for other conditions in which the stomach makes too much acid, such as heartburn or acid indigestion. It is available both with and without a prescription.

Ranitidine is a type of drug known as a histamine H_2 antagonist or blocker. It works by decreasing the amount of acid produced by the stomach.

SIDE EFFECTS

Inform your health-care practitioner if you experience any severe or persistent side effects. If symptoms such as heartburn and acid indigestion last for 2 weeks while you are taking ranitidine, consult your health-care practitioner. Only he or she can determine whether or not you should continue to take this drug.

- *Common:* nausea, vomiting, abdominal pain, gas, indigestion, headache, fatigue, nasal inflammation, sore throat, dizziness, increased sweating, weakness
- *Less Common or Rare:* chest pain, back pain, muscle pain, stomach or intestinal problems, constipation, appetite loss, visual disturbances, teeth problems, anxiety, nervousness, trouble sleeping, sleepiness, cough, fever, dry mouth, infection, rash

IMPORTANT PRECAUTIONS

Always tell your health-care practitioner about any other medical conditions that you may have, especially kidney or liver disease, acute porphyria, or phenylketonuria. Also inform your health-care practitioner if you have ever experienced an allergic reaction to this or similar drugs, such as cimetidine.

Ranitidine is intended for the treatment of noncancerous stomach ulcers, and may conceal warning signs of a malignancy. Contact your health-care practitioner if you experience any problems while taking this drug.

DRUG INTERACTIONS

Inform your health-care practitioner and pharmacist if you are taking any other prescription or over-the-counter drugs, as well as any vitamins, herbs, or other supplements. Possible drug interactions include the following:

- ➤ Consult your health-care practitioner about combining antacids with ranitidine. You will probably be advised to separate the times you take them by half an hour to an hour.
- ➤ Ranitidine may increase the effects of procainamide and theophylline.
- ➤ Ranitidine may also interact with other drugs, such as warfarin, diazepam, diltiazem, glipizide, glyburide, phenytoin, sucralfate, triazolam, itraconazole, and ketoconazole.
- ➤ Alcohol use and cigarette smoking decrease the effect of ranitidine, by increasing the amount of acid produced by the stomach.

FOOD, VITAMIN, AND HERBAL INTERACTIONS

Certain foods—such as garlic, onions, and tomatoes—may increase stomach acid production, and spicy or deep-fried foods are likely to cause heartburn. Ask your health-care practitioner about any special dietary recommendations.

Do not use herbs such as kola and ephedra (ma huang), which may increase stomach acid.

RECOMMENDED DOSAGE

Ranitidine is available as a tablet, effervescent tablet, granule packet, and liquid. Most ulcers respond well to 4 to 8 weeks of treatment. If this drug is prescribed for longer periods (for example, to prevent duodenal ulcers), it is usually at a lower dosage. Although the doses given below are typical, only your health-care practitioner can determine the dose and schedule that are most appropriate for you.

- ➤ *Children 1 Month to 16 Years:* 2 to 4 mg per 2.2 pounds of body weight twice daily, to a maximum of 300 mg daily; preventive doses for long-term use are a maximum of 150 mg daily
- ➤ *Adults:* 300 mg once a day at bedtime, or 150 mg twice a day; lower preventive doses of 150 mg maximum daily are prescribed for long-term use

Ranitidine may be taken with or without food. Dissolve effervescent tablets in 6 to 8 ounces of water. If you miss a dose, take it as soon as you remember. However, if it is nearly time for your next scheduled dose, do not take the missed dose. Follow your regular dosing schedule. Never take a double dose.

SYMPTOMS OF OVERDOSE AND WHAT TO DO

No specific information on ranitidine overdose is available. If you suspect an overdose, seek immediate medical attention, and bring the prescription bottle to the hospital with you.

SPECIAL INFORMATION FOR PREGNANT OR NURSING WOMEN

No studies have adequately investigated the effects of ranitidine during pregnancy or breastfeeding. If you are pregnant or planning to become pregnant, or if you are breastfeeding or plan to do so, talk with your health-care practitioner before starting this drug. Only a health-care practitioner can determine whether the potential benefits outweigh the potential dangers.

SPECIAL INFORMATION FOR SENIORS

Side effects are more common in seniors, and lower dosages are usually recommended.

GENERIC NAME

Ranitidine bismuth citrate

BRAND NAME

Tritec

No generic available

ABOUT THIS DRUG

Ranitidine bismuth citrate is used to treat duodenal (upper intestinal) ulcers associated with *H. pylori* bacteria. It is prescribed with the antibiotic clarithromycin.

Ranitidine bismuth citrate is a combination of ranitidine and bismuth. Ranitidine decreases the amount of acid produced by the stomach, and bismuth disrupts the cell walls of *H. pylori* bacteria.

SIDE EFFECTS

Inform your health-care practitioner if you experience any severe or persistent side effects. Only he or she can determine whether or not you should continue to take this drug.

- *Common:* diarrhea, changes in the sense of taste
- *Less Common or Rare:* nausea, vomiting, headache, gynecological problems, abdominal discomfort, stomach pain, tremor, drug reactions, rash

IMPORTANT PRECAUTIONS

Ranitidine bismuth citrate should not be used alone for ulcers. It is always prescribed with clarithromycin. If ulcers persist despite treatment, the bacteria may be resistant to this antibiotic, and your health-care practitioner will prescribe a different one.

Always tell your health-care practitioner about any other medical conditions that you may have, especially kidney or liver disease, acute porphyria, or phenylketonuria. Also inform your health-care practitioner if you have ever experienced an allergic reaction to ranitidine, bismuth, or similar drugs.

DRUG INTERACTIONS

Inform your health-care practitioner and pharmacist if you are taking any other prescription or over-the-counter drugs, as well as any vitamins, herbs, or other supplements. Possible drug interactions include the following:

- Combining ranitidine bismuth citrate and clarithromycin enhances the effectiveness of these drugs.
- Consult your health-care practitioner about combining antacids with ranitidine bismuth citrate. You will probably be advised to separate the times you take them by half an hour to an hour.
- Alcohol use and cigarette smoking decrease the effect of ranitidine bismuth citrate, by increasing the amount of acid produced by the stomach.

FOOD, VITAMIN, AND HERBAL INTERACTIONS

Certain foods—such as garlic, onions, and tomatoes—may increase stomach acid production, and spicy or deep-fried foods are likely to cause heartburn. Ask your health-care practitioner about any special dietary recommendations.

Do not use herbs such as kola and ephedra (ma huang), which may increase stomach acid.

RECOMMENDED DOSAGE

Ranitidine bismuth citrate comes as a tablet. Most ulcers must be treated for at least 4 weeks. Although the doses given below are typical, only your health-care practitioner can determine the dose and schedule that are most appropriate for you.

- *Children:* This drug is not recommended for children.
- *Adults:* 400 mg twice a day for 4 weeks, taken with 500 mg of clarithromycin 3 times a day for the first 2 weeks

Ranitidine bismuth citrate may be taken with or without food. If you miss a dose, take it as soon as you remember. However, if it is nearly time for your next scheduled dose, do not take the missed dose. Follow your regular dosing schedule. Never take a double dose.

SYMPTOMS OF OVERDOSE AND WHAT TO DO

No specific information on ranitidine bismuth citrate overdose is available. If you suspect an overdose, seek immediate medical attention, and bring the prescription bottle to the hospital with you.

SPECIAL INFORMATION FOR PREGNANT OR NURSING WOMEN

No studies have adequately investigated the effects of ranitidine bismuth citrate during pregnancy or breastfeeding. If you are pregnant or planning to become pregnant, or if you are breastfeeding or plan to do so, talk with your health-care practitioner before starting this drug. Only a health-care practitioner can determine whether the potential benefits outweigh the potential dangers.

SPECIAL INFORMATION FOR SENIORS

There are no special instructions for seniors.

GENERIC NAME

Repaglinide

BRAND NAME

Prandin
No generic available

ABOUT THIS DRUG

Repaglinide is used to treat the form of diabetes mellitus known as type 2. Type 2 diabetes was formerly known as adult-onset, and is also referred to as noninsulin-dependent. Diet and exercise play a key role in the management of this disease. Repaglinide may be prescribed alone or with metformin.

This drug helps control diabetes by increasing insulin production. Repaglinide must be taken shortly before meals in order to stimulate the pancreas to release more insulin.

SIDE EFFECTS

Report any severe or persistent side effects to your health-care practitioner. All diabetics should learn to recognize the symptoms of low blood sugar and high blood sugar and know what to do when they occur. It is essential to control these symptoms before they progress to more serious conditions.

- *Common:* low or high blood sugar, headache, respiratory infection, back pain, urinary tract infection, sinus inflammation, indigestion, nausea, vomiting, diarrhea, constipation, skin tingling
- *Hypoglycemia (Low Blood Sugar):* "drunken" behavior, drowsiness, unusual tiredness or weakness, slurred speech, shakiness, dizziness, difficulty concentrating, headache, confusion, anxiety, nervousness, blurred vision, cold sweats, cool pale skin, excessive hunger, restless sleep, nightmares, nausea, fast heartbeat
- *Hyperglycemia (High Blood Sugar):* dry mouth, thirst, frequent urination, dry skin, flushing, appetite loss, difficulty breathing, tiredness
- *Less Common or Rare:* angina (chest pain), tooth problems, allergic reactions

IMPORTANT PRECAUTIONS

Repaglinide should not be used if you have type 1 (insulin-dependent) diabetes or diabetic ketoacidosis (a life-threatening condition caused by insufficient insulin, with symptoms such as nausea, fatigue, excessive thirst, lower chest pain, and fruity breath). Use this drug with caution if you have an active infection or a history of kidney or liver disease.

Your health-care practitioner will also most likely advise you to stop taking this drug for a short time before and after having any type of surgery or dental procedure.

Too much repaglinide can cause low blood sugar (hypoglycemia). The people most susceptible to this problem are older, weak, or malnourished, or have kidney, liver, adrenal, or hormone problems. Symptoms vary from person to person, so it is essential to learn which symptoms you usually have. As soon as you experience the characteristic signs, address and control them quickly by taking a fast-acting sugar, such as a glucose tablet, glass of fruit juice or nondiet soft drink, tablespoon of corn syrup or honey, or tablespoon of table sugar dissolved in water.

People with uncontrolled diabetes may also experience high blood sugar, or hyperglycemia. (See symptoms on previous page.) If this condition is not treated, it can lead to diabetic coma and death.

In order to prevent these types of complications, carefully follow all diet and exercise recommendations made by your health-care practitioner and nutritionist. In fact, many people with type 2 diabetes are able to successfully control this disease by making healthy lifestyle changes, cutting back on the need for medication.

To monitor the effectiveness of repaglinide, measure the amount of glucose in your urine or blood on a regular basis. Your health-care practitioner may also tell you to test your urine for ketones (substances that appear in urine when diabetes is not properly controlled). Carefully follow the instructions of your health-care practitioner and pharmacist when conducting these tests at home. If blood sugar is high or sugar or ketones are present in urine, call your health-care practitioner.

DRUG INTERACTIONS

Inform your health-care practitioner and pharmacist if you are taking any other prescription or over-the-counter drugs, as well as any vitamins, herbs, or other supplements. Possible drug interactions include the following:

- Combining repaglinide with certain drugs may increase the risk of low blood sugar. These include erythromycin, ketoconazole, and miconazole.
- Other drugs that may increase repaglinide's blood-sugar-lowering effects include beta-blockers, NSAIDs, blood thinners, and sulfa drugs.
- Many drugs may increase the risk of high blood sugar. These include barbiturates, carbamazepine, rifampin, troglitazone, calcium channel blockers, corticosteroids, estrogens, oral contraceptives, phenothiazines, thiazide diuretics, and stimulants.
- Do not drink alcohol while taking repaglinide. Alcohol alters blood sugar.

FOOD, VITAMIN, AND HERBAL INTERACTIONS

Supplements such as chromium, garlic, ginger, ginseng, hawthorn, and nettle may affect blood sugar levels. Check with your health-care practitioner before using any dietary supplement.

RECOMMENDED DOSAGE

Repaglinide comes in tablet form. Although the doses given below are typical, only your health-care practitioner can determine the dose and schedule that best fit your needs.

- *Children:* This drug is not recommended for children.
- *Adults:* 0.5 to 4 mg 15 to 30 minutes before each meal; maximum daily dose is 16 mg

It is very important to take repaglinide exactly as prescribed. If you forget to take it just prior to a meal, take it with the meal. If you don't remember until after you finish eating, skip that dose. Never take a double dose. If you skip a meal, also skip that dose of repaglinide.

SYMPTOMS OF OVERDOSE AND WHAT TO DO

An overdose of repaglinide may cause low blood sugar. (See symptoms listed in Side Effects.) If you suspect that an overdose has occurred, take a fast-acting sugar. If symptoms persist, seek immediate medical attention and take the prescription bottle to the hospital with you.

SPECIAL INFORMATION FOR PREGNANT OR NURSING WOMEN

Repaglinide should not be used during pregnancy. It is critically important to monitor and control blood sugar when you are pregnant. However, it is safer to accomplish this through diet or a combination of diet and insulin. Consult your health-care practitioner as soon as you think you may be pregnant or if you are planning to become pregnant.

If you are breastfeeding or plan to do so, talk with your health-care practitioner before starting this drug. Only a health-care practitioner can determine whether the potential benefits outweigh the potential dangers.

SPECIAL INFORMATION FOR SENIORS

Seniors may be more sensitive to the effects of repaglinide.

GENERIC NAME

Rifampin

BRAND NAMES

Rifadin, Rimactane
Generic available

ABOUT THIS DRUG

Rifampin is prescribed for tuberculosis, meningitis, and other infections. In the treatment of tuberculosis, it is always used with at least one other tuberculosis drug (such as isoniazid or pyrazinamide). This drug works by eradicating the underlying organisms responsible for infection.

SIDE EFFECTS

Inform your health-care practitioner if you experience any severe or persistent side effects. Some side effects—such as urine, feces, sweat, saliva, and tears turning reddish-brown—are startling but not a cause for concern. However, contact your health-care practitioner at once if you experience flu-like symptoms, unusual bleeding or bruising, nausea, vomiting, headache, rash, itching, or yellow skin and eyes.

➤ *Common:* nausea, vomiting, cramps, upset stomach, gas, heartburn, diarrhea, flu-like symptoms, fever, dizziness, drowsiness, confusion, menstrual disturbances, visual disturbances, numbness, drug sensitivity reactions

➤ *Less Common or Rare:* liver damage, blood or kidney effects

IMPORTANT PRECAUTIONS

Rifampin should be used with extreme caution if you have liver disease. People taking this drug should be carefully monitored for signs of liver damage.

Rifampin may suppress the immune system.

Tell your health-care practitioner if you have ever had an allergic reaction to this or similar drugs.

Because rifampin may reduce the effectiveness of oral contraceptives, use alternate means of contraception while taking this medication.

This drug may make you drowsy. Until you know how rifampin affects you, do not drive a car, operate machinery, or perform other tasks that demand concentration.

This drug should not be used for meningococcus infection.

DRUG INTERACTIONS

Inform your health-care practitioner and pharmacist if you are taking any other prescription or over-the-counter drugs, as well as any vitamins, herbs, or other supplements. Possible drug interactions include the following:

- Taking rifampin with other drugs that cause liver damage may result in liver toxicity.
- Rifampin may reduce the effectiveness of oral contraceptives.
- Rifampin may interact with many other drugs, including blood thinners, cyclosporine, estrogens, hydrocortisone, medications for heart disease and diabetes, theophylline, and verapamil.
- Do not drink alcohol while taking rifampin.

FOOD, VITAMIN, AND HERBAL INTERACTIONS

Rifampin may interfere with the body's formation of vitamin D. Vitamin supplementation may be beneficial.

RECOMMENDED DOSAGE

Rifampin comes in capsule form. Although the doses given below are typical, only your health-care practitioner can determine the dose and schedule that best fit your needs.

- *Children:* 4.5 to 9 mg per pound of body weight; maximum dose is 600 mg daily
- *Adults:* 600 mg once daily

Rifampin should be taken 1 hour before or 2 hours after meals. If you miss a dose, take it as soon as you remember. However, if it is nearly time for your next scheduled dose, do not take the missed dose. Follow your regular dosing schedule. Never take a double dose. Missing numerous doses increases the risk of side effects.

SYMPTOMS OF OVERDOSE AND WHAT TO DO

Little information is available regarding rifampin overdose. If you suspect that an overdose has occurred, seek immediate medical attention and take the prescription bottle to the hospital with you.

SPECIAL INFORMATION FOR PREGNANT OR NURSING WOMEN

Animal studies have indicated that rifampin may cause birth defects. This drug should be taken during pregnancy only if absolutely necessary. Because rifampin may pass into breast milk, your health-care practitioner may recommend that you stop breastfeeding while taking this medication.

SPECIAL INFORMATION FOR SENIORS

Seniors with liver disease may be more sensitive to side effects.

GENERIC NAME
Riluzole

BRAND NAME

Rilutek
No generic available

ABOUT THIS DRUG

Riluzole is prescribed to slow the progress of amyotrophic lateral sclerosis (ALS, which is also known as Lou Gehrig's disease). ALS is a progressive and eventually fatal disease of the nervous system. Riluzole is the only medication thus far known to treat it.

Although no one knows exactly how this drug works, it slows the release of glutamate, which is thought to damage important nerve centers. Riluzole may delay the need for a breathing tube, but it is not a cure for ALS.

SIDE EFFECTS

Side effects are extremely common, and 14% of people stop taking riluzole because of them. Inform your health-care practitioner if you experience any severe or persistent problems. Call your health-care practitioner immediately if you feel feverish and ill. Only he or she can determine whether you should continue to take this drug.

- *Common:* nausea, vomiting, diarrhea, appetite loss, dizziness, drowsiness, weakness, fainting, fatigue, a tingling sensation around the mouth, reduced lung function, pneumonia
- *Less Common or Rare:* upset stomach, gas, back pain, headache, runny or stuffy nose, cough, general feeling of unwellness, high blood pressure, swelling in the arms and legs, joint pain, mouth infection, urinary infection, rapid heartbeat

IMPORTANT PRECAUTIONS

Riluzole should be used with extreme caution if you have liver or kidney disease. People taking this drug should be carefully monitored for signs of liver inflammation.

This drug may make you dizzy or drowsy. Until you know how riluzole affects you, do not drive a car, operate machinery, or perform other tasks that demand concentration.

Women are more prone than men to side effects such as dizziness. People of Japanese descent eliminate this drug from their bodies more slowly than Caucasians.

DRUG INTERACTIONS

Inform your health-care practitioner and pharmacist if you are taking any other prescription or over-the-counter drugs, as well as any vitamins, herbs, or other supplements. Possible drug interactions include the following:

- Taking riluzole with other drugs that cause liver damage may result in liver toxicity.
- Drugs such as caffeine, quinolone antibiotics, amitriptyline, phenacetin, and theophylline increase the risk of side effects of riluzole.
- Do not drink alcohol or smoke cigarettes while taking riluzole.

FOOD, VITAMIN, AND HERBAL INTERACTIONS

Avoid charcoal-broiled foods while taking this drug. They affect its absorption.

Also avoid caffeinated beverages such as cola, coffee, and tea.

RECOMMENDED DOSAGE

Riluzole comes in tablet form. Although the doses given below are typical, only your health-care practitioner can determine the dose and schedule that best fit your needs.

- *Children:* This drug is not recommended for children.
- *Adults:* 50 mg every 12 hours

Riluzole should be taken 1 hour before or 2 hours after meals at the same time each day. If you miss a dose, take it as soon as you remember. However, if it is nearly time for your next scheduled dose, do not take the missed dose. Follow your regular dosing schedule. Never take a double dose. Taking more than 100 mg daily increases side effects and is not recommended.

SYMPTOMS OF OVERDOSE AND WHAT TO DO

Little information is available regarding riluzole overdose. If you suspect that an overdose has occurred, seek immediate medical attention and take the prescription bottle to the hospital with you.

SPECIAL INFORMATION FOR PREGNANT OR NURSING WOMEN

Animal studies have indicated that riluzole has toxic effects. This drug should be taken during pregnancy only if absolutely necessary. Because riluzole may pass into breast milk, your health-care practitioner may recommend that you stop breastfeeding while taking this medication.

SPECIAL INFORMATION FOR SENIORS
Seniors with liver or kidney disease may be more sensitive to side effects, and should use this drug with caution.

GENERIC NAME
Rimantadine

BRAND NAME
Flumadine
No generic available

ABOUT THIS DRUG
Rimantadine is an antiviral drug used to prevent and treat infections caused by influenza A virus. Although an annual flu vaccine is the best way to prevent this virus, it takes 2 to 4 weeks to work. In the meantime, rimantadine can be taken to prevent the flu in high-risk individuals. This drug can also be used to treat type A flu. It works by interfering with the reproduction of the virus.

SIDE EFFECTS
If you develop side effects while taking rimantadine, ask your health-care practitioner whether it is safe for you to continue taking this drug.

- *Common:* difficulty sleeping and concentrating, nervousness, upset stomach, abdominal pain, nausea, vomiting, appetite loss, headache, fatigue, weakness, dry mouth
- *Less Common or Rare:* dizziness, agitation, fainting, pallor, hallucinations, depression, euphoria, ringing in the ears, high blood pressure, rapid heartbeat, heart palpitations, heart failure, heart block, changes in gait, swelling of ankles and feet, breathing difficulties, changes in taste and smell, diarrhea, constipation, mouth sores, swallowing difficulties, cough, fever, tremors, convulsions

IMPORTANT PRECAUTIONS
Older people and others at risk should continue to receive yearly flu shots to prevent this virus.

Always tell your health-care practitioner about all other medical conditions from which you suffer, including kidney or liver impairment, seizures, or blood disorders. Do not use rimantadine if you have experienced an allergic reaction to this or any similar medication. People with kidney or liver disease should receive lower doses.

Rimantadine may cause side effects such as dizziness. Until you know how this drug affects you, do not drive a car, operate machinery, or engage in other actions that require concentration.

Children may receive this drug for prevention but not treatment of the flu.

The influenza virus may become resistant to rimantadine in nearly a third of the people who take this drug.

DRUG INTERACTIONS

Tell your health-care practitioner and pharmacist if you are taking any other prescription or over-the-counter drugs, as well as any vitamins, herbs, or other supplements. Drug interactions occur infrequently. Taking rimantadine with aspirin or acetaminophen may reduce the amount of rimantadine in the blood.

FOOD, VITAMIN, AND HERBAL INTERACTIONS

No food, vitamin, or herbal interactions have been noted.

RECOMMENDED DOSAGE

Rimantadine comes as a tablet or liquid. The doses given below are typical, but only your health-care practitioner can determine the dose and schedule that best fit your particular needs.

- *Children Younger than 10 Years:* 2.25 mg per pound of body weight; maximum daily dosage is 150 mg
- *Children Older than 10 Years and Adults:* 100 mg twice a day

Rimantadine should be taken 1 hour before or 2 hours after meals. If you miss a dose, take it as soon as you remember. However, if it is nearly time for your next scheduled dose, do not take the missed dose. Follow your regular dosing schedule dose. Never take a double dose.

SYMPTOMS OF OVERDOSE AND WHAT TO DO

Symptoms of rimantadine overdose may include abnormal heart rhythm, agitation, and hallucinations. If you suspect an overdose, seek immediate medical attention, and bring the prescription bottle to the hospital with you.

SPECIAL INFORMATION FOR PREGNANT OR NURSING WOMEN

Animal studies have indicated that rimantadine has toxic effects on fetuses. This drug should be taken during pregnancy only if absolutely necessary. Because rimantadine may pass into breast milk, your health-care practitioner may recommend that you stop breast-feeding while taking this medication.

SPECIAL INFORMATION FOR SENIORS

Seniors may be more sensitive to the side effects of rimantadine, and may benefit from lower doses.

GENERIC NAME

Risedronate *see Bisphosphonates, page 200*

GENERIC NAME

Risperidone

BRAND NAME

Risperdal
No generic available

ABOUT THIS DRUG

Risperidone is used to treat severe mental illnesses such as schizophrenia and bipolar disease. It helps reduce symptoms such as hallucinations, delusions, and hostility.

Risperidone works by affecting the action of two important nerve transmitters in the brain, dopamine and serotonin. This corrects an underlying imbalance believed to be responsible for a number of mental disorders.

SIDE EFFECTS

Talk to your health-care practitioner if you develop side effects while taking risperidone. Only he or she can determine whether it is safe for you to continue taking this drug and whether it is necessary to adjust your dosage.

- *Common:* headache, sleepiness, sleeplessness, agitation, anxiety, runny nose
- *Less Common or Rare:* nausea, vomiting, upset stomach, abdominal pain, constipation, rapid heart rate, dizziness, dizziness or fainting upon rising, changes in saliva, toothache, breathing difficulties, sore throat, cough, sinus infection, joint or back pain, chest pain, fever, visual disturbances, dandruff, dry skin, rash, sun sensitivity, urinary infection, difficulty swallowing, pneumonia, Parkinson-like reactions (such as uncontrollable jerking movements), symptoms of tardive

dyskinesia (such as lip smacking, wormlike movements of the tongue, and slow, rhythmical, involuntary movements), seizures

People taking antipsychotic drugs may experience a rare but life-threatening set of side effects known as neuroleptic malignant syndrome (NMS). Symptoms include fever, difficulty breathing, rapid heartbeat, rigid muscles, mental changes, increased sweating, irregular blood pressure, and convulsions. Immediate medical attention is required.

Side effects such as lip smacking, wormlike movements of the tongue, and slow, rhythmical, involuntary movements are characteristic of a disorder known as tardive dyskinesia. Older adults (especially women) are more susceptible to this condition, which may become permanent. If you experience tardive dyskinesia, your health-care practitioner will probably advise you to stop taking this drug.

IMPORTANT PRECAUTIONS

You should not take risperidone if you have neuroleptic malignant syndrome or if you have experienced a previous allergic reaction to this drug. Risperidone may cause a life-threatening abnormal heart rhythm, called *torsade de pointes.* You are at a greater risk of this problem if you have heart disease or a slow heart rate, are dehydrated, or take other medications with a risk of *torsade de pointes.*

Use risperidone with caution if you have kidney or liver disease, a seizure disorder, breast cancer, thyroid disorders, dehydration, or a history of stroke or mini-strokes. Doses are lower for older people and those with kidney or liver disease.

Risperidone raises the level of the hormone prolactin in your body. High prolactin levels are associated with an increased risk of breast, pituitary gland, and pancreas tumors.

This medication may mask the symptoms of drug overdose, intestinal obstructions, a brain tumor, or Reye's syndrome.

Tell your health-care practitioner if you have ever experienced an allergic reaction to this or similar drugs.

Before having any type of surgery or dental procedure, tell your surgeon or dentist that you are taking risperidone.

This drug may impair your physical coordination and mental alertness. Until you know how risperidone affects you, do not drive a car, operate machinery, or perform other tasks that demand concentration.

Drink plenty of fluids and avoid extreme heat. Be especially careful when you exercise in hot weather or enter a hot bath or sauna. Heavy sweating can lead to dizziness, lightheadedness, fainting, vomiting, and dehydration.

When you first start taking this drug or when the dosage is increased, you may experience dizziness or faintness when you rise quickly from a sitting or reclining position (postural hypotension). Try to get up slowly, and consult your health-care practitioner if the problem continues.

Risperidone may cause increased sun sensitivity. Wear protective clothing and apply sunscreen.

DRUG INTERACTIONS

Inform your health-care practitioner and pharmacist if you are taking any other prescription or over-the-counter drugs, as well as any vitamins, herbs, or other supplements. Possible drug interactions include the following:

- Since risperidone may cause low blood pressure, be cautious about combining this medication with high blood pressure drugs.
- Risperidone may decrease the effects of levodopa.
- Central nervous system depressants (such as sedatives, tranquilizers, narcotics, and sleeping pills) may cause increased drowsiness.
- Carbamazepine and clozapine reduce the amount of risperidone absorbed by the body.
- Avoid alcohol while taking risperidone.

FOOD, VITAMIN, AND HERBAL INTERACTIONS

Do not combine risperidone with herbs that produce sedative effects, such as catnip, elecampane, goldenseal, gotu kola, hops, kava, lemon balm, skullcap, St. John's wort, and valerian. Also do not use stimulating herbs such as ginseng, kola, or ephedra (ma huang) while taking this drug.

RECOMMENDED DOSAGE

Risperidone comes as a tablet, oral solution, and intramuscular (IM) injection (Risperdal Constra). The doses given below are typical (dosages for IM form not listed), but dosage is always carefully individualized according to a person's particular needs and reactions to therapy.

- *Children:* This drug is not recommended for children.
- *Adults:* 1 mg twice daily to start; this may be gradually increased as needed to a maximum daily dosage of 6 mg

Risperidone may be taken with or without food. If you forget a dose, take it as soon as you remember. If it is almost time for the next dose, skip it and resume your normal schedule. Never take a double dose. Call your health-care practitioner if you miss 2 doses in a row. This drug must be taken for several weeks before its full effect is felt. When you stop taking it, dosage must be decreased gradually.

SYMPTOMS OF OVERDOSE AND WHAT TO DO

The symptoms of risperidone overdose include drowsiness, rapid heartbeat, low blood pressure, and sedation. If overdose occurs, seek immediate medical attention and take the prescription bottle to the hospital with you.

SPECIAL INFORMATION FOR PREGNANT OR NURSING WOMEN

No studies have adequately investigated the effects of risperidone during pregnancy or breastfeeding. If you are pregnant or planning to become pregnant, or if you are breastfeeding or plan to do so, talk with your health-care practitioner before starting this drug. Only a health-care practitioner can determine whether the potential benefits outweigh the potential dangers.

SPECIAL INFORMATION FOR SENIORS

Seniors require lower doses of risperidone. This age group is more likely to experience effects such as tardive dyskinesia (a condition that causes lip smacking, wormlike movements of the tongue, and slow, rhythmical, involuntary movements).

GENERIC NAME

Ritonavir

BRAND NAME

Norvir

No generic available

ABOUT THIS DRUG

Ritonavir is a protease inhibitor used to treat HIV, the human immunodeficiency virus that causes acquired immune deficiency syndrome (AIDS). It is commonly prescribed in a triple-drug cocktail in combination with antiretroviral drugs such as zidovudine (AZT).

Triple-drug cocktails are credited with reducing the death rate from AIDS in the mid-1990s.

Ritonavir works by interfering with the reproduction of HIV. It disrupts the process through which proteins are formed and become mature HIV. This in turn slows the progression of the virus and the destruction of the immune system.

SIDE EFFECTS

Side effects of this drug are common. Contact your health-care practitioner if they become persistent or severe. Only he or she can determine if you should continue to take ritonavir.

➤ *Common:* nausea, vomiting, abdominal pain, appetite loss, diarrhea, gas, weakness, tiredness, tingling around the mouth, hands, and feet

➤ *Less Common or Rare:* rash, drowsiness, dizziness, headache, fever, sore throat, sweating, weight loss, insomnia, fatigue, overall feeling of unwellness, muscle and joint aches, liver inflammation, yellow skin and eyes, high blood sugar, diabetes, pancreatitis, high cholesterol, anxiety, bedwetting, incontinence, allergic reactions

Serious side effects can occur virtually anywhere in the body when you take ritonavir. This drug may affect your gastrointestinal tract, sexual function, mental state, kidneys, liver, muscles, and joints. Consult your health-care practitioner if you experience symptoms such as nausea, vomiting, increased hunger, increased thirst, increased urination, dry or itchy skin, confusion, dehydration, fatigue, and fruity mouth odor.

IMPORTANT PRECAUTIONS

Tell your health-care practitioner about any other medical conditions you suffer from, especially liver disease, a history of alcohol abuse, or diabetes. Inform your health-care practitioner if you have ever experienced an allergic reaction to this or other protease inhibitors.

If you are using oral contraceptives, practice other means of contraception while taking ritonavir.

Ritonavir does not cure HIV or AIDS, nor does it prevent you from passing the virus on to others. You may continue to experience complications including opportunistic infections. It is important to always practice safe sex while taking this drug.

Visit your health-care practitioner on a regular basis to monitor your progress. Periodic blood tests are necessary to investigate unwanted effects, such as high blood sugar.

DRUG INTERACTIONS

Check first with your health-care practitioner before taking any other medication with ritonavir. To avoid unwanted side effects, tell your health-care practitioner and pharmacist about all other prescription or over-the-counter drugs, vitamins, herbs, or other supplements that you are taking. Possible drug interactions include the following:

- Ritonavir makes AZT and other anti-HIV drugs more effective.
- Do not take ritonavir with alprazolam, bepridil, bupropion, cisapride, clorazepate, clozapine, diazepam, encainide, estazolam, flecainide, flurazepam, meperidine, midazolam, piroxicam, propafenone, propoxyphene, quinidine, rifabutin, terfenadine, triazolam, or zolpidem. These combinations are potentially life-threatening.
- Do not take ritonavir at the same time as didanosine.
- Ritonavir may cause birth control pills to be less effective.
- Tobacco decreases the effects of ritonavir.

FOOD, VITAMIN, AND HERBAL INTERACTIONS

When taking the triple-drug cocktail, it is particularly important to follow your health-care practitioner's dietary recommendations.

RECOMMENDED DOSAGE

Ritonavir is available as gelatin capsules and oral solution. The doses given below are typical. However, doses are different for different patients, and only your health-care practitioner can determine the dose and schedule that are most appropriate for you.

- *Children:* This drug is not recommended for children.
- *Adults:* 600 mg twice daily

If possible, ritonavir should be taken with food. It is essential to take this drug exactly as prescribed. If you miss a dose, take it as soon as you remember. However, if it is nearly time for your next scheduled dose, do not take the missed dose. Follow your regular dosing schedule. Never take a double dose.

SYMPTOMS OF OVERDOSE AND WHAT TO DO

No specific information on overdosing with ritonavir is available. However, if you suspect overdose, seek medical attention immediately, and bring the prescription bottle with you to the hospital so that health-care practitioners will know exactly what drug was taken.

SPECIAL INFORMATION FOR PREGNANT OR NURSING WOMEN

No studies have adequately investigated the effects of ritonavir during pregnancy or breastfeeding. If you are pregnant or plan to become pregnant, consult with your health-care practitioner before taking this medication. It is not known whether ritonavir passes into breast milk. However, HIV can be transferred by breast milk, so bottle-feeding is recommended.

SPECIAL INFORMATION FOR SENIORS

There are no special instructions for seniors.

GENERIC NAME

Rivastigmine tartrate

BRAND NAME

Exelon
No generic available

ABOUT THIS DRUG

Rivastigmine tartrate is used to treat mild-to-moderate Alzheimer's disease. This drug can improve symptoms such as thinking ability. However, it cannot cure Alzheimer's disease nor prevent the disease from growing worse. You may need to take rivastigmine for up to 12 weeks in order to experience its full benefits.

Changes in the brain associated with Alzheimer's disease include a shortage of acetylcholine (ACh), a chemical that helps the brain function properly. Rivastigmine slows the breakdown of ACh.

SIDE EFFECTS

Most side effects of rivastigmine involve the stomach and intestines. If any side effects of this drug become persistent or severe, ask your health-care practitioner whether it is safe for you to continue taking it.

- *Common:* nausea, vomiting, diarrhea, constipation, indigestion, abdominal pain, cramping, bloating, appetite loss, weight loss, headache, fatigue, dizziness, trouble sleeping, depression, confusion, hallucinations
- *Less Common or Rare:* high blood pressure, fainting, overall feeling of unwellness, increased sweating, runny nose, belching, difficulty urinating, aggression, convulsions

IMPORTANT PRECAUTIONS

Always tell your health-care practitioner about all other medical conditions from which you suffer, especially heart disease, seizures, and asthma or other breathing problems. Do not use rivastigmine if you have ever experienced an allergic reaction to it, and inform your health-care practitioner if you have ever experienced an allergic reaction to any similar medication.

This drug may make you dizzy or unsteady. Until you know how rivastigmine affects you, do not drive a car, operate machinery, or perform other tasks that demand concentration.

Visit your health-care practitioner on a regular basis to monitor your progress. Symptoms such as nausea and vomiting may be common, especially at the beginning of treatment and especially in women. This can lead to significant weight loss. Always tell your health-care practitioner if side effects are troubling or if Alzheimer's symptoms grow worse.

DRUG INTERACTIONS

Tell your health-care practitioner and pharmacist if you are taking any other prescription or over-the-counter drugs, as well as any vitamins, herbs, or other supplements. Drug interactions occur infrequently. Consult your health-care practitioner before combining rivastigmine with other drugs such as bethanechol or drugs that control spasms.

FOOD, VITAMIN, AND HERBAL INTERACTIONS

No food, vitamin, or herbal interactions have been noted.

RECOMMENDED DOSAGE

Rivastigmine comes as a capsule. The doses given below are typical, but only your health-care practitioner can determine the dose and schedule that best fit your particular needs.

- *Children:* This drug is not indicated for children.
- *Adults:* 1.5 mg twice a day to start; this may be gradually increased as needed to a maximum daily dosage of 12 mg

Rivastigmine should be taken with food in the morning and evening. If you miss a dose, take it as soon as you remember. However, if it is nearly time for your next scheduled dose, do not take the missed dose. Follow your regular dosing schedule dose. Never take a double dose. Do not stop taking medication suddenly. This may cause mental or behavioral changes.

SYMPTOMS OF OVERDOSE AND WHAT TO DO
Rivastigmine overdose may result in convulsions and shock. If you suspect an overdose, seek immediate medical attention, and bring the prescription bottle to the hospital with you.

SPECIAL INFORMATION FOR PREGNANT OR NURSING WOMEN
Rivastigmine should not be taken by women of childbearing age.

SPECIAL INFORMATION FOR SENIORS
This drug is specifically intended for seniors.

GENERIC NAME

Rizatriptan

see Triptan-Type Antimigraine Drugs, page 1083

GENERIC NAME

Ropinirole

BRAND NAME
Requip
No generic available

ABOUT THIS DRUG
Ropinirole is used to treat Parkinson's disease. It is often combined with levodopa. An advantage of ropinirole is that if you experience the "on-off" phenomenon—in which symptom-free periods alternate with periods during which medication loses its effect—ropinirole shortens the negative "off" ones.

Like other antiparkinsonian drugs, ropinirole works by correcting the dopamine deficiency that is believed to be the cause of Parkinson's disease. It stimulates dopamine receptors in the brain.

SIDE EFFECTS
Side effects from ropinirole are common. Call your health-care practitioner if they become severe or do not go away. Contact your health-care practitioner immediately if you experience alarming effects such as hallucinations, eye problems, swelling, or respiratory difficulties. Only your health-care practitioner can determine if you should continue to take this drug.

- *Common:* hallucinations, abnormal dreams, memory loss, nausea, vomiting, lack of appetite, dry mouth, constipation, confusion, fatigue, dizziness, dizziness upon standing, weakness, difficulty sleeping, involuntary or jerky body movements, increased urination, urinary tract infections, chest pain, difficulty breathing, arthritis, vision abnormalities, viral infection
- *Less Common or Rare:* overall feeling of unwellness, impotence, reduced sex drive, restlessness, muscle spasms or twitching, delusions, thinking abnormalities, difficulty swallowing, urinary incontinence, circulation problems, skin disorders, darkening of skin or eye color, eye disorders, pneumonia, blood clots, heart or lung problems, mental illness, convulsions

IMPORTANT PRECAUTIONS

Always inform your health-care practitioner of any other medical conditions you have, especially heart disease, kidney disease, or eye problems. Older people are more susceptible to side effects such as hallucinations. Contact your health-care practitioner if you experience problems such as falling asleep while going about your daily activities.

Because ropinirole may cause side effects such as dizziness and fatigue, do not drive a car, operate machinery, or perform other tasks that require concentration until you know how this drug affects you.

When you first start taking this drug or when the dosage is increased, you may experience dizziness or faintness when you rise quickly from a sitting or reclining position (postural hypotension). Try to get up slowly, and consult your health-care practitioner if the problem continues.

Ropinirole may cause dry mouth. To counteract this effect, use sugarless gum or candy, ice chips, or a saliva substitute. If the problem continues, consult your health-care practitioner or dentist.

To monitor treatment, visit your health-care practitioner on a regular basis.

DRUG INTERACTIONS

Tell your health-care practitioner and pharmacist if you are taking any other prescription or over-the-counter drugs, as well as any vitamins, herbs, or other supplements. Possible drug interactions include the following:

- Combining ropinirole with levodopa may cause twitching or jerky movements. To prevent these effects, your health-care practitioner will adjust the dosage of medications.

- Many drugs decrease the effects of ropinirole. These include haloperidol, phenothiazines, thioxanthenes, and metoclopramide.
- Other drugs increase the effects of ropinirole. These include ciprofloxacin, diltiazem, enoxacin, erythromycin, estrogen, fluvoxamine, norfloxacin, and tacrine.
- Ropinirole may increase the effects of central nervous system depressants such as tranquilizers.
- Tobacco may increase the effects of ropinirole.

FOOD, VITAMIN, AND HERBAL INTERACTIONS

Consult your health-care practitioner before combining ropinirole with any herbs with sedative effects, such as catnip, elecampane, goldenseal, gotu kola, hops, kava, lemon balm, skullcap, St. John's wort, and valerian.

RECOMMENDED DOSAGE

Ropinirole is available in tablet form. Although the doses given below are typical, only your health-care practitioner can determine the dose and schedule that are most appropriate for you.

- *Children:* This drug is not recommended for children.
- *Adults:* 0.25 mg 3 times daily to start, which can be gradually increased as needed to a maximum daily dose of 24 mg

To prevent stomach upset, take ropinirole with food. If you miss a dose, take it as soon as you remember. However, if it is almost time for the next dose, skip the one you missed and go back to your regular dosing schedule. Never take a double dose. Do not stop taking ropinirole suddenly. This may cause severe Parkinson's symptoms to return.

SYMPTOMS OF OVERDOSE AND WHAT TO DO

Symptoms of ropinirole overdose may include drowsiness, increased jerky movements, agitation, confusion, nausea, vomiting, chest pain, and dizziness upon standing. If you suspect an overdose, seek medical attention immediately, and bring the prescription bottle with you to the hospital so that health-care practitioners will know exactly what drug was used.

SPECIAL INFORMATION FOR PREGNANT OR NURSING WOMEN

No studies have adequately investigated the effects of ropinirole during pregnancy or breastfeeding. However, this drug caused birth defects in animal studies. If you are pregnant or plan to become pregnant, talk with your health-care practitioner before starting this drug. Only a health-care practitioner can determine whether the potential benefits outweigh the potential dangers.

Ropinirole may reduce milk production, and may pass into breast milk. If you must take this drug, your health-care practitioner will probably recommend bottle-feeding.

SPECIAL INFORMATION FOR SENIORS

Seniors may be more susceptible to side effects such as hallucinations.

GENERIC NAME

Rosiglitazone

BRAND NAME

Avandia
No generic available

ABOUT THIS DRUG

Rosiglitazone is used to treat the form of diabetes mellitus known as type 2. Type 2 diabetes was formerly known as adult-onset, and is also referred to as noninsulin-dependent. Diet and exercise play a key role in the management of this disease. Rosiglitazone can be used alone or with metformin or sulfonylureas.

This drug helps your body regulate the amount of glucose (sugar) in blood. It works by decreasing sugar production and making insulin work more efficiently. Rosiglitazone takes effect slowly.

SIDE EFFECTS

Report any severe or persistent side effects to your health-care practitioner. All diabetics should learn to recognize the symptoms of low blood sugar and high blood sugar and know what to do when they occur. It is essential to control these symptoms before they progress to more serious conditions.

- ➤ *Common:* respiratory infection, headache, accidental injury
- ➤ *Less Common or Rare:* low or high blood sugar, diarrhea, sinus irritation, fatigue, back pain, swelling, weight gain
- ➤ *Hypoglycemia (Low Blood Sugar):* "drunken" behavior, drowsiness, unusual tiredness or weakness, slurred speech, shakiness, dizziness, difficulty concentrating, headache, confusion, anxiety, nervousness,

blurred vision, cold sweats, cool pale skin, excessive hunger, restless sleep, nightmares, nausea, fast heartbeat

- *Hyperglycemia (High Blood Sugar):* dry mouth, thirst, frequent urination, dry skin, flushing, appetite loss, difficulty breathing, tiredness

IMPORTANT PRECAUTIONS

Rosiglitazone should not be used if you have liver disease, type 1 diabetes, or diabetic ketoacidosis (a life-threatening condition caused by insufficient insulin, with symptoms such as nausea, fatigue, excessive thirst, lower chest pain, and fruity breath). This drug may raise cholesterol levels and worsen heart failure and fluid retention. Tell your health-care practitioner if you plan to have any type of surgery or dental procedure.

Combining other antidiabetes medications with rosiglitazone may result in low blood sugar. The people most susceptible to hypoglycemia are older, weak, or malnourished, or have kidney, liver, adrenal, or hormone problems. Symptoms vary from person to person, so it is essential to learn which symptoms you usually have. As soon as you experience the characteristic signs, address and control them quickly by taking a fast-acting sugar, such as a glucose tablet, glass of fruit juice or nondiet soft drink, tablespoon of corn syrup or honey, or tablespoon of table sugar dissolved in water.

People with uncontrolled diabetes may also experience high blood sugar, or hyperglycemia. (See symptoms on previous page.) If this condition is not treated, it can lead to diabetic coma and death.

In order to prevent these types of complications, carefully follow all diet and exercise recommendations made by your health-care practitioner and nutritionist. In fact, many people with type 2 diabetes are able to successfully control this disease by making healthy lifestyle changes, cutting back on the need for medication.

To monitor the effectiveness of rosiglitazone, measure the amount of glucose in your urine or blood on a regular basis. Your health-care practitioner may also tell you to test your urine for ketones (substances that appear in urine when diabetes is not properly controlled). Carefully follow the instructions of your health-care practitioner and pharmacist when conducting these tests at home. If blood sugar is high or sugar or ketones are present in urine, call your health-care practitioner. Your health-care practitioner will also monitor your glucose levels and liver function during regular visits.

This drug may increase the possibility of conception. Use effective means of birth control.

Women may require lower doses of this drug than men.

DRUG INTERACTIONS

Inform your health-care practitioner and pharmacist if you are taking any other prescription or over-the-counter drugs, as well as any vitamins, herbs, or other supplements. Possible drug interactions include the following:

- Taking rosiglitazone with other antidiabetes drugs increases the risk of low blood sugar.
- Do not drink alcohol while taking rosiglitazone. Alcohol alters blood sugar.

FOOD, VITAMIN, AND HERBAL INTERACTIONS

Supplements such as chromium, garlic, ginger, ginseng, hawthorn, and nettle may affect blood sugar levels. Check with your health-care practitioner before using any dietary supplement.

RECOMMENDED DOSAGE

Rosiglitazone comes in tablet form. Although the doses given below are typical, only your health-care practitioner can determine the dose and schedule that best fit your needs.

- *Children:* This drug is not recommended for children.
- *Adults:* 4 to 8 mg daily in single or divided doses

This drug can be taken with or without food. If you miss a dose, take it as soon as you remember. However, if it is nearly time for your next scheduled dose, do not take the missed dose. Follow your regular dosing schedule. Never take a double dose.

SYMPTOMS OF OVERDOSE AND WHAT TO DO

Little information is available regarding rosiglitazone overdose. If you suspect that an overdose has occurred, seek immediate medical attention and take the prescription bottle to the hospital with you.

SPECIAL INFORMATION FOR PREGNANT OR NURSING WOMEN

No studies have adequately investigated the effects of rosiglitazone during pregnancy. It is critically important to monitor and control blood sugar when you are pregnant. However, it is safer to accomplish this through diet or a combination of diet and insulin. Consult your health-care practitioner as soon as you think you may be pregnant or if you are planning to become pregnant.

If you are breastfeeding or plan to do so, talk with your health-care practitioner before starting this drug. Only a health-care practitioner can determine whether the potential benefits outweigh the potential dangers.

SPECIAL INFORMATION FOR SENIORS

There are no special instructions for seniors.

GENERIC NAME

Rosiglitazone and metformin

BRAND NAME

Avandamet

No generic available

ABOUT THIS DRUG

The drug combination of rosiglitazone and metformin, along with diet and exercise, is used to reduce and maintain blood sugar (glucose) levels in people who have type 2 diabetes. Type 2 diabetes was formerly known as adult-onset, and is also referred to as non-insulin-dependent.

This drug works in two ways: The rosiglitazone portion of the drug increases insulin sensitivity, while the metformin decreases glucose production and improves glucose tolerance.

SIDE EFFECTS

Be sure to tell your health-care practitioner if you experience any side effects while taking rosiglitazone and metformin. Only your health-care practitioner can determine whether it is safe for you to continue taking this drug.

People with diabetes need to learn to recognize the symptoms of low blood sugar and high blood sugar and what to do when they occur. It is essential to control these symptoms before they progress to more serious conditions.

Rarely, people who have taken metformin have developed a life-threatening condition called lactic acidosis, an accumulation of lactic acid in the blood. In most cases, this condition occurs in people who have kidney or liver problems, and it is fatal in about 50 percent of cases. (See symptoms of lactic acidosis below.)

- *Common:* upper respiratory infection, headache, back pain, hyperglycemia, fatigue, diarrhea, viral infection, joint pain, sinusitis, anemia
- *Rare:* swelling, weight gain, shortness of breath. If these occur, contact your health-care practitioner immediately.

- *Hypoglycemia (Low Blood Sugar):* "drunken" behavior, drowsiness, unusual tiredness or weakness, slurred speech, shakiness, dizziness, difficulty concentrating, headache, confusion, anxiety, nervousness, blurred vision, cold sweats, cool pale skin, excessive hunger, restless sleep, nightmares, nausea, fast heartbeat
- *Hyperglycemia (High Blood Sugar):* dry mouth, thirst, frequent urination, dry skin, flushing, appetite loss, difficulty breathing, tiredness
- *Lactic Acidosis:* diarrhea, stomach discomfort, unusual tiredness or sleepiness, feeling cold, dizziness, lightheadedness, weakness, muscle pain and cramping, fast shallow breathing, slow or irregular heartbeat

IMPORTANT PRECAUTIONS

Tell your health-care practitioner if you are sensitive or allergic to rosiglitazone or metformin or to any other drugs.

Do not use this combination medication if you have liver disease, kidney disease, lung disease, heart failure that requires drug treatment, or if you drink alcohol in excess. Your health-care practitioner may conduct blood tests to monitor your liver while you take this drug. Also inform your health-care practitioner if you have other medical conditions such as pituitary or thyroid disease, adrenal insufficiency, or hormone problems. This drug is not approved for use with insulin.

This drug combination may cause swelling which, if not addressed, could worsen or lead to heart failure. If you notice swelling, dark urine, yellowing of the skin, unusual tiredness, or stomach problems while taking this drug, contact your health-care practitioner immediately.

Do not take this drug combination 2 days before or after having an X-ray using an injectable iodinated contrast agent (e.g., Omnipaque). Your health-care practitioner will also most likely advise you to stop taking this drug for a short time before and after having any type of surgery or dental procedure.

Hyperglycemia is a possible side effect of this drug combination (see symptoms above). If this condition is not treated, it can lead to diabetic coma and death. Another possible side effect is lactic acidosis (see symptoms above). In order to prevent these types of complications, carefully follow all diet and exercise recommendations made by your health-care practitioner and nutritionist. In fact, many people with type 2 diabetes are able to successfully control this disease by making healthy lifestyle changes, cutting back on the need for medication.

DRUG INTERACTIONS

Tell your health-care practitioner and pharmacist if you are taking any prescription or nonprescription drugs, as well as any vitamins, herbs, or other supplements. Possible drug interactions include the following:

- Taking rosiglitazone with other antidiabetes drugs increases the risk of low blood sugar.
- Metformin increases the blood-sugar-lowering effects of insulin.
- ACE inhibitors, amiloride, beta-blockers, cimetidine, clotrimazole, digoxin, furosemide, morphine, procainamide, quinidine, quinine, ranitidine, triamterene, trimethoprim, and vancomycin may increase the risk of side effects of this drug.
- Metformin may reduce the effect of glyburide, a sulfonylurea.
- Do not drink alcohol while taking this drug combination, as alcohol alters blood sugar levels.

FOOD, VITAMIN, AND HERBAL INTERACTIONS

Supplements such as chromium, garlic, ginger, ginseng, hawthorn, and nettle may affect blood sugar levels. Check with your health-care practitioner before using any dietary supplements.

Metformin is associated with malabsorption of vitamin B_{12}. Supplementation with vitamin B_{12} and calcium (which helps your body absorb B_{12}) may be helpful; consult with your health-care practitioner.

RECOMMENDED DOSAGE

The combination of rosiglitazone/metformin is available in tablets in the following formulas (the first number is rosiglitazone, the second, metformin): 1 mg/500 mg, 2 mg/500 mg, 4 mg/500 mg, 2 mg/1,000 mg, and 4 mg/1,000 mg. The dosages given here are typical. However, your health-care practitioner will determine the most appropriate dose and schedule for your needs.

- *Children:* not recommended for children
- *Adults:* Your health-care practitioner will decide which formulation is right for your needs, but dosage should not exceed 8 mg/2,000 mg per day, taken in divided doses.

The combination of rosiglitazone/metformin should be taken with meals. If you forget a dose, take it as soon as you remember. If it is almost time for the next dose, skip the missed dose and resume your normal dosing schedule. Never take a double dose.

SYMPTOMS OF OVERDOSE AND WHAT TO DO
An overdose of this drug combination may cause lactic acidosis. (See symptoms under "Side Effects.") If you suspect that an overdose has occurred, seek immediate medical attention and take the prescription bottle to the hospital with you.

SPECIAL INFORMATION FOR PREGNANT OR NURSING WOMEN
This drug should not be used during pregnancy. It is critically important to monitor and control blood sugar during pregnancy. However, it is safer to accomplish this through diet or a combination of diet and insulin. Consult your health-care practitioner as soon as you think you may be pregnant or if you are planning to become pregnant.

If you are breastfeeding or plan to do so, talk with your health-care practitioner before starting this drug. Only a health-care practitioner can determine whether the potential benefits outweigh the potential dangers.

SPECIAL INFORMATION FOR SENIORS
Adults 65 years and older are at increased risk of developing lactic acidosis when taking this drug because of a natural decline in kidney function. Your health-care practitioner should assess kidney function before prescribing this drug.

GENERIC NAME

Salmeterol

BRAND NAME
Serevent
No generic available

ABOUT THIS DRUG
Salmeterol is a long-acting bronchodilator medication used to prevent wheezing, shortness of breath, and troubled breathing caused by asthma, chronic bronchitis, emphysema, and other lung diseases. This drug is different from many other bronchodilators in that it does not work quickly enough to treat an asthma attack that has already begun.

Salmeterol works by relaxing the walls of the bronchial tubes. This opens air passages in the lungs, making it easier to breathe.

SIDE EFFECTS

Speak to your health-care practitioner if you develop side effects while taking this drug. Only he or she can determine whether you should continue taking salmeterol.

- *Common:* dry mouth, sore throat, changes in taste, nervousness, chest congestion, fast or irregular heartbeat, heart palpitations, nervousness, trembling
- *Less Common or Rare:* bad taste in mouth, cough, dizziness, tiredness, headache, stomach upset, nausea, vomiting, diarrhea, tremors, insomnia, heart rhythm disturbances, high blood pressure, worsening of asthma

IMPORTANT PRECAUTIONS

Salmeterol has a weaker effect on nerve receptors in the heart and blood vessels, which makes it safer to use if you have heart problems. However, large doses can still cause difficulties such as heart rhythm disturbances. Always tell your health-care practitioner about any other medical conditions you may have, especially heart disease, an irregular heartbeat, increased heart rate, high blood pressure, an overactive thyroid, glaucoma, diabetes, or seizures.

Keep in mind that salmeterol is for prevention only. Do not attempt to use it to treat acute asthma attacks. If asthma worsens, do not use more medication. See your health-care practitioner.

Inform your health-care practitioner if you have experienced allergies to this or similar medications in the past.

Because salmeterol may cause side effects such as nervousness and dizziness, do not drive a car, operate machinery, or perform other tasks that require concentration until you know how this drug affects you.

To relieve dry mouth or throat irritation, use sugarless gum or hard candy, or rinse your mouth with water.

DRUG INTERACTIONS

Tell your health-care practitioner if you are taking any other prescription or over-the-counter drugs, as well as any vitamins, herbs, or supplements. Possible drug interactions include the following:

- Taking salmeterol at the same time as or within 14 days of monoamine oxidase inhibitor (MAOI) antidepressants can cause a dangerous increase in blood pressure.
- Do not use other asthma medications without consulting your health-care practitioner. This can result in increased cardiovascular side effects.

- Salmeterol may reduce the effects of antihypertensive medications.
- Use tricyclic antidepressants with caution while taking this drug.
- Check with your health-care practitioner before using over-the-counter drugs. Many cold, cough, allergy, sinus, and weight loss remedies can raise blood pressure.

FOOD, VITAMIN, AND HERBAL INTERACTIONS

Do not take herbs that increase blood pressure, such as ephedra (ma huang), ginseng, goldenseal, licorice, and saw palmetto. Combining salmeterol with kola can cause nervousness. Avoid caffeinated beverages such as coffee, tea, and cola while you are taking this drug.

RECOMMENDED DOSAGE

Salmeterol comes as a powder for inhalation. Although the doses given below are typical, only your health-care practitioner can determine the dose and schedule that best fit your individual needs.

- *Children:* Powder for inhalation is not recommended for children under the age of 4.
- *Children 4 Years and Older and Adults:* 1 inhalation twice daily; or 1 inhalation at least 30 minutes before exercise

It is important to take salmeterol exactly as prescribed. Taking it more often than recommended can result in a loss in effectiveness and heart rhythm disturbances. If you forget a dose, take it as soon as you remember. Take the rest of the day's doses at evenly spaced intervals, and resume your normal schedule the next day. Never take a double dose. If you need to use 4 or more inhalations a day, consult your health-care practitioner.

SYMPTOMS OF OVERDOSE AND WHAT TO DO

Symptoms of salmeterol overdose include chest pain, rapid heart rate, high blood pressure, nervousness, tremor, dizziness, dry mouth, and headache. If overdose occurs, seek immediate medical attention and take the prescription bottle to the hospital with you.

SPECIAL INFORMATION FOR PREGNANT OR NURSING WOMEN

No studies have adequately investigated the effects of salmeterol during pregnancy or breastfeeding. If you are pregnant or plan to become pregnant, or if you are breastfeeding or plan to do so, talk with your health-care practitioner before starting this drug. Only a

health-care practitioner can determine whether the potential benefits outweigh the potential dangers.

SPECIAL INFORMATION FOR SENIORS

There are no special instructions for seniors.

GENERIC NAME

Selegiline

BRAND NAMES

Atapryl, Carbex, Eldepryl
Generic available

ABOUT THIS DRUG

Selegiline is used to treat Parkinson's disease. It is always combined with levodopa and carbidopa, and by itself has no effect. This drug is generally prescribed when levodopa and carbidopa alone grow less effective in controlling the symptoms of Parkinson's disease.

Like other antiparkinsonian drugs, selegiline works by correcting the dopamine deficiency that is believed to be the cause of Parkinson's disease. It stimulates dopamine receptors and blocks the effects of the enzyme monoamine oxidase (MAO).

SIDE EFFECTS

Taking more than 10 mg of selegiline daily has been associated with potentially fatal high blood pressure. Stop taking medication and contact your health-care practitioner immediately if you experience symptoms such as a severe headache, chest pain, heart palpitations, nausea, vomiting, muscle spasms, or unusual jerking body movements. Also inform your health-care practitioner of other side effects, particularly if they are severe or prolonged. Only your health-care practitioner can determine whether it is safe for you to continue taking this drug.

- *Common:* nausea, vomiting, abdominal or stomach pain, dizziness, lightheadedness, fainting, dry mouth, trouble sleeping, mood or other mental changes, increase in unusual body movements
- *Less Common or Rare:* anxiety, sweating, chills, diarrhea, constipation, body aches, muscle cramps, heart rhythm disturbances, fast heartbeat, false sense of well-being, delusions, depression, irritability, memory problems, blurred or double vision, involuntary movements, tremor, numbness of fingers and toes, restlessness, ringing in

the ears, taste changes, loss of appetite, weight loss, dizziness upon standing, increased sensitivity to light, rash, itching, inability to urinate, heartburn, headache, migraine, heart palpitations, high blood pressure, convulsions

IMPORTANT PRECAUTIONS

Always inform your health-care practitioner of any other medical conditions you have, especially ulcers. Tell your health-care practitioner if you have ever experienced an allergic reaction to this or any other MAO inhibitor.

Because selegiline may cause side effects such as dizziness and fatigue, do not drive a car, operate machinery, or perform other tasks that require concentration until you know how this drug affects you.

When you first start taking this drug or when the dosage is increased, you may experience dizziness or faintness when you rise quickly from a sitting or reclining position (postural hypotension). Try to get up slowly, and consult your health-care practitioner if the problem continues.

Selegiline may cause dry mouth. To counteract this effect, use sugarless gum or candy, ice chips, or a saliva substitute. If the problem continues, consult your health-care practitioner or dentist.

Selegiline may cause increased sensitivity to sunlight. When you take this drug, avoid direct sunlight and wear sunscreen.

To monitor treatment, visit your health-care practitioner on a regular basis.

DRUG INTERACTIONS

Selegiline may have dangerous interactions with many drugs. Always tell your health-care practitioner and pharmacist if you are taking any other prescription or over-the-counter drugs, as well as any vitamins, herbs, or other supplements. Possible drug interactions include the following:

- Do not take selegiline with tricyclic antidepressants, fluoxetine, fluvoxamine, meperidine, nefazodone, paroxetine, sertraline, or venlafaxine. These combinations may increase the risk of serious side effects. If you have been taking any of these drugs, your health-care practitioner will advise you to wait from 14 days to 5 weeks in order to clear them completely from your system before beginning to take selegiline.
- Do not combine selegiline with over-the-counter remedies such as cold, sinus, asthma, hay fever, allergy, or appetite control remedies. Many of these medications affect blood pressure.

- Selegiline is typically combined with levodopa or carbidopa to control symptoms.
- Avoid alcohol while taking this drug.

FOOD, VITAMIN, AND HERBAL INTERACTIONS

If you are using doses of more than 10 mg daily, it is essential to avoid foods that are rich in the amino acid tyramine while taking and for 2 weeks after taking selegiline. This combination may result in an excessive and potentially fatal rise in blood pressure. Tyramine-rich foods include (but are not limited to) aged cheeses, bologna, chicken liver, chocolate, figs, pickled herring, pepperoni, raisins, salami, soy sauce, and yeast extracts. Also avoid beverages that contain meat or meat tenderizers, and alcoholic beverages that may contain tyramine, which include some beers, vermouth, and Chianti wines.

Herbs that affect the central nervous system—including St. John's wort, guarana, ephedra (ma huang), ginseng, scotch broom, and kola—must also be avoided when taking selegiline. In addition, avoid caffeinated beverages, such as coffee, tea, and cola.

RECOMMENDED DOSAGE

Selegiline is available in capsule or tablet form. Dosage is particularly important with this drug, since doses of more than 10 mg are associated with dangerous side effects. Although the doses given below are typical, only your health-care practitioner can determine the dose and schedule that are most appropriate for you.

- *Children:* This drug is not recommended for children.
- *Adults:* 5 mg twice daily, with breakfast and lunch

To prevent stomach upset, take selegiline with food. If you miss a dose, take it as soon as you remember. However, if it is almost time for the next dose, skip the one you missed and go back to your regular dosing schedule. Never take a double dose. Do not stop taking selegiline suddenly.

SYMPTOMS OF OVERDOSE AND WHAT TO DO

Overdose may be fatal. Symptoms include chest pain, dizziness, agitation, fainting, high fever, changes in blood pressure, sweating, difficulty breathing, and convulsions. If you suspect an overdose, seek medical attention immediately, and bring the prescription bottle with you to the hospital so that health-care practitioners will know exactly what drug was used.

SPECIAL INFORMATION FOR PREGNANT OR NURSING WOMEN

No studies have adequately investigated the effects of selegiline during pregnancy or breastfeeding. If you are pregnant or plan to become pregnant, or if you are breastfeeding or plan to do so, talk with your health-care practitioner before starting this drug. Only a health-care practitioner can determine whether the potential benefits outweigh the potential dangers.

SPECIAL INFORMATION FOR SENIORS

Seniors may be more susceptible to side effects and should take the lowest effective dosage.

GENERIC NAME

Sertraline

BRAND NAME

Zoloft

No generic available

ABOUT THIS DRUG

Sertraline is used to treat mental depression. Symptoms include sleep disturbances, appetite changes, sadness, guilt, shame, low self-esteem, anxiety, and extreme fatigue that last for over two weeks. It is also prescribed for obsessive-compulsive disorder, panic disorder, and posttraumatic stress disorder.

Sertraline is a type of drug known as a selective serotonin reuptake inhibitor (SSRI). It works by making more serotonin available in the brain.

SIDE EFFECTS

Inform your health-care practitioner if you develop side effects while taking sertraline. If symptoms are severe or prolonged, ask your health-care practitioner whether your dosage requires adjustment, and whether it is safe for you to continue taking this drug.

- *Common:* decreased sexual desire or ability, drowsiness, dizziness, weakness, trembling, shaking, increased sweating, decreased appetite, weight loss, dry mouth, nausea, diarrhea, constipation, gas, nervousness, male genital disorders
- *Less Common or Rare:* agitation, blurred vision, drugged feeling, pounding heartbeat, flushing, increased appetite, breast tender-

ness, vaginal inflammation, persistent and painful erection, muscle tenderness or weakness, upset stomach, vomiting, yawning, twitching, tightness in throat, altered sense of taste, burning or tingling sensation, urinary disorders, rash, sensitivity to light, changes in blood pressure, restlessness, inability to sit still, mania

IMPORTANT PRECAUTIONS

Always inform your health-care practitioner about any other medical conditions you may have, especially a history of convulsions or seizures, brain disease, mental retardation, kidney or liver impairment, or mania (a type of mental illness). Tell your health-care practitioner if you have ever experienced an allergic reaction to this or similar drugs. Lower doses are appropriate for seniors and those with liver or kidney disease.

If you plan to undergo surgery or a dental procedure, tell your health-care practitioner or dentist that you are taking sertraline.

This drug can make you dizzy and less alert than usual. Until you know how sertraline affects you, do not drive a car, operate machinery, or perform other tasks that require concentration.

If this drug causes dry mouth, use sugarless gum or candy, ice chips, or artificial saliva. If the problem continues, consult your health-care practitioner or dentist.

Sertraline may cause excessive sweating. If you work or exercise in hot weather, drink plenty of fluids to prevent dehydration.

Sertraline may cause increased sensitivity to sunlight. When you take this drug, avoid direct sunlight and wear sunscreen.

You may have to take this drug for 4 or more weeks before it takes effect. You should be regularly monitored by your health-care practitioner while taking sertraline.

DRUG INTERACTIONS

Tell your health-care practitioner and pharmacist if you are taking any other prescription or over-the-counter drugs, as well as any vitamins, herbs, or other supplements. Possible drug interactions include the following:

- Do not take monoamine oxidase inhibitor (MAOI) antidepressants at the same time as or within 14 days of sertraline. This combination can cause potentially fatal serotonin syndrome (racing heartbeat, restlessness, increased sweating, mood or behavior changes, overactive reflexes, shivering, shaking, diarrhea, and fever).
- Other drugs that may lead to serotonin syndrome include buspirone, dextromethorphan (an ingredient in many over-the-counter cough suppressants), levodopa, lithium, meperidine, nefazodone, pentazocine, sumatriptan, tricyclic antidepressants, and venlafaxine.

- Taking other central nervous system depressants along with sertraline can result in more drowsiness.
- Taking sertraline with warfarin may result in increased bleeding.
- Cimetidine may increase the effects of sertraline.
- The combination of lithium and sertraline may cause increased adverse effects.
- Do not drink alcohol while taking sertraline.

FOOD, VITAMIN, AND HERBAL INTERACTIONS

Do not combine sertraline with herbs such as hops, kava, passionflower, and valerian. These can increase effects such as drowsiness. Do not take St. John's wort with sertraline, since both affect serotonin. Other inappropriate herbs include ginseng, ephedra (ma huang), and yohimbe.

RECOMMENDED DOSAGE

Sertraline comes as a tablet or an oral concentrate. Although the doses given below are typical, only your health-care practitioner can determine the dose and schedule that best fit your needs.

- *Children:* 25 to 50 mg once daily, which may be gradually increased as needed to a maximum daily dose of 200 mg
- *Adults:* 50 to 200 mg once daily

Sertraline can be taken with or without food. It must be taken regularly for several weeks before its full effect is felt. The oral concentrate may be mixed with 4 ounces of water, ginger ale, orange juice, or lemonade. If you forget a dose, take it as soon as you remember. If it is almost time for the next dose, skip the missed one and resume your normal schedule. Never take a double dose. Do not stop taking this drug suddenly, especially if you have been taking it a long time. Your health-care practitioner will gradually reduce dosage.

SYMPTOMS OF OVERDOSE AND WHAT TO DO

The symptoms of sertraline overdose include anxiety, drowsiness, nausea, vomiting, dilated pupils, and rapid heartbeat. If overdose occurs, seek immediate medical attention and take the prescription bottle to the hospital with you.

SPECIAL INFORMATION FOR PREGNANT OR NURSING WOMEN

No studies have adequately investigated the effects of sertraline during pregnancy or breastfeeding. If you are pregnant or plan to become pregnant, or if you are breastfeeding or plan to do so, talk with your health-care practitioner before starting this drug. Only a health-care practitioner can determine whether the potential benefits outweigh the potential dangers.

SPECIAL INFORMATION FOR SENIORS

Seniors may benefit from smaller doses.

OPEN QUESTIONS OR CONTROVERSIES

In June 2004, the Food and Drug Administration asked manufacturers of sertraline to include in their labeling a warning statement that recommends close observation of adult and pediatric patients for clinical worsening of depression or the emergence of suicidality when being treated with this drug, especially when beginning the drug, or at the time of dose changes, either increases or decreases.

GENERIC NAME

Sevelamer polysulfate sodium

BRAND NAME

Renagel

No generic available

ABOUT THIS DRUG

Sevelamer polysulfate sodium is used to treat high blood phosphate levels in people with end-stage renal disease (ESRD). People with ESRD, a form of kidney disease, retain phosphorus. This can accumulate and have a negative impact on calcium levels. Sevelamer works by reducing the amount of phosphorus absorbed by the body through food.

SIDE EFFECTS

Inform your health-care practitioner if you develop side effects while taking sevelamer. If symptoms are severe or prolonged, ask your health-care practitioner whether your dosage requires adjustment, and whether it is safe for you to continue taking this drug.

- *Common:* nausea, vomiting, diarrhea, pain, stomach upset, headache, changes in blood pressure, blood clotting problems
- *Less Common or Rare:* bloating, gas, constipation, cough

IMPORTANT PRECAUTIONS

Always inform your health-care practitioner about any other medical conditions you may have, especially stomach or intestinal problems, intestinal blockage, difficulty swallowing, a history of gastrointestinal surgery, or a low phosphate level.

If you plan to undergo surgery or a dental procedure, tell your health-care practitioner or dentist that you are taking sevelamer.

DRUG INTERACTIONS

Tell your health-care practitioner and pharmacist if you are taking any other prescription or over-the-counter drugs, as well as any vitamins, herbs, or other supplements. Drug-drug interactions may occur. Generally, take sevelamer 1 hour before or 3 hours after other drugs.

FOOD, VITAMIN, AND HERBAL INTERACTIONS

Take a daily multivitamin, and follow any special dietary instructions recommended by your health-care practitioner or nutritionist.

RECOMMENDED DOSAGE

Sevelamer comes as a capsule or tablet. Although the doses given below are typical, only your health-care practitioner can determine the dose and schedule that best fit your needs.

- *Children:* This drug is not recommended for children.
- *Adults:* 2 to 4 capsules 3 times daily with meals, or 1 to 4 tablets 3 times daily with meals

Sevelamer should be taken with meals. Swallow the capsules whole. If you forget a dose, skip it and take the next dose with your next meal. Never take a double dose.

SYMPTOMS OF OVERDOSE AND WHAT TO DO

No specific information on overdosing with sevelamer is available. If you suspect an overdose, seek immediate medical attention and take the prescription bottle to the hospital with you.

SPECIAL INFORMATION FOR PREGNANT OR NURSING WOMEN

No studies have adequately investigated the effects of sevelamer during pregnancy or breastfeeding. However, in animal studies, it has affected bone development. If you are pregnant or plan to become pregnant, or if you are breastfeeding or plan to do so, talk with your health-care practitioner before starting this drug. Only a health-care practitioner can determine whether the potential benefits outweigh the potential dangers.

SPECIAL INFORMATION FOR SENIORS

There are no special instructions for seniors.

GENERIC NAME

Sibutramine

BRAND NAME

Meridia
No generic available

ABOUT THIS DRUG

Sibutramine is an appetite suppressant used in the treatment of obesity. This drug should be used on a short-term basis only and under a health-care practitioner's close supervision. Appetite suppressants are not a substitute for a sensible, healthy, overall weight loss program. Sibutramine works by stimulating the activity of norepinephrine and serotonin in the brain.

SIDE EFFECTS

If you develop side effects while taking sibutramine, ask your health-care practitioner whether it is safe for you to continue taking this drug.

➤ *Common:* nervousness, anxiety, restlessness, irritability, impatience, difficulty sleeping, headache, dizziness, dry mouth, stuffy or runny nose, constipation

➤ *Less Common or Rare:* high blood pressure, throbbing heartbeat, nausea, vomiting, diarrhea, thirst, aches, chills, emotional changes, mental depression, painful menstruation, swelling of feet and ankles, abdominal or back pain, tingling, itching, flushing, increased sweating, changes in taste, drowsiness, increase in appetite, reduced vision, vaginal or urinary infection

IMPORTANT PRECAUTIONS

This drug is not an appropriate remedy for people who have anorexia, heart disease, high blood pressure, glaucoma, or a history of stroke. Also tell your health-care practitioner about any other medical conditions you may have, such as brain disease, mental retardation, seizures, gallstones, thyroid problems, or kidney or liver disease. Do not use sibutramine if you have ever experienced an allergic reaction to this or other appetite suppressants. Because appetite suppressants have habit-forming potential, inform your health-care practitioner if you have a history of mental illness or substance abuse. If you have diabetes, sibutramine may alter the amount of medication you require.

In order to lose weight, follow a reduced-calorie diet and an exercise program while taking sibutramine. To keep weight off after you stop taking this drug, continue to follow a sensible program of diet and exercise under the supervision of your health-care practitioner.

Sibutramine makes some people dizzy and nervous. Until you know how this drug affects you, do not drive a car, operate machinery, or engage in other actions that require concentration.

Because sibutramine may cause dry mouth, use sugarless candy or gum, ice chips, or a saliva substitute. If the problem continues, consult your health-care practitioner or dentist.

Before having surgery or a dental procedure, tell your health-care practitioner or dentist that you take sibutramine.

Because sibutramine may cause serious side effects such as high blood pressure, your health-care practitioner will carefully monitor your condition while you take it. Notify your health-care practitioner at once if you experience an allergic reaction such as a rash or hives.

DRUG INTERACTIONS

Tell your health-care practitioner and pharmacist if you are taking any other prescription or over-the-counter drugs, as well as any vitamins, herbs, or other supplements. Possible drug interactions include the following:

➤ Do not take sibutramine with or within 14 days of taking a monoamine oxidase (MAO) inhibitor. This combination can cause dangerous and potentially life-threatening effects such as seizures or very high blood pressure.

➤ Combining sibutramine with other stimulants (such as other appetite suppressants, amphetamines, methylphenidate, caffeine, or cocaine) can result in unwanted effects ranging from overstimulation to heart problems.

➤ Other medications that may cause unwanted effects when combined with sibutramine include tricyclic antidepressants, SSRIs such as paroxetine, buspirone, levodopa, meperidine, nefazodone, pentazocine, sumatriptan, tramadol, tryptophan, and venlafaxine.

- Be careful when you use over-the-counter remedies while taking sibutramine. Many decongestant, cough, cold, sinus, and allergy remedies raise blood pressure.
- Avoid alcohol while taking this drug.

FOOD, VITAMIN, AND HERBAL INTERACTIONS

Do not take sibutramine with herbs that raise blood pressure, such as ephedra (ma huang), ginseng, goldenseal, licorice, or saw palmetto. Avoid taking with St. John's wort as both this herb and sibutramine affect serotonin.

Moderate your consumption of caffeinated beverages such as coffee, tea, and cola.

RECOMMENDED DOSAGE

Sibutramine comes as a capsule. The doses given below are typical, but only your health-care practitioner can determine the dose and schedule that best fit your particular needs.

- *Children:* This drug is not recommended for children under the age of 16.
- *Adults:* 10 to 15 mg once daily in the morning

Sibutramine may be taken with or without food. If you forget a dose and remember it within 2 or 3 hours, take it. Otherwise skip that dose and return to your normal schedule. Never take double doses.

SYMPTOMS OF OVERDOSE AND WHAT TO DO

Little is known about sibutramine overdose. If overdose occurs, seek immediate medical attention and take the bottle of sibutramine to the hospital with you.

SPECIAL INFORMATION FOR PREGNANT OR NURSING WOMEN

Do not use sibutramine during pregnancy. If you are of childbearing age, use an effective means of contraception while taking this drug. It is not known whether sibutramine passes into breast milk. However, if you are breastfeeding, your health-care practitioner will likely advise you to stop until your treatment is done.

SPECIAL INFORMATION FOR SENIORS

Sibutramine may aggravate many diseases associated with old age, including heart disease and high blood pressure.

OPEN QUESTIONS OR CONTROVERSIES

Appetite suppressants can cause dependence. They should be used on a short-term basis only, and should be avoided by those with a history of mental illness or drug or alcohol abuse. Signs of dependence include a strong need for medication, a desire to increase the dosage, and withdrawal symptoms (such as depression, cramps, nausea, and fatigue) when you stop taking sibutramineg.

GENERIC NAME

Sildenafil citrate

BRAND NAME

Viagra

No generic available

ABOUT THIS DRUG

Sildenafil citrate is used to treat men who have erectile dysfunction, or sexual impotence. This is the first oral drug for impotence. It works by controlling the enzyme phosphodiesterase. This helps maintain an erection when the penis is stimulated. Sildenafil does not work in the absence of stimulation.

SIDE EFFECTS

If you experience a prolonged or painful erection for 4 hours or more, contact your health-care practitioner at once. Also inform him or her if any other side effects are severe or prolonged. Only your health-care practitioner can determine whether it is safe for you to continue taking this drug.

- *Common:* headache, flushing, nasal congestion, stomach discomfort following meals
- *Less Common or Rare:* diarrhea, visual disturbances, sensitivity to light, dizziness, bladder pain, bloody or cloudy urine, increased frequency of urination, pain upon urination

Men taking sildenafil have experienced sharp rises in blood pressure, heart attacks, other heart irregularities, and strokes. These problems occur more frequently in men who have risk factors for cardiovascular disease.

IMPORTANT PRECAUTIONS

Do not take sildenafil if you have heart problems severe enough to limit sexual activity. Use this drug with extreme caution (if at all) if you have coronary artery disease, an irregular heartbeat, blood pressure abnormalities, a history of heart attack or stroke in the last 6 months, penis abnormalities, a blood disorder, bleeding problems, kidney or liver impairment, or retinitis pigmentosa. Do not use this drug if you have experienced an allergic reaction to it in the past.

Possible side effects of sildenafil include blurred vision and dizziness. Until you know how this drug affects you, do not drive a car, operate machinery, or perform other tasks that require concentration.

DRUG INTERACTIONS

Tell your health-care practitioner and pharmacist if you are taking any other prescription or over-the-counter drugs, as well as any vitamins, herbs, or other supplements. Possible drug interactions include the following:

- Do not combine sildenafil with nitrates such as nitroglycerin. Sildenafil increases their blood-pressure-lowering effects.
- Consult your health-care practitioner before taking sildenafil with any other drugs that lower blood pressure.
- Certain drugs can increase the unwanted effects of sildenafil. These include cimetidine, erythromycin, itraconazole, ritonavir, and saquinavir.
- Rifampin may reduce the effects of sildenafil.

FOOD, VITAMIN, AND HERBAL INTERACTIONS

Do not combine sildenafil with herbal remedies for impotence, such as ginseng.

RECOMMENDED DOSAGE

Sildenafil comes as a tablet. The doses given below are typical. However, only your health-care practitioner can determine the dose and schedule that best fit your individual needs.

- *Children:* This drug is not recommended for children.
- *Adults:* 50 to 100 mg as a single dose once daily, 1 hour before sexual activity

Sildenafil usually begins to work within 30 minutes. It may continue to work for up to 4 hours, although it usually begins to lose effectiveness after 2 hours.

SYMPTOMS OF OVERDOSE AND WHAT TO DO

No information is available regarding sildenafil overdose. However, if you suspect an overdose, seek immediate medical attention and take the prescription bottle to the hospital with you so the health-care practitioner will know exactly what medication was taken.

SPECIAL INFORMATION FOR PREGNANT OR NURSING WOMEN

Sildenafil is approved for use by men only.

SPECIAL INFORMATION FOR SENIORS

The recommended dosage for men over age 65 is 25 mg as a single dose no more than once daily.

GENERIC NAME

Simvastatin

see *Statin Cholesterol-Lowering Drugs, page 959*

GENERIC NAME

Sparfloxacin

see *Fluoroquinolone Antibiotics, page 468*

GENERIC NAME

Spironolactone

BRAND NAMES

Aldactone, Dyrenium, Midamor
Generic available

ABOUT THIS DRUG

Spironolactone is a potassium-sparing diuretic used to reduce the amount of water in the body. Also known as a "water pill," this drug is prescribed for high blood pressure and fluid retention caused by conditions such as heart disease.

Spironolactone helps reduce the amount of water and salt in the body. Unlike many other diuretics, this medication does not cause your body to lose potassium. It works by interfering with the action of aldosterone, a hormone that helps regulate the body's salt and potassium levels.

SIDE EFFECTS

Consult your health-care practitioner if you develop side effects while taking spirolactone. Only he or she can determine whether it is safe for you to continue taking this drug.

- *Common:* nausea, vomiting, stomach cramps, diarrhea, tiredness, frequent urination (especially at first)
- *Less Common or Rare:* dizziness, headache, sweating, decreased sexual ability, breast tenderness and deepening of voice in females, irregular menstrual periods, breast enlargement in males, rash, itching, shortness of breath, cough, hoarseness, fever, chills, lower back or side pain, painful or difficult urination

Beware of symptoms of high blood potassium (hyperkalemia), which may include shortness of breath, nervousness, numbness or tingling, confusion, tiredness, weakness, and heaviness in legs.

IMPORTANT PRECAUTIONS

Do not use spironolactone if you have high blood potassium, difficulty urinating, or kidney failure. Tell your health-care practitioner if you have or have ever had medical conditions such as diabetes, liver disease, menstrual problems, or dehydration.

Before having any type of surgery or dental procedure, tell your surgeon or dentist that you are taking spironolactone. Your health-care practitioner will monitor your blood pressure, potassium level, and kidneys while you take this medication.

Treatment of high blood pressure also entails certain lifestyle changes, such as weight control, smoking cessation, and close attention to diet.

Spironolactone may cause side effects such as dizziness. Do not drive a car, operate machinery, or perform other tasks that require concentration until you know how the drug you are taking affects you.

Alert your health-care practitioner if you experience an illness accompanied by diarrhea, vomiting, and sweating. This may cause the loss of too much water and potassium.

Be careful when you exercise in hot weather or enter a hot bath or sauna. Heavy sweating can lead to dizziness, lightheadedness, fainting, vomiting, dehydration, and low blood pressure.

DRUG INTERACTIONS

Tell your health-care practitioner and pharmacist if you are taking any other prescription or over-the-counter drugs, as well as any vitamins, herbs, or other supplements. Possible drug interactions include the following:

- Spironolactone enhances the effectiveness of certain other blood pressure medications.
- Do not take ACE inhibitors in combination with spironolactone.
- Spironolactone may interfere with blood thinners such as warfarin.
- Taking this drug with barbiturates or narcotics may increase the risk of dizziness and fainting.
- NSAIDs such as indomethacin may result in dangerous elevations of potassium.
- Consult your health-care practitioner before taking over-the-counter cough, cold, sinus, allergy, or weight loss medications. Many of these can raise blood pressure.
- Other medications that may interact with spironolactone include digoxin, lithium, mitotane, and corticosteroids.
- Limit your alcohol intake. You are more likely to experience effects such as dizziness, lightheadedness, and fainting if you use alcohol.

FOOD, VITAMIN, AND HERBAL INTERACTIONS

Do not take herbs that increase blood pressure, such as ephedra (ma huang), ginseng, goldenseal, licorice, and saw palmetto. Consult your health-care practitioner before taking substances that may lower blood pressure, such as calcium, soy, or garlic.

Do not take potassium supplements with spironolactone unless they are prescribed by your health-care practitioner. Consult your health-care practitioner before making any dietary changes. Do not use salt substitutes or low-sodium milk, which often contain potassium.

RECOMMENDED DOSAGE

Spironolactone comes in tablet form. Although the doses given below are typical, only your health-care practitioner can determine the dose and schedule that are most appropriate for you.

- *Children:* 1 to 2 mg per pound of body weight daily
- *Adults:* 25 to 400 mg daily in single or divided doses

Take spironolactone doses at the same time every day with food. If you miss a dose, take it as soon as you remember. However, if it is nearly time for your next scheduled dose, do not take the missed dose. Follow your regular dosing schedule. Never take a double dose.

SYMPTOMS OF OVERDOSE AND WHAT TO DO

Symptoms of overdose may include nausea, vomiting, drowsiness, dizziness, confusion, rash, and diarrhea. If overdose occurs, seek immediate medical attention, and bring the prescription bottle with you to the hospital so that health-care practitioners will know exactly what drug was used.

SPECIAL INFORMATION FOR PREGNANT OR NURSING WOMEN

No studies have adequately investigated the effects of this drug during pregnancy or breastfeeding. If you are pregnant or plan to become pregnant, or if you are breastfeeding or plan to do so, talk with your health-care practitioner before starting spironolactone. Only a health-care practitioner can determine whether the potential benefits outweigh the risks.

SPECIAL INFORMATION FOR SENIORS

Because seniors are more sensitive to the effects of this drug, lower doses are usually prescribed.

GENERIC NAME

Class: Statin cholesterol-lowering drugs

Generics: (1) atorvastatin; (2) fluvastatin; (3) lovastatin; (4) pravastatin; (5) rosuvastatin; (6) simvastatin

BRAND NAMES

(1) Lipitor; (2) Lescol; (3) Altocor, Mevacor; (4) Pravachol; (5) Crestor; (6) Zocor

No generic available

ABOUT THESE DRUGS

Statin cholesterol-lowering drugs are used to reduce the amount of cholesterol and fatty substances called triglycerides in the body. They are used in combination with dietary adjustments. Accumulation of cholesterol and fats along the walls of arteries decreases blood flow and oxygen supply to the heart, brain, and other parts of the body. Lowering cholesterol and triglyceride levels helps prevent heart disease, angina (chest pain), heart attacks, and strokes.

These drugs work by blocking the effects of an enzyme known as HMG-CoA reductase. Cholesterol levels are improved in as little as 1 to 2 weeks after you begin taking a statin drug, but the full effect may take up to 6 weeks.

SIDE EFFECTS

Consult your health-care practitioner if you develop side effects while taking one of these drugs. Only he or she can determine whether it is safe for you to continue taking it.

- *Common:* headache, muscle aches, diarrhea, constipation, stomach pain, cramps, gas, nausea, vomiting, common cold symptoms, generalized pain, changes in taste
- *Less Common or Rare:* dizziness, sleepiness, joint pain, arthritis, runny nose, sinus irritation, tooth problems, chest pain, sore throat, cough, infection, urinary difficulties, blurred vision, rash, itching, allergic reactions

If you experience muscle pain, stop taking medication and contact your health-care practitioner at once. This may be a sign of a rare but extremely dangerous muscle problem called rhabdomyolysis.

IMPORTANT PRECAUTIONS

Tell your health-care practitioner if you have or have ever had medical conditions such as kidney or liver disease, a dependence on alcohol, low blood pressure, or seizures. Inform your health-care practitioner if you have ever experienced an allergic reaction to a statin drug.

Before having any type of surgery or dental procedure, tell your surgeon or dentist that you are taking a statin drug. Your health-care practitioner will monitor your condition while you take statins, especially your liver function.

Statin drugs may cause side effects such as dizziness and sleepiness. Do not drive a car, operate machinery, or perform other tasks that require concentration until you know how the drug you are taking affects you.

Statin drugs may cause increased sensitivity to sunlight. Avoid direct sunlight, wear protective clothing, and apply sunscreen.

Treatment of high blood pressure also entails certain lifestyle changes, such as weight control, smoking cessation, and close attention to diet.

DRUG INTERACTIONS

Tell your health-care practitioner and pharmacist if you are taking any other prescription or over-the-counter drugs, as well as any vitamins, herbs, or other supplements. Possible drug interactions include the following:

- Statins should be taken with caution, if at all, with cyclosporine, erythromycin, gemfibrozil, or niacin. These combinations increase the risk of muscle problems.

- Statins increase the absorption of digoxin.
- Itraconazole and cholestyramine may increase the effects of statins.
- Propranolol may reduce the effects of statins.
- Statins may increase the effects of warfarin.
- Separate doses of antacids and atorvastatin by at least an hour.
- Atorvastatin increases blood levels of oral contraceptives.
- Using alcohol with statins increases the risk of liver damage.

FOOD, VITAMIN, AND HERBAL INTERACTIONS

It is very important to follow your health-care practitioner's dietary recommendations. A low-fat, low-cholesterol diet will help control cholesterol and triglyceride levels.

Do not take herbs that increase blood pressure, such as ephedra (ma huang), ginseng, goldenseal, licorice, and saw palmetto. Consult your health-care practitioner before taking substances that may lower blood pressure, such as calcium, soy, or garlic. Do not combine statins with St. John's wort, since both cause heightened sensitivity to the sun.

RECOMMENDED DOSAGE

Statin cholesterol-lowering drugs come primarily in tablet form. (Fluvastatin comes as a capsule.) Although the doses given below are typical, only your health-care practitioner can determine the dose and schedule that are most appropriate for you.

Atorvastatin

- *Children:* This drug is not recommended for children.
- *Adults:* 10 to 80 mg daily

Fluvastatin

- *Children:* This drug is not recommended for children.
- *Adults:* 20 to 40 mg daily at bedtime

Lovastatin

- *Children:* This drug is not recommended for children.
- *Adults:* 20 to 80 mg daily, in 1 or 2 doses; for Mevacor, starting dose is 20 to 60 mg once at bedtime.

Pravastatin

- *Children:* This drug is not recommended for children.
- *Adults:* 10 to 40 mg daily at bedtime

Rosuvastatin

- *Children:* This drug is not recommended for children.
- *Adults:* 5 to 40 mg daily in one dose

Simvastatin

- *Children:* This drug is not recommended for children.
- *Adults:* 5 to 40 mg daily at bedtime

Take lovastatin with meals. Other statins may be taken with or without food. If you miss a dose of a statin, take it as soon as you remember. However, if it is nearly time for your next scheduled dose, do not take the missed dose. Follow your regular dosing schedule. Never take a double dose.

SYMPTOMS OF OVERDOSE AND WHAT TO DO

No specific information is available regarding overdose. However, if you suspect an overdose, seek immediate medical attention, and bring the prescription bottle with you to the hospital so that health-care practitioners will know exactly what drug was used.

SPECIAL INFORMATION FOR PREGNANT OR NURSING WOMEN

These drugs should not be used if you are pregnant or breastfeeding.

SPECIAL INFORMATION FOR SENIORS

Because seniors are more sensitive to the effects of these drugs, lower doses are prescribed.

OPEN QUESTIONS OR CONTROVERSIES

In August 2001, a statin drug known as cerivastatin was withdrawn from the U.S. market. All statins may in rare cases be associated with dangerous muscle cell damage. However, this problem appeared to be much more common with cerivastatin, which was linked with 31 deaths.

GENERIC NAME

Stavudine

BRAND NAME

Zerit
No generic available

ABOUT THIS DRUG

Stavudine is an antiviral drug prescribed to treat advanced HIV, the human immunodeficiency virus that causes acquired immune deficiency syndrome (AIDS). This drug has many serious side effects, and is only used when other AIDS treatments aren't working or can't be tolerated. Stavudine, which is also known as d4T, interferes with viral DNA duplication, which helps to keep the HIV virus from reproducing.

SIDE EFFECTS

Side effects from this drug are common and can be life-threatening. Contact your health-care practitioner at once if you develop any new persistent or severe symptoms. Only he or she can determine if you should continue to take stavudine.

- *Common:* peripheral neuropathy (tingling, burning, numbness, or pain in the hands or feet), nausea, vomiting, upset stomach, diarrhea, constipation, headache, dizziness, weakness, an overall feeling of unwellness, depression, anxiety, nervousness, insomnia, abdominal or back pain, chest pain, joint and muscle aches, generalized pain, appetite and weight loss, swollen glands, flu-like symptoms, chills, sweating, fever, rash, itching, allergic reactions
- *Less Common or Rare:* pancreatitis (inflammation of the pancreas), high blood pressure, flushing, tumors, stomach ulcers, asthma, tremors, pelvic pain, painful urination, genital pain, painful menstruation, visual disturbances, confusion, migraine headaches, pneumonia

IMPORTANT PRECAUTIONS

Always tell your health-care practitioner about any other medical conditions you suffer from, especially peripheral neuropathy (which is the most common side effect of stavudine), kidney problems, liver disease, or a history of alcohol abuse. If you have kidney disease, your health-care practitioner will prescribe a lower dosage. Tell your health-care practitioner if you have ever experienced an allergic reaction to this or other AIDS drugs.

Potentially life-threatening pancreatitis (inflammation of the pancreas) may develop when you are taking this drug. Call your health-care practitioner immediately if you develop symptoms such as severe abdominal pain, tense abdominal muscles, fever, sweating, shallow breathing, nausea, and vomiting.

Stavudine does not cure HIV, nor does it prevent you from passing on these infectious viruses to others. Therefore it is important to always practice safe sex while taking this drug.

Opportunistic infections may continue to occur while you are taking this drug. Frequent health-care practitioner visits and blood counts are necessary.

Stavudine may cause side effects such as dizziness and visual disturbances. Do not drive a car, operate machinery, or perform other tasks that require concentration until you know how the drug you are taking affects you.

DRUG INTERACTIONS

Tell your health-care practitioner and pharmacist if you are taking any other prescription or over-the-counter drugs, as well as any vitamins, herbs, or other supplements. Possible drug interactions include the following:

- Taking stavudine with certain other medications increases the risk of peripheral neuropathy. These include chloramphenicol, cisplatin, dapsone, didanosine, ethambutol, ethionamide, hydralazine, isoniazid, lithium, metronidazole, nitrofurantoin, phenytoin, vincristine, and zalcitabine.
- Combining stavudine with didanosine or hydroxyurea increases the risk of pancreatitis and liver toxicity.
- Do not take stavudine at the same time as zidovudine.

FOOD, VITAMIN, AND HERBAL INTERACTIONS

HIV infection may deplete the body of many nutrients. Ask your health-care practitioner about vitamin and mineral supplementation.

RECOMMENDED DOSAGE

Stavudine comes as a capsule or oral solution. Although the doses given below are typical, only your health-care practitioner can determine the dose and schedule that are most appropriate for you.

- *Children:* Consult your health-care practitioner.
- *Adults:* 30 to 40 mg every 12 hours

Stavudine can be taken with or without food. It is essential to take stavudine exactly as prescribed. If you miss a dose, take it as soon as you remember. However, if it is nearly time for your next scheduled dose, do not take the missed dose. Follow your regular dosing schedule. Never take a double dose.

SYMPTOMS OF OVERDOSE AND WHAT TO DO

Symptoms of stavudine overdose may include those of peripheral neuropathy (tingling, burning, numbness, or pain in the hands or feet). If overdose occurs, seek medical attention immediately, and bring the prescription bottle with you to the hospital so that health-care practitioners will know exactly what drug was used.

SPECIAL INFORMATION FOR PREGNANT OR NURSING WOMEN

Stavudine is known to cross the placenta, and high doses have caused birth defects in animals. Do not use this drug unless the benefits of therapy clearly outweigh the potential risks to the fetus.

Stavudine may pass into breast milk, and HIV can be transferred by breast milk. Bottle-feeding is preferable.

SPECIAL INFORMATION FOR SENIORS

Smaller doses of stavudine are usually appropriate for seniors, due to their lower levels of kidney function.

OPEN QUESTIONS OR CONTROVERSIES

It has not been definitively established that stavudine improves survival from AIDS or reduces the risk of opportunistic infections. Moreover, this drug can cause serious side effects such as peripheral neuropathy and life-threatening pancreatic inflammation. It should only be taken when other drugs prove ineffective or cannot be tolerated.

GENERIC NAME

Sucralfate

BRAND NAME

Carafate

Generic available

ABOUT THIS DRUG

Sucralfate is used to prevent and treat duodenal (upper intestinal) ulcers. This drug should only be used for up to 8 weeks at a time.

Sucralfate works by forming a protective coating over the ulcer. This protects the ulcer from stomach acid and allows it to heal.

SIDE EFFECTS

Side effects are usually mild. However, if they become prolonged or severe, contact your health-care practitioner. Only he or she can determine whether or not you should continue to take this drug.

- *Common:* constipation
- *Less Common or Rare:* nausea, diarrhea, upset stomach, indigestion, sleepiness, dizziness, dry mouth, back pain, rash, itching

IMPORTANT PRECAUTIONS

Sucralfate should be used with caution if you have gastrointestinal obstruction or kidney failure, or are on dialysis. Always tell your health-care practitioner about any other medical conditions that you may have.

Sucralfate may cause dizziness, so limit activities such as driving as necessary.

DRUG INTERACTIONS

Inform your health-care practitioner and pharmacist if you are taking any other prescription or over-the-counter drugs, as well as any vitamins, herbs, or other supplements. Possible drug interactions with sucralfate may include the following:

- Antacids may inhibit the absorption and benefits of sucralfate. Separate doses of antacids and sucralfate by at least 1/2 hour.
- Do not combine sucralfate with antacids that contain aluminum.
- Sucralfate may alter the absorption of digoxin, ketoconazole, phenytoin, quinidine, tetracycline, theophylline, warfarin, and quinolone antibiotics.

FOOD, VITAMIN, AND HERBAL INTERACTIONS

High-fat meals may reduce the absorption and effects of sucralfate.

RECOMMENDED DOSAGE

Sucralfate is available as a tablet. Although the doses given below are typical, only your health-care practitioner can determine the dose and schedule that are most appropriate for you.

- *Children:* This drug is not recommended for children.
- *Adults:* 1 tablet 4 times a day for active ulcers; 1 tablet 2 times a day for prevention

Sucralfate should be taken on an empty stomach 1 hour before or 2 hours after meals. If you miss a dose, take it as soon as you remember. However, if it is nearly time for your next scheduled dose, do not take the missed dose. Follow your regular dosing schedule. Never take a double dose.

SYMPTOMS OF OVERDOSE AND WHAT TO DO

Little information is available regarding sucralfate overdose. If you suspect an overdose, seek immediate medical attention, and bring the prescription bottle to the hospital with you.

SPECIAL INFORMATION FOR PREGNANT OR NURSING WOMEN

No studies have adequately investigated the effects of sucralfate during pregnancy or breastfeeding. If you are pregnant or plan to become pregnant, or if you are breastfeeding or plan to do so, talk with your health-care practitioner before starting one of these medications. Only a health-care practitioner can determine whether the potential benefits outweigh the risks.

SPECIAL INFORMATION FOR SENIORS

There are no special instructions for seniors.

GENERIC NAME

Class: Sulfa drugs

Generics: (1) sulfadiazine; (2) sulfamethizole; (3) sulfamethoxazole; (4) sulfasalazine; (5) sulfisoxazole; (6) sulfathiazole, sulfacetamide, and sulfabenzamide (triple sulfa)

BRAND NAMES

(1) available as generic only; (2) Thiosulfil Forte; (3) Protrin, Septra, Sulfatrim, among many others; (4) Azulfidine; (5) Gantrisin; (6) Dayto Sulf, Gyne-Sulf, Sultrin, Trysul, V.V.S.

All available as generic except sulfamethizole

ABOUT THESE DRUGS

Also known as sulfonamides, sulfa drugs are used to treat a variety of bacterial and protozoal infections. They have no impact on viral infections such as colds and flu. Triple sulfa is prescribed only for vaginal infections.

Sulfa drugs work by killing bacteria and other microorganisms. Sulfasalazine differs from other sulfa drugs in that more of it remains in the intestines; as a result, this drug is also prescribed for inflammatory conditions such as colitis.

SIDE EFFECTS

Consult your health-care practitioner if you develop side effects while taking one of these drugs. Only he or she can determine whether it is safe for you to continue taking a sulfa drug.

- *Common:* increased sensitivity of skin to sunlight, rash, itching, nausea, vomiting, appetite loss, diarrhea, dizziness, headache, tiredness
- *Less Common or Rare:* joint and muscle aches, blood diseases, change in blood composition, unusual bleeding or bruising, blistering or peeling skin, pallor, extreme weakness or fatigue, difficulty swallowing, sore throat, fever, yellow eyes or skin, severe abdominal pain, bloody diarrhea, blood in urine, reduced sperm count (sulfasalazine)

IMPORTANT PRECAUTIONS

Tell your health-care practitioner if you have ever experienced an allergic reaction to any sulfa drug. Also report allergies to any other medications, including aspirin, anesthetics, diuretics, and sulfonylurea drugs.

Inform your health-care practitioner about all medical conditions you have, especially blood problems such as anemia or G6PD deficiency, porphyria, or liver or kidney disease.

Promptly report any symptoms of skin, blood, liver, or nervous system problems to your health-care practitioner. You should be monitored on a regular basis while taking a sulfa drug.

Sulfa drugs may cause blood problems. Pay special attention to dental hygiene while taking these medications, and if possible postpone dental work until your blood count returns to normal.

Before having any type of surgery or dental procedure, tell your surgeon or dentist that you are taking a sulfa drug.

Sulfa drugs may cause side effects such as dizziness. Do not drive a car, operate machinery, or perform other tasks that require concentration until you know how the drug you are taking affects you.

Sulfa drugs may cause increased sensitivity to sunlight. When you take one of these drugs, avoid direct sunlight, wear protective clothing, and apply sunscreen.

DRUG INTERACTIONS

Tell your health-care practitioner and pharmacist if you are taking any other prescription or over-the-counter drugs, as well as any vitamins, herbs, or other supplements. Possible drug interactions include the following:

- Sulfa drugs may increase the effects of sulfonylurea drugs. Your health-care practitioner may need to adjust your dosage.
- Sulfa drugs may also increase the effects of aspirin, indomethacin, methotrexate, warfarin, and hydantoin antiseizure drugs such as phenytoin.
- Taking sulfa drugs with dapsone, methyldopa, nitrofurantoin, procainamide, quinidine, and quinine may increase the risk of side effects affecting the blood.
- Liver side effects are more likely when sulfa drugs are combined with disulfiram, divalproex, estrogens, methyldopa, naltrexone, oral contraceptives, phenothiazines, valproic acid, and other anti-infective drugs.

FOOD, VITAMIN, AND HERBAL INTERACTIONS

Taking vitamin K with sulfa drugs increases the risk of blood-related side effects.

RECOMMENDED DOSAGE

Sulfa drugs come in a variety of oral forms, including tablets, suspension, and syrup. Triple sulfa is for vaginal application. These medications work best when you take doses evenly spaced throughout the day. Ask your health-care practitioner to help you plan the best way to take your medication. Although the doses given below are typical, only your health-care practitioner can determine the dose and schedule that are most appropriate for you.

Sulfadiazine

- *Children Older than 2 Months:* 34 to 68 mg per pound of body weight daily
- *Adults:* 2 to 4 grams daily

Sulfamethizole

- *Children Older than 2 Months:* 13 to 20 mg per pound of body weight daily
- *Adults:* 1.5 to 4 grams daily

Sulfamethoxazole

- *Children Older than 2 Months:* 23 to 27 mg per pound of body weight daily
- *Adults:* 2 to 3 grams daily

Sulfasalazine

- *Children Older than Age 2:* 18 to 27 mg per pound of body weight daily
- *Adults:* 1 to 4 grams daily

Sulfisoxazole

- *Children Older than 2 Months:* 34 to 68 mg per pound of body weight daily
- *Adults:* 2 to 8 grams daily

Triple Sulfa

- *Children:* This drug is not recommended for children.
- *Adults:* 1 intravaginal tablet twice a day for 10 days

Oral sulfa drugs should be taken with a full glass (8 ounces) of water. If they cause stomach upset, these drugs can be taken with food or milk. Drinking extra water throughout the day will help prevent side effects. If you miss a dose, take it as soon as you remember. However, if it is nearly time for your next scheduled dose, do not take the missed dose. Follow your regular dosing schedule. Never take a double dose. Continue to take medication even if you feel better.

SYMPTOMS OF OVERDOSE AND WHAT TO DO

Symptoms of overdose may include nausea, vomiting, dizziness, colic, appetite loss, high fever, and drowsiness progressing to unconsciousness. If overdose occurs, seek immediate medical attention, and bring the prescription bottle with you to the hospital so that health-care practitioners will know exactly what drug was used.

SPECIAL INFORMATION FOR PREGNANT OR NURSING WOMEN

No studies have adequately investigated the effects of these drugs during pregnancy or breastfeeding. However, sulfa drugs have caused birth defects in animal studies. If you are pregnant or plan to become pregnant, or if you are breastfeeding or plan to do so, talk with your health-care practitioner before starting one of these medications. Only a health-care practitioner can determine whether the potential benefits outweigh the risks.

SPECIAL INFORMATION FOR SENIORS

Seniors are more sensitive to effects such as skin and blood problems. These problems are more likely to occur in people who are taking diuretics.

GENERIC NAMES

Sulfabenzamide *see Sulfa Drugs, page 967*

Sulfacetamide *see Sulfa Drugs, page 967*

Sulfadiazine *see Sulfa Drugs, page 967*

Sulfamethizole *see Sulfa Drugs, page 967*

Sulfamethoxazole *see Sulfa Drugs, page 967*

Sulfasalazine *see Sulfa Drugs, page 967*

Sulfisoxazole *see Sulfa Drugs, page 967*

GENERIC NAME

Class: Sulfonylurea antidiabetes drugs

Generics: (1) acetohexamide; (2) chlorpropamide; (3) glimepiride; (4) glipizide; (5) glyburide; (6) tolazamide; (7) tolbutamide

BRAND NAMES

(1) Dymelor; (2) Diabinese; (3) Amaryl; (4) Glucotrol, Glucotrol XL; (5) DiaBeta, Glynase Pres Tab, Micronase; (6) Tolinase; (7) Orinase
All available as generic except glimepiride

ABOUT THESE DRUGS

Sulfonylurea antidiabetes drugs are used to treat the form of diabetes mellitus known as type 2. Type 2 diabetes was formerly known as adult-onset, and is also referred to as noninsulin-dependent. Diet and exercise play a key role in the management of this disease.

The various sulfonylurea drugs differ from one another in how long they take to work, how long their effects last, and how much medication must be taken. They are not used for type 1 diabetes.

Sulfonylurea drugs help your body regulate the amount of glucose (sugar) in blood. They lower blood sugar by stimulating the pancreas to secrete insulin and making insulin work more efficiently. The pancreas must produce insulin in order for these medications to work.

SIDE EFFECTS

Report any severe or persistent side effects to your health-care practitioner. All diabetics should learn to recognize the symptoms of low blood sugar and high blood sugar and know what to do when they occur. It is essential to control these symptoms before they progress to more serious conditions.

- *Common:* nausea, vomiting, loss of appetite, stomach upset, weakness, tingling in hands or feet, increased sun sensitivity
- *Less Common or Rare:* low blood sugar, yellow eyes or skin, rash, itching
- *Hypoglycemia (Low Blood Sugar):* "drunken" behavior, drowsiness, unusual tiredness or weakness, slurred speech, shakiness, dizziness, difficulty concentrating, headache, confusion, anxiety, nervousness, blurred vision, cold sweats, cool pale skin, excessive hunger, restless sleep, nightmares, nausea, fast heartbeat

IMPORTANT PRECAUTIONS

Sulfonylurea drugs have been associated with an increased risk of potentially fatal cardiovascular problems. Tell your health-care practitioner if you have any heart or circulation problems. These drugs should be used with caution if you have kidney or liver impairment or endocrine disease. If you are ill or under stress, or plan to have any type of surgery or dental procedure, inform your health-care practitioner. These circumstances may reduce the effectiveness of sulfonylurea drugs. Also tell your health-care practitioner if you have ever experienced an allergic reaction to any of these medications.

Combining other antidiabetes medications with sulfonylurea drugs may result in low blood sugar. The people most susceptible to hypoglycemia are older, weak, or malnourished, or have kidney, liver, adrenal, or hormone problems. Symptoms vary from person to person, so it is essential to learn which symptoms you usually have.

As soon as you experience the characteristic signs, address and control them quickly by taking a fast-acting sugar, such as a glucose tablet, glass of fruit juice or nondiet soft drink, tablespoon of corn syrup or honey, or tablespoon of table sugar dissolved in water.

People with uncontrolled diabetes may also experience high blood sugar, or hyperglycemia. Symptoms include dry mouth, thirst, frequent urination, dry skin, flushing, appetite loss, difficulty breathing, and tiredness. If this condition is not treated, it can lead to diabetic coma and death.

In order to prevent these types of complications, carefully follow all diet and exercise recommendations made by your health-care practitioner and nutritionist. In fact, many people with type 2 diabetes are able to successfully control this disease by making healthy lifestyle changes, cutting back on the need for medication.

To monitor the effectiveness of sulfonylurea drugs, measure the amount of glucose in your urine or blood on a regular basis. Your health-care practitioner may also tell you to test your urine for ketones (substances that appear in urine when diabetes is not properly controlled). Carefully follow the instructions of your health-care practitioner and pharmacist when conducting these tests at home. If blood sugar is high or sugar or ketones are present in urine, call your health-care practitioner. Your health-care practitioner will also monitor your glucose levels and liver function during regular visits.

Sulfonylurea drugs may cause increased sun sensitivity. Wear protective clothing and sunscreen.

DRUG INTERACTIONS

Inform your health-care practitioner and pharmacist if you are taking any other prescription or over-the-counter drugs, as well as any vitamins, herbs, or other supplements. Drug interactions may include the following:

- Taking sulfonylurea drugs with other antidiabetes drugs increases the risk of low blood sugar. Your health-care practitioner may need to adjust your dosages.
- Many drugs may increase your need for sulfonylurea drugs. These include beta-blockers, calcium channel blockers, cholestyramine, corticosteroids, estrogens, isoniazid, nicotinic acid, oral contraceptives, phenothiazines, hydantoin drugs such as phenytoin, rifampin, stimulants, thiazide diuretics, and thyroid replacement drugs.
- Other drugs may decrease your need for sulfonylurea drugs. These include aspirin, sulfa drugs, androgens, chloramphenicol, cimetidine, clofibrate, famotidine, fenfluramine, fluconazole, itraconazole, ketoconazole, ranitidine, magnesium, methyldopa, miconazole,

MAOI or tricyclic antidepressants, nizatidine, phenylbutazone, and warfarin.

- Cigarette smoking may reduce the effectiveness of sulfonylurea drugs.
- Limit your alcohol intake. You are more likely to experience effects such as low blood sugar if you use alcohol.

FOOD, VITAMIN, AND HERBAL INTERACTIONS

Supplements such as chromium, garlic, ginger, ginseng, hawthorn, and nettle may affect blood sugar levels. Check with your health-care practitioner before using any dietary supplement.

RECOMMENDED DOSAGE

Sulfonylurea drugs come as tablets. Ask your health-care practitioner to help you plan the best way to take your medication. Although the doses given below are typical, only your health-care practitioner can determine the dose and schedule that are most appropriate for you.

Acetohexamide

- *Children:* This drug is not recommended for children.
- *Adults:* 250 to 1,500 mg daily

Chlorpropamide

- *Children:* This drug is not recommended for children.
- *Adults:* 100 to 750 mg daily

Glimepiride

- *Children:* This drug is not recommended for children.
- *Adults:* 1 to 8 mg daily

Glipizide

- *Children:* This drug is not recommended for children.
- *Adults:* 5 to 40 mg daily; the maximum daily dose of Glucotrol XL is 20 mg

Tolazamide

- *Children:* This drug is not recommended for children.
- *Adults:* 100 to 1,000 mg daily

Tolbutamide

- *Children:* This drug is not recommended for children.
- *Adults:* 1 to 3 grams daily

All sulfonylurea drugs except glipizide may be taken with food. If you miss a dose, take it as soon as you remember. However, if it is nearly time for your next scheduled dose, do not take the missed dose. Follow your regular dosing schedule. Never take a double dose.

SYMPTOMS OF OVERDOSE AND WHAT TO DO

An overdose may cause low blood sugar. (See symptoms listed under Side Effects.) If overdose occurs, seek immediate medical attention, and bring the prescription bottle with you to the hospital so that health-care practitioners will know exactly what drug was used.

SPECIAL INFORMATION FOR PREGNANT OR NURSING WOMEN

Sulfonylurea drugs have caused birth defects in animal studies. It is critically important to monitor and control blood sugar during pregnancy. However, it is safer to accomplish this through diet or a combination of diet and insulin. Consult your health-care practitioner as soon as you think you may be pregnant or if you are planning to become pregnant.

These drugs may pass into breast milk and lower blood sugar in infants. If you are breastfeeding or plan to do so, talk with your health-care practitioner before starting one of these drugs. Only a health-care practitioner can determine whether the potential benefits outweigh the potential dangers.

SPECIAL INFORMATION FOR SENIORS

Older adults—especially those who are debilitated or malnourished, or who have kidney or liver impairment—are more susceptible to effects such as low blood sugar. Lower doses are recommended.

OPEN QUESTIONS OR CONTROVERSIES

Sulfonylurea drugs have been associated with an increased risk of fatal heart trouble. Before taking any of these medications, speak to your health-care practitioner about the possible risks, benefits, and treatment alternatives for diabetes.

GENERIC NAME
Sulindac

BRAND NAME
Clinoril
Generic available

ABOUT THIS DRUG
Sulindac is a nonsteroidal anti-inflammatory drug (NSAID) used to relieve the pain and inflammation of rheumatoid arthritis, osteoarthritis, ankylosing spondylitis, and gout. This drug works by reducing the level of prostaglandins, chemicals in the body that produce inflammation and pain.

SIDE EFFECTS
Sulindac may cause potentially serious side effects, especially when used for a long time and in large doses. If you develop severe or persistent side effects, ask your health-care practitioner whether it is safe for you to continue taking this drug.

- *Common:* diarrhea, constipation, stomach upset or pain, gas, nausea, vomiting, fluid retention, ringing in the ears, appetite loss
- *Less Common or Rare:* headache, dizziness, blurred vision, sensitivity to light, confusion, fainting, tingling in the hands or feet, mouth sores, fatigue, weakness, abnormal bleeding or bruising, rash, hives, itching, heart palpitations, difficulty breathing, gastrointestinal bleeding, pancreatitis, ulcers, painful urination, kidney damage

Stop taking sulindac and consult your health-care practitioner immediately if you experience symptoms such as abdominal pain, stomach cramps, diarrhea, nausea, heartburn, indigestion, visual disturbances, vomiting of blood or material that looks like coffee grounds, or black, tarry stools. These may be signs of dangerous reactions such as ulcers or internal bleeding.

IMPORTANT PRECAUTIONS
Sulindac can cause gastrointestinal bleeding, ulcers, and stomach perforation. If you take this drug on a regular basis, these types of side effects can occur at any time, with or without warning. People with a history of ulcers, colitis, or any type of gastrointestinal bleeding should be extremely careful when taking this drug.

Do not take sulindac if you have a bleeding disorder or asthma or nasal polyps associated with aspirin use. Use this drug with caution if you have high blood pressure or other heart problems, or impaired liver or kidney function. Tell your health-care practitioner if you have ever experienced an allergic reaction to aspirin or related drugs.

Drinking 3 or more alcoholic beverages a day increases the risk of side effects such as bleeding.

Other possible side effects of sulindac include blurred vision and dizziness. Until you know how this drug affects you, do not drive a car, operate machinery, or perform other tasks that require concentration.

Sulindac may cause increased sun sensitivity. Wear protective clothing and apply sunscreen when using this drug.

Before undergoing any type of surgery or dental procedure, inform your health-care practitioner or dentist that you are taking sulindac. Visit your health-care practitioner on a regular basis while taking this drug.

DRUG INTERACTIONS

Tell your health-care practitioner and pharmacist if you are taking any other prescription or over-the-counter drugs, as well as any vitamins, herbs, or other supplements. Possible drug interactions include the following:

- Do not combine with aspirin, ibuprofen, or other prescription or over-the-counter NSAIDs. This increases the risk of bleeding.
- Other drugs that may increase the risk of bleeding include dipyridamole, sulfinpyrazone, valproic acid, and blood thinners such as warfarin.
- Taking sulindac with antihypertensive medications such as ACE inhibitors, beta-blockers, and diuretics decreases their blood-pressure-lowering effects.
- Mixing sulindac with cyclosporine may increase the negative kidney effects of both drugs.
- Taking sulindac with lithium or methotrexate can lead to toxic levels of lithium or methotrexate in the body.
- Do not use alcohol when you are taking sulindac. Both are stomach irritants, and using them together can increase the risk of stomach bleeding and ulcers.

FOOD, VITAMIN, AND HERBAL INTERACTIONS

Do not combine sulindac with herbal remedies such as clove oil, feverfew, garlic, ginkgo, and ginseng. These herbs may affect clotting.

RECOMMENDED DOSAGE

Sulindac comes as a tablet. The doses given below are typical. However, only your health-care practitioner can determine the dose and schedule that best fit your individual needs.

- *Children:* This drug is not recommended for children.
- *Adults:* 300 to 400 mg daily in divided doses

Sulindac may be taken with food, milk, or an antacid to prevent stomach upset. Your health-care practitioner may also advise you to take medication with a full (8-ounce) glass of water, and remain upright (do not lie down) for 15 to 30 minutes afterward. If you forget to take a dose, take it as soon as you remember. But if it is almost time for the next dose, skip the one you missed and resume your normal schedule. Never take a double dose.

SYMPTOMS OF OVERDOSE AND WHAT TO DO

Symptoms of overdose may include nausea, vomiting, diarrhea, abdominal pain, drowsiness, rapid breathing, rapid heartbeat, agitation, confusion, disorientation, sweating, ringing in the ears, stupor, and seizures. If an overdose occurs, seek immediate medical attention and take the prescription bottle to the hospital with you so the health-care practitioner will know exactly what medication was taken.

SPECIAL INFORMATION FOR PREGNANT OR NURSING WOMEN

Use of sulindac should be avoided in late pregnancy. If you want to take this drug in early pregnancy, ask your health-care practitioner whether the potential benefits outweigh the risks. Because sulindac may pass into breast milk, it is best to stop breastfeeding while you take this drug.

SPECIAL INFORMATION FOR SENIORS

Smaller doses are recommended for seniors, who are more susceptible to side effects such as confusion, fluid retention, swelling of the feet and lower legs, stomach ulcers, and kidney or liver effects.

GENERIC NAME

Sumatriptan

see Triptan-Type Antimigraine Drugs, page 1083

GENERIC NAME
Tacrine

BRAND NAME
Cognex
No generic available

ABOUT THIS DRUG
Tacrine is used to treat mild-to-moderate Alzheimer's disease. This drug can improve symptoms such as thinking ability. However, it cannot cure Alzheimer's disease nor prevent the disease from growing worse. You may need to take tacrine for several weeks before you begin to experience its full benefits.

Changes in the brain associated with Alzheimer's disease include a shortage of acetylcholine (ACh), a chemical that helps the brain function properly. Tacrine was the first drug found to raise ACh levels.

SIDE EFFECTS
Many people stop taking tacrine because of the side effects. Immediately report problems such as nausea, vomiting, loose stools, rash, fever, yellow eyes or skin, or seizures. If any side effects become persistent or severe, ask your health-care practitioner whether it is safe for you to continue taking this drug.

- *Common:* nausea, vomiting, diarrhea, constipation, indigestion, gas, abdominal pain, appetite loss, weight loss, headache, fatigue, dizziness, flushing, trouble sleeping, depression, confusion, agitation, anxiety, abnormal thinking, clumsiness, unsteadiness, rash, frequent urination, urinary tract infection, chest pain, upper respiratory infection, liver inflammation
- *Less Common or Rare:* hallucinations, tremor, weakness, hostile attitude, back pain, skin discoloration, purple or red spots on the skin, fever, yellow eyes or skin, seizures

IMPORTANT PRECAUTIONS
Always tell your health-care practitioner about all other medical conditions from which you suffer, especially heart or blood vessel disease, a liver or kidney disorder, bladder obstruction, stomach ulcers, seizures, and asthma or other breathing problems. Tacrine may slow heart rate and increase the production of stomach acid. Do not use tacrine if you have ever experienced an allergic reaction to it, and inform your health-care practitioner if you have ever experienced an allergic reaction to any similar medication.

This drug may make you dizzy or unsteady. Until you know how tacrine affects you, do not drive a car, operate machinery, or perform other tasks that demand concentration.

Visit your health-care practitioner on a regular basis to monitor your progress. Regular blood tests are necessary because of risks such as liver problems. Women may be more susceptible to these side effects. Always tell your health-care practitioner if side effects are troubling or if Alzheimer's symptoms grow worse. Inform your health-care practitioner before you have any type of surgery, including dental procedures.

DRUG INTERACTIONS

Tell your health-care practitioner and pharmacist if you are taking any other prescription or over-the-counter drugs, as well as any vitamins, herbs, or other supplements. Possible drug interactions include the following:

- Tacrine may increase the effects of theophylline and of certain muscle relaxants used during surgery.
- Cimetidine may increase the effects of tacrine.
- Tacrine may interfere with the effects of anticholinergic drugs.
- Alcohol may add to the drowsiness caused by this drug.

FOOD, VITAMIN, AND HERBAL INTERACTIONS

No food, vitamin, or herbal interactions have been noted.

RECOMMENDED DOSAGE

Tacrine comes as a capsule. The doses given below are typical, but only your health-care practitioner can determine the dose and schedule that best fit your particular needs.

- *Children:* This drug is not indicated for children.
- *Adults:* 10 to 40 mg 4 times daily

Tacrine is best taken on an empty stomach 1 hour before or 2 hours after meals. However, if it upsets your stomach, ask your health-care practitioner about taking it with food. If you miss a dose, take it as soon as you remember. However, if it is nearly time for your next scheduled dose, do not take the missed dose. Follow your regular dosing schedule dose. Never take a double dose. Do not stop taking medication suddenly. This may cause mental or behavioral changes.

SYMPTOMS OF OVERDOSE AND WHAT TO DO

Tacrine overdose can be fatal. Symptoms may include nausea, vomiting, sweating, extreme muscle weakness, collapse, and convulsions. If you suspect an overdose, seek immediate medical attention, and bring the prescription bottle to the hospital with you.

SPECIAL INFORMATION FOR PREGNANT OR NURSING WOMEN

Tacrine should not be taken by women of childbearing age.

SPECIAL INFORMATION FOR SENIORS

Seniors with liver disease are more susceptible to side effects.

GENERIC NAME

Tacrolimus

BRAND NAME

Prograf
No generic available

ABOUT THIS DRUG

Tacrolimus is used to prevent the rejection of transplanted organs. Once known as FK 506, this drug is used primarily in liver transplants.

Tacrolimus works by suppressing the immune activity of T-cells. These cells ordinarily protect the body by attacking foreign substances.

SIDE EFFECTS

Side effects of tacrolimus can be extremely serious, and must be promptly reported to your health-care practitioner. They include kidney damage, seizures, tremors, headache, and muscle function changes. Call your health-care practitioner at the first sign of fever, and promptly report any other severe or persistent effects.

- *Common:* nausea, vomiting, diarrhea, stomach upset, appetite loss, pain, fever, weakness, dizziness, reduced platelet count, other blood changes, rash, itchiness, increased risk of infection, breathing difficulties, liver and kidney problems
- *Less Common or Rare:* headache, fatigue, sore throat, chills, frequent or painful urination, decreased urination, bruises, unusual bleeding, muscle or joint pain, hives, lung disease, wheezing, stomach bleeding, infection, diabetes, swelling of the feet and ankles,

tremor, anxiety, depression, confusion, abnormal dreaming, weight gain, yellow eyes and skin, kidney damage, seizures

IMPORTANT PRECAUTIONS

Always tell your health-care practitioner about any other medical conditions you may have, especially heart or kidney disease or diabetes. Inform your health-care practitioner if you have ever experienced an allergic reaction to this or similar drugs.

Tacrolimus suppresses the immune system, and may decrease the body's ability to combat infection. You may be at risk for opportunistic infections.

This drug may cause dizziness and fatigue. Until you know how tacrolimus affects you, do not drive a car, operate machinery, or perform other tasks that require concentration.

People taking tacrolimus must be closely monitored with regular complete blood counts and other tests.

DRUG INTERACTIONS

Inform your health-care practitioner and pharmacist if you are taking any other prescription or over-the-counter drugs, as well as any vitamins, herbs, or other supplements. Possible drug interactions include the following:

- Do not have live-virus immunizations while taking this drug without your health-care practitioner's approval. You are at risk of opportunistic infections.
- Tacrolimus should not be taken at the same time as other immune suppressants.
- Taking cyclosporine with this drug increases the risk of kidney damage.
- A number of drugs may increase the effects of tacrolimus. These include antifungals, calcium channel blockers, cimetidine, clarithromycin, danazol, erythromycin, and metoclopramide.
- Drugs such as phenobarbital and phenytoin may reduce the effects of tacrolimus.

FOOD, VITAMIN, AND HERBAL INTERACTIONS

Drink plenty of fluids while taking this drug, so it will pass through your body more quickly and prevent kidney problems.

RECOMMENDED DOSAGE

Tacrolimus comes in capsule and injectable form. The doses below are typical. However, dosage is highly individualized and must be determined by your health-care practitioner.

➤ *Children and Adults:* 0.075 to 0.15 mg per pound of body weight daily

It is essential to follow the schedule prescribed by your health-care practitioner. If you miss a dose, take it as soon as you remember. If it is almost time for the next dose, skip it and resume your regular schedule. Never take a double dose. Call your health-care practitioner if you forget 2 doses in a row.

SYMPTOMS OF OVERDOSE AND WHAT TO DO

Symptoms of tacrolimus overdose may consist of severe side effects. If you suspect that an overdose has occurred, seek immediate medical attention and take the prescription bottle to the hospital with you.

SPECIAL INFORMATION FOR PREGNANT OR NURSING WOMEN

Do not take this drug if you are pregnant or think you may be pregnant. Tacrolimus may cause birth defects and miscarriage. Because of the possibility of serious side effects, breastfeeding is not recommended while you take this drug.

SPECIAL INFORMATION FOR SENIORS

Side effects are more likely to occur in seniors. Kidney function must be closely monitored throughout treatment.

GENERIC NAME

Tadalafil

BRAND NAME

Cialis

No generic available

ABOUT THIS DRUG

Tadalafil is used to treat men who have erectile dysfunction, or sexual impotence.

This drug works by relaxing the muscles in the penis, which allows increased blood flow into the penis, which is necessary to achieve and maintain an erection. Tadalafil does not work in the absence of stimulation.

SIDE EFFECTS

If you experience a prolonged or painful erection for 4 hours or more, contact your health-care practitioner at once. Also inform him or her if any other side effects are severe or prolonged. Only your health-care practitioner can determine whether it is safe for you to continue using this drug.

- *Most Common:* diarrhea, facial flushing, flu-like symptoms, headache, nausea, stomach upset
- *Less Common:* abnormal ejaculation, blurred vision, changes in color vision, chest pain, low blood pressure, priapism (prolonged, painful erection)

Men taking tadalafil have experienced increases in heart rate and sharp rises in blood pressure. These problems occur more frequently in men who have risk factors for cardiovascular disease.

IMPORTANT PRECAUTIONS

Tell your health-care practitioner if you are sensitive or allergic to tadalafil or to any other drugs.

Do not take tadalafil if you have heart problems severe enough to limit sexual activity. Use this drug with extreme caution (if at all) if you have coronary artery disease, an irregular heartbeat, blood pressure abnormalities, a history of heart attack or stroke in the last 6 months, penis abnormalities, a blood disorder, bleeding problems, kidney or liver impairment, or retinitis pigmentosa. Do not use this drug if you have experienced an allergic reaction to it in the past.

Do not use tadalafil with excessive amounts of alcohol (5 or more drinks daily).

Do not use tadalafil if you are taking any form of nitrates; if medically necessary, nitrates may be administered greater than 48 hours after the last dose of tadalafil, under medical supervision. Tadalafil should not be given with any alpha-blocker, other than tamsulosin.

DRUG INTERACTIONS

Tell your health-care practitioner and pharmacist if you are taking any prescription or nonprescription drugs, as well as any vitamins, herbs, or other supplements. Possible drug interactions include the following:

- Do not combine tadalafil with nitrates such as nitroglycerin, as tadalafil increases their blood-pressure-lowering effects.

- Consult your health-care practitioner before taking tadalafil with any other drugs that lower blood pressure, especially alpha-blockers (e.g., doxazosin).
- Certain drugs can increase the unwanted effects of tadalafil. These include erythromycin, indinavir, itraconazole, ketoconazole, and ritonavir.

FOOD, VITAMIN, AND HERBAL INTERACTIONS

Do not combine tadalafil with herbal remedies for impotence, such as ginseng and yohimbine. Do not take this drug with grapefruit or grapefruit juice, as dangerous interactions may occur.

RECOMMENDED DOSAGE

Tadalafil is available in 5-, 10- and 20-mg tablets. The dosages given here are typical. However, your health-care practitioner will determine the most appropriate dose and schedule for your needs.

- *Children:* This drug is not for use in children.
- *Adults:* 10 mg as a single dose once daily, 1 hour before sexual activity. Your health-care practitioner may increase or decrease the dose, depending on adequacy of response and side effects.

SYMPTOMS OF OVERDOSE AND WHAT TO DO

No information is available regarding tadalafil overdose. However, if you suspect an overdose, seek immediate medical attention and take the prescription bottle to the hospital with you.

SPECIAL INFORMATION FOR PREGNANT OR NURSING WOMEN

Tadalafil is approved for use by men only.

SPECIAL INFORMATION FOR SENIORS

The recommended dosage for men over age 65 is 5 mg as a single dose no more than once daily.

GENERIC NAME

Tamoxifen

BRAND NAME

Nolvadex

Generic available

Note: The information in this profile also applies to toremifene citrate. However, toremifene is used only to treat (not prevent) breast cancer.

ABOUT THIS DRUG

Tamoxifen is an anticancer drug used primarily in the treatment of breast cancer. It may also be prescribed for breast cancer that has metastasized or spread, and women at high risk may take this drug to prevent breast cancer.

Tamoxifen works by blocking the effects of estrogen on cancer cell growth. This drug is most effective in combating the type of breast cancer that is stimulated to estrogen.

SIDE EFFECTS

Side effects of tamoxifen are generally mild. However, several can be serious. Promptly report effects such as abnormal vaginal bleeding, pelvic pain, hot flashes, weakness, dizziness, or visual problems to your health-care practitioner. Only your health-care practitioner can determine whether it is safe for you to continue taking this medication.

- *Common:* nausea, vomiting, hot flashes
- *Less Common or Rare:* menstrual irregularities, vaginal bleeding, vaginal discharge, tumor pain, bone pain, diarrhea, rash, depression, dizziness, lightheadedness, headache, hair loss, blood clots, visual problems, swelling of arms and legs, liver disorders, yellow eyes or skin

IMPORTANT PRECAUTIONS

Always tell your health-care practitioner about any other medical conditions you may have, especially liver disease. Inform your health-care practitioner if you have ever experienced an allergic reaction to this or similar medications.

People taking tamoxifen must be closely monitored with a thorough physical examination. This drug increases the risk of endometrial cancer and uterine sarcoma, stroke, and blood clots. It can also cause liver damage, high cholesterol, and vision problems.

Tamoxifen may cause birth defects, and oral contraceptives should not be taken with this drug. Use alternate means of contraception.

This medication may cause side effects such as visual problems, dizziness, and lightheadedness. Until you know how tamoxifen affects you, do not drive a car, operate machinery, or perform other tasks that require concentration.

DRUG INTERACTIONS

Inform your health-care practitioner and pharmacist if you are taking any other prescription or over-the-counter drugs, as well as any vita-

mins, herbs, or other supplements. Possible drug interactions include the following:

- The effects of blood thinners such as warfarin may be increased by tamoxifen.
- Bromocriptine may increase the effects of tamoxifen.
- Do not take oral contraceptives while using this medication.
- Do not drink alcohol while taking tamoxifen. This increases the possibility of undesirable liver effects.

FOOD, VITAMIN, AND HERBAL INTERACTIONS

Tamoxifen may cause abnormally high levels of calcium. Symptoms include muscle pain and weakness and appetite loss. Severe cases can lead to kidney failure.

Gammalinolenic acid—an omega-6 fatty acid present in borage and evening primrose oils—may enhance the action of tamoxifen in women with breast cancer.

RECOMMENDED DOSAGE

Tamoxifen comes as a tablet. The doses given below are typical, but only your health-care practitioner can determine the dose and schedule that best fit your particular needs.

- *Children:* This drug is not recommended for children.
- *Adults:* 20 to 40 mg daily

If tamoxifen upsets your stomach, take it with food or milk. If you miss a dose or vomit shortly after taking a dose, call your health-care practitioner for instructions. Never take a double dose.

SYMPTOMS OF OVERDOSE AND WHAT TO DO

Symptoms of tamoxifen overdose may include dizziness, unsteadiness, breathing difficulties, tremors, and convulsions. If you suspect that an overdose has occurred, seek immediate medical attention and take the prescription bottle to the hospital with you.

SPECIAL INFORMATION FOR PREGNANT OR NURSING WOMEN

Do not take this drug if you are pregnant or think you may be pregnant. Tamoxifen may cause birth defects. Because of the possibility of serious side effects, breastfeeding is not recommended while you take this drug.

SPECIAL INFORMATION FOR SENIORS

There are no special instructions for seniors.

GENERIC NAME

Tamsulosin

BRAND NAME

Flomax
No generic available

ABOUT THIS DRUG

Tamsulosin is used to treat benign prostatic hyperplasia (BPH) in men. Also known as an enlarged prostate, this condition causes difficulties with urination.

Tamsulosin, an alpha blocker, works by blocking nerve endings called alpha1 receptors. This relaxes smooth muscles in the prostate and bladder.

SIDE EFFECTS

Side effects such as dizziness, headache, and sleepiness are most common after the first few doses. Promptly report severe or persistent effects such as heart palpitations or dizziness. Only your health-care practitioner can determine whether or not it is safe for you to continue taking this drug.

- *Common:* dizziness, sleepiness, weakness, headache, diarrhea, abnormal ejaculation, back pain, chest pain, runny nose, cough, sinus problems, sore throat, infection
- *Less Common or Rare:* sexual dysfunction, decreased sex drive, persistent and painful erection, vision problems, dental problems, insomnia, low blood pressure upon standing, fainting, vertigo, vomiting, palpitations, constipation

IMPORTANT PRECAUTIONS

Always tell your health-care practitioner about any other medical conditions you may have, and if you have ever experienced an allergic reaction to this or similar medications.

People taking this drug must be closely monitored with regular complete blood counts and other tests.

This drug may cause drowsiness, especially when you first start using it. Do not drive a car, operate machinery, or perform other tasks that demand concentration for 12 hours after the first dose.

When you first start taking this drug or when the dosage is increased, you may experience dizziness or faintness when you rise quickly from a sitting or reclining position (postural hypotension). Try to get up slowly, and consult your health-care practitioner if the problem continues.

DRUG INTERACTIONS

Inform your health-care practitioner and pharmacist if you are taking any other prescription or over-the-counter drugs, as well as any vitamins, herbs, or other supplements. Drug interactions occur infrequently. Taking antihypertensive drugs such as beta-blockers with tamsulosin may increase effects such as dizziness and fainting, and result in a severe reduction in blood pressure.

FOOD, VITAMIN, AND HERBAL INTERACTIONS

No food, vitamin, or herbal interactions have been noted.

RECOMMENDED DOSAGE

Tamsulosin comes in capsule form. Although the doses given below are typical, doses are different for different patients. Only your health-care practitioner can determine the dose and schedule that best fit your particular needs. This drug is only for use by men.

- *Adults:* 0.4 to 0.8 mg daily

This drug should be taken once daily, 1/2 hour before the same meal each day. If you miss a dose, take it as soon as you remember. However, if it is nearly time for your next scheduled dose, do not take the missed dose. Follow your regular dosing schedule. Never take a double dose.

SYMPTOMS OF OVERDOSE AND WHAT TO DO

Symptoms of tamsulosin overdose may include headache, dizziness, and fainting. If you suspect that an overdose has occurred, seek immediate medical attention and take the prescription bottle to the hospital with you.

SPECIAL INFORMATION FOR PREGNANT OR NURSING WOMEN

This drug is for men only.

SPECIAL INFORMATION FOR SENIORS

Seniors may be more sensitive to the effects of tamsulosin.

GENERIC NAME
Tazarotene

BRAND NAME
Tazorac
No generic available

ABOUT THIS DRUG
Tazarotene is used to treat mild-to-moderate acne. It may also be prescribed for other skin conditions, such as psoriasis. This drug is for topical application only. Like other acne medications, it is chemically related to vitamin A.

SIDE EFFECTS
Consult your health-care practitioner if you develop side effects while using tazarotene. Only he or she can determine whether it is safe for you to continue using this drug.

➤ *Common:* itching, burning, stinging, dryness, redness, peeling skin

➤ *Less Common or Rare:* irritation, pain, cracking, swelling, discoloration

IMPORTANT PRECAUTIONS
Keep tazarotene away from your eyes. Always tell your health-care practitioner about all other medical conditions you have, and if you have ever experienced an allergic reaction to this or similar medications. If skin irritation is excessive, stop using tazarotene until it heals. Wind and cold may worsen irritation. Avoid excessive exposure to the sun while using this medication.

DRUG INTERACTIONS
Although no specific interactions are known, always inform your health-care practitioner and pharmacist if you are taking any other prescription or over-the-counter drugs, as well as any vitamins, herbs, or other supplements.

FOOD, VITAMIN, AND HERBAL INTERACTIONS
Do not use tazarotene with other skin products that have drying effects.

RECOMMENDED DOSAGE
Tazarotene comes in gel form. The doses given below are typical. However, consult your health-care practitioner for the exact dose and schedule that are most appropriate for you.

- *Children:* This drug is not recommended for children.
- *Adults:* Apply a thin layer to affected skin areas once daily in the evening.

Wash your face before applying medication. If you forget a dose, use it as soon as you remember. If it is almost time for the next dose, skip the forgotten one, and resume your normal schedule. Never take double doses.

SYMPTOMS OF OVERDOSE AND WHAT TO DO

Tazarotene is for external use only. Accidental ingestion may cause dizziness and vomiting. If overdose occurs, seek immediate medical attention and take the prescription container to the hospital with you.

SPECIAL INFORMATION FOR PREGNANT OR NURSING WOMEN

Do not take tazarotene if you are pregnant. This drug may cause birth defects. Because tazarotene may pass into breast milk, ask your health-care practitioner if it is appropriate to use while breast-feeding.

SPECIAL INFORMATION FOR SENIORS

There are no special instructions for seniors.

GENERIC NAME

Tegaserod

BRAND NAME

Zelnorm
No generic available

ABOUT THIS DRUG

Tegaserod is used for short-term treatment of women who have irritable bowel syndrome with constipation. This medication has not been shown to work in men who have this same disorder.

This drug works by increasing the action of serotonin in the intestinal tract, which in turn stimulates and speeds up bowel movements.

SIDE EFFECTS

Be sure to tell your health-care practitioner if you experience any side effects while taking tegaserod. Only your health-care practi-

tioner can determine whether it is safe for you to continue taking this drug.

- *Most Common:* diarrhea (a single episode is common; see "Important Precautions"); abdominal pain, flatulence, headache, nausea
- *Less Common:* back pain, dizziness, joint inflammation, leg pain, migraine

IMPORTANT PRECAUTIONS

Tell your health-care practitioner if you are sensitive or allergic to tegaserod or to any other drugs.

Discontinue use of tegaserod immediately if you experience any new or sudden worsening of abdominal pain.

Contact your health-care practitioner immediately if you experience significant diarrhea along with lightheadedness, dizziness, or faintness.

Avoid use of tegaserod if you have a history of diarrhea, poor kidney function, liver disease, gallbladder disease, or intestinal blockage or adhesions.

DRUG INTERACTIONS

Tell your health-care practitioner and pharmacist if you are taking any prescription or nonprescription drugs, as well as any vitamins, herbs, or other supplements. No specific drug-drug interactions have been reported. However, other drugs that increase intestinal contractions (e.g., some laxatives) will likely cause more diarrhea if they are taken with tegaserod.

FOOD, VITAMIN, AND HERBAL INTERACTIONS

No food, vitamin, or herbal interactions have been noted. However, you should talk to your health-care practitioner before using any herbal laxatives, such as psyllium or fenugreek, or other natural laxatives, such as oat bran.

RECOMMENDED DOSAGE

Tegaserod is available in 2- and 6-mg tablets. The dosages given here are typical. However, your health-care practitioner will determine the most appropriate dose and schedule for your needs.

- *Children:* Not recommended for children
- *Adults:* 6 mg twice daily for 4 to 6 weeks

You may experience improvement in some or all symptoms within one to two weeks of beginning treatment. If you don't see any improvement after four to six weeks, talk to your doctor about extending treatment.

Tegaserod should be taken on an empty stomach, before meals. If you miss a dose, take it as soon as you remember. If it is nearly time for your next dose, do not take the missed dose. Continue with your regular dosing schedule. Never take a double dose.

SYMPTOMS OF OVERDOSE AND WHAT TO DO

Symptoms of overdose include abdominal pain, diarrhea, headache, nausea, and vomiting. If overdose occurs, seek immediate medical attention and bring the prescription container with you to the hospital.

SPECIAL INFORMATION FOR PREGNANT OR NURSING WOMEN

Adequate studies of the effects of tegaserod on pregnant or nursing women have not been done. If you are pregnant or plan to become pregnant, you and your health-care practitioner should weigh the potential benefits against the potential risks.

Tegaserod may pass into breast milk. If you are breastfeeding, your health-care practitioner will likely advise you to switch to bottle feeding.

SPECIAL INFORMATION FOR SENIORS

No special precautions for seniors have been noted.

GENERIC NAME

Telithromycin

BRAND NAME

Ketek

No generic available

ABOUT THIS DRUG

Telithromycin is an antibiotic that is used to fight bacterial infections in the lungs and sinuses, including acute sinusitis, acute worsening of chronic bronchitis, and community-acquired pneumonia (all in adults).

This drug inhibits the production of protein that bacteria need to grow and reproduce.

SIDE EFFECTS

Be sure to tell your health-care practitioner if you experience any side effects while taking telithromycin. Only your health-care practitioner can determine whether it is safe for you to continue taking this drug.

- *Most Common:* diarrhea, dizziness, headache, loose stools, nausea, vomiting
- *Less Common:* vision problems (blurred vision, difficulty focusing, double vision)
- *Rare:* allergic reaction (closed throat, difficulty breathing, hives, swollen tongue, lips, or face), fainting, irregular heartbeat, unusual bleeding or bruising, yellow skin or eyes

IMPORTANT PRECAUTIONS

Tell your health-care practitioner if you are sensitive or allergic to telithromycin or to any other drugs.

Telithromycin should be used with caution if you have myasthenia gravis, coronary heart disease, decreased kidney or liver function, a history of arrhythmia (irregular heartbeat), low blood potassium or magnesium levels, bradycardia (slow heartbeat, less than 50 beats per minute), or if you or a close family member have a rare heart condition called congenital prolongation of the QT interval.

Telithromycin must not be taken if you are receiving cisapride or pimozide.

Telithromycin may cause vision problems, including blurred vision, difficulty focusing, and double vision. Although most events are mild to moderate, severe cases have occurred. Vision problems most occur after the first or second dose and may last several hours. Therefore, use caution when driving or engaging in hazardous activities.

DRUG INTERACTIONS

Tell your health-care practitioner and pharmacist if you are taking any prescription or nonprescription drugs, as well as any vitamins, herbs, or other supplements. Possible drug interactions include the following:

- Carbamazepine, phenytoin, phenobarbital, and rifamin use should be avoided during and for two weeks after use of telithromycin, as they may make the antibiotic less effective.
- Antifungals (e.g., itraconazole, ketoconazole), cimetidine, and HIV protease inhibitors (e.g., ritonavir) may increase the blood level of telithromycin.

- Antiarrhythmics (e.g., amiodarone, disopyramide, procainamide, metoprolol, sotalol), antidepressants (e.g., amitriptyline, imipramine, maprotiline), antimalarials (e.g., chloroquine, halofantrine, quinine), antipsychotics (e.g., chlorpromazine, haloperidol, sertindole, thioridazine), pimozide, cisapride, and erythromycin may increase the risk of abnormal heart rhythms.
- Telithromycin may increase the blood levels of statins (e.g., atorvastatin, lovastatin, simvastatin). Statins should be discontinued during therapy with telithromycin.
- Telithromycin may increase the blood levels of benzodiazepines (e.g., alprazolam, midazolam, triazolam), digoxin, and immunosuppressants (e.g., ciclosporin, sirolimus, tacrolimus).
- Theophylline should be taken at least one hour before or after use of telithromycin to avoid nausea and vomiting.

FOOD, VITAMIN, AND HERBAL INTERACTIONS

Use of St. John's wort should be avoided during and for two weeks after use of telithromycin because this herb can make the antibiotic less effective.

RECOMMENDED DOSAGE

Telithromycin is available in 400-mg tablets. The dosages given here are typical. However, your health-care practitioner will determine the most appropriate dose and schedule for your needs.

- *Children:* Efficacy and dosing in children 12 years old and younger has not been established.
- *Adults:* 800 mg (two 400-mg tablets) taken once daily

Telithromycin should be taken at the same time each day with 8 ounces of water, with or without food.

If you miss a dose, take it as soon as you remember. If it is nearly time for your next dose, do not take the missed dose. Continue with your regular dosing schedule. Never take a double dose.

Complete the entire course of treatment that your health-care practitioner prescribes for you, even if you feel better before you take all the medication. Your symptoms may begin to improve before the infection is completely treated.

SYMPTOMS OF OVERDOSE AND WHAT TO DO

Symptoms of an overdose with telithromycin have not been reported. If overdose occurs, seek immediate medical attention and bring the prescription container with you to the hospital.

SPECIAL INFORMATION FOR PREGNANT OR NURSING WOMEN

Adequate studies of the effects of telithromycin on pregnant or nursing women have not been done. If you are pregnant or plan to become pregnant, talk to your health-care practitioner. You and your health-care practitioner should weigh the potential benefits against the potential risks.

It is not known whether telithromycin passes into breast milk. Your health-care practitioner may recommend you switch to bottle feeding until you complete treatment with telithromycin.

SPECIAL INFORMATION FOR SENIORS

No special information is needed for seniors.

GENERIC NAME

Telmisartan

see Angiotensin II Blockers, page 123

GENERIC NAME

Temazepam

BRAND NAME

Restoril

Generic available

ABOUT THIS DRUG

Temazepam is used on a short-term basis to treat insomnia. It belongs to a class of central nervous system depressant drugs known as benzodiazepines. Temazepam works by attaching to a site in the brain that results in decreased activity of nervous tissue.

SIDE EFFECTS

Consult your health-care practitioner if you develop side effects while using temazepam. Only he or she can determine whether it is safe for you to continue using this drug.

- *Common:* sedation, dizziness, drowsiness, fatigue, headache, nausea, weakness, sluggishness, a hangover sensation on the day after bedtime use, nervousness
- *Less Common or Rare:* sleep disturbances, increased dreaming, nightmares, loss of memory, overstimulation, agitation, hallucinations, vertigo, dry mouth, loss of equilibrium, diarrhea, heartbeat changes, anxiety, depression, appetite loss, eye problems, vomiting

IMPORTANT PRECAUTIONS

Inform your health-care practitioner about any other medical conditions you may have, especially kidney or liver disease, heart disease, glaucoma, chronic lung disease, or depression. Tell your health-care practitioner if you have ever experienced an allergic reaction to this drug or another benzodiazepine.

Temazepam is recommended for short-term use only. If you need to take this drug for longer than 7 to 10 days, consult your health-care practitioner. Temazepam should not be taken for more than 5 weeks. Long-term use can lead to physical and/or psychological addiction. This drug should be used with caution in anyone with a history of drug or alcohol abuse or depression.

Temazepam can make you drowsy and less alert than usual. Until you know how this drug affects you, do not drive a car, operate machinery, or perform other tasks that require concentration.

DRUG INTERACTIONS

Tell your health-care practitioner and pharmacist if you are taking any other prescription or over-the-counter drugs, as well as any vitamins, herbs, or other supplements. Dosage adjustments may be necessary when you begin taking temazepam. Possible drug interactions include the following:

- Many drugs may add to drowsiness and other effects of temazepam. These include other central nervous system depressants (such as antidepressants, antihistamines, muscle relaxants, and sedatives), oral contraceptives, seizure medications, and digoxin.
- Do not drink alcohol while taking temazepam. This combination worsens coordination and impairs mental function.
- Cigarette smoking may decrease the effectiveness of this drug.

FOOD, VITAMIN, AND HERBAL INTERACTIONS

Do not drink grapefruit juice while taking temazepam. Grapefruit juice slows the body's breakdown of benzodiazepine drugs, which can lead to their potentially dangerous concentration in the blood.

Do not take temazepam with hops, kava, passionflower, and valerian. These can increase its sedative effects. Temazepam should not be combined with hawthorn.

Avoid caffeinated beverages such as coffee, tea, and cola.

RECOMMENDED DOSAGE

Temazepam comes as a capsule. Although the doses given below are typical, only your health-care practitioner can determine the dose and schedule that best fit your needs.

- *Children:* Temazepam is not recommended for children.
- *Adults:* 7.5 to 30 mg at bedtime

Temazepam can be taken with or without food. If you forget a dose, skip it and resume your normal schedule. Never take a double dose. If you have been taking temazepam for a few weeks, do not stop taking it suddenly. Abrupt withdrawal can lead to symptoms such as cramps, vomiting, sweating, tremor, ringing in the ears, sleep disturbances, depression, and convulsions. Speak to your health-care practitioner about gradually reducing dosage. You may experience sleeping difficulties the first night or two after stopping this medication.

SYMPTOMS OF OVERDOSE AND WHAT TO DO

The symptoms of temazepam overdose include drowsiness, sluggishness, confusion, lack of coordination, low blood pressure, and coma. If overdose occurs, seek immediate medical attention and take the prescription bottle to the hospital with you.

SPECIAL INFORMATION FOR PREGNANT OR NURSING WOMEN

Do not take temazepam if you are pregnant or planning to become pregnant. This drug is associated with an increased risk of birth effects. Since temazepam may pass into breast milk, breastfeeding is not advisable while taking this medication.

SPECIAL INFORMATION FOR SENIORS

Side effects such as lethargy, fatigue, and weakness are more likely to occur in older people. Smaller doses are recommended.

OPEN QUESTIONS OR CONTROVERSIES

Temazepam can cause psychological and/or physical dependence. Tolerance may develop with long-term use, making it less effective. Do not take a larger dose of temazepam, take it more often, or use it for a longer period than your health-care practitioner recommends.

GENERIC NAME
Terazosin

BRAND NAME
Hytrin
Generic available

ABOUT THIS DRUG
Terazosin is used to treat high blood pressure (hypertension) and benign prostatic hyperplasia (BPH). BPH—more commonly known as an enlarged prostate—causes difficulties with urination.

Terazosin, an alpha blocker, works by blocking nerve endings called alpha1 receptors. This action relaxes and expands blood vessels, thus lowering blood pressure. It also relaxes smooth muscles in the prostate and bladder.

SIDE EFFECTS
Side effects such as dizziness and fainting are most common when you first start taking terazosin. Call your health-care practitioner at once if you experience a painful, persistent erection. If any other side effects become persistent or severe, speak to your health-care practitioner. Only he or she can determine whether it is safe for you to continue taking this drug.

- *Common:* drowsiness, dizziness, headache, weakness, lack of energy, nausea, heart palpitations
- *Less Common or Rare:* dizziness upon standing, fainting, vertigo, shortness of breath, confusion, nervousness, depression, blurred vision, red eyes, constipation, diarrhea, dry mouth, nasal congestion, fluid retention, frequent urination, nosebleeds, rash, ringing in ears, pins and needles, painful and persistent erection, impotence, urinary problems, joint pain, rapid heartbeat, weight gain, changes in blood count

IMPORTANT PRECAUTIONS
Always inform your health-care practitioner about any other medical conditions you suffer from, such as heart, liver, or kidney disease. Tell your health-care practitioner if you have ever experienced an allergic reaction to this or similar medications.

This drug may make you dizzy or drowsy. Until you know how terazosin affects you, do not drive a car, operate machinery, or perform other tasks that demand concentration. This is especially important in the 12 to 24 hours after your first dose.

When you first start taking this drug, you may experience dizziness or faintness when you rise quickly from a sitting or reclining position (postural hypotension). Try to get up slowly, and consult your health-care practitioner if the problem continues.

Be extremely careful when you exercise in hot weather. Heavy sweating can lead to dizziness, lightheadedness, fainting, vomiting, dehydration, and low blood pressure.

Terazosin may cause dry mouth. To counteract this effect, use sugarless gum or candy, ice chips, or a saliva substitute. If the problem continues, consult your health-care practitioner or dentist.

Treatment of high blood pressure also entails certain lifestyle changes, such as weight control, smoking cessation, and close attention to diet. Before having any type of surgery or dental procedure, tell your surgeon or dentist that you are taking terazosin.

DRUG INTERACTIONS

Tell your health-care practitioner and pharmacist if you are taking any other prescription or over-the-counter drugs, as well as any vitamins, herbs, or other supplements. The following drug interactions may occur:

➤ Terazosin adds to the effects of other blood-pressure-lowering medications.

➤ Indomethacin may decrease the effects of terazosin.

➤ Alcohol may further lower blood pressure and increase the risk of side effects such as dizziness and lightheadedness.

➤ Consult your health-care practitioner before taking over-the-counter cough, cold, sinus, allergy, or weight loss medications. Many of these can raise blood pressure.

FOOD, VITAMIN, AND HERBAL INTERACTIONS

Do not take herbs that increase blood pressure, such as ephedra (ma huang), ginseng, goldenseal, licorice, and saw palmetto. Consult your health-care practitioner before taking substances that may lower blood pressure, such as calcium, soy, or garlic. Talk to your health-care practitioner about diet and salt intake.

RECOMMENDED DOSAGE

Terazosin is available in tablet or capsule form. Although the doses given below are typical, only your health-care practitioner can determine the dose and schedule that best fit your needs.

Hypertension

- *Children:* This drug is not recommended for children.
- *Adults:* 1 to 5 mg at bedtime; the maximum daily dose is 20 mg

Benign Prostatic Hyperplasia

- *Children:* This drug is not recommended for children.
- *Adults:* 1 to 10 mg at bedtime for 4 to 6 weeks; the maximum daily dose is 20 mg

Terazosin can be taken with or without food. Continue to take this drug even if you feel well. Do not discontinue use without consulting your health-care practitioner. If you miss a dose, take it as soon as you remember. If it is almost time for the next dose, skip the forgotten one, and resume your normal schedule. Never take a double dose.

SYMPTOMS OF OVERDOSE AND WHAT TO DO

The symptoms of terazosin overdose include drowsiness and low blood pressure. If overdose occurs, seek immediate medical attention and take the prescription bottle to the hospital with you.

SPECIAL INFORMATION FOR PREGNANT OR NURSING WOMEN

No studies have adequately investigated the effects of terazosin during pregnancy or breastfeeding. If you are pregnant or plan to become pregnant, or if you are breastfeeding or plan to do so, talk with your health-care practitioner before starting this drug. Only a health-care practitioner can determine whether the potential benefits outweigh the potential dangers.

SPECIAL INFORMATION FOR SENIORS

Seniors are more susceptible to side effects such as drowsiness, lightheadedness, and dizziness upon rising. Lower doses are recommended.

GENERIC NAME

Terbinafine

BRAND NAME

Lamisil
No generic available

ABOUT THIS DRUG

Terbinafine is used to treat fungal infections of the skin, fingernails, and toenails. This medication comes in topical and oral form. It works by killing the fungi responsible for infections such as ringworm, athlete's foot, or jock itch.

SIDE EFFECTS

Consult your health-care practitioner if you develop side effects while taking terbinafine. Only he or she can determine whether it is safe for you to continue taking this drug.

- *Common (oral):* rash, headache, diarrhea; *(topical):* irritation, burning sensation, rash
- *Less Common or Rare (oral):* nausea, vomiting, upset stomach, abdominal pain, taste changes, temporary vision changes, infection, fever, drop in white blood cell count, severe skin reactions

IMPORTANT PRECAUTIONS

Always tell your health-care practitioner about all other medical conditions you have, especially kidney or liver disease. Terbinafine has been associated with rare cases of liver damage. Inform your health-care practitioner if you have ever experienced an allergic reaction to this or similar medications.

DRUG INTERACTIONS

Always inform your health-care practitioner and pharmacist if you are taking any other prescription or over-the-counter drugs, as well as any vitamins, herbs, or other supplements. Possible drug interactions with the oral form include the following:

- Terfenadine and cimetidine may increase the effects of terbinafine.
- Terbinafine may reduce the effects of cyclosporine.
- Terbinafine should not be combined with rifampin.

FOOD, VITAMIN, AND HERBAL INTERACTIONS

Terbinafine may increase the effects of caffeine. Consult your health-care practitioner before combining this drug with caffeinated beverages such as coffee, tea, or cola.

RECOMMENDED DOSAGE

Terbinafine comes as a topical cream or oral tablet. Treatment ranges in length from 1 to 12 weeks. The doses given below are typical. However, consult your health-care practitioner for the exact dose and schedule that are most appropriate for you.

Cream

- ➤ *Children:* This drug is not recommended for children.
- ➤ *Adults:* Apply a small amount to affected areas twice daily for 1 to 4 weeks.

Tablets

- ➤ *Children:* This drug is not recommended for children.
- ➤ *Adults:* 250 mg once daily for 6 to 12 weeks

If you forget to take a dose, take it as soon as you remember. If it is almost time for the next dose, skip the forgotten one, and resume your normal schedule. Never take double doses. To cure your infection, continue to take this drug even if you feel well. Do not discontinue use without consulting your health-care practitioner.

SYMPTOMS OF OVERDOSE AND WHAT TO DO

Symptoms of overdose may include nausea, vomiting, abdominal pain, dizziness, frequent urination, and headache. If you suspect that an overdose has occurred, seek immediate medical attention and take the prescription bottle to the hospital with you.

SPECIAL INFORMATION FOR PREGNANT OR NURSING WOMEN

Terbinafine tablets should not be started during pregnancy. If you are breastfeeding or plan to do so, talk with your health-care practitioner before starting this drug. Only a health-care practitioner can determine whether the potential benefits outweigh the potential dangers.

SPECIAL INFORMATION FOR SENIORS

There are no special instructions for seniors.

GENERIC NAME

Terbutaline

BRAND NAMES

Brethaire, Brethine, Bricanyl
No generic available

ABOUT THIS DRUG

Terbutaline is a bronchodilator medication used to prevent and treat wheezing, shortness of breath, and troubled breathing caused by asthma, chronic bronchitis, emphysema, and other lung diseases. It has a weaker effect on the heart and blood vessels than other bronchodilators such as metaproterenol. This makes it a relatively safer choice for people with heart disease.

Terbutaline works by relaxing and opening air passages in the lungs, making it easier to breathe. It also dilates bronchial tubes that are in constriction.

SIDE EFFECTS

Speak to your health-care practitioner if you develop side effects while taking this drug. Only he or she can determine whether you should continue taking terbutaline.

- *Common:* nervousness, fast or irregular heartbeat, heart palpitations, increased heart rate, trembling, flushing, headache, nausea, vomiting, dizziness, drowsiness, chest discomfort, difficulty breathing, weakness
- *Less Common or Rare:* dry mouth, sore throat, sweating, sleeplessness, changes in smell and taste, anxiety, muscle cramps, inflamed blood vessels

IMPORTANT PRECAUTIONS

Tell your health-care practitioner about any other medical conditions you may have, especially angina (chest pain), heart disease, an irregular heartbeat, increased heart rate, high blood pressure, an overactive thyroid, glaucoma, prostate disease, diabetes, or seizures.

Inform your health-care practitioner if you have experienced allergies to this or similar medications in the past.

Because terbutaline may cause side effects such as nervousness and dizziness, do not drive a car, operate machinery, or perform other tasks that require concentration until you know how this drug affects you.

To relieve dry mouth or throat irritation, use sugarless gum or hard candy, or rinse your mouth with water. Consult your health-care practitioner if the problem persists.

DRUG INTERACTIONS

Tell your health-care practitioner if you are taking any other prescription or over-the-counter drugs, as well as any vitamins, herbs, or supplements. Possible drug interactions include the following:

- Taking terbutaline at the same time as or within 14 days of monoamine oxidase inhibitor (MAOI) antidepressants can cause a dangerous increase in blood pressure.

- Do not use other inhaled medications without consulting your health-care practitioner. This can result in increased cardiovascular side effects.
- Do not take terbutaline at the same time as theophylline.
- Medications such as beta-blockers may decrease the effects of terbutaline.
- Use tricyclic antidepressants with caution.
- Check with your health-care practitioner before using over-the-counter drugs. Many cold, cough, allergy, sinus, and weight loss remedies can raise blood pressure.

FOOD, VITAMIN, AND HERBAL INTERACTIONS

Do not take herbs that increase blood pressure, such as ephedra (ma huang), ginseng, goldenseal, licorice, and saw palmetto. Combining terbutaline with kola can cause nervousness. Avoid caffeinated beverages such as coffee, tea, and cola while you are taking this drug.

RECOMMENDED DOSAGE

Terbutaline comes as a tablet to take by mouth and as an aerosol to inhale by mouth. The tablets are taken to prevent symptoms, while the aerosol is taken to prevent or relieve symptoms. Although the doses given below are typical, only your health-care practitioner can determine the dose and schedule that best fit your individual needs.

Aerosol

- *Children Up to 12 Years:* This drug is not recommended for children under the age of 12.
- *Children 12 Years and Older and Adults:* 1 or 2 puffs every 4 to 6 hours

Tablets

- *Children Up to 12 Years:* This drug is not recommended for children under the age of 12.
- *Children 12 to 14 Years:* 2.5 mg 3 times daily
- *Children 15 Years and Older and Adults:* 2.5 to 5 mg 3 times daily

It is important to take terbutaline exactly as prescribed. Taking it more often than recommended can result in increased difficulty breathing and heart rhythm disturbances. Oral medication is more effective when taken on an empty stomach. If you forget a dose, take it as soon as you remember. Take the rest of the day's doses at evenly spaced intervals, and resume your normal schedule the next day. Never take a double dose.

SYMPTOMS OF OVERDOSE AND WHAT TO DO

Symptoms of terbutaline overdose include chest pain, rapid heart rate, heart palpitations, nervousness, tremor, sweating, vomiting, and headache. If overdose occurs, seek immediate medical attention and take the prescription bottle to the hospital with you.

SPECIAL INFORMATION FOR PREGNANT OR NURSING WOMEN

Terbutaline should not be taken after the first 3 months of pregnancy; however, in special situations it is sometimes prescribed to prevent premature labor. If you are breastfeeding or plan to do so, talk with your health-care practitioner before starting this drug. Only a health-care practitioner can determine whether the potential benefits outweigh the potential dangers.

SPECIAL INFORMATION FOR SENIORS

Seniors are more susceptible to side effects such as nervousness, heart rhythm disturbances, heart palpitations, and muscle tremors. Terbutaline should be used with extreme caution in older people who have heart problems or high blood pressure.

GENERIC NAME

Terconazole

BRAND NAMES

Terazol 3, Terazol 7
No generic available

ABOUT THIS DRUG

Terconazole is an antifungal agent used to treat fungal and yeast infections of the vagina such as candidiasis. It is for topical application only.

SIDE EFFECTS

Consult your health-care practitioner if you develop side effects such as burning or itching while using terconazole. Only he or she can determine whether it is safe for you to continue using this drug.

- *Common:* headache
- *Less Common or Rare:* missed menstrual periods, painful menstruation, genital pain, abdominal pain, fever, chills, vaginal irritation and itching, burning sensation

IMPORTANT PRECAUTIONS

To avoid reinfection, refrain from sexual intercourse or use a condom. Sanitary napkins will protect your clothing while you use this drug.

If a vaginal infection does not respond to treatment, see your health-care practitioner. The problem may be a different type of infection that does not respond to terconazole.

Always tell your health-care practitioner about all other medical conditions you have.

DRUG INTERACTIONS

Although no specific interactions are known, always inform your health-care practitioner and pharmacist if you are taking any other prescription or over-the-counter drugs, as well as any vitamins, herbs, or other supplements.

FOOD, VITAMIN, AND HERBAL INTERACTIONS

No food, vitamin, or herbal interactions have been noted.

RECOMMENDED DOSAGE

Terconazole comes in cream and suppositories for vaginal insertion. The doses given below are typical. However, consult your health-care practitioner for the exact dose and schedule that are most appropriate for you.

- *Children:* This drug is not recommended for children.
- *Adults:* Insert 1 applicatorful or suppository into the vagina at bedtime for 3 to 7 days.

If you forget a dose, use it as soon as you remember. If it is almost time for the next dose, skip the forgotten one, and resume your normal schedule. Never take double doses. To cure your infection, continue to take this drug even if you feel well. Do not discontinue use without consulting your health-care practitioner.

SYMPTOMS OF OVERDOSE AND WHAT TO DO

Terconazole is for external use only. Accidental ingestion may cause stomach upset. If overdose occurs, seek immediate medical attention and take the terconazole container to the hospital with you.

SPECIAL INFORMATION FOR PREGNANT OR NURSING WOMEN

Pregnant women should not use terconazole in the first trimester. If you are pregnant or plan to become pregnant, or if you are breast-feeding or plan to do so, talk with your health-care practitioner before starting this drug. Only a health-care practitioner can determine whether the potential benefits outweigh the potential dangers.

SPECIAL INFORMATION FOR SENIORS

There are no special instructions for seniors.

GENERIC NAME

Teriparatide

BRAND NAME

Forteo

No generic available

ABOUT THIS DRUG

Teriparatide is a synthetic form of human parathyroid hormone, which is the main substance that regulates calcium and phosphate metabolism in bone. This drug is for treatment of osteoporosis in postmenopausal women who are at high risk for having a fracture, and for men who have osteoporosis who are at high risk for fracture.

This drug helps form new bone, which in turn increases bone mineral density and bone strength.

SIDE EFFECTS

Be sure to tell your health-care practitioner if you experience any side effects while taking teriparatide. Only your health-care practitioner can determine whether it is safe for you to continue taking this drug.

- *Most Common:* dizziness, headache, fast heartbeat after injection, leg cramps
- *Rare:* constipation, muscle weakness, nausea, vomiting, all of which may indicate high calcium levels (hyperkalcemia) in the blood.

IMPORTANT PRECAUTIONS

Tell your health-care practitioner if you are sensitive or allergic to teriparatide, mannitol, or to any other drugs.

This drug should not be taken if you have Paget's disease, if you are younger than 18 years old, if you have high levels of calcium in the blood, or if you have bone cancer. Also inform your health-care practitioner if you have any condition that causes high levels of calcium in the blood, such as parathyroid gland disease, kidney stones, urinary tract stones, and liver, kidney, or heart disease.

Because teriparatide can cause dizziness, make sure you know how you react to this drug before you drive or operate dangerous equipment.

Rats given teriparatide developed osteosarcoma, a very rare type of cancer. It is not known if this drug will increase the risk of osteosarcoma in humans.

Teriparatide may cause dizziness, lightheadedness, and fainting when you get up too quickly from a lying position. This response is more common when you first begin treatment. To avoid this problem, get out of bed slowly and rest your feet on the floor for a few minutes before you stand up. Be seated or have a chair nearby when you give yourself an injection.

The safe use and efficacy of teriparatide has not been evaluated for use greater than 2 years; therefore use for longer than this period is not recommended.

DRUG INTERACTIONS

Tell your health-care practitioner and pharmacist if you are taking any prescription or nonprescription drugs, as well as any vitamins, herbs, or other supplements. Possible drug interactions include the following:

- ➤ Digoxin and hydrochlorothiazide may require your health-care practitioner to adjust your dosage of teriparatide and/or monitor you for side effects.

FOOD, VITAMIN, AND HERBAL INTERACTIONS

Because it is important to get enough calcium and vitamin D while you take teriparatide, your health-care practitioner may recommend your taking supplements of these nutrients if your dietary intake is not sufficient.

RECOMMENDED DOSAGE

Teriparatide is available as a dose-regulated injection (in a preassembled penlike device) which is administered by the patient into the thigh or abdomen. The dosage given here is typical. However, your health-care practitioner will determine the most appropriate dose and schedule for your needs.

- *Children:* Not recommended for children younger than 18
- *Adults:* One pre-measured dose, delivered in a pre-assembled pen-like device, daily in the thigh or abdomen. The recommended dose is 20 mcg daily.

Teriparatide should be refrigerated until use. The drug comes in a pen-injection device that contains enough medication for 28 doses. You will use a new needle for each injection, and needles should be disposed of in a puncture-resistant container. Recap the pen and put it back into the refrigerator after each use. The same pen can be used for up to 28 days after the first injection, then thrown away, even if the device is not empty. Do not use teriparatide if it is discolored or cloudy.

If you miss a dose, take it as soon as you remember if it is within the same day. If it is nearly time for your next dose, do not take the missed dose and continue with your regular dosing schedule. Never take a double dose.

SYMPTOMS OF OVERDOSE AND WHAT TO DO

Symptoms of overdose include nausea, vomiting, dizziness, lightheadedness and fainting upon standing, constipation, lack of energy, muscle weakness, and headache. If overdose occurs, seek immediate medical attention and bring the prescription container with you to the hospital.

SPECIAL INFORMATION FOR PREGNANT OR NURSING WOMEN

Teriparatide is for use in postmenopausal women only, and should not be used by women who are pregnant or breastfeeding.

SPECIAL INFORMATION FOR SENIORS

No special precautions have been noted for older adults.

GENERIC NAME

Testosterone

BRAND NAMES

Androderm, Testim, Testoderm

No generic available

Note: The information in this profile also applies to methyltestosterone (Android, Oreton Methyl, Testred, Virilon).

ABOUT THIS DRUG

Testosterone is used to replace natural testosterone in males who have impotence or a delayed onset of puberty due to hormone deficiency. Testosterone is the principal male hormone, or androgen, produced by the body. It is needed for the normal growth and development of male sex organs. Testosterone may also be used to treat metastatic cancer (cancer that has spread) in women.

SIDE EFFECTS

Consult your health-care practitioner if you develop side effects while using testosterone. Only he or she can determine whether it is safe for you to continue using this drug.

- *Common:* headache, dizziness, confusion, tiredness, depression, upset stomach, rapid weight gain, nausea, vomiting, flushing, fluid retention, ankle swelling, thirst, increased urination, increased blood pressure and cholesterol, enlargement of the breasts in women and men, menstrual irregularities and deepening voice in women, increased number and/or duration of erections in men, decreased sperm production, local irritation at patch site
- *Less Common or Rare:* acne, diarrhea, difficulty breathing, difficulty sleeping, increase in pubic hair, male pattern baldness, yellow eyes and skin, unusual bleeding, rash, hives, itching, decreased testicle size, impotence

IMPORTANT PRECAUTIONS

Testosterone is not an appropriate drug for everyone. It should be avoided by anyone with heart or kidney disease, pregnant women, and men with prostate or breast cancer. Do not use this drug if you have experienced an allergic reaction to it in the past.

Possible side effects of testosterone include dizziness. Until you know how this drug affects you, do not drive a car, operate machinery, or perform other tasks that require concentration.

Long-term use of large doses of this hormone has been associated with potentially life-threatening liver damage. Other serious consequences may include high cholesterol, decreased sperm count, enlarged breasts in men, and acute intermittent porphyria (a condition characterized by nausea, vomiting, abdominal pain, constipation, nerve irritation, and neurotic behavior). You should be closely monitored by your health-care practitioner while taking testosterone.

A man using a patch on his scrotum may inadvertently transfer hormones to a sexual partner, which may result in the development of unwanted secondary sex characteristics.

DRUG INTERACTIONS

Tell your health-care practitioner and pharmacist if you are taking any other prescription or over-the-counter drugs, as well as any vitamins, herbs, or other supplements. Possible drug interactions include the following:

- Do not combine testosterone with imipramine. This may lead to paranoid reactions.
- Testosterone may increase the effects of blood thinners such as warfarin.
- Testosterone may alter the results of thyroid tests.

FOOD, VITAMIN, AND HERBAL INTERACTIONS

Do not combine testosterone with herbal remedies for impotence, such as ginseng.

RECOMMENDED DOSAGE

Testosterone substitutes come as oral tablets or skin patches. The doses given below are typical. However, only your health-care practitioner can determine the dose and schedule that best fit your individual needs.

Gel

- *Children:* Consult your health-care practitioner.
- *Men:* Apply contents of one 5-g packet or tube daily to a clean, dry, hairless site on the skin.

Tablets

- *Children:* Consult your health-care practitioner.
- *Women:* 50 to 200 mg daily
- *Men:* 10 to 30 mg daily

Skin Patches

- *Children:* This drug is not indicated for children.
- *Women:* Consult your health-care practitioner.
- *Men:* Apply 1 patch nightly to a clean, dry, hairless site on the skin.

If you forget a dose, take it as soon as you remember. If it is almost time for the next dose, skip the forgotten one, and resume your normal schedule. Never take double doses.

SYMPTOMS OF OVERDOSE AND WHAT TO DO

Symptoms of testosterone overdose may include exaggerated side effects. If you suspect an overdose, seek immediate medical attention and take the prescription bottle to the hospital with you so the health-care practitioner will know exactly what medication was taken.

SPECIAL INFORMATION FOR PREGNANT OR NURSING WOMEN

Testosterone should not be used during pregnancy. Because this hormone may pass into breast milk, your health-care practitioner may recommend bottle-feeding.

SPECIAL INFORMATION FOR SENIORS

Seniors who take testosterone may be at increased risk of prostate problems.

GENERIC NAME

Class: Tetracycline antibiotics

Generics: (1) demeclocycline; (2) doxycycline; (3) meclocycline sulfosalicylate; (4) minocycline; (5) oxytetracycline; (6) tetracycline

BRAND NAMES

(1) Declomycin; (2) Bio-Tab, Doryx, Doxy Caps, Doxychel Hyclate, Monodox, Periostat, Vibramycin, Vibra-Tabs; (3) Meclan; (4) Dynacin, Minocin, Vectrin; (5) Terramycin, Uri-Tet; (6) Ala-Tet, Nor-Tet, Panmycin, Sumycin, Tetracap, Tetracyn, Tetralan, Topicycline

All available as generic except demeclocycline and meclocycline

ABOUT THESE DRUGS

Tetracycline antibiotics are broad-spectrum antibiotics used to treat a wide variety of infections, including acne, amebic dysentery, anthrax, cholera, Lyme disease, plague, respiratory infections such as pneumonia, Rocky Mountain spotted fever, and urinary tract infections. When penicillin cannot be taken, they are prescribed for gonorrhea and syphilis.

Tetracycline antibiotics work by preventing the reproduction of invading bacteria. These drugs are not effective against other types of microorganisms, such as viruses, fungi, and parasites. Antibiotics should not be prescribed for colds or flu. Numerous bacteria are also resistant to tetracycline antibiotics.

SIDE EFFECTS

Consult your health-care practitioner if you develop side effects while taking one of these drugs. Only he or she can determine whether it is safe for you to continue taking a tetracycline antibiotic.

- *Common:* diarrhea, upset stomach, nausea, vomiting, rash
- *Less Common or Rare:* superinfection, headache, blurred vision, fluid retention, sensitivity to light, appetite loss, yellow eyes and skin, anemia, hairy tongue, excessive thirst or urination, vaginal or anal itching, thyroid gland problems, liver or kidney problems

IMPORTANT PRECAUTIONS

Tell your health-care practitioner if you have ever experienced an allergic reaction to a tetracycline antibiotic. If so, he or she will most likely prescribe a different antibiotic for you.

Always inform your health-care practitioner about any other medical conditions you suffer from, especially kidney or liver disease, or urinary problems.

Do not use tetracyclines after their expiration date. This may cause kidney damage.

Tetracycline antibiotics should not be given to children 8 years old or younger. These drugs may discolor developing teeth.

If you are using oral contraceptives, practice other means of contraception while taking tetracycline antibiotics.

Because these drugs may cause side effects such as nervousness and dizziness, do not drive a car, operate machinery, or perform other tasks that require concentration until you know how they affect you.

Tetracycline antibiotics may cause increased sensitivity to the sun. Wear protective clothing and apply sunscreen while taking them.

DRUG INTERACTIONS

Check first with your health-care practitioner before taking any other medication with a tetracycline antibiotic. To avoid unwanted side effects, tell your health-care practitioner and pharmacist about all other prescription or over-the-counter drugs, vitamins, herbs, or other supplements that you are taking. Possible drug interactions include the following:

- Tetracycline antibiotics may decrease the effects of oral contraceptives.
- Avoid using antacids that contain aluminum, magnesium, or calcium. If you must take them, separate them from tetracycline antibiotics by 2 to 3 hours.

- A number of drugs may decrease the effects of tetracycline antibiotics. These include cimetidine and ranitidine.
- Tetracyclines may alter the effects of insulin, digoxin, and lithium.
- These drugs may increase the effects of blood thinners such as warfarin.
- Tetracyclines should not be taken with penicillin antibiotics.

FOOD, VITAMIN, AND HERBAL INTERACTIONS

When taking these antibiotics, you also destroy friendly bacteria such as *Lactobacillus acidophilus* that normally reside in the intestine. This can result in yeast infections. To prevent this problem, eat yogurt with live cultures or take *Lactobacillus acidophilus* supplements.

Take tetracycline antibiotics 1 hour before or 2 hours after calcium supplements, and 2 hours before or 3 hours after iron preparations.

RECOMMENDED DOSAGE

Tetracycline antibiotics are available in a wide variety of forms, including oral tablets, capsules, and suspension, and a topical solution to be applied to the skin. Take only the exact type, brand, and strength of medication prescribed by your health-care practitioner. Different forms are not interchangeable. Your health-care practitioner will most likely advise you to divide doses evenly throughout the day. The doses given below are average. However, doses vary from person to person, and according to the condition being treated. Only your health-care practitioner can determine the dose and schedule that are most appropriate for you.

Demeclocycline

- *Children Older than 8 Years:* 3 to 6 mg per pound of body weight daily
- *Adults:* 600 mg daily

Doxycycline

- *Children Older than 8 Years (under 100 pounds):* 1 to 2 mg per pound of body weight daily
- *Children Older than 8 Years and Adults (over 100 pounds):* 100 to 200 mg daily; dosage is higher for gonorrhea and syphilis

Meclocycline Sulfosalicylate

- *Children:* Consult your health-care practitioner.
- *Adults:* Apply to affected skin twice daily.

Minocycline hydrochloride

- *Children Older than 8 Years:* 2 mg per pound of body weight daily
- *Adults:* 200 mg daily

Oxytetracycline

- *Children Older than 8 Years:* 10 to 20 mg per pound of body weight daily
- *Adults:* 1 to 2 grams daily

Tetracycline

- *Children Older than 8 Years:* 10 to 20 mg per pound of body weight daily
- *Adults:* 1 to 2 grams daily

Most tetracycline antibiotics are best absorbed on an empty stomach, and should be taken 1 hour before or 2 hours after meals. Exceptions are doxycycline and minocycline, which may be taken with food (but not milk). However, if an antibiotic upsets your stomach, ask your health-care practitioner about taking it with a snack such as crackers. These antibiotics should not be taken with dairy products. Drink a full (8-ounce) glass of water with each dose.

If you miss a dose, take it as soon as you remember. If it is nearly time for your next scheduled dose, do not take the missed dose. Follow your regular dosing schedule. Never take a double dose.

It is essential to take tetracycline antibiotics exactly as your health-care practitioner instructs you. In order to receive their full benefits, continue to take antibiotics for the full number of days prescribed. Failing to do so can result in even more serious and drug-resistant infection.

SYMPTOMS OF OVERDOSE AND WHAT TO DO

Symptoms of overdose may include diarrhea and stomach upset. If you suspect overdose, seek medical attention immediately, and bring the prescription bottle with you to the hospital so that health-care practitioners will know exactly what drug was taken.

SPECIAL INFORMATION FOR PREGNANT OR NURSING WOMEN

Tetracycline antibiotics should not be used during pregnancy. They may interfere with the development of your baby's bones and teeth. Because tetracycline antibiotics may pass into breast milk, your health-care practitioner will most likely advise you to stop breast-feeding while you take these drugs.

SPECIAL INFORMATION FOR SENIORS

Seniors may be more susceptible to side effects, especially if they have poor kidney function.

GENERIC NAME

Thalidomide

BRAND NAME

Thalomid
No generic available

ABOUT THIS DRUG

Thalidomide is used to treat erythema nodosum leprosum (ENL), a skin condition associated with leprosy. When this drug was first prescribed in Europe in the early 1960s, it caused a number of severe birth defects. It was only approved for use in the United States in 1998, and is very strictly regulated. Thalidomide is also being used in the treatment of certain cancers. It slows cancer cell growth by preventing the formation of new blood vessels.

Thalidomide works by suppressing the immune system. It affects white blood cells and tumor necrosis factor (TNF).

SIDE EFFECTS

Side effects of thalidomide can be extremely serious, and must be promptly reported to your health-care practitioner. Even a single dose can cause birth defects, and side effects can occur anywhere in the body.

➤ *Common:* stomach pain, nausea, diarrhea, constipation, headache, tiredness, an overall feeling of unwellness, fainting, dizziness, muscle weakness, back pain, rash, fever, chills, sore throat, sinus irritation, infection, tingling, burning, numbness, or pain in the extremities

➤ *Less Common or Rare:* mood changes, agitation, dry mouth, dry skin, acne, nail problems, fungal skin infections, blistering skin, itching, sweating, gas, abdominal pain, loss of appetite, runny nose, tooth pain, rigid neck, swollen lymph glands, blood problems, anemia, blood in urine, decreased urination, impotence, liver inflammation, low blood pressure, irregular heartbeat, accidental injuries, convulsions

IMPORTANT PRECAUTIONS

Always tell your health-care practitioner about any other medical conditions you may have, especially decreased white blood cell counts, peripheral neuropathy, epilepsy, or a risk of seizures.

Thalidomide can cause serious birth defects if either a man or woman is taking it at the time of conception. It is also associated with impotence.

Thalidomide suppresses the immune system, causes a drop in white blood cells, and may decrease the body's ability to combat infection.

Thalidomide frequently causes nerve damage and irritation. An allergic reaction to this drug may include symptoms such as rapid heartbeat, fever, low blood pressure, and rash. People taking any dose of thalidomide must be closely monitored with regular complete blood counts and other tests.

This drug may cause tiredness and drowsiness. Until you know how thalidomide affects you, do not drive a car, operate machinery, or perform other tasks that require concentration.

Thalidomide may cause sun sensitivity. Wear protective clothing and apply sunscreen.

DRUG INTERACTIONS

Inform your health-care practitioner and pharmacist if you are taking any other prescription or over-the-counter drugs, as well as any vitamins, herbs, or other supplements. Possible drug interactions include the following:

- Thalidomide may add to the sedative effects of central nervous system depressants. These include antihistamines, allergy and cold medications, antidepressants, sedatives, tranquilizers, sleeping pills, barbiturates, narcotics, seizure medications, muscle relaxants, and anesthetics.
- Many drugs may increase the risk of peripheral neuropathy (tingling, burning, pain, and numbness in the hands and feet) when combined with thalidomide. These include chloramphenicol, cisplatin, dapsone, didanosine, ethambutol, ethionamide, hydralazine, isoniazid, lithium, metronidazole, nitrofurantoin, nitrous oxide, phenytoin, stavudine, vincristine, and zalcitabine.

- Avoid medications that interfere with oral contraceptives.
- Do not drink alcohol while taking thalidomide.

FOOD, VITAMIN, AND HERBAL INTERACTIONS
Do not take thalidomide with supplements such as St. John's wort, which may also cause increased sun sensitivity.

RECOMMENDED DOSAGE
Thalidomide comes as a capsule. The doses given below are typical. However, only your health-care practitioner can determine the dose and schedule that best fit your individual needs.

- *Children:* This drug is not recommended for children.
- *Adults:* 100 to 400 mg daily

Do not take thalidomide with high-fat meals. If you miss a dose, take it as soon as you remember. If it is almost time for the next dose, skip it and resume your regular schedule. Never take a double dose.

SYMPTOMS OF OVERDOSE AND WHAT TO DO
Symptoms of thalidomide overdose may include exaggerated side effects. If you suspect that an overdose has occurred, seek immediate medical attention and take the prescription bottle to the hospital with you.

SPECIAL INFORMATION FOR PREGNANT OR NURSING WOMEN
Do not under any circumstances take this drug if you are pregnant or think you may be pregnant. Thalidomide may cause severe birth defects. Use 2 reliable means of contraception while taking this drug, and take weekly pregnancy tests. Because of the possibility of serious side effects, breastfeeding is not recommended while you take this drug.

SPECIAL INFORMATION FOR SENIORS
There are no special instructions for seniors.

GENERIC NAME

Theophylline

see Xanthine Bronchodilators, page 1116

GENERIC NAME
Class: Thiazide diuretics

Generics: (1) bendroflumethiazide; (2) benzthiazide; (3) chlorothiazide; (4) chlorthalidone; (5) hydrochlorothiazide; (6) hydroflumethiazide; (7) indapamide; (8) methyclothiazide; (9) metolazone; (10) polythiazide; (11) quinethazone; (12) trichlormethiazide

BRAND NAMES

(1) Naturetin; (2) Exna; (3) Diurigen, Diuril; (4) Hygroton, Thalitone; (5) Esidrix, Ezide, HydroDIURIL, Hydro-Par, Oretic; (6) Diucardin, Saluron; (7) Lozol; (8) Aquatensen, Enduron; (9) Mykrox, Zaroxolyn; (10) Renese; (11) Hydromox; (12) Diurese, Metahydrin, Naqua
All available as generic except bendroflumethiazide, benzthiazide, metolazone, and polythiazide

ABOUT THIS DRUG

Thiazide diuretics are used to reduce the amount of water in the body. Also known as "water pills," these drugs are prescribed for congestive heart failure, high blood pressure, cirrhosis, kidney problems, fluid accumulation in the lungs, and other conditions that require the removal of excess fluid from the body. They are often prescribed with other drugs to treat these conditions.

Thiazide diuretics cause the kidneys to get rid of unneeded water and salt from the body into the urine. They increase urine production by altering the movement of sodium and chloride through the kidneys.

SIDE EFFECTS

The most common side effect of these drugs is excessive potassium loss. Consult your health-care practitioner if you develop side effects while taking one of these drugs. Only he or she can determine whether it is safe for you to continue taking a thiazide diuretic.

- *Common:* frequent urination, dizziness or lightheadedness when getting up from a sitting or lying down position, changes in blood levels of potassium and possibly other electrolytes, dry mouth, increased thirst, irregular heartbeat, mood or mental changes, muscle cramps or pain, nausea, vomiting, weakness, tiredness, weak pulse, a decrease in magnesium, an increase in blood sugar or blood uric acid levels
- *Less Common or Rare:* appetite loss, abdominal discomfort, fever, diarrhea, constipation, headache, sensitivity to the sun, rash, dizziness, lightheadedness, blurred vision, tingling in the fingers and

toes, jaundice, abdominal pain, bloating, breathing difficulties, muscle spasms, impotence

Beware of symptoms of low blood potassium (hypokalemia), which may include excessive thirst, dry mouth, decreased urination, drowsiness, weakness, lethargy, muscle pain or cramps, abnormal heart rate, upset stomach, nausea, vomiting, and low blood pressure.

IMPORTANT PRECAUTIONS

Tell your health-care practitioner if you have or have ever had medical conditions such as diabetes, gout, heart or blood vessel disease, lupus, kidney or liver disease, pancreatitis, or low blood potassium or other electrolytes.

Thiazide diuretics may affect blood sugar levels. If you have diabetes, be careful when testing your glucose levels, and closely monitor your diet.

Before having any type of surgery or dental procedure, tell your surgeon or dentist that you are taking a thiazide diuretic.

Treatment of high blood pressure also entails certain lifestyle changes, such as weight control, smoking cessation, and close attention to diet.

When you first start taking this drug or when the dosage is increased, you may experience dizziness or faintness when you rise quickly from a sitting or reclining position (postural hypotension). Try to get up slowly, and consult your health-care practitioner if the problem continues.

Thiazide diuretics may cause side effects such as dizziness and tiredness. Do not drive a car, operate machinery, or perform other tasks that require concentration until you know how the drug you are taking affects you.

Alert your health-care practitioner if you experience an illness accompanied by diarrhea, vomiting, and sweating. This may cause the loss of too much water and potassium.

Be careful when you exercise in hot weather or enter a hot bath or sauna. Heavy sweating can lead to dizziness, lightheadedness, fainting, vomiting, dehydration, and low blood pressure.

Thiazide diuretics may cause increased sensitivity to sunlight. When you take this drug, avoid direct sunlight and wear sunscreen.

DRUG INTERACTIONS

Tell your health-care practitioner and pharmacist if you are taking any other prescription or over-the-counter drugs, as well as any vita-

mins, herbs, or other supplements. Possible drug interactions include the following:

- Thiazide diuretics enhance the effectiveness of other blood pressure medications.
- These drugs should be taken more than 2 hours before cholestyramine and colestipol.
- Thiazide diuretics increase the risk of lithium side effects.
- NSAIDs (especially indomethacin) may lessen the effectiveness of thiazide diuretics.
- Combining a thiazide diuretic with digoxin may result in increased blood levels and effects of digoxin.
- Thiazide diuretics may increase the absorption of blood thinners such as warfarin, leading to an increased risk of bleeding.
- Consult your health-care practitioner before taking over-the-counter cough, cold, sinus, allergy, or weight loss medications. Many of these can raise blood pressure.
- It may be necessary to adjust the dosages of oral diabetes drugs taken along with thiazide diuretics.
- Your health-care practitioner may recommend medication to prevent potassium loss.
- Limit your alcohol intake. Alcohol makes you more likely to experience effects such as dizziness and lightheadedness.

FOOD, VITAMIN, AND HERBAL INTERACTIONS

Do not take herbs that increase blood pressure, such as ephedra (ma huang), ginseng, goldenseal, licorice, and saw palmetto. Gingko biloba, when combined with a thiazide diuretic, may increase blood pressure. Consult your health-care practitioner before taking substances that may lower blood pressure, such as calcium, soy, or garlic. Do not combine these drugs with St. John's wort, since both may cause heightened sensitivity to the sun.

Because thiazide diuretics may deplete your body's supply of potassium, consult your health-care practitioner about possible dietary changes. However, do not change your diet on your own (especially if you have other health issues such as diabetes). Your health-care practitioner may recommend a higher intake of potassium-rich foods such as bananas, prunes, raisins, citrus fruits, orange juice, melons, and tomatoes. Magnesium levels may also be affected, so inquire about a daily nutritional supplement. A low-sodium diet may be advised.

RECOMMENDED DOSAGE

Thiazide diuretics come in tablet, capsule, or suspension form. Ask your health-care practitioner to help you plan the best way to take this medication. If you are prescribed a single dose, it is best to take it in the morning to avoid nighttime urination. If you take more than one dose a day, take the last dose before 6 p.m. Although the doses given below are typical, only your health-care practitioner can determine the dose and schedule that are most appropriate for you. For example, sometimes doses are taken on alternate days.

Bendroflumethiazide

- *Children:* Consult your health-care practitioner.
- *Adults:* 2.5 to 20 mg daily

Benzthiazide

- *Children:* Consult your health-care practitioner.
- *Adults:* 50 to 200 mg daily

Chlorothiazide

- *Children:* Consult your health-care practitioner.
- *Adults:* 250 to 1,000 mg daily

Chlorthalidone

- *Children:* Consult your health-care practitioner.
- *Adults:* 25 to 100 mg daily

Hydrochlorothiazide

- *Children:* Consult your health-care practitioner.
- *Adults:* 25 to 200 mg daily

Hydroflumethiazide

- *Children:* Consult your health-care practitioner.
- *Adults:* 25 to 200 mg daily

Indapamide

- *Children:* Consult your health-care practitioner.
- *Adults:* 1.25 to 2.5 mg daily

Methyclothiazide

- *Children:* Consult your health-care practitioner.
- *Adults:* 2.5 to 10 mg daily

Metolazone

- *Children:* Consult your health-care practitioner.
- *Adults:* 2.5 to 20 mg daily

Polythiazide

- *Children:* Consult your health-care practitioner.
- *Adults:* 1 to 4 mg daily

Quinethazone

- *Children:* Consult your health-care practitioner.
- *Adults:* 50 to 200 mg daily

Trichlormethiazide

- *Children:* Consult your health-care practitioner.
- *Adults:* 1 to 4 mg daily

If they cause stomach upset, thiazide diuretics can be taken with food. If you miss a dose of a thiazide diuretic, take it as soon as you remember. However, if it is nearly time for your next scheduled dose, do not take the missed dose. Follow your regular dosing schedule. Never take a double dose.

SYMPTOMS OF OVERDOSE AND WHAT TO DO

Symptoms of overdose may include nausea, vomiting, weakness, lethargy, dizziness, tingling in the arms and legs, heartbeat changes, urinary difficulties, dry mouth, restlessness, muscle cramps, and drowsiness progressing to coma. If overdose occurs, seek immediate medical attention, and bring the prescription bottle with you to the hospital so that health-care practitioners will know exactly what drug was used.

SPECIAL INFORMATION FOR PREGNANT OR NURSING WOMEN

Thiazide diuretics may cause low potassium, blood problems, and jaundice in newborns. They may also pass into breast milk. If you are pregnant or plan to become pregnant, or if you are breastfeeding or plan to do so, talk with your health-care practitioner before starting one of these medications. Only a health-care practitioner can determine whether the potential benefits outweigh the risks.

SPECIAL INFORMATION FOR SENIORS

Seniors are more sensitive to side effects such as dizziness, lightheadedness, and signs of potassium loss. Lower doses are usually prescribed.

GENERIC NAME

Thioridazine

BRAND NAME

Mellaril
Generic available

ABOUT THIS DRUG

Thioridazine is used to treat schizophrenia and symptoms such as hostility, delusions, and hallucinations. It may also be prescribed for depression and anxiety in adults, and severe behavioral problems in children.

This drug is known as a phenothiazine. It works by affecting a part of the brain called the hypothalamus, which controls vital functions such as alertness, hormone balance, body temperature, metabolism, muscle tone, and vomiting.

SIDE EFFECTS

Side effects are common. If they become persistent or severe, consult your health-care practitioner. Only he or she can determine whether it is safe for you to continue taking this drug and whether it is necessary to readjust your dosage.

- *Common:* drowsiness, dizziness, dizziness upon rising, fainting, loss of balance, mask-like face, headache, blurred vision, change in color vision, difficulty seeing at night, dry mouth, decreased sweating, nasal congestion, upset stomach, constipation, diarrhea, vomiting, weight gain, restlessness, shuffling walk, stiffness of arms and legs, trembling and shaking of hands, symptoms of tardive dyskinesia (such as lip smacking or puckering, wormlike movements of the tongue, inability to move eyes, trouble speaking, difficulty breathing or swallowing, tics, twitching, and slow, rhythmical, involuntary movements)

- *Less Common or Rare:* difficulty urinating, rash, skin discoloration, itchy skin, sensitivity to the sun, sunburn, irregular or slow heart rate, recurrent fainting, abdominal or stomach pain, aching muscles and joints, muscle weakness, unusual bleeding or bruising, mouth sores, rough or fuzzy tongue, fever, chills, dark urine, agitation, strange dreams, trouble sleeping, hair loss, chest pain, menstrual irregularities, change in sexual desire, prolonged and painful erection, yellow eyes or skin, weight gain

People taking antipsychotic drugs may experience a rare but life-threatening set of side effects known as neuroleptic malignant syndrome (NMS). Symptoms include fever, difficulty breathing, rapid heartbeat, rigid muscles, mental changes, increased sweating, irregular blood pressure, and convulsions. Immediate medical attention is required.

Side effects such as lip smacking, wormlike movements of the tongue, and slow, rhythmical, involuntary movements are characteristic of a disorder known as tardive dyskinesia. Older adults (especially women) are more susceptible to this condition, which may become permanent. If you experience tardive dyskinesia, your health-care practitioner will probably advise you to stop taking this drug.

IMPORTANT PRECAUTIONS

You should not take thioridazine if you have neuroleptic malignant syndrome or if you have experienced a previous allergic reaction to this drug or other phenothiazines.

Tell your health-care practitioner if you have other medical conditions, especially kidney or liver disease, a seizure disorder, brain damage, breast cancer, heart or blood vessel disease, high or low blood pressure, a blood disorder, glaucoma, difficult urination, an enlarged prostate, asthma or other lung disease, Parkinson's disease, stomach ulcers, pheochromocytoma, or Reye's syndrome.

Before having any type of surgery, dental procedure, emergency treatment, or medical test, tell your health-care practitioner or dentist that you are taking thioridazine.

This drug may impair your vision and physical coordination. Until you know how thioridazine affects you, do not drive a car, operate machinery, or perform other tasks that demand concentration.

This medicine may make you sweat less. Drink plenty of fluids and avoid extreme heat. Be especially careful when you exercise in hot weather or enter a hot bath or sauna. Overheating may result in heatstroke.

When you first start taking this drug or when the dosage is increased, you may experience dizziness or faintness when you rise quickly from a sitting or reclining position (postural hypotension). Try to get up slowly, and consult your health-care practitioner if the problem continues.

This drug may cause heightened sun sensitivity. Wear sunglasses and protective clothing, and apply sunscreen.

If thioridazine causes dry mouth, use sugarless gum or hard candy, ice chips, or a saliva substitute. Consult your health-care practitioner or dentist if the problem continues.

DRUG INTERACTIONS

Inform your health-care practitioner and pharmacist if you are taking any other prescription or over-the-counter drugs, as well as any vitamins, herbs, or other supplements. Possible drug interactions include the following:

- Taking central nervous system depressants such as tranquilizers, sleep aids, or antidepressants increases the effects of thioridazine.
- This drug may increase the effects of tricyclic antidepressants.
- Since thioridazine may cause low blood pressure, be cautious about combining this medication with antihypertensive drugs such as propranolol.
- Do not take this drug within 2 hours of antacids or medicine for diarrhea.
- Combining thioridazine with lithium increases the risk of serious nerve side effects.
- Taking metoclopramide with thioridazine increases the risk of Parkinson-like reactions.
- This drug may cause false positive results in pregnancy tests.
- Avoid alcohol while taking thioridazine.

FOOD, VITAMIN, AND HERBAL INTERACTIONS

Do not combine thioridazine with herbs that produce sedative effects, such as catnip, elecampane, goldenseal, gotu kola, hops, kava, lemon balm, skullcap, St. John's wort, and valerian. Stimulants such as ginseng, ephedra (ma huang), or caffeine may reduce the effectiveness of this drug.

RECOMMENDED DOSAGE

Thioridazine comes as a tablet, oral solution, and oral suspension. The doses given below are typical, but dosage is always carefully individualized according to a person's particular needs and reactions to therapy.

- *Children 2 Years and Older:* 20 to 30 mg daily, in divided doses
- *Adults:* 75 to 300 mg daily, in divided doses; maximum dosage is 800 mg daily

Liquid medication may be diluted with water or fruit juice. Do not allow liquid medication to touch your skin. If you take multiple doses daily and remember a forgotten dose within an hour of the time you normally take it, go ahead and take it. Otherwise skip it and resume your normal schedule. Never take a double dose. Although this drug is not habit-forming, dosage must be reduced gradually.

SYMPTOMS OF OVERDOSE AND WHAT TO DO

The symptoms of thioridazine overdose may include agitation, confusion, blurred vision, low blood pressure, heart abnormalities, fluid in the lungs, difficulty breathing, convulsions, and coma. If overdose occurs, seek immediate medical attention and take the prescription bottle to the hospital with you.

SPECIAL INFORMATION FOR PREGNANT OR NURSING WOMEN

Thioridazine is not recommended during pregnancy. This drug may pass into breast milk, so breastfeeding is not advised while you take it.

SPECIAL INFORMATION FOR SENIORS

Seniors require lower doses of thioridazine. Older people (especially women) are more likely to experience side effects such as drowsiness, dizziness, low blood pressure, and tardive dyskinesia (with symptoms such as lip smacking, wormlike movements of the tongue, and slow, rhythmical, involuntary movements).

GENERIC NAME

Thyroglobulin

see Thyroid Hormone Replacements, page 1029

GENERIC NAME

Class: Thyroid hormone replacements

Generics: (1) levothyroxine sodium; (2) liothyronine sodium; (3) liotrix; (4) thyroglobulin; (5) thyroid hormone

BRAND NAMES

(1) Eltroxin, Levo-T, Levothroid, Levoxine, Levoxyl, Novothyrox, Synthroid; (2) Cytomel; (3) Thyrolar; (4) available as generic only; (5) Alti-Thyroxine, Armour Thyroid, S-P-T, Thyroid Strong, Thyrar
Generic available

ABOUT THESE DRUGS

Thyroid hormone replacements are used to treat an underactive thyroid gland, or hypothyroidism. These drugs are prescribed when your thyroid gland cannot produce sufficient hormone. Symptoms include low energy, sluggishness, and weight gain. Thyroid hormones are also taken for the prevention or treatment of goiter (an enlarged thyroid gland).

The major differences among thyroid hormone replacements lie in their sources and hormone content. Thyroid hormone is manufactured from beef and pork thyroid, while other thyroid drugs are synthetic. Currently levothyroxine is considered the drug of choice for hypothyroidism.

These medications work by speeding up your metabolism and making more energy available. Thyroid hormones play a key role in normal growth and development.

SIDE EFFECTS

Side effects are uncommon when your dosage is adjusted correctly. However, always consult your health-care practitioner if you develop persistent or severe side effects while taking one of these drugs. Only he or she can determine whether it is safe for you to continue taking a thyroid hormone replacement.

- *Common:* headache, hair loss
- *Less Common or Rare:* angina (chest pain), heart palpitations, rapid heartbeat, weight loss, hand tremor, diarrhea, sweating, heat intolerance, nervousness, insomnia, menstrual irregularities, rash, hives

IMPORTANT PRECAUTIONS

Tell your health-care practitioner if you have ever experienced an allergic reaction to any thyroid replacement drug. Always inform your health-care practitioner about any other medical conditions you suffer from, especially diabetes, Addison's disease, adrenal insufficiency, high blood pressure, a recent heart attack, or any form of heart disease.

If you have angina, use caution when you exercise. Thyroid replacements may worsen chest pain during physical activity.

These drugs may increase your sensitivity to heat. Consult your health-care practitioner if you experience effects such as headache, nervousness, and sweating during hot months of the year.

Thyroid replacements should not be used for weight loss unless you also have hypothyroidism. They are also not an appropriate remedy for nonspecific fatigue.

DRUG INTERACTIONS

Check first with your health-care practitioner before taking any other medication with a thyroid medication. To avoid unwanted side effects, tell your health-care practitioner and pharmacist about all other prescription or over-the-counter drugs, vitamins, herbs, or other supplements that you are taking. Possible drug interactions include the following:

- Thyroid hormone replacements may decrease the effects of digoxin.
- Combining these drugs with amphetamines may result in life-threatening toxicity.
- Antacids may decrease the absorption and effects of thyroid medications.
- Beta-blockers may block warning signs of insufficient thyroid hormone replacement.
- These drugs may increase the effects of blood thinners such as warfarin.
- Thyroid hormone replacements may require an increase in insulin dosage for diabetics.
- Certain drugs may decrease the effects of thyroid drugs. These include cholestyramine, colestipol, iron salts, lovastatin, phenytoin, ritonavir, and sucralfate.
- Estrogen drugs may increase the need for thyroid hormone replacements.
- Combining thyroid hormones with benzodiazepines or tricyclic antidepressants may increase the effects of both medications.

- Your health-care practitioner may need to adjust your dosage of antiasthma medications.
- Consult your health-care practitioner before taking over-the-counter drugs such as allergy or cold medications, decongestants, and appetite suppressants. Many of these are stimulants.

FOOD, VITAMIN, AND HERBAL INTERACTIONS

Take thyroid hormone replacements 4 hours before or after calcium supplements. Iodine and cabbage may worsen hypothyroidism and goiter. Speak to your health-care practitioner before taking any dietary supplement with thyroid hormones. Horseradish root may aggravate hypothyroidism, and gamma oryzanol may lower thyroid stimulating hormone (TSH).

RECOMMENDED DOSAGE

Thyroid hormone replacements are available primarily in tablet form. Take only the exact type, brand, and strength of medication prescribed by your health-care practitioner. Different forms are not interchangeable. Children may require higher doses than adults.

Levothyroxine Sodium

- *Children and Adults:* 25 to 400 mcg daily

Liothyronine Sodium

- *Children and Adults:* 5 to 100 mcg daily

Liotrix

- *Children and Adults:* 1½ to 2 tablets daily

Thyroglobulin

- *Children and Adults:* 15 to 180 mg daily

Thyroid Hormone

- *Children and Adults:* 15 to 180 mg daily

Thyroid hormone replacements are best taken once a day in the morning on an empty stomach. If you miss a dose, take it as soon as you remember. If it is nearly time for your next scheduled dose, do not take the missed dose. Follow your regular dosing schedule. Never take a double dose. Call your health-care practitioner for advice if you miss 2 consecutive doses.

Thyroid hormone replacements must be taken on a regular basis in order to be effective. Treatment may need to be lifelong. Never stop taking this medication without your health-care practitioner's approval.

SYMPTOMS OF OVERDOSE AND WHAT TO DO

Symptoms of overdose may include diarrhea, headache, nervousness, insomnia, sweating, increased body heat, rapid heartbeat, muscle cramps, and heart attack. If you suspect overdose, seek medical attention immediately, and bring the prescription bottle with you to the hospital so that health-care practitioners will know exactly what drug was taken.

SPECIAL INFORMATION FOR PREGNANT OR NURSING WOMEN

Pregnant women have used thyroid hormone replacements with no adverse effects on the fetus. These drugs may pass into breast milk. However, when doses are carefully adjusted, thyroid medications are considered safe to use while breastfeeding.

SPECIAL INFORMATION FOR SENIORS

Seniors are more sensitive to the effects of these drugs, and generally require lower doses.

OPEN QUESTIONS OR CONTROVERSIES

Thyroid hormone replacements should not be used to treat conditions such as infertility or obesity in people who do not have hypothyroidism. If you have normal thyroid function and take these drugs for weight loss, serious side effects may result. Combining thyroid drugs with appetite suppressants such as amphetamines can be fatal.

GENERIC NAME

Tiagabine

BRAND NAME

Gabitril

No generic available

ABOUT THIS DRUG

Tiagabine is an anticonvulsant used to relieve epileptic seizures. Although it cannot cure epilepsy, this drug will help control seizures while you take it. Tiagabine is believed to work by affecting GABA, a substance that inhibits nerve activity in the part of the brain and central nervous system.

SIDE EFFECTS

Consult your health-care practitioner at once if you experience problems such as extreme weakness, changes in vision, blue or purple spots on the skin, or a severe rash. Always report any side effects that are severe or prolonged. Ask your health-care practitioner whether your dosage should be altered, and whether it is safe for you to continue taking this drug.

- *Common:* dizziness, drowsiness, tiredness, weakness, diarrhea, nausea, vomiting, fever, chills, sore throat, muscle aches or pain, confusion, nervousness, difficulty concentrating, blue or purple spots on the skin
- *Less Common or Rare:* abdominal pain, increased appetite, mouth ulcers, cough, flushing, rolling of eyeballs, visual impairment, speech or language problems, depression, agitation, hostility, muscle weakness, trouble sleeping, numbness and tingling, clumsiness, unsteadiness, rash, itching

IMPORTANT PRECAUTIONS

Always inform your health-care practitioner about any other medical conditions you may have, especially liver disease or status epilepticus. Tell your health-care practitioner if you have ever experienced an allergic reaction to this or similar drugs.

This drug may affect your vision and can make you drowsy and less alert than usual. Until you know how tiagabine affects you, do not drive a car, operate machinery, or perform other tasks that require concentration.

Regular blood tests are necessary to monitor your reaction to tiagabine. People with liver damage require lower doses.

DRUG INTERACTIONS

Tell your health-care practitioner and pharmacist if you are taking any other prescription or over-the-counter drugs, as well as any vitamins, herbs, or other supplements. Possible drug interactions include the following:

- Tiagabine may alter the absorption of other anticonvulsants, such as phenobarbital, phenytoin, and carbamazepine. Your health-care practitioner may need to adjust dosages.

- Taking other central nervous system depressants (such as sedatives, antidepressants, narcotics, or tranquilizers) with tiagabine can result in increased drowsiness and excessive sedation.
- Avoid alcohol while you are taking tiagabine.

FOOD, VITAMIN, AND HERBAL INTERACTIONS

Do not combine tiagabine with herbs such as hops, kava, passionflower, and valerian. These can increase tiagabine's sedative effects.

RECOMMENDED DOSAGE

Tiagabine comes as tablets. The doses given below are average. However, doses vary from person to person, and only your health-care practitioner can determine the dose and schedule that are most appropriate for you.

- *Children:* This drug is not recommended for children under age 12.
- *Adults:* 4 mg once daily to start; dosage may be gradually increased as needed to 56 mg daily in divided doses

To prevent stomach upset, tiagabine may be taken with food. However, avoid high-fat meals. If you forget a dose, take it as soon as you remember. If it is almost time for the next dose, skip the missed one and resume your normal schedule. Never take a double dose. If you have been taking tiagabine for a long period of time, to prevent seizures you must stop taking it gradually.

SYMPTOMS OF OVERDOSE AND WHAT TO DO

The symptoms of tiagabine overdose may include confusion, slurred speech, agitation, unsteadiness, clumsiness, muscle twitching, sluggishness, weakness, increase in seizures, and coma. If overdose occurs, seek immediate medical attention and take the prescription bottle to the hospital with you.

SPECIAL INFORMATION FOR PREGNANT OR NURSING WOMEN

Tiagabine has caused birth defects in animal studies and may pass into breast milk. If you are pregnant or plan to become pregnant, or if you are breastfeeding or plan to do so, talk with your health-care practitioner before starting this medication. Only a health-care practitioner can determine whether the potential benefits outweigh the risks.

SPECIAL INFORMATION FOR SENIORS

There are no special instructions for seniors.

GENERIC NAME

Ticlopidine

BRAND NAME

Ticlid
Generic available

ABOUT THIS DRUG

Ticlopidine is an antiplatelet drug used to reduce the risk of having a stroke. This drug has a number of serious side effects, and is no longer widely prescribed today. It has largely been replaced by clopidogrel. Ticlopidine works by preventing platelets from sticking or clumping together and causing clots.

SIDE EFFECTS

Side effects of ticlopidine occur in more than half the people who take this drug, and cause more than one in ten people to stop taking it. Effects can be extremely serious, and must be promptly reported to your health-care practitioner. Contact your health-care practitioner at once if you experience any unusual bleeding, black or tarry stools, signs of infection (such as fever and chills), mouth ulcers, dark or bloody urine, yellow eyes or skin, or pinpoint red spots on skin. Always report any other side effects that are severe or prolonged. Ask your health-care practitioner whether it is safe for you to continue taking this drug.

- *Common:* stomach pain or upset, nausea, diarrhea, rash
- *Less Common or Rare:* bruising, reduced white blood cell counts, bloating, gas, dizziness, vomiting, itching, liver function changes

IMPORTANT PRECAUTIONS

Always tell your health-care practitioner about any other medical conditions you may have, especially blood clotting problems such as hemophilia, blood disease, stomach ulcers, and liver or kidney disease. This drug increases the risk of serious bleeding, especially after an injury.

Regular blood tests are essential while you take ticlopidine. In addition, tell your health-care practitioner or dentist that you are taking this medication before undergoing any procedure. Serious bleeding can occur during surgery or dental work.

This drug may cause side effects such as dizziness. Until you know how ticlopidine affects you, do not drive a car, operate machinery, or perform other tasks that require concentration.

DRUG INTERACTIONS

Inform your health-care practitioner and pharmacist if you are taking any other prescription or over-the-counter drugs, as well as any vitamins, herbs, or other supplements. Possible drug interactions include the following:

- Combining ticlopidine with aspirin and other NSAIDs or blood thinners such as warfarin increases the risk of bleeding.
- Many other drugs may also interact with ticlopidine, including antacids, antiasthma medications, and phenytoin.

FOOD, VITAMIN, AND HERBAL INTERACTIONS

Do not take ticlopidine with herbs that affect blood clotting, such as garlic and ginkgo.

RECOMMENDED DOSAGE

Ticlopidine comes as a tablet. The doses given below are typical. However, only your health-care practitioner can determine the dose and schedule that best fit your individual needs.

- *Children:* This drug is not recommended for children.
- *Adults:* 250 mg twice daily

Ticlopidine should be taken with food. If you miss a dose, take it as soon as you remember. If it is almost time for the next dose, skip it and resume your regular schedule. Never take a double dose.

SYMPTOMS OF OVERDOSE AND WHAT TO DO

Symptoms of ticlopidine overdose may include bleeding and liver inflammation. If you suspect that an overdose has occurred, seek immediate medical attention and take the prescription bottle to the hospital with you.

SPECIAL INFORMATION FOR PREGNANT OR NURSING WOMEN

Ticlopidine has caused unwanted effects in animal studies. If you are pregnant or plan to become pregnant, or if you are breastfeeding or plan to do so, talk with your health-care practitioner before starting this medication. Only a health-care practitioner can determine whether the potential benefits outweigh the risks.

SPECIAL INFORMATION FOR SENIORS

Seniors may be more sensitive to the effects of this drug.

GENERIC NAME

Tiludronate *see Bisphosphates, page 200*

GENERIC NAME

Timolol

BRAND NAMES

Betimol, Blocadren, Timoptic, Timoptic-XE
Generic available

ABOUT THIS DRUG

Timolol is a beta-adrenergic blocking agent (beta-blocker) prescribed for mild-to-moderate high blood pressure (hypertension). It is also taken for angina (chest pain). This drug is available in combination with a diuretic (another type of high blood pressure medication). Timolol eye solution is used to treat glaucoma.

Timolol works by decreasing the force and rate of heart contractions. This reduces angina and lowers blood pressure. Timolol eyedrops reduce pressure in the eye.

SIDE EFFECTS

Speak to your health-care practitioner if you develop side effects while taking this drug. Only he or she can determine whether it is safe for you to continue taking timolol.

- *Common:* dizziness, drowsiness, tiredness, weakness, changes in heartbeat
- *Less Common or Rare:* lightheadedness, cold hands and feet, fainting, nausea, upset stomach, indigestion, vomiting, diarrhea, cramps, sweating, fatigue, urinary difficulties, impotence, muscle weakness, vivid dreams, excessive tiredness or weakness, constipation, breathing difficulties, cough, fever, blurred vision, dry eyes, rash, stuffy nose, chest pain, slow heartbeat, heart failure

IMPORTANT PRECAUTIONS

Inform your health-care practitioner about any other medical conditions you suffer from, especially a slow heart rate or serious heart block, congestive heart failure, angina, asthma or other lung ailments, liver or kidney problems, diabetes or hypoglycemia, or a thyroid condition.

Before having any type of surgery or dental procedure, inform your surgeon or dentist that you are taking timolol.

This drug may make you more sensitive to the cold. Beta-blockers can decrease blood circulation in the fingers, toes, and skin. Be sure to dress warmly in low temperatures, especially if you already have blood circulation problems.

This drug may make you drowsy. Until you know how timolol affects you, do not drive a car, operate machinery, or perform other tasks that demand concentration.

Treatment of high blood pressure also entails certain lifestyle changes, such as weight control, smoking cessation, and a low-sodium diet.

Be extremely careful when you exercise in hot weather. Heavy sweating can lead to dizziness, lightheadedness, vomiting, fainting, dehydration, and a drop in blood pressure.

When you first start taking this drug or when the dosage is increased, you may experience dizziness or faintness when you rise quickly from a sitting or reclining position (postural hypotension). Try to get up slowly, and consult your health-care practitioner if the problem continues.

DRUG INTERACTIONS

Tell your health-care practitioner and pharmacist if you are taking any other prescription or over-the-counter drugs, as well as any vitamins, herbs, or other supplements. Possible drug interactions include the following:

- Drugs that contain aspirin can lessen the blood-pressure-lowering effects of timolol.
- Taking other blood pressure medications (including clonidine, reserpine, and calcium channel blockers) can increase the effects of timolol.
- Timolol can interfere with the action of oral antidiabetes medications. It may also change blood glucose levels.
- Timolol may interfere with the effectiveness of certain asthma medications, including aminophylline, epinephrine, isoproterenol, and theophylline.
- Timolol may increase the effect of antianxiety benzodiazepine drugs.
- If you are also taking ergot alkaloids for migraines, timolol may worsen side effects such as cold hands and feet. In rare cases, this drug combination may lead to gangrene.
- Timolol may interact with anesthetics during surgery, increasing the risk of heart problems. As a result, your health-care practitioner will instruct you to stop taking this drug at least two days before surgery.

- Alcohol intensifies the drowsiness caused by this drug.
- Cocaine and cigarette smoking may reduce the effectiveness of timolol.
- Ask your health-care practitioner about taking over-the-counter cough, cold, sinus, allergy, and weight loss remedies. Many of these can raise blood pressure.

FOOD, VITAMIN, AND HERBAL INTERACTIONS

Do not take herbs that increase blood pressure, including ephedra (ma huang), ginseng, goldenseal, licorice, and saw palmetto. Consult your health-care practitioner before taking substances that may lower blood pressure, such as calcium, soy, or garlic. Your health-care practitioner will probably recommend a low-sodium diet.

RECOMMENDED DOSAGE

Timolol comes as a tablet or eye solution. Although the doses given below are typical, only your health-care practitioner can determine the dose and schedule that are most appropriate for you.

Tablets

- *Children:* This drug is not recommended for children.
- *Adults:* 20 to 60 mg in single or divided doses

Eye Solution

- *Children:* This drug is not recommended for children.
- *Adults:* 1 drop twice daily

If timolol tablets upset your stomach, take them with food. If you forget to take a dose, take it as soon as you remember. If it is almost time for the next dose, skip the forgotten one, and resume your normal schedule. Never take double doses.

Continue to take this drug even if you feel well. Do not discontinue use without consulting your health-care practitioner. Abrupt withdrawal can cause chest pain, breathing difficulties, increased sweating, irregular heartbeat, and even heart attack in some people. To end treatment, in most cases your health-care practitioner will reduce dosage gradually over a 2-week period.

SYMPTOMS OF OVERDOSE AND WHAT TO DO

The symptoms of timolol overdose include slow heart rate, low blood pressure, dizziness, fainting, difficulty breathing, bluish fingernails and palms, and seizures. If overdose occurs, seek immediate medical attention and take the prescription bottle to the hospital with you.

SPECIAL INFORMATION FOR PREGNANT OR NURSING WOMEN

Some studies have shown that women who take beta-blockers during pregnancy give birth to babies with lower birth weight, heart rate, and blood pressure. As a result, timolol should be avoided if you are pregnant.

Small amounts of timolol can pass into breast milk and cause problems such as slow heart rate, low blood pressure, and trouble breathing. If you must take timolol, your health-care practitioner may recommend bottle-feeding.

SPECIAL INFORMATION FOR SENIORS

Seniors usually require lower doses of timolol. Older people are more apt to experience side effects such as heightened sensitivity to the cold, a general feeling of unwellness, chest pain, breathing difficulties, sweating, and variations in heartbeat.

GENERIC NAME

Tioconazole *see Miconazole, page 694*

GENERIC NAME

Tiotropium

BRAND NAME

Spiriva HandiHaler

No generic available

ABOUT THIS DRUG

Tiotropium is an anticholinergic drug that is used to treat bronchospasm associated with chronic obstructive pulmonary disease, such as chronic bronchitis and emphysema.

This drug prevents narrowing of airway passages and allows freer exchange of air in the lungs. Tiotropium is used as a once-daily maintenance medication.

SIDE EFFECTS

Be sure to tell your health-care practitioner if you experience any side effects while using tiotropium. Only your health-care practitioner can determine whether it is safe for you to continue using this drug.

- *Most Common:* constipation, difficult urination, dry mouth, increased heart rate
- *Rare:* allergic reaction (closing of the throat, difficulty breathing, hives, swelling of the tongue, lips, or face), narrow-angle glaucoma (blurred vision, color distortion, eye pain, red eyes)

IMPORTANT PRECAUTIONS

Tell your health-care practitioner if you are sensitive or allergic to tiotropium or to any other drugs.

Tiotropium should not be used during acute bronchospastic attacks; it is only for use to prevent attacks.

Tiotropium should not be used if you have urinary retention, gastric retention, or uncontrolled narrow-angle glaucoma.

Before using tiotropium, talk to your health-care practitioner if you have an enlarged prostate or experience difficult urination.

Tiotropium is available as a powder contained in a capsule, which is then inserted into an inhaler for use. Exercise caution when handling the capsules; do not open or crush them. Do not let the powder contact your eyes, as it may cause blurry vision. If you do get tiotropium in your eyes, flush them with water and seek medical attention if side effects occur.

DRUG INTERACTIONS

Tell your health-care practitioner and pharmacist if you are taking any prescription or nonprescription drugs, as well as any vitamins, herbs, or other supplements. Possible drug interactions include the following:

- Before using albuterol, dicyclomine, ipratropium, mepenzolate, methscopolamine, propantheline, or scopolamine, talk to your health-care practitioner, as your dosage of tiotropium may need to be adjusted or your health-care practitioner may need to monitor you during drug usage.

FOOD, VITAMIN, AND HERBAL INTERACTIONS

No food, vitamin, or herbal interactions have been reported.

RECOMMENDED DOSAGE

Tiotropium is available in capsules containing 18 micrograms of active drug that are inserted into an inhaler. The dosages given here are typical. However, your health-care practitioner will determine the most appropriate dose and schedule for your needs.

- *Children:* To be determined by your health-care practitioner
- *Adults:* 1 capsule per day

The capsules are for use in the inhaler; they should not be swallowed. If you miss a dose, take it as soon as you remember. If it is nearly time for your next dose, do not take the missed dose. Continue with your regular dosing schedule. Never take a double dose.

SYMPTOMS OF OVERDOSE AND WHAT TO DO

Symptoms of overdose include abdominal pain, altered mental state, constipation, and shaking. If overdose occurs, seek immediate medical attention and bring the prescription container with you to the hospital.

SPECIAL INFORMATION FOR PREGNANT OR NURSING WOMEN

Adequate studies of the effects of tiotropium on pregnant or nursing women have not been done. If you are pregnant or plan to become pregnant, talk to your health-care practitioner.

It is not known whether tiotropium passes into breast milk. If you are breastfeeding, your health-care practitioner may advise you to switch to bottle feeding until your treatment is complete.

SPECIAL INFORMATION FOR SENIORS

Inserting the capsule into the inhaler may be difficult for some seniors to do, especially if they have arthritis in their hands. A health-care practitioner should demonstrate the process and make sure individuals can use the inhaler properly.

GENERIC NAME

Tizanidine

BRAND NAME

Zanaflex
Generic available

ABOUT THIS DRUG

Tizanidine is an antispastic drug prescribed to relax muscles in the body. This drug relieves the spasms, tightness, and cramping of muscles that are associated with multiple sclerosis and spine injuries. It is used along with rest, physical therapy, and other treatment. Tizanidine works by acting on the central nervous system.

SIDE EFFECTS

Inform your health-care practitioner if you develop side effects while taking tizanidine. If symptoms are severe or prolonged, ask your health-care practitioner whether your dosage requires adjustment, and whether it is safe for you to continue taking this drug.

➤ *Common:* drowsiness, tiredness, dizziness, weakness, dry mouth

➤ *Less Common or Rare:* fainting, lightheadedness, flu symptoms, fever, sweating, loss of appetite, runny nose, sore throat, abdominal pain, upset stomach, nausea, vomiting, diarrhea, constipation, blurred vision, eye pain, increased muscle spasms or tone, joint or muscle pain or stiffness, uncontrolled body movements, mood changes, excitement, nervousness, anxiety, depression, difficulty speaking, hallucinations, delusions, psychotic symptoms, pain or burning while urinating, urinary infection, skin sores, tingling or prickling sensations, rash, weight gain or loss, yellow eyes or skin, liver inflammation, irregular heartbeat

Seek immediate medical attention if you experience symptoms such as blood in your urine, convulsions, yellow skin or eyes, extreme fatigue, fever, chills, black, tarry stools, vomiting blood, or hallucinations.

IMPORTANT PRECAUTIONS

Always inform your health-care practitioner about any other medical conditions you may have, especially kidney or liver impairment, or seizures. Tizanidine can cause liver damage, and several people taking it have died of liver failure.

This drug can make you drowsy and less alert than usual. Until you know how tizanidine affects you, do not drive a car, operate machinery, or perform other tasks that require concentration.

When you first start taking this drug or when the dosage is increased, you may experience dizziness or faintness when you rise quickly from a sitting or reclining position (postural hypotension). Try to get up slowly, and consult your health-care practitioner if the problem continues.

If tizanidine causes dry mouth, use sugarless gum or hard candy, ice chips, or a saliva substitute. Consult your health-care practitioner or dentist if the problem continues.

Visit your health-care practitioner on a regular basis while taking this medication, especially during the first weeks of treatment.

DRUG INTERACTIONS

Tell your health-care practitioner and pharmacist if you are taking any other prescription or over-the-counter drugs, as well as any vita-

mins, herbs, or other supplements. Possible drug interactions include the following:

- Consult your health-care practitioner before combining tizanidine with other central nervous system depressants, including tranquilizers, sedatives, sleep aids, antihistamines, narcotics or other pain medication, barbiturates, seizure medications, and anesthesia. These can result in increased effects such as drowsiness and dizziness.
- Combining tizanidine with antihypertensive drugs may result in severe low blood pressure.
- Tizanidine may increase the effects of phenytoin.
- This drug may increase the risk of side effects of oral contraceptives.
- Do not drink alcohol while taking tizanidine. This combination can add to drowsiness.

FOOD, VITAMIN, AND HERBAL INTERACTIONS

Do not take tizanidine with herbs such as hops, kava, passionflower, and valerian. These can increase effects such as drowsiness.

RECOMMENDED DOSAGE

Tizanidine comes in tablet form. Although the doses given below are typical, only your health-care practitioner can determine the dose and schedule that best fit your needs.

- *Children:* This drug is not recommended for children.
- *Adults:* initial dose is 4 mg every 6 to 8 hours, which may be increased by 2 to 4 mg, up to 8 mg every 6 to 8 hours as needed; maximum daily dosage is 36 mg

Tizanidine may be taken with or without food. If you forget a dose, take it as soon as you remember. If it is almost time for the next dose, skip the missed one and resume your normal schedule. Never take a double dose. Do not stop taking this medication without consulting your health-care practitioner.

SYMPTOMS OF OVERDOSE AND WHAT TO DO

No specific information on overdosing with tizanidine is available. However, if you suspect that an overdose has occurred, seek immediate medical attention and take the prescription bottle to the hospital with you.

SPECIAL INFORMATION FOR PREGNANT OR NURSING WOMEN

Tizanidine has caused birth defects in animal studies. If you are pregnant or plan to become pregnant, or if you are breastfeeding or plan to do so, talk with your health-care practitioner before starting this drug. Only a health-care practitioner can determine whether the potential benefits outweigh the potential dangers.

SPECIAL INFORMATION FOR SENIORS

Altered doses may be prescribed for seniors.

GENERIC NAME

Tocainide

BRAND NAME

Tonocard

No generic available

ABOUT THIS DRUG

Tocainide is used to treat severe abnormal heart rhythms (arrhythmias). There are two types of arrhythmias. In tachycardia, heartbeats are faster than normal. In bradycardia, they are slower than normal.

This drug works similarly to injectable lidocaine, rather than oral medications such as quinidine or procainamide. It slows the transmission of nerve impulses through the heart and makes the heart tissue less sensitive.

SIDE EFFECTS

Because this drug may cause a number of serious side effects, you should be closely monitored by your health-care practitioner while taking it. Only your health-care practitioner can determine whether it is safe for you to continue taking tocainide.

- *Common:* nausea, loss of appetite, dizziness, lightheadedness
- *Less Common or Rare:* blurred vision, confusion, anxiety, headache, nervousness, trembling, shaking, hallucinations, visual disturbances, diarrhea, sweating, vomiting, numbness or tingling in fingers and toes, cough, shortness of breath, chest pain, fever, chills, unusual bleeding or bruising, mouth sores, irregular heartbeat, skin blisters, rash, peeling or scaling skin, weakness, yellow eyes and skin, changes in blood count, reduced levels of white blood cells and platelets

Immediately report any signs of blood and lung disorders, which are most likely to occur during the first 3 months of treatment. Symptoms include fever, chills, sore throat, easy bleeding or bruising, cough, wheezing, tremor, palpitations, and mouth ulcers.

IMPORTANT PRECAUTIONS

Always inform your health-care practitioner about any other medical conditions you suffer from, especially a heart block, heart failure, or liver or kidney problems. Tell your health-care practitioner if you have ever experienced an allergic reaction to tocainide or similar drugs or to anesthetics.

This drug may make you dizzy and weak. Until you know how tocainide affects you, do not drive a car, operate machinery, or perform other tasks that demand concentration.

Before having any type of surgery or dental procedure, inform your surgeon or dentist that you are taking tocainide. See your health-care practitioner on a regular basis while taking this medication.

DRUG INTERACTIONS

Tell your health-care practitioner and pharmacist if you are taking any other prescription or over-the-counter drugs, as well as any vitamins, herbs, or other supplements. Possible drug interactions include the following:

- ➤ Taking other antiarrhythmic drugs with tocainide may depress heart function.
- ➤ Combining tocainide with blood pressure medications (such as beta-blockers) increases the risk of side effects of tocainide.
- ➤ Cimetidine and rifampin reduce the effects of tocainide.
- ➤ Tocainide may increase the effects of other medications that affect bone marrow function and lead to reductions in white blood cells and platelets.
- ➤ Consult your health-care practitioner before taking over-the-counter cough, cold, sinus, allergy, or weight loss medications. Many of these are stimulants.

FOOD, VITAMIN, AND HERBAL INTERACTIONS

Consult your health-care practitioner before taking herbal remedies that may affect the cardiovascular system, such as ephedra (ma huang), ginseng, goldenseal, licorice, and saw palmetto.

RECOMMENDED DOSAGE

Tocainide comes as a tablet. Although the doses given below are typical, real doses are highly individualized according to the nature of your particular heart problem, age, and levels of kidney and liver function.

➤ *Children:* This drug is not recommended for children.

➤ *Adults:* 400 to 600 mg every 8 hours

If tocainide upsets your stomach, ask your health-care practitioner about taking it with food. It is particularly important to take tocainide on a regular basis at evenly spaced times. Try not to forget any doses. Tocainide works best when there is a constant amount in the blood. If you forget to take a dose and remember it within 4 hours, take it as soon as you remember. Otherwise skip the forgotten dose, and resume your normal schedule. Never take double doses.

Continue to take tocainide even if you feel well. Do not discontinue use without consulting your health-care practitioner. Abrupt withdrawal can cause potentially serious changes in heart activity. To end treatment, in most cases your health-care practitioner will reduce dosage gradually.

SYMPTOMS OF OVERDOSE AND WHAT TO DO

The symptoms of tocainide overdose may include central nervous system effects such as tremors. If overdose occurs, seek immediate medical attention and take the bottle of tocainide to the hospital with you.

SPECIAL INFORMATION FOR PREGNANT OR NURSING WOMEN

Tocainide has caused spontaneous abortions and stillbirths in animal studies. This drug should not be used during pregnancy unless absolutely necessary. Because tocainide may pass into breast milk, your health-care practitioner may recommend bottle-feeding.

SPECIAL INFORMATION FOR SENIORS

Seniors are more apt to experience side effects such as dizziness or lightheadedness.

GENERIC NAME

Tolazamide

see Sulfonylurea Antidiabetes Drugs, page 971

GENERIC NAME
Tolbutamide *see Sulfonylurea Antidiabetes Drugs, page 971*

GENERIC NAME
Tolcapone

BRAND NAME
Tasmar
No generic available

ABOUT THIS DRUG
Tolcapone is used in combination with levodopa and carbidopa to treat Parkinson's disease. Because this drug may cause liver failure, it is only prescribed when other medications fail to control symptoms such as muscle stiffness, tremor, and weakness. Tolcapone works by extending the therapeutic effects of levodopa and carbidopa.

SIDE EFFECTS
Side effects from tolcapone are common, especially in the first weeks of therapy. Severe low blood pressure, accompanied by dizziness, fainting, nausea, and sweating, may occur. Hallucinations are also common in the first 2 weeks, and severe diarrhea may develop after 6 to 12 weeks. At any time during treatment, contact your health-care practitioner at once if you experience symptoms of liver damage, such as yellow eyes and skin, pale stools, dark urine, loss of appetite, fatigue, itching, and pain in the upper right abdomen. Call your health-care practitioner about any other persistent or severe effects, because only he or she can determine if you should continue to take this drug.

- *Common:* hallucinations, low blood pressure, dizziness, fainting, nausea, excessive dreaming, headache, diarrhea, constipation, abdominal pain, vomiting, lack of appetite, fatigue, nasal congestion, runny nose, sneezing, sore throat, cough, dry mouth, confusion, dizziness upon standing, difficulty sleeping, decreased muscle movement, twisting or twitching, respiratory infections
- *Less Common or Rare:* overall feeling of unwellness, agitation, irritability, hyperactivity, loss of balance, falling, blood in urine, chest pain, burning or tingling sensation, burning of feet, muscle cramps, neck pain, stiffness, chills, difficulty breathing, trouble thinking or concentrating, yellow eyes and skin, pale stools, dark urine, loss of appetite, fatigue, itching, pain in the upper right abdomen

IMPORTANT PRECAUTIONS

Because this drug may cause liver failure, it should not be taken by people with liver disease. Also inform your health-care practitioner of any other medical conditions you have, especially kidney problems, low blood pressure, orthostatic or postural low blood pressure (dizziness and fainting when getting up suddenly from a lying or sitting position), or hallucinations. Older people are more susceptible to side effects such as hallucinations.

Because tolcapone may cause side effects such as dizziness and fainting (especially at the start of therapy), do not drive a car, operate machinery, or perform other tasks that require concentration until you know how this drug affects you.

When you first start taking this drug or when the dosage is increased, you may experience dizziness or faintness when you rise quickly from a sitting or reclining position (postural hypotension). Try to get up slowly, and consult your health-care practitioner if the problem continues.

Tolcapone may cause mouth dryness. To counteract this effect, use sugarless gum or candy, ice chips, or a saliva substitute. If the problem continues, consult your health-care practitioner or dentist.

To monitor treatment, visit your health-care practitioner on a regular basis. Regular liver function tests are required.

DRUG INTERACTIONS

Tell your health-care practitioner and pharmacist if you are taking any other prescription or over-the-counter drugs, as well as any vitamins, herbs, or other supplements. Possible drug interactions include the following:

- Tolcapone is prescribed in combination with levodopa and carbidopa in order to extend the effects of these drugs.
- Do not take tolcapone at the same time as or within 14 days of monoamine oxidase inhibitor (MAOI) antidepressants.
- Tolcapone may increase the effects of blood thinners such as warfarin.
- Tolcapone may increase the effects of central nervous system depressants such as alcohol and sedatives.

FOOD, VITAMIN, AND HERBAL INTERACTIONS

Consult your health-care practitioner before combining tolcapone with any herbs with sedative effects, such as catnip, elecampane, goldenseal, gotu kola, hops, kava, lemon balm, skullcap, St. John's wort, and valerian.

RECOMMENDED DOSAGE

Tolcapone is available in tablet form. Although the doses given below are typical, only your health-care practitioner can determine the dose and schedule that are most appropriate for you.

- *Children:* This drug is not recommended for children.
- *Adults:* 100 mg 3 times daily in addition to levodopa and carbidopa

Take this drug at least 1 hour before or 2 hours after meals. If you miss a dose, take it as soon as you remember. However, if it is almost time for the next dose, skip the one you missed and go back to your regular dosing schedule. Never take a double dose. Do not stop taking tolcapone suddenly. This may cause severe Parkinson's symptoms to return.

SYMPTOMS OF OVERDOSE AND WHAT TO DO

Symptoms of tolcapone overdose may include nausea, vomiting, and dizziness. If you suspect an overdose, seek medical attention immediately, and bring the prescription bottle with you to the hospital so that health-care practitioners will know exactly what drug was used.

SPECIAL INFORMATION FOR PREGNANT OR NURSING WOMEN

Tolcapone has caused birth defects in animal studies. If you are pregnant or plan to become pregnant, or if you are breastfeeding or plan to do so, talk with your health-care practitioner before starting this drug. Only a health-care practitioner can determine whether the potential benefits outweigh the potential dangers.

SPECIAL INFORMATION FOR SENIORS

Seniors may be more susceptible to side effects such as hallucinations.

GENERIC NAME

Tolmetin sodium

BRAND NAME

Tolectin
Generic available

ABOUT THIS DRUG

Tolmetin is a nonsteroidal anti-inflammatory drug (NSAID) used to relieve the pain and inflammation of rheumatoid arthritis and osteoarthritis. This drug works by reducing the level of prostaglandins, chemicals in the body that produce inflammation and pain.

SIDE EFFECTS

Tolmetin may cause potentially serious side effects, especially when used for a long time and in large doses. If you develop severe or persistent side effects, ask your health-care practitioner whether it is safe for you to continue taking this drug.

- *Common:* diarrhea, constipation, stomach upset or pain, gas, nausea, vomiting, fluid retention, ringing in the ears, appetite loss
- *Less Common or Rare:* headache, dizziness, blurred vision, sensitivity to light, confusion, fainting, tingling in the hands or feet, mouth sores, fatigue, weakness, abnormal bleeding or bruising, rash, hives, itching, heart palpitations, difficulty breathing, water retention, gastrointestinal bleeding, ulcers, painful urination, kidney damage

Stop taking tolmetin and consult your health-care practitioner immediately if you experience symptoms such as abdominal pain, stomach cramps, diarrhea, nausea, heartburn, indigestion, visual disturbances, vomiting of blood or material that looks like coffee grounds, or black, tarry stools. These may be signs of dangerous reactions such as ulcers or internal bleeding.

IMPORTANT PRECAUTIONS

Tolmetin can cause gastrointestinal bleeding, ulcers, and stomach perforation. If you take this drug on a regular basis, these types of side effects can occur at any time, with or without warning. People with a history of ulcers, colitis, or any type of gastrointestinal bleeding should be extremely careful when taking this drug.

Do not take tolmetin if you have a bleeding disorder or asthma or nasal polyps associated with aspirin use. Use this drug with caution if you have high blood pressure or other heart problems, or impaired liver or kidney function. Tell your health-care practitioner if you have ever experienced an allergic reaction to aspirin or related drugs.

Drinking 3 or more alcoholic beverages a day increases the risk of side effects such as bleeding.

Other possible side effects of tolmetin include blurred vision and dizziness. Until you know how this drug affects you, do not drive a car, operate machinery, or perform other tasks that require concentration.

Tolmetin may cause increased sensitivity to the sun. Wear protective clothing and apply sunscreen while you take this drug.

Before undergoing any type of surgery or dental procedure, inform your health-care practitioner or dentist that you are taking tolmetin. Visit your health-care practitioner on a regular basis while taking this drug.

DRUG INTERACTIONS

Tell your health-care practitioner and pharmacist if you are taking any other prescription or over-the-counter drugs, as well as any vitamins, herbs, or other supplements. Possible drug interactions include the following:

- Do not combine tolmetin with aspirin, ibuprofen, or other prescription or over-the-counter NSAIDs. This increases the risk of bleeding.
- Other drugs that may increase the risk of bleeding include dipyridamole, sulfinpyrazone, valproic acid, and blood thinners such as warfarin.
- Taking tolmetin with antihypertensive medications such as ACE inhibitors, beta-blockers, and diuretics decreases their blood-pressure-lowering effects.
- Mixing tolmetin with cyclosporine may increase the negative kidney effects of both drugs.
- Taking tolmetin with lithium or methotrexate can lead to toxic levels of lithium or methotrexate in the body.
- Do not use alcohol when you are taking tolmetin. Both are stomach irritants, and using them together can increase the risk of stomach bleeding and ulcers.

FOOD, VITAMIN, AND HERBAL INTERACTIONS

Do not combine tolmetin with herbal remedies such as clove oil, feverfew, garlic, ginkgo, and ginseng. These herbs may affect clotting.

RECOMMENDED DOSAGE

Tolmetin comes as a tablet or capsule. The doses given below are typical. However, only your health-care practitioner can determine the dose and schedule that best fit your individual needs.

- *Children Older than 2 Years:* 9 mg per pound of body weight daily
- *Adults:* 1,200 to 1,800 mg daily in divided doses

Tolmetin may be taken with food, milk, or an antacid to prevent stomach upset. Your health-care practitioner may also advise you to take medication with a full (8-ounce) glass of water, and remain upright (do not lie down) for 15 to 30 minutes afterward. If you forget to take a dose, take it as soon as you remember. But if it is almost time for the next dose, skip the one you missed and resume your normal schedule. Never take a double dose.

SYMPTOMS OF OVERDOSE AND WHAT TO DO
No specific information is available regarding overdose. If an overdose occurs, seek immediate medical attention and take the prescription bottle to the hospital with you so the health-care practitioner will know exactly what medication was taken.

SPECIAL INFORMATION FOR PREGNANT OR NURSING WOMEN
Use of tolmetin should be avoided in late pregnancy. If you want to take this drug in early pregnancy, ask your health-care practitioner whether the potential benefits outweigh the risks. Because tolmetin may pass into breast milk, it is best to stop breastfeeding while you take this drug.

SPECIAL INFORMATION FOR SENIORS
Smaller doses are recommended for seniors, who are more susceptible to side effects such as confusion, fluid retention, swelling of the feet and lower legs, stomach ulcers, and kidney or liver effects.

GENERIC NAME
Tolterodine

BRAND NAME
Detrol
No generic available

ABOUT THIS DRUG
Tolterodine is an anticholinergic drug used to treat an overactive bladder. It controls the urge to urinate, lowers frequency of urination, and decreases the unexpected and urgent need to urinate. This drug works by interfering with the nerve receptors that control the muscles in the bladder.

SIDE EFFECTS

Speak to your health-care practitioner if you develop side effects while using tolterodine. Only he or she can determine whether or not you should continue taking this drug.

- *Common:* dry mouth, headache, nasal congestion, constipation, diarrhea, stomach upset, abdominal pain, drowsiness, tiredness, dizziness, blurred vision
- *Less Common or Rare:* difficulty urinating, incomplete bladder emptying, photosensitivity, dry skin or eyes, skin tingling or burning, vertigo, falling, inflamed nose or throat, infection, respiratory tract infection, high blood pressure, rash

IMPORTANT PRECAUTIONS

Do not use this drug if you have urinary retention, gastric retention, or poorly controlled narrow-angle glaucoma. Take it with caution if you suffer from urinary tract problems or blockage, a digestive disorder, a history of bowel obstruction, heart or blood vessel disease, controlled glaucoma, or constipation. If you have liver or kidney disease, your health-care practitioner will probably prescribe a lower dosage. Also inform your health-care practitioner if you have ever experienced an allergic reaction to this or similar medications.

This drug may cause blurred vision. Until you know how tolterodine affects you, do not drive a car, operate machinery, or perform other tasks that demand concentration.

Tolterodine may lead to mouth dryness. To counteract this effect, use sugarless gum or candy, ice chips, or a saliva substitute. If the problem continues, consult your health-care practitioner or dentist.

This drug may make you sweat less, which can cause your temperature to rise. Be extremely careful when you exercise in hot weather or enter a sauna. Heavy sweating can lead to fever, dizziness, lightheadedness, vomiting, fainting, dehydration, and heat stroke.

Tolterodine may cause increased sensitivity to the sun. Wear protective clothing and apply sunscreen while you take this drug.

DRUG INTERACTIONS

Inform your health-care practitioner and pharmacist if you are taking any other prescription or over-the-counter drugs, as well as any vitamins, herbs, or other supplements. Possible drug interactions include the following:

- Combining tolterodine with warfarin may increase the risk of bleeding.

- Taking fluoxetine with tolterodine can lead to toxic levels of tolterodine.
- Combining tolterodine with erythromycin, clarithromycin, ketoconazole, itraconazole, and miconazole may result in increased effects of tolterodine.
- Avoid alcohol and tobacco while taking this drug.

FOOD, VITAMIN, AND HERBAL INTERACTIONS

Consult your health-care practitioner before combining tolterodine with any herbs with photosensitivity effects, such as St. John's wort. Do not take this drug with grapefruit juice. Ask your health-care practitioner about moderating your consumption of caffeinated beverages such as cola, coffee, and tea.

RECOMMENDED DOSAGE

Tolterodine comes as a tablet. The doses given below are typical. However, consult your health-care practitioner for the exact dose and schedule that are most appropriate for you.

- *Children:* This drug is not recommended for children.
- *Adults:* 1 to 2 mg twice daily

Tolterodine may be taken with or without food. If you forget a dose, take it as soon as you remember. If it is almost time for the next dose, skip the forgotten one, and resume your normal schedule. Never take double doses.

SYMPTOMS OF OVERDOSE AND WHAT TO DO

Symptoms of tolterodine overdose may include drowsiness, dry eyes and mouth, blurred vision, and constipation. If overdose occurs, seek immediate medical attention and take the prescription container to the hospital with you.

SPECIAL INFORMATION FOR PREGNANT OR NURSING WOMEN

No studies have adequately investigated the effects of tolterodine during pregnancy. If you are pregnant or plan to become pregnant, talk with your health-care practitioner before starting this drug. Only a health-care practitioner can determine whether the potential benefits outweigh the potential dangers. Because tolterodine passes into breast milk, breastfeeding is not recommended while taking this drug.

SPECIAL INFORMATION FOR SENIORS

There are no special instructions for seniors.

GENERIC NAME

Topiramate

BRAND NAME

Topamax
No generic available

ABOUT THIS DRUG

Topiramate is an anticonvulsant drug used to relieve epileptic seizures. It is prescribed for both mild partial seizures and severe tonic-clonic (grand mal) seizures.

Topiramate works by inhibiting epileptic activity in the brain. This drug is usually prescribed when other medications fail to control seizures.

SIDE EFFECTS

Side effects are usually most common at the beginning of therapy, and many disappear after the first 8 weeks. However, anytime that effects are severe or prolonged, ask your health-care practitioner whether adjusting your dosage would be helpful, and whether it is safe for you to continue taking this drug. Promptly report any unusual problems.

- *Common:* constipation, nausea, weight loss, dizziness, drowsiness, fatigue, impaired coordination, slowing of movements, tingling or burning sensations, tremor, weakness, confusion, nervousness, agitation, anxiety, memory problems, language or speech problems, difficulty concentrating, double vision, sinusitis, sore throat, chest pain, breast pain, menstrual problems
- *Less Common or Rare:* heart palpitations, hyperactivity, emotional instability, suicidal tendencies, mood swings, feeling of unreality, apathy, aggressiveness, decreased awareness, exaggerated sense of well-being, insomnia, overall sense of unwellness, eye pain, hearing difficulties, changes in taste, gum inflammation, dry mouth, ringing in ears, sensitivity to touch, severe itching, leg pain, fever, fluid retention, gas, vomiting, weight gain, increased sweating, body odor, frequent or painful urination, bladder infection, kidney stones, urinary incontinence, decreased sex drive, impotence, acne, abnormal walk, involuntary muscle movements, muscle weakness, loss of balance, shortness of breath, infections, allergic reactions

IMPORTANT PRECAUTIONS

Always inform your health-care practitioner about any other medical conditions you may have. If you have kidney disease or are on dialysis, your health-care practitioner will adjust your dosage of topiramate. This drug must be used with caution if you have liver disease. Tell your health-care practitioner if you have ever experienced an allergic reaction to this or similar drugs.

This drug can make you drowsy and less alert than usual. Until you know how topiramate affects you, do not drive a car, operate machinery, or perform other tasks that require concentration.

Because topiramate may reduce the effectiveness of oral contraceptives, use alternate means of contraception.

Topiramate may affect the gums, so good oral hygiene and regular visits to the dentist are essential.

Regular blood tests are necessary to monitor the absorption of topiramate, especially during the first months of treatment.

DRUG INTERACTIONS

Tell your health-care practitioner and pharmacist if you are taking any other prescription or over-the-counter drugs, as well as any vitamins, herbs, or other supplements. Possible drug interactions include the following:

- Other anticonvulsants, such as phenytoin and carbamazepine, may reduce levels of topiramate. Dosages must be adjusted.
- Taking other central nervous system depressants (such as sedatives, antidepressants, narcotics, or tranquilizers) with topiramate can result in increased drowsiness and excessive sedation.
- Topiramate reduces the effectiveness of many other drugs, such as oral contraceptives and digoxin.
- Do not drink alcohol while taking topiramate.

FOOD, VITAMIN, AND HERBAL INTERACTIONS

Drink several glasses of water a day to help prevent kidney stones. Do not combine this drug with herbs such as hops, kava, passionflower, and valerian. These can increase topiramate's sedative effects.

RECOMMENDED DOSAGE

Topiramate comes as a tablet. The doses below are typical, but only your health-care practitioner can determine the best dose and schedule for you.

- *Children:* Consult your health-care practitioner.
- *Adults:* 50 mg once daily to start, which is gradually increased as needed to an average dose of 200 mg twice daily

Topiramate may be taken with or without food. If you forget a dose, take it as soon as you remember. If it is within 4 hours of the next dose, skip the missed one and resume your normal schedule. Never take a double dose. If you have been taking topiramate for a long period of time, to prevent seizures you must stop taking it gradually.

SYMPTOMS OF OVERDOSE AND WHAT TO DO

Topiramate overdose may cause nervous system depression. If overdose occurs, seek immediate medical attention and take the prescription bottle to the hospital with you.

SPECIAL INFORMATION FOR PREGNANT OR NURSING WOMEN

Antiepileptic drugs are associated with an increased risk of birth defects, and whenever possible should not be used during pregnancy. Because topiramate may pass into breast milk, breastfeeding is not advisable while taking this drug.

SPECIAL INFORMATION FOR SENIORS

Seniors with impaired kidney function require lower doses.

GENERIC NAME

Toremifene

see Tamoxifen, page 985

GENERIC NAME

Torsemide

see Loop Diuretics, page 622

GENERIC NAME

Tramadol

BRAND NAME

Ultram
No generic available

ABOUT THIS DRUG

Tramadol is an analgesic prescribed to relieve pain. This drug has minimal side effects in comparison to pain relievers such as morphine.

Tramadol acts on the central nervous system. It works by increasing the availability of the neurotransmitters norepinephrine and serotonin.

SIDE EFFECTS

Inform your health-care practitioner if you develop side effects while taking tramadol. If effects are severe or prolonged, ask your health-care practitioner whether your dosage requires adjustment, and whether it is safe for you to continue taking this drug.

- *Common:* drowsiness, lightheadedness, dry mouth, constipation, blurred vision
- *Less Common or Rare:* nausea, vomiting, diarrhea, headache, dizziness, agitation, confusion, mental sluggishness, rapid heart rate, heart palpitations, flushing, sweating, hallucinations, suicidal tendencies, restlessness, rash, urinary retention, low blood pressure, dizziness upon standing, seizures

IMPORTANT PRECAUTIONS

Always inform your health-care practitioner about any other medical conditions you may have. Tramadol should not be taken if you are allergic to this or similar drugs, such as codeine or morphine. It should be used with caution if you have a head injury, liver or kidney disease, a history of convulsions or seizures, ulcers, or constipation.

Tramadol can lead to physical and/or psychological addiction. This drug should be used with caution in anyone with a history of drug or alcohol abuse.

If you plan to undergo surgery or a dental procedure, tell your health-care practitioner or dentist that you are taking tramadol.

This drug can make you drowsy and less alert than usual. Until you know how tramadol affects you, do not drive a car, operate machinery, or perform other tasks that require concentration.

When you first start taking this drug, you may feel lightheaded, and experience dizziness or faintness when you rise quickly from a sitting or reclining position (postural hypotension). Try to get up slowly, and consult your health-care practitioner if the problem continues.

DRUG INTERACTIONS

Tell your health-care practitioner and pharmacist if you are taking any other prescription or over-the-counter drugs, as well as any vita-

mins, herbs, or other supplements. Possible drug interactions include the following:

- Do not take monoamine oxidase inhibitor (MAOI) antidepressants at the same time as or within 14 days of tramadol.
- Combining tramadol with drugs such as tricyclic antidepressants, fluoxetine, fluvoxamine, and sertraline may increase the risk of seizures.
- Taking other central nervous system depressants along with tramadol can result in increased sedation.
- Carbamazepine may reduce the effects of tramadol.
- Combining digoxin with tramadol may cause digoxin toxicity.
- Drugs such as phenothiazines increase blood levels and thus effects of tramadol.
- Do not drink alcohol while taking tramadol.

FOOD, VITAMIN, AND HERBAL INTERACTIONS

Do not take tramadol with herbs such as hops, kava, passionflower, and valerian. These can increase its sedative effects. Do not use ginseng or St. John's wort.

RECOMMENDED DOSAGE

Tramadol comes as a tablet. Although the doses given below are typical, only your health-care practitioner can determine the dose and schedule that best fit your needs.

- *Children:* This drug is not recommended for children.
- *Adults:* 50 to 100 mg every 4 to 6 hours, with a maximum daily dose of 300 mg

Tramadol may be taken with or without food. This drug must be taken exactly as directed. Too much medication can be habit-forming and can possibly lead to overdose. If you forget a dose, take it as soon as you remember. If it is almost time for the next dose, skip the missed one and resume your normal schedule. Never take a double dose. If you have been taking tramadol for several weeks and you feel it is not working, do not take a higher dose. Consult your health-care practitioner.

SYMPTOMS OF OVERDOSE AND WHAT TO DO

The symptoms of tramadol overdose may include breathing problems and seizures. If overdose occurs, seek immediate medical attention and take the prescription bottle to the hospital with you.

SPECIAL INFORMATION FOR PREGNANT OR NURSING WOMEN

Tramadol has caused birth defects in animal studies. This medication should be avoided in pregnancy, especially during the first 3 months. Because tramadol may pass into breast milk, breastfeeding is not advisable while taking it.

SPECIAL INFORMATION FOR SENIORS

Seniors are at higher risk of side effects and should take smaller doses.

OPEN QUESTIONS OR CONTROVERSIES

Tramadol can cause psychological and/or physical dependence. Tolerance may develop with long-term use, making it less effective. Do not take a larger dose of tramadol, take it more often, or use it for a longer period than your health-care practitioner recommends.

GENERIC NAME

Trandolapril

BRAND NAME

Mavik
No generic available

ABOUT THIS DRUG

Trandolapril is an angiotensin-converting enzyme (ACE) inhibitor used to treat high blood pressure (hypertension). This drug may be prescribed alone or with other high blood pressure medications, such as thiazide diuretics. It works by blocking an enzyme in the body, which relaxes blood vessels and lowers blood pressure.

SIDE EFFECTS

Stop taking this drug and seek immediate medical attention if you experience allergic reactions such as swelling of the face, lips, hands, or feet. Report any other persistent or severe side effects that develop while taking trandolapril. Only your health-care practitioner can determine whether you should continue taking this drug.

➤ *Common:* dizziness, lightheadedness, headache, cough, tiredness

➤ *Less Common or Rare:* angina (chest pain), faintness, vertigo, upset stomach, abdominal pain, nausea, vomiting, bleeding in the stomach or intestines, overall feeling of unwellness, dizziness upon standing, insomnia, constipation, pins and needles, skin disease, urinary tract infection, low blood pressure, palpitations, allergic reactions, swelling of the face, lips, hands, or feet

IMPORTANT PRECAUTIONS

Always inform your health-care practitioner about any other medical conditions you suffer from, especially congestive heart failure, heart or circulatory problems, diabetes, lupus, or kidney or liver disease.

Trandolapril can affect your kidneys, especially if you have congestive heart failure. If you already have kidney disease, your dosage should be lower than usual. Your kidneys must be monitored while you take this drug.

Before having any type of surgery, anesthesia, or dental procedure, tell your surgeon or dentist that you are taking trandolapril.

This drug may make you dizzy or drowsy. Until you know how trandolapril affects you, do not drive a car, operate machinery, or perform other tasks that demand concentration.

Treatment of high blood pressure also entails certain lifestyle changes, such as weight control, smoking cessation, and close attention to diet.

When you first start taking this drug, you may feel lightheaded, and experience dizziness or faintness when you rise quickly from a sitting or reclining position (postural hypotension). Try to get up slowly, and consult your health-care practitioner if the problem continues.

Be extremely careful when you exercise in hot weather. Heavy sweating can lead to dizziness, lightheadedness, fainting, vomiting, dehydration, and low blood pressure.

Do not take this drug if you have ever experienced an allergic reaction to it or to other ACE inhibitors. If you have an allergic reaction such as swelling of the face and mouth and a sudden problem with breathing, seek immediate medical attention. Also contact your health-care practitioner immediately if you develop a sore throat and fever, or yellow eyes or skin.

Your health-care practitioner will monitor your response to this drug with regular blood counts and other tests.

DRUG INTERACTIONS

Tell your health-care practitioner and pharmacist if you are taking any other prescription or over-the-counter drugs, as well as any vita-

mins, herbs, or other supplements. Possible drug interactions include the following:

- Taking other blood pressure medications can increase the blood-pressure-lowering effects of trandolapril.
- If you are already taking a diuretic, when possible your health-care practitioner will have you stop taking it 2 to 3 days before starting trandolapril.
- Trandolapril may increase blood levels of potassium, particularly when taken with potassium-sparing diuretics. Too much potassium can cause heart rhythm disturbances.
- Combining trandolapril with allopurinol increases the risk of side effects.
- Taking trandolapril with lithium can result in toxic levels of lithium in the blood.
- Phenothiazine tranquilizers and antiemetics may increase the effects of trandolapril.
- Indomethacin may reduce the blood-pressure-lowering effects of trandolapril.
- Separate doses of antacids and trandolapril by 2 hours.
- Trandolapril increases blood levels of digoxin.
- Avoid alcoholic beverages. Alcohol may further lower blood pressure, and increase the risk of dizziness and fainting.
- Consult your health-care practitioner before taking over-the-counter cough, cold, sinus, allergy, or weight loss medications. Many of these can raise blood pressure.

FOOD, VITAMIN, AND HERBAL INTERACTIONS

Do not take herbs that increase blood pressure, such as ephedra (ma huang), ginseng, goldenseal, licorice, and saw palmetto. Consult your health-care practitioner before taking substances that may lower blood pressure, such as calcium, soy, or garlic. To minimize possible interactions, take trandolapril and iron supplements 2 to 3 hours apart. Because ACE inhibitors raise potassium levels in the body, *do not* take potassium supplements or use salt substitutes containing potassium, and ask your health-care practitioner how many potassium-rich foods (such as bananas, prunes, raisins, melons, tomatoes, citrus fruit, and orange juice) you can safely include in your diet. Also talk to your health-care practitioner about salt intake.

RECOMMENDED DOSAGE

Trandolapril is available as tablets. African Americans require higher doses, while lower doses are recommended for those with kidney or liver disease. Although the doses given below are typical, only your health-care practitioner can determine the dose and schedule that best fit your needs.

- *Children:* This drug is not recommended for children.
- *Adults:* 1 to 4 mg once daily

If trandolapril upsets your stomach, take it with food. Continue to take this drug even if you feel well. Do not discontinue use without consulting your health-care practitioner. If you miss a dose, take it as soon as you remember. If it is almost time for the next dose, skip the forgotten one, and resume your normal schedule. Never take a double dose.

SYMPTOMS OF OVERDOSE AND WHAT TO DO

The symptoms of trandolapril overdose may include dizziness and fainting caused by a severe drop in blood pressure. If overdose occurs, seek immediate medical attention and take the prescription bottle to the hospital with you.

SPECIAL INFORMATION FOR PREGNANT OR NURSING WOMEN

Do not take trandolapril if you are pregnant (especially during the final six months). This drug can cause fetal injury and death. If you become pregnant while taking trandolapril, call your health-care practitioner immediately.

Small amounts of trandolapril may pass into breast milk. If you are breastfeeding, your health-care practitioner will likely advise you to stop until your treatment is done.

SPECIAL INFORMATION FOR SENIORS

Seniors usually require lower doses of trandolapril.

GENERIC NAME

Trastuzumab

BRAND NAME

Herceptin

No generic available

ABOUT THIS DRUG

Trastuzumab is a monoclonal antibody used in the treatment of breast cancer that has metastasized (spread) to other parts of the body. Even low doses of this drug can prove toxic, so it is prescribed with extreme care.

Trastuzumab works by blocking the activation of breast cancer cells that express receptors for HER2. The presence of this receptor on cancer cells leads to uncontrolled cell growth.

SIDE EFFECTS

Side effects of trastuzumab can be extremely serious, and must be promptly reported to your health-care practitioner. Rare side effects may occur anywhere in the body. Report any other persistent or severe side effects that develop while taking trastuzumab. Only your health-care practitioner can determine whether you should continue taking this drug.

- *Common:* fever, chills, nausea, vomiting, diarrhea, constipation, stomach pain, headache, dizziness, depression, sleeplessness, appetite loss, flu-like symptoms, sinus irritation, cough, sore throat, runny nose, shortness of breath, infection, pain, swelling in the arms and legs, fluid retention, tingling in the hands and feet
- *Less Common or Rare:* cold sores, acne, anemia, low white blood cell count, nerve inflammation and pain, joint pain, bone pain, urinary infection, fatigue, rapid heartbeat, heart failure

IMPORTANT PRECAUTIONS

Always tell your health-care practitioner about any other medical conditions you may have, especially heart problems. Trastuzumab may cause congestive heart failure and heart ventricle disorders.

This drug may cause a number of distressing side effects. Until you know how trastuzumab affects you, do not drive a car, operate machinery, or perform other tasks that require concentration.

People taking any dose of trastuzumab must be closely monitored with complete blood counts and other tests, including test of heart function. This drug may cause anemia and low white blood cell counts.

DRUG INTERACTIONS

Inform your health-care practitioner and pharmacist if you are taking any other prescription or over-the-counter drugs, as well as any vitamins, herbs, or other supplements. In terms of drug interactions, trastuzumab should not be combined with other drugs during intravenous injection.

FOOD, VITAMIN, AND HERBAL INTERACTIONS

No food, vitamin, or herbal interactions have been noted.

RECOMMENDED DOSAGE

Trastuzumab is available by injection and is administered in a health-care facility. Dosage is highly individualized and must be determined by your health-care practitioner.

SYMPTOMS OF OVERDOSE AND WHAT TO DO

Symptoms of trastuzumab overdose may include chills, fever, headache, nausea, vomiting, shaking, fainting, dizziness, trouble breathing, pain, rash, and weakness. If you suspect that an overdose has occurred, seek immediate medical attention.

SPECIAL INFORMATION FOR PREGNANT OR NURSING WOMEN

This drug may affect the fetus. If you are pregnant or think you may be pregnant, carefully discuss the risks versus benefits of taking trastuzumab. Because of the possibility of serious side effects, breastfeeding is not recommended while you are taking this drug or for 6 months afterward.

SPECIAL INFORMATION FOR SENIORS

Seniors are more susceptible to side effects such as those that affect the heart.

GENERIC NAME

Travoprost

BRAND NAME

Travatan

No generic available

ABOUT THIS DRUG

Travoprost ophthalmic eye solution is used to treat glaucoma and ocular hypertension (high blood pressure within the eye). This drug lowers pressure in the eye by increasing the outflow of eye fluid.

SIDE EFFECTS

Consult your health-care practitioner if you experience side effects while taking travoprost. Only he or she can determine whether or not you should continue to take this drug.

- *Common:* eye discomfort or pain, itchy eye, red eye, feeling of having something in the eye, decreased vision
- *Less Common or Rare:* blurred vision, eye burning, darkening of eyelid skin color, increased pigmentation of the iris, lengthening and darkening of eyelashes, dry eye, excessive tearing, eyelid pain or swelling, eye discharge, increased sensitivity of the eyes to sunlight, mood or mental changes, dizziness, dizziness upon rising, fainting, pelvic pain, chest pain or tightness, slow or irregular heartbeat, sudden sweating, muscle and joint pain or stiffness, cough, difficulty breathing, wheezing, loss of bladder control, runny nose, sore throat, pounding in the ears

IMPORTANT PRECAUTIONS

Before taking this drug, tell your health-care practitioner if you have eye disease (such as iritis or uveitis) or problems such as loss of the lens of the eye. Travoprost should be used with caution if you have kidney or liver disease. Tell your health-care practitioner if you have ever experienced an allergic reaction to this or similar medications.

Travoprost may cause blurred vision. Until you know how this medication affects you, do not drive a car, operate machinery, or perform other tasks that demand concentration.

See your health-care practitioner on a regular basis to have your eye pressure monitored.

DRUG INTERACTIONS

Tell your health-care practitioner and pharmacist if you are taking any other prescription or over-the-counter drugs, as well as any vitamins, herbs, or other supplements.

FOOD, VITAMIN, AND HERBAL INTERACTIONS

Do not take the herb scopolia root, which has glaucoma as a possible side effect.

RECOMMENDED DOSAGE

Travoprost comes as an eyedrop solution. Although the dosage below is typical, consult your health-care practitioner for exact instructions.

- *Children:* This drug is not recommended for children.
- *Adults:* Apply 1 drop of travoprost once daily in the evening.

Remove contact lenses before using travoprost, and do not reinsert them for at least 15 minutes. Be careful not to touch the dropper to the eye. To limit absorption into the body, press your finger to the inner corner of the eye during and for one minute after administration.

If you miss a dose of travoprost, administer it as soon as you remember. However, if it is nearly time for your next scheduled dose, do not administer the missed dose. Follow your regular dosing schedule. Never use a double dose.

SYMPTOMS OF OVERDOSE AND WHAT TO DO

Symptoms of overdose may include bloodshot eyes and eye irritation, which can progress to abdominal pain, nausea, sweating, flushing, dizziness, and fatigue. Seek immediate medical attention, and bring the prescription bottle to the hospital with you.

SPECIAL INFORMATION FOR PREGNANT OR NURSING WOMEN

No studies have adequately investigated the effects of travoprost during pregnancy or breastfeeding. If you are pregnant or plan to become pregnant, or if you are breastfeeding or plan to do so, talk with your health-care practitioner before starting this drug. Only a health-care practitioner can determine whether the potential benefits outweigh the potential dangers.

SPECIAL INFORMATION FOR SENIORS

No special instructions are provided for seniors.

GENERIC NAME

Trazodone

BRAND NAME

Desyrel

Generic available

ABOUT THIS DRUG

Trazodone is used to treat mental depression. The symptoms of depression include sleep and appetite changes, sadness, guilt, shame, low self-esteem, anxiety, and extreme fatigue that last for over two weeks. This drug works by making more serotonin available in the brain.

SIDE EFFECTS

Inform your health-care practitioner if you develop side effects while taking trazodone. If symptoms are severe or prolonged, ask your health-care practitioner whether your dosage requires adjustment, and whether it is safe for you to continue taking this drug.

- *Common:* drowsiness, dizziness, lightheadedness, dry mouth, constipation, blurred vision, weight gain
- *Less Common or Rare:* abnormal dreams, confusion, anger, hostility, hallucinations, delusions, diarrhea, nausea, headache, nervousness, fatigue, difficulty concentrating, tremors, urinary retention, blood in urine, decreased sex drive in men, a persistent and painful erection, increased sex drive in women, altered menstruation, muscle aches and pains, breathing difficulties, seizures, liver damage, irregular heartbeat

IMPORTANT PRECAUTIONS

Do not take this drug if you have had a recent heart attack or if you have carcinoid syndrome. Always inform your health-care practitioner about any other medical conditions you may have, especially heart disease, alcoholism, epilepsy, or kidney or liver impairment. Tell your health-care practitioner if you have ever experienced an allergic reaction to this or similar drugs.

If you plan to undergo surgery or a dental procedure, tell your health-care practitioner or dentist that you are taking trazodone.

This drug can make you drowsy and less alert than usual. Until you know how trazodone affects you, do not drive a car, operate machinery, or perform other tasks that require concentration.

If this drug causes dry mouth, use sugarless gum or candy, ice chips, or artificial saliva. If the problem continues, consult your health-care practitioner or dentist.

DRUG INTERACTIONS

Tell your health-care practitioner and pharmacist if you are taking any other prescription or over-the-counter drugs, as well as any vitamins, herbs, or other supplements. Possible drug interactions include the following:

- Do not take monoamine oxidase inhibitor (MAOI) antidepressants at the same time as or within 14 days of trazodone. This combination can cause reactions ranging from confusion to seizures, and is potentially fatal.
- Combining this drug with antihypertensive medications may cause a dangerous drop in blood pressure.
- Taking other central nervous system depressants along with trazodone can result in increased drowsiness and other effects.
- Trazodone can increase blood levels and effects of digoxin and phenytoin.
- Do not drink alcohol while taking trazodone.

FOOD, VITAMIN, AND HERBAL INTERACTIONS

Do not combine this drug with herbs such as hops, kava, passionflower, and valerian. These can increase effects such as drowsiness. Do not take St. John's wort with trazodone, since both affect serotonin. Other inappropriate herbs include ginseng, ephedra (ma huang), and yohimbe.

RECOMMENDED DOSAGE

Trazodone comes as a tablet. Although the doses given below are typical, only your health-care practitioner can determine the dose and schedule that best fit your needs.

- *Children:* This drug is not recommended for children.
- *Adults:* 150 to 400 mg daily in divided doses

Trazodone should be taken with food to prevent side effects such as lightheadedness and dizziness. It must be taken regularly for several weeks before its full effect is felt. If you forget a dose, take it as soon as you remember. If it is almost time for the next dose, skip the missed one and resume your normal schedule. Never take a double dose. Do not stop taking this drug suddenly, especially if you have been taking it a long time. Your health-care practitioner will gradually reduce dosage.

SYMPTOMS OF OVERDOSE AND WHAT TO DO

The symptoms of trazodone overdose include vomiting, sleepiness, an irregular heartbeat, and difficulty breathing. If overdose occurs, seek immediate medical attention and take the prescription bottle to the hospital with you.

SPECIAL INFORMATION FOR PREGNANT OR NURSING WOMEN

No studies have adequately investigated the effects of trazodone during pregnancy or breastfeeding. However, decreased fertility and fetal damage occurred in animal studies. If you are pregnant or plan to become pregnant, or if you are breastfeeding or plan to do so, talk with your health-care practitioner before starting this drug. Only a health-care practitioner can determine whether the potential benefits outweigh the potential dangers.

SPECIAL INFORMATION FOR SENIORS

Seniors are at higher risk of side effects, and usually require smaller doses.

GENERIC NAME
Tretinoin

BRAND NAMES
Avita, Renova, Retin-A
Generic available

ABOUT THIS DRUG
Tretinoin is used to treat acne. It may also be prescribed for other skin conditions, such as fine wrinkles and liver spots on aging skin. Like other acne medications, this drug is chemically related to vitamin A. Tretinoin helps to keep the skin pores clear.

SIDE EFFECTS
Consult your health-care practitioner if you develop side effects while using tretinoin. Only he or she can determine whether it is safe for you to continue using this drug.

- *Common:* itching, burning, stinging, tingling, swelling, blistering, peeling, chapping, redness, dryness, lightening of skin, increased sensitivity to the sun
- *Less Common or Rare:* darkening of treated skin

IMPORTANT PRECAUTIONS
Keep tretinoin away from your eyes, lips, and the inside of your nose. Do not apply to windburned or sunburned skin or open wounds. Always tell your health-care practitioner about all other medical conditions you have, especially eczema, dermatitis, or sunburn. Inform your health-care practitioner if you have ever experienced an allergic reaction to this or similar medications. If skin irritation is excessive, stop using tretinoin until it heals. Wind and cold may worsen irritation. Avoid excessive exposure to the sun while using this medication. When you are exposed to the sun, wear protective clothing and hats, and apply sunblock. Do not use a sunlamp.

DRUG INTERACTIONS
Tell your health-care practitioner and pharmacist if you are taking any other prescription or over-the-counter drugs, as well as any vitamins, herbs, or other supplements. Possible drug interactions include the following:

- Do not combine tretinoin with other skin care products that contain peeling agents (such as benzoyl peroxide or salicylic acid).

- Avoid irritating hair products such as dyes.
- Avoid drying or abrasive skin care products and those that contain alcohol.

FOOD, VITAMIN, AND HERBAL INTERACTIONS

Do not use tretinoin with other skin care products that have drying effects.

RECOMMENDED DOSAGE

Tretinoin comes as a cream, gel, or solution. The doses given below are typical. However, consult your health-care practitioner for the exact dose and schedule that are most appropriate for you.

- *Children:* This drug is not recommended for children.
- *Adults:* Apply a thin layer to affected skin areas once daily in the evening. Do not use an excessive amount.

Gently wash your face 20 to 30 minutes before applying medication. If you forget a dose, skip it. Never apply double doses.

SYMPTOMS OF OVERDOSE AND WHAT TO DO

Tretinoin is for external use only. Accidental ingestion may cause dizziness, abdominal pain, and weakness. If overdose occurs, seek immediate medical attention and take the prescription container to the hospital with you.

SPECIAL INFORMATION FOR PREGNANT OR NURSING WOMEN

Do not use tretinoin if you are pregnant. This drug may cause birth defects. Use 2 reliable forms of birth control and have regular pregnancy tests while taking this drug. Because tretinoin may pass into breast milk, ask your health-care practitioner if it is appropriate to use while breastfeeding.

SPECIAL INFORMATION FOR SENIORS

There are no special instructions for seniors.

GENERIC NAME

Triamcinolone *see Corticosteroids, Oral, page 330*

GENERIC NAME

Triamcinolone acetonide

see Corticosteroids, Nasal Inhalation, page 327; Corticosteroids, Oral Inhalers, page 334; Corticosteroids, Topical, page 337

GENERIC NAME

Triazolam

BRAND NAME

Halcion
Generic available

ABOUT THIS DRUG

Triazolam is used on a short-term basis to treat insomnia. It belongs to a class of central nervous system depressant drugs known as benzodiazepines. Triazolam attaches to a site in the brain and decreases activity of nervous tissue. This drug has less of a "hangover" effect than other benzodiazepines.

SIDE EFFECTS

Consult your health-care practitioner if you develop side effects while using triazolam. Only he or she can determine whether it is safe for you to continue using this drug. Tell your health-care practitioner at once if you experience changes in thoughts or behavior, such as anxiety or depression.

- *Common:* dizziness, lightheadedness, drowsiness, headache, nausea, vomiting, nervousness, coordination problems
- *Less Common or Rare:* sleep disturbances, increased dreaming, nightmares, loss of memory (traveler's amnesia), anxiety, depression, lost sense of reality, overstimulation, aggressiveness, agitation, behavior problems, hallucinations, vertigo, fainting, falling, dry mouth, loss of equilibrium, diarrhea, heartbeat changes, chest pain, appetite loss, eye problems, vomiting, taste changes, visual disturbances, ringing in the ears, a hangover sensation on the day after bedtime use, changes in sexual drive, incontinence, yellow eyes and skin, itching, loss of appetite, anterograde amnesia (forgetting events after an injury)

IMPORTANT PRECAUTIONS

Inform your health-care practitioner about any other medical conditions you may have, especially kidney or liver disease, respiratory disease, or sleep apnea. Tell your health-care practitioner if you have ever experienced an allergic reaction to this drug or another benzodiazepine.

Triazolam is recommended for short-term use only. If you need to take this drug for longer than 7 to 10 days, consult your health-care practitioner. Triazolam should not be taken for more than a few weeks. Long-term use can lead to physical and/or psychological addiction. This drug should be used with caution in anyone with a history of drug or alcohol abuse or depression.

Triazolam can make you drowsy and less alert than usual. Until you know how this drug affects you, do not drive a car, operate machinery, or perform other tasks that require concentration.

DRUG INTERACTIONS

Tell your health-care practitioner and pharmacist if you are taking any other prescription or over-the-counter drugs, as well as any vitamins, herbs, or other supplements. Dosage adjustments may be necessary when you begin taking triazolam. Possible drug interactions include the following:

- Many drugs may add to drowsiness and other effects of triazolam. These include other central nervous system depressants (such as antidepressants, antihistamines, muscle relaxants, and sedatives), oral contraceptives, seizure medications, and digoxin.
- Macrolide antibiotics such as azithromycin and erythromycin may also increase the effects of triazolam.
- Triazolam decreases the effects of levodopa.
- Do not drink alcohol while taking triazolam. This combination worsens coordination and impairs mental function.
- Do not take clozapine with this drug.
- Cigarette smoking, rifampin, and theophylline may decrease the effectiveness of triazolam.

FOOD, VITAMIN, AND HERBAL INTERACTIONS

Do not drink grapefruit juice while taking triazolam. Grapefruit juice slows the body's breakdown of benzodiazepine drugs, which can lead to their potentially dangerous concentration in the blood.

Do not take triazolam with hops, kava, passionflower, and valerian. These can increase its sedative effects. Triazolam should not be combined with hawthorn.

Avoid caffeinated beverages such as coffee, tea, and cola.

RECOMMENDED DOSAGE

Triazolam comes as a tablet. Although the doses given below are typical, only your health-care practitioner can determine the dose and schedule that best fit your needs.

- *Children:* Triazolam is not recommended for children.
- *Adults:* 0.125 to 0.5 mg at bedtime

Triazolam can be taken with or without food. If you forget a dose, skip it and resume your normal schedule. Never take a double dose. If you have been taking triazolam for a few weeks, do not stop taking it suddenly. Abrupt withdrawal can lead to symptoms such as cramps, vomiting, sweating, tremor, ringing in the ears, sleep disturbances, depression, and convulsions. Speak to your health-care practitioner about gradually reducing dosage. You may experience sleeping difficulties the first night or two after stopping this medication ("rebound insomnia").

SYMPTOMS OF OVERDOSE AND WHAT TO DO

Triazolam overdose can be fatal. The symptoms include sleep apnea (temporary cessation of breathing), drowsiness, sluggishness, confusion, lack of coordination, low blood pressure, and coma. If overdose occurs, seek immediate medical attention and take the prescription bottle to the hospital with you.

SPECIAL INFORMATION FOR PREGNANT OR NURSING WOMEN

Do not take triazolam if you are pregnant or planning to become pregnant. This drug is associated with an increased risk of birth defects. Since triazolam may pass into breast milk, breastfeeding is not advisable while taking this medication.

SPECIAL INFORMATION FOR SENIORS

Side effects such as lethargy, fatigue, and weakness are more likely to occur in older people. Smaller doses are recommended.

OPEN QUESTIONS OR CONTROVERSIES

Triazolam can cause psychological and/or physical dependence. Tolerance may develop with long-term use, making it less effective. Do not take a larger dose of triazolam, take it more often, or use it for a longer period than your health-care practitioner recommends.

GENERIC NAME

Trichlormethiazide *see Thiazide Diuretics, page 1020*

GENERIC NAME

Class: Tricyclic antidepressants

Generics: (1) amitriptyline; (2) amitriptyline and perphenazine; (3) amitriptyline and chlordiazepoxide; (4) amoxapine; (5) clomipramine; (6) desipramine; (7) doxepin; (8) imipramine; (9) nortriptyline; (10) protriptyline; (11) trimipramine

BRAND NAMES

(1) Elavil (discontinued December 2003); (2) Etrafon, Etrafon A, Etrafon 2-10, Etrafon Forte, Triavil 2-10, Triavil 2-25, Triavil 4-10, Triavil 4-25, Triavil 4-50; (3) Limbitrol, Limbitrol DS 10-25; (4) Asendin; (5) Anafranil; (6) Norpramin; (7) Sinequan; (8) Tofranil, Tofranil-PM; (9) Aventyl, Aventyl Pulvules, Pamelor; (10) Vivactil; (11) Surmontil
All available as generic except trimipramine

ABOUT THIS DRUG

Tricyclic antidepressants are used to treat mental depression. The symptoms of depression include sleep and appetite changes, sadness, guilt, shame, low self-esteem, anxiety, and extreme fatigue that last for over two weeks. Imipramine is also prescribed for bedwetting in children, and clomipramine is also used to treat obsessive-compulsive disorder (OCD). Amitriptyline combinations are prescribed for anxiety and depression. Tricyclic antidepressants work by making more serotonin and norepinephrine available in the brain.

SIDE EFFECTS

Side effects are common. If they become persistent or severe, consult your health-care practitioner. Only he or she can determine whether it is safe for you to continue taking a tricyclic antidepressant and whether it is necessary to readjust your dosage.

- *Common:* drowsiness, dizziness, dizziness upon rising, lightheadedness, headache, nausea, tiredness, weakness, blurred vision, dry mouth, constipation, impaired urination, unpleasant taste, increased appetite, weight gain, impaired erection or ejaculation

- *Less Common or Rare:* nervousness, anxiety, unsteadiness, disorientation, confusion, delirium, restlessness, unusual excitement, tremors, fainting, sleep disturbances, vivid dreams, ringing in the ears, numbness and tingling, poor coordination, photosensitivity, impotence, changes in sex drive, enlargement of breasts, changes in blood sugar levels, diarrhea, fever, fluid retention, allergy, heartburn, increased sweating, vomiting, abnormal heart rate, blood pressure changes, heart attack

A rare but life-threatening set of side effects known as neuroleptic malignant syndrome (NMS) may occur when you are taking a tricyclic antidepressant. Symptoms include fever, difficulty breathing, rapid heartbeat, rigid muscles, mental changes, increased sweating, irregular blood pressure, and convulsions. Immediate medical attention is required.

In rare cases, amoxapine has been associated with side effects such as lip smacking, wormlike movements of the tongue, and slow, rhythmical, involuntary movements. These are characteristic of a disorder known as tardive dyskinesia. If you experience tardive dyskinesia, your health-care practitioner will probably advise you to stop taking this drug.

IMPORTANT PRECAUTIONS

Tricyclic antidepressants may make certain conditions worse. These include asthma, bipolar disorder, blood disorders, convulsions, difficult urination, enlarged prostate, glaucoma, heart disease, high blood pressure, an overactive thyroid, schizophrenia, and stomach or intestinal problems. If you have kidney or liver disease, you may require a lower dosage.

Inform your health-care practitioner if you have ever experienced an allergic reaction to a tricyclic antidepressant, carbamazepine, maprotiline, or trazodone.

Before having any type of surgery, dental procedure, emergency treatment, or medical test, tell your health-care practitioner or dentist that you are taking tricyclic antidepressants.

These drugs may impair your vision and physical coordination. Until you know how a tricyclic antidepressant affects you, do not drive a car, operate machinery, or perform other tasks that demand concentration.

When you first start taking one of these drugs or when the dosage is increased, you may experience dizziness or faintness when you rise quickly from a sitting or reclining position (postural hypotension). Try to get up slowly, and consult your health-care practitioner if the problem continues.

These medications may cause heightened sun sensitivity. Wear sunglasses and protective clothing, and apply sunscreen.

If tricyclic antidepressants cause dry mouth, use sugarless gum or hard candy, ice chips, or a saliva substitute. Consult your health-care practitioner or dentist if the problem continues.

DRUG INTERACTIONS

Inform your health-care practitioner and pharmacist if you are taking any other prescription or over-the-counter drugs, as well as any vitamins, herbs, or other supplements. Possible drug interactions include the following:

- Do not take monoamine oxidase inhibitor (MAOI) antidepressants at the same time as or within 14 days of a tricyclic antidepressant. This combination can cause reactions ranging from confusion to seizures, and is potentially fatal.
- Taking central nervous system depressants such as tranquilizers, sleep aids, or other antidepressants increases the effects of tricyclic antidepressants.
- Many drugs may increase the risk of serious effects on the heart. These include allergy and asthma medications, amphetamines, appetite suppressants, cold and cough remedies, ephedrine, isoproterenol, and phenylephrine.
- Combining tricyclic antidepressants with cimetidine, methylphenidate, or phenothiazine drugs may lead to severe side effects.
- Tricyclic antidepressants may reduce the effects of guanethidine.
- Since tricyclic antidepressants may cause low blood pressure, be cautious about combining these medications with antihypertensive drugs.
- Oral contraceptives and tobacco may reduce the effects of tricyclic antidepressants.
- Avoid alcohol while taking tricyclic antidepressants.

FOOD, VITAMIN, AND HERBAL INTERACTIONS

Do not combine tricyclic antidepressants with dietary supplements such as dong quai, hops, kava, passionflower, St. John's wort, valerian, SAMe, or 5-HTP. Consult your health-care practitioner before taking one of these drugs with grapefruit juice.

RECOMMENDED DOSAGE

Tricyclic antidepressants come in a variety of forms, including tablets, capsules, syrup, and oral solution. The doses given below are typical, but dosage is always carefully individualized according to a person's particular needs and reactions to therapy. Do not switch types or brands of medication without consulting your health-care practitioner. Lower doses are recommended for seniors.

Amitriptyline

- *Children:* Consult your health-care practitioner.
- *Adults:* 25 mg 2 to 4 times daily; maximum daily dose is 150 mg

Amoxapine

- *Children:* Consult your health-care practitioner.
- *Adults:* 100 to 400 mg daily in divided doses

Clomipramine

- *Children:* Consult your health-care practitioner.
- *Adults:* 25 to 250 mg daily in single or divided doses; single daily doses may be given at bedtime

Desipramine

- *Children:* Consult your health-care practitioner.
- *Adults:* 100 to 200 mg daily

Doxepin

- *Children:* Consult your health-care practitioner.
- *Adults:* 25 mg 3 times daily; maximum daily dose is 300 mg

Imipramine

- *Children:* 25 mg once daily 1 hour before bedtime to prevent bed-wetting
- *Adults:* 25 mg 3 to 4 times daily; maximum daily dose is 200 mg

Nortriptyline

- *Children:* Consult your health-care practitioner.
- *Adults:* 25 mg 3 to 4 times daily; maximum daily dose is 150 mg

Protriptyline

- *Children:* Consult your health-care practitioner.
- *Adults:* 5 to 10 mg 3 to 4 times daily; maximum daily dose is 60 mg

Trimipramine

- *Children:* Consult your health-care practitioner.
- *Adults:* 75 mg daily in divided doses; maximum daily dose is 200 mg

If tricyclic antidepressants upset your stomach, they may be taken with food. If you forget to take a dose, take the forgotten dose as soon as you remember it. However, if it is almost time for the next dose, skip it and resume your normal schedule. Never take a double dose. Although these drugs are not habit-forming, dosage must be reduced gradually.

SYMPTOMS OF OVERDOSE AND WHAT TO DO

The symptoms of tricyclic antidepressant overdose may include drowsiness, confusion, inability to concentrate, hallucinations, enlarged pupils, low body temperature, low blood pressure, abnormal heart rate, heart failure, stupor, convulsions, and coma. The effects of a tricyclic antidepressant overdose can be fatal. If overdose occurs, seek immediate medical attention and take the prescription bottle to the hospital with you.

SPECIAL INFORMATION FOR PREGNANT OR NURSING WOMEN

No studies have adequately investigated the effects of tricyclic antidepressants during pregnancy or breastfeeding. However, newborns of mothers taking these drugs have experienced heart, breathing, and urinary problems. If you are pregnant or plan to become pregnant, talk with your health-care practitioner before starting one of these drugs. Only a health-care practitioner can determine whether the potential benefits outweigh the potential dangers. These drugs may pass into breast milk, so breastfeeding is not advised while you take them.

SPECIAL INFORMATION FOR SENIORS

Seniors require lower doses of tricyclic antidepressants. Older people are more likely to experience side effects such as drowsiness, dizziness, confusion, dry mouth, vision problems, constipation, and trouble urinating.

GENERIC NAME

Trimethoprim

BRAND NAMES

Proloprim, Trimpex
Generic available

ABOUT THIS DRUG

Trimethoprim is an antibiotic used to treat urinary tract and eye infections. This drug is not effective against other types of microorganisms, such as viruses, fungi, and parasites. Antibiotics should not be prescribed for colds or flu. Trimethoprim is also prescribed in combination with sulfamethoxazole. It works by preventing the growth and multiplication of invading bacteria.

SIDE EFFECTS

Side effects from short-term use are uncommon. However, consult your health-care practitioner if you develop any persistent or severe effects. Only he or she can determine whether it is safe for you to continue taking trimethoprim.

➤ *Less Common or Rare:* upset stomach, nausea, vomiting, cramping, diarrhea, rash, itching, difficulty breathing or swallowing, sore throat, fever, chills, mouth sores, unusual bruising or bleeding, yellow skin or eyes, paleness, joint aches, headache, abnormal taste in mouth, blood cell disorders

IMPORTANT PRECAUTIONS

Always inform your health-care practitioner about any other medical conditions you suffer from, especially kidney or liver disease, cardiovascular disease, anemia, or folic acid deficiency. Tell your health-care practitioner if you have ever experienced an allergic reaction to a trimethoprim or similar drugs.

DRUG INTERACTIONS

Check first with your health-care practitioner before taking any other medication with trimethoprim. To avoid unwanted side effects, tell your health-care practitioner and pharmacist about all other prescription or over-the-counter drugs, vitamins, herbs, or other supplements that you are taking. Possible drug interactions include the following:

➤ A number of drugs may decrease the effects of trimethoprim. These include cholestyramine, rifampin, and ritonavir.

- Trimethoprim may increase the absorption and effects of many drugs, including ACE inhibitors, amantadine, cyclosporine, dapsone, digoxin, lamivudine, metformin, methotrexate, phenytoin, procainamide, and zidovudine.

FOOD, VITAMIN, AND HERBAL INTERACTIONS

Pure cranberry juice may also be helpful in controlling urinary tract infections. Because trimethoprim may lower homocysteine levels, a daily multivitamin is recommended.

When taking antibiotics, you also destroy friendly bacteria such as *Lactobacillus acidophilus* that normally reside in the intestine. This can result in yeast infections. To prevent this problem, eat yogurt with live cultures or take *Lactobacillus acidophilus* supplements.

RECOMMENDED DOSAGE

Trimethoprim comes as a tablet. The doses given below are average. However, doses vary from person to person, and only your health-care practitioner can determine the dose and schedule that are most appropriate for you.

- *Children:* Consult your health-care practitioner.
- *Adults:* 100 mg every 12 hours for 10 days

Trimethoprim should be taken 1 hour before or 2 hours after meals. If you miss a dose, take it as soon as you remember. If it is nearly time for your next scheduled dose, do not take the missed dose. Follow your regular dosing schedule. Never take a double dose.

It is essential to take trimethoprim exactly as your health-care practitioner instructs. In order to receive their full benefits, always continue to take antibiotics for the full number of days prescribed. Failing to do so can result in even more serious and drug-resistant infection.

SYMPTOMS OF OVERDOSE AND WHAT TO DO

Symptoms of overdose may include nausea, vomiting, headache, dizziness, confusion, bone marrow suppression, and jaundice. If you suspect an overdose, seek medical attention immediately, and bring the prescription bottle with you to the hospital so that health-care practitioners will know exactly what drug was taken.

SPECIAL INFORMATION FOR PREGNANT OR NURSING WOMEN

Trimethoprim has caused birth defects in animal studies. If you are pregnant or plan to become pregnant, consult with your health-care practitioner before taking this medication. It should be avoided during the first 3 months and final 2 weeks of pregnancy. Because trimethoprim may pass into breast milk, your health-care practitioner may advise you to stop breastfeeding while you take this drug.

SPECIAL INFORMATION FOR SENIORS

Smaller doses may be recommended for seniors.

GENERIC NAME

Trimipramine

see Tricyclic Antidepressants, page 1076

GENERIC NAMES

Class: Triptan-type antimigraine drugs

Generics: (1) almotriptan; (2) eletriptan; (3) naratriptan; (4) rizatriptan; (5) sumatriptan; (6) zolmitriptan

BRAND NAMES

(1) Axert; (2) Relpax; (3) Amerge; (4) Maxalt; (5) Imitrex; (6) Zomig
No generic available

ABOUT THESE DRUGS

Triptan-type antimigraine drugs are used to treat migraine headaches in adults. They relieve symptoms such as pain, nausea, vomiting, and exaggerated light and sound sensitivity. These medications are only prescribed when analgesics such as aspirin and ibuprofen fail to control symptoms. Sumatriptan may also be used for cluster headaches.

Triptan-type antimigraine drugs act on the blood vessels to narrow or constrict them. Swollen or dilated blood vessels are believed to be the cause of migraines.

SIDE EFFECTS

Inform your health-care practitioner if you develop side effects while taking triptan-type antimigraine drugs. Rare effects can occur in many parts of the body. Stop taking these drugs and seek immediate medical attention if you develop symptoms such as a tight chest or throat, difficulty breathing, wheezing, heart palpitations, high blood pressure, a rash, or swelling in the face. If any other effects are severe or prolonged, ask your health-care practitioner whether your dosage requires adjustment, and whether it is safe for you to continue taking these drugs.

- *Common:* dizziness, fatigue, tiredness, nausea, nasal discomfort, tingling in the hands or feet, warm or burning sensation, tightness in the jaw or neck, excessive thirst, frequent urination, transient rises in blood pressure, taste changes
- *Less Common or Rare:* vision changes, headache, flushing, heart palpitations, chest tightness or pain, cardiac problems, throat tightness or heaviness, weakness, agitation, muscle aches, sweating, vomiting, fainting, an overall feeling of unwellness, rash, itching, erection problems in men

IMPORTANT PRECAUTIONS

Always inform your health-care practitioner about any other medical conditions you may have. Triptan-type antimigraine drugs should not be taken if you have ischemic heart disease, uncontrolled high blood pressure, or a seizure disorder. They should be used with caution if you have other types of heart disease, high blood pressure or cholesterol, angina (chest pain), diabetes, obesity, a history of smoking, liver or kidney disease, or Raynaud's phenomenon. Tell your health-care practitioner if you have ever experienced an allergic reaction to triptan-type antimigraine drugs.

These drugs may cause dizziness and fatigue. Until you know how triptan-type antimigraine drugs affect you, do not drive a car, operate machinery, or perform other tasks that require concentration.

Triptan-type antimigraine drugs may cause increased sensitivity to sunlight. Exercise precautions such as wearing protective clothing and applying sunscreen.

If your headaches change in character or worsen, see your health-care practitioner. Because of the risk of vision changes, have your eyes checked on a regular basis while taking a triptan-type antimigraine drug. These medications are not meant for everyday headaches.

DRUG INTERACTIONS

Tell your health-care practitioner and pharmacist if you are taking any other prescription or over-the-counter drugs, as well as any vitamins, herbs, or other supplements. Possible drug interactions include the following:

- Do not take monoamine oxidase inhibitor (MAOI) antidepressants at the same time as or within 14 days of triptan-type antimigraine drugs.
- Do not take more than 1 triptan-type antimigraine drug at a time.
- Taking ergotamine-containing medications with triptan-type antimigraine drugs can result in prolonged constriction of blood vessels. Do not take these drugs within 24 hours of each other.
- Do not combine these drugs with citalopram.
- Combining triptan-type antimigraine drugs with drugs such as fluoxetine, fluvoxamine, paroxetine, and sertraline may cause coordination problems.
- Other drugs that may interact with these medications include cimetidine, oral contraceptives, and propranolol.
- Do not drink alcohol while taking triptan-type antimigraine drugs.

FOOD, VITAMIN, AND HERBAL INTERACTIONS

Do not take triptan-type antimigraine drugs with herbs such as St. John's wort, ephedra (ma huang), or kola. These may trigger migraines in some people. Learn to identify and avoid foods or additives that trigger your migraines. These may include chocolate and monosodium glutamate (MSG).

RECOMMENDED DOSAGE

Triptan-type antimigraine drugs come primarily as tablets. Sumatriptan also comes as a nasal spray, and rizatriptan is available as both a regular and disintegrating tablet. Although the doses given below are typical, only your health-care practitioner can determine the dose and schedule that best fit your needs.

Almotriptan

- *Children:* This drug is not recommended for children.
- *Adults:* 6.25 or 12.5 mg as a single dose. If the migraine returns after you've had relief, you can take another dose if you do so at least two hours after the first dose. Never take more than 2 doses within any 24-hour period.

Eletriptan

- *Children:* Consult your health-care practitioner.
- *Adults:* 20 to 40 mg as a single dose; if migraine returns after being relieved, you can take another dose if it has been at least 2 hours since you took the first dose. Do not take more than 2 doses within a 24-hour period.

Naratriptan

➤ *Children:* This drug is not recommended for children.

➤ *Adults:* 1 to 2.5 mg as soon as migraine pain starts. A second dose may be taken in 4 hours if needed. The maximum daily dose is 5 mg.

Rizatriptan

➤ *Children:* This drug is not recommended for children.

➤ *Adults:* 5 to 10 mg as soon as migraine pain starts. A second dose may be taken in 2 hours if needed. The maximum daily dose is 30 mg.

Sumatriptan Tablets

➤ *Children:* This drug is not recommended for children.

➤ *Adults:* 25 to 50 mg as soon as migraine pain starts. A second dose may be taken in 2 hours if needed. The maximum daily dose is 300 mg.

Sumatriptan Nasal Spray

➤ *Children:* This drug is not recommended for children.

➤ *Adults:* 5 to 20 mg as soon as migraine pain starts. A second dose may be taken in 2 hours if needed. The maximum daily dose is 40 mg.

Zolmitriptan

➤ *Children:* This drug is not recommended for children.

➤ *Adults:* 1.25 to 5 mg as soon as migraine pain starts. A second dose may be taken in 2 hours if needed. The maximum daily dose is 10 mg.

Triptan-type antimigraine drugs may be taken with or without food. Medication should be taken at the very first sign of a migraine, such as pain or an aura.

SYMPTOMS OF OVERDOSE AND WHAT TO DO

The symptoms of triptan-type antimigraine drug overdose may include slowed breathing, bluish lips and skin, sedation, swelling, tremors, weakness, dilated pupils, changes in blood pressure, and seizures. If overdose occurs, seek immediate medical attention and take the prescription bottle to the hospital with you.

SPECIAL INFORMATION FOR PREGNANT OR NURSING WOMEN

Triptan-type antimigraine drugs have caused toxic defects on fetuses in animal studies. Your health-care practitioner must carefully consider the potential risks versus benefits of using these medications during pregnancy. Because triptan-type antimigraine drugs may pass into breast milk, your health-care practitioner may advise you to stop breastfeeding while taking them.

SPECIAL INFORMATION FOR SENIORS

Because of the higher risk of side effects, naratriptan is not recommended for seniors. There are no special instructions for other triptan-type antimigraine drugs.

GENERIC NAME

Trospium

BRAND NAME

Sanctura
No generic available

ABOUT THIS DRUG

Trospium is an antispasmodic used in the treatment of overactive bladder with symptoms of urge urinary incontinence, urgency, and urinary frequency.

Trospium relaxes the bladder muscles, which results in a reduction in bladder contractions as well as symptoms of overactive bladder.

SIDE EFFECTS

Be sure to tell your health-care practitioner if you experience any side effects while taking trospium. Only your health-care practitioner can determine whether it is safe for you to continue taking this drug.

➤ *Most Common:* constipation, dry mouth

➤ *Less Common:* abdominal pain, dry eyes, fatigue, flatulence, headache, heartburn, urinary retention

IMPORTANT PRECAUTIONS

Tell your health-care practitioner if you are sensitive or allergic to trospium or to any other drugs.

Trospium should be used with caution if you have significant bladder outflow obstruction, ulcerative colitis, intestinal atony, myasthenia gravis, narrow-angle glaucoma, or moderate to severe liver dysfunction.

Heat prostration (fever and heat stroke due to decreased sweating) may occur if you take trospium in a hot environment.

DRUG INTERACTIONS

Tell your health-care practitioner and pharmacist if you are taking any prescription or nonprescription drugs, as well as any vitamins, herbs, or other supplements. Possible drug interactions include the following:

- Taking trospium with other drugs that cause dry mouth and constipation (i.e., anticholinergic agents, such as atropine, ipratropium, meclizine, oxybutynin, scopolamine, among others) may increase the frequency and severity of these effects.
- Trospium taken with any of the following drugs may increase the concentration of trospium and/or the other drugs: digoxin, metformin, morphine, pancuronium, procainamide, tenofovir, and vancomycin.

FOOD, VITAMIN, AND HERBAL INTERACTIONS

No food, vitamin, or herbal interactions have been reported.

RECOMMENDED DOSAGE

Trospium is available in 20-mg tablets. The dosages given here are typical. However, your health-care practitioner will determine the most appropriate dose and schedule for your needs.

- *Children:* use and dose to be determined by your health-care practitioner
- *Adults:* 20 mg twice daily. Your health-care practitioner may reduce your dose to 20 mg once daily if you are 75 years or older.

Take trospium on an empty stomach or at least one hour before meals. If you miss a dose, take it as soon as you remember, as long as it is at least one hour before eating. If it is nearly time for your next dose, skip the missed dose. Return to your regular dosing schedule. Never take a double dose.

SYMPTOMS OF OVERDOSE AND WHAT TO DO

Symptoms of overdose include abnormal dilation of the pupils and abnormally rapid heartbeat (tachycardia). If overdose occurs, seek immediate medical attention and bring the prescription container with you to the hospital.

SPECIAL INFORMATION FOR PREGNANT OR NURSING WOMEN

Adequate studies of the effects of trospium on pregnant or nursing women have not been done. If you are pregnant or plan to become pregnant, talk to your health-care practitioner.

It is not known whether trospium passes into breast milk. If you are breastfeeding, your health-care practitioner will likely advise you to switch to bottle feeding until your treatment is complete.

SPECIAL INFORMATION FOR SENIORS

Seniors 75 years and older may require a lower dose of 20 mg once daily.

GENERIC NAME

Trovafloxacin *see Fluoroquinolone Antibiotics, page 468*

GENERIC NAME

Unoprostone isopropyl ophthalmic

BRAND NAME

Rescula

No generic available

ABOUT THIS DRUG

Unoprostone ophthalmic eye solution is used to treat open-angle glaucoma and ocular hypertension (high blood pressure within the eye). This drug works by lowering pressure in the eye.

SIDE EFFECTS

Consult your health-care practitioner if you experience side effects while taking unoprostone. Only he or she can determine whether or not you should continue to take this drug.

- *Common:* double vision, dry eyes, eye burning, stinging, tearing, bloodshot eyes, itchy eyes, foreign body sensation, change in length of eyelashes, chills, shivering, cough, fever, runny nose, sore throat, sweating, vomiting, unusual tiredness or weakness, headache, trouble sleeping, overall feeling of unwellness, diarrhea, muscle or joint pain
- *Less Common or Rare:* eye pain, eye swelling, eye inflammation, eye discharge, redness of eye or inside of eyelid, eyelid pain or swelling,

change in color of iris or eyelid, increase in the number of eyelashes, sensitivity to light, difficulty seeing at night

IMPORTANT PRECAUTIONS

Before taking this drug, tell your health-care practitioner if you wear contact lenses, and let him or her know if you have ever experienced an allergic reaction to this or similar drugs. Inform your health-care practitioner if you develop an eye infection, injure your eye, or plan to have eye surgery while using unoprostone. See your health-care practitioner on a regular basis to monitor your progress.

Unoprostone may cause blurred vision. Until you know how this medication affects you, do not drive a car, operate machinery, or perform other tasks that demand clear vision.

Because this drug may make your eyes more sensitive, avoid bright light and wear sunglasses.

DRUG INTERACTIONS

Tell your health-care practitioner and pharmacist if you are taking any other prescription or over-the-counter drugs, as well as any vitamins, herbs, or other supplements. Drug interactions may occur if unoprostone is used along with other eyedrops. If your health-care practitioner has prescribed other eyedrops in addition to unoprostone, use the drops at least 5 minutes apart.

FOOD, VITAMIN, AND HERBAL INTERACTIONS

Do not take the herb scopolia root, which has glaucoma as a possible side effect.

RECOMMENDED DOSAGE

Unoprostone comes as an eyedrop solution. Although the dosage below is typical, consult your health-care practitioner for exact instructions.

- *Children:* This drug is not recommended for children.
- *Adults:* Apply 1 drop of unoprostone in the affected eye twice daily.

Remove contact lenses before using unoprostone, and do not reinsert them for at least 15 minutes. Be careful not to touch the dropper to the eye. To limit absorption into the body, press your finger to the inner corner of the eye during and for one minute after administration.

If you miss a dose of unoprostone, administer it as soon as you remember. However, if it is nearly time for your next scheduled dose, do not administer the missed dose. Follow your regular dosing schedule. Never use a double dose.

SYMPTOMS OF OVERDOSE AND WHAT TO DO
Little is known about overdosing with unoprostone. However, if you suspect an overdose, seek immediate medical attention, and bring the prescription bottle to the hospital with you.

SPECIAL INFORMATION FOR PREGNANT OR NURSING WOMEN
No studies have adequately investigated the effects of unoprostone during pregnancy or breastfeeding. If you are pregnant or plan to become pregnant, or if you are breastfeeding or plan to do so, talk with your health-care practitioner before starting this drug. Only a health-care practitioner can determine whether the potential benefits outweigh the potential dangers.

SPECIAL INFORMATION FOR SENIORS
No special instructions are provided for seniors.

GENERIC NAME

Valacyclovir

BRAND NAME
Valtrex
No generic available

ABOUT THIS DRUG
Valacyclovir is an antiviral drug used to treat genital herpes and herpes zoster (shingles). It does not cure herpes infections, but decreases pain and itching, helps sores to heal, and prevents new sores from forming. Treatment must begin as soon as possible after diagnosis.

In the body, valacyclovir is rapidly converted to the antiviral drug acyclovir. Acyclovir slows the growth of existing viruses by interfering with the reproduction of viral DNA.

SIDE EFFECTS
Consult your health-care practitioner if you experience side effects while taking valacyclovir. Only he or she can determine whether or not you should continue to take this drug.

- *Common:* nausea, vomiting, abdominal pain, appetite loss, diarrhea, constipation, headache, dizziness, weakness
- *Less Common or Rare:* overall feeling of unwellness, fatigue, aching joints, tingling in the hands and feet, leg pain, sleeplessness, fever, gas, change in sense of taste, rash

IMPORTANT PRECAUTIONS

Always tell your health-care practitioner about any other medical conditions you have. Do not take this medication if you have acquired immunodeficiency syndrome (AIDS) or a seriously compromised immune system. Valacyclovir should be used with caution if you are infected with the human immunodeficiency virus (HIV), or if you have problems with your immune system or kidney or liver disease. Some people with advanced HIV or who had transplants experienced a fatal blood-clotting disorder while taking this drug. Lower doses are required if you have kidney damage. Inform your health-care practitioner if you have ever experienced an allergic reaction to this, acyclovir, or similar drugs.

Women with genital herpes face an increased risk of cervical cancer and should have regular Pap smears. Use condoms to prevent the transmission of genital herpes.

DRUG INTERACTIONS

Tell your health-care practitioner and pharmacist if you are taking any other prescription or over-the-counter drugs, as well as any vitamins, herbs, or other supplements. Possible drug interactions with valacyclovir may include the following:

- Cimetidine and probenecid may increase blood levels and effects of valacyclovir.
- The combination of acyclovir and zidovudine may cause extreme lethargy or drowsiness.

FOOD, VITAMIN, AND HERBAL INTERACTIONS

No food, vitamin, or herbal interactions have been noted.

RECOMMENDED DOSAGE

Valacyclovir comes as a tablet. Although the doses given below are typical, only your health-care practitioner can determine the dose and schedule that are most appropriate for you.

Shingles

- *Children:* This drug is not recommended for children under 12.
- *Adults:* 1,000 mg 3 times daily for 7 days

Genital Herpes

- *Children:* This drug is not recommended for children under 12.
- *Adults:* 500 mg twice daily for 5 days

Treatment must begin at the first sign of infection. If you forget to take a dose, take it as soon as you remember. If it is almost time for the next dose, skip the forgotten one, and resume your normal schedule. Never take double doses.

SYMPTOMS OF OVERDOSE AND WHAT TO DO

Little is known about overdosing with valacyclovir. However, if you suspect an overdose, seek immediate medical attention, and bring the prescription bottle to the hospital with you.

SPECIAL INFORMATION FOR PREGNANT OR NURSING WOMEN

No studies have adequately investigated the effects of valacyclovir during pregnancy or breastfeeding. If you are pregnant or plan to become pregnant, or if you are breastfeeding or plan to do so, talk with your health-care practitioner before starting this drug. Only a health-care practitioner can determine whether the potential benefits outweigh the potential dangers.

SPECIAL INFORMATION FOR SENIORS

Dosage must be lowered for seniors with reduced kidney function.

GENERIC NAME

Valdecoxib

BRAND NAME

Bextra
No generic available

ABOUT THIS DRUG

Valdecoxib is a nonsteroidal anti-inflammatory drug (NSAID) used to treat arthritis. It relieves symptoms such as pain, inflammation, swelling, and stiffness. This drug is also prescribed for menstrual pain. Valdecoxib works by reducing the level of prostaglandins, chemicals in the body that produce inflammation and pain.

SIDE EFFECTS

Valdecoxib may cause potentially serious side effects, especially when used for a long time and in large doses. If you develop side effects while taking this drug, ask your health-care practitioner whether it is safe for you to continue taking it.

- *Common:* diarrhea, stomach upset, indigestion, heartburn, headache, belching, sore throat, cough, ear congestion
- *Less Common or Rare:* back pain, tiredness, weakness, abdominal fullness or bloating, facial bloating, swelling of the extremities, tingling in hands and feet, muscle aches and pains, gas, nausea, stomach pain, weight gain, runny or stuffy nose, accidental injury, blurred vision, fever, chills, dizziness, pale skin, pounding in the ears, difficulty breathing with exertion, urinary difficulties, unusual bleeding or bruising, blood in urine, liver damage

Stop taking valdecoxib and consult your health-care practitioner immediately if you experience symptoms such as abdominal pain, stomach cramps, diarrhea, nausea, heartburn, indigestion, visual disturbances, vomiting of blood or material that looks like coffee grounds, or black, tarry stools. These may be signs of dangerous reactions such as ulcers or internal bleeding.

Another rare but life-threatening possibility is an allergic reaction called anaphylaxis. This requires immediate medical attention. Symptoms include rapid breathing, wheezing, gasping for breath, swelling around the eyes, changes in skin color, and fainting.

IMPORTANT PRECAUTIONS

Valdecoxib may cause gastrointestinal bleeding, ulcers, and stomach perforation. If you take valdecoxib on a regular basis, these types of side effects can occur at any time, with or without warning. People with a history of ulcers, colitis, or any type of gastrointestinal bleeding should be extremely careful when taking any NSAID.

Do not take valdecoxib if you have a bleeding disorder such as anemia or asthma or nasal polyps associated with aspirin use. Use this drug with caution if you have high blood pressure or other heart problems, dehydration, fluid retention, or impaired liver or kidney function. Tell your health-care practitioner if you have ever experienced an allergic reaction to aspirin or related drugs.

Drinking alcoholic beverages increases the risk of side effects such as bleeding.

Other possible side effects of valdecoxib include blurred vision and dizziness. Until you know how this drug affects you, do not drive a car, operate machinery, or perform other tasks that require concentration.

Before undergoing any type of surgery or dental procedure, inform your health-care practitioner or dentist that you are taking valdecoxib. Visit your health-care practitioner on a regular basis while taking this drug.

DRUG INTERACTIONS

Tell your health-care practitioner and pharmacist if you are taking any other prescription or over-the-counter drugs, as well as any vitamins, herbs, or other supplements. Possible drug interactions include the following:

- Do not combine valdecoxib with other NSAIDs such as aspirin. This increases the risk of bleeding.
- Taking valdecoxib with lithium, fluconazole, or ketoconazole increases the effects of valdecoxib.
- Do not use alcohol when you are taking valdecoxib. Both are stomach irritants, and using them together can increase the risk of stomach bleeding and ulcers.
- Tobacco increases the risk of side effects.

FOOD, VITAMIN, AND HERBAL INTERACTIONS

Do not combine valdecoxib with herbal remedies such as clove oil, feverfew, garlic, ginkgo, and ginseng. These herbs may affect clotting.

RECOMMENDED DOSAGE

Valdecoxib comes as a tablet. The doses given below are typical. However, only your health-care practitioner can determine the dose and schedule that best fit your individual needs.

- *Children:* This drug is not recommended for children.
- *Adults:* 10 to 40 mg daily in single or divided doses

Valdecoxib may be taken with food or milk to prevent stomach upset. If you forget to take a dose, take it as soon as you remember. If it is almost time for the next dose, skip the one you missed and resume your normal schedule. Never take a double dose.

SYMPTOMS OF OVERDOSE AND WHAT TO DO

Symptoms of valdecoxib overdose may include nausea, vomiting, stomach pain, drowsiness, and lethargy. If an overdose occurs, seek immediate medical attention and take the prescription bottle to the hospital with you so the health-care practitioner will know exactly what medication was taken.

SPECIAL INFORMATION FOR PREGNANT OR NURSING WOMEN

Do not use valdecoxib in late pregnancy. If you want to take this drug in early pregnancy, ask your health-care practitioner whether the potential benefits outweigh the risks. Because valdecoxib may pass into breast milk, it is best to stop breastfeeding while you take this drug.

SPECIAL INFORMATION FOR SENIORS

There are no special instructions for seniors.

OPEN QUESTIONS OR CONTROVERSIES

In December 2004, the producer of Bextra, Pfizer Inc., announced that it had placed a "black box" warning label on the drug because a few cases of Stevens Johnson syndrome, a painful and sometimes fatal condition, have been linked with use of the drug. Stevens Johnson syndrome occurs when the immune system attacks the body in an effort to rid itself of a drug, causing severe, painful blistering of the mucous membranes and skin. The risk is greatest during the first two weeks the drug is taken. Before taking valdecoxib, you should consult with your health-care practitioner about the latest information on this drug and any alternative medications for your health-care needs.

GENERIC NAME

Valproic acid

BRAND NAME

Depakene

Generic available

Note: The information in this profile also applies to divalproex sodium (Depakote, Depakote Sprinkle, Depakote ER).

ABOUT THIS DRUG

Valproic acid is an anticonvulsant used to relieve epileptic seizures. This drug may be prescribed for absence seizures, tonic-clonic seizures, myoclonic seizures, and psychomotor seizures. It is often taken with other antiseizure drugs.

This medication is believed to work by affecting GABA, a substance that inhibits nerve activity in the part of the brain and central nervous system. Although valproic acid cannot cure epilepsy, it will help control seizures while you take it.

SIDE EFFECTS

Consult your health-care practitioner at once if you experience problems such as extreme weakness, fatigue, loss of appetite, vomiting, dark urine, and yellow skin or eyes. Severe and potentially fatal liver damage may occur while taking this drug, especially in the first 6 months. Also report any other side effects that are severe or prolonged. Ask your health-care practitioner whether your dosage should be altered, and whether it is safe for you to continue taking this drug.

- *Common:* drowsiness, lethargy, sleepiness, sedation, nausea, vomiting, indigestion, weakness, depression, aggression, emotional upset, hyperactivity, blood disorders such as changes in platelet function
- *Less Common or Rare:* abdominal cramps, changes in appetite, constipation, cough, visual impairment, double vision, spots before the eyes, sensitivity to light, loss of eye muscle control, drooping eyelids, dizziness, headache, trouble speaking, mouth sores, muscle pain or weakness, loss of coordination, tremors, unsteadiness, rash, itching

IMPORTANT PRECAUTIONS

Always inform your health-care practitioner about any other medical conditions you may have. Do not take valproic acid if you have active liver disease or a bleeding disorder, or if you are pregnant. Use this drug with caution if you have a history of liver disease or a bleeding disorder, or myasthenia gravis. Tell your health-care practitioner if you have ever experienced an allergic reaction to this or similar medications.

This drug may affect your vision and can make you drowsy and less alert than usual. Until you know how valproic acid affects you, do not drive a car, operate machinery, or perform other tasks that require concentration.

Regular blood tests are necessary to monitor your reaction to valproic acid. Inform your health-care practitioner or dentist that you are taking this medication before undergoing any medical or dental procedure.

DRUG INTERACTIONS

Tell your health-care practitioner and pharmacist if you are taking any other prescription or over-the-counter drugs, as well as any vitamins, herbs, or other supplements. Possible drug interactions include the following:

- Valproic acid may alter the absorption of other anticonvulsants, such as phenobarbital, phenytoin, and carbamazepine. Your health-care practitioner may need to adjust dosages.
- Taking other central nervous system depressants (such as sedatives, antidepressants, narcotics, or tranquilizers) with valproic acid can result in increased drowsiness and excessive sedation.
- Drugs such as aspirin, cimetidine, chlorpromazine, erythromycin, and felbamate may increase the risk of side effects of valproic acid.
- Combining valproic acid with aspirin, dipyridamole, and sulfinpyrazone may increase the risk of bleeding.
- Medications including acyclovir and ritonavir may reduce the effects of valproic acid.
- Antacids may decrease absorption and effects of valproic acid.
- Valproic acid may increase the effects of antidepressants, benzodiazepines, and blood thinners such as warfarin.
- Avoid alcohol while you are taking valproic acid.

FOOD, VITAMIN, AND HERBAL INTERACTIONS

Do not combine valproic acid with herbs such as hops, kava, passionflower, and valerian. These can increase valproic acid's sedative effects. Herbs such as ephedra (ma huang) and kola may cause overstimulation; ginkgo may lead to bleeding; and St. John's wort, like valproic acid, is associated with increased sun sensitivity. Supplementation is recommended to replace depleted zinc, selenium, and carnitine.

RECOMMENDED DOSAGE

This drug comes as a capsule, extended-release capsule, capsule containing sprinkles, tablet, and liquid. The doses given below are average. However, doses vary from person to person, and only your health-care practitioner can determine the dose and schedule that are most appropriate for you.

- *Children:* Consult your health-care practitioner.
- *Adults:* 7 mg per pound of body weight to start. The average daily dosage is 1,000 to 1,600 mg daily in divided doses.

If valproic acid upsets your stomach, it may be taken with food. Take medication with a full (8-ounce) glass of water. The sprinkle capsule may be swallowed whole, or sprinkled on a teaspoon of applesauce or pudding. Do not take the liquid with carbonated beverages.

If you forget a dose, take it as soon as you remember. If it is almost time for the next dose, skip the missed one and resume your normal schedule. Never take a double dose. If you have been taking valproic acid for a long period of time, you must stop taking it gradually to prevent seizures from recurring.

SYMPTOMS OF OVERDOSE AND WHAT TO DO

The symptoms of valproic acid overdose may include drowsiness, confusion, unsteadiness, weakness, stupor, and coma. If overdose occurs, seek immediate medical attention and take the prescription bottle to the hospital with you.

SPECIAL INFORMATION FOR PREGNANT OR NURSING WOMEN

Valproic acid has caused birth defects in animal studies and may pass into breast milk. If this drug is considered crucial for your health, carefully discuss the potential benefits versus risks with your health-care practitioner.

SPECIAL INFORMATION FOR SENIORS

Smaller doses are recommended for seniors.

GENERIC NAME

Valsartan *see Angiotensin II Blockers, page 123*

GENERIC NAME

Vardenafil

BRAND NAME

Levitra

No generic available

ABOUT THIS DRUG

Vardenafil is used to treat men who have erectile dysfunction, or sexual impotence. This drug inhibits the enzyme phosphodiesterase and helps maintain an erection when the penis is stimulated. Vardenafil does not work in the absence of stimulation.

SIDE EFFECTS

Be sure to tell your health-care practitioner if you experience any side effects while taking vardenafil. Only your health-care practitioner can determine whether it is safe for you to continue taking this drug. If you experience a prolonged or painful erection for 4 hours or more, contact your health-care practitioner at once.

- *Most Common:* diarrhea, flushing, headache, heartburn, runny nose
- *Less Common:* back pain, dizziness, low blood pressure, nausea

IMPORTANT PRECAUTIONS

Tell your health-care practitioner if you are sensitive or allergic to vardenafil or to any other drugs.

Do not use vardenafil if you use nitrate therapy, nitric oxide, or alpha-blockers, or if your health-care practitioner has recommended you not engage in sexual activity because of underlying heart conditions.

Prolonged erections (more than 4 hours) and priapism (painful erection for more than 6 hours) have been reported. If either of these symptoms occur, seek immediate medical attention.

Before using vardenafil, consult your health-care practitioner if you currently have or have ever had a heart attack, stroke, irregular heartbeat, angina, congestive heart failure, high or low blood pressure, personal or family history of long QT syndrome, liver impairment, kidney problems, blood disease (e.g., sickle cell anemia, multiple myeloma, leukemia), clotting disorder, stomach ulcer, degenerative eye disease (e.g., retinitis pigmentosa), or a physical abnormality of the penis (e.g., Peyronie's disease).

Use of vardenafil does not provide any protection against sexually transmitted diseases.

DRUG INTERACTIONS

Tell your health-care practitioner and pharmacist if you are taking any prescription or nonprescription drugs, as well as any vitamins, herbs, or other supplements. Possible drug interactions include the following:

- Erythromycin, ketoconazole, indinavir, and ritonavir may increase blood levels of vardenafil.

- Vardenafil reduces the concentration of ritonavir and indinavir and thus may reduce the effectiveness of these drugs.
- Vardenafil enhances the blood pressure lowering effects of nitrates (e.g., nitroglycerine) and alpha-blocking drugs (e.g., terazosin).
- Drugs used to treat impotence, such as alprostadil, should not be taken along with vardenafil.

FOOD, VITAMIN, AND HERBAL INTERACTIONS

Do not take any herbal remedies to treat impotence, such as yohimbine, without first consulting your health-care practitioner. Also, do not take vardenafil with grapefruit or grapefruit juice, as the interaction can have dangerous consequences.

RECOMMENDED DOSAGE

Vardenafil is available in 2.5-, 5-, 10-, and 20-mg tablets. The dosages given here are typical. However, your health-care practitioner will determine the most appropriate dose and schedule for your needs.

- *Children:* not for use in children
- *Adults:* starting dose is generally 10 mg taken 60 minutes before sexual activity. Your health-care practitioner may reduce this dose to 2.5 or 5 mg if you are taking certain medications that increase the blood levels of vardenafil (see "Drug Interactions").

Vardenafil should be taken 60 minutes before sexual activity, with or without food. This drug should be taken only once per day and in some cases, only once every three days. Consult your health-care practitioner about dosing.

SYMPTOMS OF OVERDOSE AND WHAT TO DO

Symptoms of overdose are not known but may include abnormal vision, back pain, chest pain, dizziness, irregular heartbeat, muscle pain, and swelling of the ankles or legs. If overdose occurs, seek immediate medical attention and bring the prescription container with you to the hospital.

SPECIAL INFORMATION FOR PREGNANT OR NURSING WOMEN

Vardenafil is approved for use by men only.

SPECIAL INFORMATION FOR SENIORS

The recommended dosage for men older than age 65 is 5 mg as a single dose.

GENERIC NAME
Venlafaxine

BRAND NAMES
Effexor, Effexor XR
No generic available

ABOUT THIS DRUG
Venlafaxine is used to treat mental depression. The symptoms of depression include sleep and appetite changes, sadness, guilt, shame, low self-esteem, anxiety, and extreme fatigue that last for over two weeks. Venlafaxine may also be prescribed for generalized anxiety disorder.

This drug works by inhibiting the reuptake (return) of nerves transmitters, making more serotonin, norepinephrine, and dopamine available in the brain. It has fewer side effects and takes effect more quickly than tricyclic antidepressants.

SIDE EFFECTS
Inform your health-care practitioner if you develop side effects while taking venlafaxine. If effects are severe or prolonged, ask your health-care practitioner whether your dosage requires adjustment, and whether it is safe for you to continue taking this drug.

- *Common:* constipation, headache, dizziness, fatigue, dry mouth, weight loss, small increase in cholesterol levels
- *Less Common or Rare:* blurred vision, dilated pupils, changes in taste, ringing in ears, high blood pressure, rapid heartbeat, palpitations, agitation, anxiety, nervousness, insomnia, nausea, vomiting, appetite loss, tremors, sweating, weakness, abnormal ejaculation, prolonged erection, impotence, reduced sex drive, delayed orgasm, chills, yawning, fluid retention, rash, hives

IMPORTANT PRECAUTIONS
Always inform your health-care practitioner about any other medical conditions you may have, especially high blood pressure or cholesterol, a recent heart attack, glaucoma, seizures, suicidal tendencies, a history of drug addiction, insomnia, or mania (extreme excitability). Tell your health-care practitioner if you have ever experienced an allergic reaction to this or similar drugs.

This drug may cause side effects such as dizziness and blurred vision. Until you know how venlafaxine affects you, do not drive a car, operate machinery, or perform other tasks that require concentration.

If this drug causes mouth dryness, use sugarless gum or candy, ice chips, or artificial saliva. If the problem continues, consult your health-care practitioner or dentist.

DRUG INTERACTIONS

Tell your health-care practitioner and pharmacist if you are taking any other prescription or over-the-counter drugs, as well as any vitamins, herbs, or other supplements. Possible drug interactions include the following:

- Do not take monoamine oxidase inhibitor (MAOI) antidepressants at the same time as or within 14 days of venlafaxine. This combination can cause reactions ranging from confusion to seizures, and is potentially fatal.
- Combining this drug with antihypertensive medications may cause a dangerous drop in blood pressure.
- Do not take venlafaxine with SSRIs such as paroxetine without consulting your health-care practitioner.
- Other drugs that may lead to severe side effects or toxicity include cimetidine, tramadol, tricyclic antidepressants, dextromethorphan, warfarin, zolmitriptan, and zolpidem.
- Avoid alcohol while taking venlafaxine.

FOOD, VITAMIN, AND HERBAL INTERACTIONS

Do not combine this drug with herbs such as hops, kava, passionflower, and valerian. These can increase effects such as drowsiness. Do not take St. John's wort with venlafaxine, since both affect serotonin. Other inappropriate herbs include ginseng, ephedra (ma huang), and yohimbe. Do not take this medication with grapefruit juice.

RECOMMENDED DOSAGE

Venlafaxine comes as a tablet. Although the doses given below are typical, only your health-care practitioner can determine the dose and schedule that best fit your needs.

- *Children:* This drug is not recommended for children.
- *Adults:* 37.5 to 225 mg daily in divided doses

Venlafaxine should be taken with food. It must be taken regularly for several weeks before its full effect is felt. If you forget a dose, take it as soon as you remember. If it is almost time for the next dose, skip the missed one and resume your normal schedule. Never take a double dose. Do not stop taking this drug suddenly, especially if you have been taking it a long time. Your health-care practitioner will gradually reduce dosage.

SYMPTOMS OF OVERDOSE AND WHAT TO DO

The symptoms of venlafaxine overdose include sleepiness, an irregular heartbeat, low blood pressure, vertigo, seizures, and coma. If overdose occurs, seek immediate medical attention and take the prescription bottle to the hospital with you.

SPECIAL INFORMATION FOR PREGNANT OR NURSING WOMEN

No studies have adequately investigated the effects of venlafaxine during pregnancy or breastfeeding. However, decreased fertility and fetal damage occurred in animal studies. If you are pregnant or plan to become pregnant, or if you are breastfeeding or plan to do so, talk with your health-care practitioner before starting this drug. Only a health-care practitioner can determine whether the potential benefits outweigh the potential dangers.

SPECIAL INFORMATION FOR SENIORS

Seniors face a higher risk of side effects, and usually require smaller doses.

OPEN QUESTIONS OR CONTROVERSIES

In June 2004, the Food and Drug Administration asked manufacturers of venlafaxine to include in their labeling a warning statement that recommends close observation of adult and pediatric patients for clinical worsening of depression or the emergence of suicidality when being treated with this drug, especially when beginning the drug, or at the time of dose changes, either increases or decreases.

GENERIC NAME

Verapamil

BRAND NAMES

Calan, Calan SR, Covera HS, Isoptin, Isoptin SR, Verelan, Verelan PM
Generic available

ABOUT THIS DRUG

Verapamil is a calcium channel blocker used to treat angina (chest pain), irregular heartbeats (arrhythmias), and mild-to-moderate high blood pressure (hypertension). This drug may be prescribed both for chest pain that occurs spontaneously (Prinzmetal's angina) and chest pain that develops as a result of exertion.

In the treatment of high blood pressure, verapamil can be used alone or in combination with other antihypertensive medication (especially trandolapril). The sustained-release forms of this medication are recommended for high blood pressure only.

Calcium channel blockers including verapamil work by blocking the passage of calcium into the heart and smooth muscles. This reduces the heart's workload, relaxes blood vessels, and increases the supply of oxygen and blood to the heart.

SIDE EFFECTS

Consult your health-care practitioner if you develop side effects while taking this drug. Only he or she can determine whether it is safe for you to continue taking verapamil.

- *Common:* headache, low blood pressure, dizziness, nausea, constipation, weakness, slow heartbeat, fluid retention, swelling of feet, tiredness, increased chest pain at the start of treatment, congestive heart failure, rash, shortness of breath, lung congestion, upper respiratory infection
- *Less Common or Rare:* chest pain, rapid or irregular heartbeat, dizziness upon rising, bleeding or tender gums, flushing and feeling of warmth, faintness, drowsiness, difficulty sleeping, dry mouth, impotence, breast development in males, increased urination, menstrual changes, upset stomach, diarrhea, sweating, pins and needles, numbness or coldness in the extremities, muscle cramps, abnormal growth of the gums, photosensitivity, antiplatelet effect

IMPORTANT PRECAUTIONS

Verapamil should not be taken if you have active liver disease, sick sinus syndrome, ventricular tachycardia, atrial fibrillation, heart block, congestive heart failure, or low blood pressure, or if you have ever experienced an allergic reaction to this drug in the past. Use verapamil with caution if you have aortic stenosis, liver or kidney impairment, impaired circulation to the fingers, a recent history of heart attack or stroke, muscular dystrophy, a narrowing of the stomach or intestines, or a previous allergic reaction to another calcium channel blocker.

This drug may cause side effects such as drowsiness and dizziness. Until you know how verapamil affects you, do not drive a car, operate machinery, or perform other tasks that require concentration.

When you first start taking this drug or when the dosage is increased, you may experience dizziness or faintness when you rise quickly from a sitting or reclining position (postural hypotension). Try to get up slowly, and consult your health-care practitioner if the problem continues.

Chest pain resulting from exercise is usually prevented by this drug. This may tempt you to be more active than you should. Ask your health-care practitioner what amount of exercise is appropriate. When you exercise in hot weather, use even greater care. Heavy sweating can lead to dizziness, lightheadedness, fainting, vomiting, dehydration, and low blood pressure.

Treatment for high blood pressure also entails careful attention to other aspects of your lifestyle. Your health-care practitioner will most likely recommend a diet that is low in salt and saturated fat. It is also important to maintain a healthy weight and to refrain from smoking. People taking verapamil must be closely monitored with regular blood tests, and should learn to check their pulses to monitor heart rate.

Before having any type of surgery or dental procedure, tell your surgeon or dentist that you are taking verapamil.

DRUG INTERACTIONS

Inform your health-care practitioner and pharmacist if you are taking any other prescription or over-the-counter drugs, as well as any vitamins, herbs, or other supplements. Drug interactions may include the following:

➤ Taking other blood pressure medications such as beta-blockers and digitalis can excessively increase the blood-pressure-lowering effects of verapamil. This type of combination must be carefully monitored by your health-care practitioner.

➤ Taking amiodarone with this drug may cause the heart to stop.

➤ Medications such as cimetidine, ranitidine, and ritonavir may increase the effects of verapamil.

➤ Antacids may reduce the effects of verapamil.

➤ Rifampin, barbiturates, antiseizure medications such as phenytoin, NSAIDs including aspirin, and sulfinpyrazone may reduce the blood-pressure-lowering effects of verapamil.

➤ Verapamil can increase blood levels of carbamazepine, cyclosporine, lithium, and theophylline to toxic levels.

- Combining verapamil with blood thinners such as warfarin may increase the risk of bleeding.
- Alcohol may further lower blood pressure. Use with caution.
- Tobacco may reduce the effectiveness of verapamil.
- Consult your health-care practitioner before taking over-the-counter cough, cold, sinus, allergy, or weight loss medications. Many of these can raise blood pressure.

FOOD, VITAMIN, AND HERBAL INTERACTIONS

Do not take verapamil with grapefruit juice or with high-fat meals. Do not take herbs that increase blood pressure, such as ephedra (ma huang), ginseng, goldenseal, licorice, and saw palmetto. Consult your health-care practitioner before taking substances that may lower blood pressure, such as magnesium, calcium, soy, or garlic.

RECOMMENDED DOSAGE

Verapamil is available as regular tablets and extended-release tablets or capsules. The doses given below are typical. However, doses are different for different patients, and only your health-care practitioner can determine the dose and schedule that are most appropriate for you.

- *Children:* This drug is not recommended for children.
- *Adults:* 120 to 480 mg daily in single or divided doses

Immediate-release verapamil products should be taken 1 hour before or 2 hours after meals. If they upset your stomach, sustained-release products may be taken with food or milk. Swallow them whole. If you miss a dose, take it as soon as you remember. However, if it is nearly time for your next scheduled dose, do not take the missed dose. Follow your regular dosing schedule. Never take a double dose. Do not suddenly stop taking verapamil without consulting your health-care practitioner. A gradual reduction in dosage is safest.

SYMPTOMS OF OVERDOSE AND WHAT TO DO

Symptoms of verapamil overdose may include low blood pressure, an irregular heartbeat, weakness, lightheadedness, flushed skin, sweating, fluid build-up in the lungs, and loss of consciousness. If you suspect that an overdose has occurred, seek immediate medical attention and take the prescription bottle to the hospital with you.

SPECIAL INFORMATION FOR PREGNANT OR NURSING WOMEN

No studies have adequately investigated the effects of verapamil during pregnancy or breastfeeding. However, birth defects have occurred in animal studies. Avoid taking verapamil during the first three months of pregnancy, and consult your health-care practitioner before taking this medication in your second or third trimester. Only a health-care practitioner can determine whether the potential benefits outweigh the risks. Since verapamil may pass into breast milk, your health-care practitioner may advise you to stop breastfeeding while taking this drug.

SPECIAL INFORMATION FOR SENIORS

Seniors may be more prone to side effects such as weakness, dizziness, and fainting, and may benefit from a lower dosage.

OPEN QUESTIONS OR CONTROVERSIES

Some studies have suggested that people taking calcium channel blockers several times a day (rather than once a day) are more likely to have a heart attack than those who take beta-blockers or similar medications. Ask your health-care practitioner which drug is the best choice for you.

GENERIC NAME

Verteporfin

BRAND NAME

Visudyne
No generic available

ABOUT THIS DRUG

Verteporfin is used to treat abnormal blood vessel formation in the eye. It is prescribed for conditions such as pathologic myopia, ocular histoplasmosis, and macular degeneration. Left untreated, these problems can lead to a loss of vision.

Verteporfin works in combination with a special laser light in a technique known as photodynamic therapy. This drug makes you more sensitive to the effects of all types of light.

SIDE EFFECTS

Consult your health-care practitioner if you develop side effects while taking this drug. Only he or she can determine whether it is safe for you to continue taking verteporfin.

- *Common:* blurred vision, other visual disturbances, headache, itching, pain, or other reactions at the injection site
- *Less Common or Rare:* potentially severe decrease in vision, eye pain or irritation, eye redness or itching, pounding in the ears, changes in heartbeat, pale skin, dizziness, tiredness, weakness, fainting, nervousness, difficulty breathing upon exertion, unusual bleeding or bruising, photosensitivity, skin redness, sunburn, sore throat, fever, trouble sleeping, cloudy urine, constipation, diarrhea, difficult urination, overall feeling of unwellness

IMPORTANT PRECAUTIONS

Always tell your health-care practitioner about any other medical conditions you may have, especially impaired liver function or porphyria. Inform your health-care practitioner if you have ever experienced an allergic reaction to this or similar medications.

You will be extra sensitive to sunlight and bright indoor lights for 5 days after a verteporfin injection. During this time, your health-care practitioner will instruct you to wear special sunglasses and avoid exposure to sunlight, sun lamps, halogen lighting, and lights in operating rooms or dentists' offices. Sunscreen *cannot* protect you from effects such as burning and blistering during this period. However, exposure to normal shaded lamps in your home should not be a problem.

This drug may cause side effects such as blurred vision. Until you know how verteporfin affects you, do not drive a car, operate machinery, or perform other tasks that require accurate vision.

People taking verteporfin should be closely monitored by their health-care practitioners.

DRUG INTERACTIONS

Inform your health-care practitioner and pharmacist if you are taking any other prescription or over-the-counter drugs, as well as any vitamins, herbs, or other supplements. Possible drug interactions include the following:

- Certain drugs may increase the effects of verteporfin. These include calcium channel blockers, polymyxin B, and medicines used in radiation therapy.

- Other drugs decrease the effects of verteporfin. These include dimethyl sulfoxide, medications that decrease blood clotting and blood vessel constriction, and alcohol.
- Drugs such as oral antidiabetes medications, griseofulvin, phenothiazines, sulfonamides, tetracycline antibiotics, and thiazide diuretics increase your skin's sensitivity to sunlight.

FOOD, VITAMIN, AND HERBAL INTERACTIONS

Consult your health-care practitioner before taking verteporfin with antioxidant vitamins or minerals. These may decrease the effects of verteporfin. Avoid herbs such as St. John's wort, which increases your skin's sensitivity to sunlight.

RECOMMENDED DOSAGE

Verteporfin is available by injection. Dosage is highly individualized and must be determined by your health-care practitioner. The injection is typically administered 15 minutes before exposure to laser light.

SYMPTOMS OF OVERDOSE AND WHAT TO DO

No specific information is available regarding verteporfin overdose. If you suspect that an overdose has occurred, seek immediate medical attention.

SPECIAL INFORMATION FOR PREGNANT OR NURSING WOMEN

No studies have adequately investigated the effects of verteporfin during pregnancy or breastfeeding. However, fetal damage has occurred in animal studies. If you are pregnant or plan to become pregnant, or if you are breastfeeding or plan to do so, talk with your health-care practitioner before starting this drug. Only a health-care practitioner can determine whether the potential benefits outweigh the potential dangers.

SPECIAL INFORMATION FOR SENIORS

The effects of verteporfin may be reduced in those over 75 years of age.

GENERIC NAME
Class: Vitamins

BRAND NAMES
Adeflor, Cari-Tab, Centrum, Florvite, Mulvidren-F, Polytabs-F, Poly-Vi-Flor, Soluvite, Theragran, Tri-Vi-Flor, Vi-Daylin, Vi-Daylin/F
Generic available

ABOUT THESE DRUGS
Vitamins are natural substances that your body needs for normal growth and development. Vitamin supplements are available both over-the-counter and by prescription. Normally a well-balanced diet containing a variety of foods provides all the vitamins required by most healthy people. (The body can also synthesize vitamin D from sunshine, and the intestines also produce vitamin K.) However, there are periods during which you may need extra vitamins. These include pregnancy, childhood, illness, and advancing age. People with poor diets also benefit from supplementation.

Thirteen vitamins are required by the body. These include the fat-soluble vitamins A, D, E, and K, and the water-soluble vitamin C (ascorbic acid) and the B vitamins (thiamine, riboflavin, niacin, pantothenic acid, biotin, vitamin B_6, vitamin B_{12}, and folate). Vitamins are required for essential functions such as growth, normal digestion, mental alertness, and resistance to infection. When the body is deficient in vitamins, disease results. For example, vitamin B_{12} deficiency can lead to pernicious anemia, and vitamin A deficiency can cause night blindness.

Vitamins are available in a wide variety of formulations. Many are combined with iron, calcium, and minerals. Vitamin supplements should never be used as a substitute for a healthy diet and lifestyle.

SIDE EFFECTS
Side effects are not common. However, consult your health-care practitioner if any effects are persistent or severe. Only he or she can determine whether it is safe for you to continue taking a vitamin supplement.

- *Common:* unpleasant taste
- *Less Common or Rare:* upset stomach

IMPORTANT PRECAUTIONS
Always tell your health-care practitioner about any other medical conditions you may have. These may call for special vitamin requirements.

Many vitamins are available in high-dose formulations. Do not take any special formulations without consulting your health-care practitioner.

DRUG INTERACTIONS

Inform your health-care practitioner and pharmacist if you are taking any other prescription or over-the-counter drugs, as well as any vitamins, herbs, or other supplements. In terms of drug interactions, consult your health-care practitioner before combining blood thinners such as warfarin with a multivitamin.

FOOD, VITAMIN, AND HERBAL INTERACTIONS

Do not use vitamin supplements as a substitute for a healthy, well-balanced diet. Only whole foods provide the ideal complex mix of vitamins, minerals, fiber, and other important food substances for optimal nutrition.

RECOMMENDED DOSAGE

Multivitamins come in regular tablets, chewable tablets, capsules, and liquid. They are typically taken once a day. Carefully follow your health-care practitioner's instructions and the directions on the prescription or package label on how to take them. If vitamins come in a dropper bottle, use the specially marked dropper to measure each dose. Do not take higher than recommended doses of vitamins.

SYMPTOMS OF OVERDOSE AND WHAT TO DO

Megadoses of vitamins can lead to serious problems. For example, high doses of niacin can aggravate stomach ulcers. If you develop any unusual symptoms while taking a vitamin supplement and suspect that an overdose has occurred, seek immediate medical attention and take the bottle to the hospital with you.

SPECIAL INFORMATION FOR PREGNANT OR NURSING WOMEN

Consult your health-care practitioner if you are or are planning to become pregnant. Obstetricians usually prescribe special formulations of vitamins to meet the nutritional needs of pregnant and nursing women.

SPECIAL INFORMATION FOR SENIORS

Seniors may benefit from special formulations of vitamins designed to meet the nutritional requirements of older people.

GENERIC NAME
Warfarin

BRAND NAMES
Carfin, Coumadin, Panwarfin, Sofarin
Generic available

ABOUT THIS DRUG
Warfarin is an anticoagulant or blood thinner used to prevent blood clots from forming or growing larger. It is prescribed for the prevention or treatment of blood clots in veins or arteries; to prevent or treat blood clots that may arise from certain heart disorders or heart valve replacement; to prevent blood clots that may form anywhere in the body after a heart attack; to prevent another heart attack or a stroke after a heart attack; and to prevent blood clots from forming in the lungs after hip replacement surgery.

Warfarin works by inhibiting the production of 4 vitamin K–dependent blood-clotting factors. This drug must be used with extreme caution, because even at correct therapeutic doses it may cause minor bleeding episodes.

SIDE EFFECTS
The most serious side effect of warfarin is bleeding or hemorrhaging. Less frequently, treatment can lead to skin tissue damage or death (necrosis). Contact your health-care practitioner at once if you experience symptoms such as pain (which may occur anywhere in the body), swelling, black or bloody stools, blood in urine, nose bleeds, excessive bleeding from the gums, vomiting blood, excessive bruising, skin inflammation or rash, purple toes, headache, dizziness, weakness, numbness and tingling, unusually heavy menstrual bleeding, low blood pressure, shortness of breath, paralysis, or shock. Always report any other side effects that are severe or prolonged, and ask your health-care practitioner whether it is safe for you to continue taking this drug.

- *Common:* minor bruising or bleeding from razor cuts or after brushing teeth
- *Less Common or Rare:* headache, stomach upset or pain, diarrhea, fever, rash, tiredness, lethargy, unexplained fever, chills, sore throat, fluid retention, taste changes, intolerance to cold, vomiting, loss of hair, overall feeling of unwellness, allergic reactions, purple toes, yellow eyes or skin, liver damage

IMPORTANT PRECAUTIONS

Always tell your health-care practitioner about any other medical conditions you may have, especially a blood clotting disorder such as hemophilia, a stomach ulcer, colitis, an arterial aneurysm, high blood pressure, congestive heart failure, infective pericarditis, endocarditis, esophageal varices, a blood disorder such as low blood platelets, preeclampsia or eclampsia, heavy menstrual bleeding, diabetes, or liver or kidney disease. Inform your health-care practitioner if you have had a recent stroke, spinal tap, or lumbar block (anesthesia).

Watch for signs of unusual bleeding, such as excessive bleeding from a minor shaving cut, bleeding gums, or blood in urine or feces. Immediately report these signs to your health-care practitioner, who may need to adjust your dosage.

Because this drug increases the risk of serious bleeding, avoid activities with a high risk of injury.

Regular blood tests are essential while you take warfarin. Your health-care practitioner must carefully monitor your prothrombin time and INR (the clotting process) while you are being treated with this medication.

Tell your health-care practitioner or dentist that you are taking warfarin before undergoing any procedure. Because serious bleeding can occur during surgery or dental work, you must stop taking this drug several days before any operation takes place.

Warfarin may cause side effects such as dizziness. Until you know how this drug affects you, do not drive a car, operate machinery, or perform other tasks that require concentration.

DRUG INTERACTIONS

Anticoagulants like warfarin have a high number of drug interactions. Always inform your health-care practitioner and pharmacist if you are taking any other prescription or over-the-counter drugs, as well as any vitamins, herbs, or other supplements. Possible drug interactions include the following:

- Combining warfarin with aspirin and other NSAIDs increases the risk of bleeding.
- Many other drugs also increase the effects of warfarin. These include acarbose, acetaminophen, allopurinol, alteplase, amiodarone, amprenavir, androgens, azithromycin, bismuth subsalicylate, calcium channel blockers, carbamazepine, cephalosporins, chloral hydrate, chloramphenicol, cimetidine, ciprofloxacin, cisapride, clarithromycin, clofibrate, clopidogrel, cloxacillin, clotrimazole, COX-2 inhibitors, disopyramide, disulfiram, enoxaparin, erythromycin, flu-

conazole, fluoxetine, fluvastatin, fluvoxamine, gemfibrozil, glucagon, heparin, influenza vaccine, isoniazid, itraconazole, ketoconazole, metronidazole, miconazole, minocycline, omeprazole, orlistat, paroxetine, pravastatin, propranolol, quinidine, quetiapine, ranitidine, sertraline, simvastatin, sulfonamides, tamoxifen, terbinafine, testosterone, tetracycline, thyroid hormones, tramadol, trastuzumab, tricyclic antidepressants, trimethoprim-sulfamethoxazole, vancomycin, zafirlukast, and zileuton.

- Many other drugs decrease the effects of warfarin. These include barbiturates, birth control pills, carbamazepine, chlordiazepoxide, cholestyramine, estrogens, glutethimide, griseofulvin, phenobarbital, primidone, rifampin, spironolactone, sucralfate, antithyroid drugs, and thiazide diuretics.
- Warfarin may increase the effects of oral hypoglycemic agents.
- Warfarin may decrease the effects of cyclosporine.
- Warfarin may increase or decrease the effects of phenytoin.

FOOD, VITAMIN, AND HERBAL INTERACTIONS

Do not take vitamin K with warfarin. Consult your health-care practitioner before taking any herb or other dietary supplement with this drug. Warfarin may interact with garlic, ginkgo, bromelain, dong quai, St. John's wort, danshen, and coenzyme Q10. St John's wort and ginseng may decrease blood levels of warfarin, whereas gingko increases bleeding risk with warfarin.

Speak to your health-care practitioner before making any dietary changes while taking warfarin. It is especially important to avoid increasing your consumption of foods that are rich in vitamin K, such as green leafy vegetables, asparagus, broccoli, and cauliflower.

RECOMMENDED DOSAGE

Warfarin comes as a tablet. The doses given below are typical. However, only your health-care practitioner can determine the dose and schedule that best fit your individual needs.

- *Children:* This drug is not recommended for children.
- *Adults:* 2 to 5 mg daily to start; average ongoing maintenance dose is 2 to 10 mg daily

Warfarin is best taken on an empty stomach. If you miss a dose, take it as soon as you remember. If it is almost time for the next dose, skip it and resume your regular schedule. Never take a double dose.

It is especially important to take warfarin exactly as directed by your health-care practitioner. Record any missed doses and report them to your health-care practitioner. Missing doses will affect your regular blood clotting tests.

SYMPTOMS OF OVERDOSE AND WHAT TO DO

Symptoms of warfarin overdose are internal or external bleeding. Signs of internal bleeding are blood in the stools or urine or excessive and unusual bruising. If you suspect that an overdose has occurred, seek immediate medical attention and take the prescription bottle to the hospital with you.

SPECIAL INFORMATION FOR PREGNANT OR NURSING WOMEN

Warfarin has caused fetal hemorrhage and death in animal studies, and there have been reports of similar problems in women. If you are pregnant or plan to become pregnant, speak to your health-care practitioner before starting this drug. Because warfarin may pass into breast milk, your health-care practitioner may advise you to stop breastfeeding while taking it.

SPECIAL INFORMATION FOR SENIORS

Seniors may be more sensitive to side effects and may benefit from lower doses.

GENERIC NAME

Class: Xanthine bronchodilators

Generics: (1) aminophylline; (2) dyphylline; (3) oxtriphylline; (4) theophylline

BRAND NAMES

(1) Phyllocontin, Truphylline; (2) Dilor, Dilor-400, Lufyllin, Lufyllin-400, Neothylline; (3) Choledyl SA; (4) Aerolate, Aquaphyllin, Asmalix, Bronkodyl, Elixomin, Elixophyllin, Lanophyllin, Quibron-T Dividose, Quibron-T/SR Dividose, Respbid, Slo-bid Gyrocaps, Slo-Phyllin, Slo-Phyllin Gyrocaps, Sustaire, T-Phyl, Theo-24, Theo-Dur, Theo-Sav, Theo-X, Theobid Duracaps, Theochron, Theoclear-80, Theoclear L.A., Theochron, Theolair, Theolair-SR, Theospan-SR, Theostat-80, Theovent, Uniphyl

Generic available

ABOUT THESE DRUGS

Xanthine bronchodilators are used to prevent and treat wheezing, shortness of breath, and troubled breathing caused by asthma, chronic bronchitis, emphysema, and other lung diseases. Dyphylline is associated with fewer drug interactions than other drugs in this group.

Xanthine bronchodilators work by relaxing and opening air passages in the lungs, making it easier to breathe. They also dilate bronchial tubes that are in constriction.

SIDE EFFECTS

Side effects are directly linked to dosage. Speak to your health-care practitioner if you develop side effects while taking one of these drugs. Only he or she can determine whether your dosage must be adjusted and if you should continue taking a xanthine bronchodilator.

- *Common:* nervousness, restlessness, irritability, headache, nausea, vomiting, upset stomach, stomach pain, diarrhea, difficulty sleeping
- *Less Common or Rare:* irregular heartbeat, heart palpitations, increased heart rate, excitability, muscle spasms and twitching, fever, headache, rash, seizures, brain damage, death

IMPORTANT PRECAUTIONS

Tell your health-care practitioner about any other medical conditions you may have, especially stomach ulcers, heart disease, congestive heart failure, high blood pressure, a heart rhythm disorder, thyroid disease, impaired liver or kidney function, or seizures. Inform your health-care practitioner if you have ever experienced an allergic reaction to one of these medications.

Because xanthine bronchodilators may cause side effects such as nervousness and restlessness, do not drive a car, operate machinery, or perform other tasks that require concentration until you know how the medication you are taking affects you.

These drugs have a very narrow therapeutic range in which they successfully treat your problem but do not cause side effects. Side effects may be severe and potentially fatal. For example, theophylline may cause or worsen heart rhythm disturbances, and in rare cases has been associated with convulsions and death. Since side effects are linked to the amount of medication in your blood, your health-care practitioner will closely monitor you with regular blood tests while you take a xanthine bronchodilator.

DRUG INTERACTIONS

Tell your health-care practitioner if you are taking any other prescription or over-the-counter drugs, as well as any vitamins, herbs, or supplements. Possible drug interactions include the following:

- Taking more than 1 xanthine bronchodilator at a time increases the risk of side effects.
- Many drugs increase the effects of xanthine bronchodilators. These include flu vaccine, allopurinol, beta-blockers, calcium channel blockers, cimetidine, oral contraceptives, corticosteroids, disulfiram, ephedrine, erythromycin, interferon, quinolone antiinfectives, and thiabendazole.
- Drugs that decrease xanthine bronchodilator effects include aminoglutethimide, barbiturates, charcoal, ketoconazole, rifampin, and phenytoin.
- Xanthine bronchodilators may interact with drugs used in anesthesia.
- Other drugs that may interact with xanthine bronchodilators include benzodiazepines, carbamazepine, isoniazid, lithium, probenecid, and loop diuretics.
- Tobacco and marijuana reduce the effectiveness of xanthine bronchodilators.
- Check with your health-care practitioner before using over-the-counter drugs. Many cold, cough, allergy, sinus, and weight loss remedies can raise blood pressure.

FOOD, VITAMIN, AND HERBAL INTERACTIONS

Do not take herbs such as ephedra (ma huang), ginseng, or kola with xanthine bronchodilators. Avoid caffeinated products such as chocolate, coffee, tea, and cola while you are taking these drugs. Caffeine is a xanthine derivative.

Consult your health-care practitioner before making any dietary changes while taking a xanthine bronchodilator. These may change the way you absorb medication. A daily B vitamin supplement may be beneficial.

RECOMMENDED DOSAGE

Xanthine bronchodilators come in many forms, including tablets, capsules, suspensions, and elixirs. Children typically require larger doses than adults. The sustained-release forms are taken to prevent symptoms, while the immediate-release forms are taken to relieve an acute attack. Do not change types or brands of medication without consulting your health-care practitioner. The doses given below are typical. However, the dose and schedule of xanthine bronchodilators are carefully calibrated to fit each individual's needs.

Aminophylline

- *Children Younger than 16 Years:* 1 to 2.5 mg per pound of body weight every 6 hours
- *Children 16 Years and Older and Adults:* 100 to 200 mg every 6 hours; dosage of sustained-release forms is 200 to 500 mg daily in divided doses

Dyphylline

- *Children:* This drug is not recommended for children.
- *Adults:* Up to 7 mg per pound of body weight up to 4 times daily

Oxtriphylline

- *Children 1 to 9 Years:* 2.8 mg per pound of body weight 4 times daily
- *Children 10 Years and Older and Adults:* 2 mg per pound of body weight 3 times daily; dosage of sustained-release forms is 400 to 600 mg every 12 hours

Theophylline

- *Children Younger than 1 Year:* Consult your health-care practitioner.
- *Children 1 to 8 Years:* Up to 10.9 mg per pound of body weight daily
- *Children 9 to 11 Years:* Up to 9 mg per pound of body weight daily
- *Children 12 to 16 Years:* Up to 8.1 mg per pound of body weight daily
- *Children Older than 16 Years and Adults:* Up to 6 mg per pound of body weight daily, to a maximum daily dosage of 900 mg

It is important to take xanthine bronchodilators exactly as prescribed. Taking even a small amount of medication in excess of the amount prescribed may constitute an overdose, resulting in dangerous side effects. Medication is more effective when taken on an empty stomach, at least 1 hour before or 2 hours after meals. If you forget a dose, take it as soon as you remember. If it is almost time for the next dose, skip the one you missed and resume your normal schedule. Never take a double dose.

SYMPTOMS OF OVERDOSE AND WHAT TO DO

Symptoms of xanthine bronchodilator overdose may include nausea, vomiting, loss of appetite, difficulty sleeping, nervousness, restlessness, and headache. These symptoms may progress to abnormal heart rhythms, convulsions, and collapse. If overdose occurs, seek immediate medical attention and take the prescription bottle to the hospital with you.

SPECIAL INFORMATION FOR PREGNANT OR NURSING WOMEN

Although xanthine bronchodilators are not believed to cause birth defects, they should be taken during pregnancy only when absolutely necessary. Infants born to mothers taking these drugs may be nervous and irritable and gag when they feed. If you are breast-feeding or plan to do so, talk with your health-care practitioner before starting one of these drugs. Xanthine bronchodilators may pass into breast milk and make babies nervous and irritable. Only a health-care practitioner can determine whether the potential benefits outweigh these dangers.

SPECIAL INFORMATION FOR SENIORS

Seniors are more susceptible to side effects and require lower doses of xanthine bronchodilators.

GENERIC NAME

Zafirlukast

see Leukotriene Antagonist/Inhibitors, page 600

GENERIC NAME

Zalcitabine

BRAND NAMES

Dideoxycytidine, ddC, Hivid

No generic available

ABOUT THIS DRUG

Zalcitabine is an antiviral drug used to treat HIV, the human immunodeficiency virus that causes acquired immune deficiency syndrome (AIDS). It is typically prescribed in combination with zidovudine (AZT) and other antiretroviral drugs.

Zalcitabine interferes with the reproduction of HIV, which slows the progression of this virus and the breakdown of the immune system.

SIDE EFFECTS

Side effects are common and may be severe (especially in those with advanced HIV). They include peripheral neuropathy, pancreatitis (inflammation of the pancreas), liver failure, weakening of the heart, and ulcers in the mouth and esophagus. Contact your health-care practitioner at once if you develop any persistent or severe side effects while taking this drug. Only he or she can determine if you should continue to take zalcitabine.

- *Common:* abdominal pain, nausea, vomiting, appetite loss, weight loss, muscle and joint pain, fatigue, headache, mouth sores, rash, hives, itching, tingling, pins and needles, numbness, and burning in the extremities
- *Less Common or Rare:* diarrhea, constipation, fever, stomach irritation and ulcers, changes in blood components, anemia, dark urine, yellow eyes or skin, pale stools, liver and pancreas damage, weakening of the heart, ulcers in the mouth and esophagus, convulsions

IMPORTANT PRECAUTIONS

Tell your health-care practitioner about any other medical conditions you suffer from, especially peripheral neuritis, peripheral nerve damage, pancreatitis, severe myelosuppression, esophageal ulcers, congestive heart failure, cardiac muscle damage, kidney or liver impairment, or a history of alcoholism. Inform your health-care practitioner if you have ever experienced an allergic reaction to this or similar drugs.

Nerve damage may occur when taking zalcitabine. One in 3 people with advanced HIV may develop peripheral neuropathy, with initial symptoms such as tingling, pins and needles, numbness, and burning in the extremities. Report these symptoms to your health-care practitioner at once. He or she may advise you to stop taking this drug to prevent further damage.

People with advanced HIV may also be more susceptible to pancreatitis when taking zalcitabine. Call your health-care practitioner immediately if you develop symptoms such as severe abdominal pain, tense abdominal muscles, fever, sweating, shallow breathing, nausea, and vomiting.

Zalcitabine does not cure HIV or AIDS. You may still develop complications such as opportunistic infections. It is important to be monitored with regular physical exams and blood tests while taking this medication.

Zalcitabine does not prevent you from passing on HIV to others. Therefore it is important to always practice safe sex while taking this drug.

DRUG INTERACTIONS

Tell your health-care practitioner and pharmacist if you are taking any other prescription or over-the-counter drugs, as well as any vitamins, herbs, or other supplements. Possible drug interactions include the following:

- Zalcitabine increases the absorption of AZT, making it more effective.
- Do not take zalcitabine with lamivudine.
- Zalcitabine should not be taken with other drugs that irritate the pancreas or are associated with peripheral neuropathy.
- Cimetidine and probenecid may lead to toxic levels of zalcitabine.
- Metoclopramide may reduce the effects of zalcitabine.

FOOD, VITAMIN, AND HERBAL INTERACTIONS

When taking HIV medications, it is especially important to follow your health-care practitioner's dietary recommendations. Do not take echinacea if you have a damaged immune system.

RECOMMENDED DOSAGE

Zalcitabine comes as a tablet. Although the doses given below are typical, only your health-care practitioner can determine the dose and schedule that are most appropriate for you. Dosage is reduced for people with impaired kidney function.

- *Children:* This drug is not recommended for children under the age of 13.
- *Children Older than 12 Years and Adults:* 0.75 mg every 8 hours

Zalcitabine should be taken on an empty stomach, 1 hour before or 2 hours after meals. It is essential to take zalcitabine exactly as prescribed. If you miss a dose, take it as soon as you remember. However, if it is nearly time for your next scheduled dose, do not take the missed dose. Follow your regular dosing schedule. Never take a double dose. Call your health-care practitioner if you forget several doses in a row.

SYMPTOMS OF OVERDOSE AND WHAT TO DO

Symptoms of zalcitabine overdose may include nausea, vomiting, diarrhea, stomach pain, drowsiness, liver toxicity, and hand and foot pain. If overdose does occur, seek medical attention immediately, and bring the prescription bottle with you to the hospital so that health-care practitioners will know exactly what drug was used.

SPECIAL INFORMATION FOR PREGNANT OR NURSING WOMEN

High doses of zalcitabine have caused birth defects in animals. Do not use this drug unless the benefits of therapy clearly outweigh the potential risks to the fetus.

Zalcitabine may pass into breast milk, and HIV can be transferred by breast milk. Bottle-feeding is preferable.

SPECIAL INFORMATION FOR SENIORS

Smaller doses of zalcitabine are usually appropriate for seniors, due to their lower levels of kidney function.

GENERIC NAME

Zaleplon

BRAND NAME

Sonata

No generic available

ABOUT THIS DRUG

Zaleplon is used on a short-term basis to treat insomnia. It works by attaching to a specific site in the brain. This drug has less of a "hang-over" effect than many other sleeping pills.

SIDE EFFECTS

Side effects are generally mild. However, consult your health-care practitioner if you develop any persistent or severe effects while using zaleplon. Only he or she can determine whether it is safe for you to continue using this drug.

- *Common:* headache, dizziness, tiredness, memory loss, abdominal pain, muscle aches, weakness
- *Less Common or Rare:* drowsiness, daytime sleepiness, weakness, tingling in the hands and feet, fever, difficulty swallowing, visual disturbances, sensitivity to light, eye pain, ear pain, sensitivity to noise, muscle pain, menstrual pain, nausea, stomach upset, anxiety, tremor, hallucinations, sensation of unreality, swelling of the hands and feet

IMPORTANT PRECAUTIONS

Inform your health-care practitioner about any other medical conditions you may have, especially kidney or liver impairment or respiratory disease. Tell your health-care practitioner if you have ever experienced an allergic reaction to this or similar drugs.

Zaleplon is recommended for short-term use only. If you need to take this drug for longer than 7 to 10 days, consult your health-care practitioner. Zaleplon should not be taken for more than a few weeks. Long-term use can lead to physical and/or psychological addiction. This drug should be used with caution in anyone with a history of drug or alcohol abuse or depression.

Zaleplon can make you drowsy and less alert than usual. Until you know how this drug affects you, do not drive a car, operate machinery, or perform other tasks that require concentration.

DRUG INTERACTIONS

Tell your health-care practitioner and pharmacist if you are taking any other prescription or over-the-counter drugs, as well as any vitamins, herbs, or other supplements. Dosage adjustments may be necessary when you begin taking zaleplon. Possible drug interactions include the following:

- Zaleplon may add to drowsiness and other effects of central nervous system depressants (such as antidepressants, antihistamines, muscle relaxants, narcotics, and sedatives).
- Cimetidine may increase the effects of zaleplon.
- Rifampin may decrease the effects of zaleplon.
- Zaleplon may increase the effects of chlorpromazine.
- Do not combine zaleplon and diphenhydramine.
- Do not drink alcohol while taking zaleplon. This combination worsens coordination and impairs mental function.

FOOD, VITAMIN, AND HERBAL INTERACTIONS

Do not take zaleplon with hops, kava, passionflower, and valerian. These can increase its sedative effects. Stimulating herbs such as ephedra (ma huang), kola, and ginseng should also be avoided, as should caffeinated products including chocolate, coffee, tea, and cola.

RECOMMENDED DOSAGE

Zaleplon comes as a tablet. Although the doses given below are typical, only your health-care practitioner can determine the dose and schedule that best fit your needs.

- *Children:* Zaleplon is not recommended for children.
- *Adults:* 5 to 10 mg at bedtime

Zaleplon should be taken on an empty stomach. If you forget a dose, skip it and resume your normal schedule. Never take a double dose. If you have been taking zaleplon for a few weeks, do not stop taking it suddenly. Abrupt withdrawal can lead to sleep disturbances and anxiety. Speak to your health-care practitioner about gradually reducing dosage. You may experience sleeping difficulties the first night or two after stopping this medication ("rebound insomnia").

SYMPTOMS OF OVERDOSE AND WHAT TO DO

Symptoms of zaleplon overdose may include dizziness, tiredness, and an inability to concentrate. If overdose occurs, seek immediate medical attention and take the prescription bottle to the hospital with you.

SPECIAL INFORMATION FOR PREGNANT OR NURSING WOMEN

Do not take zaleplon if you are pregnant or planning to become pregnant. This drug is associated with an increased risk of birth effects. Since zaleplon may pass into breast milk, breastfeeding is not advisable while taking this medication.

SPECIAL INFORMATION FOR SENIORS

Side effects are more likely to occur in older people. Smaller doses are recommended.

GENERIC NAME

Zanamivir

BRAND NAME

Relenza

No generic available

ABOUT THIS DRUG

Zanamivir is an antiviral drug used to shorten the duration of the flu. This drug is prescribed for influenza types A and B. In order to be effective, it must be taken in the first 2 days of showing symptoms of the virus. Although zanamivir cannot cure the flu, it may shorten its duration by at least a day. Zanamivir works by blocking the flu virus from making copies of itself and infecting new cells.

SIDE EFFECTS

If you develop breathing difficulties or wheezing while taking zanamivir, stop taking it and call your health-care practitioner immediately. Always report any other severe or persistent effects to your health-care practitioner. Only he or she can determine whether it is safe for you to continue taking this drug.

- *Common:* nausea, vomiting, diarrhea, headache, dizziness, nasal irritation, stuffy nose, sinus irritation, bronchitis, ear, nose, and throat infections
- *Less Common or Rare:* fatigue, joint or muscle pain, overall feeling of unwellness, fever, rash, itching, bleeding in the ear, nose, or throat, allergic reactions, heartbeat irregularities, breathing difficulties, asthma

IMPORTANT PRECAUTIONS

Zanamivir is not a cure for the flu. You are still contagious while you are taking this medicine. Older people and others at risk should continue to receive yearly flu shots to prevent this virus.

Always tell your health-care practitioner about all other medical conditions from which you suffer, especially liver disease and asthma or other lung disorders. Zanamivir should be used with extreme caution in these cases. Do not use zanamivir if you have experienced an allergic reaction to this or any similar medication in the past.

Zanamivir may cause side effects such as dizziness. Until you know how this drug affects you, do not drive a car, operate machinery, or engage in other actions that require concentration.

DRUG INTERACTIONS

Although no specific drug interactions are known, always tell your health-care practitioner and pharmacist if you are taking any other prescription or over-the-counter drugs, as well as any vitamins, herbs, or other supplements.

FOOD, VITAMIN, AND HERBAL INTERACTIONS

No food, vitamin, or herbal interactions have been noted.

RECOMMENDED DOSAGE

Zanamivir comes as an oral inhalation from a Diskhaler. The dose and schedule below are standard. You must take the first dose within 48 hours of the beginning of symptoms, and complete the entire 5-day course of treatment.

- *Children:* This drug is not recommended for children under 7.

➤ *Children 7 Years and Older and Adults:* 2 inhalations twice daily for 5 days. Allow at least 2 hours between doses on the first day, and try to allow 12 hours between doses on subsequent days.

Make sure that you do not have any food in your mouth when you inhale a dose of zanamivir. If you miss a dose, take it as soon as you remember. However, if it is nearly time for your next scheduled dose, do not take the missed dose. Follow your regular dosing schedule. Never take a double dose.

SYMPTOMS OF OVERDOSE AND WHAT TO DO

No specific information is available regarding zanamivir overdose. If you suspect an overdose, seek immediate medical attention, and bring the prescription container to the hospital with you.

SPECIAL INFORMATION FOR PREGNANT OR NURSING WOMEN

No studies have adequately investigated the effects of zanamivir during pregnancy or breastfeeding. If you are pregnant or plan to become pregnant, or if you are breastfeeding or plan to do so, talk with your health-care practitioner before starting this drug. Only a health-care practitioner can determine whether the potential benefits outweigh the potential dangers.

SPECIAL INFORMATION FOR SENIORS

There are no special instructions for seniors.

GENERIC NAME

Zidovudine

BRAND NAME

Retrovir
No generic available

ABOUT THIS DRUG

Zidovudine—more commonly known as AZT—is an antiviral drug used to treat HIV, the human immunodeficiency virus that causes acquired immune deficiency syndrome (AIDS). This drug is also prescribed to prevent the transmission of HIV from mother to infant. It is typically taken in combination with other antiretroviral drugs such as zanamivir.

Zidovudine interferes with essential enzyme systems, which slows the growth and reproduction of HIV and thus the breakdown of the immune system.

SIDE EFFECTS

Side effects are common and may be severe, especially in those with advanced HIV and people who begin treatment later in the course of their infection. Effects may include liver damage, muscle disorders, lactic acidosis (a potentially fatal metabolic imbalance), and blood diseases such as severe anemia and granulocytopenia (characterized by a sharp decrease in white blood cells known as granulocytes). Contact your health-care practitioner at once if you develop any persistent or severe side effects while taking this drug. Only he or she can determine if you should continue to take zidovudine.

➤ *Common:* nausea, vomiting, appetite loss, indigestion, stomach and intestinal pain, constipation, diarrhea, muscle pain, weakness, dizziness, fever, sweating, overall feeling of unwellness, difficulty breathing, rash, tingling, pins and needles, numbness, and burning in the extremities

➤ *Less Common or Rare:* sore throat, flu-like symptoms, headache, nervousness, anxiety, depression, moodiness, decreased mental acuity, confusion, fainting, fatigue, altered taste, acne, lip or mouth sores, bleeding gums, nosebleeds, swollen mouth or tongue, sinus inflammation, loss of speech, difficulty swallowing, hearing loss, muscle irritation and abnormalities, twitching, tremors, seizures, abnormal bleeding or bruising, changes in blood components, anemia, reduced white blood cell counts, esophageal ulcers, liver damage

IMPORTANT PRECAUTIONS

Tell your health-care practitioner about any other medical conditions you suffer from, especially bone marrow suppression, kidney or liver impairment, or a folic acid or vitamin B_{12} deficiency. Inform your health-care practitioner if you have ever experienced an allergic reaction to this or similar drugs.

Zidovudine does not cure HIV or AIDS. You may still develop complications such as opportunistic infections. It is important to be monitored with regular physical exams and blood tests while taking this medication.

Zidovudine does not prevent you from passing on HIV to others. Therefore it is important to always practice safe sex while taking this drug.

Zidovudine may cause side effects such as dizziness. Until you know how this drug affects you, do not drive a car, operate machinery, or engage in other actions that require concentration.

DRUG INTERACTIONS

Tell your health-care practitioner and pharmacist if you are taking any other prescription or over-the-counter drugs, as well as any vitamins, herbs, or other supplements. Possible drug interactions include the following:

- Zidovudine is often combined with other antiretroviral drugs in the treatment of HIV.
- Certain drugs may increase the effects and possibly the toxicity of zidovudine. These include acetaminophen, acyclovir, aspirin, benzodiazepines, cimetidine, fluconazole, ganciclovir, indomethacin, interferon, methadone, morphine, probenecid, and sulfonamides.
- Combining zidovudine with drugs such as dapsone and didanosine may increase the risk of bone marrow suppression.
- Nimodipine may increase nerve toxicity when taken with zidovudine.
- Rifampin, ritonavir, and stavudine may reduce the effects of zidovudine.

FOOD, VITAMIN, AND HERBAL INTERACTIONS

When taking HIV medications, it is especially important to follow your health-care practitioner's dietary recommendations. Do not take echinacea if you have a damaged immune system. Vitamin supplementation may be beneficial.

RECOMMENDED DOSAGE

Zidovudine comes as a capsule, tablet, and syrup. Although the doses given below are typical, only your health-care practitioner can determine the dose and schedule that are most appropriate for you. Dosage is reduced for people with liver or kidney impairment.

- *Children Older than 3 Months:* Consult your health-care practitioner.
- *Adults:* 500 to 600 mg daily in divided doses

Zidovudine should be taken on an empty stomach. However, if it upsets your stomach, ask your health-care practitioner about taking this drug with food. Take medicine with a full (8-ounce) glass of water and do not lie down for an hour afterward.

It is essential to take zidovudine exactly as prescribed. Adults with symptomatic AIDS must take doses every 4 hours around the clock, even if this means interrupting sleep.

If you miss a dose, take it as soon as you remember. However, if it is nearly time for your next scheduled dose, do not take the missed dose. Follow your regular dosing schedule. Never take a double dose. Call your health-care practitioner if you forget several doses in a row.

SYMPTOMS OF OVERDOSE AND WHAT TO DO

Symptoms of zidovudine overdose may include nausea, vomiting, diarrhea, and bone marrow suppression. If overdose occurs, seek medical attention immediately, and bring the prescription bottle with you to the hospital so that health-care practitioners will know exactly what drug was used.

SPECIAL INFORMATION FOR PREGNANT OR NURSING WOMEN

Zidovudine is given to HIV-infected pregnant women to prevent the transmission of HIV to fetuses. Treatment should begin after 14 weeks of pregnancy.

Zidovudine may pass into breast milk, and HIV can be transferred by breast milk. Bottle-feeding is preferable.

SPECIAL INFORMATION FOR SENIORS

Seniors face a greater risk of side effects of zidovudine due to their lower levels of kidney function.

GENERIC NAME

Zileuton

see Leukotriene Antagonist/Inhibitors, page 600

GENERIC NAME

Ziprasidone

BRAND NAME

Geodon
Generic available

ABOUT THIS DRUG

Ziprasidone is an antipsychotic drug used to treat schizophrenia. This is a serious disorder characterized by disturbances in thinking, behavior, and emotional reactions.

Ziprasidone works by blocking the action of serotonin and dopamine, two mood-modifying chemicals in the brain.

SIDE EFFECTS

If any effects become persistent or severe, consult your health-care practitioner. Only he or she can determine whether it is safe for you to continue taking this drug and whether it is necessary to readjust your dosage.

- *Common:* nausea, constipation, diarrhea, stomach discomfort or pain, indigestion, sour or acid stomach, heartburn, belching, restlessness, weakness, loss of strength, loss of balance, uncontrollable body movements, twisting movements, jerking, stiffness, shuffling walk, muscle trembling, difficulty speaking, drooling, rash, weight gain
- *Less Common or Rare:* fast, irregular, or pounding heartbeat or pulse, heart palpitations, loss of appetite, weight loss, dry mouth, muscle aches or tightness, dizziness upon standing, stuffy or runny nose, sneezing, increased blinking or eyelid spasms, changes in vision, cracked or scaly skin, itching or reddening of skin, swelling, unusual facial expressions, dizziness, faintness, persistent and painful erection, seizures, symptoms of tardive dyskinesia (such as lip smacking or puckering, wormlike movements of the tongue, inability to move eyes, trouble speaking, difficulty breathing or swallowing, tics, twitching, and slow, rhythmical, involuntary movements)

People taking antipsychotic drugs may experience a rare but life-threatening set of side effects known as neuroleptic malignant syndrome (NMS). Symptoms include fever, difficulty breathing, rapid heartbeat, rigid muscles, mental changes, increased sweating, irregular blood pressure, and convulsions. Immediate medical attention is required.

Side effects such as lip smacking, wormlike movements of the tongue, and slow, rhythmical, involuntary movements are characteristic of a disorder known as tardive dyskinesia. Older adults (especially women) are more susceptible to this condition, which may become permanent. If you experience tardive dyskinesia, your health-care practitioner will probably advise you to stop taking this drug.

IMPORTANT PRECAUTIONS

Always inform your health-care practitioner about all other medical conditions you suffer from, especially heart disease, an irregular heartbeat, heart failure, or a recent heart attack. Ziprasidone may worsen these conditions. Low blood levels of magnesium or potassium may also increase your risk for heart problems. Neuroleptic malignant syndrome and tardive dyskinesia may appear or worsen during treatment with ziprasidone. This drug may increase the risk of seizures and aspiration pneumonia in people who have Alzheimer's disease or a history of seizures. Tell your health-care practitioner if you have experienced a previous allergic reaction to this or similar drugs.

Before having any type of surgery, dental procedure, emergency treatment, medical test, or general or spinal anesthesia, tell your health-care practitioner or dentist that you are taking ziprasidone. You should be monitored with regular blood tests while taking this medication.

If ziprasidone causes dry mouth, use sugarless gum or hard candy, ice chips, or a saliva substitute. Consult your health-care practitioner or dentist if the problem continues.

This drug may cause side effects such as drowsiness and sleepiness. Until you know how ziprasidone affects you, do not drive a car, operate machinery, or perform other tasks that demand concentration.

This medicine may make you oversensitive to cold or heat. Drink plenty of fluids and avoid extreme heat. Be especially careful when you exercise in hot weather or enter a hot bath or sauna. Overheating may result in heatstroke.

When you first start taking ziprasidone or when the dosage is increased, you may experience dizziness or faintness when you rise quickly from a sitting or reclining position (postural hypotension). Try to get up slowly, and consult your health-care practitioner if the problem continues.

DRUG INTERACTIONS

Inform your health-care practitioner and pharmacist if you are taking any other prescription or over-the-counter drugs, as well as any vitamins, herbs, or other supplements. Possible drug interactions include the following:

- Combining ziprasidone with certain drugs may increase the risk of heart problems. These include dofetilide, moxifloxacin, pimozide, quinidine, sotalol, sparfloxacin, and thioridazine.
- Speak to your health-care practitioner before taking over-the-counter allergy and cold medications with this drug.
- Avoid alcohol while taking ziprasidone.

FOOD, VITAMIN, AND HERBAL INTERACTIONS

Avoid herbs that produce sedative effects, such as catnip, elecampane, goldenseal, gotu kola, hops, kava, lemon balm, skullcap, St. John's wort, and valerian. Stimulants such as ginseng, ephedra (ma huang), or caffeine may reduce the effectiveness of this drug. Vitamin supplementation may be beneficial.

RECOMMENDED DOSAGE

Ziprasidone comes as a capsule. The doses given below are typical, but dosage is always carefully individualized according to a person's particular needs and reactions to therapy.

- *Children:* This drug is not recommended for children.
- *Adults:* 20 mg twice daily to start; maximum dosage is 80 mg daily

Ziprasidone should be taken with food. If you miss a dose, take it as soon as you remember. If it is almost time for the next dose, skip it and resume your normal schedule. Never take a double dose.

SYMPTOMS OF OVERDOSE AND WHAT TO DO

The symptoms of ziprasidone overdose may include drowsiness, sleepiness, and slurred speech. If overdose occurs, seek immediate medical attention and take the prescription bottle to the hospital with you.

SPECIAL INFORMATION FOR PREGNANT OR NURSING WOMEN

Ziprasidone has caused birth defects in animal studies. If you are pregnant or planning to become pregnant, consult your health-care practitioner before starting this medication. Because ziprasidone may pass into breast milk, your health-care practitioner may advise you to stop breastfeeding while you take it.

SPECIAL INFORMATION FOR SENIORS

There are no special instructions for seniors.

GENERIC NAME

Zoledronic acid

BRAND NAME

Zometa

No generic available

ABOUT THIS DRUG

Zoledronic acid is used to treat hypercalcemia (high levels of blood calcium) that develops in people with some types of cancer. This drug inhibits the breakdown of bone that causes the levels of calcium in the bloodstream to rise. Zoledronic acid is also used to prevent other bone complications associated with advanced cancer, such as bone fractures and bone metastases (spread of the cancer to the bone).

SIDE EFFECTS

If any effects become persistent or severe, consult your health-care practitioner. Only he or she can determine whether it is safe for you to continue taking this drug and whether it is necessary to readjust your dosage.

- *Common:* fever, diarrhea, dehydration, constipation, abdominal pain, bone pain, fatigue, headache, sleepiness or sleeplessness, appetite loss, weight loss, swelling of legs, pain and swelling of joints
- *Less Common or Rare:* mood or mental changes, confusion, nausea, vomiting, pale skin, shortness of breath, difficulty breathing, wheezing, difficult or painful urination, muscle pain or cramps, muscle trembling or twitching, shaking hands or feet, lower back or side pain, rash, cracks in skin at corners of mouth, soreness or redness around fingernails and toenails, black and sticky stools, chest pain, tightness in chest, irregular heartbeat, convulsions, numbness and tingling around mouth, fingertips, or feet, unusual bleeding or bruising, unusual tiredness or weakness

IMPORTANT PRECAUTIONS

Always tell your health-care practitioner about any other medical conditions you may have, especially asthma, heart disease, and kidney disease. Zoledronic acid may worsen these problems. Inform your health-care practitioner if you have ever experienced an allergic reaction to this or similar drugs.

People taking zoledronic acid should be closely monitored with regular physical exams and blood tests.

This drug may cause side effects such as drowsiness. Until you know how zoledronic acid affects you, do not drive a car, operate machinery, or perform other tasks that require concentration.

DRUG INTERACTIONS

Always inform your health-care practitioner and pharmacist if you are taking any other prescription or over-the-counter drugs, as well as any vitamins, herbs, or other supplements.

FOOD, VITAMIN, AND HERBAL INTERACTIONS

No food, vitamin, or herbal interactions have been noted.

RECOMMENDED DOSAGE

Zoledronic acid is available by injection. Dosage is highly individualized and must be determined by your health-care practitioner.

SYMPTOMS OF OVERDOSE AND WHAT TO DO
No specific information is available regarding zoledronic acid overdose. If you suspect that an overdose has occurred, seek immediate medical attention.

SPECIAL INFORMATION FOR PREGNANT OR NURSING WOMEN
Zoledronic acid has caused birth defects in animal studies. If you are pregnant or planning to become pregnant, consult your health-care practitioner before starting this medication. Because zoledronic acid may pass into breast milk, your health-care practitioner may advise you to stop breastfeeding while you take it.

SPECIAL INFORMATION FOR SENIORS
There are no special guidelines for seniors.

GENERIC NAME
Zolmitriptan *see Triptan-Type Antimigraine Drugs, page 1083*

GENERIC NAME
Zolpidem

BRAND NAME
Ambien
No generic available

ABOUT THIS DRUG
Zolpidem is used on a short-term basis to treat insomnia. Occasionally this drug has been prescribed for longer periods of time. It has less of a "hangover" effect than many other sleeping pills.

Zolpidem works by attaching to a specific receptor in the brain. Its goal is to reduce the amount of time between when you go to bed and when you fall asleep.

SIDE EFFECTS
Consult your health-care practitioner if you develop any persistent or severe effects while taking zolpidem. Be sure to report any unusual or strange thoughts or behavior. Only your health-care practitioner can determine whether it is safe for you to continue taking this drug.

- *Common:* drowsiness, blurred vision, "hangover" effects after long-term use
- *Less Common or Rare:* clumsiness, unsteadiness, depression, confusion, memory problems, drugged feeling, overall feeling of unwellness, daytime sleepiness, trouble sleeping, nightmares or unusual dreams, unusual excitement or nervousness, dizziness, lightheadedness, fainting, headache, weakness, tingling in the hands and feet, fever, difficulty swallowing, trouble breathing, visual disturbances, eye pain, sensitivity to light, muscle pain, menstrual disorder, nausea, vomiting, stomach upset or pain, diarrhea, dry mouth, anxiety, tremor, hallucinations, swelling due to fluid retention, swelling of face, rash

IMPORTANT PRECAUTIONS

Inform your health-care practitioner about any other medical conditions you may have, especially liver or kidney impairment, sleep apnea, or a serious lung problem. Tell your health-care practitioner if you have ever experienced an allergic reaction to this or similar drugs.

Zolpidem is usually recommended for short-term use only. If you need to take this drug for longer than 7 to 10 days, consult your health-care practitioner. Long-term use may lead to dependence. This drug should be used with caution in anyone with a history of drug or alcohol abuse or depression.

Zolpidem can make you drowsy and less alert than usual. Until you know how this drug affects you, do not drive a car, operate machinery, or perform other tasks that require concentration.

DRUG INTERACTIONS

Tell your health-care practitioner and pharmacist if you are taking any other prescription or over-the-counter drugs, as well as any vitamins, herbs, or other supplements. Possible drug interactions include the following:

- Zolpidem may add to drowsiness and other effects of central nervous system depressants (such as antidepressants, antihistamines, muscle relaxants, narcotics, and sedatives).
- Bupropion, desipramine, and sertraline may increase the risk of hallucinations.
- Rifampin may decrease the effects of zolpidem.
- Ritonavir and antifungal drugs such as ketoconazole may lead to zolpidem toxicity.
- Zolpidem may increase the effects of chlorpromazine.
- Do not drink alcohol while taking zolpidem. This combination worsens coordination and impairs mental function.

FOOD, VITAMIN, AND HERBAL INTERACTIONS

Do not take zolpidem with hops, kava, passionflower, and valerian. These can increase its sedative effects. Stimulating herbs such as ephedra (ma huang), kola, and ginseng should also be avoided, as should caffeinated products including chocolate, coffee, tea, and cola.

RECOMMENDED DOSAGE

Zolpidem comes as a tablet. Although the doses given below are typical, only your health-care practitioner can determine the dose and schedule that best fit your needs.

- *Children:* Zolpidem is not recommended for children.
- *Adults:* 5 to 10 mg at bedtime

Zolpidem should be taken on an empty stomach. If you forget a dose, skip it and resume your normal schedule. Never take a double dose. If you have been taking zolpidem for a few weeks, do not stop taking it suddenly. Abrupt withdrawal can lead to sleep disturbances and anxiety. Speak to your health-care practitioner about gradually reducing dosage. You may experience sleeping difficulties the first night or two after stopping this medication ("rebound insomnia").

SYMPTOMS OF OVERDOSE AND WHAT TO DO

Symptoms of zolpidem overdose may include sleepiness, dizziness, unsteadiness, troubled breathing, lethargy, and coma. If overdose occurs, seek immediate medical attention and take the prescription bottle to the hospital with you.

SPECIAL INFORMATION FOR PREGNANT OR NURSING WOMEN

Do not take zolpidem if you are pregnant or planning to become pregnant. This drug is associated with an increased risk of birth effects. Since zolpidem may pass into breast milk, breastfeeding is not advisable while taking this medication.

SPECIAL INFORMATION FOR SENIORS

Side effects are more likely to occur in older people. Smaller doses are recommended.

A Primer of Drug Classifications

DRUG CLASSES

In each of the drug descriptions in this book, we have referred to various drug classes. Drugs are placed into classes based on shared potent chemical characteristics, similar side effects, and the fact that they work in the body in similar ways. Thus, if you have a negative reaction to one drug in a given class, you will likely have a negative reaction to another in the same class. Naturally, you should consult your health-care practitioner with any questions about medication use.

Some drugs fall into more than one class. Aspirin, for example, is an analgesic (pain killer) and also an antipyretic (fever-reducer). The following listing brings together the drugs that typically fall into a given class. Because there is no universal list of drug class names, some reference books may use different names for any given class. For example, anti-AIDS/HIV drugs are also referred to as anti-retrovirals; cephalosporins and antiviral drugs can also be referred to as anti-infectives. We have given some of these alternative names in parentheses after the bold class name.

This list is representative of the drugs available in each class and does not include all the drugs in each class. If you do not see a specific drug, talk to your health-care practitioner or pharmacist to get more information.

ACE (Angiotensin-Converting Enzyme) Inhibitors
benazepril (Lotensin)
captopril (Capoten)
enalapril (Vasotec)
fosinopril (Monopril)
lisinopril (Zestril)
moexipril (Univasc)
quinapril (Accupril)
ramipril (Altace)
trandolapril (Mavik)

Amphetamine-Like Drugs
dextroamphetamine (Dexedrine)
methylphenidate (Ritalin)

Analgesics
acetaminophen
aspirin
butalbital/acetaminophen/caffeine (Esgic)
butalbital/aspirin/caffeine (Fiorital)
propoxyphene (Darvon)
tramadol (Ultram)
see also: Narcotics; Nonsteroidal Anti-Inflammatory Drugs (NSAIDs)

Androgens (Male Hormones)
methyltestosterone
testosterone

Angiotensin II Blockers (Beta-Blockers)
candesartan (Atacand)
eprosartan (Teveten)
irbesartan (Avapro)
losartan (Cozaar)
telmisartan (Micardis)
valsartan (Diovan)

Anthelmintic Drugs
albendazole (Albenza)

Antiacne Drugs
adapalene (Differin)
isotretinoin (Accutane)
tazarotene (Tazorac)
tretinoin (Retin-A)

Anti-ALS Drugs
riluzole (Rilutek)

Anti-Alzheimer's Drugs
donepezil (Aricept)
galantamine (Reminyl)
memantine (Namenda)
rivastigmine (Exelon)
tacrine (Cognex)

Antiandrogens
bicalutamide (Casodex)

Antianginal Drugs
isosorbide (Imdur)
nitroglycerin (Nitrol)
see also: Beta-Blockers; Calcium Channel Blockers

Antianxiety Drugs
buspirone (BuSpar)
hydroxyzine (Atarax)
meprobamate (Miltown)
see also: Benzodiazepine Drugs; Selective Serotonin Reuptake Inhibitors

Antiarrhythmic Drugs
amiodarone (Cordarone)
disopyramide (Norpace)
flecainide (Tambocor)
procainamide (Procan)
quinidine (Cardioquin)
tocainide (Tonocard)
see also: Antihypertensive Drugs; Digitalis Preparations

Antiarthritic Drugs
anakinra (Kineret)
see also: Disease-Modifying Antirheumatic Drugs (DMARDs)

Antiasthmatic Drugs
albuterol (Proventil)
bitolterol (Tornalate)
cromolyn (Gastrocrom)
formoterol (Foradil)
ipratropium (Atrovent)
metaproterenol (Metaprel)
nedocromil (Tilade)
pirbuterol (Maxair)

salmeterol (Serevent)
terbutaline (Brethaire)
see also: Bronchodilators; Corticosteroids, Nasal Inhalants; Corticosteroids, Oral Inhalants; Leukotriene Antagonist/Inhibitors

Anti–Attention Deficit Hyperactivity Disorder (ADHD) Drugs
methylphenidate (Ritalin)
pemoline (Cylert)

Antibiotics
clindamycin (Cleocin)
mupirocin (Bactroban)
neomycin (Neosporin ophthalmic)
telithromycin (Ketek)
see also: Anti-Infectives; Cephalosporin Antibiotics; Penicillin Antibiotics; Tetracycline Antibiotics

Anticancer (Antineoplastic) Drugs
anastrozole (Arimidex)
bevacizumab (Avastin)
cetuximab (Erbitux)
exemestane (Aromasin)
fluoxymesterone (Android-F)
flutamide (Eulexin)
gefitinib (Iressa)
letrozole (Femara)
levamisole (Ergamisol)
methotrexate (Rheumatrex)
mitoxantrone (Novantrone)
nilutamide (Nilandron)
oxaliplatin (Eloxatin)
paclitaxel (Taxol)
tamoxifen (Nolvadex)
trastuzumab (Herceptin)

Anti–Canker Sore Drugs
amlexanox (Aphthasol)

Anticholinergics
tiotropium (Spiriva HandiHaler)
tolterodine (Detrol)
see also: Antiasthmatic Drugs; Antidepressants (some); Antiparkinsonism Drugs; Antispasmodic Drugs (some); Muscle Relaxants (some)

Anticoagulant Drugs
warfarin (Coumadin)

Anticonvulsant Drugs (Antiseizure Drugs)
carbamazepine (Tegretol)
clonazepam (Klonopin)
felbamate (Felbatol)
gabapentin (Neurontin)
lamotrigine (Lamictal)
levetiracetam (Keppra)
phenytoin (Dilantin)
tiagabine (Gabitril)
topiramate (Topamax)
valproic acid (Depakene)

Antidepressants
bupropion (Wellbutrin)
isocarboxazid (Marplan)
maprotiline (Ludiomil)
mirtazapine (Remeron)
nefazodone (Serzone)
paroxetine (Paxil)
trazodone (Desyrel)
see also: Antianxiety Drugs; Selective Serotonin Reuptake Inhibitors; Tricyclic Antidepressants

Antidiabetics
acarbose (Precose)
insulin (various)
metformin (Glucophage)
miglitol (Glyset)
pioglitazone (Actos)
repaglinide (Prandin)
rosiglitazone (Avandia)
see also: Sulfonylureas Antidiabetes Drugs

Antidiarrheal Drugs
difenoxin and atropine (Motofen)

Antidiuretic Drugs
desmopressin (Stimate)

Antiemetics (Antinausea)
aprepitant (Emend)
dolasetron (Anzemet)
dronabinol (Marinol)
granisetron (Kytril)
ondansetron (Zofran)

Antifungal Drugs
butenafine (Mentax)
caspofungin (Cancidas)
ciclopirox (Loprox)
clotrimazole (Lotrimin)
econazole (Spectazole)
fluconazole (Diflucan)
flucytosine (Ancobon)
griseofulvin (Grifulvin)
itraconazole (Sporanox)
ketoconazole (Nizoral)
miconazole (Monistat)
nystatin (Mycostatin)
oxiconazole (Oxistat)
terbinafine (Lamisil)
terconazole (Terazol)
see also: Anti-Infectives; Antimalarial Drugs; Antiviral Drugs

Antiglaucoma Drugs
acetazolamide (Dazamide)
apraclonidine (Iopidine)
brimonidine (Alphagan)
dipivefrin (Propine)
dorzolamide (Trusopt)
latanoprost (Xalatan)
travoprost (Travatan)
unoprostone (Rescula)

Antigout Drugs
allopurinol (Aloprim)
colchicine

Antihistamine Drugs
azelastine (Astelin)
cetirizine (Zyrtec)
clemastine (Tavist)
desloratadine (Clarinex)
diphenhydramine
emedastine (Emadine)
ketotifen (Zaditor)
meclizine (Antivert)
olopatadine (Patanol)
see also: Antihistamine/ Decongestant Drugs

Antihistamine/ Decongestant Drugs
acrivastine and pseudoephedrine
azatadine and pseudoephedrine
brompheniramine and pseudoephedrine
carbinoxamine and pseudoephedrine
chlorpheniramine and phenylephrine
chlorpheniramine and phenyltoloxamine and phenylephrine
chlorpheniramine and pseudoephedrine
chlorpheniramine and pyrilamine and phenylephrine
dexbrompheniramine and pseudoephedrine
fexofenadine and pseudoephedrine
loratadine and pseudoephedrine
promethazine and phenylephrine
see also: Antihistamine Drugs

Antihypertensive Drugs
acebutolol (Sectral)
betaxolol (Betoptic)
clonidine (Catapres)
doxazosin (Cardura)
eplerenone (Inspra)
guanabenz (Wytensin)
see also: ACE Inhibitors; Angiotensin II Blockers; Beta-Blockers; Calcium Channel Blockers; Diuretics

Anti-Impotence Drugs
alprostadil (Caverject)
sildenafil (Viagra)
tadalafil (Cialis)
vardenafil (Levitra)

Anti-Infectives
atovaquone (Mepron)
metronidazole (Flagyl)
trimethoprim (Proloprim)
see also: Antifungal Drugs;

Antimalarial Drugs; Antiviral Drugs; Cephalosporin Antibiotics; Fluoroquinolone Antibiotics; Macrolide Antibiotics; Tetracyclines

Antimalarial Drugs
halofantrine (Halfan)

Antimigraine Drugs
almotriptan (Axert)
ergotamine (Cafergot)
methysergide (Sansert)
see also: Triptan-Type Antimigraine Drugs

Antimetabolite Drugs
capecitabine (Xeloda)
methotrexate (Rheumatrex)

Anti-Osteoporotic Drugs
calcitonin (Miacalcin)
raloxifene (Evista)
teriparatide (Forteo)
see also: Bisphosphonates

Antiparkinsonism Drugs
amantadine (Symmetrel)
benztropine (Cogentin)
carbidopa (Lodosyn)
levodopa (Bendopa)
pergolide (Permax)
pramipexole (Mirapex)
ropinirole (Requip)
selegiline (Atapryl)
tolcapone (Tasmar)

Antiplatelet Drugs
cilostazol (Pletal)
clopidogrel (Plavix)
dipyridamole (Persantine)
ticlopidine (Ticlid)

Antipregnancy Drugs
mifepristone (Mifeprex)

Antiprostatism Drugs
alfuzosin (Uroxatral)
tamsulosin (Flomax)
terazosin (Hytrin)

Antipsoriatic Drugs
acitretin (Soriatane)
alefacept (Amevive)

Antipsychotic Drugs
aripiprazole (Abilify)
clozapine (Clozaril)
haloperidol (Haldol)
lithium (Eskalith)
olanzapine (Zyprexa)
quetiapine (Seroquel)
risperidone (Risperdal)
ziprasidone (Geodon)
see also: Phenothiazines

Antipyretic Drugs (Fever-Reducing Drugs)
acetaminophen
aspirin
see also: Nonsteroidal Anti-Inflammatory Drugs (NSAIDs)

Antispasmodic Drugs
dicyclomine (Bentyl)
hyoscyamine (Donnamar)
oxybutynin (Ditropan)
trospium (Sanctura)

Antitussive Drugs (Cough Suppressants)
benzonatate (Tessalon)
hydrocodone (Hycodan)

Antiulcer Drugs
misoprostol (Cytotec)
nizatidine (Axid)
see also: Gastrointestinal Drugs; Histamine 2 Blocker Drugs

Antiviral Drugs
acyclovir (Zovirax)
amantadine (Symmetrel)
atazanavir (Reyataz)
delavirdine (Rescriptor)
efavirenz (Sustiva)
famciclovir (Famvir)
ganciclovir (Cytovene)
influenza vaccine (FluMist)
lamivudine (Epivir)
nevirapine (Viramune)
oseltamivir (Tamiflu)

penciclovir (Denavir)
podofilox (Condylox)
rifampin (Rifadin)
rimantadine (Flumadine)
stavudine (Zerit)
valacyclovir (Valtrex)
zalcitabine (Hivid)
zanamivir (Relenza)

Appetite Suppressants/Weight Loss Agents
diethylpropion (Tenuate)
mazindol (Mazanor)
orlistat (Xenical)
phendimetrazine (Adipost)
phentermine (Adipex-P)
sibutramine (Meridia)

Barbiturates
phenobarbital (Bellatal)

Benzodiazepine Drugs
alprazolam (Xanax)
chlordiazepoxide (Librium)
clonazepam (Klonopin)
clorazepate (Tranxene)
diazepam (Valium)
estazolam (ProSom)
flurazepam (Dalmane)
halazepam (Paxipam)
lorazepam (Ativan)
temazepam (Restoril)
triazolam (Halcion)

Beta-Blockers (Beta-Adrenergic Blockers)
atenolol (Tenormin)
betaxolol (Betoptic)
bisoprolol (Zebeta)
carteolol (Cartrol)
carvedilol (Coreg)
labetalol (Normodyne)
metoprolol (Lopressor)
nadolol (Corgard)
penbutolol (Levatol)
pindolol (Visken)
propranolol (Inderal)
timolol (Timoptic)

Bisphosphonates
alendronate (Fosamax)
etidronate (Didronel)
risedronate (Actonel)
tiludronate (Skelid)

Bowel Anti-Inflammatory Drugs
mesalamine (Asacol)
olsalazine (Dipentum)

Bronchodilators
See Antiasthmatic Drugs

Calcium Channel Blockers
amlodipine (Norvasc)
bepridil (Vascor)
diltiazem (Cardizem)
felodipine (Plendil)
isradipine (DynaCirc)
nicardipine (Cardene)
nifedipine (Procardia)
nimodipine (Nimotop)
nisoldipine (Sular)
verapamil (Calan)

Cardiac Stimulant Drugs
nesiritide (Natrecor)

Cephalosporin Antibiotics
cefaclor (Ceclor)
cefadroxil (Duricef)
cefdinir (Omnicef)
cefixime (Suprax)
cefpodoxime (Vantin)
cefprozil (Cefzil)
ceftibuten (Cedax)
cefuroxime (Ceftin)
cephalexin (Keflex)
cephradine (Velosef)
loracarbef (Cefobid)

Cholesterol-Lowering Drugs
cholestyramine (Questran)
clofibrate (Abitrate)
colesevelam (Welchol)
colestipol (Colestid)
fenofibrate (Tricor)
gemfibrozil (Lopid)
niacin (various)

Contraceptives, Oral
See Female Sex Hormones

Corticosteroids, Nasal Inhalants
beclomethasone (Beconase)
budesonide (Rhinocort)
dexamethasone (Dexacort)
flunisolide (Nasalide)
fluticasone (Flonase)
mometasone (Nasonex)
triamcinolone (Nasacort)

Cortocosteroids, Oral
betamethasone (Celestone)
cortisone (Cortone)
dexamethasone (Decadron)
hydrocortisone (Cortef)
methylprednisolone (Medrol)
prednisolone (Delta-Cortef)
prednisone (Deltasone)
triamcinolone (Kenacort)

Cortocosteroids, Oral Inhalants
betaclomethasone (Beclodisk)
budesonide (Pulmicort Turbohaler)
dexamethasone (Decadron Respihaler)
flunisolide (AeroBid)
fluticasone (Flovent)
triamcinolone (Azmacort)

Cortocosteroids, Topical
alclometasone (Aclovate)
amcinonide (Cyclocort)
betamethasone (augmented and regular) (Betatrex)
clobetasol (Cormax)
clocortolone (Cloderm)
desonide (DesOwen)
desoximetasone (Topicort)
dexamethasone (Decadron)
diflorasone (Florone)
fluocinolone (Fluonid)
fluocinonide (Fluonex)
flurandrenolide (Cordran)
fluticasone (Cutivate)
halcinonide (Halog)
halobetasol (Ultravate)
hydrocortisone (Cetacort)
mometasone (Elocon)
prednicarbate (Dermatop)
triamcinolone (Kenalog)

COX-2 Inhibitors
celecoxib (Celebrex)
valdecoxib (Bextra)

Digitalis Preparations
digitoxin (Crystodigin)
digoxin (Lanoxin)

Dihydrotestosterone Inhibitors
finasteride (Propecia)

Disease-Modifying Antirheumatic Drugs (DMARDs)
adalimumab (Humira)
etanercept (Enbrel)
infliximab (Remicade)
leflunomide (Arava)

Diuretics
acetazolamide (Dazamide)
amiloride (Midamor)
spironolactone (Midamor)
see also: Loop Diuretics; Thiazide Diuretics

Enzyme Inhibitors
eflornithine (Vaniqa)

Female Sex Hormones
ethinyl estradiol (Desogen, Demulen, Ortho-Novum, many others)
estrogens, conjugated (Premarin)
estrogens, other

Fluoroquinolone Antibiotics
ciprofloxacin (Cipro)
enoxacin (Penetrex)
gatifloxacin (Tequin)
levofloxacin (Levaquin)
lomefloxacin (Maxaquin)
moxifloxacin (Avelox)
norfloxacin (Noroxin)
ofloxacin (Floxin)
sparfloxacin (Zagam)
see also: Anti-Infectives

Gastrointestinal Drugs
balsalazide (Colazal)
esomeprazole (Nexium)

lansoprazole (Prevacid)
loperamide (Imodium)
metoclopramide (Reglan)
omeprazole (Prilosec)
pantoprazole (Protonix)
tegaserod (Zelnorm)
see also: Antiemetic; Antiulcer Drugs

Hair Growth Stimulants
finasteride (Propecia)
minoxidil (Rogaine)

Histamine H_2 Blocker Drugs
cimetidine (Tagamet)
famotidine (Pepcid)
ranitidine (Zantac)

Hypnotics (Sedatives)
estazolam (ProSom)
flurazepam (Dalmane)
triazolam (Halcion)
zaleplon (Sonata)
zolpidem (Ambien)
see also: Benzodiazepine Drugs

Immunomodulator Drugs
glatiramer (Copaxone)
imiquimod (Aldara)
interferon alfa-2A
interferon alfa-2B
interferon alfa-3N
interferon beta 1A and 1B

Immunosuppressant Drugs
cyclosporine (Sandimmune)
tacrolimus (Prograf)

Leukotriene Antagonist/Inhibitors
montelukast (Singulair)
zafirlukast (Accolate)
zileuton (Zyflo Filmtab)

Loop Diuretics
bumetanide (Bumex)
furosemide (Lasix)
torsemide (Demadex)

Macrolide Antibiotics
azithromycin (Zithromax)
clarithromycin (Biaxin)
dirithromycin (Dynabac)
erythromycin
see also: Anti-Infectives

Monoamine Oxidase Inhibitor (MAOI) Drugs
phenelzine (Nardil)

Muscle Relaxants
baclofen (Lioresal)
carisoprodol (Soma)
chlorzoxazone (Paraflex)
cyclobenzaprine (Flexeril)
metaxalone (Skelaxin)
methocarbamol (Robaxin)
tizanidine (Zanaflex)

Narcotics (Opioids)
acetaminophen and codeine, hydrocodone, or oxycodone
butalbital/aspirin/caffeine/codeine (Fiorinal with Codeine)
codeine
hydrocodone and chlorpheniramine (Tussionex)
hydrocodone and ibuprofen (Vicoprofen)
meperidine (Demerol)
morphine (MS Contin)
oxycodone (OxyContin)
see also: Analgesics

Nonsteroidal Anti-Inflammatory Drugs (NSAIDs)
diclofenac (Voltaren)
diflunisal (Dolobid)
etodolac (Lodine)
indomethacin (Indocin)
ketorolac (Toradol)
meclofenamate (Meclomen)
mefenamic acid (Ponstel)
meloxicam (Mobic)
nabumetone (Relafen)
piroxicam (Feldene)
sulindac (Clinoril)
tolmetin (Tolectin)
see also: Cox-2 Inhibitors; Propionic Acid Drugs

Oral Contraceptives
See Female Sex Hormones

Pediculicide (Anti-Lice)
permethrin (Acticin)

Penicillin Antibiotics (Anti-Infectives)
amoxicillin (Amoxil)
ampicillin (Omnipen)
bacampicillin (Spectrobid)
carbenicillin (Geocillin)
cloxacillin (Cloxapen)
dicloxacillin (Dycill)
nafcillin (Unipen)
oxacillin (Bactocill)
penicillin V (Penicillin VK)

Phenothiazines (Antipsychotic Drugs)
chlorpromazine (Thorazine)
mesoridazine (Serentil)
prochlorperazine (Compazine)
thioridazine (Mellaril)
trifluoperazine (Stelazine)

Potassium Replacements
K-Dur

Progestins
medroxyprogesterone (Amen)
megestrol (Megace)
norethindrone (Aygestin)
progesterone (Gesterol)

Propionic Acid Drugs
fenoprofen (Nalfon)
flurbiprofen (Ansaid)
ibuprofen (Advil)
ketoprofen (Orudis)
naproxen (Naprosyn)
oxaprozin (Daypro)
see also: Nonsteroidal Anti-Inflammatory Drugs (NSAIDs)

Protease Inhibitors
amprenavir (Agenerase)
indinavir (Crixivan)
nelfinavir (Viracept)
ritonavir (Norvir)

Prostamides
bimatoprost (Lumigan)

Recombinant Human Growth Factor
becaplermin (Regranex)

Selective Norepinephrine Reuptake Inhibitors
atomoxetine (Strattera)
duloxetine (Cymbalta)

Selective Serotonin Reuptake Inhibitors
citalopram (Celexa)
escitalopram (Lexapro)
fluoxetine (Prozac)
fluvoxamine (Luvox)
sertraline (Zoloft)
venlafaxine (Effexor)
see also: Antidepressants

Smoking Cessation Drugs
bupropion (Zyban)
nicotine (Nicoderm)

Statin-Lowering Cholesterol Drugs
atorvastatin (Lipitor)
fluvastatin (Lescol)
lovastatin (Mevacor)
pravastatin (Pravachol)
simvastatin (Zocor)

Sulfa Drugs (Sulfonamides; Anti-Infectives)
sulfadiazine
sulfamethizole
sulfasalazine
sulfathiazole, sulfacetamide, and sulfabenzamide (triple sulfa)
sulfisoxazole

Sulfonylurea Antidiabetes Drugs (Oral Antidiabetic Drugs)
acetohexamide (Dymelor)
chlorpropamide (Diabinese)
glimepiride (Amaryl)
glipizide (Glucotrol)
glyburide (DiaBeta)

tolazamide (Tolinase)
tolbutamide (Orinase)
see also: Antidiabetics

Testosterone
leuprolide (Eligard)

Tetracycline Antibiotics (Anti-Infectives)
demeclocycline (Declomycin)
doxycycline (Bio-Tab)
meclocycline (Meclan)
minocycline (Dynacin)
oxytetracycline (Terramycin)
tetracycline (Tetracyn)

Thiazide Diuretics
bendroflumethiazide (Naturetin)
benzthiazide (Exna)
chlorothiazide (Diuril)
chlorthalidone (Hygroton)
hydrochlorothiazide (Esidrix)
hydroflumethiazide (Diucardin)
indapamide (Lozol)
methyclothiazide (Enduron)
metolazone (Mykrox)
polythiazide (Renese)
quinethazone (Hydromox)
trichlormethiazide (Metahydrin)

Thyroid Hormone Replacement Drugs
levothyroxine (Synthroid)
liothyronine (Cytomel)
liotrix (Thyrolar)
thyroglobulin
thyroid hormone (Armour Thyroid)

Tranquilizers
See Antianxiety Drugs; Antipsychotic Drugs

Tricyclic Antidepressants
amitriptyline (Elavil)
amitriptyline and chlordiazepoxide (Limbitrol)
amitriptyline and perphenazine (Etrafon)
amoxapine (Asendin)
clomipramine (Anafranil)
desipramine (Norpramin)
doxepin (Sinequan)
imipramine (Tofranil)
nortriptyline (Pamelor)
protriptyline (Vivactil)
trimipramine (Surmontil)

Triptan-Type Antimigraine Drugs
almotriptan (Axert)
naratriptan (Amerge)
rizatriptan (Maxalt)
sumatriptan (Imitrex)
zolmitriptan (Zomig)

Xanthine Bronchodilators
aminophylline (Phyllocontin)
dyphylline (Dilor)
oxtriphylline (Choledyl SA)
theophylline (Bronkodyl)
see also: Antiasthmatic Drugs

INDEX

Medications are listed alphabetically in *The Complete Pill Guide* by their generic names, because many medications have several brand names but only one generic name. Each entry notes whether a particular medication is available in a generic form; a generic medication is less expensive than the brand-name equivalent of the same drug, and typically performs as effectively as the brand-name drug.

The index that follows will help you find your prescription medication, whether you are searching for a brand-name or a generic drug.

- Generic names of drugs appear in boldface, followed in parentheses by the drug's most commonly known brand name.
- Brand names of drugs appear in a regular typeface, followed in parentheses by the medication's different strengths and types, if applicable, then by the generic name in boldface.
- Class names of drugs appear in italics.
- Color photographs are indicated by page letter.

E

G

H

I

J

K

N

O

P

Q

R

S

W

X

Z